Clinical Use of Pediatric Diagnostic Tests

Enid Gilbert-Barness, M.D., MBBS, FRCPA, FRCPath, Dsci(hc), M.D.(hc)
Professor of Pathology, Laboratory Medicine, Pediatrics, and Obstetrics and Gynecology
University of South Florida College of Medicine
Tampa General Hospital
Tampa, Florida

Professor Emeritus, Pathology, Laboratory Medicine, and Pediatrics
Distinguished Medical Alumni Professor Emeritus
University of Wisconsin Medical School
Madison, Wisconsin

Lewis A. Barness, M.D., Dsci(hc)
Professor of Pediatrics
Tampa General Hospital
Professor of Public Health
College of Public Health
College of Medicine and Department of Community and Family Health
University of South Florida College of Medicine
Tampa, Florida

Professor Emeritus, Pediatrics
University of Wisconsin Medical School
Madison, Wisconsin

Foreword by
Philip M. Farrell, M.D., Ph.D.
Alfred Dorrance Daniels Professor on Diseases of Children
Dean, University of Wisconsin School of Medicine
Vice Chancellor for Medical Affairs
Madison, Wisconsin

LIPPINCOTT WILLIAMS & WILKINS
A **Wolters Kluwer** Company
Philadelphia • Baltimore • New York • London
Buenos Aires • Hong Kong • Sydney • Tokyo

Acquisitions Editor: Timothy Y. Hiscock
Developmental Editor: Michelle LaPlante
Supervising Editor: Mary Ann McLaughlin
Production Editor: Amanda Yanovitch, Silverchair Science + Communications
Manufacturing Manager: Tim Reynolds
Cover Designer: Jeane Norton
Compositor: Silverchair Science + Communications
Printer: Maple Press

530 Walnut Street
Philadelphia, PA 19106 USA
LWW.com

Printed in the USA

Library of Congress Cataloging-in-Publication Data
Gilbert-Barness, Enid, 1927-
Clinical use of pediatric diagnostic tests / Enid Gilbert-Barness, Lewis A. Barness.-- 1st ed.
p. ; cm.
Includes bibliographical references and index.
ISBN 0-7817-3605-6
1. Children--Diseases--Diagnosis. 2. Children--Medical examinations. 3. Pediatrics. I. Barness, Lewis A. II. Title.
[DNLM: 1. Diagnostic Techniques and Procedures--Child. 2. Pediatrics--methods. WS 141 G464c 2002]
RJ50 .G547 2002
618.92'0075--dc21

2002069432

10 9 8 7 6 5 4 3 2 1

To our children and grandchildren,
and to all children on whom
our future depends
who may benefit from accurate
diagnosis through diagnostic testing

Contents

Color images fall after page 368.

Preface

Laboratory tests in the diagnosis of diseases in the pediatric age group are commonly an essential part of the diagnostic workup and are important for selecting the most appropriate treatment.

Many new techniques and laboratory studies have been introduced in the last few years, and many have replaced older methods that have become obsolete. It has become essential to the practice of modern pediatrics to be familiar with advances in laboratory medicine, and it has become important to meet the demands of the practicing physician. The complexity and sophistication of many tests exceed the capabilities of many office or small hospital facilities; however, when necessary, these tests can be referred to specialized reference laboratories. These laboratories or facilities we have indicated.

The database and intent of laboratory testing and the medical knowledge necessary to intelligently use laboratory tests extend beyond the capabilities of any one individual. We have, therefore, attempted to assemble this text into categories of disease with a brief outline of signs and symptoms that remain integral and essential for diagnosis. This is followed by diagnostic tests, including the most important methods for diagnosis (e.g., molecular procedures, DNA, probes, monoclonal antibodies, polymerase chain reaction, immunocytochemical and cytochemical staining, flow cytometry, and cytogenetics).

Many tables and algorithms have been included to simplify, clarify, and expedite the understanding and selection of diagnostic tests. Pertinent recent references are included.

When diagnosis is dependent on visual recognition, as for parasites, urinary crystals, and blood cells, drawings and/or pictures are included.

We have used the conventional units for measurements and biochemical levels and have omitted the Système International (SI) units, because the latter is now rarely used, and the consensus amongst physicians is to maintain the use of conventional units.

It is our hope that *Clinical Use of Pediatric Diagnostic Tests* will meet the needs of pediatricians, family practitioners, students, residents, pathologists, nurses, practitioners, and laboratory technicians. We trust that our combined expertise in clinical pathology (laboratory medicine) and pediatrics, combined with our many years of teaching, has enabled us to meet these goals.

Enid Gilbert-Barness, M.D.
Lewis A. Barness, M.D.

Foreword

It is an honor for me to introduce this timely, unique book that adds significantly to pediatric practice literature and to the extraordinary publication records of Drs. Enid Gilbert-Barness and Lewis Barness. They have created a sorely needed and unique treatise on how to use laboratory medicine in diagnosing diseases of children. Their integrated, comprehensive treatment of this important topic impressed me greatly. The cohesiveness of the book reflects the well-organized, critical thinking of the two authors. In my judgment, this pair of collaborating pediatric subspecialists has exceeded all their precedessors with respect to organizing and contributing knowledge essential for diagnosing childhood illnesses. Indeed, Enid and Lew have married their intellectual and writing talents to produce what I believe will become the "Bible" of pediatric medicine. This book adds significantly to their other recent "Bible" of biochemical genetics.[1]

In my years of pediatric practice, I have believed, as stated in a recent article,[2] that "Every physician's first duty is to diagnose—accurately and promptly. Diagnosis is the first step of treatment." This book provides what every practicing pediatrician, no matter how subspecialized, needs to practice: the art and science of diagnosis.

As a physician whose initial career interest was laboratory medicine,[2] I was eager to learn, when first perusing the manuscripts, how Enid and Lew organized the essential information to make the book practical and user friendly. I found that all the chapters are logically organized and easy to follow. It was reassuring to find the most fundamental aspects first, with excellent coverage of pregnancy, fetal medicine, and neonatology featured early in the book and followed by infection and immunology. The tables are superb and will be an extraordinary resource for medical students and residents in both pediatrics and family medicine. Scientific information is presented clearly and coherently. The organ-oriented approach is a brilliant aspect of this book. It will help readers seek information rapidly as they are seeking diagnoses in sick children.

I enjoyed reading several chapters in areas of special interest to me, such as Acid-Base Disorders, Disorders Specific to the Newborn, Pulmonary Function Tests, and Nutritional Diseases. I paid particular attention to the sections covering respiratory disorders, particularly cystic fibrosis, because of my special interest in that disorder. It is extraordinary that the essence of diagnosing and evaluating these disorders could be presented so concisely.

This book should become the standard in pediatric diagnosis and serve most of our needs for many years to come. Congratulations to Enid and Lew for sharing the value of their marriage and their encylopedic minds with all of us.

Philip M. Farrell, M.D., Ph.D.

[1]Gilbert-Barness E, Barness LA. *Metabolic diseases: foundations of clinical management, genetics and pathology.* Natick: Eaton Publishing, 2000, as reviewed by Farrell PM. *Arch Pediatr Adolesc Med* 2001;155:621–622.
[2]Farrell PM. Earlier diagnosis and improved outcome through neonatal screening. In: Doershuk C, ed. *Cystic fibrosis in the 20th century.* Cleveland: AM Publishing, 2002:120–137.

Acknowledgments

We wish to thank our many colleagues who have encouraged us to produce this volume, have generously given their time in reviewing the text, and have made invaluable suggestions. In particular, we are indebted to Dr. Irwin Browarsky and Dr. David Shields for their input into the chapters on Coagulation Disorders and Hematologic Disorders and to Dr. Alfonso Campos for his critical review of the Urinary Diseases chapter.

We express our appreciation to Dr. Philip Farrell for his invaluable suggestions and advice and to Dr. John Balis, Dr. Darlene Calhoun, Dr. Robert Christensen, Dr. John Curran, Dr. Verena Jorgenson, Dr. Richard Karl, Dr. Robert Kearney, Dr. Robert Nelson, Dr. Santa Nicosia, Dr. John M. Opitz, Dr. Herbert Pomerance, Dr. Lynn Ringenberg, and Dr. Allen Root for their encouragement.

Our thanks also to Acquisitions Editor Timothy Y. Hiscock and to Senior Developmental Editor Michelle LaPlante for superb editing, advice, and encouragement, as well as to Production Editor Amanda Yanovitch for her excellent editorial help in the final stages of the production of this volume.

Above all, we are indebted to Kathleen Lonkey for her timeless, diligent, meticulous, and dedicated work in the preparation of the entire manuscript and without whom this work could not have been completed.

Clinical Use of Pediatric Diagnostic Tests

1 Normal Values

Blood Tubes[1]

Lavender Top (Ethylenediaminetetraacetic Acid)

Complete blood cell count and differential
Reticulocyte count
Direct Coombs test
Glucose-6-phosphate dehydrogenase
Sickle cell
Malaria stain
Adrenocorticotropic hormone

Red/Gray (Tiger Top)

Sequential multiple analyzer computer (glucose)*
Cardiac enzymes
Liver enzymes
Drug concentrations (alcohol, digoxin, gentamicin, and so forth)
C-peptide/insulin
Protein electrophoresis
C3, C4 cryoglobulins
Osmolality
Pregnancy test

Red Top

Cross match
Haptoglobin
Trichloroacetic acid concentrations
Rheumatoid arthritis latex
Antinuclear antibody

Green Top

Lactate*
Ammonia*

*These specimens must be delivered to the laboratory immediately or put on ice for transportation.

Blue Top (Citrate)

Prothrombin time, activated partial thromboplastin time
Fibrinogen
Circulating anticoagulants
Coagulation factor assays

Blue Top (for Fibrin Degradation Products Only)

Fibrin degradation products

[1]Marshall SA, Ruedy J. *On call: principles and protocols.* Philadelphia: WB Saunders, 1993.

Artefactual Results Due to Problems in Specimen Collection/ Handling or to Pathologic Conditions

See Table 1.

Normal Values*†

*These values are compiled from the published literature. Normal values vary with the analytic method used. Consult your laboratory for its analytic method and range of normal values.
†Conventional units used.

Acid Phosphatase

Major sources: prostate and erythrocytes.[2]

Newborn	7.4–19.4 U/L
2–13 yr	6.4–15.2 U/L
Adult male	0.5–11.0 U/L
Adult female	0.2–9.5 U/L

Alanine Aminotransferase (Serum Glutamic Pyruvic Transaminase)

1–3 yr	5–45 U/L	
4–6 yr	10–25 U/L	
7–9 yr	10–35 U/L	
	Males	**Females**
10–11 yr	10–35 U/L	10–30 U/L
12–13 yr	10–55 U/L	10–30 U/L
14–15 yr	10–45 U/L	5–30 U/L
16–19 yr	10–40 U/L	5–35 U/L

Aldolase

Major sources: skeletal muscle and myocardium.

Infant	<32 U/L
Child	<16 U/L
Adult	<8 U/L

Alkaline Phosphatase

Major sources: liver, bone, intestinal mucosa, placenta, and kidney.

Infant	150–420 U/L
2–10 yr	100–320 U/L
11–18 yr (male)	100–390 U/L
11–18 yr (female)	100–320 U/L
Adult	30–120 U/L

α_1-Antitrypsin

93–244 mg/dL

α-Fetoprotein

>1 yr to adult	<30 ng/mL

Tumor Marker

0–10 mg/mL

Ammonia

Heparinized venous specimen on ice analyzed within 30 minutes.

Newborn	90–150 μg/dL
0–2 wk	79–129 μg/dL
>1 mo	29–70 μg/dL
Adult	0–50 μg/dL

[2]Marshall SA, Ruedy J. *On call: principles and protocols.* Philadelphia: WB Saunders, 1993.

Amylase
Major sources: pancreas, salivary glands, and ovaries.

Newborn	0–44 U/L
Adult	0–88 U/L

Antihyaluronidase Antibody
<1:256

Antinuclear Antibody

Not significant	<1:80
Likely significant	>1:320

Patterns with clinical correlation:
- Centromere—CREST (*c*alcinosis cutis, *R*aynaud's phenomenon, *e*sophageal motility disorder, *s*clerodactyly, and *t*elangiectasia)
- Nucleolar—scleroderma
- Homogeneous—native DNA, antihistone antibody

Antistreptolysin O Titer
Fourfold rise in paired serial specimens is significant.

Preschool	<1:85
School age	<1:170
Older adult	<1:85

Note: Alternatively, values up to 200 Todd units are normal.

Apolipoprotein A-I

Males	90–155 mg/dL
Females	94–172 mg/dL

Apolipoprotein B

Males	55–100 mg/dL
Females	45–110 mg/dL

Arsenic

Normal	<3 μg/dL
Acute poisoning	60–930 μg/dL
Chronic poisoning	10–50 μg/dL

Aspartate Aminotransferase
Major sources: liver, skeletal muscle, kidney, myocardium, and erythrocytes.

Newborn/infant	20–65 U/L
Child/adult	0–35 U/L

Base, Excess

Newborns	–10 to –2 mEq/L
Infants	–7 to –1 mEq/L
Children	–4 to +2 mEq/L
Adults	–3 to +3 mEq/L

Bicarbonate

Preterm	18–26 mEq/L
Full term	20–25 mEq/L
>2 yr	22–26 mEq/L

Table 1. Artefactual Results Due to Problems in Specimen Collection/Handling or to Pathologic Conditions

	Na	K	Total Calcium	Albumin	Phosphate	Creatinine	Lactate Dehydrogenase
Prolonged venous stasis during collection (tourniquet)	—	—	Increased	Increased	—	—	—
Samples collected proximal to infusion (as indicated)	Increased (saline) Decreased (dextrose)	Increased (KCl) Decreased (other)	Decreased	Increased (plasma, albumin) Decreased (other)	Decreased	Decreased	Decreased
Difficult or traumatic collection	—	Increased	—	—	—	—	Increased
Use of incorrect anticoagulant (as indicated)	Increased (Na^2 EDTA or sodium citrate)	Increased (K^2 EDTA)	Decreased (EDTA, citrate, or oxalate)	—	—	—	—
Too little blood added to anticoagulant	—	Increased (if marked discrepancy)	—	—	—	—	—
Too much blood added to anticoagulant	—	—	—	—	—	—	—
Prolonged storage or refrigeration of whole blood	Decreased (RT or 4°C)	Increased (RT or 4°C)	—	—	Increased (RT)	—	Increased (RT or 4°C)
Extreme leukocytosis	—	Increased	—	—	—	—	Increased
Extreme thrombocytosis	—	Increased	—	—	—	—	Increased
Marked erythrocytosis	—	—	—	—	—	—	—
Marked lipemia	Decreased	—	—	—	—	Possible interference with assay	—
Marked hyperglobulinemia	Decreased	—	Decreased	—	—	—	—
Marked jaundice	—	—	—	—	—	Decreased (some methods)	—

APTT/PT, activated partial thromboplastin time/prothrombin time; EDTA, ethylenediaminetetraacetic acid; K, potassium; Na, sodium; RT, room temperature (approximately 22°C); TGs, triglycerides.
From *Manual of use and interpretation of pathology tests*, 2nd ed. Sydney, Australia: Royal College of Pathologists of Australasia, 1997.

Alkaline Phosphatase	Aspartate Aminotransferase	Glucose	Lipids	APTT/PT	Hemoglobin/ Packed Cell Volume	White Cell Count	Platelet Count
—	—	—	Increased	May be shortened	Increased	Increased	Increased
Decreased	Decreased	Increased (dextrose) Decreased (other)	Increased (TGs) Decreased (other)	Prolonged (heparin)	Decreased	Decreased	Decreased
—	Increased	—	—	May be shortened, prolonged	Decreased (May be small clot in sample)	Decreased	Decreased
Decreased (EDTA)	—	—	—	Prolonged (EDTA or heparin)	—	—	Decreased (heparin)
—	—	—	—	Prolonged	Artefactual changes in cell morphology, on blood film		
—	—	—	—	May be shortened, prolonged	Decreased (May be small clot in sample)	Decreased	Decreased
—	Increased	Decreased (RT)	—	Prolonged (RT or 4°C)	— Artefactual changes in cell morphology, on blood film	Decreased	Decreased
—	—	Decreased	—	—	Hemoglobin may be increased	—	—
—	—	Decreased	—	—	—	—	—
—	—	Decreased	—	Prolonged	—	—	—
—	—	Interference with assay	—	Interference with automated methods	Hemoglobin may be increased	—	—
—	—	—	—	—	Hemoglobin may be increased	—	—
—	—	Decreased (some methods)	—	—	—	—	—

Bilirubin (Conjugated)

0.0–0.4 mg/dL

Bilirubin (Total)

Cord	Preterm	<2 mg/dL
	Term	<2 mg/dL
0–1 d	Preterm	<8 mg/dL
	Term	<6 mg/dL
1–2 d	Preterm	<12 mg/dL
	Term	<8 mg/dL
3–5 d	Preterm	<16 mg/dL
	Term	<12 mg/dL
Thereafter	Preterm	<2 mg/dL
	Term	<1 mg/dL
Adult		0.1–1.2 mg/dL

Calcium (Ionized)

Newborn <48 hr	4.0–4.7 mg/dL
Adult	4.52–5.28 mg/dL

Calcium (Total)

Preterm <1 wk	6–10 mg/dL
Full term <1 wk	7.0–12.0 mg/dL
Child	8.0–10.5 mg/dL
Adult	8.5–10.5 mg/dL

Carbon Dioxide (CO_2 Content)

Cord blood	14–22 mEq/L
Infant/child	20–24 mEq/L
Adult	24–30 mEq/L

Carbon Monoxide (Carboxyhemoglobin)

Nonsmoker	0–2% of total hemoglobin (Hb)
Smoker	2–10% of total Hb
Toxic	20–60% of total Hb
Lethal	>60% of total Hb

Carotenoids (Carotenes)

Infant	20–70 μg/dL
Child	40–130 μg/dL
Adult	50–250 μg/dL

Chloride (Serum)

Pediatric	99–111 mEq/L
Adult	96–109 mEq/L

Cholinesterase

Plasma	7–25 U/mL
Red blood cell (RBC)	0.65–1.30 pH units

Complement

Total complement	25–110 U
C1 esterase inhibitor	8–24 mg/dL
C1q complement component	7–15 mg/dL
C2 (second component of complement)	50–250% of normal
C3 (third component of complement)	70–150 mg/dL
C4 (fourth component of complement)	10–30 mg/dL
C5 (fifth component of complement)	9–18 mg/dL

Copper

0–6 mo	20–70 μg/dL
6 yr	90–190 μg/dL
12 yr	80–160 μg/dL
Adult male	70–140 μg/dL
Adult female	80–155 μg/dL

C-Reactive Protein
0.0–0.5 mg/dL

Creatine Kinase (Creatine Phosphokinase)
Major sources: myocardium, skeletal muscle, smooth muscle, and brain.

Newborn	100–200 U/L
Male	12–80 U/L
Female	10–55 U/L

Creatinine (Serum)

Cord	0.6–1.2 mg/dL
Newborn	0.3–1.0 mg/dL
Infant	0.2–0.4 mg/dL
Child	0.3–0.7 mg/dL
Adolescent	0.5–1.0 mg/dL
Male	0.6–1.3 mg/dL
Female	0.5–1.2 mg/dL

Ferritin

Newborn	25–200 ng/mL
1 mo	200–600 ng/mL
6 mo	50–200 ng/mL
6 mo–15 yr	7–140 ng/mL
Adult male	15–200 ng/mL
Adult female	12–150 ng/mL

Fibrinogen
200–400 mg/dL

Folic Acid (Folate)
3.0–17.5 ng/mL

Folic Acid (Red Blood Cells)
153–605 μg/mL RBCs

Galactose

Newborn	0–20 mg/dL
Thereafter	<5 mg/dL

γ-Glutamyltransferase
Major sources: liver (biliary tree) and kidney.

Cord	19–270 U/L
Preterm	56–233 U/L
0–3 wk	0–130 U/L
3 wk–3 mo	4–120 U/L
>3 mo (male)	5–65 U/L
>3 mo (female)	5–35 U/L
1–3 yr	6–19 U/L

4–6 yr	10–22 U/L	
7–9 yr	13–25 U/L	
	Males	**Females**
10–11 yr	17–30 U/L	17–28 U/L
12–13 yr	17–44 U/L	14–25 U/L
14–15 yr	12–33 U/L	14–26 U/L
16–19 yr	11–34 U/L	11–28 U/L

Gastrin

<100 pg/mL

Glucose (Serum)

Preterm	45–100 mg/dL
Full term	45–120 mg/dL
1 wk–16 yr	60–105 mg/dL
>16 yr	70–115 mg/dL

Homocysteine, Total

Reference range	5–15 µmol/L
Desirable	<10 µmol/L
Optimal	<12 µmol/L
Borderline	12–15 µmol/L
Moderate hyperhomocystinemia	>15–30 µmol/L
Intermediate hyperhomocystinemia	>30–100 µmol/L
Severe hyperhomocystinemia	>100 µmol/L

Immunoglobulins

	Immunoglobulin (Ig) G (mg/dL)	IgA (mg/dL)	IgM (mg/dL)
0–4 mo	141–930	5–64	14–142
5–8 mo	250–1,190	10–87	24–167
9–11 mo	320–1,250	17–94	
1–3 yr	400–1,250		
1–2 yr			35–242 (female) 35–200 (male)
2–3 yr		24–192	41–242 (female) 41–200 (male)
4–6 yr	560–1,307	26–232	
7–9 yr	598–1,379	33–258	
10–12 yr	638–1,453	45–285	
13–15 yr	680–1,531	47–317	
16–17 yr	724–1,611	55–377	
4–17 yr			56–242 (female) 47–200 (male)
≥178 yr	700–1,500	60–400	60–300

Immunoglobulin D

135–145 mEq/L

Immunoglobulin E

<1 yr	0.0–6.6 U/mL	7–8 yr	0.3–46.1 U/mL
1–2 yr	0.0–20.0 U/mL	8–9 yr	1.8–60.1 U/mL
2–3 yr	0.1–15.8 U/mL	9–10 yr	3.6–81.0 U/mL
3–4 yr	0.0–29.2 U/mL	10–11 yr	8.0–95.0 U/mL
4–5 yr	0.3–25.0 U/mL	11–12 yr	1.5–99.7 U/mL
5–6 yr	0.2–17.6 U/mL	12–13 yr	3.9–83.5 U/mL
6–7 yr	0.2–13.1 U/mL	13–16 yr	3.3–188.0 U/mL

Iron

Newborn	100–250 µg/dL
Infant	40–100 µg/dL

Child	50–120 μg/dL
Adult male	65–170 μg/dL
Adult female	50–170 μg/dL

Isocitrate Dehydrogenase
3–85 U/L

Ketones (Serum)

Qualitative	Negative
Quantitative	0.5–3.0 mg/dL

Lactate

Capillary blood	
Newborn	<27 mg/dL
Child	5–20 mg/dL
Venous	5–20 mg/dL
Arterial	5–14 mg/dL

Lactate Dehydrogenase (at 37°C)
Major sources: myocardium, liver, skeletal muscle, erythrocytes, platelets, and lymph nodes.

Neonate	160–1,500 U/L
Infant	150–360 U/L
Child	150–300 U/L
Adult	0–220 U/L

Lactate Dehydrogenase Isoenzymes (% Total)

Lactate dehydrogenase (LD)-1: heart	24–34%
LD-2: heart, erythrocytes	35–45%
LD-3: muscle	15–25%
LD-4: liver, trace muscle	4–10%
LD-5: liver, muscle	1–9%

Lead

Child	<10 μg/dL

Leptin

<15% of body fat in men and <25% in women	1–16 μg/L

Leucine Aminopeptidase
Depends on method.

Lipase
4–24 U/dL

Lipids

	Cholesterol (mg/dL)			LDL (mg/dL)			HDL (mg/dL)
	Desirable	Borderline	High	Desirable	Borderline	High	Desirable
Child/adolescent	<170	170–199	≥200	<110	110–129	≥130	>50
Adult	<200	200–239	≥240	<130	130–159	≥160	>50

Magnesium
1.3–2.0 mEq/L

Manganese (Blood)

Newborn	2.4–9.6 µg/dL
2–18 yr	0.8–2.1 µg/dL

Methemoglobin
0.0–1.3% total Hb

Myoglobin (Serum)
≤90 ng/mL

Osmolality
285–295 mOsmol/kg

Oxygen

Saturation, arterial	96–100% of capacity
Tension, partial pressure of oxygen, arterial while breathing room air	
Newborns	60–75 mm Hg
<60 yr	>85 mm Hg
60 yr	>80 mm Hg
70 yr	>70 mm Hg
80 yr	>60 mm Hg
90 yr	>50 mm Hg
While breathing 100% oxygen	>500 mm Hg
Oxygen dissociation, P^{50} (RBCs)	26–30 mm Hg

pH, Arterial
7.36–7.44

pH, Venous
7.32–7.38

Phenylalanine

Newborn	4.2–9.0 mg/dL
0–15 yr	3.2–6.3 mg/dL
Adult	2.7–4.5 mg/dL

Porcelain
0.52–1.94 mg/dL

Potassium

<10 d of age	4.0–6.0 mEq/L
>10 d of age	3.5–5.0 mEq/L

Prealbumin

Newborn to 6 wk	6.8–13.4 mg/dL
6 wk–16 yr	13–27 mg/dL
Adult	18–45 mg/dL

Proteins
Protein electrophoresis (g/dL)

Age	Total Protein	Albumin	α-1	α-2	β	γ
Cord	4.8–8.0	2.2–4.0	0.3–0.7	0.4–0.9	0.4–1.6	0.8–1.6
Newborn	4.4–7.6	3.2–4.8	0.1–0.3	0.2–0.3	0.3–0.6	0.6–1.2
1 d–1 mo	4.4–7.6	2.5–5.5	0.1–0.3	0.3–1.0	0.2–1.1	0.4–1.3
1–3 mo	3.6–7.4	2.1–4.8	0.1–0.4	0.3–1.1	0.3–1.1	0.2–1.1
4–6 mo	4.2–7.4	2.8–5.0	0.1–0.4	0.3–0.8	0.3–0.8	0.1–0.9

7–12 mo	5.1–7.5	3.2–5.7	0.1–0.6	0.3–1.5	0.4–1.0	0.2–1.2
13–24 mo	3.7–7.5	1.9–5.0	0.1–0.6	0.4–1.4	0.4–1.4	0.4–1.6
25–36 mo	5.3–8.1	3.3–5.8	0.1–0.3	0.3–1.1	0.3–1.2	0.4–1.5
3–5 yr	4.9–8.1	2.9–5.8	0.1–0.4	0.4–1.0	0.5–1.0	0.4–1.7
6–8 yr	6.0–7.9	3.3–5.0	0.1–0.5	0.5–0.8	0.5–0.9	0.7–2.0
9–11 yr	6.0–7.9	3.2–5.0	0.1–0.4	0.5–1.1	0.5–1.1	0.6–2.0
12–16 yr	6.0–7.9	3.2–5.1	0.1–0.4	0.5–1.1	0.5–1.1	0.6–2.0
Adult	6.0–8.0	3.1–5.4	0.1–0.4	0.4–1.1	0.5–1.2	0.7–1.7

Pyruvate
0.3–0.9 mg/dL

Rheumatoid Factor
<20

Rheumaton Titer
<10
(Modified Waaler-Rose slide test)

Sodium

Preterm	130–140 mEq/L
Older	135–148 mEq/L

Transaminase (Serum Glutamic Oxaloacetic Transaminase)
See Aspartate Aminotransferase.

Transaminase (Serum Glutamic Pyruvic Transaminase)
See Alanine Aminotransferase (Serum Glutamic Pyruvic Transaminase).

Transferrin

Newborn	130–275 mg/dL
Adult	200–400 mg/dL

Triglycerides (Fasting)

	Males (mg/dL)	Females (mg/dL)
Cord blood	10–98	10–98
0–5 yr	30–86	32–99
6–11 yr	31–108	35–114
12–15 yr	36–138	41–138
16–19 yr	40–163	40–128
20–29 yr	44–185	40–128
Adults	40–160	35–135

Troponin
0.03–0.15 ng/mL

Urea Nitrogen
7–22 mg/dL

Uric Acid

0–2 yr	2.4–6.4 mg/dL
2–12 yr	2.4–5.9 mg/dL
12–14 yr	2.4–6.4 mg/dL
Adult male	3.5–7.2 mg/dL
Adult female	2.4–6.4 mg/dL

Viscosity (Correlates with Fibrinogen, High-Density Lipoprotein Cholesterol)
(Viscosimeter)

Plasma	1.38 ± 0.08 relative units
Serum	1.26 ± 0.08 relative units

Vitamin A (Retinol)

Newborn	35–75 µg/dL
Child	30–80 µg/dL
Adult	30–65 µg/dL

Vitamin B_1 (Thiamine)
5.3–7.9 µg/dL
Vitamin B_2 (Riboflavin)
3.7–13.7 µg/dL
Vitamin B_{12} (Cobalamin)
130–785 pg/mL
Vitamin C (Ascorbic acid)
0.2–2.0 mg/dL
Vitamin D_3 (1,25-Dihydroxyvitamin D)
25–45 pg/mL
Vitamin E
5–20 mg/dL
Zinc
70–150 µg/dL

Causes of Increased and Decreased Routine Chemistry Tests in Pediatrics

See Table 2.

Reference Blood Values for Fetal Umbilical Blood at 18 to 40 Weeks of Pregnancy

See Table 3.

Normal Blood and Urine Hormone Levels

Adrenocorticotropic Hormone, Plasma

≤ 60 pg/mL

Aldosterone, Serum

0–3 wk	16.5–154.0 ng/dL
1–11 mo	6.5–86.0 ng/dL
1–10 yr (supine)	3.0–39.5 ng/dL
1–10 yr (upright)	3.5–124.0 ng/dL
≥11 yr (morning specimen, peripheral vein)	1–21 ng/dL

Aldosterone, Urine

0–30 d	0.7–11.0 µg/24 hr
1–11 mo	0.7–22.0 µg/24 hr
≥1 yr	2–16 µg/24 hr

Androstenedione, Serum

	Male	Female
0–7 yr	0.1–0.2 ng/mL	0.1–0.3 ng/mL
8–9 yr	0.1–0.3 ng/mL	0.2–0.5 ng/mL
10–11 yr	0.3–0.7 ng/mL	0.4–1.0 ng/mL
12–13 yr	0.4–1.0 ng/mL	0.8–1.9 ng/mL
14–17 yr	0.5–1.4 ng/mL	0.7–2.2 ng/mL
≥18 yr	0.3–3.1 ng/mL	0.2–3.1 ng/mL

Table 2. Causes of Increased and Decreased Routine Chemistry Tests in Pediatrics

Analyte	Reference Range (Serum or Plasma)	Causes of an Increased Result	Causes of a Decreased Result
Sodium	mmol/L (mEq/L) Preterm cord: 116–140 48 hr: 128–148 Newborn cord: 126–166 Newborn: 133–146 Thereafter: 136–146	Disease: • Sodium intake much greater than water intake (formula, error, and parenteral fluids) • Water loss greater than sodium loss [vomiting, diarrhea, polyuria, renal failure, diabetes insipidus (central or nephrogenic), hypothalamic hypodipsia (tumor), osmotic diuresis, burns, profuse sweating, prolonged hyperpnea] • Hyperaldosteronism, Cushing syndrome • During insulin therapy Artefact: • Loss of specimen integrity (concentration by evaporation, failure to mix after freeze-thaw)	Disease: • Excessive sodium loss from gastrointestinal tract (vomiting, diarrhea, salt-losing enteropathy), kidney (renal tubular or mineralocorticoid disorder, diuretic, polyuria), skin (sweat, burns), ketonuria, or into "third spaces" (burns) • Metabolic acidosis (Na^+–H^+ exchange) • Alkalosis or alkalinized urine • Hypothyroidism, adrenal insufficiency • Salt-losing congenital adrenal hyperplasia • Syndrome of inappropriate secretion of antidiuretic hormone • Dilution from overhydration, edema (due to renal, hepatic, or cardiac disease), ascites, malnutrition • Chronic disease Artefact: • Gross lipemia (depending on analytic method) • Hyperglycemia
Potassium	mmol/L (mEq/L) Cord: 5.0–10.2 48 hr: 3.0–6.0 Newborn cord: 5.6–12.0 Newborn: 3.7–5.9 Infant: 4.1–5.3 Child: 3.4–4.7 Thereafter: 3.5–5.1	Disease: • Shift from intracellular to extracellular fluid in acidosis, insulin deficiency, fever, hemolysis, rhabdomyolysis, tumor lysis, trauma, dehydration, shock, and burns • Increase in total body potassium in acute and chronic renal failure, congenital adrenal hyperplasia, excessive intravenous infusion, potassium-sparing diuretics Artefact: • Thrombocytosis (from platelet K^+ in clotted specimens), hemolysis, tissue lysis in capillary specimens, evaporation, failure to mix	Disease: • Shift from extracellular to intracellular fluid in alkalosis (H^+–K^+ exchange in cells), insulin therapy of hyperglycemia, starvation, periodic paralysis • Depletion of total body potassium stores with vomiting, diarrhea, and renal disorders (diuretics, diuretic phase of acute tubular necrosis, renal tubular acidosis), through skin (burns, sweating), hyperaldosteronism, Cushing syndrome, Bartter syndrome, cirrhosis Artefact: • Gross lipemia

(continued)

Table 2. (continued)

Analyte	Reference Range (Serum or Plasma)	Causes of an Increased Result	Causes of a Decreased Result
Chloride	mmol/L (mEq/L) Cord: 96–104 Newborn (0–30 d): 98–113 Thereafter: 98–107	Disease: • Metabolic acidosis due to HCO_3^- depletion in diarrhea, renal tubular acidosis, mineralocorticoid deficiency, respiratory alkalosis • Acute renal failure, diabetes insipidus, salicylate intoxication • Increased intake (parenteral nutrition) Artefact: • Evaporation or failure to mix, bromide ion	Disease: • Excessive loss in vomiting, mineralocorticoid excess, salt-losing pyelonephritis, metabolic acidosis due to organic acid accumulation, high HCO_3^- (respiratory acidosis, metabolic alkalosis), hyponatremia Artefact: • Gross lipemia
Total carbon dioxide	mmol/L (mEq/L) Cord: 14–22 Preterm (1 wk): 14–27 Newborn: 13–22 Thereafter: 20–28	Disease: • Metabolic alkalosis (prolonged vomiting, cystic fibrosis, excess glucocorticoids or mineralocorticoids, hypokalemia, alkali intake, licorice, high-dose penicillin or carbenicillin) • Respiratory acidosis	Disease: • Metabolic acidosis, gastrointestinal loss (diarrhea, ileal diversion), renal tubular acidosis, hypoaldosteronism • Respiratory alkalosis Artefact: • Delayed analysis and equilibration with air • Gross lipemia
Glucose	mg/dL Cord: 45–96 Preterm: 20–60 Neonate: 30–60 Newborn (1 d): 40–60 Newborn (>1 d): 50–80 Child: 60–100 Adult: 70–105	Disease: • Diabetes mellitus • Pancreatic inflammation • Acromegaly • Cushing syndrome • Thyrotoxicosis • Pancreatic or adrenal tumors • Chronic renal or hepatic disease Artefact: • Stress (up to 300–400 mg/dL) • Inherent inaccuracy of glucometers	Disease: • Intrauterine growth retardation • Maternal diabetes or toxemia • Islet cell tumor • Hepatic failure • Hypopituitarism • Glycogen storage • Galactosemia • Hereditary fructose intolerance • Leucine hypersensitivity • Reactive hypoglycemia Artefact: • 1–2 hr postprandial, *in vitro* glucose use by blood cells, gross lipemia

Blood urea nitrogen	mg/dL Cord: 21–40 Preterm (1 wk): 3–25 Newborn: 4–12 Infant/child: 5–18 Adult: 7–18	Disease: • Prerenal (dehydration, shock, congestive heart failure, cirrhosis) • Renal (acute or chronic renal failure) • Postrenal (urinary obstruction) • Gastrointestinal hemorrhage (hypovolemia and reabsorption of blood proteins) • Increased protein breakdown (due to glucocorticoids, thyroid hormone, tetracycline, fever, stress, burns) Artefact: • High-protein diet	Disease: • Urea cycle disorder, hepatic failure • Decreased protein breakdown (androgens and growth hormone) • Overhydration, malnutrition Artefact: • Starvation, muscle wasting, gross lipemia
Creatinine	mg/dL Cord: 0.6–1.2 1–4 d: 0.3–1.0 Infant: 0.2–0.4 Child: 0.3–0.7 Adolescent: 0.5–1.0	Disease: • Renal disease (see prerenal, renal, and postrenal causes of increased blood urea nitrogen) • Skeletal muscle necrosis (trauma, dystrophies, inflammatory myopathies) • Methyltestosterone, hyperthyroidism, diabetic ketoacidosis Artefact: • Nonspecific reactants	Disease: • Muscle-wasting diseases • Overhydration Artefact: • Gross lipemia, hyperbilirubinemia (depending on analytic method)

(continued)

Table 2. (continued)

Analyte	Reference Range (Serum or Plasma)	Causes of an Increased Result	Causes of a Decreased Result
Calcium	mg/dL Cord: 8.2–11.2 Newborn (preterm): 6.2–11.0 Newborn (0–10 d): 7.6–10.4 Newborn (10 d–24 mo): 9.0–11.0 Child (2–12 yr): 8.8–10.8 Adult: 8.4–10.2 In general, when total calcium is abnormal, measure the free ("ionized") calcium	Disease: • Idiopathic hypercalcemia of infancy • Familial hypocalciuric hypercalcemia • Hyperparathyroidism • Renal failure or increased retention due to diuretics, malignancy (bone involvement or paraneoplastic syndrome), vitamin D intoxication, milk alkali syndrome, immobilization, hyper- or hypothyroidism, acromegaly, adrenal insufficiency, pheochromocytoma, hyperproteinemia Artefact: • Prolonged venoocclusion before blood draw • Erect posture • Sleep (Hyperventilation and exercise increase free but not total calcium concentration)	Disease: • Prematurity • Asphyxia • Maternal diabetes • Neonatal hypocalcemia • Hypoparathyroidism • Vitamin D deficiency • DiGeorge syndrome • Osteomalacia • Rickets • Pancreatitis • Healing phase of bone disease • Hypoalbuminemia • Chronic renal failure • Magnesium deficiency • Large volumes of citrated blood products Artefact: • Citrate, oxalate, or EDTA anticoagulants • Recumbent posture • Hemolysis (may raise total calcium, depending on method) (Excess heparin in syringes will lower free but not total calcium)

Phosphorus, inorganic	mg/dL Cord: 3.7–8.1 0–10 d: 4.5–9.0 10 d–24 mo: 4.5–6.7 24 mo–12 yr: 4.5–5.5 Thereafter: 2.7–4.5	Disease: • Increased intake (laxatives or enemas) • Cell lysis (rhabdomyolysis, tumor or blast lysis) • Acidosis (lactic, β-OH-butyrate, or respiratory) • Decreased renal excretion (renal failure) • Hypoparathyroidism • Acromegaly • EDTA therapy Artefact: • Prolonged *in vitro* contact with erythrocytes, hemolysis	Disease: • Gastrointestinal loss (vomiting, diarrhea, antacids) • Malabsorption from vitamin D deficiency • Hyperglycemia • Nutritional recovery • Renal tubular defects (Fanconi syndrome, familial hypophosphatemia) • Burns • Hyperparathyroidism • Respiratory alkalosis Artefact: • Diurnal variation (diet), gross lipemia
Magnesium	mEq/L Newborn (2–4 d): 1.2–1.8 5 mo–20 yr: 1.3–1.9	Disease: • Increased intake (antacids, cathartics, purgatives) • Parenteral therapy (parenteral nutrition in patients who have renal failure or $MgSO_4$ infusion for pregnancy induced hypertension) • Renal failure • Rhabdomyolysis • Lithium therapy • Familial hypocalciuric hypercalcemia	Disease: • Primary hypomagnesemia • Decreased absorption (diarrhea, malabsorption, prolonged nasogastric suction, bowel resection, or fistulas) • Increased loss (pancreatitis, parenteral nutrition therapy, osmotic diuresis) • Hypercalcemia • Drugs (diuretics, aminoglycosides, cyclosporine, cardiac glycosides, amphotericin B, cisplatin, pentamidine) • Diabetes mellitus • Metabolic acidosis • Renal disease (glomerular and interstitial nephritis, diuretic phase of acute tubular necrosis, renal tubular acidosis) Artefact: • Gross lipemia

(continued)

Table 2. (continued)

Analyte	Reference Range (Serum or Plasma)	Causes of an Increased Result	Causes of a Decreased Result
Total protein	g/dL Preterm: 3.6–6.0 Newborn: 4.6–7.0 Cord: 4.8–8.0 1 wk: 4.4–7.6 7 mo–1 yr: 5.1–7.3 1–2 yr: 5.6–7.5 ≥3 yr: 6.0–8.0 Adult (ambulatory): 6.4–8.3 Adult (recumbent): 6.0–7.8	Disease: • Dehydration with hemoconcentration (vomiting, diarrhea, diabetic ketoacidosis) • Adrenal insufficiency • Inflammation with increases in acute phase reactants and immunoglobulins • Cystic fibrosis Artefact: • See Albumin	Disease: • See Albumin • Hemodilution (water intoxication, salt retention, intravenous therapy) • Increased loss (burns) • Hypogammaglobulinemia Artefact: • Recumbency lowers values approximately 0.5 g/dL
Albumin	g/dL 0–4 d: 2.8–4.4 4 d–14 yr: 3.8–5.4 Thereafter: 3.5–5.0	Disease: • Dehydration Artefact: • Prolonged tourniquet time (hydrostatic pressure results in loss of water and concentration of albumin)	Disease: • Malnutrition • Liver disease (decreased synthesis, but 17-day half-life precludes its use as a marker of rapid change in liver function) • Maldistribution (edema, ascites) • Loss in feces (protein-losing enteropathy) • Loss in urine (nephrotic syndrome, glomerulonephritis, diabetic nephropathy) • Loss from skin (burns) • Congenital absence (not usually associated with edema)

Aspartate aminotransferase (serum glutamic oxaloacetic transaminase)	U/L Newborn: 9–120 10 d–2 yr: 9–80 Thereafter: 10–40 (37°C, pyridoxal-5-phosphate added)	Disease: • Liver disease • Pulmonary embolism • Myocardial infarction • Skeletal muscle disease or injury • Hemolytic disease Artefact: • Specimen hemolysis • Platelet aspartate aminotransferase in plasma specimens that are insufficiently centrifuged	Disease: • End-stage liver disease Artefact: • See Alanine aminotransferase (serum glutamic pyruvic transaminase)
Lactate dehydrogenase	U/L 0–4 d: 290–775 4–10 d: 545–2,000 10 d–24 mo: 180–430 24 mo–12 yr: 110–295 12–60 yr: 100–190 (Lactate-to-pyruvate, 37°C)	Disease: • Liver disease • Myocardial disease • Hemolysis • Megaloblastic anemia • Anemia • Renal tubular or interstitial disease • Skeletal muscle disease • Tumor, especially with necrosis • Specimen hemolysis Artefact: • Assayed by pyruvate-to-lactate method (results are three times higher) • Hemolysis • Prolonged contact with clot *in vitro*	Disease: • Hereditary deficiency Artefact: • Refrigeration or freezing of specimen (inactivates liver isoenzyme)
Bilirubin	mg/dL Preterm: Cord: <2.0[a] 0–1 d: <8.0[a] 1–2 d: <12.0[a] 3–5 d: <14.0[a] Full-term: Cord: <2.0[a] 0–1 d: 2.0–6.0[a]	Disease: • Unconjugated (roughly equal to indirect bilirubin): • Physiologic jaundice of newborn • Hemolysis • Crigler-Najjar syndrome • Gilbert syndrome • Conjugated (roughly equal to direct bilirubin): • Biliary obstruction or inflammation • Drugs	Artefact: • Delayed analysis with photodegradation

(continued)

Table 2. (continued)

Analyte	Reference Range (Serum or Plasma)	Causes of an Increased Result	Causes of a Decreased Result
	1–2 d: 6.0–10.0[a] 3–5 d: 4.0–8.0[a] Thereafter: 0.2–1.0	• Dubin-Johnson syndrome • Rotor syndrome • Both fractions: • Hepatocellular injury Artefact: • Carotene (do not use a bilirubinometer for patients older than 3 mo) • Marked hemolysis	
Alanine aminotransferase (serum glutamic pyruvic transaminase)	U/L Newborn/Infant: 13–45 Thereafter: 7–40 (37°C, pyridoxal-5-phosphate added)	Disease: • Liver disease, especially hepatocellular injury due to viral infection or drug toxicity but less so with obstruction	Disease: • End-stage liver disease Artefact: • Coenzyme-deficient species in methods that do not add pyridoxal-5-phosphate, methods that run at a lower temperature
Alkaline phosphatase	U/L Male and female 1–3 yr: 145–320 4–6 yr: 150–380 7–9 yr: 175–420 10–11 yr: 130–560 12–13 yr: Male: 200–495 Female: 105–420 14–15 yr: Male: 130–525 Female: 70–230 16–19 yr: Male: 65–260 Female: 50–130 (37°C)	Disease: • Transient hyperphosphatasemia (benign, self-limited condition) • Liver disease, especially involving the biliary system, with the greatest increases (10- to 12-fold) seen with extra hepatic obstruction • Bone disease (rickets, osteomalacia, fracture)	Disease: • Zinc deficiency

γ-Glutamyl-transferase	U/L Male: ≤50 Female: ≤30 (37°C)	Disease: • Liver disease: most sensitive indicator of hepatobiliary obstruction, including focal obstruction with metastatic disease or cystic fibrosis • Usually higher in biliary atresia than neonatal hepatitis • Moderate increase in patients on anticonvulsants or other drugs that increase cytochrome P-450	Disease: • Acetaminophen toxicity (γ-glutamyltransferase will be normal-to-low when aspartate aminotransferase and alanine aminotransferase are markedly increased) Artefact: • Citrate, oxalate, or fluoride in collection tube
Cholesterol	mg/dL Acceptable: <170 Borderline: 170–199 High: ≥200	Disease: • Familial cholesterol disorder • Hepatocellular injury, cholestasis	Disease: • Hypothyroidism • Cirrhosis
Triglycerides	mg/dL Cord blood: Male: 13–96 Female: 11–76 0–9 yr: Male: 30–100 Female: 35–110 10–14 yr: Male: 32–125 Female: 37–131 15–19 yr: Male: 37–148 Female: 39–124	Disease: • Familial triglyceride disorder • Liver disease Artefact: • Nonfasting specimen (12-hr minimum recommended) • Intravenous lipid emulsion	

(continued)

Table 2. (continued)

Analyte	Reference Range (Serum or Plasma)	Causes of an Increased Result	Causes of a Decreased Result
Uric acid	mg/dL Child: 2.0–5.5 Adult male: 3.5–7.2 Adult female: 2.6–6.0	Disease: • Familial uric acid disorder (overproduction or underexcretion) • Tumor necrosis (high DNA turnover) • Lead poisoning • Acute or chronic renal failure • Hypothyroidism • Glycogen storage disease • Organic aciduria • Drugs Artefact: • High-protein diet	Disease: • Hepatocellular disease • Renal tubular disease (e.g., Fanconi syndrome)
Creatine kinase (CK) (creatine phosphokinase)	U/L Newborn (<6 wk): 100–600 6 wk–60 yr: Male: 52–200 Female: 35–165 (37°C)	Disease: • Skeletal muscle disease: dystrophy, viral myositis, polymyositis, rhabdomyolysis, and trauma, but not neurogenic atrophy, myasthenia gravis, multiple sclerosis, or poliomyelitis • Cardiac muscle disease: cardiogenic shock, myocardial infarction, cardiac trauma, surgery [note that to diagnose myocardial injury, total CK must be elevated and CK2 (MB) must be greater than 5–6% of total CK] • Central nervous system disease: cerebral ischemia (CK3), Reye syndrome (CK3), head injury, neonatal brain injury (CK1) • Other: acute psychosis, hypothyroidism Artefact: • Exercise	Disease: • Hyperthyroidism

EDTA, ethylenediaminetetraacetic acid.
[a]Nearly all unconjugated (indirect); any conjugated (direct) bilirubin >0.6 mg/dL requires evaluation.
From Pysher TJ, Bach PR. Interpretation of routine chemistry tests in pediatrics. *Pediatr Rev* 1996;17(10):357–369.

Table 3. Reference Blood Values for Fetal Umbilical Blood between 18 and 40 Weeks of Pregnancy

	Fetal	Infant	Adult
Bilirubin, total (mg/dL)	0.9–2.5	1.0–10.0	0.3–1.2
Bilirubin, direct (g/dL)	0.3–0.8		0.10–0.35
Calcium (mg/dL)	7.6–10.0		8.5–10.5
Chloride (mEq/L)	97–122		98–108
Cholesterol (mg/dL)	32–76		130–200
Creatinine (mg/dL)	0.4–0.9	0.3–0.7	Male: 0.7–1.4 Female: 0.6–1.1
γ-Glutamyltransferase (U/L)	22–146	5–120	5–45
Glucose (mg/dL)	54–103		65–110
Phosphorus, inorganic (mg/dL)	4.0–8.8	4.0–7.0	2.5–4.5
Potassium (mEq/L)	3.2–4.6		3.5–5.0
Lactate dehydrogenase (U/L)	259–552		230–460
Magnesium (mg/dL)	1.4–1.9	1.2–1.8	1.8–2.4
Sodium (mEq/L)	128–147		135–145
Transaminase			
Aspartate aminotransferase (U/L)	9–31		7–45
Alanine aminotransferase (U/L)	1–15		7–45
Triglycerides (mg/dL)	2–62		20–170
Blood urea nitrogen (mg/dL)	5–16	5–18	10–23
Uric acid (mg/dL)	1.0–5.5		Male: 3.5–7.0 Female: 2.4–5.7
Analytes that change with fetal age (approximate numbers taken from figure)			
Alkaline phosphatase (U/L)	From 525 to 400		
Creatine kinase (U/L)	From 2 to 20		
Total protein (mg/dL)	From 2.5 to 5.0		
Albumin (mg/dL)	From 2.0 to 3.2		

From Gozzo M, Noia G, Barbaresi G, et al. Reference intervals for 18 clinical chemistry analytes in fetal plasma samples between 18 and 40 weeks of pregnancy. *Clin Chem* 1998;44:683–685.

Angiotensin-Converting Enzyme, Serum

≤1 yr	10.9–42.1 U/L
1–2 yr	9.4–36.0 U/L
3–4 yr	7.9–29.8 U/L
5–9 yr	9.6–35.4 U/L
10–12 yr	10–37 U/L
13–16 yr	9.0–33.4 U/L
17–19 yr	7.2–26.6 U/L
≥20 yr	6.1–21.1 U/L

Calcitonin, Plasma

	Males	**Females**
Basal	≤19 pg/mL	<14 pg/mL
Calcium infusion (2.4 mg calcium/kg)	≤190 pg/mL	≤130 pg/mL
Pentagastrin infusion (0.5 μg/kg)	≤110 pg/mL	≤30 pg/mL

Catecholamine Fractionation (Free), Plasma

	Supine	Standing
Norepinephrine	70–150 pg/mL	200–1,700 pg/mL
Epinephrine	≤110 pg/mL	≤140 pg/mL
Dopamine	<30 pg/mL (any posture)	

Catecholamine Fractionation, Urine

Dopamine

<1 yr	<85 µg/24 hr
1 yr	10–140 µg/24 hr
2–3 yr	40–260 µg/24 hr
≥4 yr	65–400 µg/24 hr

Epinephrine

<1 yr	<2.5 µg/24 hr
1–2 yr	<3.5 µg/24 hr
2–3 yr	<6.0 µg/24 hr
4–9 yr	0.2–10.0 µg/24 hr
10–15 yr	0.5–20.0 µg/24 hr
≥16 yr	0–20 µg/24 hr

Norepinephrine

<1 yr	0–10 µg/24 hr
1 yr	1–17 µg/24 hr
2–3 yr	4–29 µg/24 hr
4–6 yr	8–45 µg/24 hr
7–9 yr	13–65 µg/24 hr
≥10 yr	15–80 µg/24 hr

Catecholamine Metabolite Fractionation, Urine

Homovanillic Acid, Urine

<1 yr	<35 µg/mg creatinine
>1 yr	<23 µg/mg creatinine
2–4 yr	<13.5 µg/mg creatinine
5–9 yr	<9 µg/mg creatinine
10–14 yr	<12 µg/mg creatinine
Adults	<8 mg/24 hr

Metanephrines, Urine

<1.3 mg/24 hr

Vanillylmandelic Acid, Urine

<1 yr	<27 µg/mg creatinine
1 yr	<18 µg/mg creatinine
2–4 yr	<13 µg/mg creatinine
5–9 yr	<8.5 µg/mg creatinine
10–14 yr	<7 µg/mg creatinine
15–18 yr	<5 µg/mg creatinine
Adults	<9 mg/24 hr

Chorionic Gonadotropins, β-Subunit, Serum

Females	<5 U/L
Postmenopausal females	<9 U/L
Males	<2.5 U/L
Cerebrospinal fluid (CSF)	≤1.5 U/L

Cortisol (for General Screening), Plasma

a.m.	7–25 μg/dL
p.m.	2–4 μg/dL

Cortisol, Free, Urine

24–108 μg/24 hr

Dehydroepiandrosterone Sulfate, Serum

	Males	Females
0–30 d (premature)	0.25–10.0 μg/mL	0.25–10.0 μg/mL
0–30 d (full-term)	0.25–2.0 μg/mL	0.25–2.0 μg/mL
1–16 yr	<0.5 μg/mL	<0.5 μg/mL
≥17 yr	<6.0 μg/mL	<3.0 μg/mL

Deoxycorticosteroids (for Metyrapone Test), Plasma

a.m.	0–5 μg/dL
p.m.	0–3 μg/dL

Estradiol, Serum

Children	<10 pg/mL
Adult males	10–50 pg/mL
Premenopausal adult females	30–400 pg/mL
Postmenopausal females	<30 pg/mL

Estrogen and Progesterone Receptor Assays, Tissue

Negative	<3 fmol/mg cytosol protein
Borderline	3–9 fmol/mg cytosol protein
Positive	≥10 fmol/mg cytosol protein

Follicle-Stimulating Hormone, Serum

	Males	Females
Prepuberty	<2 U/L	<2 U/L
Adult	1–10 U/L	
Follicular		1–10 U/L
Midcycle		6–30 U/L
Luteal		1–8 U/L
Postmenopausal		20–100 U/L

Follicle-Stimulating Hormone, Urine

	Males	Females
Prepuberty	<0.5 U/24 hr	<0.7 U/24 hr
Adult	7–10 U/24 hr	
Not midcycle		0.7–10.0 U/24 hr
Postmenopausal		>10 U/24 hr

Gastrin, Serum

≤200 pg/mL

Growth Hormone, Serum

Males	≤5 ng/mL
Females	≤10 ng/mL

5-Hydroxyindole Acetic Acid, Urine

≤6 mg/24 hr

17-Hydroxyprogesterone, Serum

Males	<220 ng/dL
Prepubertal	<110 ng/dL
Females	
Follicular phase	<80 ng/dL
Luteal phase	<285 ng/dL
Postmenopausal	<51 ng/dL
Prepubertal	<100 ng/dL
Newborns	<630 ng/dL

Insulin, Serum

<20 μU/mL	
Borderline	21–25 μU/mL

17-Ketogenic Steroids, Urine

Adult males	6–21 mg/24 hr
Adult females	4–17 mg/24 hr
Children, 0–10 yr	0.1–3.0 mg/24 hr
11–14 yr	2–7 mg/24 hr

Luteinizing Hormone, Serum

Prepubertal males	<0.5 U/L
Adult males	1–10 U/L
Prepubertal females	<0.2 U/L
Adult females, follicular	1–20 U/L
Adult females, midcycle	25–100 U/L
Postmenopausal females	20–100 U/L

Luteinizing Hormone, Urine

Prepubertal males	<0.8 U/24 hr
Adult males	0.2–5.0 U/24 hr
Prepubertal females	<0.8 U/24 hr
Adult females, nonmidcycle	0.5–5.0 U/24 hr
Postmenopausal females	>5.0 U/24 hr

Parathyroid Hormone, Serum (Intact + N-Terminal Parathyroid Hormone)

1.0–5.0 pmol/L

Pregnanetriol, Urine

	Males	Females
0–5 yr	<0.1 mg/24 hr	<0.1 mg/24 hr
6–9 yr	<0.3 mg/24 hr	<0.3 mg/24 hr
10–15 yr	0.2–0.6 mg/24 hr	0.1–0.6 mg/24 hr
>16 yr	0.2–2.0 mg/24 hr	0.0–1.4 mg/24 hr

Progesterone, Serum

	Males	Females
0–1 yr	0.87–3.37 ng/mL	0.87–3.37 ng/mL
2–9 yr	0.12–0.14 ng/mL	0.20–0.24 ng/mL
Postpuberty	<1.0 ng/mL	Increasing values
Follicular phase	—	≤0.7 ng/mL
Luteal phase	—	2.0–20.0 ng/mL

Prolactin, Serum

Males	0–20 ng/mL
Females	0–23 ng/mL

Renin Activity (Peripheral Vein), Plasma

Na-depleted, upright	
18–39 yr	2.9–24.0 ng/mL/hr
≥ 40 yr	2.9–10.8 ng/mL/hr
Na-replete, upright	
18–39 yr	≤0.6–4.3 ng/mL/hr
≥40 yr	≤0.6–3.0 ng/mL/hr

Sex Hormone–Binding Globulin, Serum

Adult males	10–80 nmol/L
Adult nonpregnant females	20–130 nmol/L

Somatomedin-C, Plasma

Age (yr)	Males	Females
0–5	0–103 ng/mL	0–112 ng/mL
6–8	2–118 ng/mL	5–128 ng/mL
9–10	15–148 ng/mL	24–158 ng/mL
11–13	55–216 ng/mL	65–226 ng/mL
14–15	114–232 ng/mL	124–242 ng/mL
16–17	84–221 ng/mL	94–231 ng/mL
18–19	56–177 ng/mL	66–186 ng/mL
20–24	75–142 ng/mL	64–131 ng/mL
25–29	65–131 ng/mL	55–121 ng/mL
30–34	58–122 ng/mL	47–112 ng/mL
35–39	51–115 ng/mL	40–104 ng/mL
40–44	46–109 ng/mL	35–98 ng/mL
45–49	43–104 ng/mL	32–93 ng/mL
≥50	40–100 ng/mL	29–90 ng/mL

Testosterone, Serum

	Total	Free	Percent
Males	300–1,200 ng/dL	9–30 ng/dL	2.0–4.8
Females	20–80 ng/dL	0.3–1.9 ng/dL	0.9–3.8

Thyroid Microsomal and Thyroglobulin Antibodies

<1:100

Vasoactive Intestinal Polypeptide, Plasma

<75 µg/mL

Thyroid Function Indicators By Age (Serum Concentration)

See Table 4.

17-Ketosteroids (Fractionation), Urine (mg/24 hr)

See Table 5.

Table 4. Thyroid Function Indicators by Age (Serum Concentration)[a]

Age	T_4 (nmol/L)	FT_4 (pmol/L)	TSH[b] (mIU/L)	TBG (mg/L)	T_3 (nmol/L)	rT_3 (nmol/L)	Thyroglobulin (μg/L)
1–4 d	142–277	28–68	1–39	22–42	1.5–11.4	—	2–110
1–4 wk	106–221	12–30	1.7–9.1	—	1.6–5.3	0.4–4.5	—
1–12 mo	76–210	10–23	0.8–8.2	16–36	1.6–3.8	0.17–2.00	—
1–5 yr	94–193	10–27	0.7–5.7	12–28	1.6–4.1	0.23–1.10	2–65
6–10 yr	82–171	13–27	0.7–5.7	12–28	1.4–3.7	0.26–1.20	2–65
11–15 yr	71–151	10–26	0.7–5.7	14–30	1.3–3.3	0.29–1.30	2–36
16–20 yr	54–152	10–26	0.7–5.7	14–30	1.2–3.2	0.39–1.20	2–36
21–80 yr	55–160	12–32	0.4–4.2	17–36	—	0.46–1.20	2–25
21–50 yr	—	—	—	—	1.1–3.1	—	—
51–80 yr	—	—	—	—	0.6–2.8	—	—

FT_4, free T_4; rT_3, reverse triiodothyronine; T_3, triiodothyronine; T_4, thyroxine; TBG, thyroxine-binding globulin; TSH, thyrotropin.
[a]No clinically significant difference by gender or race.
[b]Diurnal variation of TSH 50% between nadir (1500–1700 hr) and peak (2300–2400 hr).

Table 5. 17-Ketosteroids (Fractionation), Urine (mg/24 hr)

	Adult Females	Adult Males	Males 10–15 yr	Females 10–15 yr	6–9 yr	3–5 yr	1–2 yr	0–1 yr
Pregnanediol	0–4.5	0–1.9	0.1–1.2	0.1–0.7	<0.5	<0.3	<0.1	<0.1
Androsterone	0–3.1	0.9–6.1	0.2–2.0	0.5–2.5	0.1–1.0	<0.3	<0.3	<0.1
Etiocholanolone	0.1–3.5	0.9–5.2	0.1–1.6	0.7–3.1	0.3–1.0	<0.7	<0.4	<0.1
Dehydroepiandrosterone	0–1.5	0–3.1	<0.4	<0.4	<0.2	<0.1	<0.1	<0.1
Pregnanetriol	0–1.4	0.2–2.0	0.2–0.6	0.1–0.6	<0.3	<0.1	<0.1	<0.1
Δ5-Pregnanetriol	0–0.4	0–0.4	<0.3	<0.3	<0.2	<0.2	<0.1	<0.1
11-Ketoandrosterone	0–0.3	0–0.5	<0.1	<0.1	<0.1	<0.1	<0.1	<0.1
11-Ketoetiocholanolone	0–1.0	0–1.6	<0.3	0.1–0.5	0.1–0.5	<0.4	<0.1	<0.1
11-Hydroxyandrosterone	0–1.1	0.2–1.6	0.1–1.1	0.2–1.0	0.4–1.0	<0.4	<0.3	<0.3
11-Hydroxyetiocholanolone	0.1–0.8	0.1–0.9	<0.3	0.1–0.5	0.1–0.5	<0.4	<0.1	<0.1
11-Ketopregnanetriol	0–0.5	0–0.5	<0.3	<0.2	<0.2	<0.2	<0.2	<0.2

From Leavelle DE, ed. *Mayo medical laboratories handbook.* Rochester, MN: Mayo Medical Laboratories, 1995.

Normal Values for Serologic Tests for Infectious Agents

Amebiasis (*Entamoeba histolytica*)		
No invasive disease	<1:32	
Borderline	<1:32–1:64	
Active or recent infection	≥128	
Current infection	>1:256	
Aspergillosis	Negative	
Blastomycosis	Negative (positive in <50% of cases)	
Brucellosis	<1:80	
Candidosis	Negative (positive in 25% of normal persons)	
Chlamydia antigen (endocervix, male urine, male urethra)	Negative	
Chlamydia IgG	<1:10	
Cold agglutinin titer	<1:16	
Cryptococcosis antigen, serum or CSF	Negative	
Cryptosporidium antigen, feces	Negative	
Cysticercosis, serum	Negative	
Cytomegalovirus*		
IgG	Negative (<15 U/mL)	
IgM	Negative	
Echinococcosis	Negative at 1:128	
Herpes simplex, serum or CSF		
IgG	<1:5	
IgM	<1:10	
Histoplasmosis, serum or CSF	Negative	
Influenza A or B*	<1:10	
IgG or IgM		
Monospot screen	Negative	
Mumps*		
IgG	<1:5	
IgM	<1:10	
Murine typhus IgG	≤1:32	
Mycoplasma pneumoniae IgG or IgM	<1:10	
Polymerase chain reaction, CSF	Negative	
Q fever*		
Not infected	<1:10	
Previous infection	≥1:10	
Recent or active infection	≥1:160	
Respiratory syncytial virus		
IgG	<1:10	
IgM	<1:10	
Respiratory syncytial virus antigen, nasopharynx	Negative	
Rocky Mountain spotted fever*	IgG ≤1:32	
Rubella		
IgG	>1:10 confirms immunity	
IgM	Negative	
Rubeola, serum or CSF		
IgG	<1:5	
IgM	<1:10	
St. Louis encephalitis*	<1:10	
Scrub typhus	≤1:40	
Sporotrichosis	<1:80	
Streptococcal	Antistreptolysin-O	Antideoxyribonuclease-B
Preschool children	≤85 U	≤60 U
School-aged children	≤170 U	≤170 U
Adults	≤85 U	≤85 U

Toxocara canis antibody	Negative
Toxoplasmosis	
IgG	
No previous infection (except eye)	<1:16
Prevalent in general population	1:16–1:256
Suggests recent infection	>1:256
Active infection	≥1:1,024
IgM	
Adults	≥1:64 = active infection
Children	Any titer is significant
Trichinosis	Negative
Tularemia	<1:40
Varicella	
IgG	<1:10
IgM	<1:10 nonimmune 1:10 borderline immunity 1:40 immune

*Presence of IgM antibodies or at least a fourfold rise in IgG titer between acute- and convalescent-phase sera drawn within 30 d of each other indicates recent infection. Generally, presence of IgG indicates past exposure and possible immunity. Congenital infections require serial sera from both mother and infant. Passively acquired antibodies in infant will decay in 2–3 mo. Antibody levels that are unchanged or increased in 2–3 mo indicate active infection. Absence of antibody in mother rules out congenital infection in infant.

Normal Blood Antibody Levels

Acetylcholine	
Receptor-binding antibodies	≤0.02 nmol/L
Receptor-blocking antibodies	<25% blockade of acetylcholine receptors
Receptor-modulating antibodies	<20% loss of acetylcholine receptors
Antiglomerular basement membrane antibody	Negative
Antibodies to Jo 1 antigen	Negative
Antibodies to Scl 70 antigen	Negative
Anti–double-stranded DNA antibodies	
Negative	<70 U
Borderline	70–200 U
Positive	>200 U
Antiextractable nuclear antigens (Anti-RNP, anti-Sm, anti-SSB, anti-SSA)	Negative
Antimitochondrial antibodies	Negative
Antineutrophil cytoplasmic antibodies (C-ANCA and p-ANCA)	Negative
Antinuclear antibodies	Negative
Granulocyte antibodies	Negative
Human leukocyte antigen B27	
Present in:	Whites: 6–8% Blacks: 3–4% Asians: 1%
Intrinsic factor blocking antibody	Negative
Parietal cell antibodies	Negative
Rheumatoid factor	
Latex agglutination	Negative
Rate nephelometry	
Nonreactive	0–39 U/mL
Weakly reactive	40–79 U/mL
Reactive	≥80 U/mL
Smooth muscle antibody	Negative
Striated muscle antibodies	<1:60

Normal Blood Levels for Metabolic Diseases*

Acid mucopolysaccharides	U	
<14 yr old		Age dependent
Adult		≤13.3 μg glucuronic acid/mg creatinine
α_1-Antitrypsin	S	126–226 mg/dL
α-Fucosidase	F	Compare with controls
	L	0.49–1.76 U/g cellular protein
α-Galactosidase (Fabry disease)	S	0.016–0.200 U/L
	F	0.24–1.10 U/g cellular protein
	L	0.60–3.63 U/10^{10} cells
α-Glucosidase	F	0.13–1.84 U/g protein
α-L-Iduronidase (Hurler, Scheie syndromes)	F	0.44–1.04 U/g cellular protein
	L	0.17–0.54 U/10^{10} cells
α-Mannosidase (mannosidosis)	F	0.71–5.92 U/g cellular protein
	L	1.50–3.33 U/10^{10} cells
Alpha-*N*-acetylglucosaminidase (Sanfilippo syndrome type B)	S	0.09–0.58 U/L
	F	0.076–0.291 U/g cellular protein
Arylsulfatase A (mucolipidosis, types II and III)	F	2.28–15.74 U/g cellular protein
	L	≥2.5 U/10^{10} cells
	U	>1 U/L
Arylsulfatase B	F	1.6–14.9 U/g cellular protein
β-Galactosidase (G_{M1} gangliosidosis, Morquio syndrome)	F	4.7–19.1 U/g cellular protein
	L	1.01–6.52 U/10^{10} cells
β-Glucosidase (Gaucher disease)	F	3.80–8.70 U/g cellular protein
	L	0.08–0.35 U/10^{10} cells
β-Glucuronidase (mucopolysaccharidosis VII)	F	0.34–1.23 U/g cellular protein
Carbohydrate	U	Negative
Cystine	U	
<1 mo		64–451 μmol/g creatine
1–5 mo		66–375 μmol/g creatine
6–11 mo		70–316 μmol/g creatine
1–2 yr		53–244 μmol/g creatine
3–15 yr		11–53 μmol/g creatine
≥16 yr		28–155 μmol/g creatine
Fatty acid profile of serum lipids		
Linoleate		≥25% of fatty acids in serum lipids
Arachidonate		≥6% of fatty acids in serum lipids
Palmitate		18–26% of fatty acids in serum lipids
Phytanate		≤0.3% of fatty acids in serum lipids (>0.5% suggests Refsum disease; 0.3–0.5% borderline)
Free fatty acids	S	239–843 μEq/L
Galactose	U	Not detectable
Galactose 1-phosphate	RBC	
Nongalactosemic		5–49 μg/g Hb
Galactosemic (galactose-restricted diet)		80–125 μg/g Hb
Galactosemic (unrestricted diet)		>125 μg/g Hb
Galactose 1-phosphate uridyltransferase (galactosemia)	B	18.5–28.5 U/g
Galactokinase	B	
<2 yr old		20–80 mU/g Hb
≥2 yr old		12–40 mU/g Hb

Galactosylceramide–β-galactosidase	F	10.3–89.7 mU/g cellular protein
(Krabbe disease, globoid cell leukodystrophy)	L	>21.5 mU/g cellular protein
Glucose-6-phosphate dehydrogenase	B	
2–17 yr old		6.4–15.6 U/g Hb
>18 yr old		8.6–18.6 U/g Hb
Glucose phosphate isomerase	B	49–81 U/g Hb
Hexosaminidase (≥5 yr old) (Tay-Sachs disease, G_{M2} gangliosidosis)		
Total	S	10.4–23.8 U/L
Hexosaminidase A		
Normal		1.23–2.59 U/L; 56–80% of total
Indeterminate		1.16–1.22 U/L; 50–55% of total
Carrier		0.58–1.15 U/L; <50% of total
Total	L	16.4–36.2 U/g cellular protein
Hexosaminidase A		63–75% of total
Total	F	92.0–184.5 U/g cellular protein
Hexosaminidase A		41–65% of total
Homogentisic acid	U	Negative
Hydroxyproline, free	24-hr U	<1.3 mg/24 hr
Hydroxyproline, total	24-hr U	
<5 yr old		100–400 μg/mg creatinine
5–12 yr		100–150 μg/mg creatinine
Females ≥19 yr		0.4–2.9 mg/2-hr specimen
Males ≥19 yr		0.4–5.0 mg/2-hr specimen
^{35}S Mucopolysaccharide (I, II, III, VI, VII)	F	Normal or abnormal turnover
Phenylalanine	P	
≤1 wk old		0.69–2.0 mg/dL (42–124 mol/L)
<16 yr old		0.43–1.4 mg/dL (26–86 mol/L)
>16 yr old		0.68–1.1 mg/dL (41–68 mol/L)
Phytanate (phytanic acid)	S	<0.3% = normal 0.3–0.5% = borderline >0.5% suggests Refsum's disease
Porphobilinogen		Normal: ≤1.5 mg/24 hr Marginal: 1.5–2.0 mg/24 hr Excess: >2.0 mg/24 hr
Porphyrins, total	RBC	16–60 μg/dL packed cells
Uro (octacarboxylic)		≤2 μg/dL
Hepatocarboxylic		≤1 μg/dL
Hexacarboxylic		≤1 μg/dL
Pentacarboxylic		≤1 μg/dL
Copro (tetracarboxylic)		≤2 μg/dL
Porphyrins, total	P	≤1 μg/dL
Fractionation		≤1 μg/dL for any fraction
Porphyrins	St	
Coproporphyrin		≤200 μg/24 hr
Protoporphyrin		≤1,500 μg/24 hr
Uroporphyrin		≤1,000 μg/24 hr
Porphyrins, fractionation	U	
Uro (octacarboxylic)		
Males		≤46 μg/24 hr
Females		≤22 μg/24 hr
Hepatocarboxylic		
Males		≤13 μg/24 hr
Females		≤9 μg/24 hr
Hexacarboxylic		
Males		≤5 μg/24 hr
Females		≤4 μg/24 hr

Pentacarboxylic		
Males		≤4 μg/24 hr
Females		≤3 μg/24 hr
Corpo (tetracarboxylic)		
Males		≤96 μg/24 hr
Females		≤60 μg/24 hr
Protoporphyrins	RBC	
Free		1–10 μg/dL packed RBCs
Zinc-protoporphyrin		10–38 μg/dL packed RBCs
Sphingomyelinase (Niemann-Pick disease)	F	1.53–7.18 U/g cellular protein
Tyrosine	P	
≤1 wk		0.6–2.2 mg/dL (33–122 mol/L)
<16 yr		0.47–2.0 mg/dL (26–110 mol/L)
>16 yr		0.8–1.3 mg/dL (45–74 mol/L)
Uroporphyrinogen synthase	RBC	
Males		7.9–14.7 nM/sec/L
Females		8.0–16.8 nM/sec/L
		Marginal values 6.0–8.0 nM/sec/L are suggestive but indeterminate
		Values <6.0 nM/sec/L are definite for acute, intermittent porphyria

*B, whole blood; F, skin fibroblasts; L, leukocytes; P, plasma; RBC, erythrocytes; S, serum; St, stool; U, urine.

Cerebrospinal Fluid, Normal Values

Measurement of these components should always be performed on simultaneously drawn blood samples.

Appearance	Clear, colorless: no clot	
Total cell count		
Adults, children	0–6/mm³ (all mononuclear cells)	
Infants	<19/mm³	
Neonates	<30/mm³	
Glucose	45–80 mg/dL (20 mg/dL less than blood level)	
	Ventricular fluid 5–10 mg/dL higher than lumbar fluid	
Total protein		
Cisternal	15–25 mg/dL	
Ventricular	5–15 mg/dL	
Lumbar	15–45 mg/dL	3 mo–6 yr
	15–100 mg/dL	Neonates
	15–60 mg/dL	>60 yr
Albumin	10–35 mg/dL	
Protein electrophoresis		
Transthyretin	2–7%	
Albumin	56–76%	
α_1-Globulin	2–7%	
α_2-Globulin	4–12%	
β-Globulin	8–18%	
γ-Globulin	3–12%	
IgG	<4.0 mg/dL	
	<10% of total CSF protein	
Albumin index ratio	<9.0	
IgG synthesis rate	0.0–0.8 mg/d	
IgG index ratio	0.28–0.66	
CSF IgG/albumin ratio	0.09–0.25	
Oligoclonal bands	Negative	
Myelin basic protein	0.0–4.0 ng/mL	

Chloride	120–130 mEq/L (20 mEq/L above serum values)
Sodium	142–150 mEq/L
Potassium	2.2–3.3 mEq/L
Carbon dioxide	25 mEq/L
pH	7.35–7.40
Transaminase (aspartate aminotransferase)	7–49 U
LD	
LD-1	38–58% (LD-1 > LD-2)
LD-2	26–36%
LD-3	12–24%
LD-4	1–7%
LD-5	0–5%
Creatine kinase	0–5 U/L
Bilirubin	0
Urea nitrogen	5–25 mg/dL
Amino acids	30% of blood level
Xanthochromia	0
Total volume (adults)	140 mL
Generation rate	0.35 mL/min = 500 mL/d

Cerebrospinal Fluid Amino Acid Values

See Table 6.

Critical Values[3]

Hematology

	Low	High
Hematocrit (packed cell volume)	<20 vol%	>60 vol%
Hb	<7 g/dL	>20 g/dL
Platelet count (adult)	<40,000/mm^3	>1,000,000/mm^3
Platelet count (pediatric)	<20,000/mm^3	>1,000,000/mm^3
Activated partial thromboplastin time	None	>78 sec
Prothrombin time	None	>30 sec or >3× control level
Positive for fibrin split products, protamine sulfate, high heparin levels		
Fibrinogen	<100 mg/dL	>700 mg/dL
White blood cells	<2,000/mm^3	>30,000/mm^3
Presence of blast cells, sickle cells		
New diagnosis of leukemia, sickle cell anemia, aplastic crisis		

[3]Adapted from Wallach J. *Interpretation of diagnostic tests*. Philadelphia: Lippincott Williams & Wilkins, 2000.

Table 6. Cerebrospinal Fluid Amino Acid Values

Amino Acid	0–3 mo (μmol/dL)	3 mo–2 yr (μmol/dL)	2–10 yr (μmol/dL)	Adult (μmol/dL)
β-Alanine	+	+	+	+
Alanine (α-Alanine)	3.50–8.54	1.41–2.39	1.23–2.11	3.06–3.48
α-Aminoadipic acid	+	+	+	+
Amino-β-guanidinopropionic acid	+	+	+	+
γ-Aminobutyric acid	+	+	+	+
β-Aminoisobutyric acid	+	+	+	+
α-Amino-*N*-butyric acid	+	+	+	+
Anserine	+	+	+	+
Arginine	1.20–4.22	1.56–2.20	1.29–2.17	2.03–2.29
Asparagine	1.10–2.18	0.48–0.84	0.41–0.55	0.71–0.77
Aspartic acid	0.43–0.79	0.029–0.093	0.023–0.069	0.03–0.09
Carnosine	+	+	+	+
Citrulline	0.24–0.56	+	+	0.247–0.293
Cystathionine	+	+	+	+
Cystine	+	+	+	+
Glutamic acid	0.00–3.61	0.029–0.063	0.044–0.078	0.14–0.20
Glutamine	46.2–95.4	40.9–58.7	38.1–54.5	55.6–62.4
Glycine	0.68–1.52	0.28–0.68	0.31–0.61	0.55–0.61
Histidine	1.11–4.03	1.06–1.58	0.75–1.23	1.15–1.25
Homocystine	+	+	+	+
Hydroxylysine	+	+	+	+
Hydroxyproline	+	+	+	+
Isoleucine	0.46–1.18	0.41–0.65	0.28–0.44	0.48–0.58
Leucine	1.27–2.97	0.97–1.43	0.77–10.5	1.38–1.60
Lysine	1.32–3.62	0.95–1.73	1.03–1.67	2.75–3.07
Methionine	0.43–0.93	+	+	0.23–0.27
1-Methylhistidine	+	+	+	+
3-Methylhistidine	+	+	+	+
Ornithine	0.52–1.54	0.45–0.75	0.39–0.65	0.43–0.55
Phenylalanine	1.58–3.08	0.68–1.04	0.54–0.80	0.88–1.02
Phosphoethanolamine	+	+	+	+
Phosphoserine	+	+	+	+
Proline	0.50–0.84	+	+	0.33–0.43
Sarcosine	+	+	+	+
Serine	5.64–10.32	2.14–3.24	1.63–2.47	2.23–2.47
Taurine	1.16–2.30	0.42–0.50	0.38–0.52	0.59–0.69
Threonine	3.91–8.29	1.33–2.17	1.27–1.91	3.0–3.3
Tryptophan	+	0.21–0.31	0.17–0.25	0.16–0.30
Tyrosine	1.67–4.47	0.76–1.22	0.62–0.98	0.82–0.98
Valine	2.35–4.41	+	+	1.93–2.25

+, not established.
From Tietz NW, ed. *Clinical guide to laboratory tests*. Philadelphia: WB Saunders, 1995.

Blood Chemistry

	Low	High
Ammonia	None	>40 µmol/L
Amylase	None	>200 U/L
Arterial PCO_2	<20 mm Hg	>70 mm Hg
Arterial pH	<7.2 U	>7.6 U
Arterial PO_2 (adults)	<40 mm Hg	None
Arterial PO_2 (newborns)	<37 mm Hg (standard deviation = 7)	92 mm Hg (standard deviation = 12)
Bicarbonate	<10 mEq/L	>40 mEq/L
Bilirubin, total (newborns)	None	>15 mg/dL
Blood urea nitrogen (except dialysis patients)	2 mg/dL	>80 mg/dL
Calcium	<6 mg/dL	>13 mg/dL
Carbon dioxide	<10 mEq/L	>40 mEq/L
Cardiac troponin		
Cardiac troponin T	None	>0.1 µg/L
Cardiac troponin I	None	>1.6 µg/L
Chloride	<80 mEq/L	>115 mEq/L
Creatine kinase	None	>3.5× upper limit of normal
Creatine kinase-MB	None	>5% or ≥10 µg/L
Creatinine (except dialysis patients)	None	>5.0 mg/dL
Glucose	<40 mg/dL	>450 mg/dL
Glucose (newborns)	<30 mg/dL	>300 mg/dL
Magnesium	<1.0 mg/dL	>4.7 mg/dL
Phosphorus	<1 mg/dL	None
Potassium	<2.8 mEq/L	>6.2 mEq/L
Potassium (newborns)	<2.5 mEq/L	>8.0 mEq/L
Sodium	<120 mEq/L	>160 mEq/L

Cerebrospinal Fluid

	Low	High
Glucose	<80% of blood level	
Protein, total	None	>45 mg/dL
Positive bacterial stain (e.g., Gram, acid-fast), antigen detection, culture or India ink preparation		
White blood cells in CSF	None	>10/mm^3
Presence of malignant cells or blasts or any other body fluids		

Microbiology

Positive blood culture
Positive Gram stain or culture from any body fluid (e.g., pleural, peritoneal, joint)
Positive acid-fast stain or culture from any site
Positive culture or isolate for *Corynebacterium diphtheriae*, *Cryptococcus neoformans*, *Bordetella pertussis*, *Neisseria gonorrhoeae* (only nongenital sites), dimorphic fungi (*Histoplasma*, *Coccidioides*, *Blastomyces*, *Paracoccidioides*)
Presence of blood parasites (e.g., malaria organisms, *Babesia*, microfilaria)
Positive antigen detection (e.g., *Cryptococcus*, group B streptococci, *Haemophilus influenzae* type B, *Neisseria meningitidis*, *Streptococcus pneumoniae*)
Stool culture positive for *Salmonella*, *Campylobacter*, *Vibrio*, or *Yersinia*

Urinalysis

Strongly positive test for glucose and ketone
Presence of reducing sugars in infants
Presence of pathological crystals (urate, cysteine, leucine, tyrosine)

Serology

Incompatible cross match
Positive direct and indirect antiglobulin (Coombs) test on routine specimens
Positive direct antiglobulin (Coombs) test on cord blood
Titers of significant RBC alloantibodies during pregnancy
Transfusion reaction workup showing incompatible unit of transfused blood
Failure to call within 72 hr for recombinant human Ig after possible or known exposure to recombinant human–positive RBC
Positive confirmed test for hepatitis, syphilis, acquired immunodeficiency syndrome
Increased blood antibody levels for infectious agents

Therapeutic Drugs

	Blood levels
Acetaminophen	>150 μg/mL
Carbamazepine	>20 μg/mL
Chloramphenicol	>50 μg/mL (peak)
Digitoxin	>35 ng/mL
Digoxin	>2.5 ng/mL
Ethosuximide	>200 μg/mL
Gentamicin	>12 μg/mL
Imipramine	>400 ng/mL
Lidocaine	>9 μg/mL
Lithium	>2 mEq/L
Phenobarbital	>60 μg/mL
Phenytoin	>40 μg/mL
Primidone	>24 μg/mL
Quinidine	>10 μg/mL
Salicylate	>700 μg/mL
Theophylline	>25 μg/mL
Tobramycin	>12 μg/mL (peak)

In addition, the physician is promptly notified of any of the following:

Serum glucose, fasting	>130 mg/dL
Serum glucose, random	>250 mg/dL
Serum cholesterol	>300 mg/dL
Serum total protein	>9 mg/dL
Blood lead	Increased
Urinalysis	Pus, blood, or protein ≥2+
Urine colony count/culture	>50,000 colonies/mL of single organism
Respiratory culture	Heavy growth of pathogen
Peripheral blood smear	Atypical lymphocytes, plasma cells

Lipid Fractionation: Desirable Levels for Cholesterol and Triglycerides

See Table 7.

Lipid Fractionation: Desirable Levels for High-Density Lipoprotein Cholesterol and Low-Density Lipoprotein Cholesterol

See Table 8.

Determination of Body Surface Area

See Fig. 1.

Table 7. Lipid Fractionation: Desirable Levels for Cholesterol and Triglycerides[a]

	Cholesterol (mg/dL)				Triglycerides (mg/dL)	
	Males (Percentile)		Females (Percentile)		Males (Percentile)	Females (Percentile)
Age (yr)	5–95	75[b]	5–95	75[b]	5–95	5–95
5–9	126–191	172	122–209	173	27–102	34–76
10–14	130–204	179	124–217	174	30–103	33–121
15–19	114–198	167	125–212	175	31–124	32–122
20–24	128–216	185	128–209	181	34–137	32–97
25–29	140–236	202	134–218	190	40–157	33–100
30–34	150–250	216	141–229	199	43–171	35–106
35–39	156–264	226	147–240	209	45–182	38–110
40–44	162–274	235	155–253	219	48–189	40–117
45–49	166–280	242	162–265	229	50–193	41–122
50–54	170–286	246	171–278	241	50–195	43–128
55–59	173–291	250	179–291	253	51–197	45–134
60–64	175–295	253	188–306	265	51–198	47–140
65–69	176–298	255	197–320	278	51–199	50–147
70–74	177–299	256	207–336	291	51–199	52–154
>74	178–300	257	217–352	306	51–199	54–162

[a]Data have been presented recently as "desirable levels" rather than "reference ranges" or "normal values."
[b]Seventy-fifth percentile has been recommended as upper limit for serum cholesterol and low-density lipoprotein cholesterol.

Table 8. Lipid Fractionation: Desirable Levels for HDL Cholesterol and LDL Cholesterol[a]

	HDL Cholesterol (mg/dL)				LDL Cholesterol (mg/dL)			
	Males (Percentile)		Females (Percentile)		Males (Percentile)		Females (Percentile)	
Age (yr)	5–95	75[b]	5–95	75[b]	5–95	75[b]	5–95	75[b]
6–11	30–70	55	34–65	59	60–140	114	60–150	114
12–14	30–65	50	30–65	49	60–140	111	60–150	114
15–19	30–60	53	33–65	47	60–140	113	60–150	118
20–29	30–65	55	34–75	47	60–175	131	60–160	128
30–39	30–70	60	35–80	47	70–190	147	70–170	140
40–49	30–70	63	35–80	47	70–205	160	80–190	150
>50	30–70	65	35–80	47	80–220	170	80–200	164

HDL, high-density lipoprotein; LDL, low-density lipoprotein.
[a]Recently data have been presented as "desirable levels" rather than "reference ranges" or "normal values."
[b]Seventy-fifth percentile has been recommended as upper limit for serum cholesterol and LDL cholesterol.

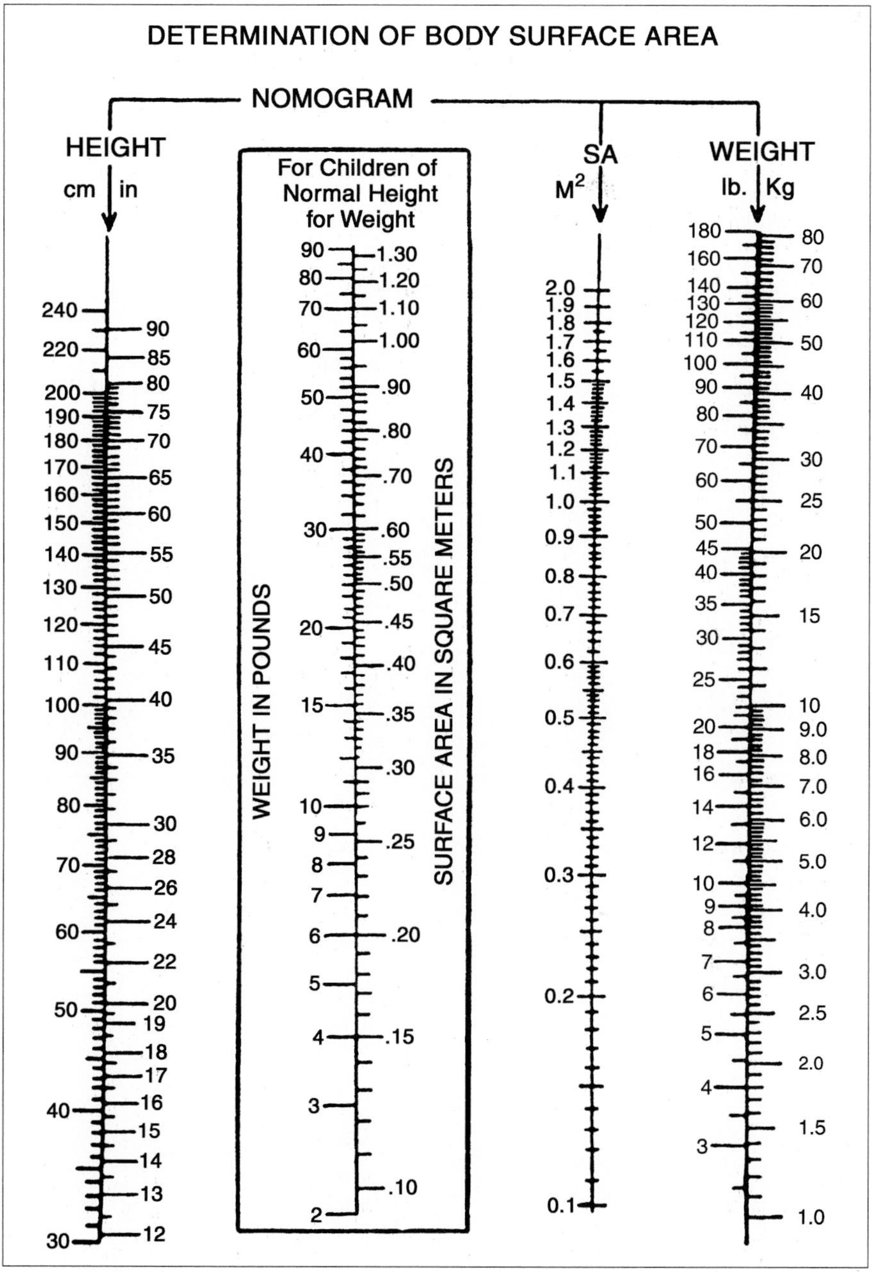

Fig. 1. Nomogram for estimation of surface area (SA). The SA is indicated where a straight line connecting the height and weight levels intersects the SA column. If the patient is approximately of average size, the SA can be estimated from the weight alone (enclosed area). (From Behrman RE, Kliegman RM, eds. *Nelson essentials of pediatrics*, 2nd ed. Philadelphia: WB Saunders, 1994, with permission.)

Bibliography

Behrman RE, Kliegman RM, Arvin AM. *Nelson textbook of pediatrics*, 16th ed. Philadelphia: WB Saunders, 2001.

Berkow R. *The Merck manual of diagnosis and therapy.* Rahway, NJ: Merck Research Laboratories, 1992.

Lundberg GD. SI unit implementation—the next step. *JAMA* 1988;260:73.

Meites S, ed. *Pediatric clinical chemistry,* 2nd and 3rd eds. American Association for Clinical Chemistry, 1981, 1989.

Oski FA. *Principles and practice of pediatrics*, 2nd ed. Philadelphia: JB Lippincott, 1994.

Scott PH, Wharton BA. Biochemical values in the newborn. In: Roberton N, ed. *Textbook of neonatology,* 2nd ed. Edinburgh: Churchill Livingstone, 1992:1213.

Siberry GK, Iannone R, eds. *The Harriet Lane handbook*, 15th ed. St. Louis: Mosby–Year Book, 2000.

Tietz NW, ed. *Textbook of clinical chemistry.* Toronto: WB Saunders, 1986.

Wallach J. *Interpretation of diagnostic tests*, 7th ed. Philadelphia: Lippincott Williams & Wilkins, 2000.

2 Acid-Base Disorders

Determination of blood pH and blood gas concentrations should be performed on arterial blood.

Determination of electrolyte levels, pH, and blood gas concentrations ideally should be performed on blood specimens obtained simultaneously, because the acid-base situation is very labile.

Blood specimens should be packed in ice immediately; delay of even a few minutes causes erroneous results, especially if white blood cell count is high.

Most laboratories measure pH and P_{CO_2} directly and calculate bicarbonate (HCO_3^-) using the modified Henderson-Hasselbalch equation:

$$\text{Arterial pH} = 6.1 + \log [(HCO_3^-) \div (0.03 \times P_{CO_2})]$$

where 6.1 is the dissociation constant for H_2CO_3 in aqueous solution and 0.03 is a constant for the solubility of CO_2 in plasma at 37°C. The pH is maintained by normal serum electrolytes and normal oxygenation (arterial P_{CO_2}, P_{CO_2}).

A normal pH does not ensure the absence of an acid-base disturbance if the P_{CO_2} is not known. Normal serum electrolyte levels are as follows:

Bases	**Acids**
Sodium, 135–145 mEq/L	Chloride, 95–105 mEq/L
Potassium, 4.0–5.5 mEq/L	Bicarbonate, 22–26 mEq/L

Decreased HCO_3^- indicates metabolic acidosis, and increased HCO_3^- indicates metabolic alkalosis. Respiratory acidosis occurs with a P_{CO_2} of >45 mm Hg, and respiratory alkalosis is associated with a P_{CO_2} of <35 mm Hg. Thus, mixed metabolic and respiratory acidosis is characterized by low pH, low HCO_3^-, and high P_{CO_2}. Mixed metabolic and respiratory alkalosis is characterized by high pH, high HCO_3^-, and low P_{CO_2}.

Base excess is a derived number that "corrects" pH to 7.40 by first adjusting P_{CO_2} to 40 mm Hg, which allows comparison of the resultant HCO_3^- value with the normal value at that pH (24 mEq/L). Base excess can be calculated from determined values for pH and HCO_3^- by the following formula:

$$\text{Base excess (mEq/L)} = HCO_3^- + 10(7.4 - \text{pH}) - 24$$

This computation does not distinguish primary from compensatory derangements. Negative base excess is an estimate of bicarbonate deficiency.

To judge hypoxemia, one must also know what the patient's hemoglobin level or hematocrit is and whether the patient was breathing room air or oxygen when the specimen was drawn.

Anion Gap

Calculated as Na – (Cl + HCO_3); typically normal level = 8–16 mEq/L; if K is included, normal = 10–20 mEq/L; reference interval varies considerably depending on instrumentation.

Increased In

Increased "unmeasured" anions

- Organic acids (e.g., lactic acidosis, ketoacidosis)

- Inorganic acids (e.g., administration of phosphate, sulfate/salicylate, formate, nitrate, penicillin, carbenicillin disodium)
- Protein (e.g., transient hyperalbuminemia)
- Exogenous
- Not completely identified (e.g., hyperosmolar hyperglycemic nonketotic coma, uremia, poisoning by ethylene glycol, methanol)
- Artefactual

Falsely increased serum sodium

Falsely decreased serum chloride or bicarbonate

Decreased In

Decreased unmeasured anion; for example, hypoalbuminemia is probably the most common cause of decreased anion gap (AG).

Artefactual

- "Hyperchloremia" in bromide intoxication (if chloride determination by colorimetric method)
- Hyponatremia due to viscous serum
- False decrease in serum sodium; false increase in serum chloride or HCO_3^-

Increased unmeasured cations

- Hyperkalemia, hypercalcemia, hypermagnesemia
- Increased proteins in multiple myeloma, paraproteinemias, polyclonal gammopathies. (These abnormal proteins are positively charged and lower the AG.)
- Increased lithium, tris(hydroxymethyl)aminomethane buffer (tromethamine)

AG >30 mEq/L almost always indicates organic acidosis even in presence of uremia.

AG of 20–29 mEq/L occurs in absence of identified organic acidosis in 25% of patients.

AG is rarely >23 mEq/L in chronic renal failure.

Simultaneous changes in ions may cancel each other out, leaving AG unchanged (e.g., increased chloride and decreased HCO_3^-).

AG may provide a clue to the presence of a mixed rather than single acid-base disturbance.

Acid-Base Changes in Blood Acidosis and Alkalosis

See Table 1.

Metabolic Acidosis

Clinical Symptoms

With Increased Anion Gap (AG >15 mEq/L)

Lactic acidosis (most common cause of metabolic acidosis with increased AG). In lactic acidosis, the increase in AG is usually greater than the decrease in HCO_3^-, in

Table 1. Acid-Base Changes in Blood Acidosis and Alkalosis

	pH	P_{CO_2}	HCO_3^-
Acidosis			
Acute metabolic	↓	N	↓
Compensated metabolic	N	↓	↓
Acute respiratory	↓	↑	N
Compensated respiratory	N	↑	↑
Alkalosis			
Acute metabolic	↑	N	↑
Chronic metabolic	↑	↑	↑
Acute respiratory	↑	↓	N
Compensated respiratory	N	↓	↓

↓, decreased; ↑, increased; N, normal.

contrast to diabetic ketoacidosis, in which the increase in AG is identical to the decrease in HCO_3^-.

Renal failure (AG)

Ketoacidosis

- Associated with diabetes mellitus (AG frequently >25 mEq/L)
- Associated with alcohol abuse (AG frequently 20–25 mEq/L)
- Associated with starvation (AG usually 5–10 mEq/L)

Drug effects

- Salicylate, methanol, ethylene glycol poisoning (AG frequently >20 mEq/L; higher in children)
- Paraldehyde treatment (AG frequently >20 mEq/L)

With Normal Anion Gap (Hyperchloremic Acidosis)

Decreased serum potassium

- Renal tubular acidosis (e.g., cystinosis, Wilson disease)

Acquired (e.g., drugs, hypercalcemia)

- Carbonic anhydrase inhibitors (e.g., acetazolamide)
- Increased loss of alkaline body fluids (e.g., diarrhea, loss of pancreatic or biliary fluids)

Normal or increased serum potassium

- Hydronephrosis
- Early renal failure
- Administration of HCl (e.g., ammonium chloride)
- Hypoadrenalism (diffuse, zona glomerulosa, or hyporeninemia)
- Renal aldosterone resistance

Diagnostic Studies

Serum pH is decreased (<7.3).

Total plasma HCO_3^- content is decreased; value <15 mEq/L rules out respiratory alkalosis.

Serum potassium is frequently increased; it is decreased in renal tubular acidosis, diarrhea, or carbonic anhydrase inhibition.

Azotemia suggests metabolic acidosis due to renal failure.

Urine is strongly acid (pH = 4.5–5.2) if renal function is normal.

Lactic Acidosis (Increased Anion Gap)

Suggests acute hypoperfusion or tissue hypoxia.

Clinical Symptoms

Should be considered in any metabolic acidosis with increased AG (>15 mEq/L).

Type A: Due to clinically apparent tissue hypoxia, for example, acute hemorrhage, severe anemia, shock, asphyxia, marathon running, seizures.

Type B: Without clinically apparent tissue hypoxia due to

- Common disorders (e.g., diabetes mellitus, uremia, liver disease, infections, malignancies)
- Drugs and toxins (e.g., ethanol, methanol, ethylene glycol, salicylates, metformin)
- Hereditary enzyme defects (e.g., methylmalonicaciduria, propionicaciduria, defects of fatty acid oxidation, pyruvate-dehydrogenase deficiency, pyruvate-carboxylase deficiency, multiple carboxylase deficiency, glycogen storage disease type 1)
- Other causes (e.g., short-bowel syndrome, poor technique in drawing blood)

With a typical clinical picture (onset after nausea and vomiting, altered state of consciousness, hyperventilation, high mortality):

- Decreased serum bicarbonate.
- Low serum pH, usually 6.98–7.25.
- Increased serum potassium, often 6–7 mEq/L.
- Serum chloride normal or low with increased AG.
- Increased white blood cell count (occasionally to leukemoid levels).
- Increased serum uric acid is frequent.
- Increased serum phosphorus. Phosphorus/creatinine ratio >3 indicates lactic acidosis, either alone or as a component of other metabolic acidosis.

Diagnostic Studies

Diagnosis is confirmed by exclusion of other causes of metabolic acidosis and serum lactate ≥ 5 mEq/L (upper limit of normal = 1.6 for plasma and 1.4 for whole blood). Considerable variation in literature in limits of serum lactate and pH to define lactic acidosis.

Laboratory tests for monitoring therapy

- Arterial pH, PCO_2, HCO_3^-, serum electrolyte levels every 1–2 hr until patient is stable
- Urine electrolyte levels every 6 hr

Associated or compensatory metabolic or respiratory disturbances (e.g., hyperventilation or respiratory alkalosis may result in normal pH)

Metabolic Acidosis with Normal Anion Gap (Hyperchloremic Acidosis)

Decreased serum potassium

- Renal tubular acidosis

Acquired (e.g., drugs, hypercalcemia)

Inherited (e.g., cystinosis, Wilson disease)

- Carbonic anhydrase inhibitors (e.g., acetazolamide, mafenide acetate)
- Increased loss of alkaline body fluids (e.g., diarrhea, loss of pancreatic or biliary fluids)
- Ureteral diversion (e.g., ileal bladder or ureter, ureterosigmoidostomy)

Normal or increased serum potassium

- Hydronephrosis
- Early renal failure
- Administration of HCl (e.g., ammonium chloride)
- Hypoadrenalism (diffuse, zona glomerulosa, or hyporeninemia)
- Renal aldosterone resistance
- Sulfur toxicity

Total plasma CO_2 content is decreased; value <15 mEq/L almost certainly rules out respiratory alkalosis.

Urine is strongly acid (pH = 4.5–5.2) if renal function is normal.

Azotemia suggests metabolic acidosis due to renal failure.

Respiratory Acidosis

Laboratory findings differ in acute and chronic conditions.

Acute

Due to decreased alveolar ventilation impairing CO_2 excretion

- Cardiopulmonary (e.g., pneumonia, pneumothorax, pulmonary edema, foreign-body aspiration, laryngospasm, bronchospasm, mechanical ventilation, cardiac arrest)
- Central nervous system (CNS) depression (e.g., general anesthesia, drug effects, brain injury, infection)
- Neuromuscular conditions (e.g., Guillain-Barré syndrome, hypokalemia, myasthenic crisis)

Acidosis is severe (pH 7.05–7.10), but HCO_3^- concentration is only 29–30 mEq/L.

Severe mixed acidosis is common in cardiac arrest when respiratory and circulatory failure cause marked respiratory acidosis and severe lactic acidosis.

Chronic

Due to chronic obstructive or restrictive conditions

- Neurologic disease
- Muscle disease
- CNS disorder
- Restriction of thorax (e.g., musculoskeletal disorders, scleroderma, pickwickian syndrome)
- Pulmonary disease (e.g., prolonged pneumonia, primary alveolar hypoventilation)

Respiratory Alkalosis

(Decreased PCO_2 <38 mm Hg)

Clinical Symptoms

Hyperventilation

- CNS disorders (e.g., infection, tumor, trauma, cerebrovascular accident)
- Salicylate intoxication
- Fever
- Bacteremia due to Gram-negative organisms
- Liver disease
- Pulmonary disease (e.g., pneumonia, pulmonary emboli, asthma)
- Mechanical overventilation
- Congestive heart failure
- Hypoxia (e.g., decreased barometric pressure, ventilation-perfusion imbalance)
- Anxiety-associated hyperventilation

Diagnostic Studies

Decreased PCO_2

Metabolic Acidosis with Respiratory Alkalosis

May be caused by rapid correction of metabolic acidosis, salicylate intoxication, septicemia due to Gram-negative organisms, initial respiratory alkalosis with subsequent development of metabolic acidosis.

Primary metabolic acidosis with primary respiratory alkalosis with an increased AG is characteristic of salicylate intoxication in absence of uremia or diabetic ketoacidosis.

Respiratory Acidosis with Metabolic Alkalosis

Clinical Symptoms

Chronic pulmonary disease with CO_2 retention in which patient develops metabolic alkalosis due to administration of diuretics, severe vomiting, or sudden improvement in ventilation ("posthypercapnic" metabolic alkalosis)

Diagnostic Studies

Decreased or absent urine chloride indicates that chloride-responsive metabolic alkalosis is present.

Respiratory acidosis but with normal blood pH or HCO_3^- higher than predicted, or both, complicates metabolic alkalosis.

Respiratory Alkalosis with Metabolic Alkalosis

Clinical Symptoms

Hepatic insufficiency with hyperventilation plus administration of diuretics or severe vomiting, metabolic alkalosis with stimulation of ventilation (e.g., sepsis, pulmonary embolism, mechanical ventilation) that causes respiratory alkalosis.

Diagnostic Studies

Marked alkalemia with decreased PCO_2 and increased HCO_3^-.

Metabolic Alkalosis

Clinical Symptoms

Loss of acid

- Vomiting, gastric suction, gastrocolic fistula

- Diarrhea in cystic fibrosis (rarely)
- Aciduria secondary to potassium depletion

Excess of base due to

- Administration of absorbable antacids (e.g., sodium bicarbonate administration; milk-alkali syndrome)
- Administration of salts of weak acids (e.g., sodium lactate, sodium or potassium citrate)
- Some vegetarian diets

Potassium depletion (causing sodium and H^+ to enter cells)

- Gastrointestinal loss (e.g., chronic diarrhea)
- Lack of potassium intake (e.g., anorexia nervosa, administration of intravenous fluids without potassium supplements for treatment of vomiting or postoperatively)
- Diuretics (e.g., mercurials, thiazides, osmotic diuresis)
- Extracellular volume depletion and chloride depletion
- All forms of mineralocorticoid excess (e.g., primary aldosteronism, Cushing's syndrome, administration of steroids, ingestion of large amount of licorice)
- Glycogen deposition
- Potassium-losing nephropathy

Hypoproteinemia per se may cause a nonrespiratory alkalosis. Decreased albumin of 1 g/dL causes an average increase in standard bicarbonate of 3.4 mEq/L, an apparent base excess of +3.7 mEq/L, and a decrease in AG of –3 mEq/L.[1]

Diagnostic Studies

Serum pH is increased (>7.60 in severe alkalemia).
Total plasma CO_2 is increased (bicarbonate >30 mEq/L).
The PCO_2 is normal or slightly increased.
Serum pH and bicarbonate level are above those predicted by the PCO_2 (by nomogram).
Hypokalemia is an almost constant feature and is the chief danger in metabolic alkalosis.
Decreased serum chloride, with level relatively lower than that of sodium.
Blood urea nitrogen may be increased.
Urine pH >7.0 (≤7.9) if potassium depletion is not severe and concomitant sodium deficiency (e.g., vomiting) is not present. With severe hypokalemia (<2.0 mEq/L), urine may be acid in presence of systemic alkalosis.
When the urine chloride level is low (<10 mEq/L) and the patient responds to chloride treatment, the cause is more likely loss of gastric juice, diuretic therapy, or rapid relief of chronic hypercapnia. Chloride replacement is complete when urine chloride remains >40 mEq/L. When the urine chloride is high (>20 mEq/L) and the patient does not respond to sodium chloride treatment, the cause is more likely hyperadrenalism or severe potassium deficiency.

Metabolic Alkalosis with Metabolic Acidosis

Clinical Symptoms

Vomiting causing alkalosis plus bicarbonate-losing diarrhea causing acidosis.

Diagnostic Studies

May be suggested by acid-base values that are too normal for clinical picture.

Summary of Pure and Mixed Acid-Base Disorders

See Table 2.

[1]Coe FL. Metabolic alkalosis. *JAMA* 1997;238:2288.

Table 2. Summary of Pure and Mixed Acid-Base Disorders

	Decreased pH	Normal pH	Increased pH
Increased PCO_2	Respiratory acidosis with or without incompletely compensated metabolic alkalosis or coexisting metabolic alkalosis	Respiratory acidosis and compensated metabolic acidosis	Metabolic alkalosis with incompletely compensated respiratory acidosis or coexisting respiratory acidosis
Normal PCO_2	Metabolic acidosis	Normal	Metabolic alkalosis
Decreased PCO_2	Metabolic acidosis with incompletely compensated respiratory alkalosis or coexisting respiratory alkalosis	Respiratory alkalosis and compensated metabolic acidosis	Respiratory alkalosis with or without incompletely compensated metabolic acidosis or coexisting metabolic alkalosis

Adapted from Friedman HH. *Problem-oriented medical diagnosis*, 3rd ed. Boston: Little, Brown and Company, 1983.

Upper Limits of Arterial Blood pH and HCO_3^- Concentration (Expected for Blood PCO_2 Values)

Arterial Blood[2]

PCO_2 (mm Hg)	pH	HCO_3^- (mEq/L)
20	7.66	22.8
30	7.53	25.6
40	7.57	27.3
60	7.29	27.9
80	7.18	28.9

Values shown are the upper limits of the 95% confidence bands.

Examples of Acidosis and Alkalosis

Pulmonary embolus: Mild to moderate respiratory alkalosis is present unless sudden death occurs. The degree of hypoxia often correlates with the size and extent of the pulmonary embolus. PO_2 of >90 mm Hg when patient breathes room air virtually excludes a lung problem.

Acute pulmonary edema: Hypoxemia is usual. CO_2 level is not increased unless the situation is grave.

Asthma: Hypoxia occurs even during a mild episode and increases as the attack becomes worse. As hyperventilation occurs, the PCO_2 falls (usually to <35 mm Hg); in a patient with true asthma (not bronchitis or emphysema), this indicates impending disaster and the need to consider intubation and ventilatory assistance.

Neurologic and neuromuscular disorders (e.g., drug overdose, Guillain-Barré syndrome, myasthenia gravis, trauma, succinylcholine administration): Acute alveolar hypoventilation causes uncompensated respiratory acidosis with high PCO_2, low pH, and normal HCO_3^-. Acidosis appears before significant hypoxemia, and rising CO_2 level indicates rapid deterioration and need for mechanical assistance.

Sepsis: Unexplained respiratory alkalosis may be the earliest sign of sepsis. It may progress to cause metabolic acidosis, and the mixed picture may produce a normal pH; low HCO_3^-. Acidosis appears before significant hypoxemia, and rising CO_2 level indicates rapid deterioration and need for mechanical assistance.

[2]Coe FL. Metabolic alkalosis. *JAMA* 1997;238:2288.

Salicylate poisoning: Characteristically, poor correlation is seen between serum salicylate level and presence or degree of acidemia (because as pH drops from 7.4 to 7.2, the proportion of nonionized to ionized salicylate doubles, and the nonionized form leaves the serum and is sequestered in the brain and other organs, where it interferes with function at a cellular level without changing blood levels of glucose, etc.). In children, this progresses rapidly to mixed respiratory alkalosis–metabolic acidosis and then to metabolic acidosis.

Isopropyl (rubbing) alcohol poisoning: Produces enough circulating acetone to produce a positive nitroprusside test (it therefore may be mistaken for diabetic ketoacidosis; thus, insulin should not be given until the blood glucose level is known). In the absence of a history of alcohol poisoning, positive serum ketone test results associated with normal AG, normal serum HCO_3^- level, and normal blood glucose level suggest rubbing alcohol intoxication.

Metabolic Acidoses of Hyperchloremia with Increased Anion Gap

(AG >15 mEq/L)

Causes

Lactic acidosis is the most common cause of metabolic acidosis with increased AG (usually >25 mEq/L).

Renal failure with uremia

Proximal renal tubular acidosis

Lactic acidosis with diarrhea

Excessive administration of sodium chloride to patient with organic acidosis

Ketoacidosis

- Diabetes mellitus (AG usually >25 mEq/L)
- Starvation (AG usually 5–10 mEq/L)

Drugs

- Salicylate poisoning (AG 10–20 mEq/L)
- Methanol poisoning (AG >20 mEq/L)
- Ethylene glycol poisoning (AG >20mEg/L)
- Paraldehyde (AG >20 mEq/L)

Diagnostic Studies

May be suspected when plasma HCO_3^- level is lower than is explained by the increase in anions (e.g., AG = 16 mEq/L and HCO_3^- = 5 mEq/L).

Anion Gap Classification

Calculated as Na – [Cl + HCO_3^-]

Increased In

Increased "unmeasured" anions

- Organic (e.g., lactic acidosis, ketoacidosis)
- Inorganic (e.g., administration of phosphate, carbenicillin)
- Protein (e.g., transient hyperalbuminemia)
- Exogenous (e.g., salicylate, formate, nitrate, penicillin, carbenicillin)
- Not completely identified (e.g., hyperosmolar, hyperglycemic nonketotic coma; uremia; poisoning by ethylene glycol, methanol, salicylates)
- Artefactual

Falsely increased serum sodium

Falsely decreased serum chloride or bicarbonate

- Decreased unmeasured cations (e.g., hypokalemia, hypocalcemia, hypomagnesemia)

When AG >12–14 mEq/L, diabetic ketoacidosis is the most common cause, uremic acidosis is the second most common cause, and drug ingestion (e.g., salicylates, methyl alcohol, ethylene glycol, ethyl alcohol) is the third most common cause; lactic acidosis should always be considered when these three causes are ruled out.

Decreased In

Decreased unmeasured anion (e.g., hypoalbuminemia, which is probably the most common cause of decreased AG).

Artefactual

- "Hyperchloremia" in bromide intoxication (if chloride determination by colorimetric method)
- Hyponatremia due to viscous serum
- False decrease in serum sodium; false increase in serum chloride or HCO_3^-

Increased unmeasured cations

- Hyperkalemia, hypercalcemia, hypermagnesemia
- Increased proteins in multiple myeloma, paraproteinemias, polyclonal gammopathies (these abnormal proteins are positively charged and lower the AG)
- Increased lithium, tris(hydroxymethyl)aminomethane buffer (tromethamine)

AG >30 mEq/L almost always indicates organic acidosis, even in presence of uremia.

AG of 20–29 mEq/L occurs in absence of identified organic acidosis in 25% of patients.

AG is rarely >23 mEq/L in chronic renal failure.

Simultaneous changes in ions may cancel each other out, leaving AG unchanged (e.g., increased chloride and decreased HCO_3^-).

AG may provide a clue to the presence of a mixed rather than simple acid-base disturbance.

Bibliography

Wallach J. *Interpretation of diagnostic tests*, 7th ed.Philadelphia: Lippincott Williams & Wilkins, 2000.

3 Pregnancy-Related Disorders and Prenatal Assessment of the Fetus

Amenorrhea

Primary amenorrhea is the absence of menses. No menses by age 14 with absence of secondary sexual characteristics, or no menses by age 16 with normal secondary characteristics.

Secondary amenorrhea is the cessation of menses for three cycles or 6 months of amenorrhea.

Signs and symptoms are the absence of periods, galactorrhea, symptoms of hypothyroidism, symptoms of early pregnancy, signs of androgen excess, and signs of estrogen deficiency.

Causes of Amenorrhea

Primary amenorrhea
- Imperforate hymen
- Agenesis of the uterus and upper two-thirds of the vagina (müllerian agenesis)
- Turner syndrome
- Constitutional delay

Secondary amenorrhea
- Physiologic causes: pregnancy, corpus luteal cyst, breast-feeding, menopause
- Suppression of the hypothalamic-pituitary axis, post–oral contraceptive pill amenorrhea, stress, intercurrent illness, weight loss, low body mass index
- Pituitary disease: ablation of the pituitary gland, Sheehan syndrome, prolactinoma
- Uncontrolled endocrinopathies: diabetes, hypo- or hyperthyroidism
- Polycystic ovary disease (Stein-Leventhal syndrome)
- Chemotherapy
- Pelvic irradiation
- Endometrial ablation (Asherman syndrome)
- Drug therapy: systemic steroids, danazol, growth-hormone–releasing factor analogs, antipsychotics, oral contraceptive pills
- Premature ovarian failure

Risk factors are overtraining (i.e., long-distance running, ballet dancing), eating disorders, psychosocial crisis.

Laboratory Tests

Pregnancy test; if results are negative, obtain levels of
- Serum prolactin
- Follicle-stimulating hormone
- Luteinizing hormone
- Thyroid-stimulating hormone
- Blood sugar

Special Diagnostic Tests

Progesterone challenge test: 10 mg of medroxyprogesterone acetate orally for 5 days.

If withdrawal bleeding occurs, amenorrhea most likely due to anovulation.

If no bleeding, evaluate estrogen status (follicle-stimulating hormone, luteinizing hormone levels).

Diagnostic Procedures

Laparoscopy: diagnosis of the streak ovaries of Turner syndrome, or polycystic ovary disease
Hysterosalpingogram to rule out Asherman syndrome

Laboratory Test Results during Menstruation

Platelet count is decreased by 50–70%; returns to normal by fourth day.
Hemoglobin (Hb) level is unchanged.
Fibrinogen level is increased.
Serum cholesterol level may increase just before menstruation.
Urine volume, sodium level, and chloride level decrease premenstrually and increase postmenstrually (diuresis).
Urine protein level may increase during premenstrual phase.
Urine porphyrin levels increase.
Urine estrogens decrease to lowest level 2–3 days after onset of menstruation.

Diagnosis of Rape

Acid Phosphatase in Vaginal Fluid

Because of high level of acid phosphatase in prostatic fluid, presence indicates recent sexual intercourse.
For diagnosis of sexual assault, rape, or recent sexual intercourse.
Normal level is <10 U/L in noncoital women.
Level of ≥50 U/sample is considered "semen positive."
Increased in 100% of women immediately after intercourse,
in 83% 8 hours after intercourse,
in 40% 24 hours after intercourse,
in 11% 72 hours after intercourse.
Low levels do not exclude recent intercourse.
In cases of possible rape, in addition to smears for sperm, specimens for identification of organisms causing sexually transmitted diseases (e.g., *Trichomonas vaginalis*, *Gonococcus*) should also be taken.
Semen specimens should be obtained for special genetic identification studies. Contact local police authorities in medicolegal cases for information on appropriate specimen types, handling, and identification.

Motile Sperm in Vaginal Fluid

May be useful in estimating time between intercourse and examination.
Presence of motile sperm in vaginal fluid usually indicates an interval of <8 hours.
Can be seen in approximately one-third of women within 6 hours.
In menstruating women, average period of motility is 4 hours.
Motile sperm are not seen in two-thirds of women examined within 6 hours.
Sperm motility in anal or oral cavity is reduced; presence indicates interval of only a few hours.

Sexually Transmitted Diseases, Prenatal Screening

All pregnant women at first prenatal visit should have
- Rapid plasma reagin test for syphilis
- Hepatitis B surface antigen test for hepatitis B virus infection
- Papanicolaou smear if not done in preceding year
- Human immunodeficiency virus test should be offered

High-risk women should have
- Test for *Neisseria gonorrhoeae* at first prenatal visit and repeat test during third trimester
- Test for *Chlamydia trachomatis* in third trimester

Table 1. Comparison of Various Causes of Vaginitis

Condition	pH	Saline Mount	10% KOH Mount	Culture	Amine Test
Normal	4.0–4.5	PMN/EC <1; rods dominant; 3+ squames	–		–
Bacterial vaginosis	>4.5	Clue cells; PMN/ED <1; D rods; I coccobacilli	–	No value	>70% +
Vulvovaginal candidiasis	4.0–4.5	PMN/EC <1; hyphae in 40%; rods dominant; 3+ squames	Hyphae in 70%	If wet mount is –	–
Trichomoniasis	5.0–6.0	Motile trichomonads in 60%; 4+ PMNs; mixed flora	–	Use if wet mount is –	Often +
Atrophic vaginitis	>6.0	1–2+ PMNs; I cocci and coliforms; D rods; parabasal cells	–		–

D, decreased; I, increased; KOH, potassium hydroxide; PMN/EC, ratio of polymorphonuclear leukocytes (PMNs) to epithelial cells; +, positive; –, negative.

Vulvovaginitis

Laboratory confirmation is necessary for reliable diagnosis.

Comparison of Various Causes of Vaginitis

See Table 1.

Due To

Fungal Infection

Especially *Candida albicans* (causes 20–25% of cases)

- Normal vaginal pH (4.0–4.5).
- Wet mount in potassium hydroxide or Gram stain of vaginal fluid may not detect 15% of cases.
- May be seen on Papanicolaou smears.
- Culture on Nickerson or Sabouraud medium is most sensitive.
- Sexual transmission plays a minor role.
- Underlying conditions may be present, especially uncontrolled diabetes mellitus, use of antibiotics, or use of vaginal sponges or intrauterine devices.

Trichomonas vaginalis Infection

- Wet-mount preparation of freshly examined vaginal fluid. Sensitivity = 50–70% compared with culture; requires 10^4 organisms/mL; specificity is almost 100%.
- Frequently an incidental finding in routine urinalysis.
- Frequently found in routine Papanicolaou smears.
- Increased polymorphonuclear leukocytes are present.
- pH is increased.
- Culture is the gold standard.
- DNA probe test kit gives prompt results; excellent method. Douching within 24 hours decreases sensitivity of tests. Do not test during first few days of menstrual cycle.
- Occasionally detected in material from male urethra in cases of nonspecific urethritis. Found in approximately 40% of male sexual partners of infected women. Prostatic fluid usually contains few organisms.

Serologic tests are not useful.

Bacterial Vaginosis

Polymicrobial infection due to increase in anaerobic organisms, including *Gardnerella vaginalis* or *Mobiluncus* or both, and concomitant decrease in lactobacilli.

Diagnosis based on presence of three or more of the following findings:
- Vaginal pH is >4.5 in >80% of these cases (found in one-third of normal women).
- Wet mount of vaginal discharge shows curved rods; "clue cells" (>20% of vaginal squamous cells coated with small coccobacilli) found in 90% of these cases.
- Positive culture results on HB or chocolate agar for *G. vaginalis* in 95% of clinical cases but not recommended for diagnosis or test of cure because may also be found in 40–50% of asymptomatic women with no signs of infection.
- DNA probe kit allows prompt results.
- Gram stain and Papanicolaou smear may also suggest this diagnosis: presence of Gram-negative curved rods and decreased to absent Gram-positive rods resembling lactobacilli.
- Local cause is most common [e.g., endocrine factors, poor hygiene, pinworms, scabies, foreign body, irritants (such as soaps, perfumes, spermicides), hypersensitivity reaction (such as to antimycotic creams, latex condoms)].

Atrophic Vaginitis

Increased pH (5.0 to 7.0).
Wet smear shows increased polymorphonuclear leukocytes and parabasal epithelial cells.
Mixed nonspecific Gram-negative rods with decreased lactobacilli.
Vaginal cytology shows atrophic pattern.

Desquamative Inflammatory Vaginitis

Purulent discharge
Increased pH
Gram stain shows absent Gram-positive bacilli replaced by Gram-positive cocci
Massive vaginal cell exfoliation with increased number of parabasal cells

Infection by Other Organisms

N. gonorrhoeae
Chlamydia
Group A Streptococcus
Staphylococcus aureus with toxic shock syndrome
Idiopathic occurrence associated with human immunodeficiency virus infection

Other Causes (Examples)

- Collagen vascular disease
- Behçet syndrome
- Pemphigus
- Lichen planus

Multiple causes may be present.

Prepartum Fetal Monitoring

Nonstress test (NST): Fetal heart rate (FHR) is monitored with the mother at rest. In a normal, reactive NST, FHR increases >15 beats per minute (bpm) for >15 seconds at least twice in 20 minutes. Reactivity can be absent in fetuses of <30 weeks' gestation because of central nervous system immaturity.

Biophysical profile: Thirty-minute ultrasonographic examination of the biophysical assessments—NST, amniotic fluid volume, fetal breathing, fetal movements and tone, and heart rate. Each parameter is scored as 2 (if normal) or 0 (if abnormal). Total scores of 8–10 are reassuring.

Intrapartum Fetal Heart Rate Monitoring

Normal baseline FHR: 120–160 bpm. Mild bradycardia: 100–200 bpm.

Normal beat-to-beat variability: Deviation from baseline of >6 bpm. Absence of variability is <2 bpm from baseline.

Early decelerations: Begin with the onset of contractions. The heart rate reaches the nadir at the peak contraction and returns to baseline as the contraction ends. Occur secondary to changes in vagal tone after brief hypoxic episodes or head compression and are benign.

Variable decelerations: Represent umbilical cord compression and have no uniform temporal relationship to the onset of the contraction. They are considered severe when the heart rate drops <60 bpm for ≥60 seconds with slow recovery to baseline.

Late decelerations: Occur after the peak of contraction, persist after the contraction stops, and show a slow return to baseline. Result from uteroplacental insufficiency and indicate fetal distress.

Laboratory Tests in Pregnancy at Term

Red blood cell (RBC) count, Hb level, and hematocrit decrease 15%.
RBC volume increases 20%, but plasma volume increases 45%.
White blood cell (WBC) count increases 66%.
Erythrocyte sedimentation rate increases markedly during pregnancy.
Serum iron level decreases 40% in patients not on iron therapy.
Serum transferrin level increases 40% and percent saturation decreases ≤70%.
Serum total protein level decreases 1 g/dL during first trimester; remains at that level.
Serum albumin level decreases 0.5 g/dL during first trimester; decreases 0.8 g/dL by term.
Serum α_1-globulin level increases 0.1 g/dL.
Serum α_2-globulin level increases 0.1 g/dL.
Serum β-globulin level increases 0.3 g/dL.
Serum ceruloplasmin level increases 70%.
Fasting blood glucose level decreases 5–10 mg/dL by end of first trimester.
Renal function changes are difficult to assess because of changes in plasma volume during pregnancy.
Blood urea nitrogen (BUN) and creatinine levels decrease 25%, especially during first half of pregnancy. BUN of 18 mg/dL and creatinine of 1.2 mg/dL represent increased (abnormal) levels in pregnancy, although these levels are normal in non-pregnant women.
Serum uric acid level decreases 35% in first trimester; returns to normal by term.
Serum cholesterol level increases 30–50%.
Serum triglyceride levels increase 100–200%.
Serum phospholipid level increases 40–60%.
Serum creatine kinase (CK) level decreases 15% by 20 weeks; increases at beginning of labor to peak at 24 hours postpartum, then gradually returns to normal. CK-MB is detected at onset of labor in 75% of patients, with peak level at 24 hours postpartum, then returns to normal.
Serum levels of lactate dehydrogenase and aspartate aminotransferase remain low.
In cases of threatened abortion during first 20 weeks of pregnancy, progressive increase in serum diamine oxidase level is usually associated with continuation of pregnancy.
Serum alkaline phosphatase (ALP) level progressively increases (200–300%) during the last trimester of normal pregnancy due to increase in heat-stable isoenzyme from the placenta.
Serum leukocyte ALP level may be moderately increased throughout pregnancy.
Serum lipase level decreases 50%.
Serum pseudocholinesterase level decreases 30%.
Serum calcium level decreases 10%.
Serum magnesium level decreases 10%.
Serum osmolality decreases 10 mOsm/kg during first trimester.
Serum vitamin B_{12} level decreases 20%.
Serum folate level decreases 50% or more. Overlap of decreased and normal range of values often makes this test useless in diagnosis of megaloblastic anemia of pregnancy.
Serum level of triiodothyronine uptake is decreased and thyroxine level is increased. T_7 (triiodothyronine × thyroxine) is normal. Level of thyroid-binding globulin is increased.
Serum aldosterone level is increased.
No changes are found in serum levels of sodium, potassium, chloride, phosphorus, amylase, aspartate aminotransferase, alanine aminotransferase, lactate dehydrogenase, acid phosphatase, and α-hydroxybutyrate dehydrogenase.
Occasionally, cold agglutinin test results may be positive and osmotic fragility increased.
Urine volume may increase ≤25% in last trimester.
Proteinuria is common (present in 20% of patients).
Glycosuria is common with decreased glucose tolerance.
Lactosuria should not be confused with glucose in urine.

Urine porphyrin levels may be increased.
Gonadotropins [human chorionic gonadotropin (hCG)] are increased.
Urine estrogen levels increase from 6 months to term (≤100 µg/24 hours).
Urine 17-ketosteroid levels rise to upper limits of normal at term.

Human Chorionic Gonadotropin

Serum β-subunit hCG assay (pregnancy test) gives positive results in 95% of patients, sensitivity of assay is <10 mU/mL; detects pregnancy 2 days earlier than urine test. Urine assays (sensitivity of 20–25 mU/mL) can detect hCG as early as 24–26 days after last menses. By 28 days after last menses, urine hCG is usually >200 mU/mL, and monoclonal antibody urine tests yield positive results. Qualitative test confirms pregnancy in 30 minutes.

- hCG level normally peaks at 100,000 mU/mL near end of first trimester, then declines to 10,000 mU/mL to end of pregnancy.
- hCG titer doubles every 2.0–3.5 days during first 40 days of normal pregnancy (at least two measurements 48–72 hours apart are needed); an abnormally slow increase in hCG (<66% in 48 hours) indicates ectopic pregnancy or abnormal intrauterine pregnancy.
- hCG level of >6,500 mU/mL (equivalent to level at 6 weeks' gestation) without visualization of an intrauterine gestational sac by transabdominal sonography favors ectopic pregnancy.
- Increase at 18–25 weeks' gestation occurs in 50% of pregnancies with Down syndrome.
- hCG of <6,000 mU/mL without a sac indicates unknown diagnosis.
- hCG of <6,300 mU with a sac suggests either ectopic pregnancy or an early normal/abnormal pregnancy.
- β-hCG >160,000 mU/mL without a sac suggests hydatidiform mole.
- β-hCG between 27,000 and 80,000 mU/mL with a sac suggests partial hydatidiform mole.
- β-hCG in choriocarcinoma is usually >150,000 mU/mL.
- Improvement in ultrasonographic instruments may change upper limits of hCG level with nonvisualization of sac to 1,500 mU/mL. Sac can be detected earlier by transvaginal sonography at a stage that is reported to correspond to an hCG level of 750 mU/mL.
- Decrease in hCG of ≥15% 12 hours after curettage is diagnostic of completed abortion, but increase or no change in hCG indicates ectopic pregnancy.

Serum hCG level is used to monitor methotrexate sodium treatment of ectopic pregnancy (testing is done weekly until hCG is undetectable).

Serum progesterone level is measured to screen patients at risk for ectopic pregnancy at time of first positive pregnancy test. Level ≥25 ng/mL indicates normal intrauterine pregnancy, and level ≤5 ng/mL confirms nonviable fetus. Diagnostic uterine curettage can be used to distinguish ectopic pregnancy from spontaneous intrauterine abortion.

WBC may be increased; usually returns to normal in 24 hours. Persistent increase may indicate recurrent bleeding. Fifty percent of patients have normal WBC; 75% of patients have WBC of <15,000 mm^3. Persistent WBC of >20,000/mm^3 may indicate pelvic inflammatory disease.

Anemia often precedes tubal pregnancy. Progressive anemia may indicate continuing bleeding into hematoma. Absorption of blood from hematoma may cause increased serum bilirubin level.

Culdocentesis fluid with a hematocrit of >15% indicates significant intraperitoneal hemorrhage.

Dilatation and curettage shows decidual changes without chorionic villi.

Algorithm for Diagnosis of Unruptured Ectopic Pregnancy

See Fig. 1.

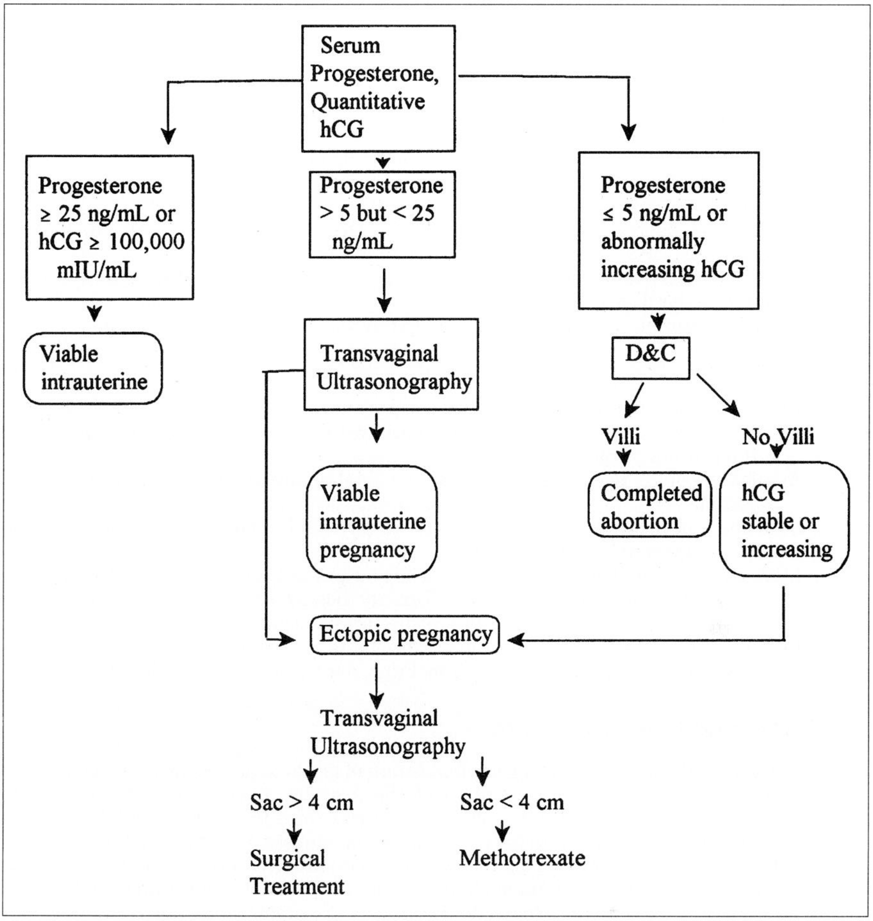

Fig. 1. Algorithm for diagnosis for unruptured ectopic pregnancy. D&C, dilatation and curettage; hCG, human chorionic gonadotropin.

Toxemia of Pregnancy

Preeclampsia

Hypertension, proteinuria, edema after 20th week of pregnancy.

Proteinuria varies from a trace to marked (≥800 mg/dL), equivalent to 15–20 g/day. Level of >150 mg/dL may indicate early toxemia.

In mild preeclampsia, proteinuria of >300 mg/dL is found in at least two random clean-catch urine specimens collected 6 hours apart.

In severe preeclampsia, significant proteinuria of ≥500 mg/24 hours (2+ on dipstick) is seen.

Oliguria: urine output <400 mL/24 hours.

Thrombocytopenia and abnormal liver function test results may be present.

RBCs and RBC casts are not abundant; hyaline and granular casts are present. BUN and renal concentrating ability are normal unless the disease is severe or a prior renal lesion is present. (BUN usually decreases during normal pregnancy because of increase in glomerular filtration rate.)
Serum uric acid level is increased (decreased renal clearance of urate) in 70% of patients. Thiazides can produce hyperuricemia independent of any disease.
Serum total protein and albumin levels commonly are markedly decreased.
Multiple clotting deficiencies may occur in severe cases. Lupus anticoagulant, antiphospholipid antibodies may be present.
Evidence of microangiopathic hemolysis, elevated liver function, and low platelet count (HELLP syndrome) occurs in 4–12% of cases.
Biopsy of kidney can establish diagnosis; rules out primary renal disease or hypertensive vascular disease.
Weekly creatinine clearance rate is used to follow renal function.

Eclampsia

Indicated by occurrence of generalized seizures.
Twenty percent of women develop eclampsia with only mild hypertension and often without proteinuria or edema.
Amniocentesis is performed to determine fetal maturity if induction of labor is required.
Usefulness of monitoring maternal levels of estriols, human placental lactogen, and other components is questionable.
Magnesium sulfate treatment requires urine output of ≥100 mL/4 hours. Therapeutic magnesium range = 4–7 mEq/L. Toxicity begins at 7–10 mEq/L; respiratory depression begins at 10–15 mEq/L; cardiac arrest begins at 30 mEq/L.
Beware of associated or underlying conditions (e.g., hydatidiform mole, twin pregnancy, prior renal disease, diabetes mellitus, nonimmune hydrops fetalis).

Amniotic Fluid Embolism

Amniotic fluid embolism is a rare complication of pregnancy. Risk factors include multiparity and premature separation of the placenta. Severe uterine contractions when the infant's head is engaged in the cervix force the amniotic fluid through a rupture in the chorion into the maternal venous sinuses, which precipitates dyspnea, tachypnea, and hypotension followed by disseminated intravascular coagulation and usually death. Amniotic fluid emboli are found in the maternal lungs at autopsy, as are disseminated fibrin thrombi in the maternal organs.

Ruptured Membranes

Diagnosis based on finding that fluid from posterior fornix is amniotic fluid rather than urine.
Detection of fetal isoform of fibronectin (by immunoassay) in vaginal secretions indicates presence of amniotic fluid. Is 5–10× greater in amniotic fluid than in maternal plasma; not present in normal vaginal secretions or urine.
Other methods for detecting amniotic fluid in the vagina include pooling, ferning, Nitrazine pH paper, ultrasonography, and dye injection. Such tests, if giving negative results, should be repeated or followed by fern tests and sterile speculum examination.

- Fern test is most reliable test (>96% accuracy). Fluid air-dried on a glass slide shows a characteristic fernlike pattern microscopically.
- Microscopic detection of fat-laden fetal squamous epithelial cells (Nile blue sulfate stain).
- Reagent strip test showing pH of ≥7 (normal vaginal pH = 4.5–5.5) and protein level of ≥100 mg/dL indicates presence of amniotic fluid.

pH alone	85%
Protein alone	90%
Either or both	95%

Presence of blood, meconium, renal disease, infection interferes with accuracy.

To detect premature rupture of membranes in any trimester, measure hCG level in saline washings of vaginal fornix; hCG levels of >50 mU/mL indicate rupture.

Measurement of α-fetoprotein (AFP) level in vaginal secretions is unreliable. Concentration is same in amniotic fluid and maternal plasma in third trimester.

Amniotic Fluid, Maternal and Fetal Serum, Normal Values

See Tables 2 and 3.

Isolation of Fetal Cells in Maternal Blood

Usual ratio = 1:1,000–1:5,000.

Prenatal Assessment of the Fetus

Routine clinical assessment by biochemical techniques and/or obtaining DNA from the fetus is possible for more than 100 possible genetic diseases. Chorionic villous sampling, amniocentesis, and fetal blood sampling are the most widely used techniques. Screening of maternal blood for fetal constituents (mainly AFP or DNA).

Obstetric Monitoring of Fetus and Placenta

Indications

Maternal age ≥35 years at delivery

Abnormal maternal serum AFP, hCG, or unconjugated estriol

Rubella, toxoplasmosis, or cytomegalovirus infection

Maternal disorder (e.g., diabetes mellitus, phenylketonuria)

Teratogen exposure (e.g., radiation, alcohol, isotretinoin, anticonvulsants, lithium)

Previous stillbirth or neonatal death

Previous child with chromosomal abnormality or structural defect

Inherited disorders (e.g., cystic fibrosis, metabolic disorders, sex-linked recessive disorders)

Either parent with balanced chromosome translocation or structural abnormality

Ethnic risk factors

- Sickle cell anemia (presence of sickling; confirmed by Hb electrophoresis)—African descent
- Tay-Sachs disease (decreased serum hexosaminidase A)—Jewish, American descent
- α and β thalassemia (decreased mean corpuscular volume; confirmed by Hb electrophoresis)—Mediterranean descent

Amniocentesis

Determination of increased bilirubin level in severe rhesus blood factor (Rh) disease.

Determination of lecithin/sphingomyelin (L/S) ratio to estimate fetal lung maturity.

Gram stain for organisms and WBC for diagnosis of amnionitis.

Prenatal diagnosis of genetic disorders

- Determination of karyotype.
- Wilms tumor may be associated with deletion of chromosome 11.

Assessment of intrauterine growth retardation.

Assessment of postdate pregnancies (>40 weeks).

Evaluation of other conditions (e.g., fetal death).

Amniotic fluid may contain abnormal metabolites (e.g., excess methylcitrate in propionicacidemia) or enzyme activity (e.g., *N*-acetyl-D-hexosaminidase A activity in Tay-Sachs disease), but usually tissue culture of amniotic fluid cells is used with analysis for specific deficient enzyme.

Amniotic Fluid Volume

At 38 weeks, normal range = 200–1,500 mL, average = 1,000 mL; progressive decrease thereafter.

Decreased (Oligohydramnios) In

Fetal anomalies

Renal agenesis (including Potter syndrome)

Table 2. Amniotic Fluid Amino Acid Reference Intervals

	9 Wk–3 Mo of Gestation (μmol/dL)	4 Mo of Gestation (μmol/dL)	5–6 Mo of Gestation (μmol/dL)	7–8 Mo of Gestation (μmol/dL)	9 Mo of Gestation (μmol/dL)	10 Mo of Gestation (μmol/dL)
β-Alanine	+	+	+	+	+	+
Alanine (α-Alanine)	26.6–61.4	32.5–83.7	28.4–53.9	15.6–30.1	9.2–25.9	10.4–29.9
α-Aminoadipic acid	+	+	+	+	+	+
Amino-β-guanidino-propionic acid	+	+	+	+	+	+
γ-Aminobutyric acid	+	+	+	+	+	+
β-Aminoisobutyric acid	+	+	+	+	+	+
α-Amino-*N*-butyric acid	+	+	+	+	+	+
Anserine	+	+	+	+	+	+
Arginine	6.0–10.5	4.0–14.3	2.8–9.6	2.1–4.8	1.4–2.8	1.1–2.6
Asparagine	0.3–3.1	1.9–3.6	0.5–5.0	0.3–0.9	0.3–0.9	0–1
Aspartic acid	0–4.1	0.3–7.7	0–4.1	0–0.8	0–0.5	0–0.4
Carnosine	+	+	+	+	+	+
Citrulline	+	+	+	+	+	+
Cystathionine	+	+	+	+	+	+
Cystine	+	+	+	+	+	+
Glutamic acid	7.7–21.2	13.7–61.0	3.8–53.3	1.7–5.6	0.9–2.3	1.4–4.4
Glutamine	7.5–41.7	3.4–29.3	9.4–36.8	16.7–57.8	11.8–39.9	11.8–36.5
Glycine	16.4–38.9	9.5–38.7	17.2–27.2	10.3–29.0	8.1–16.9	6.3–23.8
Histidine	5.5–14.2	7.1–16.9	7.5–12.9	4.5–11.1	2.5–7.2	2.8–6.3
Homocystine	+	+	+	+	+	+
Hydroxylysine	+	+	+	+	+	+

Hydroxyproline	0.3–4.3	3.1–5.1	1.9–4.8	2.2–4.7	1.1–3.8	1.0–3.7
Isoleucine	3.6–7.2	3.4–8.8	0.9–3.7	0.6–1.4	0–1.3	0.5–1.5
Leucine	9.2–18.0	7.4–19.7	2.6–15.9	1.4–3.0	0.9–2.9	1.3–2.5
Lysine	18.5–48.3	18.2–49.4	11.2–37.6	8.7–19.6	6.3–14.0	5.0–14.9
Methionine	1.4–3.8	1.8–5.8	0.9–2.8	0.3–1.1	0–0.7	0–0.9
1-Methyl-histidine	+	+	+	+	+	+
3-Methyl-histidine	+	+	+	+	+	+
Ornithine	3.6–7.1	3.8–9.7	2.1–4.5	1.5–3.9	1.3–2.4	1.0–4.2
Phenylalanine	5.0–12.1	4.9–13.7	3.0–9.9	1.1–2.8	0.9–2.6	0.8–2.5
Phosphoethanolamine	0–2.0	0.4–2.0	0–3.1	0–1.5	0–1.9	0.3–1.8
Phosphoserine	+	+	+	+	+	+
Proline	9.1–30.1	5.0–22.9	8.5–19.0	10.8–20.6	6.7–18.9	8.7–17.2
Sarcosine	+	+	+	+	+	+
Serine	3.8–8.7	2.6–9.1	2.7–6.2	2.5–5.1	1.9–4.9	2.0–5.2
Taurine	5.8–19.9	7.3–57.3	4.3–41.1	6.5–15.9	8.9–22	8.5–21.9
Threonine	10.3–23.0	13.8–33.3	15.7–27.0	9.1–19.1	6.9–15.6	4.6–16.7
Tryptophan	0–1.4	0–2	0–2	0[a]	0–0.2	0–0.2
Tyrosine	5.2–8.3	4.7–13.5	2.6–9.4	1.3–3.0	0.8–2.3	0.6–2.1
Valine	14.0–29.4	15.8–34.4	8.2–13.6	4.3–9.6	2.1–8.0	2.3–7.0

+, not established.
[a]None detected.

Table 3. Amniotic Fluid, Maternal and Fetal Serum, Normal Values

	Amniotic Fluid	Maternal Serum	Fetal Serum
Glucose (mg/dL)	10.7 (5.2)	66.6 (8.7)	48.7 (10.4)
Creatinine (mg/dL)	2.4 (0.3)	1.1 (0.2)	1.1 (0.3)
Urea (mg/dL)	33.9 (11.7)	17.1 (8.7)	16.5 (8.14)
Uric acid (mg/dL)	7.5 (0.3)	3.1 (0.8)	2.6 (0.9)
Total protein (g/dL)	0.28 (0.3)	6.5 (0.6)	5.8 (0.7)
Albumin (%)	65.2 (4.8)	46.4 (3.1)	60.8 (4.8)
Albumin/globulin ratio	1.9 (0.7)	0.8 (0.1)	1.5 (0.3)
Total cholesterol (mg/dL)	42.8 (3.2)	258.6 (47.2)	83.5 (39.7)
Triglycerides (mg/dL)	19.3 (9.4)	153.7 (51.4)	161.0 (10.7)
Lactic dehydrogenase (U/mL)	112.3 (64.8)	199.5 (46.4)	328.2 (114.0)
Aldolase (U/mL)	10.1 (7.5)	9.5 (7.0)	23.2 (9.4)

Values are mean values. Numbers in parentheses represent 1 SD.
From Castelazo-Ayala L, Karchmer S, Shor-Pinsker V. The biochemistry of amniotic fluid during normal pregnancy. Correlation with maternal and fetal blood. In: Hodari AA, Mariona F, eds. *Physiological biochemistry of the fetus. Proceedings of the international symposium.* Springfield, IL: Charles C Thomas, 1972:32–53.

Fetal obstructive uropathies
Postmaturity syndrome
Placental insufficiency (e.g., preeclampsia)
Donor-twin transfusion syndrome

Increased (Hydramnios) In

Idiopathic (35%)
Maternal diabetes (25%)
Hemolytic disease of the newborn (10%)
Multiple pregnancy (10%)
Congenital malformations (20%)

- Central nervous system malformations with exposed meninges
- Anencephaly, hydrocephaly, microcephaly
- Trisomy 21 (Down syndrome)
- Volvulus with atresia or congenital bands of upper jejunum or with common mesentery and herniation of liver
- Tracheoesophageal fistula with esophageal atresia
- Pyloric stenosis, duodenal atresia
- Imperforate anus
- Cleft palate
- Congenital heart disease
- Disease of gastrointestinal tract
- Deformity of limbs
- Agenesis of ears

Amniotic Fluid Color

May be milky or turbid (due to vernix caseosa and squamous debris) until centrifugation, which should yield a clear supernatant that is colorless to light straw color.

Yellow

- Usually due to bilirubin (normal maximum occurs at 20–28th weeks); may be increased with fetal RBC hemolysis (i.e., hemolytic disease of the newborn); increase correlates with fetal condition and prognosis.
- May also occur from fetal ascitic fluid, amniotic cysts, maternal urine (accidental puncture of mother's bladder).
- Yellow-brown color may be due to traces of meconium.

Green (may be with brown or black hue) is due to biliverdin from meconium, which may indicate fetal distress.

Red to brown is usually due to RBCs or Hb. Special staining (Betke-Kleihauer) or electrophoresis distinguishes fetal Hb from maternal blood due to trauma; or flow cytometry may be performed.

Table 4. Amniotic Fluid, Normal Chemical Components

	Second Trimester	At Term
Uric acid	3.7 mg/dL	9.9 mg/dL (due to increased muscle mass and increased output of fetus)
Creatinine	0.9 mg/dL	2.0 mg/dL (due to increased muscle mass of fetus)
Total protein	0.6 g/dL	0.3 g/dL
Albumin	0.4 g/dL	0.95 g/dL
Aspartate aminotransferase	17 U/dL	40 U/dL
Alkaline phosphatase	25 U/dL	80 U/dL (≤350 U in some cases)

Levels of glucose, bilirubin, urea nitrogen, calcium, phosphorus, cholesterol, lactic dehydrogenase do not change significantly during gestation.

Bright red indicates recent intrauterine hemorrhage or hemolysis; may be port wine color in abruptio placentae.

Brown may be due to oxidized Hb from degenerated RBCs.

Brown-black may be due to fetal maceration.

Normal Chemical Components of Amniotic Fluid

See Table 4.

Chorionic Villus Sampling

Generally done between 8 and 12 weeks of gestation; sometimes as early as 6–7 weeks. Risk of fetal loss is 0.5–2.0%.

Contamination with maternal decidua must be avoided for accurate diagnosis based on fetal chromosomes, enzyme assay, or DNA analysis.

Indications

Couples at risk for a fetus with a chromosomal disorder are the largest group to which chorionic villus sampling (CVS) is applicable. This group includes those at risk because of maternal age, the presence of chromosomal translocation in one parent, or the previous birth of a trisomic child. Chorionic villus samples can be assayed directly for enzyme activity to detect a number of metabolic disorders. Careful separation of the villi is mandatory for an accurate biochemical diagnosis with either enzymatic or DNA analysis techniques.

Advantages

There are several advantages to CVS in addition to the earlier timing of the procedure. The short culture time for the genetic studies and the direct assays performed from biochemical and DNA analysis result in a significantly shorter time to final diagnosis than is possible with amniocentesis.

Complications

A sufficient sample for diagnosis is obtained in 98% of the procedures performed. Culture failure occurs in less than 1% of cases. Immediate rupture of fetal membranes is uncommon; this reflects the benefit of sonographic guidance of the catheter.

An overall spontaneous abortion rate of 3.5–4.0% has been cited. When chromosomal aneuploidy is confined only to the villous sample and appears to represent true mosaicism within the placenta, the incidence is 1–3%. Placental mosaicism may be associated with an increased risk of pregnancy loss. In such cases, amniocentesis should be offered for confirmation.

Potential long-term complications include Rh isoimmunization, prematurity, placental abnormalities, and birth defects. Transverse limb defects and hyomandibular defects have rarely occurred when the procedure is performed at <70 days of gestation (56 days of development).

CVS is most commonly performed in a transcervical approach using a 1.5-mm (16-gauge) polyethylene catheter with a 1-mm malleable stainless steel stylet. Under direct ultrasonographic guidance, the catheter is passed transcervically and is placed within the villi of the chorion frondosum. Application of 5–15 mL of suction to the catheter by using a 20-mL syringe allows samples of 10–40 mg wet weight to be obtained. The sample is then placed into culture medium, and, under a dissecting microscope, the villi are separated from maternal decidual tissue. The villi can be analyzed for enzymatic activity and DNA, or they can be placed into culture for cytogenetic studies. Transabdominal CVS has a higher rate of successful sampling.

Risks of Second-Trimester Amniocentesis

Spontaneous abortion in up to 1% of cases.

Respiratory difficulties due to effect on developing fetal lung from sudden decrease in amniotic fluid volume.

Possibly higher rate of hip dislocation and talipes equinovarus.

Placental penetration by the amniocentesis needle.

Possibility of fetomaternal hemorrhage at the time of amniocentesis, which causes later sensitization to Rh and other antigens.

The incidence of fetal trauma is very low.

Intraamniotic Infection

Bacteria (in congenital pneumonia and chorioamnionitis, two-thirds of causative organisms are Gram negative). Most common organisms are *G. vaginalis*, *C. albicans*, group B *Streptococcus*, and diphtheroids. Most dangerous are *Escherichia coli* and group B *Streptococcus*. Twenty percent of intraamniotic infections cause two-thirds of cases of maternal or neonatal bacteremia.

Virus (e.g., rubella, virus, cytomegalovirus, herpes simplex virus).

Fetal Maturity Assessment

Menstrual history: Most accurate determination of gestational age. Nägele rule, based on a 28-day cycle, calculates expected date of confinement as 9 months (280 days) plus 7 days from the last menstrual period.

Ultrasonography: Crown-rump length obtained between 6 and 12 weeks predicts gestational age ± 3–4 days. After 12 weeks, the biparietal diameter is accurate within 10 days, and beyond 26 weeks accuracy diminishes to ± 3 weeks.

Growth: Expected birth weight (50th percentile) by gestational age is as follows:

24 wk	700 g
26 wk	900 g
28 wk	1,100 g
30 wk	1,350 g
32 wk	1,650 g
34 wk	2,100 g
36 wk	2,600 g
38 wk	3,000 g

Fetal lung maturity: Lecithin, the active component of surfactant, is present in amniotic fluid in increasing amounts throughout gestation, compared with constant levels of sphingomyelin).

- L/S ratio: >2:1 indicates fetal lung maturity in nondiabetic pregnancies. L/S ratio is generally 1:1 at 31–32 weeks' gestation, and 2:1 by 35 weeks' gestation.
- L/S ratios (determined by thin-layer chromatography) for various levels of lung maturity are shown in Table 5.

L/S ratio is single most accurate test of fetal maturity.

Determination of Preterm Delivery

Gestational age <37 weeks or 259 days; premature infant weighs <2,500 g.

Fetal fibronectin level in cervical secretions of >50 ng/mL (by immunoassay) identifies women who deliver before term.

Laboratory findings due to associated conditions (e.g., hyaline membrane disease, intraventricular hemorrhage).

Table 5. Estimation of Lung Maturity by Lecithin/Sphingomyelin Ratio

Lecithin/ Sphingomyelin Ratio	(Some Laboratories Use These Values)	Lung Maturity
<1	<2.0	Very immature lungs (up to 30th wk of gestation); severe RDS is expected; many weeks may be required to reach lung maturity; do not resample before 2 wk.
1.00–1.49		Immature lungs; moderate to severe RDS is expected; lung maturity may be reached in 2 wk; resample in 1 wk.
1.5–1.9	2.0–3.0	Lungs on threshold of maturity (within 14 d); mild to moderate RDS may occur. Test should be repeated in 1 wk.
≥2	>3.0	Mature lungs (35th wk of gestation); RDS is not expected; 80–85% sensitivity and specificity.

RDS, respiratory distress syndrome.
Adapted from Dubin SA. Assessment of fetal lung maturity. Practice parameters. *Am J Clin Pathol* 1998;110:723; Dito WR, Patrick CW, Shelly J. *Clinical pathologic correlations in amniotic fluid.* Chicago: American Society of Clinical Pathologists, 1975; and Natelson S, Scommegna A, Epstein MD, eds. Amniotic fluid. *Physiology, biochemistry and clinical chemistry.* New York: John Wiley and Sons, 1974.

Human Placental Lactogen

Appears by fifth week of gestation and increases progressively thereafter.
Values correlate better with placental than with fetal weight. Therefore useful to evaluate placental function; sudden decrease in concentration before fetal death. Use only as adjunct to other tests.

Useful In

Diabetes mellitus, severe
Hypertension
Postmaturity syndrome
Idiopathic placental failure

Not Useful In

Diabetes mellitus, mild or moderately severe
Rh sensitization disease

Prolonged Pregnancy

Amniotic fluid L/S ratio is <2. High ratio (4) can occur before 42 weeks' gestation.
Progressively falling rather than rising estriol level is usually found.
Squalene (derived from fetal sebaceous glands) is markedly increased in amniotic fluid after 39 weeks.
Squalene/cholesterol ratio in amniotic fluid:
- <0.4 before 40 weeks
- >0.4 after 40 weeks
- >1.0 after 42 weeks

Postmature Lungs

Lecithin/Sphingomyelin Ratio

In postmature lung, there is abundant lecithin with trace or no sphingomyelin.
Definite exceptions to prediction of pulmonary maturity when L/S ratio is >2.0:

- Infant of diabetic mother [L/S ratio of >2.0 has been frequently seen in cases in which respiratory distress syndrome (RDS) developed]
- Erythroblastosis fetalis

Possible exceptions

- Intrauterine growth retardation
- Toxemia of pregnancy
- Hydrops fetalis
- Placental disease
- Abruptio placentae

In twin pregnancies, L/S ratio must be determined on fluid from each amniotic sac.

Foam (Shake) Test

Reliable, simple bedside method providing qualitative expression of L/S ratio that gives prompt results. Commercial kit said to have sensitivity of 87%, specificity of 97%.

Interferences (with Lecithin/Sphingomyelin Ratio and Foam Tests)

Contamination of amniotic fluid with meconium, blood, vernix caseosa, or vaginal mucus makes L/S determinations unreliable (fluid should test negative for leukocyte esterase using urine dipstick). Whole-blood L/S ratio is 1:5.

Collection in siliconized tubes.

Dilution due to oligo- or polyhydramnios may make foam test unreliable.

Interpretation

Although an L/S ratio of >2 and positive foam test results indicate pulmonary maturity and absence of RDS in >95% of cases, a ratio of <2 and negative foam test results have a high false-negative rate in predicting RDS and therefore are unreliable.

If amniotic fluid is not available, L/S ratio or foam test can be done on gastric aspirate from infant during first 6 hours of life if no milk has been given and the trachea is not occluded by intubation. Tracheal fluid or hypopharyngeal secretion can also be used.

Other Tests

Phosphatidylglycerol content of >2% (0.5 μg/mL by immunoagglutination kit) and phosphatidylinositol content of >15% in amniotic fluid indicate fetal lung maturity; they are not affected by contamination of amniotic fluid, maternal diabetes mellitus, or hemolytic disease of the newborn and are thus more sensitive measures than L/S ratio, although more laborious to perform (commercial rapid slide agglutination test is now available). Absence of both indicates high risk of RDS for at least 3–4 weeks. Phosphatidylglycerol does not appear in amniotic fluid until after 36 weeks' gestation; therefore, absence has poor predictive value for RDS. The total profile of tests provides the most reliable results.

Measurement of optical absorbance at 650 nm to evaluate amniotic fluid turbidity; maturity criterion is a value of ≥0.1. Interference by blood, meconium, or dilution due to oligo- or polyhydramnios corresponds to the gross pearly opalescence of mature amniotic fluid and to a count of lamellar bodies (derived from fetal lung) using automated platelet counter.

Nile blue sulfate staining of amniotic fluid differentiates fetal squamous cells from anucleated fat cells. Finding of >50% fat cells indicates mature fetus (40 weeks) and also correlates with occurrence of RDS. Low counts should be interpreted with caution and correlated with other findings. Maternal diabetes may cause spurious elevation of fat cell count.

Amniotic fluid creatinine level of ≥2 mg/dL indicates muscle mass of fetus and the presence of 1 million functioning glomeruli, and corresponds to pregnancy of ≥37 weeks in >90% of cases. Values of 1.6–2.0 mg/dL are considered equivocal. Value of <1.6 mg/dL indicates fetal weight of <2,500 g and <37 weeks' gestation. May be decreased in mature but low-birth-weight infants. May be spuriously increased by hypertensive disorders of pregnancy (e.g., preeclampsia) and maternal renal disease; therefore, maternal serum creatinine should be determined. Ratio of maternal serum creatinine to amniotic creatinine ≥3 indicates gestational age of 36 weeks in 97% of cases. Urea and uric acid levels show more fluctuation and therefore are less useful than creatinine level.

Bilirubin virtually disappears from amniotic fluid by 36 weeks of gestation. May be increased due to maternal hyperbilirubinemia (e.g., hepatitis, hemolytic anemia, cholestasis) or to administration of drugs (e.g., phenothiazides), which makes the test useless. Meconium results in positive interference. Oligohydramnios may cause false-positive results, and polyhydramnios may cause false-negative results.

Amniotic fluid osmolarity of <250 mOsm/L indicates term pregnancy.

Lamellar bodies in amniotic fluid can be counted as platelets in electronic cell counter. A count of <30,000/µL has sensitivity of 100%, specificity of 64%, and negative predictive value of 100% as an indicator of lung maturity. At a count of 10,000/µL, specificity = 95%, sensitivity = 75%, and negative predictive value = 96%.

These tests are valid indicators of fetal maturity (low-false-positive rates) but less reliable indicators of immaturity (appreciable false-negative rates). In general, multiple tests give more reliable results than any single test.

A γ-glutamyl transferase/alkaline phosphatase ratio of >2.0 in amniotic fluid has been reported to indicate pulmonary maturity.

Differences between Amniotic Fluid and Urine

	Amniotic Fluid	**Urine**
Specific gravity	1.025	1.005–1.030
pH	Neutral or alkaline	Usually acid
Protein	Significant quantity	Absent
Urea	Similar to plasma	High
Bilirubin	May be present	Absent
Chloride	Moderate to high	Low to high
Creatinine	Similar to plasma	High
Uric acid	Similar to plasma	High
Alkaline phosphatase	High	Low
Ascorbic acid	Low	Low to high

Fetal Death *In Utero*

Amniotic fluid may be brown with markedly increased CK level.

Intrauterine fetal death has been said to be reliably indicated by increased CK level (usually >200 sigma U/mL; normal is <3 sigma U/mL).

Disseminated intravascular coagulation may occur, especially if gestation is >16 weeks and dead fetus is retained for ≥4 weeks.

Fetal Fibronectin

Secreted by chorionic trophoblast throughout pregnancy. Measured by enzyme-linked immunosorbent assay or rapid test using cervicovaginal sample.

Indicator of risk of preterm labor or birth (level of >50 ng/mL).

Normally absent from cervicovaginal fluid after 20 weeks. Normally present in early pregnancy and within 1–2 weeks of onset of labor at term.

For high-risk patients, sensitivity = 70%, specificity = 75%.

Hormones

Maternal Urine Estriol

Reflects both placental and fetal adrenal cortex function and fetal liver function. Monitoring is usually begun at 34 weeks but may begin at 28 weeks in high-risk pregnancy (e.g., severe maternal hypertension, intrauterine growth retardation).

Reliable evaluation requires serial (rather than isolated) determinations (at least twice a week) to detect an abrupt fall. A decrease of ≥50% is generally considered significant, but level may be affected by variable maternal renal function.

The 24-hours urine level of estriol normally shows a progressive increase during gestation. May show a 25% variation from day to day in an individual patient.
Level of >12 mg/24 hours at term indicates a healthy neonate.
Level of 4–12 mg/24 hours or decrease of >50% indicates infant in jeopardy.
Level of <4 mg/24 hours indicates fetal death or severe jeopardy.

Decreased In

Fetus

- Intrauterine death
- Fetal abnormalities (e.g., anencephaly, adrenal hypoplasia)

Placenta

- Sulfatase deficiency
- Infarcts
- Placental dysfunction
- Hydatidiform mole

Mother

- Use of oral antibiotic (values may be two-thirds of normal)
- Renal disease
- Liver disease
- Corticosteroid administration (values may be 50% of normal)
- Incomplete urine collection

Laboratory

- Mandelamine in urine (prevents bacterial splitting or reabsorption of estriol)

Plasma Progesterone and Urinary Pregnanediol (Its Chief Metabolite)

Increase progressively during pregnancy.
Reflect only adequate placental function, not fetal status.

Maternal Serum Unconjugated Estriol

Is of fetal origin from fetal adrenal, liver, and placental function. Begins to appear by seventh to ninth week of gestation.

Decreased In

Fetal Down syndrome
Low values at 35–36 weeks of gestation identify up to one-third of small-for-date infants.

Interpretation

Value >12 ng/mL rules out postmaturity in cases of prolonged gestation if no other disease is present (e.g., diabetes mellitus, isoimmunization).
Decreased value detects 45% of cases of Down syndrome with a 5.2% false-positive rate.
Value is ≤0.6 multiples of the median in 5% of unaffected pregnancies and 26% of Down syndrome cases.
Safe levels indicate fetal well-being.
Increasing serial values rule out prolonged pregnancy and postmaturity.
Constant normal values are consistent with 40–41 weeks of gestation.
Declining values are consistent with prolonged gestation.
Low or significantly falling values are seen in fetal distress and postmaturity.

Amniotic Fluid Estriol

Interpretation

Values are not meaningful before 20 weeks' gestation (<1.0 µg/dL); gradual increase to 35th week and then rapid increase to 40th week. Each laboratory must establish its own reference ranges.
Decreasing levels are associated with fetal distress, and failure to increase with fetal death.

Serum Markers for Detection of Various Prenatal Conditions

See Table 6.

Table 6. Serum Markers in Detection of Various Prenatal Conditions

Condition	α-Fetoprotein	Human Chorionic Gonadotropin	Unconjugated Estriol	Detection Rate (%)
Anencephaly	4+	–	–	95
Open spina bifida	3+	–	–	80
Abdominal wall defect	3+	–	–	75
Trisomy 21 (Down syndrome)	↓	↑	↓	60
Trisomy 18	↓↓	↓↓	↓↓	60
Other chromosomal abnormalities	↑↓	↑↓	↑↓	50

↑, increased; ↓, decreased.
From Wasserman ER. *Preventing problem pregnancies.* Advance/Laboratory Nov. 1997:53.

Maternal Serum α-Fetoprotein Screening

Screening for serum AFP level is performed as follows: Maternal serum is obtained between 16 and 18 weeks of gestation; the distributions of maternal serum AFP levels during the second trimester are given in Table 7.

Interpretation

Use of maternal serum AFP level alone is not recommended; should be combined with measurements of hCG and unconjugated estriol when maternal age is >35 years. This combination can identify 60% of cases of Down syndrome with a false-positive rate of 6.6%. Ultrasonography to verify gestational age reduces false-positive rate to 3.8%.

Finding of decreased maternal blood level of AFP in pregnancy is a valuable screening tool, but diagnosis should be confirmed by finding of increased levels in amniotic fluid and by ultrasonography (to rule out missed abortion, molar pregnancy, absent pregnancy), as well as by chromosomal studies to confirm or refute the diagnosis.

Decreased In

Down syndrome (trisomy 21) and trisomy 18
Long-standing death of fetus
Overestimation of gestational age (underestimation of age in amniotic fluid sample)
Choriocarcinoma, hydatidiform mole
Increased maternal weight (does not affect amniotic fluid concentration)
Pseudopregnancy, nonpregnancy
Use of various drugs (therefore no medications should be taken for at least 12 hours before test)

Table 7. Distributions of Maternal Serum α-Fetoprotein Levels during the Second Trimester

Week Post-Last Menstrual Period	Median (ng/mL)	2 × Median (ng/mL)	2.5 × Median (ng/mL)
15	30	60	75
16	35	70	88
17	37	74	93
18	41	82	103
19	45	90	113
20	54	108	135

From Haddow JE. *Advanced Clin Chem* NO. ACC-32, 1979.

Other unknown conditions

Women with diabetes mellitus have values 20–40% less than those of nondiabetic women.

Increased In

(Should be confirmed by increase in amniotic fluid.)

Twin pregnancy (>4.5 multiples of the median)

Increased gestational age (for which values must be adjusted)

Certain racial backgrounds (for which values must be adjusted); levels 10–15% higher in blacks.

Open neural tube defects (e.g., open spina bifida, anencephaly, encephalocele, myelocele); 80% of severe cases are detected by AFP. Women with one affected child have a 5% chance of giving birth to another; affected families make up 10% of these cases. Optimal screening is in 16th–20th week of gestation.

Hydrocephaly

Microcephaly

Ventral wall defects associated with exposed fetal membrane and blood vessel surfaces, for example,

- Omphalocele (incidence 1–3 in 10,000)
- Gastroschisis (incidence 1–10 in 10,000)

Hydrops fetalis

Intrauterine death

Fetal-maternal hemorrhage

Esophageal or duodenal atresia

Cystic hygroma

Renal disorder, for example,

- Congenital proteinuric nephropathies
- Polycystic kidneys
- Renal agenesis

Aplasia cutis

Sacrococcygeal teratoma

Tetralogy of Fallot

Turner syndrome

Oligohydramnios

Maternal disorders (e.g., neoplasm that produces AFP, hepatitis)

Very rare benign hereditary familial elevation of serum AFP

When amniotic fluid AFP level is elevated, assay of acetylcholinesterase is helpful in confirming the diagnosis of an open neural tube defect.

Maternal Serum Sampling

α-Fetoprotein

AFP is increased 4× normal in open neural tube, 7× normal in anencephaly and in ventral wall defects; associated with exposed fetal membranes and blood vessel surfaces.

Maximum serum AFP concentration is between 16–18 weeks, but sampling should not be done before 14 or after 20 weeks. If both serum and amniotic fluid show increased levels, contamination of amniotic fluid with fetal or maternal blood is ruled out by assay for fetal Hb and acetylcholinesterase. If only maternal serum AFP is increased without demonstrable defect, pregnancy is at increased risk (e.g., premature delivery, low-birth-weight baby, or fetal death).

Serum AFP levels are low in trisomy 21 (30% lower) as well as trisomy 18 (40% lower).

Triple-Screen Marker Test

The triple-screen marker test recommended by the American College of Obstetricians and Gynecologists includes the determination in the maternal serum of

AFP (2× normal in trisomy 21)

hCG

Unconjugated estriol (30% lower in trisomy 21)

This test allows for prenatal detection of 65% of cases of Down syndrome. Amniocentesis for karyotyping is then recommended for confirmation.

This triple-marker test has been improved by the addition of inhibin A—the quadruple tests. Inhibin A, like hCG, is a protein made by the placenta, and its level is twice as high in the maternal serum with a trisomy 21 fetus. The quadruple test administered in the second trimester is the best screening test available, with a detection rate of 75–80%.

Genetic Analysis

Methods for Fetal Karyotyping

	Amniocentesis	Chorionic Villus Sampling
Method	20–30 mL amniotic fluid is withdrawn under ultrasonographic guidance; results delayed as tissue culture of amniocytes required to provide sufficient sample for analysis.	Transcervical: Flexible catheter advanced under ultrasonographic guidance, small placental segment aspirated. Transabdominal: Chorionic villi obtained via needle aspiration through the abdominal wall. Results available quickly as mitotically active cells are sampled.
Indications	Detects chromosomal abnormalities, metabolic disorders, neural tube defects.	Detects chromosomal abnormalities and metabolic disorders; cannot detect neural tube defects or measure AFP.
Gestational age at testing	16–18 weeks' gestation.	8–11 weeks' gestation.
Complications	Pregnancy loss (0.5%), chorioamnionitis (<1/1,000), leakage of amniotic fluid (1/300), fetal injury (primarily superficial scars or dimpling of the skin).	Pregnancy loss (0.5–2%), maternal infection, increased risk of fetomaternal hemorrhage, fetal limb and jaw malformations.

Molecular Diagnosis of Genetic Abnormalities

Direct detection of gene deletions and mutations, and linkage analysis using cultured amniocytes or chorionic villi can make some diagnoses even when gene products are not present (e.g., adult polycystic kidney disease, sickle cell disease, α thalassemia, cystic fibrosis, Gaucher disease, Duchenne muscular dystrophy, fragile X syndrome, factor VIII and factor IX deficiencies).

Chromosome Number and Karyotype in Various Clinical Conditions

See Table 8.

Fetal Blood Sampling

Fetal blood sampling rarely stimulates uterine contractions. The cord insertion into the placenta must be clearly exposed without fetal interposition. The insertion of the cord into the placenta is its most fixed position; therefore, the cord can be punctured more easily at this point.

Once the cord insertion site has been determined, the cord must remain strictly immobile, and a 20-gauge, 9-cm spinal needle is introduced under aseptic conditions. The cord is entered approximately 1 cm from its insertion site. Use of a rigid needle is very important so that the operator will not have to reinsert the needle several times through the maternal abdominal wall. Depending on whether the placenta is anterior, lateral, or posterior, the cord insertion can be reached directly through the placenta without traversing the amniotic cavity, transplacentally and then transamniotically, or simply transamniotically.

Table 8. Chromosome Number and Karyotype in Various Clinical Conditions

	Chromosome Number and Karyotype	Incidence
Normal male	46 XY	—
Normal female	46 XX	—
Suspected autosomal syndrome		—
Down syndrome (trisomy 21)	47 XX, 21+ or 47 XY, 21+	1 in 700 live births (2% are 46 count due to translocation and have 10% risk of Down syndrome in subsequent pregnancies; 2% are 46/47 mosaics)
Trisomy 13	47 XX, 13+ or 47 XY, 13+	1 in 5,000 live births
	Translocations	Rare
	Mosaics	Rare
Trisomy 18	47 XX, 18+ or 47 XY, 18+	1 in 3,000 live births
	Translocations	Rare
	Mosaics	Rare
Trisomy 13	—	—
Trisomy 8, 9, 4p, 9p	—	—
Cri du chat syndrome	46 with partial B deletion	1 in 30,000 births
Others (e.g., 4p-, 5p-, 9p-, 13q-)		
Suspected sex chromosome syndromes		
Klinefelter syndrome	47 XXY	1 in 600 live male births
	48 XXXY	Rare
	48 XXYY	Rare
	49 XXXXY	Rare
	49 XXXYY	Rare
	Mosaics	Infrequent
Turner syndrome	45 XO	1 in 3,000 live female births
	46 XX	Rare
	Mosaics	Infrequent
Superfemale	47 XXX	1 in 1,000–2,000 live female births
	48 XXXX	Rare
	49 XXXXX	Rare
	Mosaics	Rare
Supermale	47 XXY	1 in 1,000 live male births

Fetal blood sampling can be performed from 18 weeks after the last menstrual period to term. The quantity of blood taken out during each procedure is minimal (1.5–4.0 mL, depending on the gestational age). Fetal deaths have been attributed to mechanical cord problems, major fetal malformations, or severe intrauterine growth retardation.

The apparent fetal risk is between 1% and 2%.

Indications for Fetal Blood Sampling

Infections
- Toxoplasmosis
- Rubella
- Other viral infections

Karyotyping
Coagulation disorders
- Hemophilia
- Factor deficiencies
- Platelet disorders

Rh isoimmunization
Hemoglobinopathies
Fetal welfare assessment
Metabolic diseases

Fetal Biopsy

Liver biopsy for diagnosis of deficiency of long-chain 3-hydroxyacyl-coenzyme A dehydrogenase, ornithine transcarbamylase deficiency, atypical phenylketonuria due to deficiency of glutamyl transpeptidase cyclohydrolase I, type I primary hyperoxaluria, glycogen storage disease type 1.
Skin biopsy (e.g., for certain genetic disorders such as epidermolysis bullosa).
Muscle biopsy for Duchenne muscular dystropy.

Ultrasonography and Echocardiography

Used to guide sampling process.
Used to verify gestational age.
May be abnormal.
Karyotyping is done if malformations are found.
Fifty percent of major heart, kidney, and bladder abnormalities are not detected by maternal serum AFP screening.

Bibliography

Anderson RL, Goldberg JD, Golbus MS. Prenatal diagnosis in multiple gestation: 20 years' experience with amniocentesis. *Prenat Diagn* 1991;11:263–270.
Blackstone J, Young BK. Umbilical cord blood acid-base values and other descriptors of fetal condition. *Clin Obstet Gynecol* 1993;36:33–46.
Bodurtha J, Redwine F, Jackson-Cook C. Three methods of fetal sampling in prenatal diagnosis. *Va Med Q* 1992;119:93–95.
Brambati B, Oldrini A, Ferrazzi F, et al. Chorionic villous sampling: an analysis of the obstetric experience of 1000 cases. *Prenat Diagn* 1987;7:157.
D'Alton ME, DeCherney AH. Prenatal diagnosis. *N Engl J Med* 1993;328:114–120.
Diagnostic and therapeutic technology assessment. Chorionic villous sampling: a reassessment. *JAMA* 1990;263:305–306.
Doran TA. Chorionic villous sampling as the primary diagnostic tool in prenatal diagnosis. Should it replace genetic amniocentesis? *J Reprod Med* 1990;35:935–940.
Evans MI, Koppick FC, Nemitz B, et al. Early genetic amniocentesis and chorionic villous sampling: expanding the opportunities for early prenatal diagnosis. *J Reprod Med* 1998;33:450.
Hobbins JC, Grannum PA, Romero R, et al. Percutaneous umbilical blood sampling. *Am J Obstet Gynecol* 1985;152:1–6.
Hoskins IA. Cordocentesis in isoimmunization and fetal physiologic measurement, infection and karyotyping. *Curr Opin Obstet Gynecol* 1991;3:266–271.
Hsieh FJ, Chang FM, Ko TM, et al. Percutaneous ultrasound-guided fetal blood sampling in the management of non-immune hydrops. *Am J Obstet Gynecol* 1981;156:1218.
Hurley PA, Rodeck CH. Fetal therapy. *Curr Opin Obstet Gynecol* 1992;4:4–9.
Jackson LG. Fetal genetic diagnosis by chorionic villous sampling. *Semin Perinatol* 1991;15[Suppl 1]:43–48.
Kappel B, Nielsen J, Broggard-Hansen K, et al. Spontaneous abortion after midtrimester amniocentesis: clinical significance of placental perforation and blood stained amniotic fluid. *Br J Obstet Gynaecol* 1987;94:50–54.

Ledbetter DH, Martin AI, Verlinsky Y, et al. Cytogenic results of chorionic villous sampling: high success rate and diagnostic accuracy in the United States Collaborative Study. *Am J Obstet Gynecol* 1990;162:495–501.

Loukopoulos D, Hadji A, Papadakis M, et al. Prenatal diagnosis of thalassemia and of the sickle cell syndrome in Greece. *Ann N Y Acad Sci* 1990;612:226–236.

Mastroiacovo P, Botto LD, Cavalcanti DP, et al. Limb anomalies following chorionic villous sampling: a registry based case-control study. *Am J Med Genet* 1992;44:856–864.

Maxwell DJ, Johnson P, Hurley P, et al. Fetal blood sampling and pregnancy loss in relation to indication. *Br J Obstet Gynecol* 1991;98:892–897.

McGowan KD, Blakemore KJ. Amniocentesis and chorionic villous sampling. *Curr Opin Obstet Gynecol* 1991;3:221–229.

Penso CA, Frigoletto FD Jr. Early amniocentesis. *Semin Perinatol* 1990;14:465–470.

Philip J, Smidt-Jenses S, Hilden J. The safety of chorionic villous sampling. A synthesis of literature. *Ann N Y Acad Sci* 1991;626:568–579.

Robertson AW. Amniocentesis: indications. *Nebr Med J* 1992;77:263–264.

Schulman LP, Elias S. Percutaneous umbilical blood sampling, fetal skin sampling, and fetal liver biopsy. *Semin Perinatol* 1990;14:456–464.

Silverman NS, Wapner RJ. Chorionic villus sampling and amniocentesis. *Curr Opin Obstet Gynecol* 1990;2:258–264.

Smidt-Jensen S, Permin M, Philip J, et al. Randomised comparison of amniocentesis and transabdominal and transcervical chorionic villous sampling. *Lancet* 1992;340:1237–1244.

Smith CV. Amniotic fluid assessment. *Obstet Gynecol Clin North Am* 1990;17:187–200.

Suzumori K. The role of fetal blood sampling in prenatal diagnosis. *Early Hum Dev* 1992;29:155–159.

Wallach J. *Interpretation of diagnostic tests*, 7th ed. Philadelphia: Lippincott Williams & Wilkins, 2000.

Wax JR, Blackmore KJ. What can be learned from cordocentesis? *Clin Lab Med* 1992;12:503–522.

Williams J, Wang BB, Rubin CH, et al. Chorionic villous sampling: experience with 3016 cases performed by a single operator. *Obstet Gynecol* 1992;80:1023–1029.

Young SR, Shipley CF, Wade RA, et al. Single-center comparison of results of 1000 prenatal diagnoses with chorionic villous sampling and 1000 diagnoses with amniocentesis. *Am J Obstet Gynecol* 1991;165:255–261; discussion 261–263.

4 Disorders Specific to the Newborn

Intrauterine Growth Retardation

Babies who have become growth retarded late in pregnancy due to placental dysfunction can demonstrate dramatic "catch-up" growth in 3 months postpartum, and if fed ad libitum will consume 220–250 mL/kg/day compared to the usual 150 mL/kg/day of proper formula or breast milk.

Conversely, very large babies, usually those whose mothers or grandmothers are diabetic or have glucose intolerance, grow poorly postnatally and have relatively small appetites.

Laboratory Studies for Premature Infants

Blood gas determinations (PO_2, PCO_2, and pH) as often as indicated by baby's color, condition, and respiratory symptoms.

Blood glucose level at birth and 0.5, 1, 2, and 12 hours to screen for hypoglycemia.

Blood calcium level measured on cord blood and after baby has become stable, especially if acidosis has occurred.

Nucleated Red Blood Cell Count

A value of >10 nucleated red blood cells is suggestive of fetal ischemic encephalopathy. Hematocrit in the term neonate and young infant is shown in Fig. 1.

Recommended Routine Laboratory Studies for the Well Newborn

No laboratory tests other than the newborn metabolic screen are routinely recommended for the newborn in uncomplicated circumstances. For those whose perinatal period is questionable, some tests may be recommended:

- Hematocrit, white blood cell count, and differential.
- Urinalysis.
- Standard bacteriologic tests.
- Phenylketonuria, galactosemia, 17-hydroxyprogesterone, and thyroid function tests (e.g., thyroxine or thyroid-stimulating hormone) for screening on day of discharge or follow-up at age 4 days.
- Cord blood should be saved for 2 weeks.
- Blood type and hold until or if needed, and Coombs tests if mother is Rh negative or if jaundice develops by 24 hours.
- Serologic test for syphilis and for hepatitis B virus if mother is not tested antepartum.
- Possible screening for *Toxoplasma* or viral infection if requested.
- Separated cells and plasma or serum.
- Microchemistries: Direct and total bilirubin levels and glucose, sodium, potassium, chloride, calcium levels.

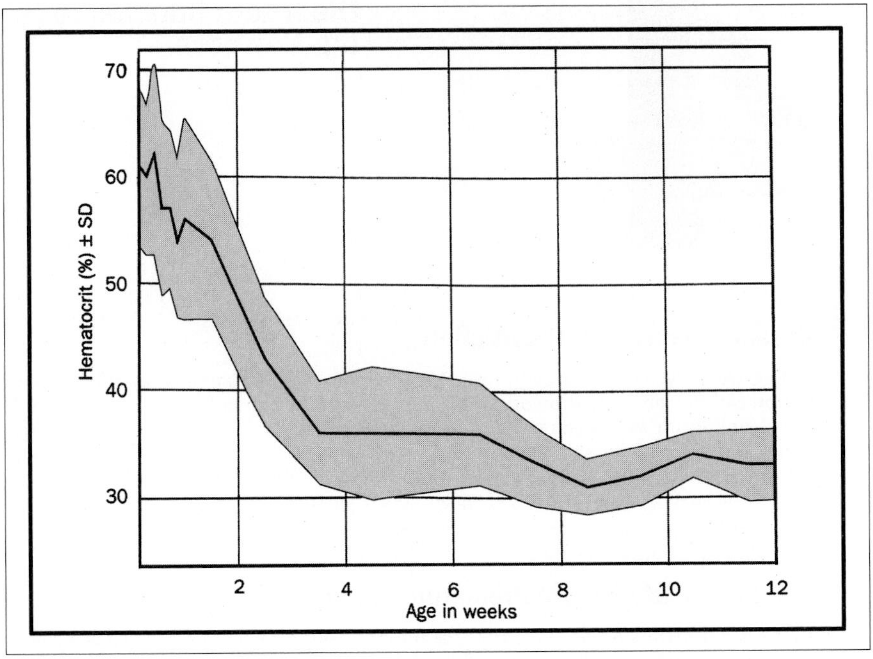

Fig. 1. Hematocrit in the term neonate and young infant. SD, standard deviation.

Recommended Laboratory Studies for High-Risk Infants

Approximately 3 infants per 100 deliveries; for example, low-birth-weight infants, high-birth-weight infants, postmaturity infants, infants of high-risk mothers (those with toxemia, diabetes, drug addiction, or cardiac or pulmonary disease), and cases involving polyhydramnios, oligohydramnios, cesarean section delivery, infection, or other major illnesses (such as hepatitis, thyrotoxicosis)
Same tests as in newborn nursery
Blood urea nitrogen level
pH, P_{O_2}, P_{CO_2}

Neonatal Monitoring for Infection

Gram staining of gastric aspirate should be performed within 6 hours of birth for any infant at risk of infection. Presence of polymorphonuclear leukocytes and bacteria raises suspicion of infection. Amniotic fluid Gram staining, culture, and tests for lung maturity in prenatal period may also indicate risk of infection.

Acid-Base Analysis

Umbilical Artery Blood Acid-Base Analysis

For symptomatic newborns assessment and newborn acid-base status. This analysis defines the presence or absence of asphyxia or hypoxia in the newborn. Carbon dioxide diffuses across the placenta very rapidly, and the rate of elimination is directly related to blood flow rates on both sides of the placenta.
The pH of blood or tissue is directly related to the concentration of base (bicarbonate) and inversely related to the concentrations of acid (H_2CO_3).

Generally, fetal or newborn acidemia is classified as respiratory, metabolic, or mixed, based on the pH and bicarbonate concentrations.

Umbilical Cord Blood Acid-Base Determinations

Umbilical cord blood pH and blood gas values are a useful adjunct to the Apgar score in assessing the immediate condition of the newborn. The technique is simple and relatively inexpensive, and the results are readily available.

Technique

A segment of umbilical cord 10–20 cm in length is doubly clamped. This should be accomplished immediately after delivery, as delays of as short as 20–30 seconds can alter the arterial blood PCO_2 and pH. Because the umbilical artery contains blood that is returning from the fetus to the placenta, values from the umbilical artery provide the most accurate information regarding fetal and newborn acid-base status. In fact, the pH and blood gas values obtained from the umbilical vein could be in the normal range. Such findings have been documented with umbilical cord prolapse. If the practitioner encounters difficulty in obtaining arterial blood from the umbilical cord (i.e., in the very premature infant), a sample from the placenta will provide accurate results. These arteries are relatively easy to identify, as they cross over the veins.

Once the umbilical cord has been clamped, blood is drawn into a 1–2-mL plastic or glass syringe that has been flushed with heparin sodium solution (1,000 U/mL) or into syringes with lyophilized heparin; any residual air or heparin should be ejected and the needle capped. Umbilical cord segments can be left at room temperature for up to 1 hour without clotting or significant changes in pH, PO_2, or PCO_2.

It has been demonstrated that a realistic pH threshold for significant or pathologic fetal acidemia (i.e., that pH associated with adverse neonatal sequelae, including death) is 7.0. An umbilical artery blood pH of less than 7.0 with a metabolic pattern appears to be an important component of a definition of birth asphyxia or hypoxia to a degree of severity that might be associated with subsequent neurologic dysfunction.

A finding of normal umbilical cord blood gas values in the premature infant virtually eliminates the diagnosis of significant intrapartum hypoxia or birth asphyxia.

Protocol for umbilical cord pH and blood gas analysis is as follows:

- Double-clamp a segment of the umbilical cord immediately after birth in all deliveries.
- If a serious abnormality that arose in the delivery process or a problem with the neonate's condition or both persist at or beyond the first 5 minutes, obtain an umbilical artery blood specimen for pH and acid-base determinations in a syringe flushed with heparin and have it analyzed.
- If a specimen cannot be obtained from the umbilical artery, obtain a specimen from an artery on the chorionic surface of the placenta.
- If the 5-minute Apgar score is satisfactory and the newborn appears stable and vigorous, the segment of umbilical cord can be discarded.

Normal Umbilical Cord Blood pH and Blood Gas Values in Term Newborns[1]

Arterial blood	
pH	7.27 (0.069)
PCO_2 (mm Hg)	50.3 (11.1)
HCO_3^- (mEq/L)	22.0 (3.6)
Base excess (mEq/L)	–2.7 (2.8)
Venous blood	
pH	7.34 (0.063)
PCO_2 (mm Hg)	40.7 (7.9)
HCO_3^- (mEq/L)	21.4 (2.5)
Base excess (mEq/L)	–2.4 (2)

Values are mean and standard deviation.

[1]Riley RJ, Johnson JWC. Collecting and analyzing cord blood gases. *Clin Obstet Gynecol* 1993;36:13–23.

Table 1. Causes of Acid-Base Disturbance in the Neonate

	pH	$[H^+]$	P_{CO_2}	$[HCO_3^-]$	Causes
Respiratory acidosis	↓	↑	↑	N	Hypoventilation
Respiratory alkalosis	↑	↓	↓	N / ↓	Overventilation
Metabolic acidosis	↓	↑	N /↓	↓	Renal impairment Poor perfusion Loss of fluid from gastrointestinal tract Metabolic disorders
Metabolic alkalosis	↑	↓	N / ↑	↑	Bicarbonate administration Pyloric stenosis Hypokalemia

↑, increased; ↓, decreased; N, normal.

Table 2. Biochemical Findings in Neonatal Hypocalcemia

Cause	Presenting Age	Plasma Phosphate	Plasma ALP	Other Plasma Investigations
Physiologic	24hr–48hr	N	N	
Vitamin D deficiency maternal	24hr–48hr[a]	N / ↓	↑	PTH ↑ / N
1-Alphahydroxylase-deficiency fat malabsorption	Infancy[b] Any			
Hypoparathyroidism	Any[b]	↑	N	PTH ↓↓
Pseudohypoparathyroidism	Any[b]	↑	N	PTH ↑ / N
Primary hypomagnesemia	>5 d	N	N	Mg^{2+} <0.4 mmol/L
Iatrogenic	>5 d	N / ↑	N	

↑, increased; ↓, decreased; ALP, alkaline phosphatase; N, normal; PTH, parathyroid hormone.
[a]Breast-feeding.
[b]Rare to present in neonate.

Acid-Base Disturbance

See Table 1.

Differential diagnosis of metabolic acidosis may be aided by calculation of the plasma anion gap $[(Na^+ + K^+) - (HCO_3^- + Cl^-)]$.

A gap of >20 mmol/L is suggestive of an organic acid disorder or lactic acidosis due to hypoxia. Biochemical investigations that may help with the differential diagnosis are measurements of urinary ketones, plasma glucose, ammonia and lactate concentrations, urine and plasma amino acids, and urinary organic acids. If plasma chloride concentration is increased, with normal amino acid distribution in serum and organic acids, then renal tubular disease should be considered.

Alkalosis

The most common cause of alkalosis is iatrogenic respiratory alkalosis in ventilated babies. Excess administration of bicarbonate can also produce alkalosis when acidosis has been overestimated clinically.

Biochemical Findings in Neonatal Hypocalcemia

See Table 2.

Pathologic Factors Aggravating Physiologic Jaundice

Prematurity	Infections	Inadequate calories
Dehydration	Hypoxia	Meconium retention
Hemolysis	Hypoglycemia	Intestinal obstruction
Polycythemia	Hypothyroidism	

Jaundice that appears unusually early (i.e., within first 24 hours) or is severe enough to require phototherapy requires investigation for the presence of hemolysis. Determination of maternal and infant blood groups, direct Coombs testing of infant blood, full blood count, and, if the baby is of Mediterranean, African, or Asian descent, measurement of glucose-6-phosphate dehydrogenase are indicated. Urine should be screened for infection, reducing sugars, and the presence of bilirubin.

Complications of Prematurity

See Table 3.

Drugs used as maternal analgesics, sedatives, or general anesthetics during labor cross the placenta and can depress the fetal respiratory center. Respiratory depression from drugs is likely to be especially important in premature infants or those with asphyxia superimposed from other causes.

Table 3. Complications of Prematurity

Conditions	Causes	Management
Anemia	Venipunctures Bone marrow refractory Increasing blood volume with growth Iron deficiency	Investigate causes
Bronchopulmonary dysplasia	Complicates respiratory distress syndrome in extreme preterm Prolonged requirement for oxygen	Monitor PO_2 Nutritional support Close monitoring of bacteriologic and cardiac status
Hypernatremia	Common in first 2–3 d in extremely preterm Dehydration	Adequate fluid intake
Hyponatremia	Renal tubular immaturity	Monitor sodium loss Adequate replacement (up to 10 mmol/kg/24 hr)
Hypocalcemia	Immature regulation Low plasma albumin	None if asymptomatic Replace in intravenous fluids if required
Hypothermia	Large surface area Immature skin Immature regulation	Clothing Warm environment ± added humidity
Infections (any)	Low immunoglobulins Ineffective localization of septic foci	High index of suspicion Early parenteral antibiotics
Intraventricular hemorrhage	Immaturity Cerebrovascular instability Postasphyxia	None possible Rarely progresses to give hydrocephalus

(continued)

Table 3. (continued)

Conditions	Causes	Management
Irregular respiration	Immature respiratory center	Monitor respiration and seek pathologic causes
Apnea	Infection Intracranial hemorrhage	Caffeine, theophylline therapy
Jaundice	Delayed food intake Bruising Hepatic immaturity	Phototherapy Exchange transfusion
Metabolic acidosis (mild)	Renal immaturity in presence of protein load (milk or total parenteral nutrition)	Reduce protein intake if deteriorating
Necrotizing enterocolitis	Infarction of gut secondary to inadequate perfusion	Supportive medical or surgical resection Generally make NPO
Osteopenia of prematurity	Progressive demineralization of bones if mineral absorption inadequate	Mineral supplements to diet
Periventricular leukomalacia	Infarction of large areas of cerebral white matter after ischemic insult	None possible
Persistent patent ductus arteriosus	Immaturity Hypoxia Acidosis	Ligation or indomethacin Diuretics for heart failure
Respiratory distress syndrome	Surfactant deficiency	Monitor blood gases Increase inspired PO_2 Continuous positive airway pressure or intermittent positive pressure ventilation Intravenous fluids/feeding Exogenous surfactant
Unable to suck reliably	Immature suck/swallow coordination	Nasogastric tube feeding if well

NPO, nothing by mouth.

Delayed Respiration and Persistent Cyanosis in the Neonate

Causes of Delayed Respiration

Intrapartum asphyxia
Drugs (causing central nervous system depression)
Prematurity
Trauma to central nervous system
Congenital abnormalities
Anemia or blood loss
Muscle weakness (prematurity or primary muscle disease)

Causes of Persistent Cyanosis

Persistent pulmonary hypertension
Cyanotic congenital heart defect
Underexpansion of lungs (surfactant deficiency)
Pneumothorax
Diaphragmatic hernia
Anatomic abnormality of airways

Hypoglycemia

Causes

Decreased Glucose Production

Preterm birth
Antenatal nutritional deficiency
Sepsis

Birth asphyxia
Hypothermia
Small for gestational age
Starvation
Congenital heart disease

Hyperinsulinism

Maternal diabetes
Beckwith-Wiedemann syndrome
Nesidioblastosis
Maternal drug therapy or glucose starvation
Erythroblastosis
Insulinoma

Inborn Errors of Metabolism

Carnitine deficiency disorders (e.g., carnitine palmitoyltransferase deficiency)
Glycogen storage disorders, especially type 1
Disorders of glyconeogenesis (e.g., pyruvate carboxylase deficiency)
Amino acid disorders (e.g., tyrosinemia type I)
Organic acid disorders (e.g., methylmalonic acidemia)
Disorders of fat oxidation (e.g., medium-chain acyl coenzyme A dehydrogenase deficiency)
Galactosemia

Hormone Deficiencies

Congenital hypopituitarism
Congenital glucagon deficiency
Congenital adrenal hyperplasia
Adrenal hypoplasia or insufficiency

Other Causes

Exchange transfusion

Diagnostic Tests for Neonatal Hypoglycemia

	Further Investigations	Diagnoses
Metabolic acidosis	Plasma lactate Plasma 3-hydroxybutyrate Plasma-free fatty acids Urine organic acids	Glycogen storage disease types 1, 3 Congenital lactic acidosis Disorders of gluconeogenesis Fatty acid oxidation defects
Liver dysfunction	Plasma and urine amino acids Galactose-1-phosphate uridyltransferase Urine sugars Urine organic acids	Tyrosinemia type I Galactosemia Hereditary fructose intolerance Fatty acid oxidation effects
Absence of acidosis and liver dysfunction	Plasma cortisol Plasma 17-hydroxyprogesterone Plasma insulin (when hypoglycemic) Plasma growth hormone and thyroid-stimulating hormone	Adrenal insufficiency Congenital adrenal hyperplasia Nesidioblastosis Hypopituitarism
Hyponatremia	Plasma 17-hydroxyprogesterone Plasma cortisol Plasma growth hormone and thyroid-stimulating hormone	Congenital adrenal hyperplasia Adrenal insufficiency Hypopituitarism

Hypocalcemia

Causes

Physiologic factors
Prematurity
Maternal diabetes mellitus
Birth asphyxia
Pathologic conditions
Vitamin D deficiency
Hypoparathyroidism

Pseudohyperparathyroidism
Maternal hypoparathyroidism
Liver disease
Renal disease
Hypomagnesemia
Organic acid disorders
Iatrogenic causes
Low calcium intake
Parenteral nutrition
High phosphate intake
Use of diuretics
Use of anticonvulsants
Exchange transfusion

Hyponatremia

Condition	Cause/Presentation	Management
Maternal influence	Reflects maternal electrolyte levels (seen especially if large volumes of dextrose given i.v. during labor)	Usually recovers with treatment.
Iatrogenic causes	Prolonged administration of i.v. dextrose without electrolyte additives	Restrict fluids. Give Na^+.
Birth injury	Inappropriate antidiuretic hormone secretion	Restrict fluids.
Meningitis	Poor urine output Weight gain Plasma osmolality <270 mmol/kg Urine osmolality increased	Usually recovers with treatment.
Diuretic administration (especially loop diuretics)	Loss of electrolyte in excess of water Drug slowly eliminated in neonates (average losses after 1 mg/kg furosemide are 28 mL/kg water, 3.6 mmol/kg Na^+, 0.3 mmol/kg K^+)	Replace Na^+. Use amiloride hydrochloride.
Acute tubular necrosis, renal failure	Increased renal fractional sodium excretion secondary to tubular damage and hyporesponsiveness to aldosterone	Measure sodium losses and replace by oral or intravenous supplements.
Salt-losing congenital adrenal hyperplasia	Mineralocorticoid deficiency Males: normal, or pigmented scrotum Females: virilization (variable) Acute illness in second or third week	Give corticosteroids.
Cystic fibrosis	Excessive sweat salt loss in high temperatures (rare presentation)	Rehydrate. Give NaCl.
Renal tubular acidosis	Loss of sodium and bicarbonate in urine	Give corticosteroids.

Hypernatremia

Condition	Cause/Presentation	Management
Overhead heater	Excessive water loss through skin, especially in preterm babies	Use heat shield, increase water administration as 5% dextrose.
Iatrogenic	Administration of $NaHCO_3$ to correct metabolic acidosis Administration of excessive supplementary salt over a short time period	Alter management.

	Use of 10% (or more) dextrose producing glycosuria and osmotic diuresis (especially in preterm babies)	
Fluid deprivation	Dehydration	Slow correction of electrolyte imbalance after initial administration of colloid to restore circulatory volume.
Starvation	Circulatory collapse	As above.
Excess gastrointestinal fluid loss	Dehydration	As above.
Nephrogenic diabetes	Failure to thrive Vomiting, constipation, episodic dehydration Persistent polyuria, unresponsive to exogenous antidiuretic hormone	Low-solute diet and diuretics.

Hypokalemia

Condition	Cause/Presentation	Management
Birth asphyxia	Part of syndrome of inappropriate secretion of antidiuretic hormone with decreased plasma osmolality (<270 mmol/kg)	Restrict fluid.
Alkalosis	Renal excretion of K^+ in place of H^+; seen in pyloric stenosis, exogenous alkali administration	Give potassium.
Drugs	Use of furosemide; seen to a lesser extent with all diuretics	Supplement or use potassium-sparing diuretics.
Renal tubular acidosis (RTA)	Proximal RTA (males)—defective proximal tubular resorption of bicarbonate Distal RTA—inability to establish H^+ ion gradient in distal tubule	Give alkali.
Iatrogenic	Use of glucose and insulin	Reconsider treatment.

Hyperkalemia

Venous or arterial, not capillary, plasma K^+ >5.5 mmol/L.

Hyperkalemia has a number of causes. Asymptomatic hyperkalemia with levels of plasma potassium that would be fatal in an adult (up to 11 mmol/L) can be tolerated in the short term in a neonate. The most important effect of hyperkalemia is on cardiac rhythm, particularly in the infant with renal failure in whom the potassium imbalance cannot be readily corrected. This effect of hyperkalemia is potentiated by hypocalcemia, even of mild degree. Electrocardiographic changes include peaked T waves, then widening of the QRS complex, bradyarrhythmias, sine waves, and eventually cardiac arrest. High potassium value obtained from a capillary sample must be replicated in a venous specimen.

Condition	Cause/Presentation	Management
Fluid deprivation	Dehydration, tissue damage.	Correct circulating volume and restore perfusion with colloid and crystalloid.
Dehydration	Dehydration and leakage from cells.	As above.

Trauma: bruising, fracture, cephalohematoma, breech delivery, intracranial hemorrhage	Release of potassium from red cell. Treat if >7 mmol/L or symptomatic.	Administer fluid or furosemide.
Acute renal failure	Associated with increased plasma and oliguria or anuria.	May require treatment with rectal resonium resin, peritoneal dialysis, or both.
Congenital adrenal hyperplasia, adrenocortical insufficiency	Mineralocorticoid deficiency. Males: normal, or pigmented scrotum. Females: virilization (variable).	Give corticosteroids.
Exchange transfusion	Citrate-phosphate-dextrose–stored blood has average potassium concentration of 12–15 mmol/L by 7 d, but can be much higher.	Avoid use of blood >5 d old.

Narcotic Withdrawal

Maternal addiction, particularly to narcotic agents, may lead to the development of withdrawal syndrome in the neonate after delivery. Presentation is generally soon after birth but can be delayed until 10 days and may last for weeks.

Symptoms are variable and are predominantly those of autonomic and cerebral irritability. Nasal congestion, sneezing, yawning, runny nose, poor suck, hiccups, and diarrhea have all been described. The cry is abnormally high-pitched with increased extensor tone, poor sleeping, tachypnea, weight loss, and seizures.

Complications of Parenteral Nutrition in Neonates

Frequent Complications	**Less Frequent Complications**
*Sodium depletion	*Hyperphenylalaninemia (± hypertyrosinemia)
*Potassium depletion	*Hyperlipidemia (cholesterol $\uparrow$, triglycerides $\uparrow$)
*Hyperglycemia	Zinc deficiency
*Glycosuria	Copper deficiency
*Jaundice	Selenium deficiency
*Hypophosphatemia	Hyperammonemia
Metabolic acidosis	
Calcium depletion	

$\uparrow$, increased.
*Particularly important in extremely preterm infants.

Fetomaternal Hemorrhage

Fetomaternal hemorrhage occurs in small amounts in approximately 75% of all pregnancies but is clinically important only in cases of large hemorrhages. Most cases of fetomaternal transfusion are spontaneous, occurring in uncomplicated term deliveries. Some may be a consequence of abdominal trauma with abruptio placentae. Hemorrhage may occur due to delivery complications when the placenta is anterior and in association with chorangioma or choriocarcinoma. There may be decreased fetal movements over a period of 24–48 hours' delivery.

The standard method of testing for fetal erythrocytes in maternal circulation is Betke-Kleihauer staining of a peripheral blood smear. The test should be done routinely in all cases of unexplained stillbirth, fetal distress, and neonatal anemia. Immediate transfusion may be lifesaving, and testing of the mother during the puerperium is important.

The size of the hemorrhage can be calculated on the basis of the percentage of fetal red cells present and estimated average maternal blood volume of 5,000 mL. For example, if 5% of the red cells in the maternal circulation are fetal in origin, the size of the hemorrhage is calculated as $0.05 \times 5{,}000 = 250$ mL of fetal blood; 80 mL (approximately one-quarter of the infant's blood volume) or greater is considered significant for fetomaternal transplacental hemorrhage. (The average blood volume of an infant is 100 mL/kg; therefore, a 3-kg term infant would have a blood volume of 300 mL.)

Fetal Blood pH

When fetal scalp blood is acidotic, maternal acidosis should be differentiated from fetal acidosis, because maternal acidosis does not have the same serious implications. Fetal pH is usually 0.04 U below maternal pH. A pH of >7.25 is normal during labor; pH of 7.20–7.25 is worrisome, and another determination should be made promptly; pH of ≤7.20 suggests significant fetal hypoxia and need for prompt delivery.

After age of 3 hours, sample of capillary blood from infant's warmed heel correlates well with arterial blood samples in measurements of acid-base status.

In uncomplicated pregnancy, umbilical cord blood pH has normal lower limit of 7.15.

Blood pH is the only objective measure available at delivery by which a diagnosis of asphyxia can be made.

In general, mean blood pH of 7.27 in the newborn is associated with an Apgar score of ≥7. Mean blood pH of 7.22 is associated with an Apgar score of ≤6. Fetal acid-base status is a valuable index of fetal asphyxia or oxygenation; it should be evaluated with other evidence of fetal distress. Fetal blood pH provides the best correlation with fetal outcome. In almost 20% of infants, the fetal acid-base status may be misleading (e.g., due to fetal scalp edema, contamination with amniotic fluid).

False Normal

Normal blood pH but depressed infant function

Due to medications administered, obstetric manipulation (e.g., difficult forceps delivery), precipitous delivery, prematurity (especially weight of <1,000 g with noncompliant lungs), congenital anomalies preventing normal onset of good lung function at birth (e.g., laryngeal web, choanal atresia, hypoplastic lungs associated with diaphragmatic hernia, edematous cyst of lung), aspiration syndromes, previous episodes of asphyxia with resuscitation, intrauterine infection

False Abnormal

Maternal acidosis is usual cause.

Base Deficit and Blood pH Measurements

	Maternal pH (mean)	Fetal pH (mean)	Base Deficit (mEq/L)
Normal mother and fetus	7.42	7.25	7.0
Normal mother and acidotic fetus	7.42	7.25	2.6
Acidotic mother and vigorous fetus	7.36	7.15	4.8

Respiratory Distress Syndrome

See Chapter 8, Pulmonary Function Tests.

Necrotizing Enterocolitis

See Chapter 9, Gastrointestinal Diseases.

Bibliography

American College of Obstetricians and Gynecologists. *An educational aid to obstetrician-gynecologists.* Washington: American College of Obstetricians and Gynecologists, November 1995. Technical Bulletin No. 216.

Wallach J. *Interpretation of diagnostic tests*, 7th ed. Philadelphia: Lippincott Williams & Wilkins, 2000.

5 Infectious Diseases[1]

Pathogens Commonly Associated with Infection in Patients with Immunosuppression (Due to Organ Transplantation, Treatment of Malignancies, Acquired Immunodeficiency Syndrome)

Immune Response Depressed	Underlying Condition	Commonly Associated Pathogens
Humoral	Lymphatic leukemia	Pneumococci
	Lymphosarcoma	*Haemophilus influenzae*
	Multiple myeloma	Streptococci
	Congenital hypogammaglobulinemias	*Pseudomonas aeruginosa*
	Nephrotic syndrome	*Pneumocystis carinii*
	Treatment with cytotoxic or antimetabolite drugs	*P. carinii*
Cellular	Terminal cancers	Tubercle bacillus
	Hodgkin disease	*Listeria*
	Sarcoidosis	*Candida* spp.
	Uremia	*Toxoplasma*
	Treatment with cytotoxic or antimetabolite drugs or corticosteroids	*P. carinii*
Leukocyte bactericidal	Myelogenous leukemia	Staphylococci
	Chronic granulomatous disease	*Serratia*
	Acidosis	*Pseudomonas* spp.
	Burns	*Candida* spp.
	Treatment with corticosteroids	*Aspergillus*
	Granulocytopenia due to drugs	*Nocardia*

Pathogens Commonly Associated with Infection in Patients with Neoplasms

Neoplasms	Infection	Commonly Associated Pathogens
Acute nonlymphocytic leukemia	Sepsis with no apparent focus, pneumonia, skin, mouth, genitourinary tract, hepatitis	Enterobacteriaceae, *Pseudomonas*, staphylococci, *Corynebacterium*, *Candida, Aspergillus*, *Mucor*, non-A, non-B hepatitis virus
Acute lymphocytic leukemia	Disseminated disease, pneumonia, pharyngitis, skin	Streptococci, *P. carinii*, herpes simplex virus, cytomegalovirus, varicella-zoster virus
Lymphoma	Disseminated disease, sepsis, genitourinary tract, pneumonia, skin	*Cryptococcus neoformans*, mucocutaneous *Candida*, herpes simplex virus, herpes zoster virus, cytomegalovirus, *P. carinii, Toxoplasma gondii*, mycobacteria, *Nocardia, Strongyloides stercoralis, Listeria monocytogenes, Brucella, Salmonella,* staphylococci, Enterobacteriaceae, *Pseudomonas*

[1]Portions of this chapter are adapted from Pickering LK, ed. *2000 Red Book: Report of the Committee on Infectious Diseases*, 25th ed. Elk Grove Village, IL: American Academy of Pediatrics, 2000, with permission.

Bacterial Diseases

Actinomycosis

Actinomyces israelii is the usual cause of actinomycosis. *A. israelii*, other *Actinomyces* species, and *Propionibacterium* (a related genus) species are slow-growing Gram-positive, anaerobic bacilli that can be part of the normal oral flora. The three major types of disease are cervicofacial, thoracic, and abdominal. Cervicofacial lesions are the most common and frequently occur after tooth extraction, oral surgery, or facial trauma or are associated with carious teeth. Localized pain and induration progress to "woody hard" nodular lesions that can be complicated by draining sinus tracts. Thoracic disease most commonly is secondary to aspiration of oropharyngeal secretions and manifests as pneumonia, which can be complicated by development of abscesses, empyema, and, rarely, pleurodermal sinuses. In abdominal infection, the appendix and cecum are the most frequent sites. Intradermal abscesses and peritoneal-dermal draining sinuses eventually occur. Chronic localized disease often forms sinus tracts that drain a purulent discharge.

Diagnostic Tests

For recovery of the organisms, specimens must be collected, transported, and cultured anaerobically on semiselective media, with microscope demonstration of beaded, branched, Gram-positive bacilli in pus or tissue. Acid-fast staining can be used to distinguish *Actinomyces* species, which are acid-fast negative, from *Nocardia* species, which are variably acid-fast positive. Sulfur granules in drainage or loculations of pus, which usually are yellow and may be visualized microscopically or macroscopically, indicate the diagnosis when present. A Gram stain of sulfur granules discloses a dense reticulum of filaments; the ends of individual filaments may project around the periphery of the granule, with or without radially arranged hyaline clubs. Immunofluorescent stains can be used for *Actinomyces* species.

Anthrax

Bacillus anthracis is an aerobic, Gram-positive, encapsulated, spore-forming, nonmotile rod, which produces several toxins responsible for the clinical manifestations of hemorrhage, edema, and necrosis. Spore size is approximately 1 μm. (See Biologic Warfare section in Chapter 25.)

Arcanobacterium haemolyticum *Infections*

Arcanobacterium haemolyticum is a Gram-positive bacillus, formerly classified as *Corynebacterium haemolyticum*.

Acute pharyngitis due to *A. hemolyticum* often is indistinguishable from that caused by group A streptococci. Fever, pharyngeal exudate, lymphadenopathy, rash, and pruritus are common, but palatal petechiae and strawberry tongue are absent. In almost half of all reported cases, a maculopapular or scarlatiniform exanthem is present, beginning on the extensor surfaces of the distal extremities, spreading centripetally to the chest and back, and sparing the face, palms, and soles.

Diagnostic Tests

A. haemolyticum can be recovered on blood-enriched agar cultures, but growth may be slow, and hemolytic colonies may not be visible for 48–72 hours after inoculation. Detection is enhanced by culture on human or rabbit blood agar, because both demonstrate larger colony growth and wider zones of hemolysis than does sheep blood agar. Growth also is enhanced by the addition of 5% carbon dioxide. Serologic tests for antibodies to *A. haemolyticum* have been used in epidemiologic investigations, but they have not been standardized and are not available commercially.

Bacillus cereus *Infections*

Bacillus cereus is an aerobic and facultatively anaerobic, spore-forming, Gram-positive bacillus. The emetic syndrome is caused by a reformed heat-stable toxin. The diarrhea syndrome is caused by *in vivo* production of a heat-labile enterotoxin. This necrotizing enterotoxin also has tissue necrotic and cytotoxic properties.

Two clinical syndromes are associated with *B. cereus* food poisoning. The first is the emetic syndrome, which has a short incubation period, similar to that of staphylococcal food poisoning, characterized by nausea, vomiting, and abdominal cramps, with diarrhea in approximately one-third of patients. The second is the diarrhea syndrome, which has a longer incubation period similar to that of *C. perfringens* food poisoning and is characterized predominantly by moderate to severe abdominal cramps and watery diarrhea, with vomiting in approximately one-fourth of patients. In both syndromes, illness is mild, usually not associated with fever, and abates within 24 hours.

Diagnostic Tests

For food-borne illness, isolation of *B. cereus* in a concentration of $>10^5$/g of epidemiologically incriminated food establishes the diagnosis. Because the organism can be recovered from stool samples from some well persons, the presence of *B. cereus* in feces or vomitus of ill persons is not definitive evidence for infection unless isolates from several ill patients are demonstrated to be the same serotype or stool cultures from a matched control group are negative. Phage typing, DNA hybridization, plasmid analysis, and enzyme electrophoresis have been used as epidemiologic tools in outbreaks of food poisoning.

In patients with risk factors for serious illness, isolation of *B. cereus* from wounds, blood, or normally sterile body fluids can be significant and should not be dismissed as contamination. Repeated cultures may help to confirm the diagnosis.

Bacteroides *and* Prevotella *Infections*

Most *Bacteroides* and *Prevotella* organisms associated with human disease are pleomorphic, non–spore-forming, facultatively anaerobic, Gram-negative bacilli.

Bacteroides and *Prevotella* species from the oral cavity can cause chronic sinusitis, chronic otitis media, dental infection, peritonitis, cervical adenitis, retropharyngeal space infection, aspiration pneumonia, lung abscess, emphysema, and necrotizing pneumonia. Species from the gastrointestinal tract flora are recovered in peritonitis, intraabdominal abscess, pelvic inflammatory disease, postoperative wound infection, and vulvovaginal and perianal infections. Soft tissue infections include synergistic bacterial gangrene and necrotizing fasciitis. Invasion of the bloodstream from the oral cavity or intestinal tract can lead to brain abscess, meningitis, endocarditis, arthritis, or osteomyelitis and decubitus ulcers. Neonatal infections, such as conjunctivitis, pneumonia, bacteremia, or meningitis, occur rarely. Most *Bacteroides* infections are polymicrobial.

Diagnostic Tests

Anaerobic cultures are necessary for recovery of *Bacteroides* and *Prevotella* species. Because infections usually are polymicrobial, aerobic cultures also should be obtained. A putrid odor of pus or other discharges is suggestive evidence of anaerobic infection. Use of anaerobic transport tubes or a sealed syringe is recommended for collection of clinical specimens. Collection of clinical material, especially from the respiratory tract, must avoid contamination of the specimen with anaerobes normally present on mucosal surfaces. Rapid identification techniques are not available.

Brucellosis

Brucella species are small, nonmotile, Gram-negative coccobacilli. The species that infect humans are *Brucella abortus, B. melitensis, B. suis*, and, rarely, *B. canis*.

Brucellosis in children frequently is a mild, self-limited disease compared with the more chronic disease observed among adults. In areas where *B. melitensis* is the endemic species, however, disease can be severe. Symptoms include fever, night sweats, weakness, malaise, anorexia, weight loss, arthralgia, myalgia, abdominal pain, and headache. Physical findings include lymphadenopathy, hepatosplenomegaly, and, occasionally, arthritis. Serious complications include meningitis, endocarditis, and osteomyelitis.

Diagnostic Tests

Brucella organisms can be recovered from blood, bone marrow, or other tissues. Incubate cultures for a minimum of 4 weeks and use proper precautions for protection against laboratory-acquired infection. Lysis-centrifugation techniques may shorten the time necessary to isolate *Brucella* organisms. A presumptive diagnosis can be made by serologic testing. The serum agglutination test, which is the most commonly used test, detects antibodies against *B. abortus, B. suis*, and *B. melitensis*, but not *B. canis*. Detection of antibodies against *B. canis* requires use of *B. canis*–specific antigen. Although a single titer is not diagnostic, most patients with active infection have titers of ≥1:160. Lower titers may be found early in the course of infection. Elevated concentrations of immunoglobulin (Ig) G agglutinins are found in acute infections, chronic infection, and relapse. When serum agglutination test titers are interpreted, the possibility of cross reactions of *Brucella* antibodies with those against other Gram-negative bacteria, such as *Yersinia enterocolitica* serotype 09, *Francisella tularensis*, and *Vibrio cholerae*, should be considered. Enzyme immunoassay (EIA) is a sensitive method for determining IgG, IgA, and IgM anti-*Brucella* antibodies, but until better standardization is established, EIA should be used for suspected cases with negative serum agglutination test titers or for evaluation of patients with suspected relapse or reinfection. The polymerase chain reaction (PCR) test has been developed but is not available in most clinical laboratories.

Burkholderia *Infections*

Burkholderia species are water- and soil-borne organisms that can survive for prolonged periods when kept moist. In most patients with and without cystic fibrosis, person-to-person spread of *B. cepacia* has been documented.

The genus *Burkholderia* was proposed in 1992 for seven species that were previously in *Pseudomonas* homology group II. Species are distinguished primarily on the basis of phenotype and biochemical characteristics. All *Burkholderia* species are animal or plant pathogens but are not significant pathogens in healthy human hosts.

Burkholderia cepacia complex has been associated with severe pulmonary infections in patients with cystic fibrosis and with fatal bacteremia in patients with chronic granulomatous disease, newborn infants, and persons with cancer. *B. cepacia* also is a nosocomial pathogen that may cause significant bacteremia in children with hemoglobinopathies or malignant neoplasms. Nosocomial infections include wound infections, urinary tract infections, and pneumonia. Pulmonary infections in persons with cystic fibrosis occur late in the course of the disease, usually after colonization with *P. aeruginosa* has been established. Colonized patients may experience no change in the rate of pulmonary decompensation, become chronically colonized, and experience a more rapid decline in pulmonary function, or experience an unexpectedly rapid deterioration in clinical status that results in death. The clinical significance of *Burkholderia gladioli* in persons with cystic fibrosis is unknown. In chronic granulomatous disease, pneumonia is the most common infection caused by *B. cepacia* complex; lymphadenitis also has been reported. Disease onset is insidious, with low-grade fever early in the course of disease and signs of systemic toxic effects occurring 3–4 weeks later. Pleural effusion is common, and lung abscess has been described.

Diagnostic Tests

Culture is the appropriate test for diagnosis of *B. cepacia* infection. In cystic fibrosis lung infection, culture of sputum on selective agar is recommended to decrease the potential for overgrowth by mucoid *P. aeruginosa*. *B. cepacia* and *B. gladioli* can be identified by PCR, but this assay is not available in most commercial laboratories. Diagnosis of melioidosis can be made by isolation of *B. pseudomallei* from blood or an infected site. The indirect hemagglutination assay is used most frequently for serologic diagnosis in young children, and a positive test result is more predictive of infection in this age group than in older children and adults because of the lower seroprevalence in young children. Other rapid assays being developed for diagnosis of melioidosis include direct fluorescent antibody (DFA) for identification of the organisms in sputum, an immunoglobulin M EIA, and DNA probes.

Cat-Scratch Disease (Bartonellosis)

Bartonella henselae is the causative organism for most cases of cat-scratch disease (CSD). This conclusion is based primarily on serologic, epidemiologic, and molecular probe rather than culture data, although *B. henselae* has been isolated from patients with classic signs of CSD, as well as from domestic cats. *B. henselae* are fastidious, slow-growing, Gram-negative bacilli that also have been identified as the causative agent of bacillary angiomatosis and peliosis hepatitis, two infections that have been reported primarily in patients infected with the human immunodeficiency virus (HIV). *B. henselae* is closely related to *Bartonella quintana*, the agent of trench fever and also a cause of bacillary angiomatosis.

Most cases occur in patients <20 years of age. Cats are the common reservoir for human disease. More than 90% of patients have a history of recent contact with cats, often kittens, which usually are healthy. No evidence of person-to-person transmission exists.

Risk factors: cats <12 months old (15×), cat bite or scratch (27×), kitten with fleas (29×).

Clinical Presentation

Lymphadenopathy: nearly 100% of cases
Fever: 28%
Inoculation lesion: 61%
Parinaud oculoglandular syndrome: 6%
Encephalopathy: 2.4%
Neuroretinitis: 1.4%
Erythema nodosum: 0.7%
Hepatosplenomegaly: 0.3%
Osteomyelitis: 0.3%
Primary atypical pneumonia: 0.1%

The predominant sign of CSD is regional lymphadenopathy in an immunocompetent person. Fever and mild systemic symptoms occur in 30% of patients. A skin papule often is found at the presumed site of bacterial inoculation and usually precedes development of lymphadenopathy by 1–2 weeks. Lymphadenopathy usually involves nodes that drain the site of inoculation and may include cervical, axillary, epitrochlear, or inguinal nodes. The area around affected lymph nodes typically is tender, warm, erythematous, and indurated. In as many as 30% of the cases of CSD, the affected nodes suppurate spontaneously. Occasionally, infection can produce Parinaud oculoglandular syndrome involving the conjunctiva and an ipsilateral preauricular lymph node. Rare clinical manifestations include encephalitis, aseptic meningitis, fever of unknown origin, neuroretinitis, osteolytic lesions, hepatitis, microabscesses in the liver and spleen, pneumonia, thrombocytopenic purpura, and erythema nodosum.

Diagnostic Tests

Obtain 2 mL serum, which should be refrigerated. Tests include the following: *B. henselae*, IgG, IgM levels; *B. quintana*, IgG level; *B. quintana*, IgM level. The indirect fluorescent antibody (IFA) test for detection of serum IgG antibody to antigens of *Bartonella* species is useful for the diagnosis of CSD. The IFA test is available through the Centers for Disease Control and Prevention (CDC), and the reagents are available to state health departments. Results of IFA tests performed in some commercial laboratories have not been reliable. There is some cross reactivity between the IgG classes of *B. henselae* and *B. quintana*. EIAs for detection of antibody to *B. henselae* have been developed; however, they have not been demonstrated to be more sensitive or specific than the IFA test. PCR assays are available in some commercial laboratories. If involved tissue is available, the putative agent of the disease may be visualized using the Warthin-Starry silver impregnation stain; however, this test is not specific for *B. henselae*. Early histologic changes consist of lymphocytic infiltrates with epithelioid granuloma formation, similar to changes in lymphomas and sarcoidosis. Later changes consist of polymorphonuclear leukocyte infiltrates with granulomas that become necrotic and resemble those of tularemia, brucellosis, and mycobacterial infections. A cat-scratch antigen skin test, prepared from aspirated pus from suppurative lymph nodes of patients with apparent CSD, has been used. This test is unlicensed and should not be used.

Causes for rejection include hemolysis, lipemia, and gross bacterial contamination.

Chancroid

Chancroid is caused by *Haemophilus ducreyi*, which is a Gram-negative coccobacillus.

Coinfection with *Treponema pallidum* or herpes simplex virus (HSV) occurs in as many as 10% of patients. Chancroid is a well-established cofactor for transmission of HIV. Because sexual contact is the only known route of transmission, the diagnosis of chancroid in infants and young children is strong evidence of sexual abuse.

Chancroid is an acute ulcerative disease that involves the genitalia. In approximately 30% of cases, chancroid is associated with a painful unilateral inguinal adenitis (bubo). An ulcer begins as a tender erythematous papule, becomes pustular, and erodes over several days, forming a sharply demarcated, somewhat superficial lesion with a serpiginous undermined border. Its base is friable and may be covered with a gray or yellow, necrotic, and purulent exudate.

Diagnostic Tests

The diagnosis of chancroid usually is made on the basis of clinical findings and the exclusion of other infections associated with genital ulcer disease, such as syphilis or HSV infection, or adenopathies, such as lymphogranuloma venereum. Direct examination of clinical material by Gram stain may strongly suggest the diagnosis if large numbers of Gram-negative coccobacilli, sometimes in "school of fish" patterns, are seen. Confirmation by recovery of *H. ducreyi* from a genital ulcer or lymph node aspirate is the more available alternative diagnostic test. Special culture media and conditions are required for isolation. Fluorescent monoclonal antibody stains and PCR tests can provide a more specific diagnosis but are not available in most laboratories.

Chlamydia *Infections*

Chlamydia pneumoniae

Chlamydia pneumoniae (formerly termed the *TWAR strain*) is a species of *Chlamydia* that is antigenically, genetically, and morphologically distinct from other *Chlamydia* species.

A variety of respiratory tract diseases are caused by the organism, including pharyngitis, sinusitis, bronchitis, and pneumonia. In some patients, a sore throat precedes the onset of cough by a week or more.

Diagnostic Tests

No reliable diagnostic test is available commercially. The organism can be isolated from nasopharyngeal swabs placed into appropriate transport media and held at 4°C (39°F) until inoculated into cell culture; prolonged nasopharyngeal shedding can occur for months after acute disease. Methods for detecting *C. pneumoniae* in clinical specimens are available in research facilities and include a fluorescent antibody test using monoclonal antibody specific for *C. pneumoniae* and a PCR test. Complement-fixing *Chlamydia* antibodies usually are present in children and adolescents with illness but often are absent in adults. The test does not distinguish among antibodies to *C. pneumoniae*, *Chlamydia trachomatis,* and *Chlamydia psittaci*. The microimmunofluorescent antibody titer increase and IgM-specific titer of ≥1:16, or an IgG-specific titer of ≥1:512 is evidence of current infection. An increase in antibody titer may be delayed for several weeks after onset of illness. Early antimicrobial therapy may suppress the antibody response.

Chlamydia psittaci

Birds are the major reservoir of *C. psittaci*. Persons in the environment of infected birds, such as workers at poultry slaughter plants, poultry farms, and pet shops, as well as pet owners, are at high risk of infection. Infections are rare in children. *C. psittaci* is antigenically and genetically distinct from the *Chlamydia* species. Illness may be caused by *Chlamydia pecorum*, a newly designated species formerly not distinguished form *C. psittaci*. Psittacosis (ornithosis) is an acute febrile respiratory tract infection with systemic symptoms and signs that often include fever, a nonproductive cough, headache, and malaise. Extensive interstitial pneumonia can occur with radiographic changes characteristically more severe than would be expected from physical examination findings. Pericarditis, myocarditis, endocarditis, superficial thrombophlebitis, hepatitis, and encephalopathy are rare complications.

Diagnostic Tests

The usual method of diagnosis is serologic, based on a fourfold increase in complement-fixation antibody titer between acute and convalescent specimens collected 2–3 weeks apart. In the presence of a compatible clinical illness, a single complement-fixation titer of ≥1:32 is considered presumptive evidence of infection. Treatment may suppress the antibody response. The complement-fixation test does not distinguish among infections caused by *C. psittaci, C. pneumoniae, C. trachomatis,* and *C. pecorum*. A microimmunofluorescence assay that is more specific for *C. psittaci* has been developed but is not available widely. Isolation of the agent from the respiratory tract should be attempted only by experienced personnel in laboratories in which strict measures to prevent spread of the organism are used during collection and handling of all specimens for culture.

Chlamydia trachomatis

C. trachomatis is a bacterial agent with at least 18 serologic variants (serovars) divided between the following two biologic variants (biovars): oculogenital (serovars A–K) and lymphogranuloma venereum (serovars L1, L2, and L3). Trachoma usually is caused by serovars A through C, and genital and perinatal infections are caused by B and D through K.

C. trachomatis is the most common reportable sexually transmitted infection in the United States with a high rate among sexually active adolescents and young adults. Possible sexual abuse should be suspected in prepubertal children beyond infancy who have vaginal, urethral, or rectal chlamydial infection, although asymptomatic infection acquired at birth can persist for as long as 3 years.

C. trachomatis is associated with (a) neonatal conjunctivitis, (b) trachoma, (c) pneumonia in young infants, (d) genital tract infection, and (e) lymphogranuloma venereum. Neonatal chlamydial conjunctivitis is characterized by ocular congestion, edema, and discharge developing a few days to several weeks after birth and lasting for 1–2 weeks, occasionally much longer. In contrast to trachoma, scars and pannus formation are rare.

Trachoma is a chronic follicular keratoconjunctivitis with neovascularization of the cornea that results from repeated and chronic infection. Blindness secondary to extensive local scarring and inflammation occurs in 1–15% of persons with trachoma. Trachoma is rare in the United States.

Pneumonia in young infants is usually an afebrile illness occurring between 2 and 19 weeks after birth. A repetitive staccato cough, tachypnea, and rales are characteristic but are not always present. Wheezing is uncommon; however, hyperinflation usually accompanies the infiltrates seen on chest radiograph. Nasal stuffiness and otitis media may occur. Untreated disease can linger or recur. Severe chlamydial pneumonia has occurred in infants and some immunocompromised adults.

Urethritis; vaginitis in prepubertal girls; cervicitis, endometritis, salpingitis, and perihepatitis in postpubertal females; epididymitis in males; and Reiter syndrome in either sex also can occur. Infection can persist for months or years. Reinfection is common. In postpubertal females, chlamydial infection can progress to acute or chronic pelvic inflammation disease and result in ectopic pregnancy or infertility.

Lymphogranuloma venereum is an invasive lymphatic infection with an initial ulceration lesion on the genitalia accompanied by tender, suppurative, regional lymphadenopathy. Anorectal infection and hemorrhagic proctitis also have been described. The disease has a chronic low-grade course.

Diagnostic Tests

Definitive diagnosis can be made by isolating the organism in tissue culture. *Chlamydia* are obligate intracellular organisms. Culture specimens must contain epithelial cells, not just exudate. Nucleic acid amplification methods, such as PCR and ligase chain reaction, are more sensitive than cell culture and more specific and sensitive than DNA probe, DFA tests, or EIAs.

Tests for detection of chlamydial antigen or nucleic acid are useful for evaluating urethral specimens from males, cervical specimens from females, and conjunctival specimens from infants. The PCR and ligase chain reaction tests are useful for evaluating urine specimens from either sex. These tests have not been evaluated adequately for detection of *C. trachomatis* in nasopharyngeal specimens. The EIA and DFA tests should not be used for testing rectal, vaginal, or urethral specimens from infants and children, because fecal bacterial flora cross-react with *C. trachomatis* antisera.

Positive DFA, EIA, or DNA probe test results should be certified if a false-positive test result is likely to have adverse medical, social, or psychological consequences. Confirmation can be accomplished by culture, a second nonculture test result different from the first, or use of a blocking antibody (e.g., Chlamydiazyme, Abbott Laboratories, Abbott Park, IL) or competitive probe. When evaluating a child for possible sexual abuse, results of rapid antigen detection of DNA tests are unacceptable, and culture of the organism is the only acceptable method of diagnosis.

In the past, neonatal *C. trachomatis* conjunctivitis was diagnosed by Giemsa staining of conjunctival scrapings. The presence of blue-stained intracytoplasmic inclusions within epithelial cells is diagnostic. The sensitivity varies from 22% to 95% depending on the technique of specimen collection and the examiner's expertise.

Serum antibody determinations are difficult to perform and available in only a few clinical laboratories. In children with pneumonia, an acute microimmunofluorescence serum titer of *C. trachomatis*–specific IgM of ≥1:32 is diagnostic. A fourfold rise in microimmunofluorescence titer to lymphogranuloma venereum antigens or a complement fixation titer of ≥1:32 is suggestive of lymphogranuloma venereum in the presence of compatible clinical findings.

Indirect laboratory evidence of chlamydial pneumonia includes hyperinflation and bilateral diffuse infiltrates on radiographs, eosinophilia of 0.3–0.4 × 10^9/L (300–400/μL) or more in peripheral blood counts, and elevated total serum IgG [5 g/L (500 mg/dL)] and IgM [1.1 g/L (110 mg/dL)] concentrations. The absence of these findings, however, does not exclude the diagnosis. Direct antigen tests and culture are now so widely available that a specific diagnosis should be based on laboratory tests.

Cholera

Vibrio cholerae, the causative organism of cholera, is a Gram-negative, motile bacillus with many serogroups. Until recently, only enterotoxin-producing organisms of serogroup 01 have caused epidemics. *V. cholerae* 01 is divided into two serotypes, Inaba and Ogawa, and two biotypes, classic and El Tor. The predominant biotype is El Tor. In 1992, a cholera epidemic due to toxigenic *V. cholerae* serogroup 0139 Bengal (a nontoxigenic strain) caused epidemic cholera in the Indian subcontinent and Southeast Asia. Serogroups of *V. cholerae* other than 01 and 0139 Bengal and nontoxigenic strains of *V. cholerae* 01 can cause sporadic diarrheal illness, but they do not cause epidemics.

Cholera is characterized by painless voluminous diarrhea without abdominal cramps or fever. Dehydration, hypokalemia, metabolic acidosis, and, occasionally, hypovolemic shock also can occur, particularly in children. Stools are colorless, with small flecks of mucus ("rice water"), and contain high concentrations of sodium, potassium, chloride, and bicarbonate. Most persons infected with toxigenic *V. cholerae* 01 have no symptoms, however, and some have only mild to moderate diarrhea, whereas <5% have severe watery diarrhea, vomiting, and dehydration (cholera gravis).

Diagnostic Tests

V. cholerae can be cultured from fecal specimens or vomitus plated on appropriate selective media. Suspect colonies are confirmed serologically by agglutination with specific antisera. Because most laboratories in the United States do not culture routinely for *V. cholerae* or other vibrios, clinicians should request appropriate cultures for clinically suspected cases. Isolates of *V. cholerae* should be sent to a state health department laboratory for serogrouping; those of serogroup 01 or 0139 Bengal are then sent to the CDC for testing for production of cholera toxin. A fourfold rise in vibriocidal antibody titers between acute and convalescent serum samples or a fourfold decline in vibriocidal titers between early and late convalescent serum samples (more than a 2-month interval) can confirm the diagnosis retrospectively.

Clostridial Infections

Botulism and Infant Botulism

Seven antigen toxin types of *Clostridium botulinum* have been identified. Human botulism almost always is caused by neurotoxins A, B, E, and F. Types C and D are associated primarily with botulism in birds and mammals. Almost all cases of infant botulism are caused by types A and B.

Botulism is a neuroparalytic disorder that can be classified into the following categories: *food-borne, infant, wound,* and *undetermined*. The latter occurs in persons >12 months of age in whom no food or wound source is implicated. Except for infant botulism, onset of symptoms occurs abruptly within a few hours or evolves gradually over several days. Symmetric, descending flaccid paralysis occurs, typically involving the bulbar musculature initially and later affecting the somatic musculature. Symmetric paralysis may progress rapidly. Patients with rapidly evolving illness may have generalized weakness and hypotonia initially. Signs and symptoms in older children or adults can include diplopia, blurred vision, dry mouth, dysphagia, dysphonia, and dysarthria. Classically, infant botulism, which occurs predominantly in infants <6 months of age, is preceded by constipation and is manifest as lethargy, poor feeding, weak cry, diminished gag reflex, subtle ocular palsies, and generalized weakness and hypotonia (e.g., "floppy infant"). A spectrum of disease ranging from rapidly progressive (e.g., apnea, sudden infant death) to mild (e.g., constipation, slow feeding) exists. Infants may be infected by ingestion of honey or corn syrups containing botulinus spores.

Diagnostic Tests

A toxin neutralization bioassay in mice is used to identify botulinum toxin in serum, stool, or suspect foods. Enriched and selective media are used to culture *C. botulinum* from stool and foods. In infant and wound botulism, the diagnosis is made by demonstrating *C. botulinum* organisms or toxin in feces or wound exudate or tissue samples. Toxin has been demonstrated in serum in approximately 1% of infants with botulism.

To increase the likelihood of diagnosis, both serum and stool should be obtained from all persons with suspected botulism. In food-borne cases, serum specimens collected >3 days after ingestion of toxin usually are negative, at which time stool and gastric aspirates are the best diagnostic specimens for culture. As obtaining a stool specimen may be difficult because of constipation, an enema using sterile nonbacteriostatic water can be given. The most prominent electromyographic finding is an incremental increase of evoked muscle potentials at high-frequency nerve stimulation (20–50 Hz). In addition, a characteristic pattern of brief, small-amplitude, overly abundant motor action potentials can be seen.

Clostridium difficile Infections

Clostridium difficile is a spore-forming, obligatory anaerobic, Gram-positive bacillus. It is the cause of pseudomembranous colitis and of a high percentage of episodes of antimicrobial-associated diarrhea. Two toxins, A and B, have been characterized.

C. difficile can be isolated from soil and frequently is present in the environment. Penicillins, clindamycin, and cephalosporins are the antimicrobial drugs most frequently associated with *C. difficile* colitis, but colitis has been associated with almost every antimicrobial agent. The organism may be recovered from stool specimens from neonates and infants who have no gastrointestinal tract illness.

Pseudomembranous colitis generally is characterized by diarrhea, abdominal cramps, fever, systemic toxic effects, abdominal tenderness, and passage of stools containing blood and mucus. The colonic mucosa often contains small (2- to 5-mm), raised, yellowish plaques. Characteristically, disease begins while the patient is in a hospital receiving antimicrobial therapy, but it may occur weeks after discharge from the hospital or after discontinuation of therapy. Severe or fatal disease is more likely to occur in severely neutropenic children with leukemia, in infants with Hirschsprung disease, and in patients with inflammatory bowel disease. Infection also may result only in mild diarrhea or asymptomatic carriage, especially in newborn infants and in children <1 year of age.

Diagnostic Tests

Endoscopic findings of pseudomembranes and hyperemic friable rectal mucosa suggest pseudomembranous colitis. To diagnose *C. difficile* infection, stool should be tested for the presence of *C. difficile* toxins. Testing for toxin is performed by EIA or cell cytotoxin assay, which has been the gold standard for toxin B. The EIAs are sensitive and easy to perform. Commercially available EIAs that detect both toxins A and B may be used, or an EIA for toxin A may be used in conjunction with cell culture cytotoxicity assay for toxin B. Latex agglutination tests should not be used.

Clostridial Myonecrosis (Gas Gangrene)

Gas gangrene usually results from contamination of open wounds involving muscle. The sources of *Clostridium* species are soil, contaminated objects, and human and animal feces. The presence of dirty surgical or traumatic wounds with significant devitalized tissue and foreign bodies predisposes to disease. Nontraumatic gas gangrene occurs occasionally from *Clostridium* organisms in a person's gastrointestinal tract.

The incubation period ranges from 6 hours to 3 weeks, but is usually 2–4 days.

C. perfringens are large, Gram-positive, anaerobic bacilli with blunt ends.

The onset is heralded by acute pain at the site of the wound, followed by edema, tenderness, exudate, and progression of pain. Systemic findings initially include tachycardia disproportionate to the degree of fever, pallor, diaphoresis, hypotension, renal failure, and, later, alterations in mental status. Crepitus is suggestive, but not pathognomonic, of *Clostridium* infection and is not always present. Diagnosis is based on clinical manifestations, including the characteristic appearance of necrotic muscle at surgery. Untreated, gas gangrene can lead to death within hours.

Diagnostic Tests

Anaerobic cultures of wound exudate, samples of involved soft tissue and muscle, and blood should be performed. Because *Clostridium* species are ubiquitous, their recovery from a wound is not diagnostic unless the appropriate clinical manifestations are present. A Gram-stained smear of wound discharge demonstrating characteristic Gram-positive bacilli and absent or sparse polymorphonuclear leukocytes suggests clostridial infection. Tissue samples and aspirates, but not swabs, are appropriate specimens for anaerobic culture. Inoculation of material into culture media in the operating room or aspiration of material into a capped syringe and rapid transport of samples to the laboratory are essential to ensure recovery of anaerobic organisms. A radiograph of the affected site may demonstrate gas in the tissue.

Clostridium perfringens Food Poisoning

Food poisoning is caused by a heat-labile toxin produced *in vivo* by *C. perfringens* type A; type C causes enteritis necroticans.

Food poisoning is characterized by the sudden onset of watery diarrhea and moderate to severe crampy midepigastric pain. Vomiting and fever are uncommon. Symptoms usually resolve within 24 hours. The absence of fever in most patients differentiates *C. perfringens* food-borne disease from shigellosis and salmonellosis, and the infrequency of vomiting and longer incubation period contrast with the clinical features of food-borne disease associated with heavy metals, *Staphylococcus aureus* enterotoxins, and fish and shellfish toxins. Diarrheal illness caused by *B. cereus* enterotoxin may be indistinguishable from that caused by *C. perfringens*. Enteritis necroticans (known locally as *pigbel*) is a cause of severe illness and death due to *C. perfringens* food poisoning among children in Papua, New Guinea.

Diagnostic Tests

Because fecal flora of healthy persons frequently includes *C. perfringens*, counts of at least 10^6 *C. perfringens* spores per gram of feces obtained within 48 hours of onset of illness are required to support the diagnosis in ill persons. The diagnosis also can be established by detection of *C. perfringens* enterotoxin in stool by commercially available kits. To confirm *C. perfringens* as the cause, the concentration of organisms should be at least 10^5 per gram in the epidemiologically implicated food. Although *C. perfringens* is an anaerobe, special transport conditions are unnecessary because the spores are durable. Stool rather than rectal swab samples should be collected.

Diphtheria

Corynebacterium diphtheriae is an irregularly staining, Gram-positive, spore-forming, nonmotile, pleomorphic bacillus with three colony types (mitis, intermedius, and gravis). Strains of *C. diphtheriae* may be toxigenic or nontoxigenic. Production of extracellular toxin consisting of an enzymatically active A domain and a binding B domain is mediated by bacteriophage infection of the bacterium and is not related to colony type.

Diphtheria usually occurs as membranous nasopharyngitis or obstructive laryngotracheitis. These local infections are associated with a low-grade fever and the gradual onset of manifestations during 1–2 days. Less commonly, the disease presents as cutaneous, vaginal, conjunctival, or otic infections. Cutaneous diphtheria is more common in tropical areas and among the homeless. Serious complications of diphtheria include upper airway obstruction caused by extensive membrane formation, myocarditis, and peripheral neuropathies.

Diagnostic Tests

Specimens for culture should be obtained from the nose, throat, or any mucosal or cutaneous lesion. Material should be obtained from beneath the membrane, or a portion of the membrane itself should be submitted for culture. Because special media are required, laboratory personnel should be notified that *C. diphtheriae* is suspected. In remote areas, throat swabs can be placed in silica gel packs or tellurite enrichment medium and sent to a reference laboratory for culture. Direct-stained smears and fluorescent antibody–stained smears are unreliable. When *C. diphtheria* is recovered, the strain should be tested for toxigenicity at a laboratory recommended by state and local authorities. All *C. diphtheria* isolates also should be sent through the state health department to the Diphtheria Laboratory, National Center for Infectious Diseases of the CDC.

Ehrlichiosis

In the United States, human ehrlichiosis may be caused by two distinct species of obligate intracellular bacteria. Human monocytic ehrlichiosis results from infection with *Ehrlichia chaffeensis*. Human granulocytic ehrlichiosis is caused by an unnamed *Ehrlichia* species closely related to *E. phagocytophila* and *E. equi*. A third human ehrlichial pathogen, *E. sennetsu*, causes Sennetsu fever, a self-limited mononucleosis-like illness that occurs in Japan and Malaysia. *Ehrlichia ewingii*, an agent reported as a cause of granulocytic ehrlichiosis in dogs, reportedly causes disease in humans.

Human ehrlichiosis in North America consists of at least two distinct diseases that are referred to as *human monocytic ehrlichiosis* and *human granulocytic ehrlichiosis*. These two diseases have different causes but similar signs, symptoms, and clinical courses. Both are acute, systemic, febrile illnesses that are similar clinically to Rocky Mountain spotted fever but with more frequent occurrence of leukopenia, anemia, and hepatitis and less frequent occurrence of rash. The febrile illness often is accompanied by headache, chills, malaise, myalgia, arthralgia, nausea, vomiting, anorexia, and acute weight loss. Rash is variable in appearance and location, typically develops approximately 1 week after onset of illness, and occurs only in approximately 50% of reported cases of monocytic ehrlichiosis and <10% of persons with granulocytic ehrlichiosis. Diarrhea, abdominal pain, and change in mental status occur infrequently. Reported complications of both diseases include pulmonary infiltrates, bone marrow hypoplasia, respiratory failure, encephalopathy, meningitis, disseminated intravascular coagulation, and renal failure. Anemia, hyponatremia, thrombocytopenia, elevated liver enzyme concentrations, and cerebrospinal fluid (CSF) abnormalities (i.e., pleocytosis with a predominance of lymphocytes and elevated total protein concentration) are common. Although both diseases typically last 1–2 weeks and recovery generally occurs without sequelae, reports suggest the occurrence of neurologic complications in some children. Fatal as well as asymptomatic infections have been reported. Secondary or opportunistic infections may occur in severe illness, which results in possible delayed recognition of ehrlichiosis and appropriate antibiotic treatment.

Diagnostic Tests

The CDC defines a confirmed case of ehrlichiosis as

1. A fourfold or greater change in antibody titer by IFA assay between acute and convalescent serum samples (ideally collected 3–6 weeks apart);
2. PCR amplification of ehrlichial DNA from a clinical sample; or
3. Detection of intraleukocytoplasmic *Ehrlichia* microcolonies (morulae) and a single IFA titer of 1:64.

The diagnosis of ehrlichiosis can be confirmed by finding cytoplasmic inclusion bodies (morulae) in granulocytes on a Wright-stained blood smear. Typically, morulae are found in 1–6% of granulocytes, although a sensitivity as high as 80% has been reported. PCR to the 16S recombinant DNA sequence has been shown to be rapid, sensitive (86%), and specific (100%).

A probable case is defined as a single IFA titer of 1:64 or the presence of morulae within infected leukocytes.

E. chaffeensis is used as the antigen for the serologic diagnosis of human monocytic ehrlichiosis, and the human granulocytic ehrlichiosis agent is used as the antigen in assays for the diagnosis of granulocytic ehrlichiosis. These tests are available in reference laboratories, some commercial laboratories and state health departments, and at the CDC. More than ten isolates of *E. chaffeensis* have been obtained from human patients. Examination of peripheral blood smears to detect morulae in peripheral blood monocytes or granulocytes is insensitive, but this test is warranted for patients for whom a high index of suspicion exists.

Escherichia Coli *Infection and Infection with Other Gram-Negative Bacilli*

Septicemia and Meningitis in Neonates

Escherichia coli strains with the K1 capsular polysaccharide antigen cause approximately 40% of cases of septicemia and 75% of cases of meningitis in the newborn. Other important Gram-negative bacilli that can cause neonatal septicemia include non-K1 strains of *E. coli* and *Klebsiella, Enterobacter, Proteus, Citrobacter, Salmonella*, and *Pseudomonas* species. Anaerobic Gram-negative bacilli are rare causes, as are nonencapsulated strains of *H. influenzae.*

Neonatal septicemia or meningitis caused by *E. coli* and other Gram-negative bacilli cannot be differentiated clinically from serious infections caused by other infectious agents. The first signs of sepsis may be minimal and similar to those observed in noninfectious processes. Clinical signs of septicemia include fever, temperature instability, apnea, cyanosis, jaundice, hepatomegaly, lethargy, irritability, anorexia, vomiting, abdominal distention, and diarrhea. Meningitis may be concomitant with septicemia without overt signs attributable to the central nervous system (CNS). Some Gram-negative bacilli such as *Citrobacter diversus* and *Enterobacter sakazakii* are associated with brain abscesses in infants with meningitis due to these organisms.

Diagnostic Tests

Growth of *E. coli* or other Gram-negative bacilli from blood, CSF, or other usually sterile sites.

Diarrhea and Hemolytic-Uremic Syndrome

Table 1 shows the classification of *E. coli* associated with diarrhea.

Table 1. Classification of *Escherichia coli* Associated with Diarrhea

E. coli Pathotype	Epidemiology	Type of Diarrhea	Mechanism of Pathogenesis
Enterohemorrhagic (EHEC)	Hemorrhagic colitis, hemolytic uremic syndrome in all ages, and postdiarrheal thrombotic thrombocytopenic purpura in adults	Bloody or nonbloody	Adherence and effacement, cytotoxin production
Enteropathogenic (EPEC)	Acute and chronic endemic and epidemic diarrhea in infants	Watery	Adherence, effacement
Enterotoxigenic (ETEC)	Infantile diarrhea in developing countries and traveler's diarrhea in all ages	Watery	Adherence, enterotoxin production
Enteroinvasive (EIEC)	Diarrhea with fever in all ages	Bloody or nonbloody diarrhea	Adherence, mucosal invasion and inflammation
Enteroaggregative (EAEC)	Acute and chronic diarrhea in infants	Watery, occasionally bloody	Adherence, mucosal damage

From Pickering LK, ed. *2000 Red Book: Report of the Committee on Infectious Diseases*, 25th ed. Section 3. Elk Grove Village, IL: American Academy of Pediatrics, 2000:243.

Illness caused by enterohemorrhagic *E. coli* (EHEC) O157:H7 occurs in a two-step process. The intestinal phase is characterized by formation of the attaching and effacing lesion, which results in secretory diarrhea. This phase is followed by elaboration of Shiga toxin, a potent cytotoxin also found in *Shigella dysenteriae* 1. The action of Shiga toxin on intestinal cells results in hemorrhagic colitis, and toxin circulation through the bloodstream is responsible for hemolytic-uremic syndrome (HUS).

Enteropathogenic *E. coli* (EPEC) belong typically to 12 O serogroups. Strains of EPEC adhere to the small bowel mucosa and, like EHEC O157:H7, produce attaching and effacing lesions.

Strains of enterotoxigenic *E. coli* (ETEC) colonize the small intestine without invading and produce heat-labile enterotoxin, heat-stable enterotoxin, or both. Heat-stable enterotoxin producers are responsible for most human illness due to ETEC.

Strains of enteroinvasive *E. coli* (EIEC) are typically lactose nonfermenting and, like *Shigella* species, invade the colonic mucosa, where they spread laterally and induce a local inflammatory response.

Strains of EHEC should be sought in the following instances: bloody diarrhea (indicated by history or inspection of stool), HUS, postdiarrheal thrombotic thrombocytopenic purpura, and any type of diarrhea in contacts of patients with HUS. Persons with presumptive diagnoses of intussusception, inflammatory bowel disease, or ischemic colitis sometimes have disease caused by EHEC O157:H7. Methods for definitive identification of EHEC that are used in reference or research laboratories include DNA probes, PCR, EIA, and phenotypic testing of strains or stool specimens for Shiga toxin. Serologic diagnosis using an EIA test to detect serum antibodies to EHEC O157:H7 lipopolysaccharide is available in reference laboratories.

The enteroaggregative (EAEC) organisms have a "stacked brick" adherence pattern in tissue culture–based assays. These organisms elaborate one or more enterotoxins and cause damage to the intestinal mucosa.

The only *E. coli* pathotype common in the United States is EHEC. Enterohemorrhagic *E. coli* O157:H7 is shed in the feces of cattle, deer, and other ruminants and is transmitted by undercooked ground beef, unpasteurized milk, and a wide variety of vehicles contaminated with bovine feces.

At least five pathotypes of diarrhea-producing *E. coli* strains have been identified. Clinical features of disease caused by each pathotype are summarized as follows:

EHEC strains, also known as Shiga-toxin producing *E. coli* or verotoxin-producing *E. coli*, are associated with diarrhea, hemorrhagic colitis, HUS, and postdiarrheal thrombotic thrombocytopenic purpura. Enterohemorrhagic *E. coli* O157:H7 is the prototype for this class of organisms. Illness caused by EHEC often begins as nonbloody diarrhea but usually progresses to diarrhea with visible or occult blood. Severe abdominal pain is typical; fever occurs in fewer than one-third of cases. Hemorrhagic colitis is the most severe intestinal infection.

Diarrhea cause by EPEC strains is characterized by watery diarrhea that often is severe and can result in dehydration. Enteropathogenic *E. coli* is a cause of chronic diarrhea that can lead to growth retardation. Illness occurs almost exclusively in neonates and children <2 years of age and predominantly in developing countries, either sporadically or in epidemics.

Infection caused by EIEC strains is similar clinically and pathogenetically to infection cause by *Shigella* species. Although dysentery can occur, diarrhea usually is watery without blood or mucus. Patients often are febrile, and stools may contain fecal leukocytes.

EAEC strains cause watery diarrhea, predominantly in infants and young children in the developing world. Enteroaggregative *E. coli* has been associated with persistent diarrhea (>14 days).

Hemolytic-Uremic Syndrome

For all patients with HUS, stool specimens should be cultured for EHEC O157:H7 and, if results are negative, for other EHEC serotypes. The absence of EHEC in feces, however, does not preclude the diagnosis of EHEC-associated HUS, because HUS typically is diagnosed a week or more after onset of diarrhea when the organisms no longer may be detectable. When EHEC infection is considered, a stool culture should be obtained as early as possible in the illness.

Table 2. Five Major Categories of Pathogenic *Escherichia coli*

Category	Abbreviation	Clinic Manifestation
Enterotoxigenic diarrhea	ETEC	Traveler's diarrhea and infant diarrhea in less-developed countries
Enteropathogenic	EPEC	Infant diarrhea
Enterohemorrhagic	EHEC	Hemorrhagic colitis Hemolytic uremic syndrome Thrombotic thrombocytopenia purpura
Enteroinvasive	EIEC	Diarrhea
	EAEC	Enterotoxins damage intestinal mucosa

Griffin PM, Ostroff SM, Tauxe RV. Illness associated with *Escherichia coli* O157:H7 infections—a broad clinical spectrum. *Ann Intern Med* 1988;109:705–712.

Traveler's Diarrhea

Traveler's diarrhea has been associated with many enteropathogens, usually is acquired by ingestion of contaminated food or water, and is a significant problem for persons traveling in developing countries.

Diagnostic Tests

Rectal swab or stool specimen in transport media.

Diagnosis of infection caused by diarrhea-associated *E. coli* usually is difficult because most clinical laboratories cannot differentiate diarrhea-associated *E. coli* strains from normal *E. coli* stool flora. The exceptions are EHEC O157:H7 and EIEC, which can be identified presumptively or specifically. For definitive identification, isolates suspected to be associated with diarrhea should be sent to reference or research laboratories.

Clinical laboratories can screen for EHEC O157:H7 by using MacConkey agar base with sorbitol substituted for lactose. Approximately 90% of human intestinal *E. coli* strains rapidly ferment sorbitol, whereas EHEC O157:H7 strains do not. These sorbitol-negative *E. coli* then can be serotyped, using commercially available antisera, to determine whether they are O157:H7. DNA probes and PCR testing are available in research and reference laboratories for identification of each *E. coli* pathotype and now are considered preferable to serotyping for identification of EPEC. If a case or outbreak due to diarrhea-associated *E. coli* other than O157:H7 is suspected, *E. coli* isolates should be referred to the state public health laboratory or another reference laboratory for serotyping and identification of pathotypes.

Major Categories of Pathogenic *Escherichia coli*

See Table 2.

Method

Cultures may be evaluated for non–sorbitol-fermenting (colorless) colonies on sorbitol-MacConkey agar or the toxin may be detected by EIA; EHEC is confirmed by an immunologic method.

Hemorrhagic colitis can be differentiated from other causes of diarrhea by its progression from watery to bloody diarrhea over a few days. Fecal leukocyte levels are markedly increased. Fever is usually absent. The disease is mediated by the production of a Shiga-like toxin that interferes with colonic brush border cells and protein synthesis, and ultimately causes cell death. Enterohemorrhagic *E. coli* (EHEC) differs from other strains of bacteria in the large amount of toxin produced. Virtually all O157:H7 organisms produce this toxin. Strains of *E. coli* other than O157 have also been shown to produce Shiga toxin.

Gonococcal Infections

Neisseria gonorrhoeae is a Gram-negative, oxidase-positive diplococcus.

Sexual abuse should be strongly considered when genital, rectal, or pharyngeal colonization or infections are diagnosed in children beyond the newborn period and before puberty and in adolescents who deny that they are sexually active. Concurrent infection with *C. trachomatis* is common.

Gonococcal infection in children occurs in three distinct age groups.

Infection in the newborn infant usually involves the eyes. Infections at other sites include scalp abscess (which can be associated with fetal monitoring), vaginitis, and disseminated disease with bacteremia, arthritis, meningitis, or endocarditis.

In prepubertal children beyond the newborn period, gonococcal infection may occur in the genital tract and is almost always sexually transmitted. Rarely, transmission from household contact can occur. Vaginitis is the most common manifestation; pelvic inflammatory disease and perihepatitis can occur but are rare. Gonococcal urethritis in the prepubertal male is uncommon. Anorectal and tonsillopharyngeal infection also can occur in prepubertal children.

In sexually active adolescents, as in adults, gonococcal infection of the genital tract in girls is most frequently asymptomatic, and common clinical syndromes are urethritis, endocervicitis, and salpingitis. In boys, infection usually is symptomatic, and the primary site is the urethra. Infection of the rectum and pharynx can occur alone or can accompany genitourinary tract infection in either sex. Rectal and pharyngeal infections often are asymptomatic. Extension from primary genital mucosal sites can lead to epididymitis, bartholinitis, pelvic inflammatory disease, and perihepatitis.

Diagnostic Tests

Microscopic examination of Gram-stained smears of exudate from the eyes, the endocervix of postpubertal girls, the vagina of prepubertal girls, male urethra, skin lesions, synovial fluid, and, when clinically warranted, CSF is useful in the initial evaluation. Identification of Gram-negative intracellular diplococci in these smears can be helpful, particularly if the organism is not recovered in culture. Gram stains of material obtained from the endocervix of postpubertal girls are less sensitive than culture for detection of infection, but they can be of immediate help in the differential diagnosis of a patient with acute abdominal pain or when immediate therapy is indicated. Organisms other than these are seldom observed within polymorphonuclear leukocytes. In prepubertal girls, vaginal specimens are adequate for diagnosis, and endocervical specimens are unnecessary.

N. gonorrhoeae can be cultured from normally sterile sites, such as blood, CSF, or synovial fluid, using nonselective chocolate agar with incubation in 5–10% carbon dioxide or specialized culture media. Selective media that inhibit normal flora and nonpathogenic *Neisseria* organisms are used for culture from nonsterile sites, such as the cervix, vagina, rectum, urethra, and pharynx. Specimens for *N. gonorrhoeae* culture from mucosal sites should be inoculated immediately onto the appropriate agar or placed in transport medium because *N. gonorrhoeae* is extremely sensitive to drying and temperature changes.

Caution should be exercised when interpreting the significance of the isolation of *Neisseria* organisms, as *N. gonorrhoeae* can be confused with other *Neisseria* species that colonize the genitourinary tract to pharynx. At least two confirmatory bacteriologic tests involving different principles (e.g., biochemical, enzyme substrate, or serology) should be performed. Interpretation of culture results from the pharynx of young children as *N. gonorrhoeae* necessitates particular caution because of the high carriage rate of nonpathogenic *Neisseria* species.

During the last few years, nucleic acid amplification methods by PCR or ligase chain reaction have become clinically available. They are highly sensitive and specific when used on urethral and cervicovaginal swab specimens. They also can be used with good sensitivity and specificity on first-void urine specimens, which has led to increased compliance with testing and follow-up in hard-to-access populations, such as adolescents. These techniques also permit dual testing of urine for *C. trachomatis* and *N. gonorrhoeae*.

Granuloma Inguinale

Granuloma inguinale is caused by *Calymmatobacterium granulomatis*, a Gram-negative bacillus.

Young children can acquire infection by contact with infected secretions.

Initial lesions are single or multiple subcutaneous nodules that progress to form painless, friable, granulomatous ulcers. Lesions usually involve genitalia, but anal infections occur in 5–10% of patients; lesions at distant sites (e.g., face, mouth, or liver) are rare. Subcutaneous extension into the inguinal area results in induration that can mimic inguinal adenopathy—that is, the "pseudobubo" of granuloma inguinale. Fibrosis manifests as sinus tracts, adhesions, and lymphedema, which result in extreme genital deformity.

Diagnostic Tests

The microscopic demonstration of intracytoplasmic Donovan bodies on Wright or Giemsa staining of a crush preparation from subsurface scrapings of a lesion or tissue is diagnostic. The microorganisms also can be detected by histologic examination of biopsy specimens. Culture of *C. granulomatis* has been accomplished using the human epidermoid larynx carcinoma cell line, but this technique is not available routinely. Lesions, however, should be cultured for *H. ducreyi* to exclude chancroid (pseudogranuloma inguinale). Granuloma inguinale frequently is misdiagnosed as carcinoma, which can be excluded by histologic examination of tissue or by response of the lesion to antibiotics. Diagnosis by PCR and serology is available.

Haemophilus influenzae *Infections*

Haemophilus influenzae is a pleomorphic Gram-negative coccobacillus. Isolates are classified into six antigenically distinct capsular types (a through f) and nonencapsulated, nontypeable strains. Before the introduction of *H. influenzae* type b (Hib) conjugate vaccination, most cases of invasive diseases in children were caused by type b. Type f is the most common other serotype causing invasive infections. Nonencapsulated strains cause upper respiratory tract infection, including otitis media, sinusitis, tracheitis, and bronchitis, and may cause pneumonia.

H. influenzae causes otitis media, sinusitis, epiglottitis, septic arthritis, occult febrile bacteremia, cellulitis, meningitis, pneumonia, and empyema. Other *H. influenzae* infections include purulent pericarditis, endocarditis, conjunctivitis, endophthalmitis, osteomyelitis, peritonitis, epididymo-orchitis, glossitis, uvulitis, and septic thrombophlebitis. Occasionally, nonencapsulated strains cause neonatal septicemia, pneumonia, and meningitis.

The incubation period is unknown.

Diagnostic Tests

CSF, blood, synovial fluid, pleural fluid, and middle ear aspirates should be cultured on a medium such as chocolate agar enriched with X and V cofactors. A Gram stain of an infected body fluid can disclose the organism and allows a presumptive diagnosis to be made. Latex particle agglutination for detection of type b capsular antigen in CSF may be helpful when antimicrobial therapy was initiated before cultures were obtained. Antigen testing of serum and urine is not recommended, however, because antigen can be detected as a result of asymptomatic nasopharyngeal carriage of Hib, recent immunization with an Hib conjugate vaccine, or contamination of urine specimens by cross-reacting fecal organisms. All *H. influenzae* isolates associated with an invasive infection should be serotyped to determine whether the strain is type b. If testing is not available, isolates should be submitted to the state health department, to the CDC, or to a reference laboratory for testing.

Helicobacter pylori *Infections*

Helicobacter pylori is a Gram-negative and spiral, curved, or U-shaped microaerophilic bacillus that has two to six polar sheathed flagellae at one end.

Acute infection is manifested by epigastric pain, nausea, vomiting, hematemesis, and guaiac-positive stools. Symptoms usually resolve within a few days despite persistence of infection for years. *H. pylori* causes chronic active gastritis and duodenal ulcer and is associated less frequently with gastric ulcer; chronic infection has a high attributable risk of gastric cancer. *H. pylori* infection is not associated with autoimmune or chemical gastritis.

Diagnostic Tests

H. pylori infection can be diagnosed as follows:

Gastric biopsy tissue can be cultured on nonselective media (e.g., chocolate agar) or selective media (e.g., Skirrow) at 37°C (98°F).

Because of production of urease by the organisms, urease testing of a gastric specimen can give a rapid and specific microbiologic diagnosis.

Each of these tests requires endoscopy and biopsy.

Organisms usually can be visualized on histologic sections with Warthin-Starry silver, Steiner, Giemsa, or Genta staining. Infection with *H. pylori* can be diagnosed but not excluded on the basis of hematoxylin-eosin stains. They cling to the mucosal surface and are frequently clumped within mucosa or epithelial surface of the biopsy specimen.

Noninvasive, commercially available tests include the breath test, which detects labeled carbon dioxide in expired air after oral administration of isotopically labeled urea, and serology for the presence of IgG to *H. pylori*. Each of the diagnostic tests has a sensitivity and specificity of 95% or more.

Helicobacter IgA, IgG, and IgM antibodies can be measured by EIA from serum to monitor the eradication of *H. pylori* after antimicrobial therapy; to identify the small percentage of *H. pylori*–infected patients who do not mount a systemic IgG response and demonstrate IgA antibodies only; and to test those patients who have chronic mucosal infection only. Antibodies to IgM may indicate an early infection. The accuracy of serologic tests is 85%.

A stool antigen test has a diagnostic accuracy of over 96% and has the advantage of being noninvasive for testing of young children. A fresh stool sample is collected and stored at –20°C for analysis. A commercial kit (HpSa Microwell EIA, Meridan Diagnostic Inc., Cincinnati, OH) is an enzyme-linked immunosorbent assay (ELISA). This is a qualitative test with a polyclonal rabbit anti–*H. pylori* antibody adsorbed to microwells. Diluted stool samples and a peroxidase-conjugated secondary polyclonal antibody are added to the microwells and incubated for 1 hour at room temperature. Reading of the results is based on spectrophotometric analysis: optical density at 450 nm of <0.14 is negative, a value of >0.16 is positive, and a value in between is equivocal. If results are equivocal, the test should be repeated.

Bacterial culture. Biopsy specimens are immediately transferred into a brain-heart infusion broth. After grinding and transformation are performed, they are streaked in the blood agar plate and incubated at 35–37°C under microaerophilic conditions (5% O_2, 10% CO_2, 85% N_2) for 3–7 days. Organisms are identified as *H. pylori* on the basis of colony structure, results of Gram stain, and the production of urease, oxidase, and catalase. This test has an accuracy of 98%.

C-urea breath test. Use of the infrared spectrophotometer (UbiT-IR200, Otsuka Electronics Co., Hirakata, Japan) has been validated and has correlated well with mass spectrometric analysis. The patient fasts overnight before the test. The procedures are done according to the manufacturer's instructions. Two bags of exhaled air are collected: one at baseline and the other 15 minutes after ingestion of a powder containing 100 mg of C-urea in 100 mL of drinking water. The two bags are inserted into the inlets of the infrared spectrophotometer, and the increased percentage of CO_2 urea is shown in 5 minutes. The cutoff point is 4.5%. This test has an accuracy of 100%.

PCR. The biopsy antrum tissues are minced, and the DNA extracted with the DNA extraction kit (Qiagen, Chatsworth, CA). Each biopsy specimen is finally adjusted to a DNA concentration of 0.1 μg/μL. The nucleotide sequences of primers (first and nested) are from *H. pylori* urease C genome as previously described. If there is no product after the first run of PCR, 1 μL of first-run PCR product is subjected to a nested PCR. A DNA fragment containing the sequences of urease C gene is cloned, expressed, and serially diluted. This is used in the sensitivity assay as a positive control. The test has an accuracy of 94%.

Legionella pneumophila *Infection*

Legionella species are fastidious aerobic bacilli that stain Gram-negative after recovery on artifical media. At least 18 different species have been implicated in human disease, but the majority of *Legionella* infections in the United States are caused by the *Legionella pneumophila* serogroup 1.

Legionellosis is associated with two clinically and epidemiologically distinct illnesses: *Legionnaires disease*, which varies in severity from a mild to a severe progressive infection characterized by fever, myalgia, cough, and pneumonia, and *Pontiac fever*, a milder illness without pneumonia. Legionnaires disease may be associated with gastrointestinal tract, CNS, and renal manifestations. Respiratory failure and death may occur. Pontiac fever is characterized by an abrupt-onset, self-limited, influenza-like illness.

Diagnostic Tests

Recovery of *L. pneumophila* from respiratory tract secretions, lung tissue, pleural fluid, or other normally sterile fluids by using special culture media provides definitive evidence of infection. The bacterium can be demonstrated by direct immunofluorescence and by DNA probes, but these tests are less sensitive and specific than culture. Detection of *L. pneumophila* serogroup 1 antigens in urine by commercially available radioimmunoassay or EIA is more sensitive and specific than immunofluorescence using respiratory tract secretions and allows rapid diagnosis, but such testing only detects infection due to this species and serogroup. For serologic diagnosis, an increase in titer of antibody to *L. pneumophila* serogroup 1 to ≥1:128, measured by an IFA test, also indicates acute infection. Antibody titers usually increase within 1–6 weeks after onset of symptoms, but the increase can be delayed for as long as 12 weeks. The positive predictive value of a single titer of ≥1:256 is low and such a result should not be used for diagnostic purposes. Newer serologic assays, such as EIA or tests using *Legionella* antigens other than serogroup 1, are available commercially but have not been standardized adequately for routine use. Antibodies to *Mycoplasma pneumoniae* and several Gram-negative organisms, including *Campylobacter jejuni, P. aeruginosa*, and *Bacteroides fragilis*, may cause false-positive IFA test results. Diagnosis of infection by detection of *L. pneumophila* DNA by PCR in respiratory tract secretions, serum, or urine is positive.

Leprosy

Leprosy (Hansen disease) is caused by *Mycobacterium leprae*.

Leprosy is a chronic disease mainly involving the skin, peripheral nerves, and mucosa of the upper respiratory tract. The clinical syndromes of leprosy represent a spectrum that reflects the cellular immune response to *M. leprae*. Characteristic features are the following.

Tuberculoid

One or few well-demarcated, hypopigmented or erythematous, hypoesthetic or anesthetic skin lesions, frequently with raised, active, spreading edges and central clearing. Cell-mediated immune responses are intact.

Lepromatous

Initial numerous, ill-defined, hypopigmented or erythematous macules that progress to papules, nodules, or plaques, and late-occurring hypesthesia. Dermal infiltration of the face, hands, and feet in a bilateral and symmetric distribution can occur without preceding maculopapular lesions. *M. leprae*–specific, cell-mediated immunity is greatly diminished, but serum antibody responses to *M. leprae*–derived antigens may occur, or titers of nonspecific antibodies (such as those used in tests for rheumatoid factor or nontreponemal tests for syphilis) may be elevated.

Indeterminate

An early form of leprosy that may develop into any of the other forms; typified by hypopigmented macules with indistinct edges and no associated dysesthesia.

Serious consequences of leprosy occur from immune reactions and nerve involvement with resulting anesthesia, which can lead to repeated unrecognized trauma, ulcerations, fractures, and bone resorption.

Diagnostic Tests

Histopathologic examination by an experienced pathologist is the best method for establishing the diagnosis and is the basis for the classification of leprosy. Acid-fast bacilli may be found in slit-smears or biopsy specimens of skin lesions but rarely from patients with the tuberculoid and indeterminate forms of disease. Organisms have not been cultured successfully *in vitro*. Drug resistance is tested by the mouse footpad inoculation test, which is performed only in specialized laboratories, and results require a period of at least 6 months. Clinically, the demonstration of morphologically normal bacilli (i.e., organisms with solid staining of the capsule on acid-fast bacillus stains) despite usually effective therapy suggests possible drug resistance (or poor compliance with therapy) and indicates the possible need for a change in therapy.

High titers of predominantly IgM serum antibodies against phenolic glycolipid-1 of *M. leprae* have been detected in untreated patients with lepromatous or borderline disease. Because elevated antibody titers frequently occur in persons without disease, this test is not diagnostic for leprosy. Titers of these antibodies slowly decrease after years of therapy. This test is experimental and available only in a few reference laboratories.

Listeriosis

Listeria monocytogenes is an aerobic, non–spore-forming, motile, Gram-positive bacillus that produces a narrow zone of hemolysis on blood agar medium.

Pregnant women and their fetuses are at high risk of infection, comprising up to 27% of all cases of *Listeria* infection. Infected women usually present with a flulike illness that may be mild and easily missed. The incubation period is long, lasting up to 2 months. If infected early, the fetus is usually aborted spontaneously. Later in the pregnancy, the fetus may show intrauterine growth retardation. If born alive, the infant may be acutely ill. Bacteremia and meningitis are the most common presentations, and the mortality rate for the infant is in the range of 50%.

The route of infection to the placenta is hematogenous, with classic parenchymal microabscesses in the parenchyma without evidence of chorioamnionitis. The organism is usually present in infected food and invades through the gastrointestinal tract. It is protected from gastric acidity by the food and the use of antacids (commonly ingested by pregnant women). Once in the gastrointestinal tract, the organism is transported to the membranous epithelial cells and then to the lymphoid tissues, where it is usually destroyed by cell-mediated immune mechanisms. Progesterone production during pregnancy decreases cell-mediated immune responses, which makes the pregnant patient especially susceptible. Hematogenous spread then ensues, with placental seeding.

L. monocytogenes infections are relatively uncommon. Those affecting children are categorized as maternal, neonatal, or childhood with or without associated predisposing conditions. The infection may be acquired from contaminated goat cheese (feta). Maternal infection can be associated with an influenza-like illness, fever, malaise, headache, gastrointestinal tract symptoms, and back pain. Neonatal illness has early-onset and late-onset syndromes similar to those of group B streptococcal infections. Prematurity, pneumonia, and septicemia are common in early-onset disease. Approximately 65% of women experience a symptomatic prodromal illness before diagnosis of listeriosis in their fetus or newborn infant. Amnionitis during labor or asymptomatic infection can occur. Granulomatosis infantisepticum, characterized clinically by an erythematous rash with small, pale nodules and histologically by disseminated granulomas, occurs less frequently. Late-onset infection occurs after the first week of life and usually results in meningitis. Infection occurs most commonly in the perinatal period and in patients with decreased cell-mediated immunity resulting from cancer chemotherapy, corticosteroid therapy, immunodeficiency, hepatic or renal disease, or HIV infection. In childhood infections, most patients have meningitis, and almost half have no underlying predisposing condition. *L. monocytogenes* rarely causes a diffuse encephalitis. The occurrence of severe disease in adults associated with contaminated meat products emphasizes that older children and adults can have systemic disease with mortality.

Diagnostic Tests

The diagnosis of listeriosis requires a high degree of suspicion and should be considered in any pregnant patient that presents with unexplained intrauterine growth retardation. Careful questioning looking for past flulike symptoms and investigating eating habits (consumption of unwashed vegetables, raw milk or milk products, or deli meats and similar products) should be undertaken.

The organisms can be recovered on blood agar media from cultures of blood, CSF, meconium, gastric washings, placental tissue, amniotic fluid, and other infected tissues, including joint, pleural, or pericardial fluid. Special techniques (e.g., enrichment and selective media) may be needed to recover *L. monocytogenes* from sites with mixed flora (e.g., vagina and rectum). Gram staining of gastric aspirate material or placental tissue, a biopsy specimen of rash of early-onset infection, or CSF from an infected newborn infant may demonstrate the organism. An isolate of *L. monocytogenes* mistakenly can be considered a contaminant or saprophyte because of morphologic similarity to diphtheroids and streptococci. Serologic tests can be useful, particularly in the setting of an epidemiologic investigation. Direct dark-field examination of blood or other body fluid specimens has pitfalls that obviate its usefulness, and it is not recommended. PCR assay for the detection of leptospires has been developed but is not available in commercial laboratories.

Meningococcal Infections

Neisseria meningitidis is a Gram-negative diplococcus with 13 serogroups (A, B, C, D, 29E, H, I, K, L, W-135, X, Y, and Z). Strains belonging to groups A, B, C, Y, and W-135 are implicated most frequently in systemic disease. The distribution of meningococcal serogroups in the United States has shifted in recent years. Serogroups B, C, and Y each account for approximately 30% of reported cases, but serogroup distribution may vary by location and time. Group A has been associated frequently with epidemics elsewhere in the world, primarily in sub-Saharan Africa.

Invasive infection usually results in meningococcemia, meningitis, or both. Onset is abrupt in meningococcemia with fever, chills, malaise, prostration, and a rash that initially may be urticarial, maculopapular, or petechial. In fulminant cases, purpura, disseminated intravascular coagulation, shock, coma, and death (Waterhouse-Friderichsen syndrome) can ensue within several hours despite appropriate therapy. The signs of meningococcal meningitis are indistinguishable from those of acute meningitis caused by *Streptococcus pneumoniae* or other meningeal pathogens. Invasive meningococcal infections can be complicated by arthritis, myocarditis, pericarditis, and endophthalmitis. Less common manifestations include pneumonia, occult febrile bacteremia, conjunctivitis, and chronic meningococcemia.

Diagnostic Tests

Cultures of blood and CSF are indicated in all patients with suspected invasive meningococcal disease. Cultures of petechial scraping, synovial fluid, sputum, and other body fluids yield positive results in some patients. A Gram stain of a petechial scraping, CSF, and buffy coat smear of blood can be helpful. Because *N. meningitidis* can be part of the nasopharyngeal flora, isolation of *N. meningitidis* from this site is not helpful. Bacterial antigen detection tests, such as latex agglutination, may be of value for rapid diagnosis. Detection of meningococcal polysaccharide antigens by a latex agglutination test on urine or serum is not helpful. In contrast, antigen detection in CSF supports the diagnosis of a probable case if the clinical illness is consistent with meningococcal disease. Rapid antigen tests for group B *N. meningitidis* may be unreliable. A PCR test has been used in research laboratories to detect *N. meningitidis* type B from clinical specimens and currently is used routinely in the United Kingdom.

Confirmed Diagnosis

Isolation of *N. meningitidis* from a usually sterile site, for example,

- Blood
- CSF
- Synovial fluid
- Pleural fluid
- Pericardial fluid
- Petechial or purpuric lesion

Presumptive Diagnosis

Gram-negative diplococci in any sterile fluid, such as CSF, synovial fluid, or aspirate from a petechial or purpuric lesion

Probable Diagnosis

A positive antigen test result for *N. meningitidis* in CSF in the absence of a positive finding in a sterile site culture in the setting of a clinical illness consistent with meningococcal disease or clinical purpura fulminans in the absence of a positive blood culture result.

Moraxella catarrhalis *Infections*

Moraxella catarrhalis is a Gram-negative diplococcus. Almost 100% of strains produce β-lactamase that mediates resistance to penicillins.

Common infections include acute otitis media and paranasal sinusitis in children. Bronchopulmonary infection, often occurring in patients with chronic lung disease, can occur. Rare manifestations are bacteremia in immunocompetent or immunocompromised children (sometimes associated with focal infections, such as osteomyelitis, septic arthritis, abscesses, or a rash indistinguishable from that observed in meningococcemia) and conjunctivitis or meningitis in neonates.

Diagnostic Tests

The organism can be isolated on blood and chocolate agar culture media after incubation in air or with increased carbon dioxide. Culture of middle ear or sinus aspirates is indicated for patients with unusually severe infection, those in whom the infection fails to respond to treatment, and neonates and other highly susceptible children. Concomitant recovery of *M. catarrhalis* with other pathogens (*S. pneumoniae or H. influenzae*) can occur and indicates a mixed infection.

Mycobacterial Infections (Due to Atypical Mycobacteria, Mycobacteria Other Than Mycobacterium tuberculosis*)*

Of the many species of nontuberculous mycobacteria (NTM) that have been identified, only a small number account for most human infections. The species most frequently encountered in children are *M. avium* complex (MAC) (including *M. avium* and *M. intracellulare*), *M. scrofulaceum, M. fortuitum, M. kansasii*, and *M. marinum*. Infection in patients with HIV usually is caused by MAC. *M. fortuitum, M. chelonae*, and *M. abscessus* frequently are referred to as "rapidly growing" mycobacteria because they grow sufficiently in the laboratory to be identified within 3–7 days, whereas other NTM and *M. tuberculosis* often require weeks to grow. Rapidly growing mycobacteria occasionally have been implicated in wound, soft tissue, bone, pulmonary, and middle ear infections. Other mycobacterial species, which are not pathogenic, have caused infections in immunocompromised hosts or have been associated with the presence of a foreign body.

Many NTM species are ubiquitous and are found in soil, food, water, and animals. Although many persons are exposed to NTM, only a few of these exposures result in chronic infection or disease. MAC in the respiratory or gastrointestinal tract is common in persons with HIV infection. Nontuberculous mycobacteria, usually MAC, also can be recovered from 10–20% of adolescents and young adults with cystic fibrosis. The usual portals of entry of NTM infection are believed to be abrasions in the skin (e.g., for the cutaneous lesions caused by *M. marinum*), the oropharyngeal mucosa (the presumed portal for cervical lymphadenitis), the gastrointestinal or respiratory tract for MAC, and the respiratory tract (including tympanostomy tubes) for otitis media and rare cases of mediastinal adenitis and of endobronchial disease. Most infections remain localized at the portal of entry or in regional lymph nodes. Severe pulmonary disease and dissemination to distal sites occur primarily in immunocompromised hosts, especially in persons with acquired immunodeficiency syndrome (AIDS). No definitive evidence for person-to-person transmission of NTM exists; however, clustering of patients with person-to-person exposure has occurred. Cases of otitis media caused by *M. abscessus* have been associated with use of contaminated equipment and water. A water-borne route of transmission has been suspected for MAC infection in immunodeficient hosts.

The incubation period is unknown.

Several syndromes are caused by NTM. In children, the most common of these syndromes is cervical lymphadenitis. Less common infections are cutaneous infection, osteomyelitis, otitis media, and pulmonary disease. Disseminated infection almost always is associated with immunodeficiency characterized by impaired cell-mediated immunity, such as congenital immune defects or HIV infection. Manifestations of disseminated NTM infections depend on the species and route of infection and include fever, night sweats, weight loss, abdominal pain, fatigue, diarrhea, and anemia.

Diagnostic Tests

Definitive diagnosis of disease caused by NTM requires isolation of the organism. Because these organisms commonly are found in the environment, however, contamination of the cultures or transient colonization can occur. Therefore, caution must be exercised in the interpretation of cultures obtained from sites that are not sterile, such as gastric washings, a draining sinus tract, a single sputum specimen, or a urine specimen. Caution in ascribing illness to NTM also is warranted if the species cultured usually is nonpathogenic (e.g., *M. gordonae*) and if only a few colonies are recovered from a single specimen. Repeated isolation of numerous colonies of a single species is more likely to indicate disease than culture contamination or transient colonization. Recovery of NTM from sites that usually are sterile, such as CSF, pleural fluid, bone marrow, blood, lymph node aspirates, middle ear or mastoid aspirates, or surgically excised tissue, is the most reliable diagnostic test. With the radiometric broth or lysis-centrifugation techniques, blood cultures are highly sensitive in recovery of MAC and other blood-borne NTM species. Disseminated MAC disease should prompt a search for underlying immunosuppression, usually HIV infection.

Patients with NTM infection can have false-positive purified protein derivative (PPD) skin test results, because this preparation, derived from *M. tuberculosis,* shares a number of antigens with NTM species. These false-positive PPD reactions usually measure <10 mm of induration and occur in otherwise healthy children who have no history of exposure to *M. tuberculosis* but have been sensitized by exposure to NTM in the environment.

Mycoplasma pneumoniae *Infections*

The mycoplasmas, including *Mycoplasma pneumoniae,* are the smallest free-living microorganisms. These organisms lack a cell wall and are pleomorphic.

Initial symptoms in patients who develop pneumonia, the most prominent manifestation of infection, are nonspecific and include malaise, fever, and, occasionally, headache. Cough, usually associated with widespread rales found on physical examination, develops within a few days and lasts for 3–4 weeks. The cough is nonproductive initially but later may become productive, particularly in older children and adolescents. Approximately 10% of children with pneumonia exhibit a rash, often maculopapular. Radiographic abnormalities vary, but bilateral diffuse infiltrates are common. The most common clinical syndromes are acute bronchitis and upper respiratory tract infections, including pharyngitis, and, occasionally, otitis media or myringitis, which may be bullous. Coryza, sinusitis, and croup are infrequent.

Diagnostic Tests

Recovery *of M. pneumoniae* in cultures requires the use of special enriched broth or agar media (which are not widely available), is successful in only 40–90% of cases, and takes 7–21 days. Isolation of *M. pneumoniae* in a patient with compatible clinical manifestations suggests causation. Because this organism can be excreted from the respiratory tract for several weeks after an acute infection despite appropriate therapy, isolation of the organism may not indicate acute infection. A PCR test for *M. pneumoniae* has been developed but is not available in most clinical microbiologic laboratories.

Serologic diagnosis can be made by demonstrating a fourfold or greater increase in antibody titer between acute and convalescent serum samples. The antibody titer peaks at approximately 1 month and persists for 2–3 months after infection. The complement fixation and immunofluorescence methods are most widely used. Several EIA antibody tests and other rapid diagnostic tests for detection of *M. pneumoniae* antibodies are also available. The immunofluorescence test is capable of detecting *Mycoplasma*-specific IgM and IgG antibodies. Although the presence of

IgM antibodies confirms recent *M. pneumoniae* infection, the antibodies persist in serum for several months and do not necessarily indicate current infection. Because *M. pneumoniae* complement fixation and EIA antibodies cross-react with some other antigens, particularly with those of other mycoplasmas, results of these tests should be interpreted cautiously when evaluating febrile illnesses of unknown origin. However, cross-reactivity with other respiratory tract pathogens causing diseases clinically similar to those caused by *M. pneumoniae* does not occur. False-negative results occur with both complement fixation and EIA assays.

Serum cold hemagglutinin titers of ≥1:32 are present in >50% of patients with pneumonia by the beginning of the second week of illness. Fourfold increases in hemagglutinin titer between acute and convalescent serum samples occur more often in patients with severe *M. pneumoniae* than in persons with less severe disease. This test has low specificity for *Mycoplasma* infection, however, and other agents, including adenoviruses, Epstein-Barr virus, and measles, can cause illnesses in infants or children associated with an increase in titer of cold hemagglutinins. A negative test result for cold agglutinins does not exclude the diagnosis of mycoplasmal infection. With the wide availability of specific antibody tests, this test is rarely used.

Because infections are common and resulting antibodies persist for months or years, measurement of antibody in a single serum sample is of little diagnostic value. A complement fixation titer of ≥1:32 during an acute respiratory tract illness, however, suggests *M. pneumoniae* infection.

Nocardiosis

Nocardia species are aerobic actinomycetes. Pulmonary or disseminated disease is caused most commonly by the *Nocardia asteroides* complex, which includes *N. farcinica* and *N. nova*. Cutaneous disease is caused most commonly by *N. brasiliensis*. *N. pseudobrasiliensis* seems to be associated with pulmonary, CNS, and systemic nocardiosis.

A common presentation in immunocompetent children is cutaneous or lymphocutaneous disease after soil contamination at the site of skin injury. Usually the pustular or ulcerative lesions remain localized. Invasive disease occurs most commonly in immunocompromised patients, particularly those with chronic granulomatous disease of HIV infection or those who are receiving long-term corticosteroid therapy. In these children, infection characteristically begins in the lungs, and the illness may be acute, subacute, or chronic. Pulmonary disease often presents as rounded nodular infiltrates that can undergo cavitation. Hematogenous spread may occur from lungs to the brain (single or multiple abscesses), skin (pustules, pyoderma, abscesses, mycetoma), and, occasionally, other organs.

Diagnostic Tests

Stained smears of sputum, body fluids, or pus can demonstrate beaded, branched, weakly Gram-positive rods that are variably acid fast. The Brown and Brenn and methenamine silver stains are recommended for demonstrating microorganisms in tissue. Growth of typical colonies occurs on 5% sheep blood, chocolate agar, and most media used for growth of organisms of the *Mycobacteria* genus, including BACTEC 12B broth. *Nocardia* organisms are slow growing; cultures from normally sterile sites should be maintained for 3 weeks in a liquid medium. Serologic tests for *Nocardia* species are hampered by a lack of specificity and sensitivity.

Pasteurella multocida *Infections*

Pasteurella multocida is a facultatively anaerobic, bipolar staining, Gram-negative coccobacillus that is a primary pathogen in animals.

The most common manifestation in children is cellulitis at the site of a scratch or bite of a cat, dog, or other animal. This finding usually occurs within 24 hours after the bite or scratch and includes swelling, erythema, tenderness, and serous or sanguinopurulent discharge. Regional lymphadenopathy, chills, and fever can occur. Local complications, such as septic arthritis, osteomyelitis, and tenosynovitis, are common. Less common complications include septicemia, meningitis, respiratory tract infections (e.g., pneumonia, pulmonary abscesses, and empyema), appendicitis, hepatic abscess, peritonitis, urinary tract infection, and ocular infection, including conjunctivitis, corneal ulcer, and endophthalmitis.

Diagnostic Tests

P. multocida can be isolated from skin lesion drainage or other sites of infection (e.g., joint fluid, CSF, sputum, pleural fluid, or samples from suppurative lymph nodes). Although *P. multocida* resembles several other organisms morphologically (such as *H. influenzae*, *Neisseria* species, and fastidious Gram-negative rods, particularly *Actinobacillus*) and grows on many culture media at 37°C (98°F), laboratory differentiation is not difficult.

Plague

Plague is caused by *Yersinia (Pasteurella) pestis*, a pleomorphic, bipolar staining, Gram-negative coccobacillus.

Plague most commonly presents as the bubonic form, with acute onset of fever and painful swollen regional lymph nodes (buboes). Buboes develop most commonly in the inguinal region but also occur in axillary or cervical areas. Less commonly, plague presents in the septicemic form (hypotension, acute respiratory distress, intravascular coagulopathy) or as pneumonic plague (cough, fever, dyspnea, and hemoptysis) and, rarely, as meningeal plague. Fever, chills, headache, and rapidly progressive weakness are characteristic in all cases. Occasionally, patients present with mild lymphadenitis or with prominent gastrointestinal tract symptoms, which may obscure the correct diagnosis.

Diagnostic Tests

Plague is characterized by massive growth of *Y. pestis* in affected tissues, especially lymph nodes, spleen, and liver. The organism has a bipolar (safety pin) appearance when stained with Wayson or Gram stain. The microbiology laboratory should be informed when plague organisms are suspected in submitted specimens to minimize risks of transmission to laboratory personnel. A positive fluorescent antibody test for the presence of *Y. pestis* in direct smears or cultures of a bubo aspirate, sputum, CSF, or blood provides presumptive evidence of *Y. pestis* infection. A single positive serologic test result by passive hemagglutination assay or EIA in an unimmunized patient who has not previously had plague also provides presumptive evidence of infection. Seroconversion or a fourfold difference in antibody titer between two serum specimens obtained 4 weeks to 3 months apart provides serologic confirmation. The diagnosis of plague usually is confirmed by culture of *Y. pestis* from blood, bubo aspirate, or other clinical specimen. PCR for rapid diagnosis of *Y. pestis* is not available in commercial laboratories. Isolates suspected to be *Y. pestis* should be reported immediately to the state health department and submitted to the Division of Vector-Borne Infectious Diseases of the CDC.

Pneumococcal Infections

Streptococcus pneumoniae (pneumococci) are lancet-shaped, Gram-positive diplococci. Ninety pneumococcal serotypes have been identified. Serotypes 4, 6B, 9V, 14, 18C, 19F, and 23F (Danish serotyping system) cause most invasive childhood pneumococcal infections in the United States. Serotypes 6B, 9V, 14, 19A, 19F, and 23F are the most frequent isolates associated with resistance to penicillin.

Pneumococci are the most common cause of acute bacterial otitis media and of invasive bacterial infections in children. Many children with bacteremia have no identifiable primary focus of infection. Pneumococci also are a frequent cause of sinusitis and of community-acquired pneumonia. Since introduction of Hib conjugate immunization, pneumococci and meningococci have become the two most common causes of bacterial meningitis in infants and young children.

Diagnostic Tests

Material obtained from a suppurative focus should be Gram stained and cultured by appropriate microbiologic techniques. Blood cultures should be obtained from all patients with suspected invasive pneumococcal disease; cultures of CSF and other body fluids (e.g., pleural fluid) also may be indicated. The white blood cell (WBC) count may be of assistance in suspected bacteremia caused by *S. pneumoniae*; young children with high fevers and leukocytosis [particularly a WBC count of >15,000 cells/μL (>15.0 × 10^9/L)] have an increased likelihood of bacteremia. Although the predictive value of an elevated WBC count for pneumococcal bacteremia is not high, a normal WBC count is highly predictive of the absence of bacteremia. Recovery of pneumococci from an upper respiratory tract culture is not useful in patients with otitis media, pneumonia, or sinusitis. Rapid methods to detect pneumococcal capsular antigen in CSF, pleural and joint fluid, and concentrated urine usually are of limited value.

Pseudomonas

Pseudomonas lives abundantly in soil and water and is widespread throughout nature. There are a large number of identified *Pseudomonas* species, but only a few are pathogenic for humans; of these, *P. aeruginosa* is by far the most common. Others, occasionally recognized as human pathogens, include *P. cepacia, P. maltophilia, P. fluorescens, P. putrefaciens*, and *P. mallei*, the cause of glanders in horses.

The pseudomonads are Gram-negative bacilli and are strict aerobes. As they can use any source of carbon, they multiply in most moist environments that contain minimal amounts of organic compounds. Strains from clinical specimens may produce beta-hemolysis on blood agar; more than 90% of stains produce a bluish-green phenazine pigment (blue pus) as well as fluorescein, which is yellow-green and fluoresces. These pigments diffuse into and color the medium surrounding the colonies. Strains of *Pseudomonas* can be differentiated from one another for epidemiologic purposes by serologic, phage, and pyocin typing.

Pseudomonas produces endotoxin that is extremely weak compared with that of other Gram-negative bacilli, but it may initiate diarrhea. *Pseudomonas* also elaborates a number of extracellular products, including lecithinase, collagenase, lipase, and hemolysins, which may be responsible for localized necrosis of skin. One of the hemolytic factors is a heat-resistant glycolipid that may dissolve and destroy lecithin (surfactant), and that may in turn contribute to producing atelectasis in pulmonary infections caused by *Pseudomonas*. The pathogenicity of *P. aeruginosa* also depends on its ability to resist phagocytosis, which seems to depend principally on the production of toxins. The host responds to infection by producing antibodies to *Pseudomonas* exotoxin (exotoxin A) and lipopolysaccharide.

The characteristic skin lesions of *Pseudomonas*, whether due to direct inoculation or secondary to septicemia, begin as pink macules and progress to hemorrhagic nodules and eventually to areas of necrosis with eschar formation, surrounded by an intense red areola (ecthyma gangrenosum).

Multiplication of bacteria occurs locally, and occasionally, septicemia, endocarditis, meningitis, corneal infections, orbital cellulitis, mastoiditis, folliculitis, pneumonia, or urinary tract infections may ensue in normal children. Rarely, *Pseudomonas* may be associated with gastroenteritis.

Otitis externa caused by *P. aeruginosa* may occur in swimmers who swim repetitively in pools contaminated by this organism.

Pseudomonas septicemia may occur with indwelling intravenous or urinary catheters; pneumonia and septicemia occur in children receiving inhalation therapy. Peritonitis and septicemia have been associated with contaminated equipment used for peritoneal dialysis. Abscesses or meningitis may be related to dermal sinus tract. *Pseudomonas* may produce acute or subacute endocarditis in children with congenital heart lesions or after cardiac surgery.

P. aeruginosa, especially the mucoid variety that produces an excessive amount of slime, can be recovered from the sputum of most children with cystic fibrosis.

The overall mortality is approximately 40%. Shock, pneumonia, and persistent neutropenia are each associated with poorer prognosis. Decreased white blood cell count during bacteremia in patients with leukemia or burns is more frequently due to *Pseudomonas* than to other Gram-negative rods.

Diagnosis

Recovery of the organism may be accomplished by culture from the blood, cerebrospinal fluid, urine, or needle aspirate of the lung or from purulent material obtained by aspiration of subcutaneous abscesses or areas of cellulitis.

Pseudomonas pseudomallei *(Melioidosis)*

P. pseudomallei infection is occasionally transmitted among narcotic addicts using needles in common.

Diagnosis

Diagnosis of *P. pseudomallei* infection may be accomplished by culture or animal inoculation of infected material (e.g., pus, urine, blood, sputum).

Serologic Tests

EIA for IgG antibodies is >90% sensitive and specific; EIA for IgM is 92% sensitive for active disease and can be used to monitor therapy.

Agglutination test results are positive in chronic disease; infection can be inactive for many years. Results may be negative in fulminant septicemic form.

Rat-Bite Fever

The causes of rat-bite fever are *Streptobacillus moniliformis*, a microaerophilic, Gram-negative, pleomorphic bacillus, and *Spirillum minus*, a small, Gram-negative, spiral organism with bipolar flagellar tufts.

Rat-bite fever is characterized by fever of abrupt onset, chills, a maculopapular or petechial rash predominantly on the extremities, muscle pain, and headache. Specific clinical manifestations depend on the infecting organism. With *S. moniliformis* infection (streptobacillary or Haverhill fever), the bite usually heals promptly, exhibits no or minimal inflammation, and is followed by nonsuppurative migratory polyarthritis or arthralgia in approximately 50% of patients. Complications include soft tissue and solid organ abscesses, arthritis, pneumonia, endocarditis, myocarditis, pericarditis, and meningitis. With *S. minus* infection, a period of initial apparent healing at the site of the bite usually is followed by ulceration, regional lymphangitis and lymphadenopathy, a distinctive rash of red or purple plaques, and, rarely, arthritic symptoms.

Diagnostic Tests

S. moniliformis can be isolated from blood, synovial fluid, aspirates from abscesses, or material from the bite lesion by inoculation into bacteriologic media enriched with blood, serum, or ascitic fluid. Because it is a fastidious organism, laboratory personnel should be notified that rat-bite fever is suspected. *S. minus* has not been recovered from artificial media. Organisms can be visualized by the use of dark-field microscopy in wet mounts of blood, exudate of the initial lesion, and lymph nodes. Blood specimens also should be stained with Giemsa or Wright stain. *S. minus* can be recovered from blood, lymph node samples, or specimens of local lesions by intraperitoneal inoculation of mice or guinea pigs.

Salmonellosis

Salmonella organisms are Gram-negative bacilli that belongs to the Enterobacteriaceae family. Most serotypes that cause human disease are in serogroups A through E. *Salmonella typhi* is classified in serogroup D. In 1997, the most frequently reported human isolates in the United States were *Salmonella typhimurium* (serogroup B), *Salmonella heidelberg* (B), *Salmonella enteritidis* (D), *Salmonella newport* (C2), *Salmonella infantis* (C1), *Salmonella agona* (B), *Salmonella thompson* (C1), and *Salmonellas montevideo* (C1).

Nontyphoidal *Salmonella* organisms cause asymptomatic carriage, gastroenteritis, bacteremia, and focal infections (such as meningitis and osteomyelitis). These disease categories are not mutually exclusive but represent a spectrum of illness caused by *Salmonella* organisms. The most common illness associated with nontyphoidal *Salmonella* organisms is gastroenteritis, in which diarrhea, abdominal cramps and tenderness, and fever are frequent manifestations. The site of infection usually is the small intestine, but colitis can occur.

Constipation may be an early feature. Diarrhea occurs more commonly in children than in adults. Enteric fever may present as a mild, nondescript febrile illness in young children. Sustained or intermittent bacteremia can occur in enteric fever and nontyphoidal *Salmonella* bacteremia. Recognizable focal infections may occur in as many as 10% of patients with *Salmonella* bacteremia. Recurrent *Salmonella* bacteremia is an AIDS-defining condition for adolescents and adults infected with HIV.

S. typhi and several other *Salmonella* serotypes cause protracted bacteremic illness referred to as *enteric* or *typhoid fever*. The onset of illness typically is gradual, with manifestations such as fever, constitutional symptoms (e.g., headache, malaise, anorexia, and lethargy), abdominal pain and tenderness, hepatomegaly, splenomegaly, rose spots, and changes in mental status.

Diagnostic Tests

Isolation of *Salmonella* organisms from cultures of stool, blood, urine, and material from foci of infection, as indicated by the suspected *Salmonella* syndrome, is diagnostic. Serologic tests for *Salmonella* agglutinins ("febrile agglutinins," the Widal test) may suggest the diagnosis of *S. typhi* infection, but because of false-positive and false-negative results, these tests are not recommended. DNA probes and monoclonal antibodies against protein antigens of *S. typhi* are being evaluated.

A new test kit (from Neogen) for *S. enteritidis* provides commercial egg producers with a quick and easy method of detecting this dangerous pathogen. *S. enteritidis* became the leading cause of salmonellosis in the United States in 1994. The foodborne illness caused by *S. enteritidis* is generally due to eating raw, incompletely cooked, or recontaminated eggs. Ingestion of *S. enteritidis*–contaminated poultry meat is the second leading cause of this illness.

The *S. enteritidis* test is based on antibodies developed by Neogen and the U.S. Department of Agriculture at the Russell Center in Athens, GA.

Shigella *Infections*

Shigella are Gram-negative bacilli in the family Enterobacteriaceae. Four species (of >40 serotypes) have been identified. *Shigella sonnei* currently accounts for almost three quarters of the cases in the United States, and *S. flexneri* accounts for a large percentage of the remainder. *S. dysenteriae* type 1 (the Shiga bacillus) is rare in the United States but widespread in rural Africa and the Indian subcontinent. *S. boydii* is uncommon in the United States.

In mild infections, manifestations consist of watery or loose stools of several days' duration, with minimal or no constitutional symptoms. Abrupt onset of fever, systemic toxic effects, headache, and profuse watery diarrhea occur in patients with small-bowel infection. Seizures can occur. Abdominal cramps, tenderness, tenesmus, and mucoid stools with or without blood characterize large-bowel disease (bacillary dysentery). Rare complications include bacteremia, Reiter syndrome (after *S. flexneri* infection), HUS (from *S. dysenteriae* type I infection), colonic perforation, and toxic encephalopathy (ekiri syndrome), which can be lethal within 4–48 hours of onset.

Diagnostic Tests

Cultures of feces or rectal swab specimens containing feces should be performed. Blood should be cultured only in severely ill, immunocompromised, or malnourished patients because bacteremia is rare. A stool smear stained with methylene blue may disclose polymorphonuclear leukocytes or erythrocytes, a finding indicative of enterocolitis, which is consistent with but not specific for *Shigella* infection.

Staphylococcal Infections

Staphylococci are Gram-positive cocci that appear microscopically as grapelike clusters. There are 32 species that are related closely on the basis of DNA base composition, but only 14 species are indigenous to humans. *S. aureus* is the only species that produces coagulase. Of the other 13 coagulase-negative species, *S. epidermidis*, *S. haemolyticus*, *S. saprophyticus*, and *S. lugdunensis* are those most often associated with infections. Staphylococci are ubiquitous and can survive extreme conditions of drying, heat, low oxygen, and high-salt environments. *S. aureus* has many surface receptors that enable it to bind to tissues and foreign bodies coated with fibronectin, fibrinogen, and collagen, which allows a low inoculum of organisms to adhere to sutures, catheters, prosthetic valves, and other devices. Coagulase-negative staphylococci produce an exopolysaccharide slime biofilm that makes these organisms relatively inaccessible to host defense and to antibiotics as they bind to medical devices (e.g., catheters).

S. aureus causes a wide variety of localized or invasive suppurative infections and three toxin-mediated syndromes: toxic shock syndrome (TSS), scalded skin syndrome, and food poisoning. Localized infections include furuncles, carbuncles, impetigo (bullous and nonbullous), paronychia, ecthyma, cellulitis, lymphadenitis, and wound infections. Infections of implanted prosthetic materials, as well as localized infections, may be associated with bacteremia.

Bacteremia can be complicated by septicemia, endocarditis, pericarditis, pneumonia, muscle or visceral abscesses, arthritis, osteomyelitis, septic thrombophlebitis of large vessels, and other foci of infection. Meningitis is rare. *S. aureus* infections can be fulminant, frequently are associated with metastatic foci, and require prolonged therapy to achieve cure. Risk factors for severe staphylococcal infections include neutropenia; chronic diseases including diabetes mellitus, cirrhosis, and nutritional disorders; transplantation; and disorders of neutrophil function. *S. aureus* also causes foreign-body infections, including those associated with intravascular catheters or grafts, pacemakers, peritoneal catheters, CSF shunts, and prosthetic joints.

Coagulase-Negative *Staphylococcus*

Most coagulase-negative staphylococci represent contamination of culture material. Of the isolates that do not represent contamination, the most common are from infections that are nosocomial, and most patients with coagulase-negative staphylococcal infections have obvious disruptions of host defense caused by surgery, catheter or prosthesis insertion, or immunosuppression. Coagulase-negative staphylococci are the single most frequent cause of late-onset septicemia among premature infants, especially infants weighing <1,500 g at birth, and of episodes of nosocomial bacteremia in all age groups. Coagulase-negative staphylococci are responsible for bacteremia in children undergoing treatment for leukemia, lymphoma, or solid tumors, as well as in bone marrow transplant recipients. Infections often are associated with intravascular catheters, CSF shunts, peritoneal or urinary catheters, vascular grafts or intracardiac patches, prosthetic cardiac valves, pacemaker wires, and prosthetic joints. Mediastinitis after open-heart surgery, endophthalmitis after intraocular trauma, and omphalitis and scalp abscesses in neonates have been described. Coagulase-negative staphylococci also may enter the bloodstream from the respiratory tracts of mechanically ventilated premature infants or from the gastrointestinal tracts of infants with necrotizing enterocolitis. Some species of coagulase-negative staphylococci are associated with urinary tract infection, including *S. saprophyticus* in adolescent girls or young adult women, often after sexual intercourse, and *S. hemolyticus* in hospitalized patients with urinary catheters. In general, coagulase-negative staphylococcal infections have an indolent clinical presentation.

Diagnostic Tests

Gram-stained smears of material from lesions can provide presumptive evidence of infection. Isolation of organisms from culture of an otherwise sterile body fluid is definitive. *S. aureus* is not a contaminant when isolated from a blood culture. Isolation of coagulase-negative staphylococci from a blood culture frequently is dismissed as "contamination." In a neonate, immunocompromised person, or patient with a prosthetic implant, repeated isolation of the same phenotypic strain of coagulase-negative staphylococci from blood cultures facilitates interpretation. For catheter-related bacteremia, quantitative cultures from the catheters will have five to ten times more organisms than cultures from a peripheral vessel. Criteria that may be used to determine whether coagulase-negative staphylococci are a contaminant or a pathogen include the following: (a) growth generally within 24 hours, (b) multiple blood cultures with positive results, (c) symptoms of infection in the patient, (d) placement of an intravascular catheter for 3 days or more, and (e) multidrug resistance of the coagulase-negative staphylococcal strain.

Quantitative antimicrobial susceptibility testing should be performed for all staphylococci isolated from normally sterile sites, including coagulase-negative staphylococci. Some community-acquired *S. aureus* and most hospital-acquired coagulase-negative staphylococci are methicillin and multidrug resistant. Detection of vancomycin hydrochloride–intermediate *S. aureus* is critical.

Staphylococci have several mechanisms mediating resistance to the β-lactam antibiotics. β-Lactamase production breaks down the nonsemisynthetic penicillins. Resistance to the β-lactamase–resistant semisynthetic penicillins (methicillin-resistant *S. aureus*) is mediated by a novel cell wall penicillin-binding protein called *PBP2a*. PBP2a has a decreased affinity for β-lactam antibiotics and cephalosporins. PBP2a is coded for by the *mecA* gene and generates widely varying resistance to methicillin based on the number of organisms of different susceptibilities and on the culture conditions [methicillin minimal inhibitory concentrations (MICs) of 4 μg/mL to 1,000 μg/mL]. This phenomenon is known as *heterogeneous resistance*. For coagulase-negative staphylococci and *S. aureus* strains with heterogeneous resistance, MICs of methicillin or vancomycin may indicate susceptibility after 24 hours of incubation. If these strains are incubated overnight on plates of increasing concentrations of methicillin or vancomycin, however, a small fraction of the total population will be able to grow at much higher antibiotic concentrations. If these highly resistant subclones are recultured, they may maintain this high level of resistance, which suggests a mutant strain. In some cases, however, the highly resistant subclone will revert to methicillin or vancomycin susceptibility when replated, even though it was grown from a single colony. There is no satisfactory model that can explain the mechanism governing heterogeneous resistance. Strains of coagulase-negative staphylococci and *S. aureus* with heterogeneous resistance are stable in the absence of antibiotic selective pressure. These strains may constitute 10–15% of any coagulase-negative staphylococci or *S. aureus* collection of isolates.

Methicillin-resistant *S. aureus* in neonatal nursery infections is extremely aggressive. It may be difficult to diagnose the presence of an infection in the intensive care unit, because the presenting signs are vague.

The MIC breakpoints for coagulase-negative staphylococci are based on the presence of the *mecA* gene and, therefore, the potential for the organism to develop methicillin resistance. The coagulase-resistant staphylococcal MICs no longer represent an interpretation of MIC breakpoints as determined by growth in medium.

The mechanism for vancomycin-intermediate resistance of *S. aureus* and coagulase-negative staphylococci is known. Vancomycin-intermediate *S. aureus* and cell walls are shown by electron microscopy. Vancomycin resistance may be related to an increased ability of these organisms to bind vancomycin at sites other than those to which they normally bind.

S. aureus and coagulase-negative staphylococcal strain typing has become a useful adjunct for determining whether several isolates from one patient or from different patients are the same or different. Typing allows accurate identification of the source, extent, and mechanism of transmission of an outbreak. Antimicrobial susceptibility testing is the most readily available method for typing using a phenotypic characteristic. Multilocus enzyme electrophoresis is another phenotypic tool for use in typing. Typing by genotype has proven to be highly discriminatory and highly effective for identifying epidemiologically related isolates.

Staphylococcal Food Poisoning

Illness is caused by ingestion of food containing a staphylococcal enterotoxin. Foods usually involved are those that come in contact with food handlers' hands, either without subsequent cooking or with inadequate heating or refrigeration, such as pastries, custards, salad dressing, sandwiches, poultry, sliced meat, and meat products. When these foods remain at room temperature for several hours before being eaten, toxin-producing staphylococci multiply and elaborate heat-stable toxin. The organisms may be of human origin from purulent discharges of an infected finger or eye, abscesses, acneiform facial eruptions, nasopharyngeal secretions, or apparently normal skin, or, less commonly, of bovine origin, such as contaminated milk or milk products, especially cheese, or eggs.

The incubation period is from 30 minutes to 8 hours, usually 2–4 hours.

Of the eight immunologically distinct heat-stable enterotoxins (A, B, C1–C3, D, E, and F), enterotoxins A and D are the most common in the United States. Enterotoxin F, which is identical to the toxin associated with TSS, has not been implicated in outbreaks of food poisoning.

Staphylococcal food poisoning is characterized by the abrupt and sometimes violent onset of severe nausea, abdominal cramps, vomiting, and prostration, often accompanied by diarrhea. Low-grade fever or subnormal temperature may occur. The duration of illness typically is 1–2 days, but the intensity of symptoms may require hospitalization. The short incubation period, brevity of illness, and usual lack of fever help distinguish staphylococcal from other types of food poisoning, except that caused by *B. cereus*. Chemical food poisoning usually has an even shorter incubation period. *C. perfringens* food poisoning usually has a longer incubation period and infrequently is accompanied by vomiting. Patients with food-borne *Salmonella* or *Shigella* infection usually have fever and longer incubation period.

Diagnostic Tests

Recovery of large numbers of staphylococci from stool or vomitus supports the diagnosis. In an outbreak setting, demonstration of enterotoxin or a large number of staphylococci ($>10^5$ colony-forming units per gram of specimen) in epidemiologically implicated food confirms the diagnosis. Identification (by pulsed-field gel electrophoresis) of the same types of *S. aureus* from stool or vomitus of two or more ill persons or from the stool or vomitus of an ill person and an implicated food or a person who handled the food also confirms the diagnosis. Local health authorities should be notified to help determine the source of the outbreak.

Streptococcal and Related Infections

Group A Streptococci

More than 100 distinct M-protein types of group A β-hemolytic streptococci (*Streptococcus pyogenes*) have been identified. Epidemiologic studies suggest an association between certain serotypes (types 1, 3, 5, 6, 18, 19, and 24) and rheumatic fever, but a specific rheumatogenic factor has not been identified. Several serotypes (types 49, 55, 57, and 50) are associated with pyoderma, and acute serotypes (types 1, 6, and 12) and groups C and G streptococci have been associated with pharyngitis and, occasionally, acute nephritis but do not cause rheumatic fever.

Streptococcal pharyngitis occurs at all ages, but it is most common among school-age children. Group A streptococcal (GAS) pharyngitis and pyoderma are less common in adults than in children except during epidemics.

Geographically, streptococcal pharyngitis and pyoderma are ubiquitous. Pyoderma is more common in tropical climates and in warm seasons, presumably in part because of antecedent insect bites and other minor skin trauma. Streptococcal pharyngitis occurs more frequently in the late autumn, winter, and spring in temperate climates, presumably because of the close person-to-person contact that occurs in schools. Communicability of patients with streptococcal pharyngitis is highest during the acute infection and, in untreated persons, gradually diminishes during a period of weeks. Patients can no longer transmit the disease within 24 hours of the initiation of appropriate antimicrobial therapy.

Throat specimen culture surveys of asymptomatic children during school outbreaks of pharyngitis have yielded GAS prevalence rates as high as 15–50%. These cases include children with asymptomatic infections and pharyngeal carriers with no subsequent immune response to GAS cellular or extracellular antigens. Carriage of GAS may persist for many months, but the risk of transmission to others is not appreciable, perhaps because of diminished numbers of organisms in the pharynx or the disappearance of bacteria from nasal secretions.

The incidence of acute rheumatic fever in the United States has decreased sharply over several decades, but outbreaks of rheumatic fever in the 1990s in school-age children in various geographic areas demonstrated that acute rheumatic fever remains a risk. Although the reason for these local outbreaks is not clear, their occurrence reemphasizes the importance of diagnosing GAS pharyngitis and of complying with the recommended duration of antimicrobial therapy.

In streptococcal impetigo, the organism usually is acquired from a person with impetigo, possibly by direct physical contact. Colonization of healthy skin by GAS usually precedes development of skin infection. Impetiginous lesions occur at the sites of open lesions (e.g., insect bites, traumatic wounds, or burns) because GAS organisms do not penetrate intact skin. After development of impetiginous lesions, the upper respiratory tract often becomes colonized. Infections of surgical wounds and postpartum (puerperal) sepsis usually result from contact transmission via hand carriage. At times, anal or vaginal carriers and persons with pyoderma or local suppurative infections can transmit GAS to surgical and obstetric patients, which results in nosocomial outbreaks. Infections in neonates can result from intrapartum or contact transmission; in the latter situation, infection often begins with omphalitis.

The most common clinical illness produced by group A streptococcal infection is acute pharyngitis or tonsillitis. In some patients, who usually are untreated, purulent complications, including otitis media, sinusitis, peritonsillar and retropharyngeal abscesses, and suppurative cervical adenitis develop. The significance of streptococcal upper respiratory tract disease relates particularly to its acute morbidity and nonsuppurative sequelae—that is, acute rheumatic fever and acute glomerulonephritis. Scarlet fever occurs most commonly in association with pharyngitis and, rarely, with pyoderma or an infected surgical or traumatic wound. Scarlet fever has a characteristic confluent erythematous sandpaper-like rash, which is caused by one or more of the several erythrogenic exotoxins produced by GAS strains. Severe scarlet fever with systemic toxic effects occurs rarely. Other than the occurrence of rash, the epidemiologic features, symptoms, sequelae, and treatment of scarlet fever are the same as those of streptococcal pharyngitis.

Toddlers (1–3 years of age) with GAS respiratory tract infection may present with moderate fever and serous rhinitis and may have a protracted illness with fever, irritability, and anorexia (streptococcal fever). The classic clinical presentation of streptococcal upper respiratory tract infection as acute pharyngitis is uncommon in children <3 years of age. Rheumatic fever also is uncommon at this age.

The second most common site of GAS infection is the skin. Streptococcal skin infections (pyoderma or impetigo) can result in acute glomerulonephritis, which occasionally occurs in epidemics, but acute rheumatic fever is not a sequela of streptococcal skin infection.

Other GAS infections include erysipelas, perianal cellulitis, vaginitis, bacteremia, pneumonia, endocarditis, pericarditis, septic arthritis, cellulitis, necrotizing fasciitis, osteomyelitis, myositis, puerperal sepsis, surgical wound infection, and neonatal omphalitis. Necrotizing fasciitis and other invasive GAS infections in children often occur as complications of varicella. Bacteremic GAS infections can be severe, with or without an identified focus of local infection, and can be associated with streptococcal TSS. The portal of entry of invasive infections often is the skin or soft tissue and may follow minor or unrecognized trauma.

Diagnostic Tests

Laboratory confirmation of GAS is recommended for children with pharyngitis because reliable clinical differentiation of viral and GAS pharyngitis is not possible. A specimen should be obtained by vigorous swabbing of the tonsils and posterior pharynx. Culture on sheep blood agar can confirm GAS infection, and latex agglutination, fluorescent antibody, coagglutination, and precipitation techniques performed on colonies growing on the agar plate can differentiate group A from other β-hemolytic streptococci. Appropriate use of bacitracin-susceptibility disks (containing 0.04 U) allows presumptive identification of GAS but is a less accurate method of diagnosis. False-negative culture results occur in <10% of symptomatic patients when a throat swab specimen is obtained properly and cultured. Recovery of GAS from the pharynx does not distinguish patients with bona fide streptococcal infection (defined by a serologic antibody response) from streptococcal carriers who have an intercurrent pharyngitis caused by a different organism (e.g., a virus). The number of colonies of GAS on the agar culture plate does not accurately differentiate bona fide infection from carriage. Cultures that are negative for GAS after 24 hours should be incubated for a second day to optimize recovery of GAS.

Several rapid diagnostic tests for GAS pharyngitis are available. Most are based on nitrous acid extraction of group A carbohydrate antigen from organisms obtained by throat swab. Although the methods for these tests vary, their sensitivities and specificities, in general, are similar when they are carefully performed, with rigorous attention to technique and use of control. The specificities of these tests generally are very high, but the reported sensitivities vary considerably. As with throat specimen cultures, the accuracy of these tests is highly dependent on the quality of the throat swab specimen, which must contain pharyngeal or tonsillar secretions or both, and on the experience of the person performing the test. Therefore, when a patient is suspected on clinical grounds of having GAS pharyngitis and the result of the rapid streptococcal test is negative, a throat specimen culture should be obtained to ensure that the patient does not have GAS infection. Because of the very high specificity of these rapid tests, a positive test result does not require confirmation by throat specimen culture. Rapid diagnostic tests using new techniques, such as optical immunoassay and chemiluminescent DNA probes, have been developed. Published data suggest that these tests may be as sensitive as other rapid tests. Some experts believe that the optical immunoassay test is sufficiently sensitive to be used without throat specimen culture backup. Physicians who use this test without culture backup may wish to compare their results with those of culture to validate adequate sensitivity in their practice.

Indications for Group A Streptococci Testing

Factors to be considered in the decision to obtain a throat swab specimen for testing in children with pharyngitis are the patient's age, clinical signs and symptoms, the season, and the family and community epidemiology, including contact with a GAS-infected person and presence in the family of a person with acute rheumatic fever, a history thereof, or poststreptococcal glomerulonephritis. Group A streptococcal infection is less common in children <3 years of age, but outbreaks of streptococcal pharyngitis rarely have been reported in young children in child care settings. The risk of acute rheumatic fever is so remote in developed countries in such young children that diagnostic studies for streptococcal pharyngitis are not recommended routinely for children <3 years of age. Children with manifestations highly suggestive of viral infection, such as coryza, conjunctivitis, hoarseness, cough, anterior stomatitis, discrete ulcerative lesions, or diarrhea, are unlikely to have GAS as the cause of their pharyngitis and should not be swabbed for GAS. Children with acute onset of sore throat, fever, headache, pain on swallowing, abdominal pain, nausea, vomiting, and enlarged tender anterior cervical lymph nodes are much more likely to have GAS as the cause of their pharyngitis and should be tested.

Indications for testing contacts of GAS-infected persons vary according to circumstances. Testing asymptomatic household contacts of GAS-infected individuals usually is not recommended except during outbreaks or when contacts are at increased risk for developing sequelae of GAS infection. Siblings and all other household contacts of a child who has acute rheumatic fever or poststreptococcal glomerulonephritis should have their throats swabbed and, if test results are positive, should be treated regardless of whether they are currently or were recently symptomatic. Household contacts of an index case with streptococcal pharyngitis who have recent or current symptoms suggestive of streptococcal infection also should be tested. Pyodermal lesion specimens should be cultured in families with one or more cases of acute nephritis or streptococcal TSS so that antibiotic therapy can be administered to eradicate GAS.

Posttreatment throat swab cultures are indicated only for patients who are at particularly high risk for rheumatic fever or who are still or again symptomatic. Repeated courses of antimicrobial therapy are not indicated for asymptomatic patients who remain GAS positive after appropriate antibiotic therapy; the exceptions are persons who have had, or whose family members have had, rheumatic fever or rheumatic heart disease or persons in other unique epidemiologic circumstances, such as in outbreaks of rheumatic fever or acute poststreptococcal glomerulonephritis.

Patients in whom repeated episodes of pharyngitis occur at short intervals with GAS infection documented by culture or antigen detection test present a special problem. Often these persons are long-term GAS carriers who are experiencing frequent viral illnesses. In assessing such patients, inadequate compliance with oral treatment also should be considered. Although rare, in some areas, erythromycin resistance may occur, which results in treatment failures. Such strains also are resistant to other macrolides, such as clarithromycin and azithromycin dihydrate. Testing asymptomatic household members usually is not helpful. However, if multiple household members have symptomatic pharyngitis or other GAS infection, such as pyoderma, simultaneous cultures of specimens from all household members and treatment of all persons with positive culture results may be of value.

In schools, child care centers, or other environments in which large numbers of persons are in close contact, the prevalence of GAS pharyngeal carriage in healthy children can be as high as 15% in the absence of an outbreak of streptococcal disease. Therefore, classroom or more widespread culture surveys are not indicated routinely and should be considered only if multiple cases of rheumatic fever, glomerulonephritis, or severe invasive GAS disease have occurred.

Cultures of material from impetiginous lesions are not indicated routinely because they often yield both streptococci and staphylococci, and determination of the primary pathogen may not be possible.

In cases of suspected invasive GAS infections, cultures of blood and specimens from focal sites of possible infection are indicated. In necrotizing fasciitis, magnetic resonance imaging (MRI) can be helpful in confirming the anatomic diagnosis.

Group B Streptococci

Group B streptococci (GBS; *Streptococcus agalactiae*) are divided into the following serotypes based on capsular polysaccharides: Ia, Ib, II, and III–VIII. All serotypes may cause infections in newborn infants and in all adults, but serotypes Ia, II, III, and V account for approximately 90% of cases in the United States. Serotype III is the predominant cause of early-onset meningitis and all late-onset infections in newborns.

Colonization during pregnancy usually is constant but can be intermittent. Prevention of early-onset GBS disease in the newborn or fetus is recommended by maternal intrapartum antibiotic prophylaxis. Transmission from mother to infant occurs shortly before or during delivery. After delivery, person-to-person transmission can occur. Although uncommon, GBS infection can be acquired in the nursery from colonized infants or hospital personnel (probably via hand contamination) or in the community. The risk of early-onset disease is increased in preterm infants born at <37 weeks of gestation, in infants born of women with high genital GBS inoculum, and in cases of intrapartum fever, chorioamnionitis, or GBS bacteriuria. A low or absent concentration of serotype-specific serum antibody also is a predisposing factor. Other risk factors are maternal age <20 years and black ethnicity. The period of communicability is unknown but may extend throughout the duration of colonization or of disease. Infants can remain colonized for several months after birth and after treatment for symptomatic infection. Recurrent GBS disease affects an estimated 1% of appropriately treated infants.

GBS pathogens occur as urinary tract infections in parturient women and are a major cause of perinatal bacterial infections, frequently associated with maternal bacteremia, endometritis, and amnionitis, and systemic and focal infections in infants from birth until ≥3 months of age. Invasive disease in young infants is categorized into two entities based on time of onset after birth. Early-onset disease usually occurs within the first 24 hours of life (range, 0–6 days) and is characterized by respiratory distress, apnea, shock, pneumonia, and, less often, meningitis (5–10% of cases). Late-onset disease, which typically occurs at 3–4 weeks of age (range, 7 days to 3 months), frequently is manifested as occult bacteremia or meningitis; other focal infections, such as osteomyelitis, septic arthritis, and cellulitis, also can occur. GBS organisms also cause chorioamnionitis and postpartum endometritis, as well as systemic infections in nonpregnant adults, particularly adults with diabetes mellitus, chronic liver or renal disease, malignant neoplasm, or other immunocompromising conditions.

Diagnostic Tests

The presence of Gram-positive cocci in fluids that ordinarily are sterile (such as cerebrospinal, pleural, or joint fluid) provides presumptive evidence of infection. Cultures of blood or body fluids are necessary to establish the diagnosis. Serotype identification is available in reference laboratories. Rapid tests that identify GBS antigen in body fluids other than CSF are not recommended.

Non–Group A, Non–Group B Streptococcal and Enterococcal Infections

Streptococci of groups C and G and *Enterococcus* species are common pathogens. The two most common enterococcal species are *Enterococcus faecalis* and *Enterococcus faecium*. Streptococci belonging to groups D, F, H, and K also can be pathogens. Nongroupable streptococci, such as streptococci of groups other than A and B, may be associated with disease in newborn infants, older children, and adults. Urinary tract infection, endocarditis, upper and lower respiratory tract infection, and meningitis are the principal clinical syndromes.

Diagnostic Tests

Microscopic examination of fluids that ordinarily are sterile can yield presumptive evidence of infections by Gram-negative cocci. The diagnosis is established by culture and serogrouping of the isolate, using group-specific antisera. Identification of the species of enterococci from sterile sites is important to determine ampicillin and vancomycin susceptibility, as well as gentamicin sulfate susceptibility for synergy. Some automated methods may not detect vancomycin resistance.

Tetanus (Lockjaw)

Clostridium tetani, the tetanus bacillus, is a spore-forming, anaerobic, Gram-positive bacillus. The vegetative form produces a potent plasmid-encoded exotoxin (tetanospasmin), which binds to gangliosides at the myoneural junction of skeletal muscle and on neuronal membranes in the spinal cord, blocking inhibitory pulses to motor neurons. The action of tetanus toxin on the brain and sympathetic nervous system is less well documented. *C. tetani* is a wound contaminant; it causes neither tissue destruction nor an inflammatory response.

Generalized tetanus (lockjaw) is a neurologic disease manifested by trismus and severe muscular spasms. Tetanus is caused by the neurotoxin produced by *C. tetani* in a contaminated wound. Onset is gradual, occurring over 1–7 days, and progresses to severe generalized muscle spasms, which frequently are aggravated by any external stimulus. Severe spasms persist for 1 week or more and subside in a period of weeks in those who recover. Neonatal tetanus, a common cause of neonatal mortality in developing countries but rare in the United States, arises from contamination of the umbilical stump.

Diagnostic Tests

A specimen from the offending wound should be cultured. However, confirmation of the causative organism is made infrequently by culture. The diagnosis is made clinically by excluding other possibilities, such as hypocalcemic tetany, phenothiazine reaction, strychnine poisoning, and hysteria.

Toxic Shock Syndrome

TSS may be caused by *S. aureus* or *S. pyogenes*. *S. aureus*–mediated TSS usually is caused by strains producing TSS toxin-1 (TSST-1). Most of these strains also produce at least one of the staphylococcal enterotoxins. Some TSST-1–negative strains of *S. aureus* have been implicated in nonmenstrual cases of TSS. Most cases of *S. pyogenes*–mediated TSS are caused by strains producing at least one of five protein superantigenic exotoxins: streptococcal pyogenic exotoxins A, B, or C; mitogenic factor; or streptococcal superantigen.

Both *S. aureus* and *S. pyogenes* cause an acute illness characterized by fever, rapid-onset hypotension, rapidly accelerated renal failure, and multisystem organ involvement. Profuse watery diarrhea, vomiting, generalized erythroderma, conjunctival infection, and severe myalgias frequently are present with *S. aureus*–mediated TSS but are less common with *S. pyogenes*–mediated TSS. Evidence of local soft tissue infection (e.g., cellulitis, abscess, myositis, or necrotizing fasciitis) associated with severe increasing pain is common with *S. pyogenes*–mediated TSS but not with *S. aureus*–mediated TSS. The presence of a foreign body at the site of infection is common with *S. aureus*–mediated TSS but not with *S. pyogenes*–mediated TSS. Both forms of TSS may occur without a readily identifiable focus of infection. Both forms of TSS also may be associated with more invasive infections, such as pneumonia, osteomyelitis, bacteremia, pyarthrosis, or endocarditis. Patients with *S. aureus*–mediated TSS, especially menses associated, are at risk for a recurrent episode of TSS. Recurrent episodes have not been reported for *S. pyogenes*–mediated TSS. TSS can be confused with meningococcemia, Rocky Mountain spotted fever, septic shock, Kawasaki disease, ehrlichiosis, scarlet fever, measles, systemic lupus erythematosus, and other febrile mucocutaneous diseases.

The incidence of *S. pyogenes*–mediated TSS seems to be highest among young children, particularly those with varicella, and the elderly. Of all cases of severe invasive streptococcal infections in children, <10% are associated with TSS, compared with almost one-third of such infections in persons >75 years of age. Other persons at increased risk include those with diabetes mellitus, chronic cardiac or pulmonary disease, HIV infection, and intravenous-drug and alcohol use. The risk of severe invasive infection in contacts has been estimated to be 200 times greater than for the general population, but such occurrences are still rare. Most contacts have asymptomatic colonization.

For *S. pyogenes*–mediated TSS, mortality rates are higher for adults than for children and depend on whether the TSS is associated only with bacteremia or with a specific organ infection (e.g., necrotizing fasciitis, myositis, or pneumonia).

The incubation period for *S. pyogenes*–mediated disease is not defined clearly and may depend on the route of inoculation. The incubation period has been as short as 14 hours in cases associated with the accidental subcutaneous inoculation of infected blood, such as during childbirth or after penetrating trauma.

Diagnostic Tests

Staphylococcus aureus*–Mediated Toxic Shock Syndrome*

Diagnosis of *S. aureus*–mediated TSS remains a clinical diagnosis. Blood cultures are positive for *S. aureus* in <5% of patients with *S. aureus*–mediated TSS. Results of cultures of specimens from the site of infection usually are positive, and such samples should be obtained as soon as the site is identified. Once *S. aureus* is isolated in the laboratory, it is important to determine antimicrobial susceptibilities because methicillin-resistant *S. aureus* strains have caused TSS, although rarely. Because 33% of isolates of *S. aureus* from nonmenstrual cases do not produce TSST-1, and TSST-1–producing organisms can be present as part of the normal flora of the anterior nares and vagina, production of TSST-1 by an isolate of *S. aureus* is not helpful diagnostically.

Streptococcus pyogenes*–Mediated Toxic Shock Syndrome*

Blood culture results are positive for *S. pyogenes* in >50% of patients with *S. pyogenes*–mediated TSS. Cultures from the site of infection usually are positive and may remain positive for several days after appropriate antibiotic therapy has been initiated. *S. pyogenes* is uniformly susceptible to β-lactam antibiotics. Antimicrobial susceptibilities should be determined for the non–β-lactam antibiotics, clindamycin, and erythromycin, to which *S. pyogenes* may be resistant. A significant increase in antibody titers to antistreptolysin-O, antideoxyribonuclease B, or other streptococcal extracellular products 4–6 weeks after infection may help confirm the diagnosis if culture results were negative.

For both forms of TSS, laboratory studies may reflect multisystem organ involvement and disseminated intravascular coagulation.

Clinical Case Definitions

Staphylococcal Toxic Shock Syndrome[2,3]

Fever: temperature 38.9°C (102.0°F)

Rash: diffuse macular erythroderma

Desquamation: 1–2 wks after onset, particularly on palms and soles

Hypotension: systolic blood pressure 90 mm Hg for adults; lower than fifth percentile by age for children <16 years of age; orthostatic drop in diastolic blood pressure of 15 mm Hg from lying to sitting; orthostatic syncope or orthostatic dizziness

Multisystem involvement: three or more of the following:

- Gastrointestinal: vomiting or diarrhea at onset of illness
- Muscular: severe myalgia or creatinine phosphokinase level greater than twice the upper limit of normal or urinary sediment with five white blood cells per high-power field in the absence of a urinary tract infection
- Hepatic: total bilirubin, aspartate aminotransferase, or alanine aminotransferase level greater than twice the upper limit of normal
- Hematologic: platelet count $<100 \times 10^9$/L ($<100 \times 10^3/\mu$L)
- CNS: disorientation or alterations in consciousness without focal neurologic signs when fever and hypotension are absent

Negative results on the following tests, if obtained:

- Blood, throat swab, or CSF cultures; blood culture may be positive for *S. aureus*
- Serologic tests for Rocky Mountain spotted fever, leptospirosis, or measles

[2]Wharton M, Chorba TL, Vogt RL, et al. Case definitions for public health surveillance. *MMWR Morb Mortal Wkly Rep* 1990;39(RR-13):1–43.

[3]Pickering LK, ed. *2000 Red Book: Report of the Committee on Infectious Diseases*, 25th ed. Section 3. Elk Grove Village, IL: American Academy of Pediatrics, 2000:577.

Case classification is as follows:

Probable: Five of the six aforementioned clinical findings.
Confirmed: All six of the clinical findings, including desquamation. If the patient dies before desquamation could have occurred, presence of the other five criteria constitutes a definitive case.

Streptococcal Toxic Shock Syndrome[4]

Isolation of group A β-hemolytic streptococci
- From a normally sterile site (e.g., blood, CSF, peritoneal fluid, tissue biopsy specimen)
- From a nonsterile site (e.g., throat, sputum, vagina)

Clinical signs of severity
- Hypotension systolic blood pressure 90 mm Hg in adults or lower than the fifth percentile for age in children

AND

Two or more of the following signs:
- Renal impairment: creatinine level, 177 μmol/L (2 mg/dL) for adults or two times or more the upper limit of normal for age
- Coagulopathy: platelet count, 100×10^9/L (100×10^3/μL), or disseminated intravascular coagulation
- Hepatic involvement: alanine aminotransferase, aspartate aminotransferase, or total bilirubin levels two times or more the upper limit of normal for age
- Acute respiratory distress syndrome
- Generalized erythematous macular rash that may desquamate
- Soft tissue necrosis, including necrotizing fasciitis or myositis, or gangrene

Risk Factors for Nonmenstrual Staphylococcal Toxic Shock Syndrome[5]

Colonization with or introduction of toxin-producing *S. aureus*
Absence of protective antitoxin antibody
Infected site
Primary *S. aureus* infection

Carbuncle	Endocarditis	Peritonitis	Pyomyositis
Cellulitis	Folliculitis	Peritonsillar abscess	Sinusitis
Dental abscess	Mastitis	Pneumonia	Tracheitis
Empyema	Osteomyelitis	Pyarthrosis	

Postoperative wound infection

Abdominal	Ear, nose, and throat	Cesarean section	Neurosurgical
Breast	Genitourinary	Dermatologic	Orthopedic

Skin or mucous membrane disruption

Burns (e.g., chemical, scald)	Viral infection
Dermatitis	Influenza
Postpartum (vaginal delivery)	Pharyngitis
Superficial or penetrating trauma (e.g., insect bite, needle stick)	Varicella

Surgical or nonsurgical foreign body placement

Breast augmentation devices	Surgical prostheses, stents, packing material, or sutures
Catheters	Tampons
Diaphragm	
Sponge (contraceptive)	

No obvious focus of infection (vaginal or pharyngeal colonization)

[4]The Working Group on Severe Streptococcal Infections. Defining the group A streptococcal toxic shock syndrome: rationale and consensus definition. *JAMA* 1993;269:390–391. An illness fulfilling criteria IA and IIB can be defined as a *definite* case. An illness fulfilling criteria IA and IB or IIA and IIB can be defined as a *probable* case if no other cause for the illness is identified.
[5]Pickering LK, ed. *2000 Red Book: Report of the Committee on Infectious Diseases*, 25th ed. Section 3. Elk Grove Village, IL: American Academy of Pediatrics, 2000:579.

Tuberculosis

The agent of tuberculosis is *Mycobacterium tuberculosis*, an acid-fast bacillus. Pulmonary or abdominal disease due to *Mycobacterium bovis*, the cause of bovine tuberculosis, occurs occasionally in the United States, whereas illness due to *Mycobacterium africanum* infection is rare.

Most tuberculosis infections in children and adolescents usually are asymptomatic when the tuberculin skin test (TST) result is positive. The primary complex of infection usually is not evident on the chest radiograph, and primary infection in most immunocompetent children does not progress rapidly to disease. Early clinical manifestations occurring 1–6 months after initial infection can include fever, weight loss, cough, night sweats, and chills. Pulmonary radiographic findings include lymphadenopathy of the hilar, mediastinal, cervical, or other nodes; involvement of a segment or lobe, occasionally with atelectasis or infiltrate; pleural effusion; cavitary lesions; and miliary disease. Meningitis also can occur. Extrapulmonary manifestations that can occur ≥12 months after the initial infection include disease of the middle ear and mastoid, bones, joints, and skin. Tuberculosis of a kidney and reactivation or adult-type pulmonary tuberculosis are rare in young children but can occur in adolescents. Manifestations in patients with drug-resistant tuberculosis are indistinguishable from the manifestations in patients with drug-susceptible disease.

Congenital Tuberculosis

Women who have only pulmonary tuberculosis are not likely to infect the fetus but may infect their infant after delivery. Congenital tuberculosis is rare, but *in utero* infections can occur after maternal *M. tuberculosis* bacillemia.

If a newborn is suspected of having congenital tuberculosis, a TST, chest radiograph, lumbar puncture, and appropriate cultures should be performed promptly. The TST result usually is negative in newborn infants with congenital or perinatally acquired infection. Hence, regardless of the TST results, treatment of the infant should be initiated promptly with isoniazid, rifampin, pyrazinamide, and streptomycin sulfate or kanamycin sulfate. The placenta should be examined histologically and a specimen cultured for *M. tuberculosis*. The mother should be evaluated for the presence of pulmonary or extrapulmonary, including uterine, tuberculosis. If the maternal physical examination or chest radiograph supports the diagnosis of tuberculous disease, the newborn infant should be treated with regimens recommended for tuberculous meningitis, excluding corticosteroids. If meningitis is confirmed, corticosteroids should be given. Drug susceptibilities of the organism recovered from the mother, infant, or both should be determined.

Diagnostic Tests

Isolation of *M. tuberculosis* by culture from gastric aspirates, sputum, pleural fluid, CSF, urine, other body fluids, or a biopsy specimen establishes the diagnosis. The best specimen for the diagnosis of pulmonary tuberculosis in any young child, or in any older child or adolescent in whom the cough is nonproductive or absent, is an early morning gastric aspirate. Gastric aspirate specimens should be obtained with a nasogastric tube on awakening the child and before ambulation or feeding. Three aspirate samples should be submitted. Regardless of the results of the smears for acid-fast bacilli, each specimen should be cultured.

Because *M. tuberculosis* is slow growing, detection of this organism may take as long as 10 weeks using solid media and 2–6 weeks by the radiometric method. Even with optimal culture techniques, organisms are isolated from <50% of children and <75% of infants with pulmonary tuberculosis. Identification of isolates by culture can be more rapid if a DNA probe is used. Attempts should be made to demonstrate acid-fast bacilli in sputum, body fluids, or both by the Ziehl-Neelsen method or by auramine-rhodamine staining and with fluorescence microscopy. Fluorescent methods are superior and, if available, preferred. Histologic examination for and demonstration of acid-fast bacilli in biopsy specimens from lymph node, pleura, liver, bone marrow, or other tissues can be valuable for diagnosis, but *M. tuberculosis* cannot be reliably distinguished from other mycobacteria in stained specimens.

Nucleic acid amplification tests for rapid diagnosis, including PCR, are of limited availability, expensive, and approved only for smear-positive respiratory tract specimens. Restriction fragment length polymorphism analysis for epidemiologic investigation is available in research and reference laboratories. Both tests should be ordered in consultation with a specialist in tuberculosis.

Identification of the source case should be actively pursued to support the presumptive diagnosis, define drug susceptibility if *M. tuberculosis* is isolated from this source case, and clarify resistance patterns that will affect the choice of drugs for the contact. These activities should be coordinated with the local health department.

Culture material should be obtained from children with evidence of tuberculosis, especially when (a) an isolate from a source case is not available, (b) the child is immunocompromised, including a child with HIV infection, and (c) the child has extrapulmonary disease.

Tuberculin Testing

The TST is the only practical tool for diagnosing tuberculous infection in asymptomatic persons. The Mantoux test containing 5 tuberculin units (TU) of PPD, administered intradermally, is the recommended TST. Other strengths of Mantoux skin tests (1 or 250 TU) should not be used. Multiple puncture tests are not recommended because they lack adequate sensitivity and specificity.

The American Academy of Pediatrics recommends a TST for children who are at increased risk of acquiring tuberculous infection and disease. Routine TST administration that has either a low yield of positive results or a large number of false-positive results, including school-based programs that include populations at low risk, represents an inefficient use of health care resources. Children without risk factors, including children who are <1 year of age, do not need routine TSTs.

A TST can be administered during the same visit that immunizations are given, including live-virus vaccines. Previous immunization with bacille Calmette-Guérin is not a contraindication to TST skin testing.

Administration of TSTs and interpretation of results should be performed by experienced health care professionals who have been trained in the proper methods, because administration and interpretation by unskilled persons are unreliable. The TST is administered by injecting 0.1 mL of 5 TU of PPD intradermally (Mantoux method) into the volar aspect of the forearm using a 27-gauge needle and a tuberculin syringe. When a physician is unavailable to interpret the TST, it can be interpreted by specifically trained staff of an after-hours clinic or local public health clinic, school-based nurses, home health care staff, or emergency department personnel. The primary care physician should be notified of the result promptly.

Interpretation of the Tuberculin Sensitivity Test

See Table 3.

Serial tuberculin testing may produce an augmented reaction (booster phenomenon) in those previously sensitized by infection or bacille Calmette-Guérin vaccination.

Definitions of Positive Tuberculin Skin Test Results in Infants, Children, and Adolescents*[6]

TST results should be read at 48–72 hours after PPD placement

Induration ≥5 mm

Children in close contact with known or suspected contagious cases of tuberculous disease

- Households with active or previously active cases if treatment cannot be verified as adequate before exposure, treatment was initiated after the child's contact, or reactivation of latent tuberculosis infection is suspected

Children suspected to have tuberculosis disease

- Chest radiograph consistent with active or previously active tuberculosis
- Clinical evidence of tuberculosis disease[†]

Children receiving immunosuppressive therapy or with immunosuppressive conditions, including HIV infection

Induration ≥10 mm

Children at increased risk of disseminated disease

- Young age: <4 years
- Other medical conditions, including Hodgkin disease, lymphoma, diabetes mellitus, chronic renal failure, or malnutrition

[6]Pickering LK, ed. *2000 Red Book: Report of the Committee on Infectious Diseases*, 25th ed. Section 3. Elk Grove Village, IL: American Academy of Pediatrics, 2000:594.

Table 3. Interpretation of the Tuberculin Sensitivity (Mantoux) Test[a]

	Induration			
Clinical Context	<5 mm	5–10 mm	10–20 mm	>25 mm
Screening, nonendemic population	Negative	Suspicious for infection[b]	90% of patients have infection	Virtually all have infection
Screening, endemic population	Negative	Consistent with past infection[b]	Suspicious for infection	Suggestive of infection
After bacille Calmette-Guérin vaccination	Negative	Expected	Suspicious for infection	Suggestive of infection
Suspicious clinical findings or contact with active tuberculosis	Negative	Suspicious for infection	90% of patients have infection	Virtually all have infection

[a]Intradermal injection of 10 tuberculin units of purified protein derivative.
[b]May also be due to cross reactivity with other mycobacterial species.

Children with increased exposure to tuberculous disease
- Children born or whose parents were born in high-prevalence regions of the world
- Children frequently exposed to adults who are HIV infected, homeless, users of illicit drugs, residents of nursing homes, incarcerated or institutional persons, or migrant farm workers
- Children who travel to or have lived in high-prevalence regions of the world

Induration ≥15 mm
Children ≥4 years of age without any risk factors

*These definitions apply regardless of previous bacille Calmette-Guérin immunization; erythema at TST site does not indicate a positive test.
†Evidence by physical examination or laboratory assessment that would include tuberculosis in the working differential diagnosis (e.g., meningitis).

Tularemia

Francisella tularensis, the causative agent of tularemia, is a Gram-negative pleomorphic coccobacillus.

Sources of the organism include approximately 100 species of wild mammals (e.g., rabbits, hares, muskrats, and voles); at least 9 species of domestic animals (e.g., sheep, cattle, and cats); blood-sucking arthropods that bite these animals (e.g., ticks, deerflies, and mosquitoes); and water and soil contaminated by infected animals. In the United States, rabbits and ticks are the major sources of human infection. Infected animals and arthropods, especially ticks, are infective for prolonged periods; frozen killed rabbits can remain infective for >3 years.

Most patients with tularemia experience an abrupt onset of fever, chills, myalgia, and headache. Illness usually conforms to one of the several tularemic syndromes. Most common is the ulceroglandular syndrome, which is characterized by the following: (a) a primary, painful, maculopapular lesion at the portal of bacterial entry, with subsequent ulceration and slow healing; (b) painful, acutely inflamed, regional lymph nodes, which may drain spontaneously; and (c) severe conjunctivitis. Less common disease syndromes are the following: (a) glandular (regional lymphadenopathy with no ulcer); (b) oculoglandular (severe conjunctivitis and preauricular lymphadenopathy); (c) oropharyngeal (severe exudative stomatitis, pharyngitis, or tonsillitis and cervical lymphadenopathy); (d) typhoidal (high fever, hepatomegaly, and splenomegaly); (e) intestinal (abdominal pain, vomiting, and diarrhea); and (f) pneumonic (primary pleuropulmonary disease).

Diagnostic Tests

Diagnosis is established most frequently by serologic testing. A fourfold or greater change in *F. tularensis* agglutinin titer frequently is evident after the second week of illness and is considered diagnostic. A single convalescent titer of >1:160 is consistent with recent or past infection. Slide agglutination tests are less reliable than plate or tube agglutination tests; nonspecific cross agglutination with *Brucella, Proteus*, and heterophil antibodies can cause false-positive antibody titers to *F. tularensis*. The IFA test of ulcer exudate or aspirate material can be useful as a rapid and specific screening test. PCR-based assays have been developed for detection of *F. tularensis* DNA in clinical materials, but this assay is not available in most clinical laboratories. Isolation of the organism from blood, skin, ulcers, lymph node drainage, gastric washings, or respiratory tract secretions is best made by inoculation of cysteine-enriched media or laboratory mice, but work with cultures should be attempted only by personnel who have been immunized against *F. tularensis*. Supplemented chocolate agar or modified charcoal-yeast agar (used for culture of *Legionella* organisms) can support growth of *F. tularensis*. Laboratory personnel always should be informed that *F. tularensis* is suspected because of the potential hazard to laboratory personnel and the need to use special media.

Ureaplasma urealyticum *Infections*

The genera *Ureaplasma* and *Mycoplasma* form the family Mycoplasmatacae. The genus *Ureaplasma* contains a single species, *urealyticum*, which includes at least 16 serotypes.

The most common syndrome associated with *U. urealyticum* infection is nongonococcal urethritis. Although nongonococcal urethritis most frequently is caused by *C. trachomatis*, *U. urealyticum* seems to be responsible for a significant proportion of the remainder of cases (20–30%). Without treatment, the disease usually resolves within 1–6 months, although asymptomatic infection may persist thereafter. In women, salpingitis, endometritis, and chorioamnionitis can occur. Prostatitis and epididymitis have been associated with *U. urealyticum* infection in men.

U. urealyticum has been isolated from the lower respiratory tract and lung biopsy specimens of preterm infants and may contribute to pneumonia and chronic lung disease of prematurity. Although the organism also has been recovered from respiratory tract secretions of infants ≤3 months of age with pneumonia, its role in the development of lower respiratory tract disease in otherwise healthy young infants is controversial. *U. urealyticum* has been isolated from CSF of newborns with meningitis, hydrocephalus, and intraventricular hemorrhage. The contribution of *U. urealyticum* to the outcome of these newborn infants is unclear given the confounding effects of prematurity and intraventricular hemorrhage.

Isolated cases of *U. urealyticum* arthritis, osteomyelitis, pericarditis, and progressive sinopulmonary disease in immunocompromised patients have been reported.

Diagnostic Tests

If a specimen for culture is obtained, specific *Ureaplasma* transport medium with refrigeration at 4°C (39°F) is necessary. The use of cotton swabs should be avoided. A rapid, sensitive, PCR test for detection of *U. urealyticum* has been developed but is not available routinely. The *U. urealyticum* organism can be cultured in urea-containing broth in 1–2 days. Serologic testing for *U. urealyticum* antibodies is of limited value and should not be used for routine diagnosis.

Vaginosis (Bacterial)

The microbiologic cause of bacterial vaginosis (BV) has not been delineated clearly. The microbial flora of the vagina are changed, with an overgrowth of *Gardnerella vaginalis, Mycoplasma hominis,* and anaerobic bacteria and a marked decrease in the concentration of hydrogen peroxide–producing lactobacilli. Despite these changes, little or no inflammation of the vaginal epithelium occurs.

BV, a syndrome primarily occurring in sexually active adolescent and adult women, is characterized by a vaginal discharge that adheres to the vaginal wall and that usually is malodorous (fishy odor), nonviscous, homogenous, and white. BV may be asymptomatic and is not associated with abdominal pain, significant pruritus, or dysuria.

Vaginitis and vulvitis in prepubertal girls usually have a nonspecific cause and are rarely manifestations of BV. In prepubertal girls, other predisposing causes for vaginal discharge include foreign bodies or other infections due to group A streptococci, *Trichomonas vaginalis*, HSV, *Neisseria gonorrhoeae, Chlamydia trachomatis,* or *Shigella* species.

Diagnostic Tests

The clinical diagnosis of BV requires the presence of three of the following symptoms or signs:

- Homogenous, white, noninflammatory, adherent vaginal discharge that smoothly coats the vaginal walls.
- Vaginal fluid pH >4.5.
- A fishy, amine-like odor from vaginal fluid before or after mixing with 10% potassium hydroxide.
- Presence of "clue cells" (squamous vaginal epithelial cells covered with bacteria, which cause a stippled or granular appearance and ragged "moth-eaten" borders). In BV, clue cells usually constitute at least 20% of vaginal epithelial cells.

A Gram stain of vaginal secretions is an alternative means of establishing a diagnosis. Numerous mixed bacteria, including small curved rods and cocci, and few of the large Gram-positive rods consistent with lactobacilli, are characteristic. Culture for *G. vaginalis* is not recommended because the organism may be found in females without BV, including those who are not sexually active.

Yersinia enterocolitica *and* Yersinia pseudotuberculosis *Infections (Enteritis and Other Illnesses)*

Yersinia enterocolitica and *Y. pseudotuberculosis* are Gram-negative bacilli; 34 serotypes of *Y. enterocolitica* and 5 serotypes of *Y. pseudotuberculosis* are recognized. Differences in virulence exist among varius serotypes of *Y. enterocolitica*; 0:3 and 0:9 are the most common causes of diarrhea.

The reservoirs of the organisms are animals, including rodents and many bird species (*Y. pseudotuberculosis*) and swine (*Y. enterocolitica*). Infection is believed to be transmitted by ingestion of contaminated food, especially uncooked pork products and unpasteurized milk, or contaminated water; by direct or indirect contact with animals; by transfusion with packed red blood cells; and possibly by fecal-oral, person-to-person transmission. Bottle-fed infants can be infected if their caregivers simultaneously are handling raw pork intestines (chitterlings). *Y. enterocolitica* is isolated more frequently in winter than in summer. Patients with excessive iron storage syndromes (e.g., thalassemia major), as well as patients receiving deferoxamine mesylate for iron overload, have unusual susceptibility to *Yersinia* bacteremia.

Y. enterocolitica and *Y. pseudotuberculosis* cause several age-specific syndromes and a variety of uncommon presentations. The most common manifestation of infection with *Y. enterocolitica* is enterocolitis with fever and diarrhea; stool often contains leukocytes, blood, and mucus. This syndrome occurs most often in young children. A pseudoappendicitis syndrome (fever, abdominal pain, tenderness in the right lower quadrant of the abdomen, and leukocytosis) occurs primarily in older children and young adults. Focal infections, abscess formation (such as hepatic and splenic), and bacteremia occur most often in patients with predisposing conditions, such as excessive iron storage. Other manifestations of infection are uncommon and include pharyngitis, meningitis, osteomyelitis, pyomyositis, conjunctivitis, pneumonia, acute proliferative glomerulonephritis, peritonitis, and primary cutaneous infection. Postinfectious sequelae observed with *Y. enterocolitica* include erythema nodosum and reactive arthritis, and occur most often in adults.

Diagnostic Tests

Y. enterocolitica and *Y. pseudotuberculosis* can be recovered from throat swabs, mesenteric lymph nodes, peritoneal fluid, and blood. Stool cultures generally yield positive results during the first 2 weeks of illness, regardless of the nature of the gastrointestinal tract manifestations. *Y. enterocolitica* also has been isolated from synovial fluid, bile, urine, CSF, sputum, and wounds. Because of the relatively low incidence *of Yersinia* infection and because laboratory identification of organisms from stool requires specific techniques, laboratory personnel should be notified that *Yersinia* infection is suspected. Pathogenic strains of *Y. enterocolitica* usually are pyrazinamidase negative. Infection can be confirmed by demonstrating increases in serum antibody titer after infection, but these tests generally are available only in reference or research laboratories. Cross reactions of these antibodies with *Brucella, Vibrio, Salmonella,* and *Rickettsia* species and *E. coli* lead to false-positive *Y. enterocolitica* and *Y. pseudotuberculosis* titers. In patients with thyroid disease, persistently elevated *Y. enterocolitica* antibody titers can result from antigenic similarity of the organism with antigens of the thyroid epithelial cell membrane.

Bacterial Specimens for Culture

Timing of Collection

Sputum, urine, stool, and so on, are best collected in early morning and sent to the laboratory the same day.

Procedure for Collection of Specific Specimens

Blood

A blood culture requires two bottles of blood—one for aerobic and one for anaerobic culture. Each blood culture specimen should be collected from a separate venipuncture.

Blood specimens should be collected before treatment is initiated, if possible.

Two or three sets should be collected early in the illness; collection should be repeated if cultures are negative after 48 hours of growth.

Organisms are continuously shed during intravascular infections such as endocarditis, but they are intermittently shed during occult infections. In some instances of occult infection, there is a predictable fever pattern. If this is the case, the blood for culture is best collected 30 minutes before the fever spike.

The yield beyond three or four cultures is minimal in most circumstances, and collection of more than this is discouraged.

Virtually any organism, including normal flora, can cause bacteremia. A negative culture result does not necessarily rule out bacteremia; false-negative results occur when pathogens fail to grow. A positive culture result does not necessarily indicate bacteremia; false-positive results occur when contaminants grow. Gram-negative bacilli, anaerobes, and fungi should be considered pathogens until proven otherwise. The most difficult interpretation problem is to determine whether an organism that is usually considered normal skin flora is a true pathogen.

Clinical Disease Suspected	Culture Recommendation	Rationale
Sepsis, meningitis, osteomyelitis, septic arthritis, bacterial pneumonia	Two sets of cultures—one from each of two prepared sampling sites, with the second sample drawn after a brief time interval; then therapy is begun.	Assures sufficient sampling in cases of intermittent or low-level bacteremia. Minimizes the confusion, caused by a positive culture result due to transient bacteremia or skin contamination.
Fever of unknown origin (e.g., occult abscess, empyema, typhoid fever, etc.)	Two sets of cultures—one from each of two prepared sampling sites, the second sample drawn after a brief time interval (30 min). If cultures are negative after 24–48 hr, obtain two more sets of specimens, preferably before an anticipated temperature rise.	The yield after four sets of cultures is minimal.

Endocarditis		
Acute	Blood culture: Neonates, 1–2 mL; Infants, 2–3 mL; Children, 3–5 mL; Adolescents, adults, 10–20 mL	For 95–99% of acute endocarditis patients (untreated), results are positive in one of the first three cultures.
Subacute	Blood culture sets as above for acute endocarditis.	Adequate sample volume despite low-level bacteremia or previous therapy should result in a positive yield.
Immunocompromised host (AIDS)		
Septicemia, fungemia, mycobacteremia	Obtain two sets of culture specimens from each of two prepared sites; consider lysis-concentration techniques to enhance recovery for fungi and mycobacteria.	Low levels of fungemia and mycobacteremia frequently encountered.

Upper Respiratory Tract Specimens

A nasopharyngeal culture is obtained by inserting a thin sterile swab gently through the nose to touch the pharynx; the swab is gently rotated and removed.

A throat culture is obtained by introducing a sterile swab into the mouth. A tongue blade should be used to avoid contaminating the specimen with oral secretions. Both tonsillar fossae, posterior pharynx, and any inflamed or ulcerated areas should be swabbed firmly.

Lower Respiratory Tract Specimens

Specimens include sputum, tracheal aspiration, and bronchial washings.

Rinsing the mouth with saline or water (but not mouthwash) may reduce contamination with normal oropharyngeal flora.

Deep cough should be encouraged, with expectoration of the sputum into a sterile specimen collection cup that is labeled with the patient's name.

Saliva should not be sent for culture.

When the patient is unable to cough productively, an alternative method should be used, such as

- Sputum induction by involuntary deep coughing produced by irritation.
- Tracheal aspiration. The trachea is gently irritated with a small-lumen suction catheter, which causes deep, productive coughing. Also, the specimen may be aspirated with a syringe.
- Bronchial washings. These are done in the operating room at the time of bronchoscopic examination.

A small amount of sputum is all that is required, but it must be sputum and not oral secretions.

Specimens of Wound Exudate

The steps for using a sterile transport swab in collecting wound exudate specimens are as follow:

- Gently cleanse the area, using dry, sterile gauze to remove any contaminants.
- Using a sterile red-stopper swab culture collection system, introduce the swab deeply enough to obtain a moist specimen; replace the swab in the container. Do not break the container.
- Store at room temperature.

Urine

When a urine culture is ordered, a clean-catch specimen should be collected as follows:

- A careful explanation should be given to patients of the mechanics of midstream collection and the importance of collecting an uncontaminated specimen. They should be taught how to handle the specimen container to keep it sterile.

- A clean-catch specimen is necessary to confirm the presence or absence of infecting organisms in urine. The specimen must be free of any contaminating matter that might be present on the genital organs; therefore, patients should be urged to follow the steps outlined below:

Instructions for female patients:

- If you are menstruating, first insert a fresh tampon or use cotton to stop the flow.
- Wash the urinary opening and its surroundings from front to back with a sterile antiseptic pad.
- Begin urinating into the toilet, making sure you keep the skin fold apart with the fingers of one hand.
- Wait until the urine stream is well established before moving the container into the path of the stream to catch the rest of the urine. Do not touch the container to the genital area.
- Refrigerate the specimen immediately. Label the container with your name and the time of collection, and deliver it as soon as possible to your physician.

Specimens for Anaerobic Culture

Specimens are to be collected from a prepared site using a sterile technique. Contamination with normal flora must be avoided. Some anaerobes are killed by contact with oxygen for only a few seconds. Ideally, pus obtained by needle aspiration through intact surface, which has been aseptically prepared, is put directly into anaerobic transport media. Sampling of open lesions is enhanced by deep aspiration using a sterile plastic catheter or needle. Curettings of the base of an open lesion may also provide a good yield. If irrigation is necessary, nonbacteriostatic sterile normal saline may be used. Pulmonary samples may be obtained by transtracheal percutaneous needle aspiration. If swabs must be used, two should be collected, one for culture and one for Gram stain. If a syringe is used to transport the specimen to the laboratory, all air should be expelled and the needle inserted into a sterile stopper.

Viral Diseases

Adenovirus Infections

Adenoviruses are DNA viruses; at least 51 distinct serotypes divided into six subgenera (A to F) cause human infections. Types 40 and 41 and, to a lesser extent, type 31 have been associated with gastroenteritis. The most common site of adenovirus infection is the upper respiratory tract. Manifestations include symptoms of the common cold, pharyngitis, pharyngoconjunctival fever, tonsillitis, otitis media, and keratoconjunctivitis, often associated with fever. Life-threatening disseminated infection may occur in young infants and immunocompromised hosts. Adenoviruses are infrequent causes of acute hemorrhagic cystitis and genitourinary tract disease.

Diagnostic Tests

Culture, antigen, or immunoassay techniques are used for diagnosis. Enteric adenovirus types 40 and 41 usually cannot be isolated in standard cell cultures. Detection can be made by electron microscopy of stool specimens and detection of viral DNA with genomic probes, synthetic oligonucleotide probes, or gene amplification by PCR.

Arbovirus Infections

[Includes western and eastern equine encephalitis, St. Louis encephalitis, Powassan encephalitis, California encephalitis (primarily La Crosse virus), Colorado tick fever, dengue, Japanese encephalitis, Venezuelan equine encephalitis, yellow fever, and West Nile encephalitis.

Arborviruses (arthropod-borne viruses) are spread by mosquitoes, ticks, or sandflies and produce four principal clinical syndromes: (a) CNS infection (including encephalitis, aseptic meningitis, or myelitis; (b) an undifferentiated febrile illness, often with rash; (c) acute polyarthropathy; and (d) acute hemorrhagic fever, usually accompanied by hepatitis. Infection with some arboviruses produces congenital malformations and spontaneous abortion or, in the prenatal period, congenital perinatal illness.

Diagnostic Tests

Serologic testing of CSF or isolation of the virus. Presence of virus-specific IgM antibody in CSF is confirmatory. PCR assays to detect several arboviruses have been developed, but they have not been introduced into routine laboratory diagnosis. Serologic testing for dengue and arboviruses transmitted in the United States is available through several commercial, state, research, and reference laboratories. During the acute phase of dengue, yellow fever, Colorado tick fever, Venezuelan equine encephalitis, and certain other arboviral infections, virus can be isolated from blood and, in Venezuelan equine encephalitis, from the throat. In patients with encephalitis, viral isolation should be attempted from CSF or from biopsied or postmortem brain tissue.

Major Arboviruses

Family	Genus	Representative Name
Bunyaviridae	Bunyavirus	California serogroup viruses (North and South America, Europe, Asia) Oropouche virus (South America)
	Phlebovirus	Sandfly fever virus (Europe, Africa, Asia) Toscana virus (Europe)
	Hantavirus	Hantavirus of hemorrhagic fever
Togaviridae	Alphavirus	Western equine encephalitis virus (North and South America); Eastern equine encephalitis virus (North and South America); Venezuelan equine encephalitis virus (North and South America); Mayaro virus (Central and South America); Chikungunya virus (Africa, Asia); Ross River virus (Australia, Oceania); O'nyong-nyong virus (Africa); Sindbis virus (Africa, Scandinavia, northern Europe, Asia, Australia)
Flaviviridae	Flavivirus	St. Louis encephalitis virus (North and South America); Japanese encephalitis virus (Asia); Dengue viruses (types 1–4) (tropics, worldwide); Yellow fever virus (South America, Africa); Murray Valley encephalitis virus (Australia); West Nile virus (Europe, Africa, Asia, North America); Tick-borne encephalitis complex viruses (Europe and Asia); Powassan virus (North America, Asia)
Reoviridae	Coltivirus	Colorado tick fever virus (United States, Canada, Asia)
Rhabdoviridae	Vesiculovirus	Vesicular stomatitis virus (Western hemisphere)

Astrovirus Infections

Astroviruses are nonenveloped single-stranded RNA viruses with a characteristic starlike appearance when visualized by electron microscopy. Eight antigenic types are known.

Illness is characterized by abdominal pain, diarrhea, vomiting, nausea, fever, and malaise. Illness in the immunocompetent host is self-limited, lasting a median of 5–6 days.

Diagnostic Tests

Commercial tests for diagnosis are not available. The following tests are available in some research and reference laboratories: electron microscopy for detection of viral particles in stool, EIA for detection of viral antigen in stool or antibody in serum, and reverse transcriptase-polymerase chain reaction (RT-PCR) for detection of viral RNA in stool. Of these tests, RT-PCR is the most sensitive.

Calicivirus Infections

Caliciviruses are nonenveloped RNA viruses. The three recognized genera that cause disease in humans are Norwalk-like and Sapporo-like caliciviruses and vesiviruses. Vesiviruses cause vesicular exanthema in humans.

Caliciviruses may be a cause of sporadic cases of gastroenteritis requiring hospitalization, but sensitive diagnostic tools have been applied only recently to study this problem. Most sporadic Calicivirus infections have been detected in children <4 years of age. Transmission is via the fecal-oral route. Prolonged excretion can occur in immunocompromised hosts.

Diarrhea and vomiting, frequently accompanied by fever, headache, malaise, myalgia, and abdominal cramps, are characteristic. Symptoms last from 1 day to 2 weeks.

Diagnostic Tests

Commercial tests for diagnosis are not available. The following tests are available in some research and reference laboratories: electron microscopy for detection of viral particles in stool, EIA for detection of viral antigen in stool or antibody in serum, and RT-PCR for detection of viral RNA in stool. The most sensitive assays are RT-PCR and serologic testing; electron microscopy is relatively insensitive.

Coronavirus Infections

Coronaviruses are RNA viruses that are large (80–160 nm), enveloped with lipid-soluble coats, and are pleomorphic (spherical or elliptical). At least two distinct antigenic groups of respiratory coronaviruses have been identified.

Coronaviruses are a common cause of upper respiratory tract infection and occasionally have been implicated in lower respiratory tract disease. Coronavirus-like particles, not confirmed as coronavirus, have been associated with several outbreaks of diarrhea in nurseries and, rarely, with neonatal necrotizing enterocolitis in infants.

Diagnostic Tests

Tests for human Coronavirus infection, including antibody assays, are not available commercially. Most strains cannot be isolated by the methods commonly used in diagnostic virology laboratories. Viral particles have been visualized by immunoelectron microscopy, and viral antigens have been detected by immunoassay.

Cytomegalovirus Infections

Human cytomegalovirus (CMV), a DNA virus, is a member of the herpesvirus group.

Manifestations of acquired human CMV infection vary with the age and immunocompetence of the host. Asymptomatic infections are the most common, particularly in children. An infectious mononucleosis–like syndrome with fever and mild hepatitis, in the absence of heterophil and antibody production, can occur in adolescents and adults. Pneumonia, colitis, and retinitis occur in immunocompromised hosts (particularly those receiving treatment for malignant neoplasms), in persons with HIV infection, and in persons receiving immunosuppressive therapy for organ transplantation.

Congenital infection has a spectrum of manifestations but is usually asymptomatic. Some congenitally infected infants who seem asymptomatic at birth are later found to have a hearing loss or learning disability. Approximately 5% of infants with congenital CMV infection have profound involvement, with intrauterine growth retardation, neonatal jaundice, purpura, hepatosplenomegaly, microcephaly, brain damage, intracerebral calcifications, and retinitis. Approximately 15% of infants born after maternal primary infection will have one or more sequelae of intrauterine infection.

Infection acquired at birth or shortly thereafter from maternal cervical secretions or human milk usually is not associated with clinical illness. Infection resulting from transfusion from CMV-seropositive donors to preterm infants has been associated with lower respiratory tract disease.

Vertical transmission of CMV to an infant occurs by one of the following methods: (a) *in utero* by transplacental passage of maternal blood-borne virus, (b) at birth by passage through an infected maternal genital tract, or (c) postnatally by ingestion of CMV-positive human milk. Approximately 1% of all live-born infants are infected *in utero* and excrete CMV at birth. Although *in utero* fetal infection can occur after reactivation of infection during pregnancy, sequelae are far more common in infants after maternal primary infection, with 10–20% diagnosed with mental retardation or sensorineural deafness in childhood and 5% having manifestations evident at birth.

Maternal cervical infection is common and results in exposure of many infants to CMV at birth.

Diagnostic Tests

The diagnosis of CMV is confounded by the ubiquity of the virus, the high rate of asymptomatic excretion, the frequency of reactivated infections, development of serum IgM CMV-specific antibody in some episodes of reactivation, and concurrent infection with other pathogens.

The virus can be isolated in cell culture from urine, pharyngeal specimens, peripheral blood leukocytes, human milk, semen, cervical secretions, and other tissues and body fluids.

Recovery of virus from a target organ provides unequivocal evidence that the disease is caused by CMV infection. However, a presumptive diagnosis can be made on the basis of a fourfold antibody titer rise in serum samples or by virus excretion. Techniques for detection of viral DNA in tissues and some fluids, especially CSF, by PCR or hybridization are available from specialty laboratories. Detection of p65 antigen in white blood cells is used to identify infection in immunocompromised hosts.

Complement fixation is the least sensitive serologic method for diagnosis of CMV infection and should not be used to establish previous infection or passively acquired maternal antibody. Various immunofluorescence assays, indirect hemagglutination, latex agglutination, and EIAs are preferred for this purpose.

Proof of congenital infection requires obtaining specimens within 3 weeks of birth. Virus isolation is considered diagnostic. Differentiation between intrauterine and perinatal infection is difficult later in infancy, unless clinical manifestations of the former, such as chorioretinitis or ventriculitis, are present. A strongly positive test result for serum IgM anti-CMV antibody is suggestive during early infancy but not diagnostic and is less useful during later infancy.

Ebola Hemorrhagic Fever

Ebola hemorrhagic fever (Ebola HF) is a severe, often fatal disease in humans and nonhuman primates (monkeys and chimpanzees) that has appeared sporadically since its initial recognition in 1976.

The disease is caused by infection with Ebola virus, named after a river in the Democratic Republic of the Congo (formerly Zaire) where it was first recognized. The virus is one of two members of a family of RNA viruses called the Filoviridae. Three of the four subtypes of Ebola virus identified so far have caused disease in humans: Ebola Zaire, Ebola Sudan, and Ebola Ivory Coast. The fourth, Ebola Reston, has caused disease in nonhuman primates but not in humans. A closely related virus with similar symptoms is Marburg virus.

The exact origin, locations, and natural habitat (known as the "natural reservoir") of Ebola virus remain unknown. However, on the basis of available evidence and the nature of similar viruses, the virus is probably zoonotic (animal borne) and is normally maintained in an animal host that is native to the African continent. A similar host is probably associated with the Ebola Reston virus subtype isolated from infected cynomolgus monkeys that were imported to the United States and Italy from the Philippines.

Cases of Ebola HF have been reported in the Democratic Republic of the Congo, Gabon, Sudan, and the Ivory Coast. Three cases have been reported in Texas in the United States.

The manner in which the virus first appears in a human at the start of an outbreak has not been determined. The first patient probably becomes infected through contact with an infected animal.

People can be exposed to Ebola virus from direct contact with the blood or secretions of an infected person. People can also be exposed to Ebola virus through contact with objects such as needles that have been contaminated with infected secretions.

Within a few days of becoming infected with the virus, the patient develops high fever, headache, muscle aches, stomach pain, fatigue, and diarrhea, and sometimes sore throat, hiccups, rash, red and itchy eyes, vomiting of blood, and bloody diarrhea.

Within 1 week of infection with the virus, chest pain, shock, bleeding, blindness, and death result.

A protein has been identified that appears to be the key to the uncontrollable bleeding that is the hallmark of Ebola virus infection. One of the Ebola virus's seven gene products, a glycoprotein that extends out from the surface of the virus, is apparently responsible for the virus's toxic effects. The glycoprotein causes the vessels to become leaky because of massive loss of endothelial cells.

There is no standard treatment for Ebola HF. Currently, patients receive supportive therapy. Diagnosing Ebola HF in an individual who has been infected for only a few days is difficult because early symptoms, such as red and itchy eyes and a skin rash, are nonspecific to the virus and are seen in other patients with diseases that occur much more frequently.

It has been suggested that glycoprotein-inhibiting drugs might be able to help counter the deadly effects of Ebola infection, which kills up to 90% of the people it infects.

Diagnostic Tests

Antigen-capture ELISA testing, IgG ELISA testing, PCR, and virus isolation can be used to diagnose a case of Ebola HF within a few days of the onset of symptoms. Persons tested later in the course of the disease or after recovery can be tested for IgM and IgG antibodies; the disease can also be diagnosed retrospectively in deceased patients by using immunohistochemistry testing, virus isolation, or PCR.

A practical diagnostic test that uses tiny samples from patients' skin has been developed to retrospectively diagnose Ebola HF in suspected cases in which the patients have died.

Enterovirus (Nonpolio) Infections

The enteroviruses are members of the picornavirus family and include groups A and B coxsackieviruses, echoviruses, and enteroviruses.

The nonpolio enteroviruses (NPEVs) are RNA viruses, which include 23 group A coxsackieviruses (types A1–A24, except type A23), 6 group B coxsackieviruses (types B1–B6), 29 echoviruses (types 1–33, except types 10, 22, 23, and 28), and 4 enteroviruses (types 68–71).

NPEVs are responsible for significant and frequent illnesses in infants and children, usually 4–12 years of age, and result in protean clinical manifestations. The most common presentation is nonspecific febrile illness, which in young infants may lead to evaluation for bacterial sepsis. Neonates who acquire infection without maternal antibody are at risk of severe disease with a high mortality rate. Manifestations can include the following: (a) respiratory—common cold, pharyngitis, herpangina, stomatitis, pneumonia, and pleurodynia; (b) skin—exanthem; (c) neurologic—aseptic meningitis, encephalitis, and paralysis; (d) gastrointestinal—vomiting, diarrhea, abdominal pain, and hepatitis; (e) eye—acute hemorrhagic conjunctivitis; and (f) heart—myopericarditis.

Clinical Manifestations

Mild Infections

Conjunctivitis
Croup
Fever with or without rash
Hand-foot-and-mouth disease
Herpangina
Pleurodynia
Pharyngitis

Serious Infections

Acute paralysis
Hepatitis
Encephalitis
Meningitis
Myocarditis and pericarditis
Neonatal sepsis

Prevalence of Nonpolio Enterovirus Illness

Prevalence of serious illnesses as reported to the CDC

Illness	Prevalence
Meningitis	35%
Respiratory diseases	21%
Encephalitis	11%
Carditis	2%
Paralytic disease	1%

Prevalence of serious illnesses as reported from private practices

Illness	Prevalence
Stomatitis	58%
Myalgia/malaise	28%
Hand-foot-and-mouth disease	8%
Rash	3%
Pleurodynia	3%

Diagnostic Tests

Viral Culture

Specimens providing the highest rate of viral isolation are obtained from the throat, stool, and rectum. Specimens also should be obtained from any sites of clinical involvement, such as CSF. Enteroviruses also may be recovered from blood during the acute febrile phase and, rarely, from biopsy material. Specimens should be sent to the laboratory at 4°C (39°F). Repeated freezing, thawing, and drying of specimens are detrimental to viral recovery. In patients with serious illness, viral isolation as a means of diagnosis is particularly important. Viral isolation from any specimen except feces usually can be considered causally related to the patient's illness. Isolation of an enterovirus from stool alone is less specific, because some asymptomatic infected persons may shed virus in feces for as long as 6–12 weeks. Most viral diagnostic laboratories use cell culture techniques that are capable of recovering echoviruses, group B coxsackieviruses, and some group A coxsackieviruses. Suckling mouse inoculation, which is not a routine procedure, is required for recovery of certain group A coxsackievirus serotypes.

PCR testing for the presence of enterovirus RNA in CSF, which is available in a few research laboratories, is more sensitive than viral isolation. Results are available in 24 hours. NPEVs share common genomic sequences—a fact that has been exploited to develop PCR-based assays that can now identify almost all NPEVs. The PCR can work on small clinical samples and is rapid, sensitive, and specific. Enterovirus PCR has been thoroughly studied with many different clinical samples and found superior to viral culture for diagnosing NPEV infection, especially aseptic meningitis. Rapid diagnosis has been shown to decrease costs by shortening the hospital stay and reducing unnecessary use of antibiotics.

Serologic Testing

Serum samples for antibody testing can be collected at the onset of illness and 4 weeks later and stored frozen. The demonstration of a rise in titer of virus-specific neutralizing antibody can be used to confirm infection, particularly when the specific virus has been identified previously during a community outbreak. Serologic screening without a suspected serotype generally is not performed. This is of limited clinical value because it is slow and requires acute and convalescent samples.

Epstein-Barr Virus Infections

Epstein-Barr virus (EBV), a DNA virus, is a B-lymphotropic herpesvirus and is the most common cause of infectious mononucleosis.

Infectious mononucleosis is manifested typically by fever, exudative pharyngitis, lymphadenopathy, hepatosplenomegaly, and atypical lymphocytosis. The spectrum of diseases is variable, ranging from asymptomatic to fatal infection. Infections frequently are unrecognized in infants and children. Rash can occur and is more frequent in patients treated with ampicillin as well as with penicillin. CNS complications include aseptic meningitis, encephalitis, and Guillain-Barré syndrome. Rare complications include splenic rupture, thrombocytopenia, agranulocytosis, hemolytic anemia, hemophagocytic syndrome, orchitis, and myocarditis. Replication of EBV in B lymphocytes and the resulting lymphoproliferation usually is inhibited by natural killer and T-cell responses, but in patients who have congenital or acquired cellular immune deficiencies, fatal disseminated infection or B-cell lymphomas can occur.

EBV causes several other distinct disorders, including the X-linked lymphoproliferative syndrome (also known as *Duncan syndrome*), posttransplantation lymphoproliferative disorders, Burkitt lymphoma, nasopharyngeal carcinoma, and undifferentiated B-cell lymphoma of the CNS. The X-linked lymphoproliferative syndrome occurs in adolescent boys with an inherited, maternally derived, recessive genetic defect characterized by several phenotypic expressions, including occurrence of infectious mononucleosis early in life, nodular B-cell lymphomas, often with CNS involvement, and profound hypogammaglobulinemia.

Diagnostic Tests

Isolation of EBV from oropharyngeal secretions is possible, but techniques for performing this procedure usually are not available in routine diagnostic laboratories, and viral isolation does not necessarily indicate acute infection.

Multiple specific serologic antibody tests for EBV are available in diagnostic virology laboratories. The most commonly performed test is for antibody against the viral capsid antigen (VCA). Because IgG antibody against VCA occurs in high titers early after onset of infection, testing of acute and convalescent serum samples for anti-VCA may not be useful for establishing the presence of infection. Testing for IgM anti-VCA antibody and for antibodies against early antigen is useful for identifying recent infections. Because serum antibody against EBV nuclear antigen is not present until several weeks to months after onset of the infection, a positive result on tests for antibody to EBV nuclear antigen excludes acute infection.

Nonspecific tests for heterophil antibody, including the Paul-Bunnell test and slide agglutination reaction, are most commonly available. The results of these tests are often negative in infants and children <4 years of age with EBV infection, but they identify approximately 90% of cases (proven by EBV-specific serology) in older children and adults. An absolute increase in atypical lymphocytes in the second week of illness with infectious mononucleosis is a characteristic but not specific finding.

Serologic tests for EBV are particularly useful for evaluating patients who have heterophil-negative infectious mononucleosis. Testing for other viral agents, especially CMV, is indicated for these patients. In research studies, culture of saliva or peripheral blood mononuclear cells for EBV, *in situ* DNA hybridization, or PCR can determine the presence of EBV or EBV DNA.

Hantavirus Cardiopulmonary Syndrome

Hantaviruses are RNA viruses of the Bunyaviridae family that in humans cause Hantavirus cardiopulmonary syndrome (HPS) or hemorrhagic fever with renal syndrome. Within the Hantavirus genus, the viruses associated with HPS in the Americas include Sin Nombre virus (SNV), a major cause of HPS in the United States, and Bayou virus, Black Creek Canal virus, and the New York virus, sporadic causes in Louisiana, Florida, and New York, respectively. In recent years, new Hantavirus serotypes, including Andes virus associated with an HPS-like syndrome, have been isolated in South America.

The prodromal illness of 3–7 days is characterized by fever; chills; headache; myalgias of the shoulders, lower back, and thighs; nausea; vomiting; diarrhea; and dizziness. Respiratory tract symptoms or signs do not occur for the first 3–7 days until pulmonary edema and severe hypoxemia appear abruptly and progress over a few hours. In severe cases, persistent hypotension caused by myocardial dysfunction is present—hence the name.

The extensive bilateral interstitial and alveolar pulmonary edema and pleural effusions are the result of a diffuse pulmonary capillary leak and seem to be immune mediated. Intubation usually is required for 2–4 days, with resolution heralded by the onset of diuresis and rapid clinical improvement. There are no necrotic pulmonary parenchymal changes.

The severe myocardial depression is different from that of septic shock; the cardiac indices and the stroke volume index are low, the pulmonary wedge pressure is normal, and the systemic vascular resistance is increased. Poor prognostic indicators include persistent hypotension, marked hemoconcentration, a cardiac index of <2, and the abrupt onset of lactic acidosis with a serum lactate level of >4 mmol/L (>36 mg/dL).

The mortality rate for patients with cardiopulmonary disease is 45%. Asymptomatic disease and mild disease are rare in adults, but limited information suggests they may be more common in children. Permanent sequelae are uncommon.

Diagnostic Tests

Characteristic laboratory values include a neutrophilic leukocytosis with immature granulocytes, >10% immunoblasts (basophilic cytoplasm, prominent nucleoli, and an increased nuclear/cytoplasmic ratio), thrombocytopenia, and elevated hematocrit. In fatal cases, SNV has been identified by immunohistochemical staining in capillary endothelial cells in almost every organ in the body.

The SNV RNA has been detected uniformly by RT-PCR in peripheral blood mononuclear cells and other clinical specimens from the first few days of hospitalization up to 10–21 days after symptom onset. Viral RNA is not detected readily in bronchoalveolar lavage fluids, and the duration of viremia is unknown.

Hantavirus-specific IgG and IgM antibodies are present when the cardiopulmonary manifestations begin. A rapid diagnostic test can facilitate early transfer to a tertiary care facility, result in immediate appropriate supportive therapy, and permit early enrollment in antiviral trials. The rapid immunoblot assay is a dipstick-like assay that takes 5 hours, requires minimal equipment, and can be used in rural laboratories. Immunohistochemical staining can identify hantaviral antigens in formalin-fixed tissues.

EIA (available through many state health departments and the CDC) and Western blot are assays that use recombinant antigens and have a high degree of specificity for detection of IgG and IgM heterologous and homologous antiviral antigens. CDC is distributing ELISA assays to state laboratories to detect IgG and IgM.

Hepatitis A

[Antibody to Hepatitis A Virus (HAV) IgM; Anti–HAV IgM; HAV Antibody IgM.]

HAV is an RNA virus classified as a member of the picornavirus group, and antibodies are made to capsid proteins.

Hepatitis A characteristically is an acute self-limited illness characterized by fever, malaise, jaundice, anorexia, and nausea. Asymptomatic hepatitis occurs in approximately 30% of infected children <6 years of age; few of these children have jaundice. Among older children and adults, infection usually is symptomatic and typically lasts several weeks, with jaundice occurring in approximately 70%. Prolonged or relapsing disease lasting as long as 6 months can occur. Fulminant hepatitis is rare but is more frequent in persons with underlying liver disease.

Diagnostic Tests

A 1-mL specimen of serum or plasma is required for EIA. Serum IgM is present at the onset of illness and usually disappears within 4 months but may persist for 6 months or longer. Presence of serum IgM indicates current or recent infection, although false-positive results can occur. Anti–HAV IgG is detectable shortly after the appearance of IgM. Fecal excretion of HAV peaks before symptoms develop. Hepatitis A antibody of IgG type indicative of old infection is found in almost 50% of adults and is not usually clinically relevant. Many cases of hepatitis A are subclinical. Presence of IgG antibody to HAV does not exclude acute hepatitis B or hepatitis C.

Hepatitis B

Hepatitis B virus (HBV) is a DNA virus with a protein coat, the surface antigen (HBsAg), and a nucleic acid core, the core antigen (HBcAg). There are eight different serotypes. Early in infection, HBsAg, HBV DNA, and DNA polymerase can all be detected in serum.

HBV causes a wide spectrum of manifestations, ranging from asymptomatic seroconversion, subacute illness with nonspecific symptoms (e.g., anorexia, nausea, or malaise) or extrahepatic symptoms, and clinical hepatitis with jaundice, to fulminant fatal hepatitis. Anicteric or asymptomatic infection is most common in young children. Arthralgias, arthritis, or macular rashes can occur early in the course of the illness.

The presence of HBsAg is the earliest indicator of acute infection. HBsAg can be detected 1–7 weeks before liver enzyme elevation or the appearance of clinical symptoms. Three weeks after the onset of acute hepatitis, approximately 50% of the patients are still positive for HBsAg, whereas at 17 weeks only 10% are positive. The best available markers for infectivity are HBsAg and hepatitis B early antigen (HBeAg). The presence of antibodies to HBsAg (anti-HBs) is associated with noninfectivity. If the infection is self-limited, HBsAg disappears in most patients before serum anti-HBs can be detected. Patients who are negative for HBsAg may still have acute type B viral hepatitis. There is sometimes a "core window" stage during which HBsAg is no longer detectable and the patient has not yet developed the antibody (anti-HBs). On such occasions, antibodies to HBcAg (anti-HBc) are usually detectable and anti-HBc IgM is the only specific marker for the diagnosis of acute infection. In cases in which there is strong clinical suspicion of viral hepatitis, serologic testing should not be limited to detecting HBsAg but should include a battery of tests to evaluate different stages of acute and convalescent hepatitis. The chronic carrier state is indicated by the persistence of HBsAg or HBeAg over long periods (6 months to years) without seroconversion to the corresponding antibodies. Chronic HBV infection with persistence of HBsAg occurs in as many as 90% of infants infected by perinatal transmission. Chronic HBV infection occurs in an average of 30% of children 1–5 years of age infected after birth and in 2–6% of older children, adolescents, and adults with HBV infection. Although <10% of new HBV infections occur in children, approximately one-third of the 1.25 million Americans with chronic HBV infection are estimated to have acquired their infection as infants or young children based on the higher risk of chronic infection during childhood. Chronically infected persons are at increased risk for developing chronic liver disease (e.g., cirrhosis, chronic active hepatitis, or chronic persistent hepatitis) or primary hepatocellular carcinoma in later life. The risk of death due to HBV-related liver cancer or cirrhosis is approximately 25% for persons who become chronically infected during early childhood.

Anti-HBc IgM is highly specific for establishing the diagnosis of acute infection because it is present early in the infection and during the window phase in older children and adults. At times this marker is the only one demonstrated for the diagnosis of a hepatitis B viral infection. The test for this marker uses the microparticle enzyme immunoassay method. However, IgM anti-HBc usually is not present in infants infected perinatally. Both anti-HBs and anti-HBc are detected in persons with resolved infection, whereas anti-HBs alone is present in persons immunized with hepatitis B vaccine.

HBeAg appears in acute hepatitis B with or shortly after HBsAg, when the patient is most infectious. HBeAg is probably a degradation product of HBcAg and is found only in HBsAg-positive sera. During the HBeAg-positive state, usually 3–6 weeks, hepatitis B patients are at increased risk of transmitting the virus to their contacts, including babies born during this period. Exposure to serum or body fluid positive for HBeAg and HBsAg is associated with a three to five times greater risk of infectivity than when HBsAg positivity occurs alone. The presence of HBeAg is associated with chronic liver disease. Tests for HBeAg and HBV DNA are useful in selecting candidates to receive antiviral therapy and in monitoring the response to therapy.

The appearance of antibodies to HBeAg (anti-HBe) in patients who have previously been HBeAg positive indicates a reduced risk of infectivity. Failure of appearance implies disease activity, but patients with anti-HBe may have chronic hepatitis. Chronic HBsAg carriers can be positive for either HBeAg or anti-HBe, but are less infectious when anti-HBe is present. Anti-HBe can persist for years but usually disappears earlier than anti-HBs or anti-HBc. HBeAb has not been found as the sole serologic marker for HBV infection.

Diagnostic Tests

Diagnostic tests for HBV antigens and antibodies are shown in Table 4.

Commercial serologic antigen tests are available to detect HBsAg and HBeAg. Assays also are available for detection of anti-HBs, total anti-HBc, and IgM anti-HBc, and

Table 4. Diagnostic Tests for Hepatitis B Virus Antigens and Antibodies

Factor to Be Tested	HBV Antigen or Antibody	Use
HBsAg	Hepatitis B surface antigen	Detection of acute or chronic infection; antigen used in hepatitis B vaccine
Anti-HBs	Antibody to HBsAg	Identification of persons who have resolved infections with HBV; determination of immunity after immunization
HBeAg	Hepatitis B early antigen	Identification of infected persons at increased risk for transmitting HBV
Anti-HBe	Antibody to HBeAg	Identification of infected persons with lower risk for transmitting HBV
Anti-HBc	Antibody to HBcAg[a]	Identification of persons with acute, resolved, or chronic HBV infection (not present after immunization)
IgM anti-HBc	IgM antibody to HBcAg	Identification of acute or recent HBV infections (including those in HBsAg-negative persons during the "window" phase of infection)

HBV, hepatitis B virus; IgM, immunoglobulin M.
[a]No test is available commercially to measure hepatitis B core antigen (HBcAg).
From Pickering LK, ed. *2000 Red Book: Report of the Committee on Infectious Diseases*, 25th ed. Section 3. Elk Grove Village, IL: American Academy of Pediatrics, 2000:291.

gene amplification techniques (e.g., PCR, branched DNA methods) are available to detect and quantitate HBV DNA. Tests are performed on serum or plasma. After separation (2 mL), the specimen is refrigerated. Blood donors should be tested (HBsAg-positive individuals are rejected).

The presence of anti-HBs is an indicator of clinical recovery and subsequent immunity to HBV. This test is useful for evaluation of possible immunity in individuals who are at risk for exposure to hepatitis B (hemodialysis unit personnel, venipuncturists, etc.). The need for hepatitis B immune globulin should be evaluated after needlestick injury; the need for hepatitis B vaccine should be evaluated, and immune status should be followed after hepatitis B vaccination.

Patients with anti-HBs are not overtly infective. Presence of the antibody without the presence of the antigen is evidence for immunity from reinfection with virus of the same subtype HBsAb.

Hepatitis B Core Antibody (Immunoglobulin G and Immunoglobulin M Differentiation)

HBcAg is detected in serum or in plasma and requires a 2-mL specimen using an EIA. It is useful in assessing hepatitis B virus infection.

Hepatitis Surface B Antigen (Hepatitis-Associated Antigen)

Persistence of HBsAg without anti-HBs, combined with positivity for anti-HBc, HBeAg, or anti-HBe, indicates infectivity and need for investigation for chronic persistent or chronic aggressive hepatitis.

Quantitative Determination of Hepatitis B Virus DNA

Method used is HBV hybrid capture or nucleic acid hybridization.

A serum specimen should be stored frozen.

Nucleic acid hybridization is used to detect and quantify HBV DNA.

A negative result does not exclude the possibility of HBV infection, because very low levels of infection or sampling error may cause a false-negative result.

Hepatitis C

Hepatitis C virus (HCV) is a small, single-stranded RNA virus and is a member of the flavivirus family. Multiple HCV genotypes exist that fail to elicit cross-neutralizing antibodies in animal models.

The signs and symptoms of HCV infection usually are indistinguishable from those of hepatitis A or B. Acute disease tends to be mild and insidious in onset, and in children, most infections are asymptomatic. Jaundice occurs in 25% of patients, and abnormalities in liver function tests generally are less pronounced than those in patients with HBV infection. Persistent infection with HCV occurs in 75–85% of infected persons, even in the absence of biochemical evidence of liver disease. Most children with chronic infection are asymptomatic. Chronic hepatitis develops in 60–70% of chronically infected patients, and cirrhosis develops in 10–20%; primary hepatocellular carcinoma can occur in these patients. Infection with HCV is the leading reason for liver transplantation in the United States. Because as many as 90% of commercial intravenous immunoglobulins test positive for HCV antibody, an artifactual positive test result can occur briefly after transfusion. A repeatedly reactive result may not necessarily constitute a diagnosis of hepatitis C (non-A, non-B hepatitis) or indicate the presence of antibody to HPC. It is suggested that a supplemental assay (*r*ecombinant *i*mmuno*b*lot *a*ssay, or RIBA, which requires 1 mL serum or plasma) be ordered to obtain stronger evidence of the presence of antibodies to HCV (anti-HCV). Since the development of sensitive and specific testing for hepatitis B, 90% of posttransfusion hepatitis is non-A, non-B hepatitis. HCV is the most common cause of non-A, non-B hepatitis in the United States. A gene product of HCV (c100) was isolated and an assay for anti-HCV developed. The assay detects antibody to a presumptive togavirus or flavivirus that may be an etiologic agent of non-A, non-B hepatitis (which may not be a unitary disease entity).

Diagnostic Tests

The two major types of tests available for the laboratory diagnosis of HCV infections are (1) antibody assays for anti-HCV and (2) assays to detect HCV RNA. Diagnosis by antibody assays involves an initial screening EIA; repeated positive results are confirmed by a RIBA, analogous to testing for HIV infection. Both assays detect IgG antibody; no IgM assays are available. The current EIA and RIBA assays are at least 97% sensitive and >95% specific. False-negative test findings early in the course of acute infection result from the prolonged interval between exposure or onset of illness and seroconversion that may occur. Within 15 weeks after exposure and within 5–6 weeks after the onset of hepatitis, 80% of patients have positive test results for serum HCV antibody.

Highly sensitive PCR assays for detection of HCV RNA are available from several commercial laboratories. HCV RNA can be detected in serum or plasma within 1–2 weeks after exposure to the virus and weeks before onset of liver enzyme abnormalities or appearance of anti-HCV. Although not approved by the U.S. Food and Drug Administration (FDA), PCR assays for HCV infection are used commonly in clinical practice for the early diagnosis of infection, for identification of infection in infants early in life (i.e., perinatal transmission) when maternal serum antibody interferes with the ability to detect antibody produced by the infant, and for monitoring patients receiving antiviral therapy. However, false-positive and false-negative results can occur from improper handling, storage, and contamination of the test samples. Viral RNA may be detected intermittently, and thus a single negative PCR assay result is not conclusive. Quantitative assays for measuring the concentration of HCV RNA also are available but are not standardized, and the clinical value of these assays is not yet established.

Although HCV is believed responsible for most or all cases of non-A, non-B hepatitis, other viruses not yet identified may also be involved in the pathogenesis of the disease. A positive test for anti-HCV indicates past or present infection but does not necessarily constitute a diagnosis. A positive anti-HCV result by EIA not confirmed by RIBA does not rule out the possibility of infection with HCV. All individuals for whom results are indeterminate should be retested and followed for at least 6–12 months.

Hepatitis C Virus Antibody Testing of Blood

An EIA is used to assess exposure to HCV and to test blood units for transfusion safety.

For blood donors, hepatitis C serologic results correlate with those of surrogate tests for non-A, non-B hepatitis (alanine aminotransferase and anti-HBc). Because hepatitis C serologic testing identifies a broader group of infected individuals than surrogate testing, its use reduces risk of HCV infection during transfusion. Studies involving hemophiliacs indicate that antibody to HCV is a reliable marker of HCV infection.

Hepatitis Panel

The hepatitis panel test includes measurement of HAV antibody, total; HBc antibody, total; HBs antibody; HBsAg; and HCV antibody, and can be used at all stages of infection.

Hepatitis D

The hepatitis D virus (HDV) is a 36- to 43-nm particle consisting of an RNA genome and a delta protein antigen (HDAg), both of which are coated with HBsAg.

HDV infection causes hepatitis only in persons with acute or chronic HBV infection; the HDV requires HBV as a helper virus and cannot produce infection in the absence of HBV. The importance of HDV infection lies in its ability to convert an asymptomatic or mild chronic HBV infection into a fulminant, more severe, or rapidly progressive disease. Acute coinfection with HBV and HDV usually causes an acute illness indistinguishable from acute HBV infection alone, except that the likelihood of fulminant hepatitis can be as high as 5%.

Diagnostic Tests

Radioimmunoassay and EIA for anti-HDV antibody are available commercially, usually at referral laboratories. Tests for IgM-specific anti-HDV antibody and HDAg are research procedures at present. If markers for HDV infection exist, coinfection with HBV usually can be differentiated from superinfection of an established HBsAg carrier by testing for IgM HBc antibody; absence of this core antibody suggests that the person is an HBsAg carrier. Methods for detection of HDV RNA are available.

Hepatitis E

The hepatitis E virus (HEV) is a spherical, nonenveloped, positive-stranded RNA virus and is the only known agent of enterally transmitted non-A, non-B hepatitis. HEV formerly was classified in the family Caliciviridae, genus Calicivirus; however, HEV has been reclassified into an unassigned genus of "hepatitis E–like" viruses because certain characteristics distinguish HEV from typical caliciviruses.

Hepatitis E is an acute illness characterized by jaundice, malaise, anorexia, fever, abdominal pain, and arthralgia. Subclinical infection also occurs.

Diagnostic Tests

The diagnosis of acute HEV infection can be made by detecting IgM antibody to HEV in serum or by detecting HEV RNA by PCR in serum or feces. Serologic and PCR-based assays for the diagnosis of acute HEV infection are available in research and commercial laboratories. However, none of these assays is approved by the FDA. Health care professionals who require information about HEV diagnostic tests may contact the Hepatitis Branch of the CDC at 404-639-3048; fax: 404-639-1538. The CDC criteria for considering whether an acute-phase serum specimen should be tested for evidence of HEV infection include a discrete onset of illness with jaundice or with a serum alanine aminotransferase level at least 2.5 times the upper limit of normal and negative test results for IgM antibody to HAV, IgM antibody to HBcAg, and antibody to HCV.

Hepatitis G

The hepatitis G virus (HGV) is a single-stranded RNA virus that is included in the Flaviviridae family and shares a 27% homology with HCV. The HGV has not yet been isolated.

Although HGV can cause chronic infection and viremia, it is a rare cause of hepatic inflammation, and most infected persons are asymptomatic. Histologic evidence of HGV infection is rare, and serum aminotransferase concentrations usually are normal. Although high levels of HGV RNA are found in blood, the liver is not a significant site of replication. Currently, no conclusive evidence indicates that HGV causes fulminant or chronic disease, and coinfection does not seem to worsen the course or severity of concurrent infection with HBV or HCV.

Diagnostic Tests

Currently, HGV infection can be diagnosed only by identifying viral genomes using PCR assay, which is not widely available. No serologic test is available.

Herpes Simplex (Human Herpesvirus 1 and 2 Infections)

In newborns, HSV infection can manifest as the following: (a) disseminated disease involving multiple organs, most prominently the liver and lungs, 25%; (b) localized CNS disease, 35%; or (c) disease localized to the skin, eyes, and mouth, 40%. Clinical overlap may occur among disease types. In many neonates with disseminated or CNS disease, skin lesions do not develop or the lesions appear late. In the absence of skin lesions, the diagnosis of neonatal HSV infection is difficult. Disseminated infection should be considered in neonates with sepsis syndrome, negative bacterial culture results, and severe liver dysfunction. HSV also should be considered as a causative agent in neonates with fever and irritability, and when other sexually transmitted diseases have been acquired.

Inoculation of skin occurs from direct contact with HSV-containing oral or genital secretions. This contact can result in herpes gladiatorum among wrestlers, herpes rugbiaforum among rugby players, or herpetic whitlow of the fingers in any exposed person.

HSV frequently is transmitted by infected persons who are shedding the virus asymptomatically. Patients with primary gingivostomatitis or genital herpes usually shed the virus for at least 1 week and occasionally for several weeks. Patients with recurrent infection shed the virus for a much shorter period, typically 3–4 days. Intermittent asymptomatic reactivation of oral and genital herpes is common and persists for life. The greatest concentration of virus is shed during symptomatic primary infections.

HSV encephalitis is the most commonly identified type of severe sporadic viral encephalitis in the United States. Its estimated annual incidence is 1 in 250,000 to 1 in 500,000 persons. HSV encephalitis accounts for approximately 20% of the reported cases of encephalitis in the United States. The peak of incidence is in late childhood and middle age. There is no seasonal incidence of HSV infection.

Neuroimaging with the head using computed tomographic (CT) scanning or MRI is generally regarded as the initial diagnostic measure. MRI is much more sensitive and often reveals highly characteristic abnormalities, including the virtually pathognomonic increased signal abnormalities on T2-weighted sequences in the medial temporal and insular cortical regions and inferior frontal cingulate gyri. The lesions are often bilateral.

Genital infection with HSV type 2 (HSV-2) usually results from sexual intercourse, whereas genital infection with HSV type 1 (HSV-1) usually results from oral-genital contact. After primary genital infection, which often is asymptomatic, some persons experience frequent clinical recurrences, whereas others have no recurrences. Genital HSV-2 infection is more likely to recur than is genital infection caused by HSV-1.

The incubation period for HSV infection occurring beyond the neonatal period ranges from 2 days to 2 weeks.

Diagnostic Tests

HSV grows readily in cell culture. Special transport media are available for specimens that cannot be inoculated immediately onto susceptible cell culture media. Cytopathogenic effects typical of HSV usually are observed 1–3 days after inoculation. Methods for culture confirmation include fluorescent antibody staining and EIA. Cultures that still show negative results by day 12 are likely to continue to remain negative. Rapid diagnostic techniques also are available, such as DFA staining of vesicle scrapings or EIA detection of HSV antigens. These techniques are as specific as culture but slightly less sensitive. Typing of HSV strains differentiates between HSV-1 and HSV-2 isolates. PCR is a sensitive method for detecting HSV DNA and is of particular value for evaluating CSF specimens from cases of suspected herpes encephalitis. Histologic examination of lesions for the presence of multinucleated giant cells and eosinophilic intranuclear inclusions typical of HSV (Tzanck preparation) has low sensitivity.

For the diagnosis of neonatal HSV infection, specimens for culture should be obtained from skin vesicles, mouth or nasopharynx, eyes, urine, blood, stool or rectum, and

CSF. Positive results for cultures obtained from any of these sites >48 hours after birth indicate viral replication, which suggests infant infection rather than colonization after intrapartum exposure.

Serologic tests generally are not helpful for the diagnosis of acute HSV infections. Serum samples often are obtained late in the clinical course, and an increase in antibody titers may be missed. Furthermore, recurrent infections may boost preexisting antibody titers. An additional problem with serologic diagnosis is the extensive cross reaction between antibodies against HSV-1 and those against HSV-2; despite claims to the contrary, most commercial assays for HSV antibody generally cannot differentiate between HSV-1 and HSV-2 infection. A new assay based on the type-specific glycoprotein G has substantially improved determination of the type and is becoming more widely available. IgM HSV antibody assays are poorly standardized and are not helpful for diagnosing acute HSV infection.

HSV DNA in CSF frequently can be detected by PCR in patients with HSV encephalitis, and PCR is the diagnostic method of choice when performed by experienced laboratory personnel. Histologic examination and viral culture of brain tissue obtained by biopsy are the most definitive methods for confirming the diagnosis of encephalitis caused by HSV. Cultures of CSF for HSV usually are negative.

Human Herpesvirus 6 and 7 Infections (Including Roseola)

Human herpesvirus 6 (HHV-6) and human herpesvirus 7 (HHV-7) are members of the family Herpesviridae, which contains a large, double-stranded DNA genome. Strains of HHV-6 belong to one of two major groups, variants A and B. Almost all primary infections in children are caused by variant B strains. HHV-7 is a member of the Betaherpesvirus subfamily and is closely related to human CMV and HHV-6.

Major clinical manifestations of primary infection with HHV-6 are variable in children <3 years of age. These manifestations include roseola (exanthem subitum, sixth disease) in approximately 20% of children, undifferentiated febrile illness without rash or localizing signs, and other acute febrile illnesses, often accompanied by cervical and postoccipital lymphadenopathy, gastrointestinal or respiratory tract signs, and inflamed tympanic membranes. Fever is characteristically high [>39.5°C (103.0°F)] and persists for 3–7 days. In roseola, fever is preceded, occurs during, or is followed by an erythematous maculopapular rash lasting hours to days. Seizures, which result in emergency department visits, occur during the febrile period in 10–15% of primary infections. A bulging anterior fontanelle and encephalopathy occur occasionally.

The virus persists and may reactivate. The clinical circumstances and manifestations of reactivation in healthy persons are unclear. Illness associated with reactivation has been described primarily in immunosuppressed hosts in association with manifestations such as fever, hepatitis, bone marrow suppression, pneumonia, and encephalitis. Recognition of the varied clinical manifestations of HHV-7 infection is evolving. Many, if not most, primary infections with HHV-7 may be asymptomatic or mild; some may present as typical roseola and may account for second or recurrent cases of roseola. Some investigators suggest that the association of HHV-7 with these clinical manifestations results from the ability of HHV-7 to reactivate HHV-6 from latency, particularly variant B, which causes roseola and other primary HHV-6 infections.

Diagnostic Tests

Clinical presentation is reliable and diagnostic in most cases. The laboratory diagnosis of primary HHV-6 infection currently necessitates use of research techniques to isolate the virus form in peripheral blood, as well as to demonstrate seroconversion. A fourfold increase in serum antibody levels alone does not necessarily indicate new infection, as an increase in titer also may occur with reactivation and in association with other infections. Commercial assays for antibody and antigen detection and PCR tests for detecting HHV-6 DNA are in development.

Diagnostic tests for HHV-7 are limited to research laboratories, and reliable differentiation between primary and reactivated infection is problematic. Serodiagnosis of HHV-7 is confounded by serologic cross reactivity with HHV-6 and by the potential ability of HHV-6 to be reactivated by HHV-7 infection and possibly by other infections.

Human Herpesvirus 8 Infections

Human herpesvirus 8 (HHV-8) is a member of the family Herpesviridae, the gammaherpesvirus subfamily closely related to herpesvirus saimiri of monkeys and to EBV.

For children, the clinical implications of this most recently discovered member of the herpesvirus family, HHV-8, are unknown. In adults, HHV-8 is the probable etiologic agent of Kaposi sarcoma. The HHV-8 DNA sequences have been detected in all forms of Kaposi sarcoma from all parts of the world in patients with and without HIV infection, in primary effusion lymphomas of the abdominal cavity, in lymphoproliferative syndrome (although less commonly than EBV), and in multicentric Castleman disease. Evidence of HHV-8 infection in children thus far seems rare, and no clinical associations are known.

Diagnostic Tests

Diagnostic tests for detection of HHV-8 infections are limited to research laboratories, and reliable differentiation of primary versus latent infection is questionable.

Human Immunodeficiency Virus Infections

HIV infection in children and adolescents causes a broad spectrum of disease and a varied clinical course. AIDS represents the most severe end of the clinical spectrum. The pediatric classification system that was established for surveillance of HIV infection emphasizes the importance of the $CD4^+$ T-lymphocyte count as an immunologic surrogate and prognosis marker but does not use information on viral load as quantitated by RNA PCR.

The manifestations of HIV infection include generalized lymphadenopathy, hepatomegaly, splenomegaly, failure to thrive, oral candidiasis, recurrent diarrhea, parotitis, cardiomyopathy, hepatitis, nephropathy, CNS disease (including developmental delay, which can be progressive), lymphoid interstitial pneumonia, recurrent invasive bacterial infections, opportunistic infections, and specific malignant neoplasms.

The risk of infection for an infant born to an HIV-seropositive mother who did not receive antiretroviral therapy during pregnancy is estimated to be between 13% and 39%. The exact timing of transmission from an infected mother to her infant is uncertain, but evidence suggests that approximately 30% of transmissions occur before birth and 70% occur around the time of delivery. Available evidence suggests that two-thirds of the infections occurring before delivery are due to transmission of virus within the last 14 days before delivery. Higher rates of perinatal transmission occur in women who seroconvert during pregnancy or during the postpartum period if they breast-feed. In vaginal deliveries, a first-born twin is at greater risk of HIV infection than a second-born twin. Prolonged rupture of membranes, even in the presence of antiretroviral therapy, is associated with an increased risk of transmission and must be considered when evaluating the mode of delivery and transmission.

Diagnostic Tests

The laboratory diagnosis of HIV infection during infancy depends on detection of virus or viral nucleic acid. The transplacental transfer of antibody complicates the serologic diagnosis of infant infection.

HIV nucleic acid detection by PCR of DNA extracted from peripheral blood mononuclear cells is the preferred test for diagnosis of HIV infection in infants, and results can be available within 24 hours of obtaining a sample of anticoagulated whole blood. Approximately 30% of infants with HIV infection have a positive DNA PCR result from samples obtained before 48 hours of age. The test can detect 1–10 DNA copies routinely. Approximately 93% of infected infants have detectable HIV DNA by 2 weeks of age, and almost all infants are HIV positive by 1 month of age. A single DNA PCR assay has a sensitivity of 95% and a specificity of 97% on samples collected from 1 to 36 months of age. DNA PCR is more sensitive on a single assay than is virus culture, and virus need not be replication competent to be detected.

Virus isolation by culture is expensive, available only in a few laboratories, and requires up to 28 days for positive results. This test has largely been replaced by DNA PCR testing.

Detection of the p24 antigen (including immune complex dissociated) is specific but significantly less sensitive than DNA PCR or culture. An additional drawback is the occurrence of false-positive test results in samples obtained from infants <1 month of age.

Plasma HIV RNA PCR may be used to diagnose HIV infection if the result is positive. However, the results of this test may be negative in HIV-infected persons. The test is licensed by the FDA only in quantitative format and currently is used for quantifying the amount of virus present as a measurement of disease progression, not for diagnosis of HIV infection in infants.

Infants born to HIV-infected women should be tested by HIV DNA PCR during the first 48 hours of life. Because of possible contamination with maternal blood, umbilical cord blood should not be used for this determination. A second test should be performed at 1–2 months of age. A third test is recommended at 3–6 months of age. Any time test results are positive for an infant, testing is repeated on a second blood sample as soon as possible to confirm the diagnosis. An infant is considered infected if two separate samples are positive. Infection can be reasonably excluded when two HIV DNA PCR assays performed at or beyond 1 month of age show negative results and at least one assay was performed on a sample obtained at ≥4 months of age. Alternatively, an infant for whom test results are negative for HIV antibody on two blood samples obtained after 6 months of age and at an interval of at least 1 month also can be considered not infected.

EIAs are used most widely as the initial test for serum HIV antibody. These tests are highly sensitive and specific. Repeated EIA testing of initially reactive specimens is required to reduce the small likelihood of laboratory error. Western blot or IFA tests should be used for confirmation, which will overcome the problem of a false-positive EIA result. A positive HIV antibody test result in a child ≥18 months of age usually indicates infection.

Serum antibodies to HIV are present in almost all infected persons, with the exception of a small minority who are hypogammaglobulinemic and the few persons with AIDS who become seronegative late in the disease. Some infants who receive combination antiretroviral therapy within 2–3 months of age also lose detectable antibody but remain infected.

The most notable finding is a high viral load (as measured by RNA PCR) that does not decline rapidly during the first year of life unless combination antiretroviral therapy is initiated. As the disease progresses, there is an increasing loss of cell-mediated immunity. The peripheral blood lymphocyte count at birth and during the first years of infection can be normal, but eventually lymphopenia develops because of a decrease in the total number of circulating CD4 lymphocytes. The T-suppressor $CD8^+$ lymphocyte count usually increases initially, and cells are not depleted until late in the course of the infection. These changes in cell populations result in a decrease of the normal $CD4^+/CD8^+$ cell ratio. This nonspecific finding, although characteristic of HIV infection, also occurs with other acute viral infections, including infections caused by CMV and EBV. The normal values for peripheral $CD4^+$ lymphocyte counts and percentages are age related.

Laboratory Diagnosis of Human Immunodeficiency Virus Infection

See Table 5.

Perinatal Human Immunodeficiency Virus Serologic Testing

The American Academy of Pediatrics (AAP) recommendations include the following:

- On the basis of recent advances in effective prophylaxis to reduce the rate of perinatal HIV transmission, the AAP recommends routinely offering counseling and testing with consent to all pregnant women in the United States. Consent for maternal HIV testing may be obtained in a variety of ways, including by right of refusal, that is, with testing to take place unless rejected in writing by the patient. The AAP supports use of consent procedures that facilitate rapid incorporation of HIV education and testing into routine medical care settings. For women who are examined by a health care professional for the first time in labor and have not been tested for HIV infection during the current pregnancy, counseling and immediate testing should be considered because administration of antiretroviral therapy during labor is recommended and may diminish transmission. Careful attention to further education about HIV infection is recommended during the perinatal period.
- Routine education about HIV infection and testing should be a part of a comprehensive program of health care for women.
- For newborn infants whose mother's HIV antibody status was not determined during pregnancy or the postpartum period, the infant's health care professional

Table 5. Laboratory Diagnosis of Human Immunodeficiency Virus Infection

Test	Comment
HIV DNA PCR	Preferred test to diagnose HIV infection in infants and children <18 mo of age; high sensitive and specific by 2 wk of age and available; performed on peripheral blood mononuclear cells.
HIV p24 Ag	Less sensitive, false-positive results during first month of life, variable results; not recommended.
ICD p24 Ag	Commonly available; negative test result does not rule out infection; not recommended.
HIV culture	Expensive, not easily available, requires up to 4 wk to do test.
HIV RNA PCR	Not recommended for routine testing of infants and children <18 mo of age because negative results cannot be used to exclude HIV infection.
CD4/CD8 ratio	Performed on whole blood and peripheral blood fibrin; determined by flow cytometry; CD4 (helper T cells) are decreased and CD4 (suppressor T cells) are increased, not specific; CD4 cell counts may be used for prognostic purposes and to monitor disease progression and antiretroviral therapy.

Ag, antigen; HIV, human immunodeficiency virus; ICD, immune complex dissociated; PCR, polymerase chain reaction.
From Pickering LK, ed. *2000 Red Book: Report of the Committee on Infectious Diseases*, 25th ed. Section 3. Elk Grove Village, IL: American Academy of Pediatrics, 2000:332.

should inform the mother about the potential benefits of HIV testing for her infant and the possible risks and benefits to herself of knowing the child's serostatus and recommend immediate HIV testing for the newborn.
- In the absence of known maternal HIV antibody status and parental availability for consent to test the newborn for HIV antibody, procedures should be established to facilitate rapid evaluation and testing of the infant.
- The health care professional for the infant should be informed of maternal HIV sterostatus so that appropriate care and testing of the infant can be accomplished. Similarly, if the infant is found to be seropositive but maternal HIV infection was unknown, the child's health care professional should ensure that this information and its significance be provided to the mother and, with her consent, to her health care professional.
- Comprehensive HIV-related medical services should be accessible to all infected mothers, their infants, and other family members.
- The AAP supports legislation and public policy directed toward eliminating any form of discrimination based on HIV serostatus.

Diagnostic Criteria for Human Immunodeficiency Virus Infection[7]

Criteria for Infection in Adults and Children Older Than Eighteen Months

In adults, adolescents, or children 18 months of age or older, a reportable case of HIV infection must meet at least one of the following criteria.

Laboratory Criteria

Positive results on a screening test for HIV antibody (e.g., repeatedly reactive EIA), followed by a positive result on a confirmatory (sensitive and more specific) test for HIV antibody (e.g., Western blot or IFA test)

OR

Positive result or report of a detectable quantity on any of the following HIV virologic (nonantibody) tests:
- HIV nucleic acid (DNA or RNA) detection (e.g., DNA PCR or plasma HIV-1 RNA)
- HIV p24 antigen test, including neutralization assay
- HIV isolation (viral culture)

[7]Centers for Disease Control and Prevention. CDC guidelines for national human immunodeficiency virus case surveillance, including monitoring for human immunodeficiency virus infection and acquired immunodeficiency syndrome. *MMWR Morb Mortal Wkly Rep* 1999;48(RR-13):29–31.

OR

Clinical or Other Criteria

(If the above laboratory criteria are not met)

- Diagnosis of HIV infection, based on the laboratory criteria, that is documented in a medical record by a physician

OR

- Conditions that meet criteria included in the case definition for AIDS

Criteria for Infection in Children Younger Than Eighteen Months

In a child aged <18 months, a reportable case of HIV infection must meet at least one of the following criteria.

Laboratory Criteria

DEFINITIVE

Positive results on two separate specimens (excluding cord blood) using one or more of the following HIV virologic (nonantibody) tests:

- HIV nucleic acid (DNA or RNA) detection
- HIV p24 antigen test, including neutralization assay, in a child 1 month of age
- HIV isolation (viral culture)

OR

PRESUMPTIVE

A child who does not meet the criteria for definitive HIV infection but who has

- Positive results on only one specimen (excluding cord blood) using the earlier HIV virologic tests and no subsequent negative HIV virologic or negative HIV antibody tests

OR

Clinical or Other Criteria

(If the earlier definitive or presumptive laboratory criteria are not met)

- Diagnosis of HIV infection, based on the laboratory criteria above, that is documented in a medical record by a physician

OR

- Conditions that meet criteria included in the 1987 pediatric surveillance case definition for AIDS

Criteria for Noninfection in Children Born to Infected Mothers

A child aged <18 months born to an HIV-infected mother is categorized for surveillance purposes as "not infected with HIV" if the child does not meet the criteria for HIV infection but meets the following criteria.

Laboratory Criteria

DEFINITIVE

At least two negative results on HIV antibody tests from separate specimens obtained at 6 months of age

OR

Negative results on at least three HIV virologic tests on separate specimens, both of which were performed at 1 month of age and one of which was performed at 4 months of age

AND

No other laboratory or clinical evidence of HIV infection (i.e., has not had any positive results on virologic tests, if performed, and has not had an AIDS-defining condition)

OR

PRESUMPTIVE

A child who does not meet the above criteria for definitive "not infected" status but who has

- One negative result on EIA HIV antibody test performed at 6 months of age and *no* positive results on HIV virologic tests, if performed

OR

- One negative result on an HIV virologic test performed at 4 months of age and *no* positive results on HIV virologic tests, if performed
- One positive result on an HIV virologic test with at least two subsequent negative results on virologic tests, at least one of which is at 4 months of age; or negative results on HIV antibody tests, at least one of which is at 6 months of age

AND

No other laboratory or clinical evidence of HIV infection (i.e., has not had any positive results on virologic tests, if performed, and has not had an AIDS-defining condition)

OR

Clinical or Other Criteria

(If the earlier definitive or presumptive laboratory criteria are not met)

- Determined by a physician to be "not infected," and a physician has noted the results of the preceding HIV diagnostic tests in the medical record

AND

No other laboratory or clinical evidence of HIV infection (i.e., has not had any positive virologic tests, if performed, and has not had an AIDS-defining condition)

Criteria for Perinatal Exposure of Children Born to Infected Mothers

A child aged <18 months born to an HIV-infected mother is categorized as having "perinatal exposure to HIV infection" if the child does not meet either the criteria for HIV infection of children <18 months or the criteria for noninfection of children born to infected mothers as listed in the previous two sections.

Criteria for Noninfection in Children Aged Eighteen Months to Thirteen Years

Children aged ≥18 months but <13 years of age are categorized as "not infected with HIV" if they meet the criteria given earlier for absence of infection in children of HIV-infected mothers.

Methods of Testing

In adults, adolescents, and children infected by other than perinatal exposure, plasma viral RNA nucleic acid tests should *not* be used in lieu of licensed HIV screening tests (e.g., repeatedly reactive EIA results). In addition, a negative (i.e., undetectable) plasma HIV-1 RNA test result does not rule out the diagnosis of HIV infection.

HIV nucleic acid (DNA or RNA) detection tests are the virologic methods of choice to exclude infection in children aged <18 months. Although HIV culture can be used for this purpose, it is more complex and expensive to perform and is less well standardized than nucleic acid detection tests. The use of p24 antigen testing to exclude infection in children aged <18 months is not recommended because of its lack of sensitivity.

Public Health Service Recommendations for Chemoprophylaxis after Occupational Exposure to Human Immunodeficiency Virus

See Table 6.

Influenza

Influenza viruses are orthomyxoviruses of three antigenic types (A, B, and C). Epidemic disease is caused by influenza virus types A and B. Influenza A viruses are subclassified by two surface antigens, hemagglutinin (H) and neuraminidase (N). Three immunologically distinct hemagglutinin subtypes (H1, H2, and H3) and two neuraminidase types (N1 and N2) have been recognized as causing global human epidemics. H5N1 and H9N2 avian-related strains have caused localized disease in Asia. Specific antibodies to these various antigens are important determinants of immunity. Major changes in the predominant strain in either of these antigens, such as H1 to H2, are called *antigenic shifts*; minor variations within the same subtypes are called *antigenic drifts*. Antigenic shift has occurred only with influenza A, usually at irregular intervals of ≥10 years. Antigenic drift occurs almost annually in influenza A and B viruses. Although influenza A and B viruses continually undergo antigenic change, influenza B viruses change more slowly and are not divided into subtypes.

Influenza is characterized by the sudden onset of fever, frequently with chills or rigors; headache; malaise; diffuse myalgia; and a nonproductive cough. In some children, influenza can appear as a simple upper respiratory tract infection or as a febrile illness with few respiratory tract signs. In young infants, influenza can produce a sepsis-like picture and occasionally can cause croup or pneumonia. Acute myositis characterized by calf tenderness and refusal to walk may develop after several days of influenza illness, particularly with type B infection. Reye syndrome has been associated with influenza infection, primarily with influenza B.

Table 6. Provisional Public Health Service Recommendations for Chemoprophylaxis after Occupational Exposure to Human Immunodeficiency Virus, by Type of Exposure and Source Material (1998)

Type of Exposure	Source Materials[a]	Antiretroviral Prophylaxis[b]	Antiretroviral Regimen[c]
Percutaneous	Blood		
	Highest risk	Recommend	Zidovudine plus lamivudine plus either indinavir sulfate or nelfinavir mesylate
	Increased risk	Recommend	Zidovudine plus lamivudine with or without either indinavir or nelfinavir
	No increased risk	Offer	Zidovudine plus lamivudine
	Fluid containing visible blood, other potentially infectious fluid,[d] or tissue	Offer	Zidovudine plus lamivudine
	Other body fluid (e.g., urine)	Do not offer	
Mucous membrane	Blood	Offer	Zidovudine plus lamivudine with or without either indinavir or nelfinavir
	Fluid containing visible blood, other potentially infectious fluid,[d] or tissue	Offer	Zidovudine with or without lamivudine
	Other body fluid (e.g., urine)	Do not offer	
Skin, increased risk[e]	Blood	Offer	Zidovudine plus lamivudine with or without either indinavir or nelfinavir
	Fluid containing visible blood, other potentially infectious fluid,[d] or tissue	Offer	Zidovudine with or without lamivudine
	Other body fluid (e.g., urine)	Do not offer	

[a]Any exposure to concentrated human immunodeficiency virus (HIV) (e.g., in a research laboratory or production facility) is treated as percutaneous exposure to blood with highest risk. Highest risk: exposure that involves *both* a larger volume of blood (e.g., deep injury with large-diameter hollow needle previously in source patient's vein or artery, especially involving an injection of source patient's blood) *and* blood containing a high titer of HIV (e.g., source with acute retroviral illness or end-stage acquired immunodeficiency syndrome; viral load measurement may be considered, but its use in relation to postexposure prophylaxis has not been evaluated). Increased risk: *either* exposure to a larger volume of blood *or* exposure to blood with a high titer of HIV. No increased risk: *neither* exposure to a larger volume of blood *nor* exposure to blood with a high titer of HIV (e.g., solid suture needle injury from source patient with asymptomatic HIV infection).

[b]Recommend: postexposure prophylaxis should be recommended to the exposed worker with counseling. Offer: postexposure prophylaxis should be offered to the exposed worker with counseling. Not offer: postexposure prophylaxis should not be offered because it is not an occupational exposure to HIV.

[c]Regimens for adults: zidovudine, 200 mg three times a day; lamivudine, 150 mg twice a day; indinavir sulfate, 800 mg three times a day (if indinavir is not available, ritonavir, 600 mg twice a day, or saquinavir mesylate, 600 mg three times a day, may be used); nelfinavir sulfate, 750 mg three times a day. Prophylaxis is given for 4 wk. For full prescribing information, see package inserts. Possible toxic effects from indinavir or nelfinavir may make their use unwarranted.

[d]Includes semen; vaginal secretions; cerebrospinal, synovial, pleural, peritoneal, pericardial, and amniotic fluids.

[e]For skin, risk is increased for exposures involving a high titer of HIV, prolonged contact, an extensive area of contact, or contact in an area in which skin integrity is visibly compromised. For skin exposures without increased risk, the risk of toxic effects of the drug outweigh the benefit of postexposure prophylaxis.

From Centers for Disease Control and Prevention. Public Health Service guidelines for the management of healthcare worker exposures to HIV and recommendations for postexposure prophylaxis. *MMWR Morb Mortal Wkly Rep* 1998;47(RR-7):1–33.

Diagnostic Tests

When viral cultures are performed, specimens should be obtained during the first 72 hours of illness because the quantity of virus shed subsequently decreases rapidly. Nasopharyngeal secretions obtained by swab or aspirate should be placed in appropriate transport media for culture. After inoculation into eggs or cell culture, virus usually can be isolated within 2–6 days. Rapid diagnostic tests for identification of influenza A and B antigens in nasopharyngeal specimens are available commercially, although their sensitivity and specificity have been variable. Serologic diagnosis can be established retrospectively by a significant change in antibody titer between acute and convalescent serum samples, as determined by complement fixation, hemagglutination inhibition, neutralization, or EIA tests.

Lassa Fever

Lassa fever is an acute viral illness that occurs in West Africa. The illness was discovered in 1969 when two missionary nurses died in Nigeria, West Africa. The cause of the illness was found to be Lassa virus, named after the town in Nigeria where the first cases originated. The virus, a member of the virus family Arenaviridae, is a single-stranded RNA virus and is zoonotic, or animal-borne.

In areas of Africa where the disease is endemic, Lassa fever is a significant cause of morbidity and mortality. Although the disease is mild or has no observable symptoms in approximately 80% of people infected with the virus, the remaining 20% have a severe multisystem disease. Lassa fever is also associated with occasional epidemics, during which the case fatality rate can reach 50%.

The reservoir, or host, of Lassa virus is a rodent known as the multimammate rat of the genus *Mastomys*. The *Mastomys* rodents shed the virus in urine and droppings. Therefore, the virus can be transmitted through direct contact with these materials, or through contamination of cuts or sores. Contact with the virus also occurs when a person inhales tiny particles in the air contaminated with rodent excretions.

Lassa fever may also spread through person-to-person contact with virus in the blood, tissue, secretions, or excretions of an individual infected with the Lassa virus. A person may also become infected by breathing in small air-borne particles from an infected person through coughing. The virus cannot be spread although casual contact (including skin-to-skin contact without exchange of body fluids). Person-to-person transmission is common in both village settings and in health care settings, where, along with the above-mentioned modes of transmission, the virus also may be spread in contaminated medical equipment, such as reused needles (nosocomial transmission).

Symptoms of Lassa fever typically occur 1–3 weeks after the patient comes into contact with the virus. These include fever, retrosternal pain, sore throat, back pain, cough, abdominal pain, vomiting, diarrhea, conjunctivitis, facial swelling, proteinuria, and mucosal bleeding. Neurologic symptoms have also been described, including hearing loss, tremors, and encephalitis. Because the symptoms of Lassa fever are so varied and nonspecific, clinical diagnosis is often difficult.

Some 15–20% of patients hospitalized for Lassa fever die from the illness. Overall, however, only approximately 1% of infections with the Lassa virus result in death. The death rates are particularly high for women in the third trimester of pregnancy and for fetuses, with an approximately 95% death rate *in utero*.

Diagnostic Tests

Lassa fever is most often diagnosed using ELISAs, which detect IgM and IgG antibodies as well as Lassa antigen. The virus itself may be cultured in 7–10 days. Immunohistochemical analysis performed on tissue specimens can be used to make a postmortem diagnosis. The virus can also be detected by RT-PCR; however, this method is primarily a research tool.

Lymphocytic Choriomeningitis

Infection with the virus causing lymphocytic choriomeningitis may result in a mild to severe nonspecific illness, which includes fever, malaise, myalgia, retroorbital headache, photophobia, anorexia, and nausea. Fever usually lasts 1–3 weeks, and rash is uncommon. A biphasic febrile course is frequent. Neurologic manifestations vary from aseptic meningitis to severe encephalitis. Arthralgia or arthritis, respiratory tract symptoms, orchitis, and leukopenia occasionally develop. Infection during pregnancy has been associated with abortion and with hydrocephalus, microcephaly, intracranial calcifications, and chorioretinitis in the fetus.

Diagnostic Tests

The CSF may contain hundreds to thousands of white blood cells, predominantly lymphocytes, and low glucose levels can occur. The lymphocytic choriomeningitis virus can be isolated from blood, CSF, urine, and, rarely, nasopharyngeal secretions. Acute and convalescent serum samples can be tested for increases in antibody titers; demonstration of virus-specific IgM antibodies in serum and CSF is useful. Infection of mice, the disease vector, trapped in or around houses may be identified by demonstrating serum antibody or viral antigen in liver impression smears.

Marburg Virus Infections

Marburg hemorrhagic fever is a rare, severe type of hemorrhagic fever that affects both humans and nonhuman primates. Caused by a genetically unique zoonotic RNA virus of the filovirus family, its recognition led to the creation of this virus family. The four species of Ebola virus are the only other known members of the filovirus family.

Marburg virus was first recognized in 1967, when outbreaks of hemorrhagic fever occurred simultaneously in laboratories in Marburg and Frankfurt, Germany, and in Belgrade, Yugoslavia. A total of 37 people became ill; they included laboratory workers as well as several medical personnel and family members who had cared for them. The first people infected had been exposed to African green monkeys or their tissues. In Marburg, the monkeys had been imported for research and to prepare polio vaccine.

Marburg virus is indigenous to Africa. Although the geographic area to which it is native is unknown, this area appears to include at least parts of Uganda and western Kenya, and perhaps Zimbabwe. As with Ebola virus, the actual animal host for Marburg virus also remains a mystery.

Spread of the virus between humans has occurred in a setting of close contact, often in a hospital. Droplets of body fluids or direct contact with persons, equipment, or other objects contaminated with infectious blood or tissues are all highly suspect as sources of disease.

After an incubation period of 5–10 days, the onset of the disease is sudden and is marked by fever, chills, headache, and myalgia. Around the fifth day after the onset of symptoms, a maculopapular rash, most prominent on the trunk (chest, back, stomach), may occur. Nausea, vomiting, chest pain, sore throat, abdominal pain, and diarrhea then may appear. Symptoms become increasingly severe and may include jaundice, inflammation of the pancreas, severe weight loss, delirium, shock, liver failure, massive hemorrhaging, and multiorgan dysfunction.

The case fatality rate for Marburg hemorrhagic fever is 25%.

Diagnostic Tests

Antigen-capture ELISA testing, IgM-capture ELISA, PCR, and virus isolation can be used to confirm a case of Marburg hemorrhagic fever within a few days of the onset of the symptoms. The IgG-capture ELISA is appropriate for testing persons later in the course of disease or after recovery. The disease is readily diagnosed by immunohistochemical analysis, virus isolation, or PCR of blood or tissue specimens from deceased patients.

Measles (Rubeola)

Measles virus is an RNA virus with one serotype, classified as a member of the genus Morbillivirus in the paramyxovirus family.

Measles is an acute disease characterized by temperature of ≥38.3°C (≥101°F), cough, coryza, conjunctivitis, an erythematous maculopapular rash, and a pathognomonic enanthem (Koplik spots). Complications, such as otitis media, bronchopneumonia, laryngotracheobronchitis (croup), and diarrhea, occur more commonly in young children. Acute encephalitis, which frequently results in permanent brain damage, occurs in approximately 1 of every 1,000 cases. Hemorrhagic measles marked by thrombocytopenia and purpura is rare and may be fatal. Death, predominantly due to respiratory and neurologic complications, occurs in 1–3 of every 1,000 cases reported in the United States. Case fatality rates are increased in children <5 years of age and in immunocompromised children, including those with leukemia and HIV infection. Sometimes the characteristic rash does not develop in immunocompromised patients.

Subacute sclerosing panencephalitis, a rare degenerative CNS disease characterized by behavioral and intellectual deterioration and seizures, is a result of a persistent measles virus infection that develops years after the original infection. Widespread measles immunization has led to its marked decrease in the United States.

Diagnostic Tests

Measles virus infection can be diagnosed by a positive serologic test result for measles IgM antibody, a significant increase in measles IgG antibody level in paired serum specimens from the acute phase (collected within 4 days of rash onset) and convalescent phase (collected 2–4 weeks later), any standard serologic assay, or isolation of measles virus from clinical specimens, such as urine, blood, or nasopharyngeal secretions. The state public health laboratory or the CDC Measles Laboratory will process these viral specimens free of charge. For more information, contact the state health department. The serum specimen is collected during the first encounter with a person suspected of having measles. The sensitivity of measles IgM assays varies and may be diminished during the first 72 hours after rash onset. If the result is negative for measles IgM and the patient has a generalized rash lasting >72 hours, the measles IgM tests should be repeated. Measles IgM is detectable for at least 1 month after rash onset. Persons with febrile rash illness who are seronegative for measles IgM should be tested for rubella using the same specimens. Virus isolation from clinical specimens is useful for tracking the distribution of different measles virus genotypes to determine patterns of importation and transmission. All cases of suspected measles should be reported immediately to the local or state health department, without waiting for the results of diagnostic tests.

Molluscum Contagiosum

The cause of molluscum contagiosum is a poxvirus, which is the sole member of the genus Molluscipoxvirus.

Molluscum contagiosum is a benign, usually asymptomatic viral infection of the skin with no systemic manifestations. It is characterized by relatively few (usually 2–20) discrete, flesh-colored to translucent, dome-shaped papules, some with central umbilication. Lesions commonly occur on the trunk, face, and extremities but may be generalized. An eczematous reaction encircles the lesions in approximately 10% of patients. Patients with eczema and immunocompromised persons, including persons with HIV infection, tend to have more intense and widespread eruptions.

Diagnostic Tests

The diagnosis usually can be made from the characteristic appearance of the lesions. Wright or Giemsa staining of material expressed from the central core of a lesion reveals characteristic intracytoplasmic inclusions. Electron microscopic examination identifies the typical poxvirus particles.

Mumps

Mumps is caused by a paramyxovirus. Other causes of bilateral parotitis include CMV and enterovirus infection, and other causes of unilateral parotitis include tumor, parotid duct obstruction, bacterial infection, and trauma from forceful blowing, for example, trumpet playing.

Mumps is a systemic disease characterized by swelling of one or more of the salivary glands, usually the parotid glands. Approximately one-third of infections do not cause clinically apparent salivary gland swelling. More than 50% of persons with mumps have CSF pleocytosis, but <10% have clinical evidence of CNS infection. Orchitis is a common complication after puberty, but sterility occurs only rarely. Other rare complications include arthritis, thyroiditis, mastitis, glomerulonephritis, myocarditis, orchitis, thrombocytopenia, cerebellar ataxia, transverse myelitis, pancreatitis, and hearing impairment.

Diagnostic Tests

Children with parotitis lasting ≥2 days without other apparent cause should undergo diagnostic testing to confirm mumps virus as the agent, because mumps is now a rare infection and parotitis may be caused by other agents. Mumps can be confirmed by isolation of the virus in cell culture inoculated with throat washings, urine, or CSF; by a significant rise between acute and convalescent titers in serum mumps IgG antibody titer determined by any standard serologic assay (e.g., by complement fixation), neutralization, or hemagglutination inhibition test; by an EIA; or by a positive result on a mumps IgM antibody test. Past infection is best assessed by EIA or a neutralization test; CF and hemagglutination inhibition tests are unreliable for this purpose. Skin tests also are unreliable and should not be used to test immune status.

Papillomavirus Infections

Human papillomaviruses (HPVs) are members of the Papovaviridae family and are DNA viruses. More than 70 types have been identified, but a small number of HPV types account for most warts. Those causing nongenital warts generally are distinct from those causing anogenital infections. Of the latter, only a small number have a strong association with malignant neoplasms.

HPVs produce epithelial tumors (warts) of the skin and mucous membranes. Cutaneous nongenital warts include common skin warts, plantar warts, flat warts, threadlike (filiform) warts, and epidermodysplasia verruciformis. Those affecting the mucous membranes produce anogenital, oral, nasal, and conjunctival warts, as well as respiratory papillomatosis.

Common skin warts are dome shaped with conical projections that give the surface a rough appearance. They usually are asymptomatic and multiple, occurring on the hands and around or under the nails. When small dermal vessels become thrombosed, black dots appear in the warts. Plantar warts on the foot may be painful and are characterized by marked hyperkeratosis, sometimes with black dots.

Flat warts ("juvenile warts") commonly are found on the face and extremities of children and adolescents. They usually are small, multiple, and flat topped; they seldom exhibit papillomatosis and rarely cause pain. Filiform warts occur on the face and neck. Cutaneous warts are benign.

The manifestations of anogenital HPV infection range from clinically inapparent infection to condylomata acuminata, which are skin-colored warts with a cauliflower-like surface that vary from a few millimeters to several centimeters in diameter. In males, such warts may be found on the shaft of the penis, the penile meatus, the scrotum, or the perianal area. In females, such warts are seen on the labia and perianal area and less commonly in the vagina and on the cervix. Clinically inapparent infections commonly occur in the vagina, on the cervix, and on the labia and perineum. Most anogenital warts are asymptomatic, but occasionally they cause itching, burning, local pain, or bleeding. Some HPV types are associated with genital dysplasia and epithelial cancers of the female and male genital tracts. Specific types of HPV are the causal agents of at least 90% of cervical cancers.

Laryngeal papillomas are rare. They are diagnosed most commonly in children between 2 and 3 years of age and are manifested by a voice change or abnormal cry. When laryngeal papillomas occur in infancy, they have been associated with respiratory tract obstruction. Adult onset also has been described.

Epidermodysplasia verruciformis is a rare, lifelong, severe papillomavirus infection, believed to be a consequence of an inherited deficiency of cell-mediated immunity. The lesions may resemble flat warts but often are similar to tinea versicolor, covering the torso and upper extremities. Most appear during the first decade of life, but malignant transformation, which occurs in approximately one-third of affected persons, usually is delayed until adulthood.

Diagnostic Tests

Most cutaneous and anogenital warts are diagnosed by clinical inspection. Detection of cervical HPV infection may be enhanced by use of colposcopy with application of 3–5% acetic acid (vinegar), which causes the lesion to turn white. This characteristic, however, is not specific for HPV infection, and false-positive test results are common. When the diagnosis is questionable, histologic examination of a biopsy specimen can be diagnostic.

HPV cannot be cultured. Tests for the detection of HPV nucleic acids in cervical cells are available commercially. Clinical indications for HPV testing are unclear.

Parainfluenza Viral Infections

Parainfluenza viruses are enveloped RNA viruses classified as paramyxoviruses. Four antigenically distinct types—1, 2, 3, and 4 (with two subtypes, 4A and 4B)—have been identified.

Parainfluenza viruses are the major cause of laryngotracheobronchitis (croup), but they also frequently cause upper respiratory tract infection, pneumonia, or bronchiolitis. Infections can be particularly severe and persistent in immunodeficient children.

Diagnostic Tests

Virus may be isolated from nasopharyngeal secretions, usually within 4–7 days of culture inoculation or earlier by using centrifugation of a specimen onto a monolayer of susceptible cells with subsequent staining for viral antigen (shell viral assay). Confirmation is by rapid antigen detection, usually immunofluorescence. Rapid antigen identification techniques, including IFAs, EIAs, and radioimmunoassays, can be used to detect the virus in nasopharyngeal secretions, but the sensitivity of the tests can vary. Serologic diagnosis, made retrospectively by a significant rise in antibody titer between serum samples obtained during acute infection and convalescence, may be confusing because increases in heterotypic antibody levels due to infections caused by other serotypes of parainfluenza and mumps viruses are common. Furthermore, infection may not always be accompanied by a significant homotypic antibody response.

Parvovirus B19 Infections (Erythema Infectiosum, Fifth Disease)

Human parvovirus B19 is a DNA-containing virus.

Infection with parvovirus B19 is recognized most often as erythema infectiosum (EI), which is characterized by mild systemic symptoms, fever in 15–30% of patients, and, frequently, a distinctive rash. Before onset of these manifestations, a brief, mild, nonspecific illness consisting of fever, malaise, myalgias, and headache, followed 7–10 days later by the characteristic exanthem, may occur in some patients. The facial rash is intensely red with a "slapped cheek" appearance and often accompanied by circumoral pallor. A symmetric, maculopapular, lacelike, and often pruritic rash also occurs on the trunk, moving peripherally to involve the arms, buttocks, and thighs. The rash can fluctuate in intensity and recur with environmental changes, such as temperature changes and exposure to sunlight, for weeks or months. Arthralgia and arthritis occur infrequently among infected children but commonly among adults, especially women.

Infection with the causative agent of EI, human parvovirus B19, also can cause asymptomatic infection, a mild respiratory tract illness with no rash, a rash atypical for EI that may be rubelliform or petechial, arthritis in adults (in the absence of manifestations of EI), chronic bone marrow failure in immunodeficient patients, transient aplastic crisis lasting 7–10 days in patients with hemolytic anemias (e.g., sickle cell disease and autoimmune hemolytic anemia), and other conditions associated with low hemoglobulin levels, including hemorrhage, severe anemia, and thalassemia. Chronic parvovirus B19 infection has been detected in some HIV-infected patients with severe anemia, at rates up to 17% in those with hematocrit values of ≤24% (0.24) and in 31% of those with hematocrit values of ≤20% (0.20). In addition, parvovirus B19 infection has been associated with thrombocytopenia and neutropenia. Patients with aplastic crisis may have a prodromal illness with fever, malaise, and myalgia, but rash usually is absent. The red blood cell aplasia is related to lytic infection in erythrocyte precursors.

Parvovirus B19 infection occurring during pregnancy can cause fetal anemia and hydrops and death but is not a proven cause of congenital anomalies. The risk of fetal death is probably between 2% and 6%, with the greatest risk when infection occurs during the first half of pregnancy.

Diagnostic Tests

The most feasible methods of diagnosis are direct detection of parvovirus B19 antigen or DNA in clinical specimens and serologic tests. In the healthy host, a test for serum parvovirus B19–specific IgM antibody is preferred, and detection indicates that infection probably occurred within the previous 2–4 months. By using a radioimmunoassay or EIA, antibody may be detected in ≥90% of patients at the time of the EI rash and by the third day of illness in patients with transient aplastic crisis. Presence of serum IgG antibody indicates previous infection and immunity. These assays are available through commercial laboratories and through some state health and research laboratories. However, their sensitivity and specificity may vary, particularly for IgM antibody. The optimal method for detecting chronic infection in the immunocompromised patient is demonstration of virus by nucleic acid hybridization or PCR assay, because parvovirus B19 antibody is variably present in persistent infection. Because parvovirus B19 DNA can be detected by PCR in serum after the acute viremic phase for up to 9 months in some patients, PCR detection of parvovirus B19 DNA does not necessarily indicate acute infection. The less sensitive nucleic acid hybridization assays usually are positive for only 2–4 days after onset of illness. For HIV-infected patients with severe anemia, dot blot hybridization of serum may be a more appropriate assay. Parvovirus B19 has not been grown in standard cell culture, but the virus has been cultivated in experimental cell culture.

Poliovirus Infections

Polioviruses are enteroviruses and consist of serotypes 1, 2, and 3.

Approximately 95% of poliovirus infections are asymptomatic. Nonspecific illness with low-grade fever and sore throat (minor illness) occurs in 4–8% of people who become infected. Aseptic meningitis, sometimes with paresthesias, occurs in 1–5% of patients a few days after the minor illness has resolved. Rapid onset of acute flaccid paralysis with areflexia of the involved limb occurs in 0.1–2.0% of infections, and residual paralytic disease involving the motor neutrons (paralytic poliomyelitis) occurs in approximately 1 in 250 infections. Cranial nerve involvement and paralysis of respiratory muscles can occur. Findings in the CSF are characteristic of those of viral meningitis with mild pleocytosis and lymphocytic predominance.

Adults who contracted paralytic poliomyelitis during childhood may develop the postpolio syndrome 30–40 years later. Postpolio syndrome is characterized by muscle pain and exacerbation of weakness.

Diagnostic Tests

Poliovirus can be recovered from the pharynx, feces, urine, and, rarely, CSF by isolation in cell culture. Two or more stool and throat swab specimens for enterovirus isolation should be obtained at least 24 hours apart from patients with suspected paralytic poliomyelitis as early in the course of the illness as possible, ideally within 14 days of onset of symptoms. Fecal material is most likely to yield virus.

If a poliovirus is isolated from a patient with paralysis, the isolate should be sent to the CDC through the state health department for testing to distinguish a wild-type virus from a vaccine strain. Because infants and children who are immunized with oral poliovirus vaccine can excrete vaccine virus in feces for several weeks, the incidental isolation of poliovirus from enteric sites in healthy young infants should be assumed to be the result of administration of or exposure to oral poliovirus vaccine unless an epidemiologic or clinical reason to suspect otherwise exists. Serologic testing of acute and convalescent serum samples should be performed when paralytic poliomyelitis is suspected, but interpretation of serologic tests results can be difficult. Hence, the diagnostic test of choice for confirming poliovirus disease is viral culture of stool specimens and throat swab samples obtained as early in the course of illness as possible.

Rabies

Rabies virus is an RNA virus classified in the rhabdovirus family.

Wildlife rabies exists throughout the United States except in Hawaii, which remains rabies free. Wildlife, including raccoons, skunks, foxes, coyotes, bats, and other species, is the most important potential source of infection for humans and domestic animals in the United States. Rabies is rare in small rodents (squirrels, hamsters, guinea pigs, gerbils, chipmunks, rats, and mice) and lagomorphs (rabbits and hares), but rabies may occur in woodchucks or other large rodents in areas where raccoon rabies is common. The virus is present in saliva and is transmitted by bites or, rarely, by contamination of mucosa or skin lesions by infectious material. Worldwide, most rabies cases in humans result from dog bites in areas where canine rabies is enzootic. Most dogs, cats, and ferrets become ill within 4–5 days of viral shedding, and no case of human rabies in the United States has been attributed to a dog, cat, or ferret that has remained healthy throughout the standard 10-day period of confinement.

The incubation period in humans averages 4–6 weeks but ranges from 5 days to >1 year. Incubation periods of up to 6 years have been confirmed by antigenic typing and nucleotide sequencing of strains.

Infection with rabies virus characteristically produces an acute illness with rapidly progressive CNS manifestations, including anxiety, dysphagia, and seizures. Illness almost invariably progresses to death. Some patients may present with paralysis. The differential diagnosis of all acute encephalitic illnesses of unknown cause with atypical focal neurologic signs or with paralysis should include rabies.

Diagnostic Tests

Infection in animals can be diagnosed by demonstration of virus-specific fluorescence antigen in brain tissue. Animals suspected of rabies should be euthanized in a manner that preserves brain tissue for appropriate examination. Virus can be isolated from saliva, brain, and other tissues in suckling mice or in tissue culture. The diagnosis in suspected human cases can be made postmortem and sometimes antemortem by fluorescent microscopy of skin biopsy specimens from the nape of the neck, by isolation of the virus from saliva, by detection of antibody in the CSF or serum in unimmunized persons, and by detection of viral nucleic acid in infected tissues. Laboratory personnel should be consulted before submission of specimens so that appropriate collection and transport of materials can be arranged.

Respiratory Syncytial Virus Infections

Respiratory syncytial virus (RSV) is an enveloped RNA paramyxovirus that lacks neuraminidase and a hemagglutinin. Two major subtypes (A and B) have been identified and often circulate concurrently. The clinical and epidemiologic significance of strain variation has not been determined, but evidence suggests that antigenic differences may affect susceptibility to infection, and some strains may be more virulent than others.

RSV causes acute respiratory tract illness in patients of all ages. In infants and young children, RSV is the most important cause of bronchiolitis and pneumonia. During the first few weeks of life, particularly among preterm infants, infection with RSV may produce minimal respiratory tract signs. Lethargy, irritability, and poor feeding, sometimes accompanied by apneic episodes, may be the major manifestations. Most previously healthy infants infected with RSV do not require hospitalization, and many who are hospitalized improve within a few days with supportive care. Conditions that increase the risk of severe or fatal RSV infection are cyanotic or complicated congenital heart disease, especially bronchopulmonary dysplasia; prematurity; and immunodeficiency disease or therapy causing immunosuppression at any age. Long-term sequelae of RSV infection among infants are difficult to assess. Some evidence suggests that in subpopulations of infected children, long-term abnormalities in pulmonary function develop that may manifest as recurrent wheezing. This, however, may reflect an underlying predisposition to reactive airway disease, rather than illness of which RSV is the sole cause.

Exacerbation of asthma or other chronic lung conditions is common.

Diagnostic Tests

Rapid diagnostic procedures, including immunofluorescent and EIA techniques for detection of viral antigen in clinical specimens, are available commercially and generally are reliable during RSV outbreaks. The sensitivity of these assays in comparison with culture varies between 53% and 96%, with most assays falling in the 80–90%

range. Viral isolation from nasopharyngeal secretions in cell cultures requires 3–5 days, but results and sensitivity vary because methods of isolation are exacting and RSV is a relatively labile virus with infectivity that decreases rapidly at room temperature and after freeze-thawing. An experienced viral laboratory should be consulted for optimal methods of collection and transport of specimens. Serologic testing of acute and convalescent serum samples can be used to confirm infection; however, the sensitivity of serologic diagnosis of infection is low among young infants. PCR technology has been applied to detection of RSV.

Rhinovirus Infections

Rhinoviruses are the most frequent causes of the common cold or rhinosinusitis. Rhinoviruses can be associated with pharyngitis and otitis media and with exacerbations of bronchitis and reactive airway disease. Nasal discharge usually is watery and clear at the onset but often becomes mucopurulent and viscous after a few days and may persist for 10–14 days. Malaise, headache, myalgias, and low-grade fever may occur.

Diagnostic Tests

Inoculation of nasal secretions in appropriate cell cultures for viral isolation is the best means of establishing a specific diagnosis. The large number of antigenic types makes serologic testing to diagnose infection impractical.

Rotavirus Infections

Rotaviruses are RNA viruses belonging to the family Reoviridae. At least seven distinct antigenic groups (A through G) are found. Group A viruses are the major causes of rotavirus diarrhea worldwide. Group B and C viruses also have been identified as causes of gastroenteritis in humans. Serotyping is based on the VP7 glycoprotein (G) and VP4 protease-cleaved hemagglutinin (P); G types 1–4 and 9, and P types 1A and 1B most commonly are associated with disease.

Infection can result in diarrhea, usually preceded or accompanied by emesis and fever. In severe cases, dehydration, electrolyte abnormalities, and acidosis may occur. In immunocompromised children, including those with HIV infection, persistent infection can develop.

Diagnostic Tests

EIA and latex agglutination assays for group A rotavirus antigen detection in stool are available commercially. However, EIAs are more sensitive for the detection of antigen late in the course of illness. Both assays have high specificity, but false-positive and nonspecific reactions can occur in neonates and in persons with underlying intestinal disease. These nonspecific reactions can be distinguished from true-positive ones by the performance of confirmatory assays. Virus also can be identified in stool by electron microscopy and by specific nucleic acid amplification techniques.

Rubella

Rubella virus is an RNA virus classified as a Rubivirus in the Togaviridae family.

The most commonly described anomalies associated with the congenital rubella syndrome are ophthalmologic (cataracts, retinopathy, and congenital glaucoma), cardiac (patent ductus arteriosis, peripheral pulmonary artery stenosis), auditory (sensorineural deafness), and neurologic (behavioral disorders, meningoencephalitis, and mental retardation). In addition, infants with congenital rubella frequently are growth retarded and may have radiolucent bone disease, hepatosplenomegaly, thrombocytopenia, and purpuric skin lesions (which give a "blueberry muffin" appearance). Mild forms of the disease can be associated with few or no obvious clinical manifestations at birth. The incidence of congenital defects is 50% or higher if infection occurs during the first month of gestation, 20–30% if during the second month, and 5% if during the third or fourth month.

Rubella usually is a mild disease characterized by a generalized erythematous maculopapular rash, generalized lymphadenopathy (commonly suboccipital, postauricular, and cervical), and slight fever. Transient polyarthralgia and polyarthritis occur rarely in children but are common in adolescents and adults, especially females. Encephalitis and thrombocytopenia are rare complications. Transient polyarthritis occurs rarely after rubella vaccination.

Diagnostic Tests

Rubella virus most consistently can be isolated from nasal specimens by inoculation of appropriate cell culture. Laboratory personnel should be notified that rubella is suspected because additional testing is required to detect the virus. Throat swab specimens, blood, urine, and CSF also can yield virus, particularly in congenitally infected infants. A fourfold or greater rise in antibody titer or seroconversion between acute and convalescent serum titers indicates infection. Detection of rubella-specific IgM antibody usually indicates recent postnatal infection or congenital infection in a newborn infant, but false-positive results occur. Congenital infection also can be confirmed by a finding of stable or increasing serum concentrations of rubella-specific IgG over several months. Every effort should be made to establish a laboratory diagnosis when rubella infection is suspected in pregnant women or newborn infants. The diagnosis of congenital rubella infection in children >1 year of age is difficult; serologic testing usually is not diagnostic, and viral isolation, although confirmatory, is possible in only a small proportion of congenitally infected children of this age. The hemagglutination inhibition rubella antibody test, which previously was the most frequently used method of serologic screening, generally has been supplanted by a number of equally or more sensitive assays for determining rubella immunity, including latex agglutination, fluorescence immunoassay, passive hemagglutination, hemolysis-in-gel, and EIA tests. Some persons in whom antibody has not been detected by hemagglutination inhibition testing have been found to be immune when their serum specimens were tested by more sensitive assays.

Varicella-Zoster Infections

Varicella-zoster virus is a member of the herpesvirus family.

Humans are the only source of infection for this highly contagious virus. Humans are infected when the virus comes in contact with the mucosa of the upper respiratory tract or the conjunctiva. Person-to-person transmission occurs primarily by direct contact with patients with varicella or herpes zoster and occasionally occurs by airborne spread from respiratory tract secretions or, rarely, from zoster lesions. *In utero* infection also can occur as a result of transplacental passage of virus during maternal varicella infection and, occasionally, herpes zoster. Varicella-zoster virus infection in a household member usually results in infection of almost all susceptible persons in that household. Children who acquire their infection at home (secondary family cases) may have more severe disease than that in the index case. Nosocomial transmission is well documented in pediatric units.

In temperate climates, varicella is a childhood disease that is most common during the late winter and early spring. In tropical climates seasonality is described less clearly, and a higher proportion of adults are susceptible to varicella compared with adults in temperate climates. Most cases of varicella in the United States occur in children <10 years of age. Immunity generally is lifelong. Cellular immunity is more important than humoral immunity, both for limiting the extent of primary infection with varicella-zoster virus and for preventing reactivation of virus in herpes zoster. Symptomatic reinfection is thought to be uncommon in immunocompetent persons, although asymptomatic reinfection occurs. Asymptomatic primary infection is unusual, but because some cases are mild, they may not be recognized.

Primary infections result in chickenpox, manifested by a generalized, pruritic, vesicular rash typically consisting of 250–500 lesions, mild fever, and systemic symptoms. Complications include bacterial superinfection of skin lesions, thrombocytopenia, arthritis, hepatitis, cerebellar ataxia, encephalitis, meningitis, and glomerulonephritis. Invasive group A streptococcal disease has been reported increasingly as a complication. The disease can be more severe in adolescents and adults. Reye syndrome can follow some cases of chickenpox, although the incidence of Reye syndrome has declined dramatically with the decline in use of aspirin during varicella or influenza-like illness. In immunocompromised children, progressive severe varicella characterized by continuing eruption of lesions and a high fever into the second week of illness, as well as encephalitis, hepatitis, or pneumonia, can develop. Hemorrhagic varicella is more common among immunocompetent children but is the most common complication in adults. In children with HIV infection, chronic or recurrent varicella (disseminated herpes zoster) can develop, with new lesions appearing for months. Varicella is one of the most important risk factors for severe invasive group A streptococcal disease. Severe and even fatal varicella has been reported in otherwise healthy children receiving intermittent courses of corticosteroids for treatment of asthma and other illnesses. The risk is especially great when corticosteroids are given during the incubation period for chickenpox.

Diagnostic Tests

Varicella virus can be isolated from scrapings from the base of vesicles during the first 3–4 days of the eruption but rarely from other sites, including respiratory tract secretions. A significant increase in serum varicella IgG antibody measured by any standard serologic assay can retrospectively confirm a diagnosis. These antibody tests are reliable for determining immune status in healthy hosts after natural infection but are not necessarily reliable in immunocompromised persons. Most commercially available tests are not sufficiently sensitive to demonstrate a vaccine-induced antibody response.

Viruses Typically Isolated from Clinical Specimens

See Table 7.

Specimens for Evaluation for Viral Infection

See Table 8.

Fungal Diseases

Aspergillosis

Aspergillus species are ubiquitous and grow on decaying vegetation and in soil. Most infected patients, other than those in whom aspergillomas or otomycosis and allergic

Table 7. Viruses Typically Isolated from Clinical Specimens

Specimen	Virus
Blood	CMV, enteroviruses,[a,b] HSV,[b] VZV,[b] dengue, VEE, YF, CTF, HIV
CSF and CNS tissue	Enteroviruses, mumps virus, HSV, CMV
Dermal lesions	HSV, VZV, adenovirus, enteroviruses
Eye	HSV, VZV, adenovirus, enteroviruses, CMV
Genitals	HSV, CMV
Mucosa	HSV, VZV
Mouth	HSV, VZV, VEE
Rectum	HSV, VZV, enterovirus
Respiratory tract	
Upper	Adenovirus, rhinovirus, influenza, parainfluenza, enteroviruses, RSV, reovirus, HSV
Lower	Adenovirus, influenza, parainfluenza, RSV, CMV[c]
Stool	Enteroviruses, adenoviruses
Tissues	CMV, HSV, enteroviruses
Urine	CMV, adenovirus, enteroviruses, mumps

CMV, cytomegalovirus; CNS, central nervous system; CSF, cerebrospinal fluid; CTF, Colorado tick; HIV, human immunodeficiency virus; HSV, herpes simplex virus; VZV, varicella-zoster virus; RSV, respiratory syncytial virus; VEE, Venezuela equine encephalitis virus; YF, yellow fever virus.
[a]Coxsackievirus, poliovirus, echovirus, and enterovirus.
[b]Rarely isolated.
[c]Usually found in immunocompromised hosts.

Table 8. Specimens for Diagnosis of Viral Diseases

Disease Site	Specimen/Site	Likely Viruses
Skin	Vesicle fluid	Herpesvirus
	Scrapings	Varicella-zoster virus
	Biopsy	Coxsackievirus
Genital area	Vesicle fluid	Herpesvirus
	Exudates	—
Respiratory system	Throat	Adenovirus
	Nasopharynx	Influenza virus
		Rhinovirus
Eye	Exudate	Herpesvirus
		Adenovirus
		Varicella-zoster virus
Gastrointestinal tract	Stool	Rotavirus
Central nervous system	Spinal fluid	Echovirus[a]
	Throat	Coxsackievirus
		Herpesvirus
		Mumps virus
		Poliovirus
		Arboviruses

Isolation of viruses is best done during the first 3 days of illness. Listed are the best specimens for numerous viral diseases.
[a]Enteric cytopathogenic human orphan (ECHO) virus.

bronchopulmonary or sinus disease develop, have impaired phagocyte function. The risk of aspergillosis is related directly to the duration of neutropenia. The principal route of transmission is inhalation of conidiospores. Nosocomial outbreaks of invasive pulmonary aspergillosis have occurred in which the probable source of the fungus was a nearby construction site or faulty ventilation system. Transmission by direct inoculation of skin abrasions or wounds is less likely. Person-to-person spread does not occur. The inoculation period is unknown.

Allergic bronchopulmonary aspergillosis manifests as episodic wheezing, expectoration of brown mucus plugs, low-grade fever, eosinophilia, and transient pulmonary infiltrates. This form of aspergillosis occurs most frequently in immunocompetent children with chronic asthma or cystic fibrosis.

Allergic sinusitis is a less common allergic response to colonization by *Aspergillus* species than is allergic bronchopulmonary syndrome. It occurs in children with nasal polyps or previous episodes of sinusitis or those who have undergone sinus surgery and is characterized by symptoms of chronic sinusitis with dark plugs of nasal discharge.

Aspergillomas and otomycosis are two syndromes of nonallergic colonization by *Aspergillus* species in immunocompetent children. Aspergillomas grow in preexisting cavities or bronchogenic cysts without invading pulmonary tissue; almost all patients have underlying lung disease, typically cystic fibrosis.

Invasive aspergillosis occurs almost exclusively in immunocompromised patients who have neutropenia or an underlying disease (e.g., chronic granulomatous disease), who use medications (e.g., corticosteroids) that cause neutrophil dysfunction, or who have undergone cytotoxic chemotherapy or immunosuppressive therapy (e.g., after organ transplantation). Invasive infection usually involves pulmonary, sinus, cerebral, or cutaneous sites, and the hallmark is angioinvasion with resulting thrombosis, dissemination to other organs, and, occasionally, erosion of the blood vessel wall and catastrophic hemorrhage. Rarely, endocarditis, osteomyelitis, meningitis, infection of the eye or orbit, and esophagitis occur.

Diagnostic Tests

Dichotomously branched and septate hyphae, identified by microscopic examination of 10% potassium hydroxide wet preparations or of Gomori methenamine–silver nitrate staining of tissue or bronchoalveolar lavage specimens, are suggestive of the diagnosis. The organism usually is not recoverable from blood but is isolated readily from lung, sinus, and skin biopsy specimens cultured on Sabouraud dextrose or brain-heart infusion media (without cycloheximide). *Aspergillus* species may be a laboratory contaminant, but when results from immunocompromised patients are being evaluated, recovery of this organism suggests etiologic significance. Biopsy of a lesion usually is required to confirm the diagnosis. Serologic tests (antigen or antibody) have no established value in the diagnosis of invasive aspergillosis. In allergic aspergillosis, diagnosis is suggested by a typical clinical syndrome and elevated concentrations of total and *Aspergillus*-specific serum IgE, eosinophilia, and a positive skin test result to *Aspergillus* antigens. In persons with cystic fibrosis, the diagnosis is more difficult because wheezing, eosinophilia, and a positive skin test result unassociated with allergic bronchopulmonary aspergillosis often are present.

Blastomycosis

Blastomycosis is caused by *Blastomyces dermatitidis*, a dimorphic fungus existing in the yeast form at 37°C (98°F) and in infected tissues, and in a mycelial form at room temperature and in the soil. Conidia, produced from hyphae of the mycelial form, are infectious for humans.

Infection is acquired through inhalation of conidia from soil. Person-to-person transmission does not occur. Endemic areas in the United States are the southeastern and central states and the midwestern states bordering the Great Lakes.

Infection may be asymptomatic or may be associated with acute, chronic, or fulminant disease. The major clinical manifestations of blastomycosis are pulmonary, cutaneous, and disseminated disease. Children commonly have pulmonary disease that can be associated with a variety of symptoms and radiographic appearances that may be misdiagnosed as bacterial pneumonia, tuberculosis, sarcoidosis, or malignant neoplasm. Skin lesions can be nodular, verrucous, or ulcerative, often with minimal inflammation.

Diagnostic Tests

Thick-walled, figure-of-eight, broad-based, single-budding yeast forms may be seen in sputum, tracheal aspirates, CSF, urine, or material from lesions processed with 10% potassium hydroxide or a fungal stain. Children with pneumonia who are unable to produce sputum may require an invasive procedure (e.g., open biopsy or bronchoalveolar lavage) to establish the diagnosis. Organisms can be cultured on brain-heart infusion and Sabouraud dextrose agar at room temperature. Chemiluminescent DNA probes are available for identification of *B. dermatitidis*. Because there is no skin test available for blastomycosis and available serologic tests lack adequate sensitivity, effort should be made to obtain appropriate specimens for culture.

Candidiasis

Candida albicans causes most infection (60–80%). Other *Candida* species such as *C. tropicalis*, *C. parapsilosis*, *C. glabrata*, *C. krusei*, *C. guilliermondii*, *C. lusitaniae*, *C. lipolytica,* and *C. stella-toidea* also can cause serious infections in immunocompromised hosts. Approximately 200 species of *Candida* have been identified.

Mucocutaneous infection results in oral candidiasis (thrush) or vaginal candidiasis; intertriginous lesions of the gluteal folds, neck, groin, and axilla; paronychia; and onychia. Chronic mucocutaneous candidiasis can be associated with endocrinologic diseases or progressive immunodeficiency, particularly T-cell lymphocyte deficiency, and may be the presenting sign of HIV infection. Esophagitis and laryngitis may occur in immunocompromised patients. Disseminated or invasive candidiasis occurs in very-low-birth-weight newborns and in immunocompromised or debilitated hosts. It can involve virtually any organ or anatomic site and may be rapidly fatal. The presence of typical retinal lesions may be useful in diagnosis. Candidemia can occur with or without systemic disease in patients with indwelling catheters or inpatients receiving prolonged intravenous infusions, especially parenteral alimentation and lipids. Candiduria can occur in patients with indwelling catheters or disseminated disease.

Diagnostic Tests

The presumptive diagnosis of mucocutaneous candidiasis or thrush usually can be made clinically, but thrushlike lesions also can be caused by other organisms or trauma. Both yeast and pseudohyphae can be found in *C. albicans*–infected tissue and are identified by microscopic examination of scrapings stained by Gram stain, suspended in 10–20% potassium hydroxide, or stained with methenamine silver or periodic acid–Schiff stains. Endoscopy is most useful for the diagnosis of esophagitis. Ophthalmologic examination is required to identify retinal lesions, and lesions in the brain, kidney, liver, or spleen may be detected by ultrasonography or CT.

A definitive diagnosis of invasive candidiasis requires isolation of the organism from an otherwise sterile body fluid or tissue (e.g., blood, CSF, bone marrow, or biopsy specimen) or demonstration of organisms in a tissue biopsy specimen stained with methenamine silver or periodic acid–Schiff. The hyphae have a Chinese-checker pattern admixed with yeast forms. Negativity of cultures for *Candida* species, however, does not exclude invasive infection in immunocompromised hosts. Recovery of the organism is easier and faster by blood culture using biphasic or lysis-centrifugation systems. A presumptive species identification of *C. albicans* can be made by demonstrating germ-tube formation.

Coccidioidomycosis

Coccidioides immitis is found extensively in soil and is endemic in the southwestern United States, northern Mexico, and certain areas of Central and South America.

C. immitis is a dimorphic fungus. In soil, it exists in the hyphal phase. In tissues of the infected host, spores enlarge to form spherules. Mature spherules release endospores that develop into new spherules and continue the tissue cycle.

The primary infection is acquired by the respiratory route and is asymptomatic or inapparent in 60% of children. Symptomatic disease may resemble influenza, with malaise, fever, cough, myalgia, headache, and chest pain. A diffuse erythematous maculopapular rash, erythema multiforme, erythema nodosum, and arthralgias frequently occur and may be the only clinical manifestations in some children. Chronic pulmonary lesions are rare.

Diagnostic Tests

Serologic tests are useful to confirm diagnoses and provide prognostic information. The IgM response can be detected by latex agglutination, EIA, immunodiffusion, or tube precipitin. Latex agglutination is a rapid, sensitive test that lacks specificity; hence, positive results should be confirmed by other tests. An IgM response is detectable 1–3 weeks after symptoms appear and lasts 3–4 months in most cases.

The IgG response can be detected by immunodiffusion, EIA, or complement fixation. Complement fixation antibodies in serum usually are of low titer and transient if the disease is asymptomatic or mild. High (≥1:32) persistent titers occur in severe disease and almost always in disseminated infection. CSF antibodies also are detectable by complement fixation. The concentration and persistence of antibody titers in serum from patients with disseminated severe disease and in CSF specimens from patients with meningitis are useful prognostically and for guiding treatment. Increasing serum and CSF titers indicate progressive disease, whereas decreasing titers suggest improvement. Low or nondetectable titers in immunocompromised patients should be interpreted with caution.

Skin tests may be useful for diagnosis. A delayed hypersensitivity reaction to a coccidioidin or spherulin skin test is indicative of past or current infection.

Spherules as large as 80 µm in diameter, in selected instances, can be visualized in infected body fluids and biopsy specimens of skin lesions or organs. Culture of the organism is possible but is potentially hazardous to laboratory personnel, because spherules can convert to arthroconidia-bearing mycelia on culture plates. Cultures suspected of carrying the organism should be sealed at the outset and thereafter handled only by trained personnel using appropriate safety equipment and procedures. A DNA probe can identify *C. immitis* in cultures and thereby reduce the risk of exposure to infectious fungi.

Cryptococcus neoformans *Infections*

Cryptococcus neoformans var *neoformans* is isolated primarily from soil contaminated with bird droppings and causes most human infection, especially infections in immunocompromised hosts. *Cryptococcus* species infect 5–10% of adults with AIDS, but infection is uncommon in HIV-infected children.

C. neoformans, an encapsulated yeast that grows at 37°C (98°F), is the only species of the genus *Cryptococcus* considered to be a human pathogen.

Primary infection is acquired by inhalation of aerosolized fungal elements and often is inapparent or mild. Pulmonary disease, when symptomatic, is characterized by cough, hemoptysis, chest pain, and constitutional symptoms. Hematogenous dissemination to the CNS, bones and joints, skin, and mucous membranes can occur, but dissemination is rare in children without defects in cell-mediated immunity (e.g., transplantation, malignant neoplasm, collagen-vascular disease, long-term corticosteroid administration, or sarcoidosis). Cryptococcal meningitis is the most common and serious form of cryptococcal disease.

Diagnostic Tests

Encapsulated yeast cells can be visualized by India ink or other stains of CSF containing $\geq 10^3$ colony-forming units of yeast per milliliter. Definitive diagnosis requires isolation of the organism from body fluid or tissue. The lysis-centrifugation method is the most sensitive technique for recovery of *C. neoformans* from blood cultures. Media containing cycloheximide, which inhibits growth of *C. neoformans*, should not be used. Sabouraud glucose agar is optimal for isolation of *Cryptococcus* from sputum, bronchopulmonary lavage fluid, tissue, or CSF specimens. Few organisms may be present in the CSF, and large quantities of CSF may be needed to recover the organism. The latex agglutination and EIA tests for detection of cryptococcal capsular polysaccharide antigen in serum or CSF are excellent, rapid diagnostic tests. Antigen is detected in CSF or serum in 90% of patients with cryptococcal meningitis. Cryptococcal antibody testing is useful, but skin testing is of no value.

Histoplasmosis

Histoplasma capsulatum var *capsulatum* is a dimorphic fungus. In soil, it grows as a spore-bearing mold with macroconidia, but it converts to a yeast phase at body temperature 37°C (98°F).

Histoplasmosis encompasses a spectrum of clinical manifestations in the <5% of infected persons who are symptomatic. Clinical manifestations may be classified according to site (pulmonary, extrapulmonary, or disseminated), duration of infection (acute, chronic), and pattern of infection (primary versus reactivated). Acute pulmonary histoplasmosis is an influenza-like illness with nonpleuritic chest pain, pulmonary infiltrates, and hilar adenopathy; symptoms persist for 2–3 days to 2 weeks. Erythema nodosum can occur in adolescents, but erythema nodosum and chronic pulmonary histoplasmosis are uncommon in children. Primary cutaneous infections can occur after trauma.

Acute disseminated histoplasmosis is most frequent in children with impaired cell-mediated immunity, including patients with HIV infection and solid-organ transplant recipients, and infants <1 year of age. Features include prolonged fever, failure to thrive, cough, hepatosplenomegaly, adenopathy, pneumonia, skin lesions, and pancytopenia. CNS involvement is common. Chronic disseminated infection is rare. Histoplasmosis may reactivate years after primary infection in isolated tissues, particularly in the CNS, adrenal glands, and mucocutaneous surfaces, as well as in other sites. Disseminated or extrapulmonary histoplasmosis is an AIDS-defining condition in an HIV-infected person.

Diagnostic Tests

Culture is the definitive method of diagnosis. *H. capsulatum* from bone marrow, blood, sputum, and biopsy specimens grows on standard mycologic media, but growth usually requires 2–6 weeks. The lysis-centrifugation method is preferred for blood cultures. Use of a DNA probe for *H. capsulatum* significantly shortens the time required for identification in cultures. This procedure can be applied to nonsporulating cultures, which thereby reduces the risk of exposure of laboratory personnel to infectious spores.

Direct demonstration of intracellular yeast by Gomori methenamine silver or other stains in smears of bone marrow or biopsy material from infected tissues is helpful for diagnosing disseminated or chronic histoplasmosis.

Detection of *H. capsulatum* polysaccharide antigen in serum, urine, and bronchoalveolar lavage fluid by radioimmunoassay is a specific, sensitive, and rapid method for the diagnosis of disseminated histoplasmosis, and it can be used to monitor treatment response. Cross-reacting antigens have been detected in persons with disseminated infection due to blastomycosis, coccidioidomycosis, paracoccidioidomycosis, and *Penicillium marneffei* infection.

Both mycelial-phase (histoplasmin) and yeast-phase antigens are used in serologic testing for complement-fixing antibodies to *H. capsulatum*. A fourfold increase in yeast-phase titers or a single titer of ≥1:32 is presumptive evidence of active infection. Cross-reacting antibodies can result from *B. dermatitidis* and *C. immitis* infections. In the immunodiffusion antibody test, H bands, although rarely encountered, are highly suggestive of active infection. The immunodiffusion test is more specific than the complement fixation test, but the complement fixation test is more sensitive.

The histoplasmin skin test is not recommended for diagnostic purposes but is useful for epidemiologic studies.

Paracoccidioidomycosis

Paracoccidioides brasiliensis is a dimorphic fungus with a yeast and a mycelial phase.

Disease occurs primarily in adults and is rare in children. The site of primary infection is the lungs. Clinical patterns of disease include acute pneumonia, chronic pneumonia, and dissemination to skin, mucous membranes, lymph nodes, liver, spleen, bone, CNS, gastrointestinal tract, and adrenal glands. Chronic granulomatous lesions of the mucous membranes, especially of the mouth and palate, are typical but infrequent findings. Infection may be latent for years before causing illness.

Diagnostic Tests

Round, multiple-budding cells may be seen in 10% potassium hydroxide preparations of sputum specimens, bronchoalveolar lavage specimens, scrapings from ulcers, and material from lesions or in tissue biopsy specimens. The organism can be cultured easily on most enriched media, including blood agar at 37°C (98°F) and Sabouraud dextrose agar (with cycloheximide) at 24°C (75°F). Complement fixation, EIA, and immunodiffusion methods are useful for detecting specific antibodies. Skin testing is not reliable for diagnosis because nonreactivity is common and false-positive tests can occur. Skin test positivity developing during therapy, however, portends a good prognosis.

Pneumocystis carinii *Infections*

Pneumocystis carinii seems to be an unusual or primitive fungus, based on DNA sequence homologies.

In infants and children, a subacute diffuse pneumonitis with dyspnea at rest, tachypnea, oxygen desaturation, nonproductive cough, and fever develop. The magnitude of these signs and symptoms may vary, however, and in some immunocompromised children and adults, the onset can be acute and fulminant. The chest radiograph often shows bilateral diffuse interstitial or alveolar disease; rarely, lobar, miliary, and nodular lesions occur as well. Occasionally, the chest radiograph at the time of diagnosis appears normal. Mortality in immunocompromised patients is high, ranging from 5–40% if the disease is treated, and almost 100% if it is untreated.

Diagnostic Tests

A definitive diagnosis of *P. carinii* pneumonia (PCP) is made by demonstration of organisms in lung tissue or respiratory tract secretions. The most sensitive and specific diagnostic procedures have been open lung biopsy and transbronchial biopsy. However, bronchoscopy with bronchoalveolar lavage, induction of sputum in older children and adolescents, and intubation with deep endotracheal aspiration are less invasive and often diagnostic and have been sufficiently sensitive in patients with HIV infection, who have an increased number of organisms compared with non–HIV-infected patients with PCP. Methenamine silver, toluidine blue I, calcofluor white, and fluorescein-conjugated monoclonal antibody are the most useful stains for identifying the thick-walled cysts of *P. carinii*. Extracystic trophozoite forms are identified with Giemsa stain, modified Wright-Giemsa stain, and fluorescein-conjugated monoclonal antibody. Serologic tests and PCR assays for detecting *P. carinii* infection are experimental and are not recommended for diagnosis. Many children and adults with HIV infection and PCP have elevated serum concentrations of lactate dehydrogenase, but this abnormality is not specific for PCP.

Sporotrichosis

Sporothrix schenckii is a dimorphic fungus that grows as an oval or cigar-shaped yeast at 37°C (98°F).

Sporotrichosis manifests most commonly as cutaneous infection, although pulmonary and disseminated forms occur. Inoculation occurs at a site of minor trauma, causing an ulcerative subcutaneous nodule that is firm and slightly tender but often painless. Secondary lesions may spread along lymphatic channels to form multiple nodules that ulcerate and suppurate. The extremities and face are the most common sites of infection in children.

Extracutaneous sporotrichosis commonly affects bones and joints, particularly those of the hands, elbows, ankles, or knees, but any organ can be affected. Disseminated disease generally occurs after hematogenous spread from primary skin to lung infection and is uncommon in children.

Diagnostic Tests

A culture positive for *S. schenckii* from tissue, wound drainage, or sputum is diagnostic of infection. A positive blood culture result suggests the multifocal form of sporotrichosis associated with immunodeficiency. Histopathologic examination of tissue can be helpful, but the organism is difficult to detect in biopsy samples. No standardized serologic test is available.

Tinea Capitis (Ringworm of the Scalp)

Trichophyton tonsurans is the cause of tinea capitis in >90% of cases in North and Central America. *Microsporum canis*, *Microsporum audouinii*, and *Trichophyton mentagrophytes* infections are less common. The causative agents may vary in different geographic areas.

Fungal infection of the scalp may present with one of the following distinct clinical syndromes:

- Patchy areas of dandruff-like scaling, with subtle or extensive hair loss, which easily is confused with dandruff, seborrheic dermatitis, or atopic dermatitis.
- Discrete areas of hair loss studded by the stubs of broken hairs, referred to as *black-dot ringworm*.
- Numerous discrete pustules or excoriations with little hair loss or scaling.
- Kerion, a boggy inflammatory mass surrounded by follicular pustules, is a hypersensitivity reaction to the fungal infection. Kerion may be accompanied by fever and local lymphadenopathy and frequently is misdiagnosed as impetigo, cellulitis, or an abscess of the scalp.

A pruritic, fine, papulovesicular eruption (dermatophytid or id reaction) involving the trunk, hands, or face, caused by a hypersensitivity response to the infecting fungus, may accompany the scalp lesions.

Tinea capitis may be confused with many other diseases, including seborrheic dermatitis, atopic dermatitis, psoriasis, alopecia areata, trichotillomania, folliculitis, impetigo, and lupus erythematosus.

Diagnostic Tests

Hairs may be obtained by gentle scraping of a moistened area of the scalp with a curved scalpel, toothbrush, or cotton-tip applicator for potassium hydroxide wet-mount examination and for culture. In black-dot ringworm, broken hairs should be obtained for diagnosis. In cases of *T. tonsurans* infection, microscopic examination of a potassium hydroxide wet-mount preparation will disclose numerous arthroconidia within the hair shaft. In *Microsporum* infection, spores surround the hair shaft. Use of dermatophyte test medium also is a reliable, simple, and inexpensive method of diagnosing tinea capitis. Skin scrapings, brushings, or hairs from lesions are inoculated directly onto the culture medium and incubated at room temperature. After 1–2 weeks, a phenol red indicator in the agar will turn from yellow to red in the area surrounding a dermatophyte colony. When necessary, the diagnosis also may be confirmed by culture on Sabouraud dextrose sugar.

Wood light examination of the hair of patients with *Microsporum* infection results in brilliant green fluorescence. Because *T. tonsurans* does not fluoresce under Wood light, however, this diagnostic test is not helpful for most patients with tinea capitis.

Tinea Corporis (Ringworm of the Body)

The prime causes of tinea corporis are fungi of the genus *Trichophyton*, especially *T. rubrum, T. mentagrophytes,* and *T. tonsurans*; fungi of the genus *Microsporum*, especially *M. canis*; and *Epidermophyton floccosum*.

Superficial tinea infections of the nonhairy (glabrous) skin may involve the face, trunk, or limbs but not the scalp, beard, groin, hands, or feet. The lesion generally is circular (hence, the term *ringworm*), slightly erythematous, and well demarcated with a scaly, vesicular, or pustular border. Pruritus is common. Lesions often are mistaken for atopic dermatitis, seborrheic dermatitis, or contact dermatitis. A frequent source of confusion in diagnosis is an alteration in the appearance of lesions resulting from application of a topical corticosteroid preparation. This atypical presentation has been termed *tinea incognita*. In patients with diminished T-lymphocyte function (e.g., HIV infection), the rash may appear as grouped papules or pustules unaccompanied by scaling or erythema.

A pruritic, fine, papulovesicular eruption (dermatophytid or id reaction) involving the trunk, hands, or face, caused by a hypersensitivity response to the infecting fungus, may accompany the rash.

Diagnostic Tests

The fungi responsible for tinea corporis can be detected by microscopic examination of a potassium hydroxide wet mount of skin scrapings. Use of dermatophyte test medium also is a reliable, simple, and inexpensive method of diagnosis. Skin scrapings from lesions are inoculated directly onto the culture medium and incubated at room temperature. After 1–2 weeks, a phenol red indicator in the agar will turn from yellow to red in the area surrounding a dermatophyte colony. When necessary, the diagnosis also can be confirmed by culture on Sabouraud dextrose agar.

Tinea Cruris ("Jock Itch")

The fungi *E. floccosum*, *T. rubrum*, and *T. mentagrophytes* are the most common causes of tinea cruris, a common superficial fungal disorder.

Tinea cruris affects the groin and upper thighs. The eruption is sharply marginated and usually is bilaterally symmetric. Involved skin is erythematous and scaly and varies from red to brown; occasionally, the eruption is accompanied by central clearing and a vesiculopapular border. In chronic infections, the margin may be subtle, and lichenification may be present. Tinea cruris skin lesions may be extremely pruritic. These lesions should be differentiated from intertrigo, seborrheic dermatitis, psoriasis, primary irritant dermatitis, allergic contact dermatitis (generally caused by the therapeutic agents applied to the area), or erythrasma, which is a superficial bacterial infection of the skin caused by *Corynebacterium minutissimum*.

Diagnostic Tests

The fungi responsible for tinea cruris may be detected by microscopic examination of a potassium hydroxide wet mount of scales. Use of dermatophyte test medium also is a reliable, simple, and inexpensive method of diagnosing tinea cruris. Skin scrapings from lesions are inoculated directly onto the culture medium and incubated at room temperature. After 1–2 weeks, a phenol red indicator in the agar will turn from yellow to red in the area surrounding a dermatophyte colony. When necessary, the diagnosis also can be confirmed by culture on Sabouraud dextrose agar. A characteristic coral-red fluorescence under Wood light can identify the presence of erythrasma and thus exclude tinea cruris.

Tinea Pedis (Athlete's Foot, Ringworm of the Feet)

The fungi *T. rubrum*, *T. mentagrophytes*, and *E. floccosum* are the most common causes of tinea pedis.

Tinea pedis is manifest by fine vesiculopustular or scaly lesions that frequently are pruritic. The lesions can involve all areas of the foot, but usually they are patchy in distribution, with a predisposition to fissures and scaling between the toes, particularly in the third and fourth interdigital spaces. Toenails may be infected and can be dystrophic (tinea unguium). Tinea pedis must be differentiated from dyshidrotic eczema, atopic dermatitis, contact dermatitis, juvenile plantar dermatosis, and erythrasma (a superficial bacterial infection caused by *C. minutissimum*). Tinea pedis commonly occurs in association with tinea cruris.

Diagnostic Tests

Tinea pedis usually is diagnosed by clinical manifestation and may be confirmed by microscopic examination of a potassium hydroxide wet mount of the cutaneous scrapings. Use of dermatophyte test medium is a reliable, simple, and inexpensive method of diagnosis in complicated or unresponsive cases. Skin scrapings or nail clippings are inoculated directly onto the culture medium and incubated at room temperature. After 1–2 weeks, a phenol red indicator in the agar will turn from yellow to red in the area surrounding a dermatophyte colony. When necessary, the diagnosis also can be confirmed by culture on Sabouraud dextrose agar. Infection of the nail can be certified by fungal culture of desquamated subungual material.

Tinea Versicolor (Pityriasis Versicolor)

Tinea (pityriasis) versicolor is a common superficial yeast infection of the skin characterized by multiple scaling, oval, and patchy macular lesions, usually distributed over the upper portions of the trunk, proximal areas of the arms, and neck. Facial involvement is particularly common in children. The lesions may be hypopigmented or hyperpigmented (fawn colored or brown) and may be somewhat lighter than the surrounding skin. The lesions fail to tan during the summer and during the winter are relatively darker—hence the term *versicolor.* Common conditions confused with this disorder include pityriasis alba, postinflammatory hypopigmentation, vitiligo, melasma, seborrheic dermatitis, pityriasis rosea, and secondary syphilis.

Malassezia furfur is the cause. This dimorphic lipid-dependent yeast exists on healthy skin in the yeast phase and causes clinical lesions only when substantial growth of hyphae occurs. Moist heat and lipid-containing sebaceous secretions encourage rapid overgrowth.

Diagnostic Tests

The clinical appearance usually is diagnostic. Involved areas are yellow fluorescent under Wood light. Scale scrapings examined microscopically in a potassium hydroxide wet-mount preparation or stained with methylene blue or May-Grünwald-Giemsa stain disclose the pathognomonic clusters of yeast cells and hyphae ("spaghetti and meatball" appearance). Growth of this yeast in culture requires a source of long-chain fatty acids, which may be accomplished by overlaying Sabouraud dextrose agar medium with sterile olive oil.

Other Fungal Diseases

In addition to the common mycoses, infants and children can have infections cause by infrequently encountered fungi. Infections caused by these agents usually occur in children with immunosuppression or other underlying conditions predisposing to infection. Children who are immunocompetent can acquire infection with these fungi through inhalation via the respiratory tract or direct inoculation after traumatic disruption of cutaneous barriers. A list of these fungal agents and the pertinent underlying host conditions, route of entry, clinical manifestations, diagnostic tests, and treatment for each is found in Table 9.

Summary of Fungal Diseases

Figure 1 provides a summary of organisms causing deep mycosis.

Summary of Diagnostic Methods and Specimen Collection

See Table 10.

Table 9. Additional Fungal Diseases

Disease and Agent	Underlying Condition(s)	Reservoir(s) or Route(s) of Entry	Common Clinical Manifestations	Diagnostic Laboratory Test(s)	Treatment
Fusariosis					
Fusarium spp.	Granulocytopenia; marrow disorders	Respiratory tract, sinuses, skin, eyes	Pulmonary infiltrates, cutaneous lesions, sinusitis; disseminated under eye contact lens	Culture of blood or tissue specimen	High-dose amphotericin B deoxycholate (AmB) (1.0–1.5 mg/kg/d)[a,b]
Malassezia spp.	Prematurity, exposure to parenteral nutrition that includes fat emulsions	Skin	Catheter-associated bloodstream infection, interstitial pneumonitis, urinary tract infection, meningitis	Culture of blood, catheter tip, or tissue specimen; olive oil overlay of Sabouraud dextrose agar is an effective culture medium	Removal of catheters and temporary cessation of lipid infusions; AmB; imidazoles
Penicilliosis					
Penicillium marneffei	Human immunodeficiency virus infection	Respiratory tract	Pneumonitis, invasive dermatitis, disseminated infection	Culture of blood, bone marrow, or tissue; histopathologic examination of tissue	Itraconazole or AmB with or without flucytosine
Phaeohyphomycosis					
Curvularia spp.	Prematurity, altered skin integrity, asthma or nasal polyps, chronic cough	Environment	Allergic fungal sinusitis, invasive dermatitis, disseminated infection with or without solid organ involvement	Culture and histopathologic examination of tissue	Allergic fungal sinusitis: surgery and corticosteroids Invasive disease: itraconazole[c] or AmB
Exserohilum spp.	Immunosuppression, altered skin integrity	Environment	Sinusitis, pneumonia, ocular infection, cutaneous lesions	Culture and histopathologic examination of tissue	AmB[a] or itraconazole; surgical excision

Pseudallescheria boydii	Immunosuppression	Environment	Pneumonia, disseminated infection, mycetoma (immunocompetent patients)	Culture and histopathologic examination of tissue	Itraconazole[d]; surgical excision for pulmonary infection, as feasible
Scedosporium spp.	Immunosuppression	Environment	Pneumonia, disseminated infection, osteomyelitis or septic arthritis (immunocompetent patients)	Culture and histopathologic examination of tissue	Itraconazole[b] or AmB
Trichosporin beigelii	Immunosuppression	Normal flora of skin; stool or urine cultures	Bloodstream infection, endocarditis pneumonitis	Blood culture, histopathologic examination of tissue	AmB and flucytosine
Bipolaris spp.	None or organ transplantation	Environment	Sinusitis	Culture and histopathologic examination of tissue	Itraconazole or AmB; surgical excision
Torulopsis glabrata	Immunosuppression	Blood, indwelling catheter	Fungemia	Blood, urine culture	
Zygomycosis					
Rhizopus, Absidia	Immunosuppression, hematologic malignant neoplasm, renal failure, diabetes mellitus, exposure to multiple antimicrobial agents, exposure to construction activity, use of nonsterile adhesive dressings	Respiratory tract, skin	Rhinocerebral infection, pulmonary infection, disseminated infection; skin and gastrointestinal tract less frequently	Histopathologic examination of tissue	High dose of AmB (1.0–1.5 mg/kg/d)[a] and surgical excision, as feasible

[a]Use of a lipid formulation of AmB should be considered.
[b]Infection may be refractory to AmB; use of investigational antifungal compounds may be required.
[c]Itraconazole is the treatment of choice, but data on use in children are limited.
[d]Immunocompromised patients may not respond. AmB has activity against some strains. Enhanced fungal activity may be observed when AmB is combined with itraconazole or fluconazole.

Mycosis	Fungus	Structure	Tissue	Size[1]	Culture 20°C
Cryptococcosis	*Cryptococcus neoformans*	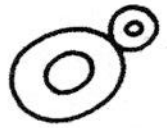	Encapsulated yeast	4–20 µ	Encapsulated yeast 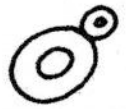
Blastomycosis	*Blastomyces dermatitidis*	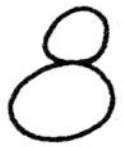	Yeast	8–15 µ	Mycelium with spores 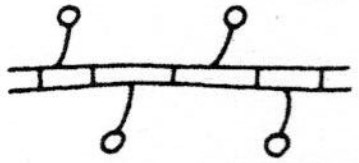
Paracoccidioido-mycosis	*Paracoccidioides brasiliensis*	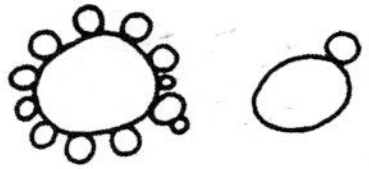	Yeast	5–30 µ	Mycelium with spores 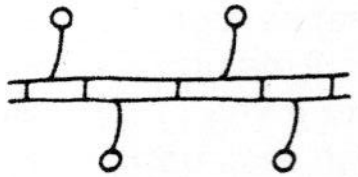
Lobomycosis	*Loboa loboi*	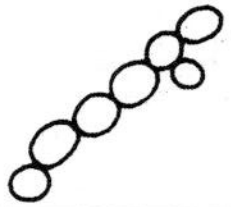	Yeast	8–12 µ	Does *not* grow
Histoplasmosis	*Histoplasma capsulatum*[2]	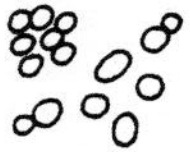	Yeast	2–5 µ	Mycelium with spores 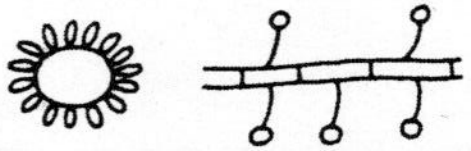
African histo-plasmosis	*H. capsulatum*, var. *duboisii*	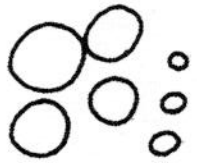	Yeast	8–15 µ 2–5 µ	Like *H. capsulatum*
Epizootic lym-phangitis	*H. farciminosum*	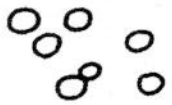	Yeast	2–5 µ	Mycelium with spores

Fig. 1. Summary of deep mycoses. [1]Diameter in microns. [2]Preferentially intracellular. [3]Width of hyphae in microns. [4]More frequent in the United States: *Petriellidum boydii*.

Mycosis	Fungus	Structure	Tissue	Size[1]	Culture 20°C
Coccidioidomycosis	*Coccidioides immitis*	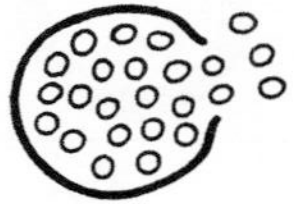	Spherule	30–60 μ	Mycelium with arthrospores 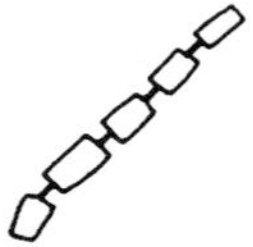
Candidiasis	*Candida albicans*, etc.	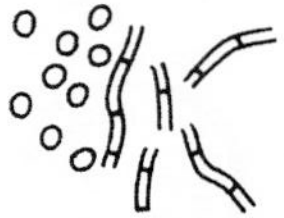	Yeast mixed with mycelium	2–4 μ 2–4 μ[3]	Yeast and/or mycelium 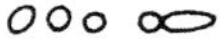
Aspergillosis	*Aspergillus fumigatus*, etc.	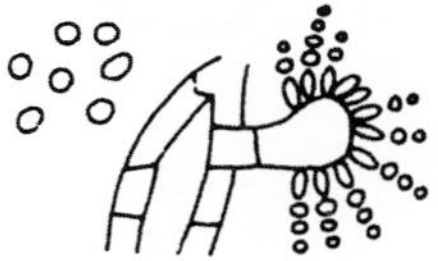	Mycelium	3–5 μ 4–6 μ[3]	Mycelium with spores 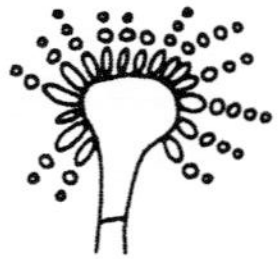
Basidiomycosis	*Schizophyllum commune* *Coprinus* sp.	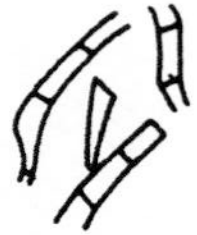	Mycelium	Variable	
Bagassosis	Varied fungi and actinomycetes	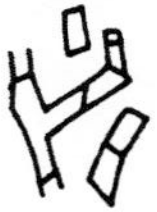	Varied debris		

Fig. 1. (continued)

Mycosis	Fungus	Structure	Tissue	Size[1]	Culture 20°C
Zygomycoses	Mucorales and Entomophthorales sp., Oomycetes (e.g., *Mucor, Absidia, Rhizopus*)	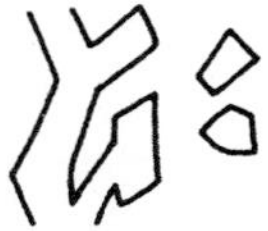	Nonseptate mycelium	6–15 μ[3]	Mycelium with spores 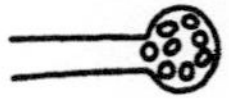
Chromomycosis	Various dematiaceous fungi	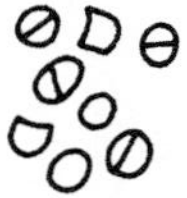		5–12 μ Brown color, round to elongate cells	Cl. 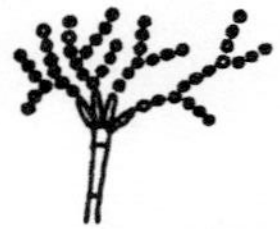
Sporotrichosis	*Sporothrix schenckii*	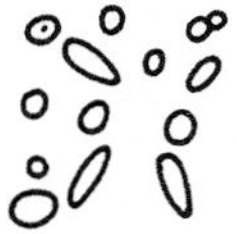		2–8 μ Pleomorphic	Mycelium with spores 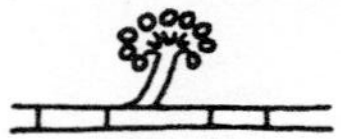
Rhinosporidiosis	*Rhinosporidium seeberi*	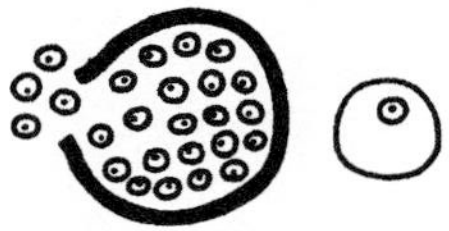	Spherule	10–200 μ	Does *not* grow
Torulopsiosis	*Torulopsis glabrata*[2]	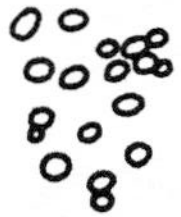	Yeast	2.5–5.0 μ	Yeast 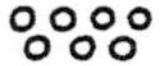
Adiaspiromycosis	*Chrysosporium parvum*, var. *crescens*	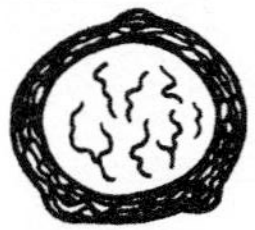	Spherule	20–40 μ 200–700 μ	Mycelium with spores 

Fig. 1. (continued)

Mycosis	Fungus	Structure	Tissue	Size[1]	Culture 20°C
Mycetomas					
Eumycetomas[4]	Various fungi	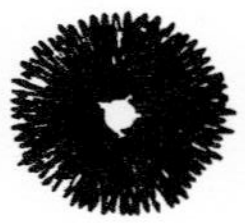		Granules up to 2 mm	Mycelium with spores 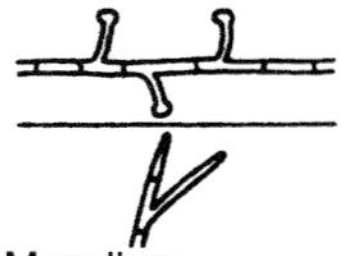 Mycelium
Actinomycetomas	Various actinomycetes				
Algoses	*Protothecus* sp. *Chorella* sp.	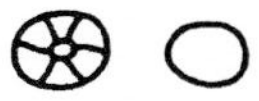	Spherule (theca)	10–30 μ	

Fig. 1. (continued)

Table 10. Fungal Infections

	Source of Material									
Disease	Blood	CSF	Stool	Urine	Naso-pharynx, Throat	Sputum, Lung	Gastric Washings	Vagina, Cervix	Exudates, Lesions, Sinus Tracts, Etc.	Skin, Nails, Hair
Cryptococcosis (*Cryptococcus neoformans*)	*	*	*	*		*				*
Coccidioidomycosis (*Coccidioides immitis*)	*	*	*			*	*			*
Histoplasmosis (*Histoplasma capsulatum*)	*					*	*			*
Actinomycosis (*Actinomyces israelii*)						*			*	
Nocardiosis (*Nocardia asteroides*)						*				*
North American blastomycosis (*Blastomyces dermatitidis*)						*				*
South American blastomycosis (*Paracoccidioides brasiliensis*)					*					*
Moniliasis (*Candida albicans*)	*				*			*		*
Aspergillosis (*Aspergillus fumigatus*, others)						*				
Chromoblastomycosis (*Fonsecaea pedrosoi, Phialophora verrucosa, compactum*, etc.)										*
Sporotrichosis (*Sporothrix schenckii*)										*
Rhinosporidiosis (*Rhinosporidium seeberi*)					*					

CSF, cerebrospinal fluid.

		Diagnostic Methods						
Bone Marrow	Lymph Node	Microscopic Examination	Fresh Unstained Material	Stained Material	Culture	Animal Inoculation	Serologic Tests	Histologic Examination
*				*	*	*	*	*
*	*		*		*	*	*	*
*	*			*	*	*	*	*
				*	*			*
				*	*	*	*	*
			*		*		*	*
	*		*		*		*	*
				*	*		*	
			*		*		*	*
			*		*			*
					*	*	*	*
								*

Superficial Mycoses

Diagnosis	Specimen of Choice
Piedra	Hair
Tinea nigra	Skin scraping
Pityriasis versicolor	Skin scraping

Dermatomycoses (Cutaneous Mycoses)

Diagnosis	Specimen of Choice
Onychomycosis	Nail scrapings
Tinea capitis	Hair (black dot)
Tinea corporis	Skin scrapings
Tinea pedis	Skin scrapings
Tinea cruris	Skin scrapings

Candidiasis

Diagnosis	Specimen of Choice
Diaper dermatitis	Scraping of pustules at margin
Paronychia	Scraping of skin around nail
Cutaneous candidiasis	Scraping of pustules at margin
Erosio interdigitalis blastomycetica (coinfection with Gram-negative rods)	Scrapings of interdigital space (routine culture also)
Congenital candidiasis	Scraping of scales, pustules, and cutaneous debris, cultures of umbilical stump, mouth scrapings, urine, and stool
Mucocutaneous candidiasis	Scraping of affected area

Systemic Mycoses

Diagnosis	Specimen of Choice in Order of Usefulness
Aspergillosis	Sputum Bronchial aspirate Biopsy specimen (lung)
Blastomycosis	Skin scrapings Abscess drainage (pus) Urine Sputum Bronchial aspirate
Candidiasis	Sputum Bronchial aspirate Blood CSF Urine Stool
Coccidioidomycosis	Sputum Bronchial aspirate CSF Urine Skin scrapings Abscess drainage (pus)
Cryptococcosis	CSF Sputum Abscess drainage (pus) Skin scraping Urine
Mycomycosis/phycomycosis	Sputum Bronchial aspirate Biopsy (lung)

Paracoccidioidomycosis (South American blastomycosis)	Skin scrapings Mucosal scrapings Biopsy specimen (lymph node) Sputum Bronchial aspirate

For sputum, deeply coughed sputum, transtracheal aspirate, bronchial washing or brushing, and deep tracheal aspirate are preferred specimens. Oncology patients, transplant patients, and patients with AIDS are particularly prone to infection with fungi.

Subcutaneous Mycoses

Diagnosis	Specimen of Choice in Order of Usefulness
Chromoblastomycosis	Skin scrapings Biopsy specimen (skin) Drainage (pus)
Maduromycosis (mycetoma)	Abscess drainage
Sporotrichosis	Biopsy specimen (lesion) Drainage (pus) Abscess drainage Biopsy (skin, lymph node)

Specimens for Examination for Fungus Infection

Abscess Material, Pus, Aspirate

Aspiration with a sterile needle and syringe should be attempted. The aspirated material should be placed in a sterile container. If a very small amount of material is collected, it may be washed from the syringe into 1 mL of sterile water or saline in a sterile container.

If a swab is used, it should be extended into the depths of the wound without touching the adjacent skin margins. It may be placed in bacterial transport medium or in a sterile container with 1 mL sterile water or saline.

Blood

Five to 10 mL blood in heparin sodium or Isolator should be submitted.

The skin should be prepared for venipuncture as follows:

- First the venipuncture site should be cleansed with isopropanol. Then tincture of iodine should be used to disinfect the site using in a pattern of progressively larger concentric circles. Iodine should remain in contact with skin for approximately 1 minute to ensure disinfection.
- The venipuncture site must not be palpated after preparation. Blood is then drawn.

After venipuncture, alcohol is used to remove the iodine from the site.

Room temperature storage is sufficient if there is to be any delay in transport.

Bone Marrow

Approximately 0.3 mL bone marrow should be submitted in a heparinized tube. A syringe with needle should not be sent.

Room temperature storage is recommended if there is to be any delay in transport.

Bronchial Brush Specimen

The brush should be inserted into 2 mL sterile saline or water in a sterile screw-cap container.

Room temperature storage is recommended if there is to be any delay in transport.

Cerebrospinal Fluid

At least 3 mL of CSF is required but at least 5 mL is recommended as optimal for test of cure for cryptococcal infections.

The specimen should be incubated at 37°C (98°F) if possible if there is to be any delay in transport. If an incubator is not available, the specimen should be maintained at room temperature.

Cutaneous Specimens

Skin scrapings are taken from an area previously cleansed with 70% alcohol on gauze sponges (sterile water or broth should be used if alcohol is not available). The entire periphery of the lesion(s) should be scraped with a sterile scalpel or the edge of a glass slide. The scrapings should be placed in a sterile screw-cap container or between clean glass slides in a slide holder, or inoculated into fungal medium. Lesions should remain untreated with topical antifungal agents for at least 1 week before culturing.

A skin biopsy specimen or punch biopsy specimen should be placed between two gauze squares moistened with sterile water or saline. These should be placed in a sterile screw-cap container.

Nails should be cleansed with 70% alcohol and then scraped deeply enough to obtain recently invaded nail tissue. Debris under the nail may be removed with a scalpel and placed between clean glass slides. If the dorsal plate appears diseased, the outer surface should be scraped and discarded, then scrapings collected through the diseased portion.

An evulsed nail should be placed in a sterile screw-cap container.

Scalp and hair specimens may be selected by placing the patient under an ultraviolet light (Wood lamp). Hairs that are fluorescent, distorted, or fractured should be cultured. Culture of the basal portion of infected hair is recommended. At least 10–12 hairs should be placed in a sterile screw-cap container.

Room temperature storage of these specimens is sufficient if there is to be any delay in transport.

Ear Specimens

The ear specimen should be submitted on a swab in red-stopper bacterial transport medium.

Room temperature storage is recommended if there is to be any delay in transport.

Eye Specimens

Ocular specimens are usually collected and immediately inoculated to the medium. If this is not possible, a swab or scraping of the corneal or conjunctival material may be submitted in a red-stopper bacterial transport medium. Fluid or pus should be collected with needle and syringe and inoculated into a bacterial transport device.

Room temperature storage is recommended if there is to be any delay in transport.

Feces

Stool specimens may be submitted in sterile screw-cap containers, but swabs of stool in red-stopper bacterial transport medium are preferred. Rectal swab specimens are not recommended because they are easily contaminated by yeast from the perianal region or the vagina.

Stool specimens should be refrigerated if there is to be any delay in transport.

Fluids

Fluids (e.g., pleural, peritoneal, joint) should be aspirated and placed into a sterile screw-cap container. For large volumes (i.e., thoracic, pleural, or abdominal fluids), a well-mixed aliquot of 50–100 mL may be submitted.

Room temperature storage is recommended if there is to be any delay in transport.

Genitourinary Tract Specimens

Urine must be collected in such a manner as to prevent contamination with yeast from the external urinary tract. First-morning clean-catch specimens or specimens obtained by catheterization are acceptable if proper cleansing procedures are used before collection.

Urine specimens should be refrigerated if there is a delay in transport.

Two swabs containing material from the vagina, cervix, or uterus should be inserted into a bacterial transport device. Refrigerated storage is recommended if there is to be any delay in transport.

Lower Respiratory Tract Specimens

Sputum should be collected as a first- or early-morning sample; a series of three to six specimens is recommended. Patients should brush the teeth, rinse out the mouth with water, then produce material from a deep cough.

Bronchial washings are usually placed in a sterile leakproof container for transport to the laboratory.

Induced specimens are recommended from patients who are not coughing. Transtracheal aspirations and bronchoscopy biopsies may be helpful.

Respiratory secretions should be refrigerated if delay in transportation is necessary.

Tissue

Tissue containing a portion of the wall, base, and center of the lesion should be obtained and placed between sterile moist gauze squares in a sterile container. Sterile saline or sterile water should be used to moisten the gauze. [Liver biopsy tissue should be placed directly into a tube of beef heart infusion (BHI) broth.]

A small amount of tissue should be placed directly into 1–2 mL sterile saline or water in a sterile screw-cap container.

Room temperature storage is recommended if there is to be any delay in transport.

Thrush Lesions of Oral Cavity

Swabs should not be used for collection. A tongue depressor that has been split in half along its long axis should be used. The lesion should be gently scraped with one-half of the tongue depressor. The material should be scraped onto a sterile swab and placed into a red-stopper bacterial transport medium.

Room temperature storage is recommended if there is to be any delay in transport.

Recommended Amounts of Specimen to Be Collected for Mycologic Studies

Specimen	Amount
Aspirated body fluids	50–100 mL
Blood	Adults: 5–10 mL Infants: 1–5 mL
Bone marrow	0.3 mL (use sterile heparin sodium anticoagulant)
Bronchial washing	10 mL
CSF	3–10 mL
Ear specimen	As many scrapings as possible, two swabs
Eye specimen	2–3 drops of fluid, as much scrapings as possible, two swabs
Gastric lavage	10–20 mL
Hair	10–12 hairs
Nails	Clippings
Mucous membranes	Washings, swabs
Prostatic secretion	0.5–1.0 mL
Pus and exudates	3–5 mL
Skin specimen	As many scrapings as possible
Sputum	5–10 mL
Stool	Swab in bacterial transport
Tissue	Half cubic inch, as much biopsy tissue as possible
Urine	10–50 mL
Vaginal/cervical/uterine specimens	Washing, swabs, aspirates

Spirochetal Diseases

Borrelia Relapsing Fever

Relapsing fever is caused by certain spirochetes of the genus *Borrelia*. *Borrelia recurrentis* is the only species that causes louse-borne (epidemic) relapsing fever. Worldwide, at least 15 *Borrelia* species cause tick-borne (endemic) relapsing fever, including *B. hermsii* and *B. turicatae* in North America.

Relapsing fever is characterized by the sudden onset of high fever, shaking, chills, sweats, headache, muscle and joint pains, and progressive weakness. A fleeting macular rash of the trunk and petechiae of the skin and mucous membranes sometimes occur. Complications include hepatosplenomegaly, jaundice, epistaxis, cough with pleuritic pain, pneumonitis, meningitis, and myocarditis. In untreated infections, an initial febrile period of 3–7 days terminates spontaneously by crisis. The initial febrile episode is followed by an afebrile period of several days to weeks, then by one or more relapses. Relapses typically become progressively shorter and milder as the afebrile periods lengthen. Infection during pregnancy often is severe and can result in abortion, stillbirth, or neonatal infection.

Incubation period is 4–18 days with a mean of 7 days.

Diagnostic Tests

Spirochetes are seen by dark-field microscopy; in Wright-, Giemsa-, or acridine orange–stained preparations of thin or dehemoglobinized thick smears of peripheral blood; or in stained buffy-coat preparations. Organisms are found in blood most frequently during the febrile stage of the illness. Spirochetes are cultured from blood by inoculating Barbour-Stoenner-Kelly medium or by intraperitoneal inoculation of immature laboratory mice. Serum antibodies to *Borrelia* species can be detected by EIA and Western immunoblotting, but the tests are not standardized and are affected by antigenic variations between and within *Borrelia* species and strains. Serologic cross reactions occur with other spirochetes, including *Borrelia burgdorferi*, the agent causing Lyme disease. Biologic specimens for laboratory testing can be sent to the Division of Vector-Borne Infectious Diseases, CDC, Fort Collins, CO 80522.

Leptospirosis

All leptospires are spirochetes that are similar in appearance and culture. Historically, they were classified into serovars and serogroups. Members of the genus *Leptospira* are classified by genetic relationships into distinct species (genospecies). The species *L. borgpetersenii*, *L. inadai*, *L. interrogans*, *L. kirschneri*, *L. noguchii*, *L. santarosai*, and *L. weilii* include almost all the pathogenic leptospires.

Leptospirosis occurs as two clinically recognizable syndromes: *anicteric* and *icteric*. The onset of leptospirosis usually is abrupt, with nonspecific, influenza-like, constitutional symptoms of fever, chills, headache, severe myalgia, malaise, and conjunctival suffusion. Gastrointestinal symptoms can occur. Of infected patients, 90% present with anicteric illness; however, 10% are severely ill, with jaundice, renal dysfunction, and CNS symptoms (Weil syndrome). This initial "septicemic" phase may be followed by a second, immune-mediated phase, classically known as the *biphasic clinical course*. Fever and other constitutional symptoms may recur, as may neurologic symptoms. The icteric or severe form of clinical presentation is associated with jaundice, abnormal liver function test results, hepatomegaly, and liver failure; renal involvement includes azotemia, abnormal urine analysis results, and renal failure. CNS involvement occurs most commonly as septic meningitis, and complications such as neuritis and uveitis occur more commonly in the immune phase. Conjunctival suffusion, the most characteristic physical finding, occurs in fewer than half of patients. The duration of symptoms varies from <1 week to 3 weeks.

Diagnostic Tests

Blood and CSF in the first 7–10 days of illness and urine after the first week and during convalescence should be cultured on special media that are now available. Laboratory personnel should be consulted in cases of suspected leptospirosis. The organism also can be recovered by inoculation of body fluids into guinea pigs. Serum antibodies, measured by EIA or agglutination reactions, develop during the second week of illness, but increases in antibody titer can be delayed or absent in some patients. Microscopic agglutination, the confirmatory serologic test, is performed in reference laboratories. Direct dark-field examination of blood or other body fluid specimens has pitfalls that obviate its usefulness, and it is not recommended. PCR assay for the detection of leptospires has been developed.

Lyme Disease

Lyme disease is a multisystem disease caused by infection with the spirochete *Borrelia burgdorferi*. The organism is injected by tick bite. The primary tick vector is *Ixodes dammini* in northeastern United States and *Ixodes pacificus* in the western United States (Fig. 2).

Stage 1: Approximately 1 week after tick bite (varies from 3 to 33 days); nonspecific febrile "viral syndrome"; 85% of patients have characteristic erythema migrans rash. Serologic test is not helpful or necessary because it is only 40–60% sensitive at this stage, and diagnosis is not ruled out by a negative test result. Early antibiotic treatment often prevents antibody response. Antibiotic therapy is critical to prevent long-term involvement of various organs.

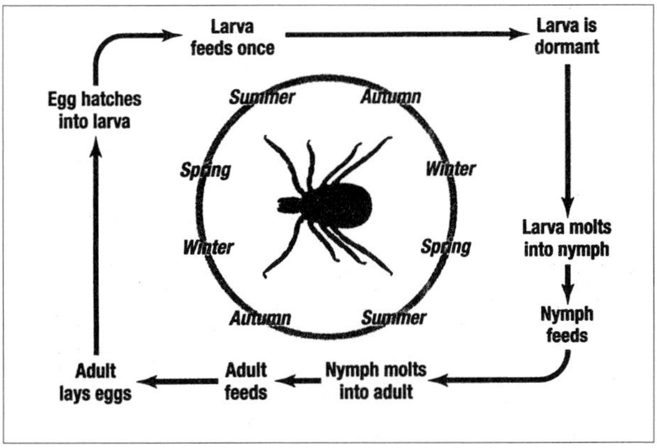

Fig. 2. The life cycle of the deer tick: The deer tick has three hosts over 2 years. The cycle starts when the female ticks deposit fertilized eggs in the soil, which hatch into larvae in late spring and early summer. Larvae feed once in summer, then lie dormant during the fall and winter and molt into nymphs the following spring. Nymphs feed in the spring and early summer, then molt into adults, which feed, mate, and lay eggs to complete the cycle.

Stage 2: Four weeks after tick bite; 10% of patients develop cardiac involvement (causes most deaths); 15% have neurologic findings (triad of aseptic meningitis, Bell palsy, and peripheral neuropathy is very suggestive).

Stage 3: Six weeks to several years after tick bite; occurs in 60% of untreated cases; characterized principally by arthritis, frequently mistaken for juvenile rheumatoid arthritis, and by fever, malaise, headache.

Clinical Manifestations

Stage	Manifestations
Stage 1 (early localized)	Cutaneous: erythema migrans Nonspecific: fever, headache, stiff neck, arthralgia, myalgia, malaise, fatigue
Stage 2 (early disseminated)	Cutaneous: secondary erythema migrans lesions, lymphocytoma Musculoskeletal: monoarticular or oligoarticular arthritis, polyarthralgia Neurologic: facial (or other cranial) nerve palsy, lymphocytic meningitis, peripheral neuropathy and radiculoneuropathy, encephalitis Cardiac: atrioventricular conduction disturbances, myopericarditis
Stage 3 (late disseminated)	Cutaneous: acrodermatitis chronica atrophicans Musculoskeletal: intermittent or chronic arthritis Neurologic: encephalopathy, polyneuropathy, leukoencephalitis

Reinfection causing recurrence of clinical disease is recognized.

Diagnostic Criteria

Isolation of organisms from clinical specimen *or*

Diagnostic titers of IgG and IgM in serum or CSF *or*

Significant change in serum titers of IgG or IgM in paired acute- and convalescent-phase sera

Serologic Tests

Recommended protocol is ELISA (sensitivity of 89%, specificity of 72%) or IFA, which should be confirmed by Western blot (immunoblot). Assays for IgM, IgG, or both.

Serologic tests should be ordered only to support clinical diagnosis, not for screening or in persons with nonspecific symptoms. Serologic testing generally is not clinically useful if pretest probability is <0.20 or >0.80. If probability is <0.20, positive ELISA result is more likely to be false-positive than true-positive. If probability is >0.20, positive ELISA result rules in diagnosis of Lyme disease.

A positive serologic test result does not necessarily indicate current infection or establish the diagnosis, and a negative serologic test result, especially within 2 weeks of onset of symptoms, should not be the only basis for excluding diagnosis.

Specific IgM antibodies usually appear 2–4 weeks after erythema migrans, peak after 3–6 weeks of illness, and decline to normal after 4–6 months; positive antibody test results are seen in only 40–60% of stage 1 cases. In some patients, IgM levels remain elevated for many months or IgM antibodies reappear late in illness, which predicts continued infection. IgM titer of 1:200 is considered positive. IgM titer of 1:100 is considered indeterminate. IgM titer of <1:100 is considered negative. A negative test result within 2 weeks of onset of symptoms does not rule out infection.

IgG titers rise more slowly (appearing 4–8 weeks after rash), peak after 4–6 months, and may remain high for months or years, even with successful antibiotic therapy. Almost all patients with complications of stages 2 and 3 have positive IgG results on first specimen. A single increased IgG titer indicates only previous exposure. An IgG titer of 1:800 is considered positive, a titer of 1:200 to 1:400 is indeterminate, and a titer of <1:100 is considered negative.

Paired acute- and convalescent-phase serum samples drawn at a 4–6 week interval showing conversion or significant rise in titer indicate infection and are principally useful in evaluating ill patients who have no known tick bite or rash who have been in an area where the disease is endemic.

False-positive high IgG titers may be due to antibodies from spirochetal diseases (syphilis, relapsing fever, yaws, pinta); false-positive low titers may be found in patients with infectious mononucleosis, hepatitis B, autoimmune diseases (e.g., systemic lupus erythematosus, rheumatoid arthritis), periodontal disease, ehrlichiosis, rickettsial infection, or other bacterial infections (e.g., with *H. pylori*), and in 5–15% of healthy persons in areas of endemic disease.

Low concordance between results using different test kits causes confusion.

The Western blot test is more sensitive and specific than ELISA and is used to distinguish true-positive and false-positive ELISA results, to confirm an indeterminate ELISA result, or to evaluate an undiagnosed antibiotic-treated patient, and it is the present gold standard; positive results on the Western blot test indicate past or current infection. Western blot results may not become positive until the patient has been ill for many months, however; when Western blot results are negative, the test should be repeated in 2–4 weeks if Lyme disease is strongly suspected. The test is expensive, limited in availability, technically difficult, and not standardized, and there are many cross-reacting antibodies.

False-positive EIA results may arise form cross reactivity caused by other spirochetal diseases (syphilis, borrelial relapsing fever, periodontal disease) and infectious diseases (ehrlichiosis, infectious mononucleosis, subacute bacterial endocarditis, and mumps meningitis) as well as rheumatologic illness (juvenile rheumatoid arthritis, rheumatoid arthritis, and systemic lupus erythematosus). The CDC has recommended a two-tier approach to laboratory confirmation of disease. The first tier is use of a sensitive EIA and the second tier is performance of a Western blot test for cases in which EIA results are either indeterminate or positive. It has been suggested that the presence of five bands for IgG and two bands for IgM on the Western blot be used to determine positive status.

Although CSF can be examined for antibodies, CSF testing generally is not necessary to diagnose CNS involvement because almost all patients with CNS involvement have positive serologic test findings. PCR testing of synovial fluid to detect *B. burgdorferi* may prove useful in differentiating between patients with continued joint infection and those with postinfectious inflammation, some investigators suggest.

True seronegativity is uncommon with disseminated or chronic Lyme disease. Serologic tests cannot judge therapeutic efficacy or provide test of cure (unlike the VRDL test for syphilis). Absence of positive titer results do not rule out Lyme disease.

Antigen can be detected in urine, blood, and tissue, and PCR can identify specific DNA in blood, CSF, joint fluid, skin biopsy specimens, and urine. Reported sensitivity is 35%, specificity is 100%; these tests have not yet been widely evaluated.

Culture may take several weeks; organisms are infrequently found even when special stains are used in known positive tissues. There is a low yield except in specimens from biopsy of erythema migrans lesions (60–80% sensitivity), which is rarely necessary. (T-cell proliferative assay needs further evaluation.) Organisms are not detected in peripheral smears.

Laboratory findings are related to organ involvement:

- *Neurologic involvement:* Eighty percent of patients with meningitis may show increased lymphocyte levels (up to 450/mm^3), increased protein and IgG levels, presence of oligoclonal bands. Encephalitis with involvement of white matter, myelitis, radiculitis, and cranial or peripheral neuritis may occur in various combinations. Intrathecal antibody may be demonstrated by findings of a higher titer in CSF than in serum. IgG and IgM may be present in CSF but not in serum. Almost all of these patients have positive serologic test results.
- *Arthritis:* Joint fluid may show increased white blood cell count (up to 34,000/mm^3), polymorphonuclear cells (96%), and protein (up to 6.6 g/dL). Lyme antibodies in fluid differentiate this from other arthritides.
- Diffuse fasciitis with eosinophilia: This is a rare finding.
- *Nonspecific findings:* Mild increase in erythrocyte sedimentation rate, lymphopenia, cryoglobulinemia, mild increase in aspartate aminotransferase level, increased serum IgM level.

Fluorescent treponemal antibody absorption test (FTA-ABS) results may be positive but nontreponemal tests (VDRL, rapid plasma reagin test) should show nonreactivity.

Morphologic changes in tissues are not specific. Coinfection with *Babesia* may occur.

Syphilis

Treponema pallidum is a thin motile spirochete that is extremely fragile, surviving only briefly outside the host. The organism has not been cultivated successfully on artificial media.

Congenital Syphilis

Infection can result in stillbirth, hydrops fetalis, or prematurity; at birth infants may or may not have signs of disease or they may present up to 2 years of age with hepatosplenomegaly, snuffles, lymphadenopathy, mucocutaneous lesions, osteochondritis and pseudoparalysis, edema, rash, hemolytic anemia, and thrombocytopenia. Some infected infants who are asymptomatic, if untreated or inadequately treated, may develop these signs within the first weeks of life. A generalized salmon-colored rash maybe present. Desquamation of the palms and soles occurs. Untreated infants, regardless of whether they have early manifestations, may develop late manifestations, which usually appear after 2 years of age and involve the CNS, bones and joints, teeth, eyes, and skin. Some consequences are anterior bowing of the shins (saber shins), frontal bossing, mulberry molars, Hutchinson teeth, saddle nose, rhagades, and Clutton joints.

Acquired Syphilis

Infection can be divided into three stages. The primary stage is characterized by one or more painless indurated ulcers (chancres) of the skin and mucous membranes at the site of inoculation, most commonly on the genitalia. The secondary stage, beginning 1–2 months later, is characterized by a polymorphic rash that most frequently is maculopapular and generalized and classically includes the palms and soles. In moist areas around the vulva or anus, hypertrophic papular lesions (condyloma latum) can occur. Generalized lymphadenopathy, fever, malaise, splenomegaly, sore throat, headache, and arthralgia can be present. A variable latent period follows but sometimes is interrupted during the first few years by recurrences of symptoms of secondary syphilis. Latent syphilis is defined as the periods after infection when patients are seroreactive but demonstrate no other evidence of disease. Latent syphilis acquired within the preceding year is referred to as *early latent syphilis*; all other cases of latent syphilis are late latent syphilis of disease of unknown duration. The tertiary stage refers to gumma and cardiovascular syphilis but not to neurosyphilis. The tertiary stage can be marked by aortitis or gummatous changes of the skin, bone, or viscera occurring years to decades after the primary infection. Neurosyphilis occurs when there is evidence of CNS infection with *T. pallidum*. The various manifestations of neurosyphilis can occur in any stage, especially in persons infected with HIV.

Diagnostic Tests

Definitive diagnosis is achieved by identifying spirochetes by microscopic dark-field examination or DFA tests of lesion exudate or tissue, such as placenta or umbilical cord. Specimens should be scraped from moist mucocutaneous lesions or aspirated from a regional lymph node. Because false-negative microscopic results are common, serologic testing, follow-up, and, often, repeated testing are necessary. Specimens from mouth lesions require DFA techniques to distinguish *T. pallidum* from nonpathogenic treponemes. PCR tests and IgM immunoblotting have been developed.

Presumptive diagnosis is possible using two types of serologic tests: (a) nontreponemal tests and (b) treponemal tests. The use of only one type of test is insufficient for diagnosis because of false-positive nontreponemal test results that occur in various medical conditions and false-positive treponemal test results that occur in other spirochetal diseases.

The standard nontreponemal tests for syphilis include the VDRL slide test, the rapid plasma reagin test, and the automated reagin test. These tests measure antibody directed against lipoidal antigen from *T. pallidum*, antibody interaction with host tissues, or both. These tests are inexpensive, are rapidly performed, and provide quantitative results, which are helpful indicators of disease activity and useful in monitoring the response to treatment. Nontreponemal test results may be falsely negative—that is, nonreactive—in early primary syphilis, latent acquired syphilis of long duration, and late congenital syphilis. Occasionally, a nontreponemal test performed on serum samples containing high concentrations of antibody against *T. pallidum* will be weakly reactive or falsely negative, a reaction termed the *prozone phenomenon*. This reaction usually can be detected by experienced laboratory technicians, and diluting the serum yields a positive test result. When these tests are used to monitor treatment response, the same type of test (e.g., VDRL, rapid plasma reagin test, or automated reagin test) must be used throughout the follow-up period, preferably performed by the same laboratory, so that results can be compared appropriately.

A reactive nontreponemal test result from a patient with typical lesions indicates the need for treatment. However, any reactive nontreponemal test finding must be confirmed by one of the specific treponemal tests to exclude a false-positive test result, which can be caused by certain viral infections (e.g., infectious mononucleosis, hepatitis, varicella, and measles), lymphoma, tuberculosis, malaria, endocarditis, connective tissue disease, pregnancy, drug abuse, or laboratory or technical error, or by Wharton jelly contamination when cord blood specimens are used. Treatment should not be delayed pending the treponemal test results in symptomatic patients or patients at high risk of infection. A sustained fourfold decrease in titer of the nontreponemal test usually becomes a nonreactive test result after successful therapy within 1 year in low-titer ($<$1:8) early (primary or secondary) syphilis and within 2 years in high-titer early and congenital syphilis, but results may remain positive despite treatment in latent or tertiary syphilis (the "serofast" state).

Treponemal tests currently in use are the FTA-ABS test and the microhemagglutination test for *T. pallidum* (MHA-TP). Positive FTA-ABS and MHA-TP test results usually remain reactive for life, even after successful therapy. Treponemal test antibody titers correlate poorly with disease activity and should not be used to assess treatment response.

Treponemal tests also are not 100% specific for syphilis; positive reactions variably occur in patients with other spirochetal diseases, such as yaws, pinta, leptospirosis, rat-bite fever, relapsing fever, and Lyme disease. Nontreponemal tests can be used to differentiate Lyme disease from syphilis because the VDRL yields uniformly nonreactive results in Lyme disease.

Usually a serum nontreponemal test is obtained initially, and, if it gives a reactive result, a treponemal test is performed. The probability of syphilis is high in a sexually active person whose serum is reactive to both nontreponemal and treponemal tests. Differentiating syphilis treated in the past from reinfection often is difficult unless the nontreponemal titer is known to be rising.

In summary, the nontreponemal antibody tests (VDRL, reactive plasma reagin test, and automated reagin test) are useful for screening; the treponemal tests (FTA-ABS and MHA-TP) are used to establish a presumptive diagnosis. Quantitative nontreponemal antibody tests are used to assess the adequacy of therapy and to detect reinfection and relapse.

Rickettsial Diseases

The rickettsiae are pleomorphic bacteria, most of which have arthropod vectors. Humans are incidental hosts, except in epidemic (louse-borne) typhus, for which humans are the principal reservoir for the disease organism and the human body louse is the vector. Rickettsiae are obligate intracellular parasites and cannot be grown in cell-free media. They have typical bacterial cell walls and cytoplasmic membranes and divide by binary fusion. Their natural life cycles typically involve mammalian reservoirs, and animal-to-human or vector-to-human transmission occurs as a result of environmental or occupational exposure.

Ticks are the vector for many rickettsial diseases. Thus, control measures involve prevention of tick transmission of rickettsial agents to humans.

Rickettsial infections have many features in common, including the following:

- The organism multiplies in an arthropod host.
- Replication is intracellular.
- Limited geographic and seasonal outbreaks occur related to arthropod life cycles, activity, and distribution.
- Diseases are zoonotic.
- Humans are incidental hosts (except in the case of louse-borne typhus).
- Local primary lesions occur with some rickettsial diseases.
- Fever, rash (especially in spotted fever and typhus group rickettsiae), headache, myalgias, and respiratory tract symptoms are prominent features.
- Systemic capillary and small-vessel endothelial damage is the primary pathologic feature of spotted fever and typhus group rickettsial infections.
- With the exception of Q fever, rickettsialpox, and ehrlichiosis, nonspecific serum *Proteus vulgaris* agglutinins (Weil-Felix test) develop during infection. However, their presence frequently is unreliable for diagnosis. Specific serologic assays for rickettsial illnesses are available and should replace the nonspecific Weil-Felix test.
- Group-specific antibodies are detectable in the serum of most patients within 7–14 days after onset of illness.
- Various serologic tests exist for detecting these antibodies. The IFA assay is recommended in most cases because of its relative simplicity, sensitivity, and specificity.
- The PCR test to detect rickettsiae in blood or tissue is promising for early diagnosis of many rickettsial diseases.
- In experienced laboratories, immunohistologic or PCR testing of skin biopsy specimens of patients with rash can be used to diagnose rickettsial infections.
- Treatment early in the course of the illness can blunt or delay serologic responses.
- Rickettsial diseases can be severe and fatal, so prompt and specific therapy is important for successful patient outcome. Appropriate antimicrobial treatment is most effective for patients who are treated during the first week of illness. If the disease remains untreated in the second week, even optimal therapy is less effective at preventing complications of the illness.
- Immunity against reinfection by the same agent after natural infection usually is of long duration, except in the case of scrub typhus caused by *Rickettsia tsutsugamushi*. Among the four groups of rickettsial diseases, partial or complete cross immunity usually is conferred by infections within groups but not among groups. Reinfection with *Ehrlichia* organisms has been reported.
- Many rickettsial diseases, including Rocky Mountain spotted fever, ehrlichiosis, and Q fever, may be reportable to state and local health departments.

A number of other epidemiologically distinct but clinically similar tick-borne spotted fever infections caused by rickettsiae have been recognized. The causative agents of some of these infections share the same group antigen as *Rickettsia rickettsii*. These include *Rickettsia conorii*, the causative agent of boutonneuse fever (also known as *Kenya tick-bite fever, African tick typhus, Mediterranean spotted fever, India tick typhus*, and *Marseilles fever*), which is endemic in southern Europe, Africa, and the Middle East; *Rickettsia sibirica*, the causative agent of Siberian tick typhus, endemic in central Asia; *Rickettsia australis*, the causative agent of North Queensland tick typhus, endemic in eastern Australia; and *Rickettsia japonica*, the causative agent of a spotted fever rickettsiosis, endemic in Japan. All of these infections have clinical, pathologic, and epidemiologic features similar to those of Rocky Mountain spotted fever and are treated similarly. The specific diagnosis is confirmed serologically. These conditions are of importance for persons traveling to endemic areas.

Rickettsialpox

Rickettsialpox is characterized by generalized erythematous papulovesicular eruptions on the trunk, face, extremities (including palms and soles), and mucous membranes after the appearance of a primary lesion at the site of the bite of the mouse mite vector. An eschar develops at the site about the time of fever onset. Regional lymph nodes in the area of the primary eschar typically become enlarged. Systemic disease lasts approximately 1 week; manifestations can include chills, fever, headache, drenching sweats, myalgias, anorexia, and photophobia. The disease is self-limited and rarely associated with complications.

Diagnostic Tests

Rickettsia akari can be isolated from blood during the acute stage of disease, but culture is not attempted routinely and is available only in specialized laboratories. An IFA or complement fixation test for *R. rickettsii* (the cause of Rocky Mountain spotted fever) demonstrates a fourfold change in antibody titers between acute and convalescent serum samples, because antibodies to *R. akari* have extensive cross reactivity with those against *R. rickettsii*. Absorption of serum samples before IFA testing can distinguish between antibody responses to *R. rickettsii* and *R. akari*. Results of the Weil-Felix test for all *P. vulgaris* OX agglutinins is negative. DFA testing of paraffin-embedded eschars and histopathologic examination of papulovesicles for distinctive features are useful diagnostic techniques.

Parasitic Diseases

Amebiasis

Amebic Dysentery

Entamoeba histolytica (Fig. 3) is an enteric protozoan that has been reclassified into two species that are morphologically identical but genetically distinct. *E. histolytica* and *Entamoeba dispar* organisms are excreted as cysts or trophozoites in stools of infected persons.

Syndromes associated with *E. histolytica* infection include noninvasive intestinal infection, which may be asymptomatic (and is more likely due to *E. dispar*), intestinal amebiasis, acute fulminant or necrotizing colitis, ameboma, and liver abscess. Disease is more severe in the very young. Persons with intestinal amebiasis (amebic colitis) generally have 1–3 weeks of increasing diarrhea progressing to grossly bloody dysenteric stools with lower abdominal pain and tenesmus. Common symptoms may be chronic and mimic symptoms of inflammatory bowel disease, toxic megacolon, fulminant colitis, ulceration of the colon and perianal area and, rarely, perforation.

In a small percentage of patients, extraintestinal disease may occur with involvement of the lungs, pericardium, brain, skin, and genitourinary tract, but the liver is the most common site. Liver abscess may be acute with fever and abdominal pain, tachypneas, and liver tenderness and hepatomegaly.

Diagnostic Tests

Trophozoites are identified by wet mount within 30 minutes of collection and fixation in formalin and polyvinyl alcohol. PCR, isoenzyme analysis, and antigen detection assays can differentiate *E. histolytica* and *E. dispar*. Ultrasonography and CT identify liver abscesses. Aspirates from a liver abscess usually show neither trophozoites nor leukocytes.

Amebic Meningoencephalitis and Keratitis

Naegleria fowleri, *Acanthamoeba* species, and *Balamuthia mandrillaris* are small, free-living amebas. *N. fowleri* can cause a rapidly progressive, almost always fatal,

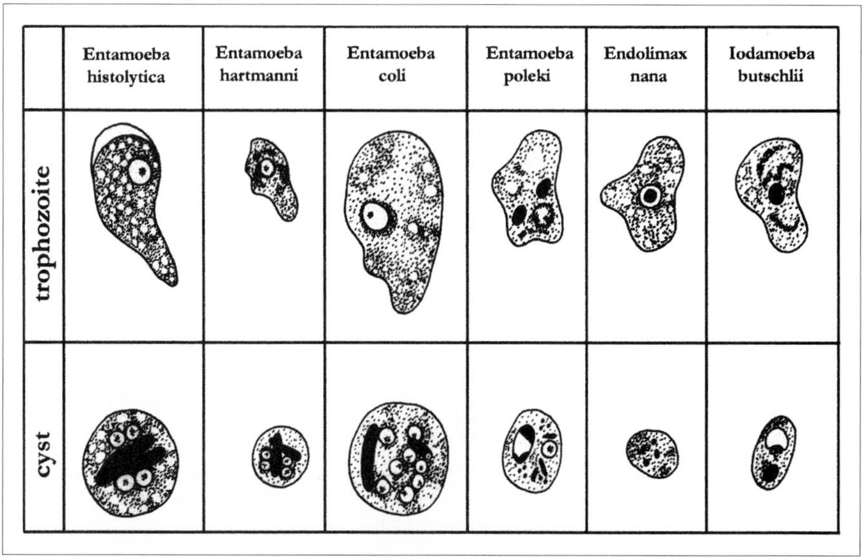

Fig. 3. Amebas.

primary amebic meningoencephalitis. Early symptoms include fever, headache, and, sometimes, disturbances of smell and taste. The illness rapidly progresses to signs of meningoencephalitis, including nuchal rigidity, lethargy, confusion, and altered level of consciousness. Seizures are common. Death may occur soon after the onset of symptoms.

Granulomatous amebic encephalitis caused by *Acanthamoeba* species and *Balamuthia* (leptomyxid) species has a more insidious onset and progression of manifestations occurring weeks to months after exposure. Signs and symptoms may include personality changes, seizures, headaches, nuchal rigidity, ataxia, cranial nerve palsies, hemiparesis, and other focal deficits. Fever is often low grade and intermittent. Skin lesions (pustules, nodules, ulcers) may be present without CNS involvement, particularly in patients with AIDS.

Amebic keratitis, usually due to *Acanthamoeba* species and rarely to other species, occurs primarily in persons who wear contact lenses and resembles keratitis caused by herpes simplex, bacteria, or fungi, except for a usually more indolent course. Corneal inflammation, photophobia, and secondary uveitis are the predominant features.

Diagnostic Tests

N. fowleri infection can be documented by microscopic demonstration of the motile trophozoites on a wet mount of centrifuged CSF. The organism also can be cultured on 1.5% nonnutrient agar layered with enteric bacteria held in Page saline. Immunofluorescent tests to determine the species of the organism are available through the CDC. The CSF shows polymorphonuclear pleocytosis, an elevated protein level, a slightly reduced glucose level, and no bacteria.

In infection with *Acanthamoeba* species, cysts can be visualized in sections of brain or corneal tissue and may be present in brain biopsy specimens. The CSF typically shows a mononuclear pleocytosis, and an elevated protein level, but no organisms or parasites, a slightly reduced glucose level, and no bacteria.

Ascaris lumbricoides *Infections*

Ascaris lumbricoides is the largest and, globally, the most widespread of all human intestinal roundworms.

Most infections are asymptomatic. During the larval migratory phase, an acute transient pneumonitis (Löffler syndrome) associated with fever and marked eosino-

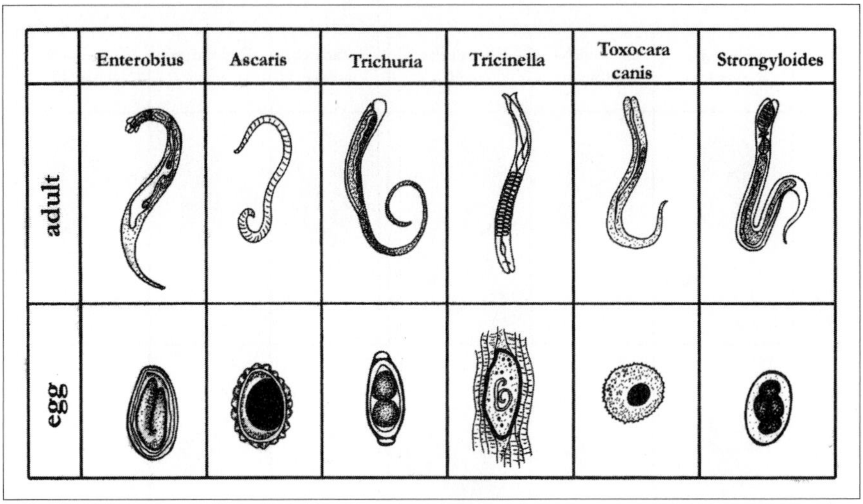

Fig. 4. Worms.

philia may occur. Acute intestinal obstruction may develop in patients with heavy infections. Worm migration can cause peritonitis, secondary to intestinal wall penetration, and common bile duct obstruction resulting in acute obstructive jaundice.

Diagnostic Tests

Ova can be detected by microscopic examination of stool. Occasionally, patients pass adult worms from the rectum, from the nose after migration through the nares in febrile patients, and from the mouth in vomitus (Fig. 4).

Babesiosis

Babesia species that cause babesiosis are intraerythrocytic protozoa. *Babesia microti* and one or more related but genetically and antigenetically distinct organisms are responsible for disease in the United States.

Gradual onset of malaise, anorexia, and fatigue typically occur, followed by intermittent fever with temperatures as high as 40°C (104°F) and one or more of the following symptoms: chills, sweats, myalgias, arthralgias, nausea, and vomiting. Less common findings are emotional lability and depression, hyperesthesia, headache, sore throat, abdominal pain, conjunctival infection, photophobia, weight loss, and nonproductive cough. Signs on physical examination generally are minimal, often consisting of fever and splenomegaly or hepatomegaly, or both. Many clinical features are similar to those of malaria. The illness can last for a few weeks to several months with a prolonged recovery of as long as 18 months. Severe illness is most likely to occur in persons >40 years of age, persons who are asplenic, and persons who are immunocompromised. Some individuals, especially those who have had a splenectomy, can suffer fulminant illness resulting in death or prolonged convalescence.

Diagnostic Tests

Babesiosis is diagnosed by microscopic identification of the organism on Giemsa- or Wright-stained thick or thin blood smears. Multiple thick and thin blood smears should be examined in suspected cases or when the initial examination result is negative. Serologic tests for detection of *Babesia* antibodies are available at the CDC and at several state reference and research laboratories.

Balantidiasis

Pigs are believed to be the primary reservoir of *Balantidium coli*. Cysts excreted in feces can be transmitted directly from hand to mouth or indirectly through fecally

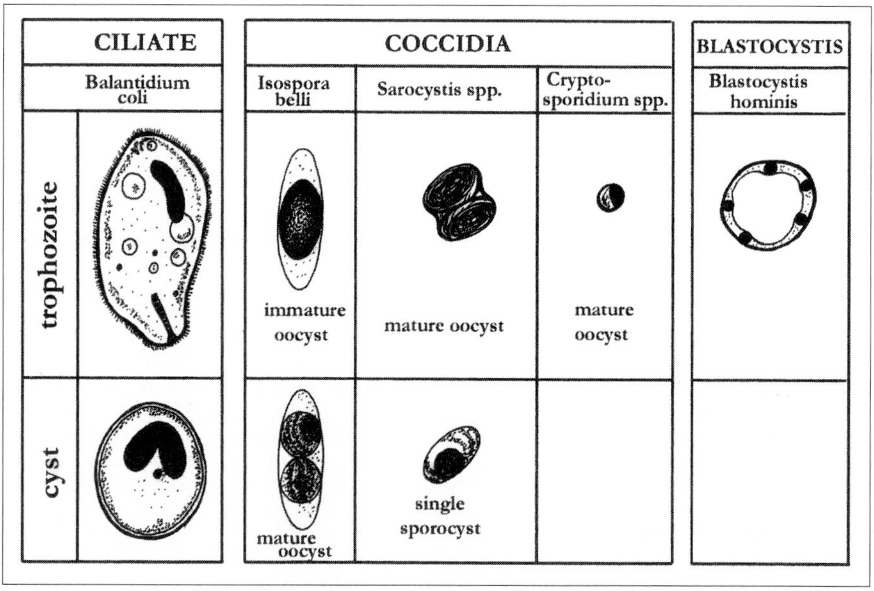

Fig. 5. Ciliates, coccidia, and *Blastocystis*.

contaminated water or food. The excysted trophozoites infect the colon. The cysts may remain viable in the environment for months.

Most human infections are asymptomatic. Acute infection is characterized by the rapid onset of nausea, vomiting, abdominal discomfort or pain, and bloody or watery mucoid diarrhea. Infected patients can develop chronic intermittent episodes of diarrhea.

Diagnostic Tests

Diagnosis of infection is established by examination of specimens scraped from lesions during sigmoidoscopy, histologic examination of intestinal biopsy specimens, or examination of stool for ova and parasites. Stool examination is less sensitive, and repeated stool examinations may be necessary to diagnose infection, because shedding of organisms can be intermittent. The diagnosis can be established only by demonstrating trophozoites in stool or tissue specimens (Fig. 5). Microscopic examination of fresh diarrheal stools must be performed promptly because trophozoites quickly degenerate.

Blastocystis hominis *Infections*

The importance of *Blastocystic hominis* as a cause of gastrointestinal tract disease is controversial. The asymptomatic carrier state is well documented. *B. hominis* infection has been associated with symptoms of bloating, flatulence, mild to moderate diarrhea without fecal leukocytes or blood, abdominal pain, and nausea. When *B. hominis* is identified in stool from symptomatic patients, other causes of this symptom complex, particularly *Giardia lamblia* and *Cryptosporidium parvum*, should be investigated before assuming that *B. hominis* is the cause of the signs and symptoms.

B. hominis is recovered from 1–20% of stool samples examined for ova and parasites (Fig. 5). Because transmission is believed to be via the fecal-oral route, the presence of the organism may be a marker for fecal contamination with other pathogens. Transmission from animals also may occur.

The incubation period is unknown.

Diagnostic Tests

Stool specimens should be preserved in polyvinyl alcohol and stained with hematoxylin or trichrome before microscopic examination. The parasite occurs in varying numbers, and infections may be reported as light to heavy. The presence of five or more organisms per high-power field (×400 magnification) suggests heavy infection.

Cryptosporidiosis

Cryptosporidium parvum is a spore-forming coccidian protozoan.

C. parvum has been found in a variety of hosts, including mammals, birds, and reptiles. *C. parvum* also causes traveler's diarrhea. Because the parasite is resistant to chlorine, appropriately functioning water-filtration systems are critical for the safety of public water supplies. In most people, shedding of *C. parvum* stops within 2 weeks, but in a few, shedding continues for up to 2 months.

Frequent nonbloody, watery diarrhea is the most common presenting symptom, although infection can be asymptomatic. Other symptoms include abdominal cramps, fatigue, vomiting, anorexia, and weight loss. Fever and vomiting are relatively common among children and often lead to a misdiagnosis of viral gastroenteritis. In infected immunocompetent persons, including children, the diarrheal illness is self-limited, usually lasting 1–20 days (mean, 10 days). In immunocompromised persons, chronic severe diarrhea can develop that results in malnutrition, dehydration, and death. Pulmonary, biliary tract, or disseminated infection can occur in immunocompromised persons, although infection usually is limited to the gastrointestinal tract.

Diagnostic Tests

On microscopic examination, the finding of oocysts in stool specimens is diagnostic (Fig. 5). The sucrose flotation method or formalin–ethyl acetate method is used to concentrate oocysts in stool before staining with a modified Kinyoun acid-fast stain. Monoclonal antibody–based fluorescein-conjugated stain for oocysts in stool and an EIA for detecting antigen in stool are available commercially. With EIA methods, false-positive results may occur, and confirmation by microscopy may be necessary. Because shedding can be intermittent, at least three stool specimens collected on separate days should be examined before considering the test results to be negative. Oocysts are small (4–6 μm in diameter) and can be missed in a rapid scan of a slide. Organisms also can be identified in intestinal biopsy tissue or intestinal fluid.

Cutaneous Larva Migrans

Cutaneous larva migrans is a disease of children, utility workers, gardeners, sunbathers, and others who come in contact with soil contaminated with cat and dog feces. In the United States, the disease is most prevalent in the Southeast.

Nematode larvae produce pruritic, reddish papules at the site of the skin entry. Intensely pruritic, serpiginous tracks are formed. Occasionally, the larvae reach the intestine and may cause eosinophilic enteritis.

Infective larvae of cat and dog hookworms (Fig. 6)—that is, *Ancylostoma braziliense* and *Ancylostoma caninum*—are the usual causes.

Diagnostic Tests

The diagnosis usually is made clinically. Biopsy specimens typically demonstrate an eosinophilic inflammatory infiltrate, but the migrating parasite is not visualized. Eosinophilia occurs in some cases. Larvae have been detected in sputum and gastric washings in patients with the rare complication of pneumonitis. Serologic testing with an EIA or Western blot using antigens of *A. caninum* may help detect occult infections. These tests, however, generally are available only in research laboratories and are not warranted routinely.

Filariasis

Filariasis is caused by the following three filarial nematodes: *Wuchereria bancrofti, Brugia malayi,* and *Brugia timori*.

Most filarial infections are asymptomatic. Early in infection, symptoms are often caused by an acute inflammatory response that can lead to dysfunction of the lymphatics in which the adult worm develops. Fever, headache, myalgia, and lymphadenitis develop with acute inflammation. The acute disease may manifest as early as 3 months after acquisition. Over time, moderate lymphadenopathy occurs, particu-

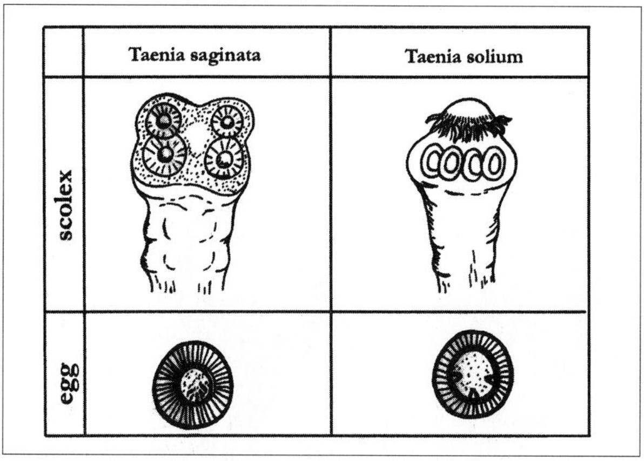

Fig. 6. Hookworms.

larly involving the inguinal lymph nodes. Inflammation of the lymphatics of the extremities and genitalia leads to adenolymphangitis that is characteristically retrograde. Epididymitis, orchitis, and funiculitis also can occur with fever, chills, and other nonspecific systemic symptoms. Lymphatic dysfunction, with resulting chronically progressive edema of the limbs and genitalia, is relatively infrequent in children. In a few persons, elephantiasis can result from fibrosis caused by chronic dysfunction of the lymphatic channels. Chyluria can occur as a manifestation of bancroftian filariasis.

Cough, fever, marked eosinophilia, and high serum IgE concentrations are the manifestations of the tropical pulmonary eosinophilia syndrome.

Disease is transmitted by the bite of the infected species of various genera of mosquitoes, including *Culex, Aedes, Anopheles,* and *Mansonia. Wuchereria bancrofti* is found in many scattered areas of the Caribbean, Venezuela, Columbia, the Guianas, Brazil, Central America, sub-Saharan Africa, North Africa, Turkey, and Asia. Because the adult worms are long-lived (5–8 years on average), reinfection is common. Microfilariae infective for mosquitoes may remain in the patient's blood for decades and may be transmitted by transfusion.

Diagnostic Tests

Microfilariae can be detected microscopically on routine blood smears obtained at night (10 p.m. to 4 a.m.) or after concentration of blood preserved in formalin or by membrane filtration. Adult worms can be identified in tissue specimens obtained at biopsy. Serologic EIA tests are available, but interpretation of results is affected by cross reactions of filarial antibodies with antibodies against other helminths. Assays for circulating parasite antigen of *W. bancrofti* are now available commercially. Lymphatic filariasis often must be diagnosed clinically because dependable serologic assays are not uniformly available, and in elephantiasis, the microfilariae may no longer be present.

Giardiasis

Giardia lamblia is a flagellate protozoan that exists in trophozoite and cyst forms; the infective form is the cyst. Infection is limited to the small intestine and biliary tract. Persons become infected directly (by hand-to-mouth transfer of cysts from feces of an infected person) or indirectly (by ingestion of fecally contaminated water or food). Most community-wide epidemics result from a contaminated water supply. Humoral immunodeficiencies predispose to chronic symptomatic *G. lamblia* infections. The disease is communicable for as long as the infected person excretes cysts.

Acute watery diarrhea with abdominal pain may develop in patients with clinical illness, or they may experience a protracted, intermittent, often debilitating disease,

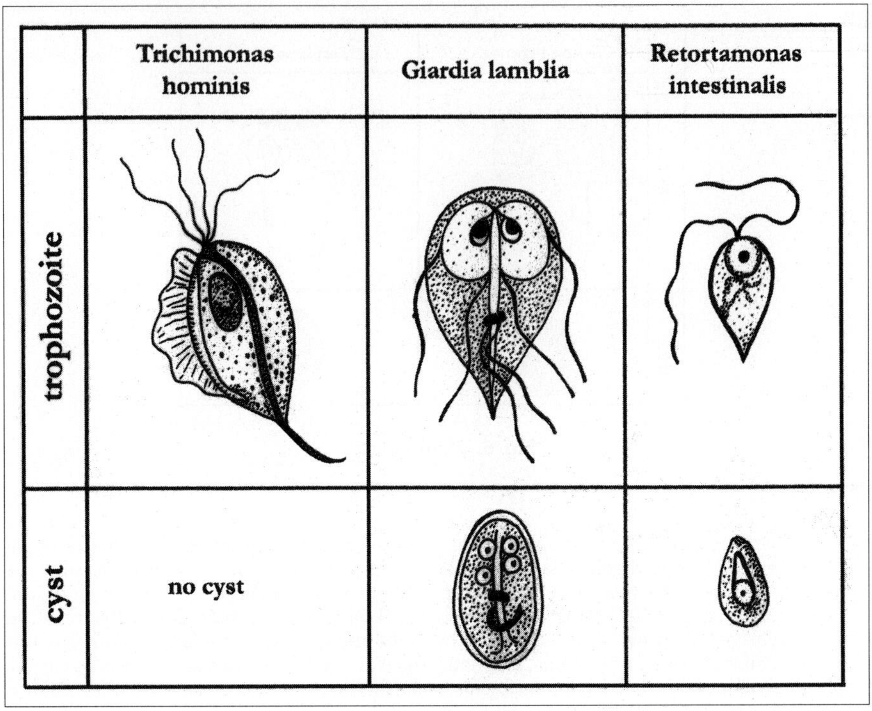

Fig. 7. Flagellates.

which is characterized by passage of foul-smelling stools associated with flatulence, abdominal distention, and anorexia. Anorexia combined with malabsorption can lead to significant weight loss, failure to thrive, and anemia. Asymptomatic infection is common.

Diagnostic Tests

Identification of trophozoites or cysts (Fig. 7) on direct smear examination, or IFA testing of stool specimens or duodenal fluid or detection of *G. lamblia* antigens in these specimens has greater sensitivity than microscopy but fails to detect other parasites. One commercially available IFA test allows microscopic detection of *Giardia* and *Cryptosporidium* species in stool with a sensitivity of approximately 75%. A single direct smear examination of the stool has a sensitivity of 50–75%, which is increased to approximately 95% by testing three specimens. To enhance detection, microscopic examination of stool specimens or duodenal fluid should be performed soon after they are obtained, or stool should be mixed, placed in fixative, concentrated, and examined by wet mount and permanent stain. Commercially available stool collection kits containing a vial of 10% formalin and a vial of polyvinyl alcohol fixative in childproof containers are convenient for preserving stool specimens collected at home. Laboratories can reduce reagent and personnel costs by pooling specimens before evaluation by microscopy or EIA. Examination of duodenal contents obtained by direct aspiration or by using a commercially available string test (Entero-Test, HDC Corporation, San Jose, CA) is a more sensitive procedure than examination of a single stool specimen. Rarely, duodenal biopsy is required for diagnosis.

Fecal specimens for parasitic examination should be collected before initiation of antidiarrheal therapy or antiparasitic therapy. The highest yield from hospitalized patients occurs when diarrhea is present on admission or within 72 hours of admission. The onset of diarrhea >72 hours after admission is usually caused by *C. difficile* toxin rather than parasites or the usual stool pathogens. The following recommendations are made for efficient and cost-effective diagnosis of diarrheal disease in patients admitted with gastroenteritis.

- One or two specimens per diarrheal illness should be submitted immediately. Requesting the EIA for *Giardia* should be considered if that is the primary suspected organism.
- If the results for these samples are negative, an additional specimen should be submitted after 5 days.
- Patients who are immunocompromised by AIDS, malignancy, or immunosuppressive therapy may require additional testing for unusual stool pathogens (e.g., *Cyclospora* or *Cryptosporidium*).

The specimen should be maintained at room temperature. The organisms are most readily demonstrated in diarrheal stools rather than formed stools.

Modified Kinyoun stain or autofluorescence or both are used in evaluating stool smears.

Specimens should not be collected for 1 week after barium or laxative administration.

Isosporiasis

Isospora belli is a coccidian protozoan.

Protracted foul-smelling, watery diarrhea is the most common presenting symptom. Manifestations are similar to those caused by *Cryptosporidium* and *Cyclospora* infection and include abdominal pain, anorexia, and weight loss. Fever, malaise, vomiting, and headache have been reported. Severity of infection ranges from self-limiting in immunocompetent hosts to life-threatening in immunocompromised patients.

Diagnostic Tests

Demonstration of oocysts in feces or in duodenal aspirates or identification of developmental stages of the parasite in biopsy specimens of the small intestine is diagnostic (Fig. 5). Oocysts in stool can be distinguished by their size, which is five times larger than that of *Cryptosporidium* organisms, and by their oval shape. Oocysts can be detected by modified Kinyoun carbol-fuchsin and auramine-rhodamine stains. Concentration techniques may be needed before staining because the organisms often are present in small numbers.

Leishmaniasis

In the human host, *Leishmania* species are obligate intracellular parasites of mononuclear phagocytes. A single *Leishmania* species can produce different clinical syndromes, and each syndrome can be caused by different species, for example, cutaneous *L. tropica*, *L. major*, *L. aethiopica* (Old World species), and *L. mexicana, L. amazonensis, L. braziliensis, L. panamensis, L. guyanensis, L. peruviana, L. chagasi*, and other New World species. Mucosal leishmaniasis is caused by *L. braziliensis* and other related species. Visceral leishmaniasis is caused by *L. donovani, L. infantum*, and *L. chagasi*, as well as *L. tropica* and *L. amazonensis*. *L. donovani* and *L. infantum* also can cause Old World cutaneous leishmaniasis.

The three major clinical syndromes are as follows:

- *Cutaneous leishmaniasis:* After inoculation by the bite of an infected sandfly, parasites proliferate locally in mononuclear phagocytes, which leads to an erythematous macule or nodule that typically forms a shallow ulcer with raised borders. Lesions commonly are located on exposed areas of the face and extremities and may be accompanied by satellite lesions and regional adenopathy. The clinical manifestations of Old World and New World cutaneous leishmaniasis are similar. Spontaneous resolution of lesions may take from weeks to years and usually results in a flat atrophic scar.
- *Mucosal leishmaniasis (espundia):* From the initial cutaneous infection by *L. braziliensis* or related New World species, parasites may disseminate to midline facial structures, including the oral and nasopharyngeal mucosa. In some patients, granulomatous ulceration follows, which leads to facial disfigurement, secondary infection, and mucosal perforation months to years after the cutaneous lesion heals.
- *Visceral leishmaniasis (kala-azar):* After cutaneous inoculation of parasites, organisms spread throughout the mononuclear macrophage system and are concentrated in the spleen, liver, and bone marrow. The resulting clinical illness is marked by

fever, anorexia, weight loss, splenomegaly, hepatomegaly, lymphadenopathy (in some geographic areas), anemia, leukopenia, thrombocytopenia with hemorrhage, and hypergammaglobulinemia. Secondary pyogenic, Gram-negative enteric, and mycobacterial infections are common. Active untreated visceral disease is nearly always fatal. Reactivation of latent visceral leishmaniasis is common in patients with concurrent HIV infection or other immunocompromising conditions.

Diagnostic Tests

Definitive diagnosis is by microscopic identification of intracellular leishmanial organisms on Wright or Giemsa stains of smears or histologic sections of infected tissues. In cutaneous disease, tissue can be obtained by a 3-mm punch biopsy, lesion scrapings, or needle aspiration of the raised nonnecrotic edge (not the center) of the lesion. In visceral leishmaniasis, the organisms can be identified in the spleen and, less commonly, in bone marrow and liver; in East Africa, the organisms also can be identified in the lymph nodes. Blood cultures have yielded positive findings in some Indian patients, and in HIV-infected patients, organisms sometimes may be observed in blood smears or buffy-coat preparations. Isolation of parasites by culture of appropriate tissue specimens in specialized media should be attempted when possible. Culture media and further information can be provided by the CDC.

The diagnosis of visceral leishmaniasis and some cases of cutaneous infection can also be aided by serologic or PCR testing, which is available at the CDC. However, a negative serologic test result should never be interpreted as excluding the possibility of a leishmanial infection. In addition, occasional false-positive serologic results may occur in serum samples of patients with other infectious diseases, especially American trypanosomiasis (Chagas disease).

Malaria

The *Plasmodium* species infecting humans in malaria are *P. falciparum*, *P. vivax*, *P. ovale*, and *P. malariae.*

The classic symptoms are high fever and chills, rigor, sweats, and headache, which may be paroxysmal. As the infection becomes synchronized, the fever and paroxysms generally occur in a cyclic pattern. Depending on the infecting species, fever appears every other or every third day. Other manifestations can include nausea, vomiting, diarrhea, cough, arthralgia, and abdominal and back pain. Anemia and thrombocytopenia are common, and pallor and jaundice caused by hemolysis may occur. Hepatosplenomegaly may be present.

Infection by *P. falciparum* is potentially fatal and most commonly manifests as a nonspecific febrile influenza-like illness without localizing signs. With more severe disease, however, *P. falciparum* infection may be manifest by one of the following clinical syndromes:

- Cerebral malaria, which may have variable neurologic manifestations, including seizures, signs of increased intracranial pressure, confusion, and progression to stupor, coma, and death
- Severe anemia due to high parasitemia and consequent hemolysis
- Hypoglycemia, sometimes associated with quinine treatment, which requires urgent correction
- Respiratory failure and metabolic acidosis, without pulmonary edema
- Noncardiogenic pulmonary edema, which is difficult to manage and may be fatal (rare in children)
- Renal failure caused by acute tubular necrosis (rare in children <8 years of age)
- Vascular collapse and shock associated with hypothermia and adrenal insufficiency

Children with asplenia are at high risk of death due to malaria.

Syndromes primarily associated with *P. vivax* and *P. ovale* infections are

- Hypersplenism with danger of late splenic rupture
- Anemia due to acute parasitemia
- Relapse, for as long as 3–5 years after the primary infection, due to latent hepatic stages

Syndromes primarily associated with *P. malariae* infection are

- Nephrotic syndrome from the deposition of immune complexes in the kidney
- Chronic asymptomatic parasitemia for as long as several years after the last exposure

Congenital malaria secondary to perinatal transmission may occur rarely. Most congenital cases are caused by *P. vivax* and *P. falciparum*; *P. malariae* and *P. ovale* account for <20% of such cases. Manifestations can resemble those of neonatal sepsis, including fever and nonspecific symptoms of poor appetite, irritability, and lethargy.

Diagnostic Tests

Definitive diagnosis relies on identification of the parasite on stained blood films. Both thick and thin blood films should be examined. The thick film allows for concentration of the blood to expose the parasite, which may be present in small numbers, whereas the thin film is most useful for species identification and determination of the level of parasitemia (the percentage of erythrocytes harboring parasites). If the initial blood smears are negative for *Plasmodium* species but malaria remains a possibility, smear examination should be repeated every 12–24 hours during a 72-hour period. Although rapid screening tests for malarial parasites are being evaluated, blood smear findings are not conclusive evidence of malaria as a cause of the presenting illness because other infections often are superimposed on low-concentration parasitemia in children with partial immunity. Confirmation and identification of the species of malarial parasites on the blood smear are important in guiding therapy. Serologic testing generally is not helpful except in epidemiologic surveys. New diagnostic tests in development, including those using PCR, DNA probes, and malarial ribosomal RNA, may provide rapid and accurate diagnosis.

Microsporidia Infections

Microsporidia are obligate, intracellular, spore-forming protozoa. The genera *Encephalitozoon, Enterocytozoon, Nosema, Pleistophora, Trachipleistophora*, and *Vittaforma*, as well as unclassified "*Microsporidium*" species, have been implicated in human infection. *Enterocytozoon bieneusi* and *Enterocytozoon* (*Septata*) *intestinalis* are important causes of chronic diarrhea in HIV-infected persons.

Patients with intestinal infection have watery, nonbloody diarrhea. Fever is uncommon. Intestinal infection, often resulting in chronic diarrhea, is most common in immunocompromised persons. The clinical course is complicated by malnutrition and progressive weight loss. Chronic infection in immunocompetent persons is rare. Other clinical syndromes that can occur in HIV-infected and immunoincompetent patients include keratoconjunctivitis, myositis, nephritis, hepatitis, cholangitis, peritonitis, and disseminated disease, but they occur infrequently.

Diagnostic Tests

Infection with microsporidia organisms can be documented by identification of organisms in biopsy specimens from the small intestine. Microsporidia spores also can be detected in formalin-fixed stool specimens or duodenal aspirates stained with a chromotrope-based stain, which is a modification of the trichrome stain, and viewed by light microscopy. Gram, acid-fast, periodic acid–Schiff, and Giemsa stains also can be used to detect organisms in tissue sections. The organisms often are not noticed because they are small, stain poorly, and evoke minimal inflammatory response. Use of one of the stool concentration techniques does not seem to improve the ability to detect *E. bieneusi* spores. Identification for classification purposes and diagnostic confirmation of species requires electron microscopy. Reliable serologic tests for the diagnosis of human microsporidiosis are lacking.

Onchocerciasis (River Blindness, Filariasis)

Onchocerca volvulus is a filarial nematode.

Infection with the organism causes disease that involves the skin, subcutaneous tissues, lymphatics, and eyes. Subcutaneous nodules of varying sizes, containing adult worms, develop 6–12 months after the initial infection. In patients in Africa, the nodules tend to be found on the lower torso, pelvis, and lower extremities, whereas in patients in Central America, the nodules more often are located on the upper body (the head and trunk) but may occur on the extremities. After the worms mature, microfilariae are produced and migrate in the tissues, and they may cause a chronic, generalized, pruritic dermatitis. After a period of years, the skin can

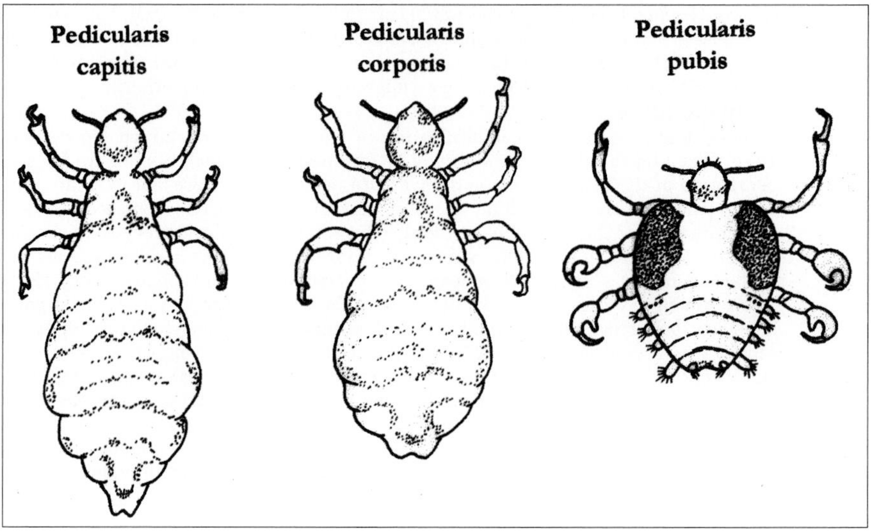

Fig. 8. Organisms causing pediculosis.

become lichenified and hypopigmented or hyperpigmented. The presence of microfilariae, living or dead, in the ocular structures, leads to photophobia and inflammation of the cornea, iris, ciliary body, retina, choroid, and optic nerve. Blindness can result if the disease is untreated.

Diagnostic Tests

Direct examination of a 1- to 2-mg shave or punch biopsy specimen of the epidermis and upper dermis (taken from the scapular or iliac crest area) usually reveals microfilariae. Adult worms may be demonstrated in excised nodules that have been sectioned and stained. A slit-lamp examination of the anterior chamber of an involved eye may reveal motile microfilariae or corneal lesions typical of onchocerciasis. Microfilariae rarely are found in blood. Eosinophilia is common. Specific serologic tests and PCR techniques for detection of microfilariae in skin are available only at selected research laboratories.

Pediculosis Capitis

Pediculus humanus var *capitis* (Fig. 8) is the head louse. Both nymphs and adult lice feed on human blood.

Itching is the most common symptom of head lice infestation, but many children are asymptomatic. Adult lice or eggs (nits) are found in the hair, usually behind the ears and near the nape of the neck. Excoriations and crusting caused by secondary bacterial infection may occur and often are associated with regional lymphadenopathy. In temperate climates, head lice deposits are associated with regional lymphadenopathy. In temperate climates, head lice deposit their eggs on a hair shaft 3–4 mm from the scalp. Because hair grows at a rate of approximately 1 cm/month, the duration of infestation can be estimated by the distance of the nit from the scalp. Lice can live only about a day outside a scalp. Any nits that remain can reinfect a child in a matter of days. Careful nitpicking is important.

Lice look like tiny crabs, and nits are tiny gray pearls cemented to the hair shaft near the root. The only sure way to eliminate lice and their eggs is to examine the hair carefully; use of a good nit comb or a good magnifying glass can help. Dr. Sydney Spiesel at Yale University is developing a shampoo containing Blankophor, which adheres to lice and nits, and makes them visible under ultraviolet light.

Diagnostic Tests

Eggs, nymphs, and lice can be identified with the naked eye; the diagnosis can be confirmed by using a hand lens or microscope. Adult lice seldom are seen because they move rapidly and conceal themselves effectively.

Pediculosis Corporis

Pediculus humanus var *corporis* (or *humanus*) is the body louse (Fig. 8). Both nymphs and adult lice feed on human blood.

Intense itching, particularly at night, is common with body lice infestations. Body lice and their eggs live in the seams of clothing. Infrequently, a louse can be seen feeding on the skin. Secondary bacterial infection of the skin caused by scratching is common.

Diagnostic Tests

Eggs, nymphs, and lice can be identified with the naked eye; the diagnosis can be confirmed by using a hand lens or microscope. Adult lice seldom are seen because they move rapidly and conceal themselves effectively.

Pediculosis Pubis

Phthirus pubis is the pubic or crab louse (Fig. 8). Both nymphs and adult lice feed on human blood. Pruritus of the anogenital area is a common symptom in pubic lice infestations ("crabs"). Many hairy areas of the body can be infested, including the eyelashes, eyebrows, beard, axilla, perianal area, and, rarely, the scalp. A characteristic sign of heavy pubic lice infestation is the presence of bluish or slate-colored maculae on the chest, abdomen, or thighs, known as maculae ceruleae.

Diagnostic Tests

Eggs, nymphs, and lice can be identified with the naked eye; the diagnosis can be confirmed by using a hand lens or microscope. Adult lice seldom are seen because they move rapidly and conceal themselves effectively.

Pinworm Infections (Enterobiasis)

Enterobius vermicularis is a nematode, or roundworm (Fig. 4).

Pinworm infection (enterobiasis) causes pruritus ani and, rarely, pruritus vulvae. Although pinworms have been found in the lumen of the appendix, most evidence indicates that they are not related causally to acute appendicitis. Many clinical findings, such as grinding of the teeth at night, weight loss, and enuresis, have been attributed to pinworm infections, but proof of a causal relationship has not been established. Urethritis, vaginitis, salpingitis, or pelvic peritonitis may occur from aberrant migration of the adult worm from the perineum.

Diagnostic Tests

Diagnosis usually is made when adult worms are visualized in the perianal region, which is best examined 2–3 hours after the child is asleep, or in the stool. Alternatively, transparent (not translucent) adhesive tape can be applied to the perianal skin to collect any eggs that may be present; the tape is then applied to a glass slide and examined under a low-power microscope lens. Three consecutively collected specimens should be obtained when the patient first awakens in the morning and before washing. The incubation period from ingestion of an egg until an adult gravid female migrates to the perianal region is 1–2 months or longer. Inspection of the perianal region while the child is asleep frequently reveals the pinworms emerging from the anus.

Scabies

The mite *Sarcoptes scabiei* subsp *hominis* (Fig. 9) is the cause of scabies. *Sarcoptes scabiei* subsp *canis*, acquired from dogs, can cause a self-limited and mild infestation, usually involving the area in direct contact with the infested animal.

Scabies is characterized by an intensely pruritic, erythematous, papular eruption caused by burrowing of adult female mites into the upper layers of the epidermis, where they create serpiginous burrows. Itching is most intense at night. In older children and adults, the sites of predilection are the interdigital folds, flexor aspects

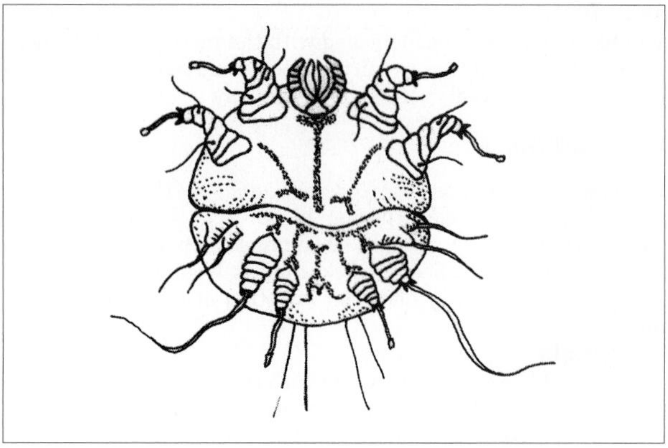

Fig. 9. *Sarcoptes scabiei*.

of the wrists, extensor surfaces of the elbows, anterior axillary folds, belt line, thighs, navel, genitalia, areolae, abdomen, intergluteal cleft, and buttocks. In children <2 years of age, the eruption generally is vesicular and often occurs in areas usually spared in older children and adults, such as the head, neck, palms, and soles. The eruption is caused by a hypersensitivity reaction to the proteins of the parasite.

The characteristic scabies burrow appears as a gray or white, tortuous, threadlike line. Excoriations are common, and most burrows are obliterated by scratching before a patient is seen by a physician. Occasionally, 2- to 5-mm red-brown nodules are present, particularly on covered parts of the body such as the genitalia, groin, and axilla. These scabies nodules are a granulomatous response to the dead mite antigens and feces. The nodules can persist for weeks and even months after effective treatment. Cutaneous secondary bacterial infection can occur and usually is caused by *S. pyogenes* or *S. aureus*.

Norwegian scabies is an uncommon form of infestation characterized by a large number of mites and widespread crusted, hyperkeratotic lesions. Norwegian scabies usually occurs in debilitated, developmentally disabled, or immunologically compromised persons.

Diagnostic Tests

Diagnosis is confirmed by identification of the mite or mite eggs, or scybala (feces) from scraping of papules or intact burrows, preferably from the terminal portion where the mite generally is found. Application of mineral oil, microscope immersion oil, or water to the skin facilitates the collection of scrapings. A No. 15 scalpel is used to scrape the burrow. The scrapings and oil are then placed on a slide under a glass coverslip and examined microscopically under low power. Adult female mites average 330–450 μm in length.

Schistosomiasis

The trematodes (flukes) (Fig. 10) *Schistosoma mansoni*, *S. japonicum*, *S. haematobium* (Fig. 11), and, rarely, *S. mekongi* and *S. intercalatum* cause disease. All species have similar life cycles. Swimmer's itch is caused by multiple avian and mammalian species of *Schistosoma*.

Initial entry of the infecting larvae (cercariae) through the skin frequently is accompanied by a transient pruritic, papular rash (cercarial dermatitis). After penetration, the organism enters the bloodstream and migrates through the lungs. Each of the three major human schistosome parasites lives in some part of the venous plexus that drains the intestines or the bladder, with the exact location depending on the *Schistosoma* species. Four to 8 weeks after exposure, an acute illness may develop, manifested by fever, malaise, cough, rash, abdominal pain, diarrhea, nau-

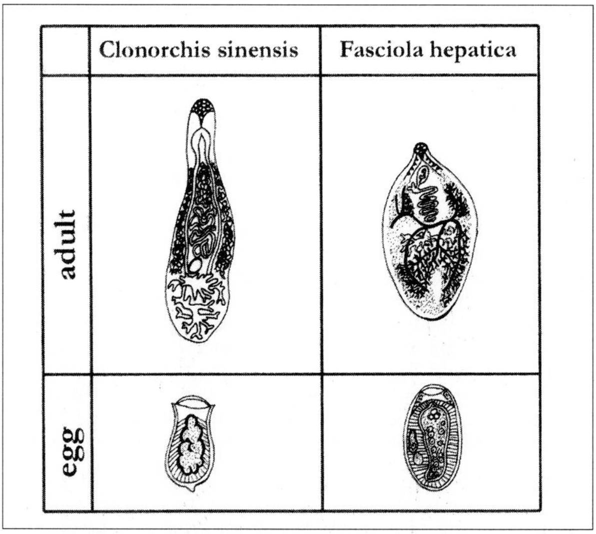

Fig. 10. Flukes.

sea, lymphadenopathy, and eosinophilia (Katayama fever). In acute infections due to heavy infestations of *S. mansoni* or *S. japonicum*, mucoid bloody diarrhea accompanied by tender hepatomegaly occurs. The severity of symptoms associated with chronic disease is related to the worm burden. Persons with low to moderate worm burdens can be asymptomatic; heavily infected persons can have a range of symptoms caused primarily by inflammation and fibrosis triggered by eggs produced by adult worms. Portal hypertension can develop and cause hepatosplenomegaly, ascites, and esophageal varices. Long-term involvement of the colon produces abdominal pain and bloody diarrhea. Other organ systems can be involved due to embolization of the eggs, for example, embolization to the lungs causing pulmonary hypertension or embolization to the CNS, notably the spinal cord. In *S. mansoni* or *S. haematobium* infections, the bladder becomes inflamed and fibrotic. Symptoms and signs include dysuria, urgency, ter-

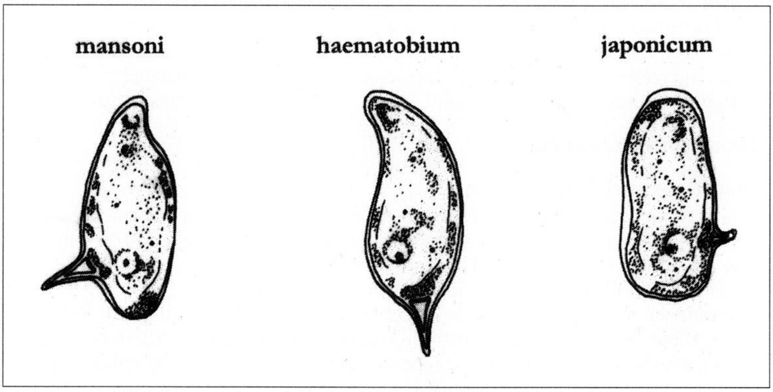

Fig. 11. Schistosoma.

minal microscopic and gross hematuria, secondary urinary tract infections, and nonspecific pelvic pain.

Swimmer's itch (cercarial dermatitis) is caused by the larvae of other avian and mammalian schistosome species that penetrate human skin but do not complete the life cycle and do not cause chronic fibrotic disease. Manifestations include mild to moderate pruritus at the penetration site a few hours after exposure, followed in 5–14 days by an intermittent pruritic, sometimes papular, eruption. In previously sensitized persons, more intense papular eruptions may occur for 7–10 days after exposure.

Diagnostic Tests

Infection with *S. mansoni* and other species (except *S. haematobium*) is determined by microscopic examination of concentrated stool specimens to detect characteristic eggs. In light infections, several specimens may need to be examined before eggs are found, and a biopsy of the rectal mucosa may be necessary. The fresh tissue obtained should be compressed between two glass slides and examined under low power (unstained) for eggs. *S. haematobium* infection is diagnosed by examining filtered urine for eggs. Egg excretion often peaks between noon and 3 p.m. Biopsy of the bladder mucosa may be necessary. Serologic tests, available through the CDC and some commercial laboratories, may be particularly helpful for detecting light infection or identifying the disease before eggs appear in the stool or urine.

Strongyloidiasis

Strongyloides stercoralis is a nematode (roundworm) that infects humans (Fig. 4).

Eosinophilia can be the only manifestation of infection. Hence, strongyloidiasis warrants consideration whenever eosinophilia (>500 cells/μL) without an obvious clinical correlation occurs in a patient who has resided in an endemic area. Infective larvae first entering the body can produce transient pruritic papules at the site of penetration of the skin, usually on the feet. Larval migration through the lungs can cause pneumonitis with a cough productive of blood-streaked sputum. The intestinal phase of infection can be accompanied by vague abdominal pain, distention, vomiting, and diarrhea that consists of voluminous mucoid stools. Malabsorption has been reported. Larval migration from defecated stool can result in pruritic skin lesions in the perianal area, buttocks, and upper thighs. The lesions may present as migrating, pruritic, serpiginous, erythematous tracks called *cutaneous larva currens*. In immunocompromised patients, particularly those receiving corticosteroids, those who are malnourished, and those who are alcoholic, complications include disseminated strongyloidiasis (caused by hyperinfection), diffuse pulmonary infiltrates, and septicemia from concurrent infection with Gram-negative bacilli.

Diagnostic Tests

Stool examination may disclose the characteristic larvae, but several fresh stool specimens may need to be examined before the organism is found. Stool concentration procedures may be required. Examination of duodenal contents obtained using the commercially available string test (Entero-Test) or of a direct aspirate may demonstrate larvae. Serodiagnosis can be helpful but is available only in a few reference laboratories, and false-negative results occur. The EIA test for antibodies gives positive results in approximately 85% of infected people; however, cross reaction with the antigens of filarial worms also occurs and limits the specificity of serodiagnosis. In disseminated strongyloidiasis, larvae can be found in the sputum.

Tapeworm Diseases

Taeniasis and Cysticercosis

Taeniasis is caused by intestinal infection by the adult tapeworm, *Taenia saginata* (beef tapeworm) or *Taenia solium* (pork tapeworm). Usually only one adult worm is present in the intestine. Human cysticercosis is caused only by the larvae of *Taenia solium* (*Cysticercus cellulosae*).

In taeniasis, mild gastrointestinal tract symptoms such as nausea, diarrhea, and pain can occur. Tapeworm segments can be seen migrating from the anus or feces.

In cysticercosis, manifestations depend on the location and numbers of pork tapeworm cysts and the host response. Cysts may be found anywhere in the body. The most common and serious manifestations usually are caused by those in the CNS.

Cysts of *T. solium* in the brain (neurocysticercosis) can cause seizures, behavioral disturbances, obstructive hydrocephalus, and other neurologic signs and symptoms. Neurocysticercosis can be a leading cause of epilepsy, depending on epidemiologic circumstances. The host reaction to degenerating cysts can produce signs and symptoms of meningitis. Cysts in the spinal column can cause gait disturbance, pain, or transverse myelitis. Subcutaneous cysts produce palpable nodules, and ocular involvement can cause visual impairment.

Diagnostic Tests

Diagnosis of taeniasis (adult tapeworm infection) is based on demonstration of the proglottids or ova in feces or the perianal region. Species identification of the parasite is based on the different structures of the terminal gravid segments. Diagnosis of neurocysticercosis is based primarily on CT or MRI. Enhanced CT may be helpful for identifying spinal and intraventricular lesions. The enzyme immunotransfer blot assay to detect serum and CSF antibody to *T. solium* is the antibody test of choice and is available through the CDC. The test is more sensitive with serum samples than with CSF specimens. The serum antibody assay results often are negative in children with solitary parenchymal lesions but usually are positive in patients with multiple inflamed lesions.

Hydatid Disease (Echinococcosis)

The larval forms of the tapeworms *Echinococcus granulosus* and *Echinococcus multilocularis* are the causes of hydatid disease. The distribution of *E. granulosus* is related to the location of sheep or cattle herding. Countries with the highest prevalence include Argentina, Australia, China, Greece, Italy, Lebanon, Romania, South Africa, Spain, Syria, Turkey, and the countries in the former Soviet Union. In the United States, small endemic foci exist in Arizona, California, New Mexico, and Utah, and a strain adapted to wolves, dingoes, and jackals can infect these animals when they swallow protoscolices of the parasite within hydatid cysts in the organs of sheep or other intermediate hosts. Dogs pass embryonated eggs in their stools, and sheep become infected by swallowing the eggs. If humans swallow *Echinococcus* eggs, they can become inadvertent intermediate hosts, and cysts can develop in various organs, particularly the liver but also the lungs, kidneys, and spleen. These cysts grow slowly (1 cm in diameter per year) and eventually can contain several liters of fluid. If a cyst ruptures, anaphylaxis and origination of multiple secondary cysts from seeding of protoscolices can result. Clinical diagnosis frequently is difficult. A history of contact with dogs in an endemic area is helpful. Space-occupying lesions can be demonstrated by radiographs, ultrasonography, or CT of various organs. Serologic tests, available at the CDC, are helpful, but false-negative results can occur.

E. multilocularis, a species for which the life cycle involves foxes and rodents, causes the alveolar form of hydatid disease, which is characterized by invasive growth of the larvae in the liver with occasional metastatic spread. The alveolar form of hydatid disease is limited to the northern hemisphere and usually is diagnosed in persons ≥50 years of age.

Other Tapeworm Diseases

Hymenolepis nana

Hymenolepis nana, also called *dwarf tapeworm* because it is the smallest of the adult tapeworms, has its entire cycle within humans. Therefore, person-to-person transmission is possible. More problematic is autoinfection, which tends to perpetuate the infection in the host because the eggs can hatch within the intestine and reinitiate the cycle; this leads to development of new worms and a large worm burden. This cycle makes eradicating the infection difficult.

Dipylidium caninum

Dipylidium caninum is the most common and widespread adult tapeworm of dogs and cats. *Dipylidium caninum* infects children when they inadvertently swallow a dog or cat flea, which serves as the intermediate host. Diagnosis is made by finding the characteristic eggs or tapeworm segments in stool. Treatment with praziquantel or niclosamide is effective.

Diphyllobothrium latum *(and Related Species)*

Diphyllobothrium latum, also called *fish tapeworm*, has fish as one of its intermediate hosts. Consumption of infected raw freshwater fish (including salmon) leads to the infection. Three to 5 weeks are needed for the adult tapeworm to mature and begin to lay eggs. The worm sometimes causes mechanical obstruction of the bowel, diarrhea, abdominal pain, or megaloblastic anemia secondary to vitamin B_{12} deficiency. The diagnosis is made by recognition of the characteristic eggs or proglottids passed in stool.

Trichomoniasis

Trichomonas vaginalis is a flagellated protozoan, slightly larger than a granulocyte.

Infection with *T. vaginalis* frequently is asymptomatic. The usual clinical picture in symptomatic postmenarcheal female patients consists of a frothy vaginal discharge and mild vulvovaginal itching. Dysuria and, rarely, lower abdominal pain can occur. The vaginal discharge usually is a pale yellow to gray-green and has a musty odor. Symptoms frequently are more severe just before or after menstruation. The vaginal mucosa often is deeply erythematous, and the cervix is friable and diffusely inflamed, sometimes covered with numerous petechiae ("strawberry cervix"). Urethritis and, more rarely, epididymitis or prostatitis can develop in infected males, but the majority of cases are asymptomatic. Reinfection is common.

Diagnostic Tests

Diagnosis is usually established by examination of a wet-mount preparation of the vaginal discharge. Lashing of the flagella and jerky motility of the organism are distinctive. Positivity of the preparations, found more frequently in women who have symptoms, is related directly to the number of organisms, but the protozoa are identified in only 40–80% of cases. Culture of the organism and antibody tests using an EIA and immunofluorescence techniques for demonstration of the organism are more sensitive than wet-mount preparations but generally are not required for diagnosis. Culture for *T. vaginalis* is positive in >95% of cases. PCR test for *T. vaginalis* is sensitive and specific but is available only as a research diagnostic test.

Trichuriasis (Whipworm Infections)

Abdominal pain, tenesmus, and bloody diarrhea with mucus can occur with *Trichuris trichiura*, the whipworm, as the causative agent (Fig. 4). Adult worms are 30–50 mm long with a large, threadlike anterior end that is embedded in the mucosa of the large intestine. Children with heavy infections can develop a *T. trichiura* dysentery syndrome or chronic *T. trichiura* colitis. *T. trichiura* colitis can mimic other forms of inflammatory bowel disease and lead to physical growth retardation. Chronic infection associated with heavy infestation also can lead to rectal prolapse.

Diagnostic Tests

Eggs may be found on direct examination of the stool or by using concentration techniques.

Trypanosomiasis

African

The West African (Gambian) form of sleeping sickness is caused by *Trypanosoma brucei gambiense*, whereas the East African (Rhodesian) form is caused by *Trypanosoma brucei rhodesiense*. Both are extracellular protozoan hemoflagellates that live in the blood and tissue of the human host.

The rapidity and severity of clinical manifestations vary with the infecting species. With *T. brucei gambiense* (West African) infection, a cutaneous nodule or chancre may appear at the site of parasite inoculation within a few days of a bite by an infected tsetse fly. Systemic illness is chronic, occurring months to years later, and is characterized by intermittent fever, posterior cervical lymphadenopathy (Winterbottom sign), and multiple nonspecific complaints, including malaise, weight loss, arthralgia, rash, pruritus, and edema. If the CNS is involved, chronic meningoencephalitis with behavioral changes, cachexia, headache, hallucinations, delusions, and somnolence can occur. In contrast, *T. brucei rhodesiense* (East African) infection is acute; generalized illness develops days to weeks after parasite inoculation, with acute manifestations including high fever, cutaneous chancre, myocarditis, hepatitis, anemia, thrombocytopenia, and laboratory evidence of disseminated intravascular coagulation. Clinical meningoencephalitis can develop as early as 3 weeks after onset of the untreated systemic illness. *T. brucei rhodesiense* infection has a high fatality rate; without treatment, infected patients usually die within days to months after clinical onset of disease.

Diagnostic Tests

Diagnosis is made by identification of trypomastigotes in blood, CSF, or fluid aspirated from a chancre or lymph node or by inoculation of susceptible laboratory animals (mice) with heparinized blood. Examination of the CSF is critical to management and should be performed using the double-centrifugation technique. Concentration and Giemsa staining of the buffy-coat layer of peripheral blood also can be helpful. *T. brucei gambiense* is more likely to be found in lymph node aspirates. Although an increased concentration of IgM in serum or CSF is considered characteristic of African trypanosomiasis, polyclonal hyperglobulinemia is common.

American (Chagas Disease)

Trypanosoma cruzi, a protozoan hemoflagellate, is the cause of American trypanosomiasis.

Patients can present with acute or chronic disease. The early phase of this disease frequently is asymptomatic. However, children are more likely to exhibit symptoms than are adults. In some patients, a red nodule known as a *chagoma* develops at the site of the original inoculation, usually on the face or arms. The surrounding skin becomes indurated and, later, hypopigmented. Unilateral firm edema of the eyelids, known as Romaña sign, is the earliest indication of the infection but is not always present. The edematous skin is violaceous and associated with conjunctivitis and enlargement of the ipsilateral preauricular lymph node. A few days after the appearance of Romaña sign, fever, generalized lymphadenopathy, and malaise can develop. Acute myocarditis, hepatosplenomegaly, edema, and meningoencephalitis can follow. Serious sequelae, consisting of cardiomyopathy and heart failure (the major cause of death), and megaesophagus, megacolon, or both, can develop many years after the initial manifestations in the chronic phase of disease. Congenital disease is characterized by low birth weight, hepatomegaly, and meningoencephalitis, with seizures and tremors.

Diagnostic Tests

During the acute disease, the parasite is demonstrable in blood, either by Giemsa staining or by direct wet-mount preparation. In chronic infections, which are characterized by low-level parasitemia, recovery of the parasite by culture on special media or identification by xenodiagnosis should be undertaken. Serologic tests include indirect hemagglutination, indirect immunofluorescence, and EIA.

Identification of Parasitic Worms

Specimen

Worm or segment of worm from urine, stool, sputum, or other clinical specimen.

Worms, or portions of them, must be submitted in formalin; the ova and parasite vial may be used. Specimen should be maintained at room temperature.

Parasitic infestation should be diagnosed; worms recovered from patient should be identified; possibility of parasite presence should be eliminated.

Method

Macroscopic and microscopic evaluation

Organisms Commonly Present in Various Sites

Site	Normal Flora	Pathogens
External ear	*Staphylococcus epidermidis* α-Hemolytic streptococci Aerobic corynebacteria *Enterobacteriaceae* spp. *Corynebacterium acnes* *Candida* spp. *Bacillus* spp.	*Pseudomonas* species *Staphylococcus aureus* Coliform bacilli α-Hemolytic streptococci *Proteus* spp. *Streptococcus pneumoniae* *Corynebacterium diphtheriae* *Aspergillus* spp. *Candida* spp. Varicella-zoster virus HSV Papovavirus Molluscum contagiosum

Middle ear	Sterile	Acute otitis media *Haemophilus influenzae* *Streptococcus pneumoniae* *Moraxella catarrhalis* β-Hemolytic streptococci Respiratory syncytial virus (RSV) Influenza viruses Enteroviruses Adenoviruses Chronic otitis media *S. aureus* *Proteus* spp. *Pseudomonas* spp. Other Gram-negative bacilli α-Hemolytic streptococci RSV Influenza virus
Nasal passages	*S. epidermidis* *S. aureus* Diphtheroids *S. pneumoniae* α-Hemolytic streptococci Nonpathogenic *Neisseria* spp. Aerobic corynebacteria	**Acute Sinusitis** *S. aureus* *S. pneumoniae* *Klebsiella-Enterobacter* spp. α-Hemolytic streptococci β-Hemolytic streptococci *M. catarrhalis* Chronic sinusitis *S. aureus* α-Hemolytic streptococci *S. pneumoniae* β-Hemolytic streptococci *Mucor, Aspergillus* spp. (especially in diabetics)
Pharynx and tonsils	α-Hemolytic streptococci *Neisseria* spp. *S. epidermidis* *S. aureus* (small numbers) *S. pneumoniae* Nonhemolytic (γ) streptococci Diphtheroids Coliforms β-Hemolytic streptococci (not group A) *Actinomyces israelii* *Haemophilus* spp. Marked predominance of one organism may be clinically significant even if it is a normal inhabitant	β-Hemolytic streptococci *C. diphtheriae* *Bordetella pertussis* *Neisseria meningitidis* *H. influenzae* *S. aureus* *Candida albicans* Respiratory viruses *Mycoplasma pneumoniae* *Neisseria gonorrhoeae* *Chlamydia pneumoniae*
Epiglottis Larynx		*H. influenzae* Respiratory viruses *C. diphtheriae* Epstein-Barr virus (infectious mononucleosis) *C. albicans*
Bronchioli Bronchi		RSV *M. pneumoniae* Viruses (e.g., influenza, rhinovirus, coronavirus, adenovirus) *C. diphtheriae* *S. pneumoniae*

Lungs		Bacteria *Pseudomonas aeruginosa* *Escherichia coli* *Klebsiella pneumoniae* *Serratia marcescens* *Enterobacter* spp. *S. aureus* *Proteus mirabilis* *S. pneumoniae* *H. influenzae* *B. pertussis* *M. pneumoniae* *C. pneumoniae* *Chlamydia psittaci* *Legionella pneumophila* *Pneumocystis carinii* Tubercle bacilli *Francisella tularensis* *Yersinia pestis* Fungi Viruses [e.g., influenza, parainfluenza, adenoviruses, RSV, echovirus, coxsackievirus, reovirus, cytomegalovirus (CMV), viruses of exanthems, HSV, hantavirus] Rickettsiae (e.g., typhus, *Coxiella burnetii*) Protozoans (e.g., *Toxoplasma*, *P. carinii*)
Gastrointestinal tract		
Mouth	α-Hemolytic streptococci Enterococci Lactobacilli Staphylococci Fusobacteria *Bacteroides* spp. Diphtheroids *Neisseria* spp. (except *N. gonorrhoeae*)	*C. albicans* *Borrelia vincentii* with *Fusobacterium fusiforme*
Esophagus		*C. albicans* CMV HSV
Stomach	Sterile	*Helicobacter pylori*
Small intestine	Sterile in one-third Scant bacteria in two-thirds *E. coli* *Klebsiella-Enterobacter* Enterococci α-Hemolytic streptococci *S. epidermidis* Diphtheroids	*Campylobacter jejuni* *H. pylori*
Colon	Abundant bacteria *Bacteroides* spp. *E. coli* *Klebsiella-Enterobacter* Paracolons *Proteus* spp. Enterococci (group D streptococci)	Enteropathogenic *E. coli* *C. albicans* *Aeromonas* spp. *Salmonella* spp. *Shigella* spp. *C. jejuni* *Yersinia enterocolitica*

	Yeasts	*S. aureus* *Clostridium difficile* *Vibrio cholerae* *Vibrio parahaemolyticus* Amebas and parasites (Fig. 2) Viruses (e.g., rotavirus, CMV, HSV, Norwalk)
Rectum		*Chlamydia* spp. *N. gonorrhoeae* *Treponema pallidum* *Chlamydia trachomatis* *Enterobius vermicularis* (anus)
Gallbladder	Sterile	*E. coli* *Enterococci* *Klebsiella-Enterobacter-Serratia* Occasionally: Coliforms *Proteus* spp. *Pseudomonas* spp.
Blood	Sterile	*S. epidermidis* *S. aureus* *E. coli* Enterococci *Pseudomonas* spp. α- and β-Hemolytic streptococci *S. pneumoniae* *H. influenzae* *Clostridium perfringens* *Proteus* spp. *Bacteroides* and related anaerobes *Neisseria meningitidis* *Brucella* spp. *Pasteurella tularensis* *Listeria monocytogenes* *Achromobacter* (*Herellea*) spp. *Streptobacillus moniliformis* *Leptospira* spp. *Vibrio fetus* *Salmonella* spp. *Nocardia* spp. Opportunistic fungi *Candida* spp. *Blastomyces dermatitidis* *Histoplasma capsulatum*
Eye	Usually sterile Occasionally small numbers of diphtheroids and coagulase-negative staphylococci	*S. aureus* *Haemophilus* spp. *S. pneumoniae* *N. gonorrhoeae* α- and β-Hemolytic streptococci *Achromobacter* (*Herellea*) spp. Coliform bacilli *P. aeruginosa* Other enteric bacilli Morax-Axenfeld bacillus *Bacillus subtilis* (occasionally) *Chlamydia* spp.
Spinal fluid	Sterile	*H. influenzae* *N. meningitidis* *S. pneumoniae* *Mycobacterium tuberculosis* Staphylococci, streptococci *Cryptococcus neoformans*

		Coliform bacilli *Pseudomonas* and *Proteus* spp. *Bacteroides* spp. *L. monocytogenes* *Leptospira* *Treponema* *Borrelia burgdorferi* Viruses (e.g., coxsackie A and B, echovirus, HSV, mumps, human immunodeficiency virus, varicella-zoster virus, lymphocytic, choriomeningitis, CMV, adenovirus) Fungi (e.g., *H. capsulatum, C. neoformans, Coccidioides immitis*) Free amebas (e.g., *Naegleria, Acanthamoeba*)
Urethra, male	*S. aureus* *S. epidermidis* Enterococci Diphtheroids *Achromobacter wolffi* (Mima) *Bacillus subtilis*	*N. gonorrhoeae* *Chlamydia* spp. *U. urealyticum* Enterococci *G. vaginalis* β-Hemolytic streptococci (usually group B) Anaerobic and microaerophilic streptococci *Bacteroides* spp. *H. ducreyi* *E. coli, Klebsiella- Enterobacter* *S. aureus*
Urethra, female, and vagina	Lactobacillus (large numbers) *E. coli, Enterobacter aerogenes* Staphylococci Streptococci (aerobic and anaerobic) Candida albicans *Bacteroides* spp. Achromobacter wolffi (Mima)	Yeast and *C. albicans* *C. perfringens* *L. monocytogenes* *G. vaginalis* *T. vaginalis* *N. gonorrhoeae* *Chlamydia* spp. (See also Urethra, male) *U. urealyticum*
Prostate	Sterile	*S. faecalis* *S. epidermis* *E. coli* *P. mirabilis* *Pseudomonas* spp. *Klebsiella* spp. Anaerobic and microaerophilic streptococci (α, β, γ types) *Bacteroides* spp. Enterococci β-Hemolytic streptococci (usually group B) Staphylococci *Proteus* spp. *C. perfringens* *E. coli* and *Klebsiella-Enterobacter-Serratia* *L. monocytogenes*

Urine	Staphylococci, coagulase negative Diphtheroids Coliform bacilli Enterococci *Proteus* spp. Lactobacilli α- and β-Hemolytic streptococci	*E. coli* *Klebsiella-Enterobacter-Serratia* *Proteus* spp. *Pseudomonas* spp. *Enterococci* *Staphylococci,* coagulase positive and negative *Providencia* spp. *M. morganii* *Alcaligenes* spp. *Achromobacter* (*Herellea*) spp. *C. albicans* β-Hemolytic streptococci *N. gonorrhoeae* *M. tuberculosis* *Salmonella* and *Shigella* spp.
Wound		*S. aureus* *S. epidermidis* *C. bacilli* *Pseudomonas* spp. *Enterococci* *S. pyogenes* *Clostridium* spp. *Bacteroides* spp.; other Gram-negative rods *Proteus* spp. *Achromobacter* (*Herellea*) spp. *Serratia* spp.
Pleura	Sterile	*S. aureus* *S. epidermidis* *S. pneumoniae* *H. influenza* *M. tuberculosis* Anaerobic streptococci *S. pyogenes* *E. coli* *K. pneumoniae* *Actinomyces* spp. *Nocardia* spp.
Pericardium	Sterile	*S. aureus* *S. pneumoniae* Enterobacteriaceae *Pseudomonas* spp. *H. influenza* *N. meningitidis* *Streptococcus* spp. Anaerobic bacteria *C. immitis* *Actinomyces* spp. *Candida* spp.
Peritoneum	Sterile	*E. coli* Enterococci *S. pneumoniae* *Bacteroides* spp.; other Gram-negative rods Anaerobic streptococci *Clostridium* spp. *S. epidermidis* *S. aureus* *Pseudomonas* spp. α-Hemolytic streptococci *K. pneumoniae*

Bones	Sterile	Acute hematogenous *S. aureus* *H. influenza* Streptococci (groups A and B) *N. gonorrhoeae* Gram-negative bacilli (e.g., *P. aeruginosa, S. marcescens, E. coli*) *M. tuberculosis* *Salmonella* spp. in sickle cell disease Contiguous Anaerobic bacteria (e.g., *Bacteroides*, Fusobacteria, anaerobic cocci) *S. aureus*
Joints	Sterile	*S. epidermidis* β-Hemolytic streptococci *S. pneumoniae* *H. influenza* *K. pneumoniae*
Skin	*S. aureus* *S. epidermidis*	*S. aureus* (impetigo, folliculitis, furunculosis) Group A streptococcus (impetigo, erysipelas) *C. diphtheriae* *Bacillus anthracis* *F. tularensis* *Mycobacterium ulcerans* *Mycobacterium marinum* Anaerobic bacteria Viruses (e.g., papillomavirus, varicella-zoster, HSV, molluscum contagiosum) Fungi (e.g., *Trichophyton, Microsporum, Epidermophytin, Actinomyces, Nocardia*)

Gram-Negative Pathogens in Newborns

Salmonella spp. in sickle cell disease
N. gonorrhoeae
M. tuberculosis
Mycobacterium kansasii
Mycobacterium intracellulare
B. burgdorferi
Viruses (e.g., mumps, rubella, HBV, parvovirus B19)
Fungi (e.g., *Candida, Sporothrix schenckii, C. immitis, B. dermatitidis*)

Bibliography

Allain JP, Dailey SH, Laurain Y, et al. Evidence for persistent hepatitis C virus (HCV) infection in hemophiliacs. *J Clin Invest* 1991;88(5):1762–1769.

Alter HJ, Tegtmeier GE, Sett BW, et al. The use of a recombinant immunoblot assay in the interpretation of antihepatitis C virus reactivity among prospectively followed patients, implicated donors, and random donors. *Transfusion* 1991;31:771–776.

Alter MJ, Hadler SC, Judson FN, et al. Risk factors for acute non-A, non-B hepatitis in the United States and association with hepatitis C Virus infection. *JAMA* 1990;264(17):2231–2235.

Anderson BE, Neumann MA. *Bartonella* spp as emerging human pathogens. *Clin Microbiol Rev* 1997;10:203–209.
Bakken JS, Dumler S, Chen SM, et al. Human granulocytic ehrlichiosis in the upper Midwest United States: a new species emerging? *JAMA* 1994;272:212–218.
Bakken JS, Krueth J, Wilson-Nordskog C, et al. Clinical and laboratory characteristics of human granulocytic ehrlichiosis. *JAMA* 1996;275:199–205.
Bass JW, Freitas BC, Freitas AD, et al. Prospective randomized double blind placebo-controlled evaluation of azithromycin for treatment of cat-scratch disease. *Pediatr Infect Dis J* 1998;17:447–452.
Bass JW, Vincent JM, Person DA. The expanding spectrum of *Bartonella* infections. *Pediatr Infect Dis J* 1997;16:163–179.
Batra P. Pulmonary coccidioidomycosis. *J Thorac Imaging* 1992;7(4):29–38.
Bortolottis F, Calzia R, Cadrobbi P, et al. Long-term evolution of chronic hepatitis B in children with antibody to hepatitis Be antigen. *J Pediatr* 1990;116(4):552–555.
Boyars MC, Zwischenberger JB, Cox CS Jr. Clinical manifestations of pulmonary fungal infections. *J Thorac Imaging* 1992;7(4):12–22.
Busch MP, Tobier L, Quan S, et al. A pattern of 5-1-1 and C100-2 only on hepatitis C virus (HCV) recombinant immunoblot assay does not reflect infection in blood donors. *Transfusion* 1993;33(1):84–88.
Centers for Disease Control. *Enterovirus surveillance summary 1970–1979*. Atlanta, GA: Centers for Disease Control, 1981.
Chomel BB, Abbott RC, Kasten RW, et al. *Bartonella henselae* prevalence in domestic cats in California: risk factors and association between bacteremia and antibody titers. *J Clin Microbiol* 1995;33:2445–2450.
Choo QL, Kuo G, Weiner AJ, et al. Isolation of a cDNA clone derived from a blood-borne non-A, non-B viral hepatitis genome. *Science* 1989;244(4902):359–362.
Chretien JH, Garagusi VF. Current management of fungal enteritis. *Med Clin North Am* 1982;66:675–687.
Clemens JM, Taskar S, Chau K, et al. IgM antibody response in acute hepatitis C viral infection. *Blood* 1992;79(1):169–172.
Devine P, Taswell HF, Moore SB, et al. Passively acquired antibody to hepatitis B surface antigen. Pitfall in evaluating immunity to hepatitis B viral infections. *Arch Pathol Lab Med* 1989;113(5):529–531.
Diamond RD. The growing problem of mycoses in patients infected with the human immunodeficiency virus. *Rev Infect Dis* 1991;13(3):480–486.
Dodd LG, McBride JH, Gitnick GL, et al. Prevalence of non-A, non-B hepatitis/hepatitis C virus antibody in human immunoglobulins. *Am J Clin Pathol* 1992;97(1):108–113.
Edelman DC, Dumler JS. Evaluation of an improved PCR diagnostic assay for human granulocytic ehrlichiosis. *Mol Diagn* 1996;1:1–49.
Edwards MS. Hepatitis B serology—help in interpretation. *Pediatr Clin North Am* 1988;35:503–515.
Fraser RS. Pulmonary aspergillosis: pathologic and pathogenic features. *Pathol Annu* 1993;28(Pt 1):231–277.
Giacoia GP, Kasprisin DO. Transfusion-acquired hepatitis A. *South Med J* 1989;82(11):1357–1360.
Gray LD, Roberts GD. Laboratory diagnosis of systemic fungal diseases. *Med Clin North Am* 1988;2:779–803.
Gupta TP, Ehrinpreis MN. Candida-associated diarrhea in hospitalized patients. *Gastroenterology* 1990;98(3):780–785.
Hay RJ. Fungal skin infections. *Arch Dis Child* 1992;67(9):1065–1067.
Lee HS, Vyas GN. Diagnosis of viral hepatitis. *Clin Lab Med* 1987;7:741–757.
Margileth AM. Recent advances in diagnosis and treatment of cat scratch disease. *Curr Infect Dis Rep* 2000;2:141–146.
Mushahwar IK, et al. Interpretation of hepatitis B virus and hepatitis delta virus serologic profiles. *Pathologist* 1984;38:648–650.
Mushahwar IK, McGrath LC, Dmec J, et al. Radioimmunoassay for detection of hepatitis Be Antigen and its antibody. Results of clinical evaluation. *Am J Clin Pathol* 1981;76:692–697.
Nath N, et al. Antibodies to delta antigen among asymptomatic HBsAg positive volunteer blood donors in the U.S. In: Vyas GN, Dienstag JL, Hoofnagle JH, eds. *Viral hepatitis and liver disease*. New York: Grune & Stratton, 1984:617.

Pichichero ME, McLinn S, Rotbart HA, et al. Clinical and economic impact of enterovirus illness in private pediatric practice. *Pediatrics* 1998;102:1126–1134.
Rasmussen JE. Cutaneous fungus infections in children. *Pediatr Rev* 1992;13(4):152–156.
Regnery RL, Anderson BE, Claridge JE, et al. Characterization of a novel *Rockalimaea* species, *R. henselae* sp nov, isolated from blood of a febrile human immunodeficiency virus-positive patient. *J Clin Microbiol* 1992;30:265–274.
Regnery RL, Tappero J. Unraveling mysteries associated with cat scratch disease, bacillary angiomatosis and related syndromes. *Emerg Infect Dis* 1995;1:1–13.
Schuyler MR. Allergic bronchopulmonary aspergillosis. *Clin Chest Med* 1983;4:15–22.
Skidmore S. Recombinant immunoblot assay for hepatitis C antibody. *Lancet* 1990;336:63.
Smedile A, Farci P, Verme G, et al. Influence of delta infection on severity of hepatitis B. *Lancet* 1982;2(8305):945–947.
Tang CM, Cohen J. Diagnosing fungal infections in immunocompromised hosts. *J Clin Pathol* 1992;45(1):1–5.
Telenti A, Steckelberg JM, Stockman L, et al. Quantitative blood cultures in candidemia. *Mayo Clin Proc* 1991;66(11):1120–1123.
Van der Poel CL, Cuypers HTM, Reesink HW, et al. Confirmation of hepatitis C virus infection by new four-antigen recombinant immunoblot assay. *Lancet* 1991;337: 317–319.
Wallach J. *Interpretation of diagnostic tests*, 7th ed. Philadelphia: Lippincott Williams & Wilkins, 2000.
Welch DF, Pickett DA, Slater LN, et al. *Rochalimaea* sp nov: a case of septicemia, bacillary angiomatosis, and parenchymal bacillary peliosis. *J Clin Microbiol* 1992; 30:275–280.
Wheat LJ. Histoplasmosis. *Med Clin North Am* 1988;2:841–859.

6 Immunologic Disorders

Normal levels of immunoglobulins G, A, and M are as follows:

	Immunoglobulin G (g/L)	Immunoglobulin A (g/L)	Immunoglobulin M (g/L)
Cord blood	6.4–16.1	0.01–0.04	0.06–0.26
1 mo	2.5–9.1	0.01–0.53	0.20–0.87
2 mo	2.1–6.0	0.03–0.47	0.17–1.10
3 mo	1.8–5.8	0.05–0.46	0.24–0.89
4 mo	2.0–5.6	0.04–0.73	0.27–1.00
5 mo	1.7–8.1	0.08–0.88	0.33–1.10
6 mo	2.2–7.0	0.08–0.84	0.35–1.00
7–9 mo	2.2–7.0	0.11–0.90	0.34–1.30
10–12 mo	2.9–11.0	0.16–0.84	0.41–1.50
1 yr	3.5–12.0	0.14–1.10	0.43–1.70
2 yr	4.2–11.0	0.14–1.20	0.48–1.70
3 yr	4.4–11.0	0.22–1.60	0.47–2.00
4–5 yr	4.6–12.0	0.25–1.50	0.43–2.00
6–8 yr	6.3–13.0	0.33–2.00	0.48–2.10
9–10 yr	6.1–16.0	0.45–2.40	0.52–2.40
Adult	6.5–16.0	0.6–4.0	0.5–3.0

Reference levels may vary with methodology and with the racial composition of the population.

The primary symptom of a patient with an immunodeficiency is increased susceptibility to infection. Patients usually suffer from recurrent or chronic infections, often caused by opportunistic organisms. These infections can involve multiple organs or multiple sites of the same organ, and the outcome can be severe and sometimes fatal. The types of infectious agents and the location of the infection often give valuable insight into the nature of the immunologic defect. For example, individuals with B-cell deficiencies characteristically have increased susceptibility to infections with encapsulated pyogenic bacteria such as *Staphylococcus*, *Haemophilus influenzae*, and *Streptococcus pneumoniae*. They are also susceptible to enterovirus infection. Patients with T-cell deficiencies often suffer from fungal and viral infections; *Pneumocystis* infections are also common. Important clinical manifestations are chronic diarrhea, malabsorption, and sometimes malnutrition, especially in infants and young children. These symptoms can be caused by infectious organisms such as *Giardia*, rotavirus, and *Cryptosporidium* but can be due to autoimmune or chronic inflammatory conditions such as inflammatory bowel disease and gluten-sensitive enteropathy. Hematologic abnormalities such as anemia, thrombocytopenia, and leukopenia are common in immunodeficient patients. These abnormalities can be intrinsic to the immunologic defect; for example, thrombocytopenia exhibited by patients with Wiskott-Aldrich syndrome (WAS) is the result of abnormal platelet structure. It is not unusual to find autoimmune or rheumatic complications as part of the clinical presentation.

Tests for Primary Immunodeficiency Diseases

Initial Tests for Immunodeficiency Diseases

White blood cell count and differential
Absolute neutrophil count
Absolute lymphocyte count
Platelet count
Serum immunoglobulin (Ig) levels
  IgG
  IgA
  IgM
Protein electrophoresis
Functional antibody concentrations
  Blood group antibodies
  Antibodies to vaccine antigens
Delayed-type hypersensitivity skin tests

Humoral immunity is evaluated by assessment of the activity of specific antibodies, which includes ABO blood group isohemagglutinins; antibodies to vaccine antigens such as diphtheria, pertussis, tetanus; and *H. influenzae* and *Neisseria* meningitis polysaccharides, bacteriophage ΦX174, and monomeric flagellin.

Cell-mediated immunity (CMI) is assessed by a complete blood count, which indicates lymphopenia, granulocytopenia, thrombocytopenia, or leukemia. An intradermal skin test is the only practical *in vivo* test available for determining the patient's CMI. This test measures delayed-type hypersensitivity reactions. Antigens used are *Candida albicans*, tetanus, diphtheria, streptokinase/streptodornase, tuberculin (purified protein derivative), trichophyton, and proteus. Reactions are read for induration 48–72 hours after inoculation. Many hospitals prefer to use the preloaded multipuncture device (multitest CMI) for performing skin tests. The advantages of the multitest CMI are standardized antigen dose and ease of use. The major disadvantage is the limited number of antigens available for testing. For infants and very young children, skin testing is not recommended because of the high frequency of false-negative responses as a result of insufficient antigenic exposure. A negative skin test result is not necessarily indicative of T-cell dysfunction, because anergy can be induced in many disease and pathologic states.

Specific Tests for Evaluation of Immunodeficiency Diseases

B Cells

B-lymphocyte quantitation
In vitro antibody production induced by pokeweed mitogen, protein A, or Epstein-Barr virus
IgG subclass quantitation
Antibody response to polysaccharide antigens, e.g., pneumococcal antigen
Isolation and biochemical analysis of defective molecules

T Cells

T-lymphocyte quantitation
  Total T cells
  T helper cells
  T suppressor/cytotoxic cells
Proliferative responses to mitogens, antigens, and allogeneic cells
Cytokine quantitation
Calcium (Ca^{2+}) flux, protein phosphorylation, and phosphatidylinositol turnover
Isolation and biochemical analysis of defective molecules

Flow cytometry provides information on the distribution of lymphocyte subsets as well as their immunologic state and stage of maturation.

In vitro lymphocyte proliferation assay is based on H-thymidine uptake into DNA of activated lymphocytes after stimulation with mitogen(s) or antigen(s). Mitogens are phytohemagglutinin, concanavalin A, and pokeweed mitogen. Other nonspecific activators are phorbol myristate acetate and superantigens such as staphylococcal enterotoxins. Phorbol myristate acetate triggers T cells by activation of protein kinase C and bypass

T-cell receptor (TCR)/CD3 receptor system. Superantigens stimulate T cells by direct binding to the Vβ chain of the TCR and the conserved regions of the HLA class II molecule. T cells can also be activated using anti-CD3 anti-TCR monoclonal antibodies; this method can detect dysfunctional or abnormal TCR/CD3 receptor complexes.

In cases of suspected chronic mucocutaneous candidiasis, stimulation with *Candida* is the crucial definitive test. Antigens commonly used in the laboratory are tetanus toxoid, *Candida* extract, pure protein derivative, and streptolysin-streptodornase. Proliferation to allogeneic cells as in mixed lymphocyte cultures is a good method for assessing T-cell function. Due to the complexity of this assay, it is not usually available in standard laboratories. Instead of using H-thymidine uptake as an indicator of activation, surface activation markers (interleukin-2R, CD69, and HLA-DR) can be quantitated on stimulated T lymphocytes using flow cytometry. Other less commonly used methods for quantitation of activation include measurement of surface interleukin-2 receptor in the culture supernatant by enzyme-linked immunoassay or detection of interleukin-2 messenger RNA by Northern blot technique or by *in situ* hybridization on activated cells.

Defects in cytotoxic T-cell function can be assayed by release of chromium from lysed target cells by specific cytotoxic T cells. This test is not routinely used because of technical difficulty and the requirement of *in vitro-in vivo* priming.

For evaluation of B-cell function, pokeweed mitogen, staphylococcus protein A, and Epstein-Barr virus (EBV) are often used *in vitro* to induce polyclonal B-cell proliferation and antibody production. Pokeweed mitogen requires the presence of T cells, whereas the other two do not. B-cell proliferation is measured by H-thymidine uptake, and production of immunoglobulins in the culture supernatants is quantitated by enzyme-linked immunoassay. An alternative method is the reverse or direct plaque-forming cell assay, which enumerates the number of antibody-producing cells.

Other tests include cytokine production, signal transduction determination, and biochemical analysis.

Detection of signal transduction defects involves the measurement of Ca^{2+} flux, protein phosphorylation, and phosphatidylinositol turnover. The Ca^{2+} method uses Indo-1 or Fluo-3 fluorescent dyes. Protein phosphorylation is measured by binding of antiphosphorylated tyrosines to multiple substrates in whole-cell lysates after electrophoresis, and phosphatidylinositol turnover is quantitated using radioactive phosphatidylinositol 4,5-diphosphate after cell activation.

If the suspected immunodeficiency is due to structural changes in cellular molecules, isolation and biochemical analysis of the abnormal molecules confirm the diagnosis.

Clinical Uses of *In Vitro* Lymphocyte Activation and Proliferation Assays

Evaluate immune competence in patients with recurrent infection.

- Monitor the efficacy of immunosuppressive drugs in transplantation patients.
- Assess functional capacity of CMI in patients with human immunodeficiency virus infection.
- Determine vaccine efficacy.
- Assess cellular aspects of autoimmune disease.
- Evaluate the capacity for CMI in shock, stress, malnutrition, and aging.
- Aid in the diagnosis of type IV hypersensitivities (e.g., beryllium disease).
- Serve as surrogate marker in monitoring allergen immunotherapy.

Laboratory Methods to Assess Activation and Proliferation

- Lymphocyte proliferation assay with H-thymidine incorporation
- Measurement of cytokine synthesis by flow cytometry
- Immunoassay for cytokines released into culture supernatants
- ELISPOT single-cell cytokine secretion test
- Polymerase chain reaction–based assay for interleukin-2 messenger RNA expression
- Flow cytometry assay for the cell surface expression of activation markers
- Measurement of increases in the intracellular nucleotide adenosine triphosphate (*in vitro* CMI)

Advantages of the *In Vitro* Cell–Mediated Immunity Method

- Test uses small volumes (<2 mL) of whole blood.
- No purification of lymphocytes is required.
- A specific subset (e.g., CD4) can be evaluated.
- No isotope is used.
- Test time is <24 hours.

T-Cell Functional Testing

Both congenital and acquired immune deficiencies require thorough assessment of immune function. Functional lymphocyte testing (T-cell proliferation) is frequently used to assess the abnormalities associated with congenital immunodeficiency (e.g., severe combined immune deficiency) and the immunodeficiencies secondary to other medical conditions (cancer, infectious disease, stress, etc.). B-cell immunity is usually assessed by challenging with both protein and polysaccharide antigens (e.g., tetanus and pneumococcal vaccines). T-cell function is evaluated by measuring the activation and proliferation responses to mitogens and recall antigens.

Low phytohemagglutinin responses are associated with poorer clinical outcomes in patients with human immunodeficiency virus infection. Because the CD4 count and viral load may be discordant, another monitoring-type test (i.e., T-cell activation and proliferation) can often be helpful in assessing clinical status and adjusting therapy.

The *in vitro* CMI Method (Cylex, Inc., Columbia, MD) measures the early events in activation and proliferation without the requirement of long-term cell culture or the use of radioactive isotopes. Blood cells are stimulated with antigens or mitogen, then incubated at 37°; then CD4 cells are separated from the blood matrix with a monoclonal antibody–coated paramagnetic particle. After the cells are washed and lysed, the nucleotide produced during activation (adenosine triphosphate) is quantified with a luminometer. This bioluminescent detection of adenosine triphosphate provides an early indicator of lymphocyte activation.

The method commonly used to measure T-cell activation and proliferation requires specialized isotope techniques, necessitates long-term cell culture, and has been difficult to standardize.

Selected Primary Immunodeficiency Diseases

See Table 1.

X-linked Agammaglobulinemia

X-linked agammaglobulinemia (XLA) is an X-linked recessive disease that occurs in 1 in 100,000 live births. The gene has been mapped to the long arm of the X chromosome at q21.2 to q22 by linkage analysis. Female heterozygous carriers are normal. Their B cells show a nonrandom X chromosome inactivation pattern with their affected X chromosome being preferentially inactivated.

Affected XLA male infants usually are well for the first 6–12 months of life. During this period, they are protected by passively transferred maternal IgG. Clinically, they often present with recurrent pneumonia, otitis media, sinusitis, and pyoderma. These infections are mainly caused by pyogenic encapsulated bacteria and can be controlled by antibiotics. Approximately 20% of patients suffer severe diarrhea, usually caused by *Giardia*, *Campylobacter*, and, in some cases, cryptosporidia. Infections by enteroviruses, particularly echoviruses, can cause fatal encephalitis.

XLA is diagnosed by the absence of, or presence of very few, B lymphocytes in the peripheral blood. The small number of B cells found are of an immature phenotype $CD19^+$ $CD38^+$. T cells are normal, but $CD4^+$ T cells are of naïve phenotype ($CD45RA^+$). The bone marrow contains an increased number of pre–B cells. Lymph nodes from XLA patients are small, with no germinal follicles in the cortex and no

Table 1. Selected Primary Immunodeficiency Diseases

Disease	Immune Defect	Mode of Inheritance	Specific Abnormality
X-linked agammaglobulinemia	No B cells	X-linked	Defective or no Btk tyrosine kinase
Transient hypogammaglobulinemia of infancy	Defective immunoglobulin production	Unknown	Unknown
X-linked hyper-IgM syndrome	No isotype switching	X-linked	Defective CD40 ligand
Common variable immunodeficiency	Defective antibody production	Autosomal recessive, autosomal dominant, unknown	Unknown
IgA deficiency	No IgA synthesis	Autosomal recessive, autosomal dominant, unknown	Unknown; isotype switch defect?
Selective IgG subclass deficiencies	No or low synthesis of specific IgG subclasses	Unknown	Unknown; isotype switch defect?
DiGeorge syndrome	No or low T cells	Autosomal dominant, autosomal recessive, unknown	Thymic aplasia
Chronic mucocutaneous candidiasis	No T-cell response to *Candida*	Autosomal dominant, autosomal recessive, unknown	Unknown
X-linked SCID deficiency	No T and B cells	X-linked	IL-2Rγ chain
Alymphocytosis	No T and B cells	Autosomal recessive	Unknown
ADA deficiency	No T and B cells	Autosomal recessive	ADA deficiency
PNP deficiency	No T cells	Autosomal recessive	PNP deficiency
Omenn syndrome	Abnormal T and low B cells	Autosomal recessive	Autoreactive T cells
Reticular dysgenesis	No T and B cells and granulocytes	Autosomal recessive	Unknown
CD3-chain deficiencies	Defective T cells	Unknown	Defective CD3γ and ε chains
MHC class II deficiency	No CD4 T cells	Autosomal recessive	TAP mutations
Ataxia telangiectasia	Defective cellular and antibody responses	Autosomal recessive	DNA fragility
Wiskott-Aldrich syndrome	Defective polysaccharide antibody response	X-linked	Defective O-glycosylation

ADA, adenosine deaminase; Ig, immunoglobulin; IL-2R, interleukin-2 receptor; MHC, major histocompatibility class; PNP, urine nucleoside phosphorylase; SCID, severe combined immunodeficiency; TAP, transporter associated with antigen processing.
Reproduced with permission from Soldin SJ, Rifai N, Hicks JM. *Biochemical bases of pediatric diseases*, 3rd ed. Washington: American Association for Clinical Chemistry Press, 1998.

plasma cells in the medulla. The lymph nodes contain primarily T lymphocytes. Serum IgA and IgM concentrations are undetectable, and serum IgG is usually <100 mg/dL. T-cell functions such as delayed-type hypersensitivity and *in vitro* response to mitogens and specific antigens are normal.

With the identification of the Btk gene, asymptomatic female carriers can be identified using DNA-based analyses such as restriction fragment length polymorphism, polymerase chain reaction, and single-strand conformation polymorphism. XLA can be directly ascertained in patients by assaying Btk enzyme activity or identifying mutations in the Btk gene.

Transient Hypogammaglobulinemia of Infancy

Transient hypogammaglobulinemia of infancy (THI) is a disorder affecting up to 20% of infants at 5–6 months of age. Infants show a delay in their immunoglobulin production with marked decrease in serum antibody. The condition persists beyond 6 months of age, and the patient usually recovers by 1–2 years of age. Children with THI may develop respiratory tract infections and fever, which are generally not life threatening.

Laboratory findings that can distinguish THI from XLA include normal IgM concentrations, good antibody responses to immunized antigens such as tetanus and diphtheria, and a normal number of circulating B cells. The number of CD4 lymphocytes is decreased in some patients.

Hyperimmunoglobulin M Immunodeficiency Syndrome

Patients with the primary immune disorder hyper-IgM immunodeficiency syndrome usually present with recurrent bacterial infections and other opportunistic infections, most often *Pneumocystis carinii* pneumonia, in the first 2 years of life. Other clinical symptoms include recurrent neutropenia, lymphoid hyperplasia diarrhea, and, in some cases, autoimmune diseases.

There are two forms of hyper-IgM syndrome, one an inherited X-linked disorder and the other an autosomal-recessive disorder. The underlying cause of the X-linked form is deficiency of expression or function, or both, of the T-cell molecule CD40 ligand (CD40L). The interaction between CD40L and CD40 receptor on B cells induces B cells to proliferate.

Hyper-IgM syndrome is diagnosed as a finding of normal or increased serum IgM and IgD concentrations but diminished concentrations or absence of IgG, IgA, and IgE. Patients have an apparently normal number of T and B lymphocytes, but B cells express only surface IgM and IgD and no IgG^+ or IgA^+ cells. Activated T cells from patients do not bind soluble CD40 antigen or anti-CD40L antibodies as determined by flow cytometry. Surface marker analyses confirm the presence of B cells with surface IgM and IgD but not IgG or IgA. The diagnosis of hyper-IgM can now be confirmed by analysis of dinucleotide repeat polymorphism in the 3' untranslated region of the CD40L gene.

Prenatal diagnosis of X-linked hyper-IgM syndrome has been accomplished in an affected fetus at 12 weeks of gestation.

Common Variable Immunodeficiency (Acquired Hypogammaglobulinemia)

Common variable immunodeficiency is a heterogenous group of immunologic disorders with similar clinical presentation. Common variable immunodeficiency can occur in childhood but most often presents in early adult life. Patients suffer from recurrent bacterial infections and opportunistic infection such as *P. carinii* pneumonia and recurrent herpes zoster. Other clinical features are autoimmune diseases, lymphopenia, splenomegaly, lymphadenopathy, lymphoid hyperplasia in the bowel, and a high incidence of lymphoid and stomach malignancy. Multiple granulomas can be found in the spleen, abdominal lymph nodes, or lungs of some patients.

There are a normal number of B cells in the peripheral blood, but plasma cells are reduced in number in the spleen and gut, and the lymph nodes are usually small.

The serum immunoglobulin concentrations are variable. Usually, IgG is <500 mg/dL and IgA is <50 mg/dL; IgM can be normal or slightly decreased. Some patients have decreased $CD4^+$ levels with normal $CD8^+$ levels, whereas others have normal numbers of $CD4^+$ cells and increased numbers of $CD8^+$ cells.

Selective Immunoglobulin A Deficiency

IgA deficiency is the most common immunodeficiency disease. The incidence is approximately 1 in 700 in whites, but it is rare in Africans and Japanese. Patients are usually clinically asymptomatic. Approximately 20% of IgA-deficient patients have concomitant IgG subclass deficiency, especially of IgG_2. This patient subgroup is more prone to recurrent respiratory infections. Allergy and autoimmune diseases, particularly rheumatoid arthritis, are common in IgA-deficient patients. A subset of patients also suffers from celiac disease. Skin disorders include pyoderma gangrenosum, vitiligo, and trachyonychia. Patients with IgA deficiency reportedly have an increased risk of malignancies, especially gastric and colonic adenocarcinomas. Some 50–70% of patients with hereditary ataxia telangiectasia (AT) are IgA deficient. Patients with IgA deficiency make antibodies to IgA, which can result in an adverse reaction to transfusion.

Laboratory evaluation shows serum IgA concentrations of <5 mg/dL with normal concentrations of IgG and IgM. Secretions are also deficient in IgA. Patients have normal T- and B-cell phenotypes. IgA^+ B cells coexpress surface IgM and IgD, however, which suggests failure of IgA^+ B cells to mature. The disorder is possibly autosomal recessive.

Congenital infections such as rubella, cytomegalovirus infection, and toxoplasmosis, and drugs (e.g., phenytoin) can cause transient IgA deficiency.

Immunoglobulin G Subclass Deficiencies

Deficiencies of some subclasses of IgG may lead to increased respiratory tract infections. Total serum IgG concentrations may be normal or elevated. Significance of deficiencies of IgG subclass is confusing. Patients with low concentrations of IgG_2 may have associated IgA deficiency. Deficiency of antibodies to multiple antigens should be determined in patients with IgG subclass deficiencies who are symptomatic.

T-Cell Immunodeficiencies

Thymic Aplasia (DiGeorge Syndrome)

DiGeorge syndrome is characterized by hypoparathyroidism and thymic aplasia as a result of congenital malformation of the third and fourth pharyngeal pouches, which results in congenital malformations of the heart, most often interrupted aortic arch, right-sided aortic arch, truncus arteriosis, and tetralogy of Fallot. Patients can have characteristic facial features with hypertelorism, micrognathia, low-set ears, and shortened philtrum of the upper lip. The thymus shadow may be absent from chest radiograph. Affected infants are hypocalcemic. Immunologic findings are heterogenous. In most cases, there are absent or decreased numbers of circulating mature T lymphocytes, particularly in the $CD8^+$ subset. B cells are normal or increased in number, and natural killer (NK) cells are normal. Patients respond poorly to mitogen and allogeneic cell stimulation. Even though B cells can make antibodies, these antibodies are often not functional. Incidence of chronic cytomegalovirus and varicella infection is increased. Recurrent bacterial infections are unusual. Autoimmune diseases may be present.

DiGeorge syndrome usually occurs sporadically, but it may be inherited as an autosomal-dominant, autosomal-recessive, and X-linked condition. The incidence has been estimated at 1 in 20,000. Microdeletion in chromosome region 22q11 is present. Patients with velocardiofacial syndrome have phenotypic characteristics that overlap those of DiGeorge syndrome. They are differentiated with specific DNA probes using fluorescent *in situ* hybridization analysis.

Chronic Mucocutaneous Candidiasis

Chronic mucocutaneous candidiasis is characterized by recurrent *Candida* infections of the skin and superficial mucous membranes. Symptoms can occur in the first 2–3 months of life. The most common feature is oral lesions. Infections with other organisms can also be present. Recurrent upper and lower respiratory tract infections are common. Systemic candidiasis is unusual. Approximately 50% of patients have an endocrinopathy, including hypoadrenalism and hypothyroidism. Autoimmune hemolytic anemia and idiopathic thrombocytopenia occur.

Chronic mucocutaneous candidiasis with endocrinopathy appears to be transmitted in an autosomal-recessive manner, whereas those forms without endocrinopathy are inherited as a dominant trait.

The patient's T lymphocytes respond normally to mitogens and allogeneic cells. Responses to antigens other than *Candida* are also normal. Similarly, the skin test to *Candida* is negative. B-cell immunity is intact, as demonstrated by normal or increased concentrations of immunoglobulins. Increased concentrations of antibody to *Candida* are often found. Selective IgA deficiency may be present. T and B cells are normal. Addison disease is the major cause of death.

Severe Combined Immunodeficiency

Infants with severe combined immunodeficiency (SCID) have no cellular and humoral immunity. By 3 months of age, affected infants present with opportunistic infections. Other common symptoms are thrush, interstitial pneumonitis, persistent diarrhea, and failure to thrive. Affected infants are lymphopenic, with <3,000 lymphocytes/mm^3. Mature T cells (CD3$^+$) are usually absent or depressed. In some infants, T cells are of maternal origin. Patient's lymphocytes are unresponsive to stimulation by mitogens, antigens, and allogeneic cells. The thymus may be absent or, if present, not well developed. All lymphoid tissue is poorly developed.

SCID can be inherited as an X-linked or autosomal-recessive disorder. SCID can be further subdivided into X-linked SCID (XSCID), Janus kinase 3 (Jak3) deficiency, alymphocytosis of unknown origin, adenosine deaminase (ADA) deficiency, purine nucleoside phosphorylase deficiency, zeta-associated protein 70 deficiency, Omenn syndrome, reticular dysgenesis, CD3-chain deficiencies, and major histocompatibility complex (MHC) class II deficiency.

X-Linked Severe Combined Immunodeficiency

XSCID is the most frequent form of SCID, accounting for 50–60% of cases. It is characterized by absence of mature T cells but with an increased or normal number of B cells. Even though SCID patients have a normal phenotype, their B cells and NK cells exhibit functional abnormalities. Serum concentrations of IgG and IgA are low, and IgM levels can be normal or low. Obligate carriers exhibit a skewed pattern of X-chromosome inactivation only in their lymphocytes; other hematopoietic cell lineages are not affected.

The gene locus is the long arm of the X chromosome at Xq13–13.3.

Janus Kinase 3 Deficiency

Jak3 deficiency is a non–X-linked form of SCID characterized by a phenotype similar to that of XSCID; it is also known as *SCID with B cells*. Mutations of the Jak3 kinase gene have been associated with the autosomal form of SCID. The gene for Jak3 is located on chromosome band 19p13.1.

Alymphocytosis of Unknown Origin

In 20–25% of SCID patients, mature T and B lymphocytes are absent, whereas NK cells are functional and ADA activity is normal. This form of SCID is inherited as an autosomal-recessive trait.

Adenosine Deaminase Deficiency

Deficiency of the enzyme ADA accounts for 20% of SCID cases. ADA deficiency can range from complete lack of ADA activity to partial deficiency. Patients with no ADA activity have very early onset of the disease and profound T and B lymphopenia, whereas those with residual activity have later onset and mild decrease in T-cell number, with normal numbers of B-cell and humoral responses. NK cell numbers can be decreased, normal, or increased. Serum IgE level is increased. Eosinophilia is common. Autoimmune symptoms such as autoimmune hypothyroidism and insulin-dependent diabetes mellitus have been described in some patients. Patients excrete large amounts of deoxyadenosine and adenosine in their urine, and quantitation of these substances is used as a diagnostic test for ADA deficiency. Approximately 50% of patients with ADA deficiency have bone abnormalities with cupping and flaring of the costochondral junctions. Renal and adrenal lesions as well as neurologic abnormalities may also be present.

ZAP-70 Deficiency

The gene for ADA is mapped to human chromosome band 20q13.11. Untreated ADA deficiency is usually fatal.

ZAP-70 deficiency is characterized by a normal number of peripheral T cells with a deficiency of $CD8^+$ T cells and TCR signal transduction defect in peripheral $CD4^+$ cells. Although there are normal immunoglobulin levels, specific antibody formation may be impaired. $CD8^+$ cells are absent in the thymus and peripheral blood. Peripheral $CD4^+$ T cells lacking ZAP-70 fail to transmit signal from the TCR normally.

Prenatal diagnosis is possible.

Purine Nucleoside Phosphorylase Deficiency

Purine nucleoside phosphorylase deficiency accounts for approximately 4% of SCID cases and is characterized by recurrent infections, failure to thrive, autoimmune disease, neurologic impairment, and malignancies. The total white blood cell count is usually within the normal range, but the percentage of lymphocytes is very low (<10%). T-cell numbers are very low, and T-cell responses to mitogens and allogeneic cells are very poor. The skin test to *Candida* is unreactive. B-cell numbers are normal, and function can be normal or hyperactive.

The gene for purine nucleoside phosphorylase is mapped to human chromosome band 14q13.1 and is inherited in an autosomal-recessive manner.

Omenn Syndrome

Infants affected with Omenn syndrome present with erythroderma, hepatosplenomegaly, histiocytosis, hypereosinophilia, protracted diarrhea, failure to thrive, and life-threatening infections. Serum IgE level is increased, with a normal or increased number of circulating T cells but deficiency in B cells. In contrast, the lymph nodes and the thymus contain no lymphocytes. It is an autosomal-recessive trait.

Reticular Dysgenesis

Reticular dysgenesis is a form of SCID in which granulocytes are also absent. It is autosomal recessive and accounts for <1% of SCID cases. It is caused by defective production or assembly of the CD3 antigen complex. Patients with CD3γ chain defect experience fatal viral infections, probably due to impaired CD8 cell function.

Major Histocompatibility Complex Class II Deficiency and Bare Lymphocyte Syndrome

MHC class II deficiency and bare lymphocyte syndrome is an autosomal-recessive disorder in which no CD4 cells are present. The genetic defect is due to mutation in a TAP (transporter associated with antigen processing) gene. In the thymus, MHC class I molecules are involved for the proper selection of CD8 T cells. The lack of MHC class I molecules results in defective selection of CD8 T cells.

These patients have a normal number of T and B lymphocytes but abnormal cellular and humoral antigenic responses. Patients usually present with severe bacterial and viral infections, protracted diarrhea, malabsorption with osteoporosis, and failure to thrive within the first year of life. Fungal infection by *Candida* and *P. carinii* pneumonia are frequent. Autoimmune cytopenia is present in some patients. Laboratory findings by flow cytometry show surface expression of HLA class I and β_2-microglobulin on leukocytes and platelets of all patients.

Numbers of $CD4^+$ lymphocytes are decreased, and the $CD8^+$ subset is increased. Levels of other surface markers are within the normal range. The majority of patients are hypogammaglobulinemic or agammaglobulinemic. Normal immunoglobulin concentrations and increased IgM have been reported. Mapping of the gene(s) is to the short arm of chromosome 19.

Hereditary Ataxia Telangiectasia

AT is an autosomal-recessive disease. Oculocutaneous telangiectasias, progressive cerebellar ataxia, and Purkinje cell degeneration as well as recurrent respiratory infections, autoimmune disease, and malignancies (particularly T-cell leukemia) are common. In 80% of patients, IgA, IgG_2, and IgE concentrations are decreased, and cellular responses are poor. The level of α-fetoprotein is increased, and its measurement is the most useful diagnostic test for AT. A hallmark of AT is DNA fragility with abnormal chromosomal translocation in lymphocytes, mainly involving T-cell receptor and immunoglobulin gene loci. The patient's DNA is abnormally sensitive to ionizing radiation, which could be the cause of malignancies.

T cells are decreased with a decrease in the CD4/CD8 ratio, cutaneous anergy, and an increase in immature T cells. The number of B cells is usually normal; however, approximately 70% of patients have a selective IgA deficiency, and more than half also have IgG_2 subclass deficiency. NK cells are usually normal. Progressive ataxia becomes apparent when the child begins to walk. Telangiectasias develop on the bulbar conjunctivae, sun-exposed areas, and flexor surfaces of the arms at 2–8 years of age.

Wiskott-Aldrich Syndrome

Boys affected by WAS, an X-linked genetic disorder, display combined immunodeficiency, thrombocytopenia, and eczema, which lead to life-threatening infections and bleeding complications. The average life span is 11 years. The syndrome has variable expression. X-linked thrombocytopenia is a related but milder form with mostly platelet defects.

There is a family history in >60% of cases. It is an X-linked recessive trait. Rarely, girls develop WAS. Some carriers express disease; other have a different but related gene defect.

Signs and Symptoms

Neonatal
- Excessive bleeding from circumcision
- Bloody diarrhea
- Petechiae and purpura

Childhood
- Eczema with secondary skin infections
- Recurrent bacterial infections
- Viral infections
- Hepatosplenomegaly
- Autoimmune vasculitis and hemolytic anemia

Causes

Hematopoietic cells express WAS.
Defective WAS fails to organize membrane activation.
Altered motility and inability to change cell shapes inhibit normal functions.
Platelets are intrinsically abnormal with accelerated destruction and are sequestered in spleen.
T cells show decreased responsiveness to antigens.
B cells show abnormal antibody production.

Risk Factors

Family history of WAS
History of congenital defects

Laboratory Studies

Small platelet size (average diameter of 1.82 μm compared to normal diameter of 2.23 μm), but platelet counts can be variable, ranging from $<10{,}000/mm^3$ to $>100{,}000/mm^3$. Lymphopenia and eosinophilia can be found in 20–30% of patients. Serum IgA and IgE levels are increased with decreased levels of IgM and normal IgG. Patients are unable to make antibodies to polysaccharide antigens such as blood group substances or capsular polysaccharides of pneumococci and *H. influenzae*. T-cell quantitation shows a gradual decline in T-cell numbers, and CD8 cell counts are usually below normal. On scanning electron microscopy, T lymphocytes appear bald with lack of villous projections with defective expression of CD43, asialophorin (leucosialin is found on platelets and nucleated blood cells). The synthesis of CD43 is normal in WAS T cells, but it is more rapidly degraded. The gene is mapped to band Xp11.22–p11.23. Diagnosis of WAS still depends on a constellation of findings, including small platelets and altered T- or B-cell function.

Pathologic Findings

Hyperplasia of lymphoreticular system
Vasculitic changes with multiple thromboses of small arterioles of kidney, lung, pancreas, brain

X-Linked Lymphoproliferative Disease

X-linked lymphoproliferative disease is characterized by failure to control the proliferation of cytotoxic T cells that is evoked by EBV infection. Onset is usually under 15 years when, after exposure to EBV, severe mononucleosis occurs that is fatal in 80% of patients because of extensive liver necrosis caused by activated cytotoxic T cells. Most boys who survive EBV infection develop lymphomas, aplastic anemia, and hypogammaglobulinemia. The gene locus is at Xq25.

Bibliography

Buckley RH. Immunodeficiency diseases. *JAMA* 1992;268:2797–2806.

Buckley RH. Primary immunodeficiency diseases due to defects in lymphocytes. *N Engl J Med* 2001;343:1313–1324.

Demaze C, Scambler P, Prieur M, et al. Routine diagnosis of DiGeorge syndrome by fluorescent in situ hybridization. *Hum Genet* 1992;93:663–665.

Derry JM, Ochs HD, Francke U. Isolation of a novel gene mutated in Wiskott-Aldrich syndrome. *Cell* 1994;78:635–644.

DiSanto JP, Bonnefoy JY, Gauchat JF, et al. CD40 ligand mutations in X-linked immunodeficiency with hyper-IgM. *Nature* 1993;361:541–543.

DiSanto JP, Markiewicz S, Gauchat JF, et al. Brief report: prenatal diagnosis of X-linked hyper-IgM syndrome. *N Engl J Med* 1994;330:969–973.

Gilbert-Barness E, Good R, Pollaro B. Immunodeficiency diseases. In: Gilbert-Barness E, ed. *Potter's atlas of fetal and infant pathology.* St. Louis, MO: Mosby, 1998.

Good R, Anderson V. Immunodeficiency diseases. In: Gilbert-Barness E, ed. *Potter's pathology of the fetus and infant*. St. Louis, MO: Mosby, 1997.

Hirschhorn R. Overview of biochemical abnormalities and molecular genetics of adenosine deaminase deficiency. *Pediatr Res* 1993;33:535–541.

Kapp LN, Painer RB, Yu LC, et al. Cloning of a candidate gene for ataxia telangiectasia group. *Am J Hum Genet* 1992;51:45–54.

Leonard WJ, Noguchi M, Russell SM, et al. The molecular basis of X-linked severe combined immunodeficiency: the role of the interleukin-2 receptor γ chain as a common γ chain, γ_e. *Immunol Rev* 1994;138:61–86.

Rawlings DJ, Witte ON. Bruton's tyrosine kinase is key regulator in B cell development. *Immunol Rev* 1994;138:105–119.

Rischer A, Cavazzana-Calvo M, De Saint Vasille G, et al. Naturally occurring primary deficiencies of the immune system. *Annu Rev Immunol* 1997;15:93–124.

Shyur SD, Hill HR. Recent advances in the genetics of primary immunodeficiency syndrome. *J Pediatr* 1996;129:8–24.

Smart BA, Ochs HD. The molecular basis and treatment of primary immunodeficiency disorders. *Curr Opin Pediatr* 1997;9:570–556.

Soldin SJ, Rifai N, Hicks JM. *Biochemical basis of pediatric disease*, 3rd ed. Washington: American Association for Clinical Chemistry Press, 1998.

Thomas JD, Sideras P, Smith CIE, et al. Colocalization of X-linked agammaglobulinemia and X-linked immunodeficiency genes. *Science* 1993;261:355–358.

Tsukada S, Rawlings DJ, Witte ON. Role of Burton's tyrosine kinase in immunodeficiency. *Curr Opin Immunol* 1994;6:623–630.

Tsukada S, Saffron DC, Rawlings DJ, et al. Deficient expression of a B cell cytoplasmic tyrosine kinase in human X-linked agammaglobulinemia. *Cell* 1993;72:279–290.

Vetrie D, Vorechovsky I, Sidreas P, et al. The gene involved in X-linked agammaglobulinemia is a member of the Src family of protein-tyrosine kinases. *Nature* 1993;361: 226–233.

Wallach J. *Interpretation of diagnostic tests*, 7th ed. Philadelphia: Lippincott Williams & Wilkins, 2000.

7 Cardiovascular Diseases

Heart Rate

Pulse Rates at Rest[1]

Age	Lower Limits of Normal (beats/min)		Average (beats/min)		Upper Limits of Normal (beats/min)	
Newborn	70		125		190	
1–11 mo	80		120		160	
2 yr	80		110		130	
4 yr	80		100		120	
6 yr	75		100		115	
8 yr	70		90		110	
10 yr	70		90		110	
	Girls	**Boys**	**Girls**	**Boys**	**Girls**	**Boys**
12 yr	70	65	90	85	110	105
14 yr	65	60	85	80	105	100
16 yr	60	55	80	75	100	95
18 yr	55	50	75	70	95	90

Causes of Rapid Heart Rates

Regular supraventricular tachycardias (SVTs)	Sinus tachycardia Reentrant SVT Atrial flutter Junctional ectopic tachycardia
Irregular SVTs	Multifocal atrial tachycardia Sinus tachycardia with premature atrial contractions Sinus tachycardia with premature ventricular contractions Atrial flutter with variable blockage
Ventricular tachycardia	Atrial fibrillation

Blood Pressure

Normal Blood Pressure

See Fig. 1.

[1]Behram RE, Kleigman RM, Arvin AM. *Nelson textbook of pediatrics*, 14th ed. Philadelphia: WB Saunders, 1996.

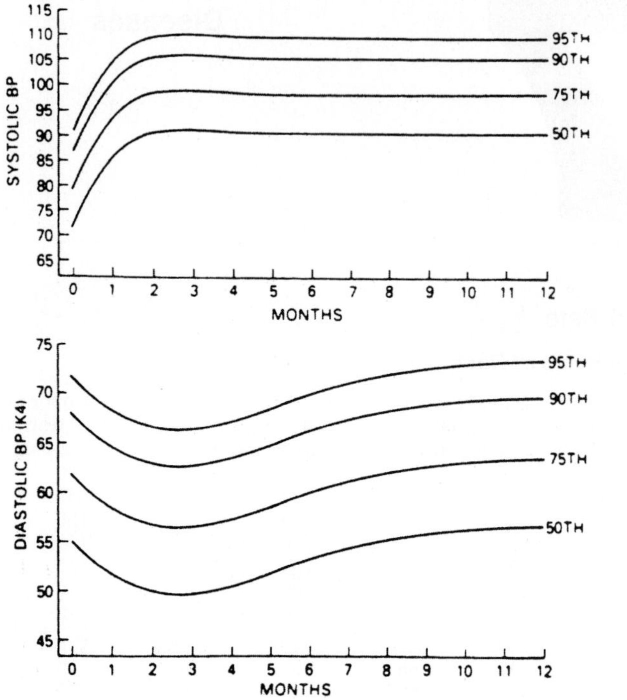

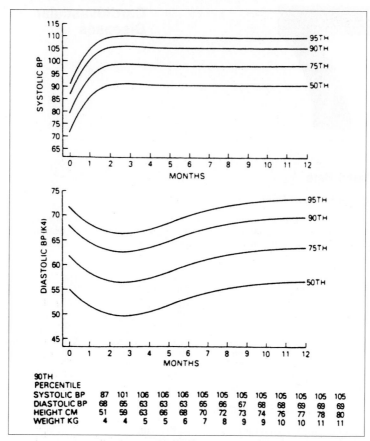

90TH PERCENTILE													
SYSTOLIC BP	87	101	106	106	106	105	105	105	105	105	105	105	105
DIASTOLIC BP	68	65	63	63	63	65	66	67	68	68	69	69	69
HEIGHT CM	51	59	63	66	68	70	72	73	74	76	77	78	80
WEIGHT KG	4	4	5	5	6	7	8	9	9	10	10	11	11

Fig. 1. Blood pressure (BP) nomogram. Age-specific percentiles of BP measurements in boys from birth to 12 months of age. Korotkoff phase IV (K4) used for diastolic BP. (From Report of the second task force on blood pressure control in children: 1987. Task force on blood pressure control in children. National Heart, Lung, and Blood Institute, Bethesda, MD. *Pediatrics* 1987;79:1.)

Etiology and Classification of Hypertension

Essential (primary) hypertension
Secondary hypertension
- Renal diseases
  - Renal vascular diseases
  - Renal artery stenosis (atherosclerosis, fibromuscular hyperplasia, posttransplantation)
  - Arteritis, polyarteritis nodosa
  - Renal artery embolism
- Renal parenchymal diseases
  - Acute glomerulonephritis
  - Chronic glomerulonephritis
  - Chronic pyelonephritis
  - Polycystic disease of the kidney
- Renal neoplasms
  - Juxtaglomerular apparatus neoplasm
  - Renal carcinoma
  - Wilms tumor

- Endocrine diseases
  - Pheochromocytoma
  - Primary aldosteronism (Conn syndrome)
  - Cushing syndrome
  - Congenital adrenal hyperplasia due to 11-hydroxylase deficiency
- Coarctation of the aorta
- Drug-induced hypertension
  - Corticosteroid use
  - Amphetamine use
  - Long-term licorice ingestion*
  - Oral contraceptive use
- Neurologic diseases
  - Raised intracranial pressure
- Hypercalcemia

Malignant (accelerated) hypertension

- Rarely seen in children.
- Characterized by very severe hypertension (diastolic pressure >110 mm Hg).
- Affected vessels show fibrinoid necrosis of the media with marked intimal fibrosis and extreme narrowing.
- Tissues supplied by affected vessels show acute ischemia with microinfarcts and hemorrhage.
- Frequently associated with elevated serum renin levels.
- Clinical features:
  - Early hypertension is asymptomatic, and the diagnosis can be made only by detecting the elevation of blood pressure.
  - Hypertensive heart disease is characterized by left ventricular hypertrophy.

*Licorice has an aldosterone-like effect ("pseudoaldosteronism").

Cyanosis

See Fig. 2.

Cyanosis in the Older Child

Cyanosis in the older child is most often due to lung disease, such as pneumonia, reactive airway disease, or cystic fibrosis. A neurologic cause may result in hypoventilation and secondary cyanosis.

Differential Diagnosis of Neonatal Cyanosis

Disease	Mechanism
Pulmonary	
Respiratory distress syndrome	Surfactant deficiency
Sepsis, pneumonia	Inflammation, pulmonary hypertension, shunting R→L
Meconium aspiration pneumonia	Mechanical obstruction, inflammation, pulmonary hypertension, shunting R→L
Persistent fetal circulation	Pulmonary hypertension, shunting R→L
Diaphragmatic hernia	Pulmonary hypoplasia, pulmonary hypertension
Transient tachypnea	Retained lung fluid
Cardiovascular	
Cyanotic heart disease with decreased pulmonary blood flow	R→L shunt as in pulmonary atresia, tetralogy of Fallot
Cyanotic heart disease with increased pulmonary blood flow	R→L shunt as in D-transposition, truncus arteriosus
Cyanotic heart disease with congestive heart failure	R→L shunt with pulmonary edema and poor cardiac output, as in sepsis, myocarditis, supraventricular tachycardia, or complete heart block; high-output failure, as in patent ductus arteriosus, vein of Galen, or other arteriovenous malformation

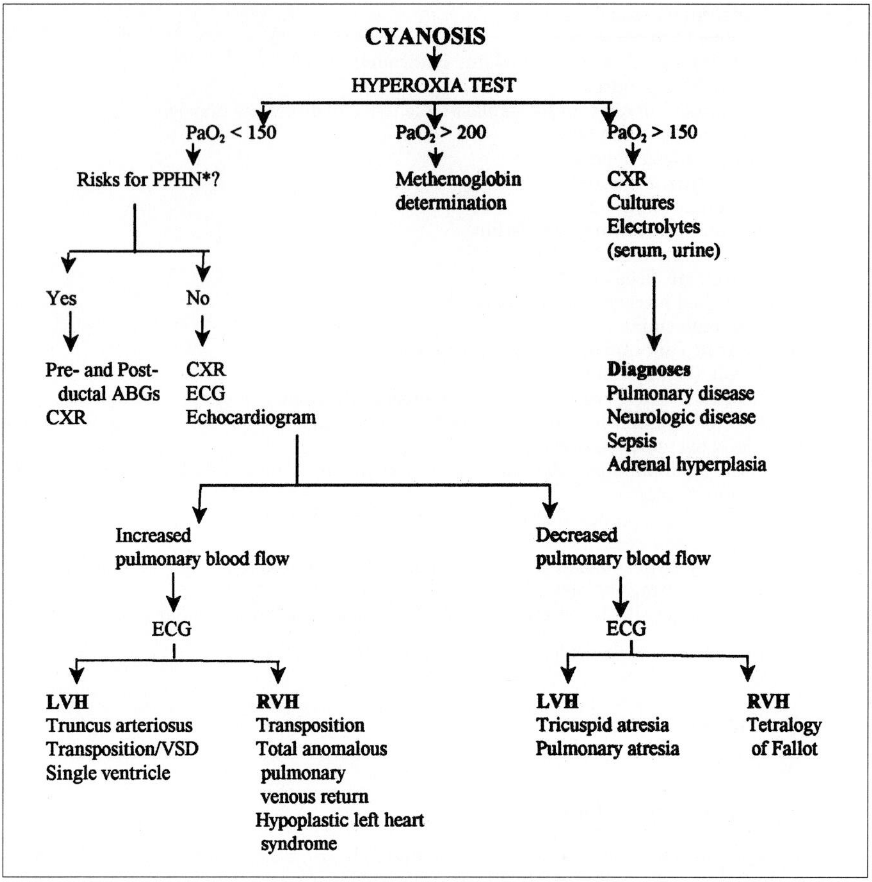

Fig. 2. Evaluation of cyanosis. *Persistent pulmonary hypertension (also known as *persistent fetal circulation*). ABG, arterial blood gases; CXR, chest radiograph; ECG, electrocardiography; LVH, left ventricular hypertrophy; RVH, right ventricular hypertrophy; VSD, ventricular septal defect.

Congenital Heart Disease

Classification and Frequency

Without shunt (20%)	
Right-sided	
Pulmonary stenosis	10%
Ebstein anomaly	Rare
Left-sided	
Coarctation of the aorta	10%
Aortic stenosis	Rare
Dextrocardia	Rare
With shunt (80%)	
Acyanotic	
Atrial septal defect	15%
Ventricular septal defect	25%
Patent ductus arteriosus	15%
Cyanotic	
Tetralogy of Fallot	10%

Transposition of great vessels	10%
Truncus arteriosus	Rare
Tricuspid atresia	Rare
Total anomalous pulmonary venous return	Rare
Hypoplastic left heart syndrome	Rare
Eisenmenger syndrome*	Rare

*The term *Eisenmenger syndrome* is applied to the development of pulmonary hypertension and reversal of shunt direction in patients with atrial septal defect, ventricular septal defect, and patent ductus arteriosus. Surgery to close the defect in the presence of this degree of pulmonary hypertension has a high mortality rate.

Thromboembolic Complications

General Information

Congenital heart disease (CHD) of a wide spectrum of severity affects approximately 1% of all live-born infants. The majority of congenital cardiac structural abnormalities occur in otherwise healthy children, and total correction of the cardiac lesion usually results in a normal, productive life span. One of the most frequent complications seen in survivors of CHD is thromboemboli, which include venous thrombus emboli (VTE), pulmonary emboli, and embolism to the central nervous system. Many thromboemboli related to CHD occur secondary to right-to-left intracardiac shunts or on the arterial side of the circulation.

Venous Thromboembolic Disease

The Canadian Childhood Thrombophilia Registry has provided the largest prospective database defining the epidemiology of VTE in children, with a mean follow-up of 2.36 years. CHD was the underlying disease process in 75 of 405 children (19%) reported with VTE and had an associated mortality of 7%. Morbidity in the form of postphlebitic syndrome and recurrent VTE occurred in 23% of children.

Childhood Stroke

The Canadian Childhood Stroke Registry identified CHD as the single most common identifiable cause of arterial ischemic stroke (AIS) in a prospectively and consecutively selected cohort of 165 children with AIS. Thirty-six percent of children with AIS had underlying CHD. In the entire stroke registry cohort, only 22% of children fully recovered, whereas two-thirds had residual neurologic defects or seizures. The contribution of CHD to AIS in children is important, because this is a cause that can likely be prevented in many children by the use of anticoagulants.

Right Atrial Thrombosis

The presence of a right atrial thrombosis is frequently clinically "asymptomatic" and is identified on routine echocardiogram in children with CHD or children receiving cardiotoxic agents for the treatment of their primary disease (e.g., acute lymphoblastic leukemia). Right atrial thrombosis also seems to occur more frequently in neonates with central venous lines. Clinically overt symptoms of right atrial thrombosis include cardiac failure, central venous line malfunction, persistent sepsis, and appearance of a new cardiac murmur. Optimal approaches to right atrial thrombosis are uncertain at this time and will likely differ, depending on the patient population.

Cardiac Arrhythmias

Classification

Altered activity of the sinoatrial node
Sinus tachycardia
Sinus bradycardia
Sinus arrhythmia
Ectopic rhythms
Supraventricular (atrial or atrioventricular nodal) arrhythmia
Supraventricular extrasystoles
Paroxysmal supraventricular tachycardia
Atrial flutter
Atrial fibrillation

Ventricular arrhythmia
Ventricular extrasystoles
Ventricular tachycardia
Ventricular fibrillation
Heart block
Sinoatrial block (partial or complete)
Atrioventricular block (partial or complete)
Bundle-branch block

Long QT Syndrome

Congenital Causes[2]

Autosomal Dominant (Romano-Ward Syndrome)

Isolated susceptibility to ventricular arrhythmias, normal hearing

- LQT1 (30–50%)—chromosome band 11p15.5, KVLQT1, potassium channel (I_{KS})
- LQT2 (20–30%)—chromosome band 7q35–36, HERG, potassium channel (I_{Kr})
- LQT3 (5–10%)—chromosome band 3p21–24, SCN5A, sodium channel (I_{Na})
- LQT4 (?%)—chromosome band 4q25–27, gene?
- LQT5 (?%)—chromosome band 21q22.1–22.2, KCNE1, β-subunit (minK) of potassium channel (I_{Kr} and I_{Ks})
- LTQ6 (?%)—chromosome?

Autosomal Recessive (Jervell and Lange-Nielsen Syndrome)

Associated with sensorineural hearing loss

- JLN1—chromosome band 11p15.5, KVLQT1
- JLN2—chromosome band 21q22.1–22.2, KCME1 (minK)

Acquired Causes of Long QT Syndrome[3]

Drugs

- Antianginals
- Antiarrhythmics
- Class IA drugs: disopyramide phosphate, procainamide hydrochloride, quinidine
- Class III drugs: amiodarone hydrochloride (rare), bretylium tosylate, dofetilide, *N*-acetylprocainamide, sotalol hydrochloride
- Antibiotics (erythromycin, pentamidine isethionate, trimethoprim-sulfamethoxazole)
- Antidepressants (tricyclics such as amitriptyline hydrochloride and desipramine hydrochloride)
- Antihistamines [astemizole, terfenadine (removed from the market for this reason)]
- Antipsychotics (haloperidol, risperidone, phenothiazines such as thioridazine hydrochloride)
- Lipid-lowering agents (probucol)
- Oral hypoglycemics (glibenclamide, glyburide)
- Organophosphate insecticides
- Promotility agents (cisapride)

Electrolyte Disturbances

- Acute hypokalemia (associated with diuretic use and hyperventilation)
- Chronic hypocalcemia
- Chronic hypokalemia
- Chronic hypomagnesemia

Underlying Medical Conditions

- Arrhythmic (complete atrioventricular block, severe bradycardia, sick sinus syndrome)
- Cardiac (anthracycline cardiotoxicity, congestive heart failure, myocarditis, tumors)
- Endocrine (hyperparathyroidism, hypothyroidism, pheochromocytoma)
- Neurologic (encephalitis, head trauma, stroke, subarachnoid hemorrhage)
- Nutritional (alcoholism, anorexia nervosa, liquid protein diet, starvation)

[2]Gilbert-Barness E, Barness L. *Metabolic diseases: foundations of clinical management, genetics and pathology.* Natick, MA: Eaton Publishing, 2000:715.
[3]Gilbert-Barness E, Barness L. *Metabolic diseases: foundations of clinical management, genetics and pathology.* Natick, MA: Eaton Publishing, 2000:714.

Heart Failure: Causes

Primary left-sided
- Hypertensive heart disease
- Aortic valve disease (stenosis, incompetence)
- Mitral valve disease (stenosis,* incompetence)
- Myocarditis
- Cardiomyopathy
- High-output states (thyrotoxicosis, anemia, arteriovenous fistula)

Primary right-sided
- Left-sided heart failure†
- Chronic pulmonary disease (cor pulmonale)
- Pulmonary valve stenosis
- Tricuspid valve disease (stenosis, incompetence)
- Congenital heart disease (ventricular septal defect, patent ductus arteriosus)
- Pulmonary hypertension (primary and secondary)
- Massive pulmonary embolism

*Mitral stenosis produces functional failure on the left side of the heart; although the left ventricle itself is not in failure, the left atrium is.
†Left heart failure is the most common cause of right heart failure because of back-pressure effects via the pulmonary circulation.

Acquired Pediatric Heart Disease

The major forms of acquired heart disease in the pediatric population include Kawasaki syndrome, rheumatic fever, infective endocarditis, cardiomyopathies, myocardial ischemia and infarction, arrhythmias, lipid disorders, and systemic arterial hypertension.

Kawasaki Syndrome

Kawasaki syndrome, a leading cause of acquired heart disease in children, is a disease of unknown etiology marked by acute vasculitis. The syndrome occurs predominantly in infancy and early childhood and is characterized by fever, bilateral nonexudative conjunctivitis, erythema of the lips and oral mucosa, changes in the extremities, rash, and cervical lymphadenopathy. Coronary artery aneurysms or ectasia develop in 15–25% of children with the disease and may lead to myocardial infarction, sudden death, or chronic coronary artery insufficiency.

The cause of Kawasaki syndrome is unknown. Antecedent viral infection of the upper respiratory tract and exposure to freshly cleaned carpets have been associated with the disease. Immunoregulatory abnormalities may contribute to the pathogenesis of Kawasaki syndrome.

During the acute phase, there is a marked deficiency of suppressor T cells, helper T cells become activated, and there are increased numbers of B cells spontaneously secreting immunoglobulin G (IgG) and immunoglobulin M (IgM) antibodies. This high level of immune activation may be associated with endothelial damage. IgM antibodies in the sera of children with acute Kawasaki syndrome cause complement-mediated killing of interferon-γ–treated, cultured, human vascular endothelial cells. In addition, IgG and IgM antibodies in sera from patients with acute disease have been reported to cause lysis of cultured human vascular endothelial cells stimulated with interleukin-1 or tumor necrosis factor. These observations suggest that mediator secretion by activated T cells and macrophages could promote vascular injury in Kawasaki syndrome.

By definition of the Centers for Disease Control and Prevention, the child with Kawasaki syndrome must have fever lasting ≥5 days without other reasonable explanation and satisfy at least four of the following five criteria:

1. Bilateral conjunctival injection (associated with anterior uveitis)
2. At least one of the following mucous membrane changes: injected or fissured lips, injected pharynx, or strawberry tongue

3. At least one of the following extremity changes: erythema of the palms and soles, edema of the hands or feet, or periungual desquamation
4. Polymorphous exanthem that is rarely vesicular or bullous and is often accentuated in the perineum, where it may be associated with local desquamation
5. Acute nonsuppurative cervical lymphadenopathy (at least one node ≥1.5 cm in diameter)

In addition to these principle signs, many other significant symptoms and signs frequently are present in children with Kawasaki syndrome, including arthralgia and arthritis, urethritis associated with sterile pyuria (mononuclear white cells rather than polymorphonuclear cells), aseptic meningitis associated with a mild mononuclear cerebrospinal fluid pleocytosis with normal glucose and protein, hydrops of the gallbladder with or without obstructive jaundice, diarrhea, vomiting, and abdominal pain. Cardiovascular manifestations during the acute phase include tachycardia, gallop rhythm, pericardial effusion, and congestive heart failure due to a myopericarditis. Transient mitral and aortic regurgitation also can be seen. During the subacute phase, congestive heart failure may result from myocardial dysfunction secondary to ischemia or infarction, with or without valvular regurgitation. Clinical symptoms and signs of Kawasaki syndrome may be particularly subtle or absent in infants <6 months of age—the subgroup at highest risk for coronary lesions.

Coronary artery ectasia or aneurysms occur in 15–25% of children with Kawasaki syndrome. Risk factors for formation of coronary artery abnormalities include male gender, age <1 year, hemoglobin <10 g/dL, a white cell count >30,000/mm^3, an erythrocyte sedimentation rate >101 mm/hour (Westergren), increased C-reactive protein level, and persistence of elevation of C-reactive protein or sedimentation rate for >30 days. The coronary artery dilatation usually peaks 3–4 weeks after onset of the illness. Partial or total regression of aneurysms may occur but sometimes may progress to the development of stenosis or occlusions.

Laboratory findings in the acute stage of Kawasaki syndrome include

1. Abdominal pain is common. It may be severe.
2. Epistaxis (historically important, but rarely seen in acute rheumatic fever).
3. Facial tics.

Causes

- Autoimmune mechanisms.
- A preceding upper respiratory tract infection with group A *Streptococcus* is a prerequisite.

Laboratory Findings

- Increase in acute-phase reactants, including sedimentation rate and level of C-reactive protein
- Bacteriologic or serologic evidence of group A streptococcal infection, antistreptolysin-O, streptozyme, or anti–deoxyribonuclease B
- Anemia

Pathologic Findings

- Subcutaneous nodules of a characteristic histologic appearance with central fibrinoid necrosis and palisading of epithelioid cells
- Pericardial effusion
- Fibrinous pericardium

Imaging Studies

- Chest radiograph
- Echocardiogram (reveals pericardial effusion and documents valvular disease)

Diagnostic Procedures

- Throat cultures for β-hemolytic streptococci.
- Diagnosis is dependent on fulfilling the modified Jones criteria of two major manifestations or one major and two minor manifestations. In either case, there must be evidence of preceding group A streptococcal infection.

Jones Criteria (Revised) for Guidance in the Diagnosis of Rheumatic Fever

Major Manifestations	Minor Manifestations
Carditis	*Clinical*
Polyarthritis	Previous rheumatic fever or rheumatic heart disease
Chorea	Arthralgia

Erythema marginatum
Subcutaneous nodules

Fever
Laboratory
Acute-phase reactions
Prolonged erythrocyte sedimentation rate, increased level of C-reactive protein, leukocytosis
Prolonged P-R interval on electrocardiogram

Plus: Supporting evidence of preceding streptococcal infections (increased levels of antistreptolysin-O or other streptococcal antibodies; positive throat culture results for group A *Streptococcus*; recent scarlet fever. The presence of two major criteria, or of one major and two minor criteria, indicates a high probability of rheumatic fever and is supported by evidence of a preceding streptococcal infection. The absence of the latter should make the diagnosis doubtful, except in situations in which rheumatic fever is first discovered after a long latent period from the antecedent infection (e.g., Sydenham chorea or low-grade carditis).

The revised Jones criteria provide guidance for the diagnosis of rheumatic fever. Laboratory data support but do not confirm the diagnosis of rheumatic fever. A throat culture from an untreated patient often grows hemolytic streptococci. The antistreptolysin-O titer is increased and may continue to rise, sometimes to remarkably high levels. Levels of other streptococcal antibodies may be increased. The erythrocyte sedimentation rate and C-reactive protein levels are almost invariably increased. The sedimentation rate may be normal in an affected child with severe liver congestion, but this is rarely seen in practice. The sedimentation rate must be corrected for anemia, because anemia is common in these patients.

Infective Endocarditis

The characteristic lesion of infective endocarditis, a vegetation, is composed of a collection of platelets, fibrin, microorganisms, and inflammatory cells. It most commonly involves heart valves but may also occur at the site of a septal defect, on the chordae tendineae, or on the mural endocardium.

Other conditions associated with an increased incidence of infective endocarditis include poor dental hygiene, long-term hemodialysis, and diabetes mellitus. Infection with the human immunodeficiency virus (HIV) may independently increase the risk of infective endocarditis. Among HIV-infected patients, however, infective endocarditis is usually associated with injection drug use or long-term use of indwelling intravenous catheters. *Staphylococcus aureus* is the most frequent pathogen in these patients, and mortality is higher among those with advanced HIV disease.

Mitral valve prolapse is now the most common cardiovascular diagnosis predisposing patients to infective endocarditis.

Diagnosis of infective endocarditis requires that one of the following three criteria be met:

1. Pathologic evidence of endocarditis (e.g., at cardiac surgery)
2. Results of at least two sets of blood cultures obtained by separate venipunctures positive for the same organism with no source of bacteremia other than the heart
3. A clinical course compatible with infective endocarditis

Symptoms may include fever, anorexia, weight loss, pallor, night sweats, malaise, arthralgias, and myalgias. Changing murmurs and development of congestive heart failure result from infection and consequent destruction of intracardiac structures. Physical signs attributable to embolic or immunologic phenomena include splinter hemorrhages, Janeway lesions, Osler nodes, splenomegaly, clubbing, arthritis, glomerulonephritis, and aseptic meningitis. There may be neurologic complications, including emboli, hemorrhage, meningitis, toxic encephalopathy, and headache. Arterial embolization may affect the lungs, kidneys, spleen, brain, and large vessels.

In the pathogenesis of infective endocarditis, local turbulence is believed to promote the formation of a network of fibrin and platelets on the endocardial surface, which is colonized later by microorganisms entering the bloodstream from a distant site.

Streptococcus viridans is the most common causative organism of infective endocarditis in children and adults. One species of community-acquired coagulase-negative

Staphylococcus, *S. lugdunensis*, is commonly associated with valve destruction and the requirement for valve replacement. Among patients without preexisting heart disease, *S. aureus* in the most common causative organism and also is the most common causative organism in endocarditis associated with intravenous injection of drugs in addicts, which typically involves the right side of the heart, and in neonates. Gram-negative organism and fungal endocarditis occur most often after cardiac surgery or in debilitated patients. Blood culture results are negative in 10–15% of cases of infective endocarditis.

Microbiologic Features of Native-Valve and Prosthetic-Valve Endocarditis

Pathogen	Neonates (%)	2 Mo to 15 Yr (%)
Streptococcus species	15–20	40–50
S. aureus	40–50	22–27
Coagulase-negative staphylococci	8–12	4–7
Enterococcus species	<1	3–6
Gram-negative bacilli	8–12	4–6
Fungi	8–12	1–3
Culture-negative and HACEK organisms*	2–6	0–15
Diphtheroids	<1	<1
Polymicrobial	3–5	<1

*Patients whose blood cultures were rendered negative by prior antibiotic treatment are excluded. HACEK denotes *Haemophilus* species (*Haemophilus parainfluenzae*, *H. aphrophilus*, and *H. paraphrophilus*), *Actinobacillus actinomycetemcomitans*, *Cardiobacterium hominis*, *Eikenella corrodens*, and *Kingella kingae*.

In addition to positive blood culture results, abnormal laboratory findings in infective endocarditis often include anemia, leukocytosis, increased erythrocyte sedimentation rate and C-reactive protein level, hematuria, diminished level of complement component 3, and mildly increased bilirubin level. Echocardiography may demonstrate vegetations and myocardial abscesses.

Polymerase chain reaction can be used to identify unculturable organisms in excised vegetations or systemic emboli. This approach has been used to diagnose infective endocarditis due to *Tropheryma whipplei* and *Bartonella* species and is a promising tool for establishing a microbiologic diagnosis in selected patients with blood culture–negative infective endocarditis.

When blood cultures from patients with suspected infective endocarditis remain sterile after 48–72 hours of incubation, the clinician must advise the laboratory of the suspected diagnosis. This allows the laboratory, if the blood cultures remain negative after 5–7 days, to intensify efforts to recover fastidious organisms and initiate serologic assessment of causation. These efforts could include prolonged incubation and the plating of subcultures on more enriched media. Use of the lysis centrifugation system for blood cultures allows direct plating to special supportive media, with the potential to increase the speed of recovery of more fastidious organisms. When blood cultures from patients with clinical symptoms of infective endocarditis are sterile after 48–72 hours of incubation, prolonged incubation and plating of subcultures on enriched media should be done.

See Table 1 for laboratory diagnosis of common causes of culture-negative endocarditis.

See Table 2 for modified Duke criteria for the diagnosis of infective endocarditis.

Diagnosis

The diagnosis of infective endocarditis requires the integration of clinical, laboratory, and echocardiographic data. Nonspecific laboratory abnormalities may be present, including anemia, leukocytosis, abnormal urinalysis results, and an elevated erythrocyte sedimentation rate and C-reactive protein level.

Patients with suspected infective endocarditis should have electrocardiography performed on admission (and repeated during their course as appropriate). New atrioventricular, fascicular, or bundle-branch block, particularly in the setting of aortic valve endocarditis, suggests perivalvular invasion, and such patients may need cardiac monitoring until they are stable. New atrioventricular block carries a moder-

Table 1. Laboratory Diagnosis of Common Causes of Culture-Negative Endocarditis

Organism	Approach
Abiotrophia species (previously classified as nutritionally variant streptococci)	Grow in thioglycolate medium of blood culture and as satellite colonies around *Staphylococcus aureus* on blood agar or on medium supplemented with pyridoxal hydrochloride or L-cysteine.
Bartonella species (usually *B. henselae* or *B. quintana*)	Serologic tests. Lysis-centrifugation system for blood cultures. PCR of valve or embolized vegetations; special culture techniques available, but organisms are slow growing and may require a month or more for isolation.
Coxiella burnetii (Q fever)	Serologic tests. PCR, Giemsa stain, or immunohistologic techniques on operative specimens.
HACEK organisms	Blood cultures positive by day 7; occasionally require prolonged incubation and subculturing.
Chlamydia species (usually *C. psittaci*)	Culture from blood has been described. Serologic tests. Direct staining of tissue with use of fluorescent monoclonal antibody.
Tropheryma whipplei	Histologic examination (silver and PAS stains) of excised heart valve. PCR or culture of vegetation.
Legionella species	Subculture from blood cultures, lysis-centrifugation pellet from blood cultures, or operative specimens on BCYE agar; direct detection on heart valves with fluorescent antibody. Serologic tests.
Brucella species (usually *B. melitensis* or *B. abortus*)	Prolonged incubation of standard or lysis-centrifugation blood cultures.
Fungi	Regular blood cultures often positive for *Candida* species; lysis-centrifugation system with specific fungal medium can increase yield. Testing urine for *Histoplasma capsulatum* antigen or serum for *Cryptococcus neoformans* polysaccharide capsular antigen can be helpful. Accessible lesions (such as emboli) should be cultured and examined histologically for fungi.

BCYE, buffered charcoal yeast extract; HACEK, *Haemophilus* species (*H. parainfluenzae*, *H. aphrophilus*, and *H. paraphrophilus*), *Actinobacillus actinomycetemcomitans*, *Cardiobacterium hominis*, *Eikenella corrodens*, and *Kingella kingae*; PAS, periodic acid–Schiff; PCR, polymerase chain reaction.

ately high positive predictive value for the formation of a myocardial abscess, but the sensitivity is low.

Pathogenesis

Bacteremia (or fungemia) is the first requirement for the onset of infective encarditis and commonly occurs in the following circumstances:

- After oral surgical procedures, including dentistry (usually *S. viridans*)
- After urologic procedures such as bladder catheterization (commonly *Streptococcus faecalis* and Gram-negative enteric bacilli)
- During long-term hemodialysis
- In patients with diabetes mellitus
- In intravenous drug abusers (commonly *S. aureus*) with right heart lesions

Table 2. Modified Duke Criteria for the Diagnosis of Infective Endocarditis

Criteria	Comments
Major criteria	
Microbiologic	
Typical microorganism isolated from two separate blood cultures; *viridans* streptococci, *Streptococcus bovis*, HACEK group, *Staphylococcus aureus*, or community-acquired enterococcal bacteremia without a primary focus	In patients with possible infective endocarditis, at least two sets of cultures of blood collected by separated venipunctures should be obtained within the first 1–2 hr of presentation. Patients with cardiovascular collapse should have three cultures of blood obtained at 5- to 10-min intervals and thereafter receive empiric antibiotic therapy.
or	
Microorganism consistent with infective endocarditis isolated from persistently positive blood cultures	
or	
Single positive blood culture for *Coxiella burnetii* or phase I immunoglobulin G antibody titer to *C. burnetii* >1:800	*C. burnetii* is not readily cultivated in most clinical microbiology laboratories.
Evidence of endocardial involvement	
New valvular regurgitation (increase or change in preexisting murmur not sufficient)	
or	
Positive echocardiogram (transesophageal echocardiogram recommended in patients who have a prosthetic valve, who are rated as having at least possible infective endocarditis by clinical criteria, or who have complicated infective endocarditis)	Three echocardiographic findings qualify as major criteria: a discrete, echogenic, oscillating intracardiac mass located at a site of endocardial injury; a periannular abscess; and a new dehiscence of a prosthetic valve.
Minor criteria	
Predisposition to infective endocarditis that includes certain cardiac conditions and injection-drug use	Cardiac abnormalities that are associated with infective endocarditis are classified into three groups: High-risk conditions: previous infective endocarditis, aortic valve disease, rheumatic heart disease, prosthetic heart valve, coarctation of the aorta, and complex cyanotic congenital heart disease. Moderate-risk conditions: mitral valve prolapse with valvular regurgitation or leaflet thickening, isolated mitral stenosis, tricuspid valve disease, pulmonary stenosis, and hypertrophic cardiomyopathy. Low- or no-risk conditions: secundum atrial septal defect, ischemic heart disease, previous coronary artery bypass graft surgery, and mitral valve prolapse with thin leaflets in the absence of regurgitation.
Fever	Temperature >38.0°C (>100.4°F).
Vascular phenomena	Petechiae and splinter hemorrhages are excluded. None of the peripheral lesions is pathognomonic for infective endocarditis.

(continued)

Table 2. (continued)

Criteria	Comments
Immunologic phenomena	Presence of rheumatoid factor, glomerulonephritis, Osler nodes, or Roth spots.
Microbiologic findings	Positive blood cultures that do not meet the major criteria.
	Serologic evidence of active infection; single isolates of coagulase-negative staphylococci and organisms that very rarely cause infective endocarditis are excluded from this category.

HACEK, *Haemophilus* species (*H. parainfluenzae*, *H. aphrophilus*, and *H. paraphrophilus*), *Actinobacillus actinomycetemcomitans*, *Cardiobacterium hominis*, *Eikenella corrodens*, and *Kingella kingae*.
Cases are defined clinically as "definite" if they fulfill two major criteria, one major criterion plus three minor criteria, or five minor criteria; they are defined as "possible" if they fulfill one major and one minor criterion, or three minor criteria.

Endocardial injury is necessary for infection by less virulent organisms, which can only infect previously abnormal endocardium. Precursor diseases are the following:

- Chronic rheumatic heart disease, most commonly mitral incompetence and aortic valve disease. Most cases of subacute endocarditis occur in patients with chronic rheumatic heart disease.
- Congenital heart disease, most often a small ventricular septal or bicuspid aortic valve.
- Degenerative valvular disease, such as calcific valves and mitral valve prolapse syndrome, is rarely complicated by infective endocarditis.
- Prosthetic cardiac valves frequently become infected. *Candida albicans* and staphylococci are common causes of prosthetic valve endocarditis.
- Mitral valve prolapse is now the most common cardiovascular diagnosis predisposing to infective endocarditis.

Pathology

Infected thrombi (vegetations) on the endocardial surface, often on valves, are the characteristic findings in infective endocarditis.

- Vegetations of infective endocarditis are multiple, large, friable, and loosely attached. They commonly become detached from the valve as emboli.

Metabolic Cardiomyopathies[4]

Disorders of Amino Acid Metabolism

Alkaptonuria
Homocystinuria
Oxalosis
Hyperglycinemia
Carnitine deficiency
  Primary
  Secondary

Mitochondrial Disorders (with or without Morphologically Abnormal Mitochondria)

Respiratory chain disorders
Cytochrome *c* reductase coenzyme deficiency
Cytochrome *c* oxidase deficiency
Cytochrome *c* oxidase deficiency with histiocytoid cardiomyopathy
Kearns-Sayre syndrome

[4]Gilbert-Barness E, Barness L. *Metabolic diseases: foundations of clinical management, genetics and pathology.* Natick, MA: Eaton Publishing, 2000:686. Reproduced with permission.

MELAS (mitochondrial, encephalopathy, lactic acidosis, and stroke) syndrome
MERRF (myoclonic epilepsy with ragged red fiber myopathy) syndrome
X-linked mitochondrial myopathy (Barth syndrome)

Neuromuscular Diseases

Duchenne muscular dystrophy
Becker muscular dystrophy
Nemaline myopathy
Malignant hyperthermia
Familial periodic paralysis
Friedreich ataxia
Kugelberg-Welander syndrome
Myotubular myopathy

Connective Tissue Disorders

Marfan syndrome
Ehlers-Danlos syndrome
Osteogenesis imperfecta
Pseudoxanthoma elasticum

Maternal Disorders with Neonatal Effects

Thyrotoxic cardiomyopathy
Lupus erythematosus
Catecholamine cardiomyopathy

Storage Disease

Glycogen storage disease types 2, 3, 4
Mucopolysaccharidoses
Mucolipidoses
I-cell disease
Gangliosidosis: G_{M1}, types I and II; G_{M2}, types I and II
Lipid storage diseases
Fabry disease
Gaucher disease
Neuronal ceroid lipofuscinosis
Multisystem triglyceride storage disease
Disseminated lipogranulomatosis (Farber disease)

Disorders of Metal and Pigment Metabolism

Hemosiderosis and hemochromatosis
Wilson disease
Menkes kinky hair syndrome
Dubin-Johnson syndrome

Hyperlipoproteinemias

Tangier disease

Obstructive Cardiomyopathy

Hypertrophic cardiomyopathy
Maternal diabetes
Hereditary hypertrophic cardiomyopathy with mitochondrial myopathy of skeletal muscle and cataracts
Leigh disease (subacute necrotizing encephalomyelopathy)

Myopathic Disorders

Genetic Myopathic Disorders[5]

Duchenne muscular dystrophy
Becker muscular dystrophy
Emery-Dreifuss muscular dystrophy
Limb-girdle muscular dystrophy

[5]Gilbert-Barness E, Barness L. *Metabolic diseases: foundations of clinical management, genetics and pathology.* Natick, MA: Eaton Publishing, 2000:709.

Fascioscapulohumeral muscular dystrophy
Myopathic scapuloperoneal syndrome
Congenital myotonic dystrophy (Steinert disease)
Nemaline myopathy
Kearns-Sayre syndrome

Acquired Myopathic Disorders

Polymyositis and other inflammatory myopathies
Scleroderma
Lupus erythematosus

Genetic Neurogenic Disorders

Friedreich ataxia

Acquired Neurogenic Disorders

Guillain-Barré syndrome
Diphtheria

Diagnostic Approach to Cardiomyopathies[6]

- Cardiologic investigations
  - Electrocardiography
  - Echocardiography
  - Hemodynamic studies
- Muscle biopsy
  - Morphologic analysis (histochemical, histoenzymologic analyses)
  - Biochemical analysis
  - Molecular genetic analysis
- Hematologic tests (overnight fasting)
  - Glucose
  - Lactate (acetate/pyruvate ratio)
  - Pyruvate
  - Free fatty acids
  - Ketone bodies (β-hydroxybutyrate/acetoacetate ratio)
  - Carnitine
- Other investigations
  - Creatinine kinase level
  - Transaminase levels
  - Plasma carnitine level (total and free)
  - Urine gas chromatography–mass spectrometry for organic acids
  - Fibroblast cultures for enzyme assays

Myocardial Ischemia and Infarction

Although myocardial ischemia and infarction are relatively rare in children, there are a number of important congenital and acquired causes. The most common congenital cause is anomalous origin of the left coronary artery from the pulmonary artery. Early studies suggested that this lesion alone may account for 25% of all cases of myocardial infarction in childhood. Kawasaki syndrome, a vasculitis of unknown etiology, has its most profound effects when it involves the coronary arteries. It is the most common acquired cause of myocardial ischemia and infarction in children. Aneurysmal dilation of the coronary arteries occurs in 15–25% of cases; however, the incidence has been significantly reduced since the initiation of intravenous γ-globulin therapy in the early stages of the disease. Myocardial infarction occurs in a small proportion of cases of Kawasaki syndrome, particularly those with giant aneurysms.

[6]Gilbert-Barness E, Barness L. *Metabolic diseases: foundations of clinical management, genetics and pathology.* Natick, MA: Eaton Publishing, 2000:716.

Increases in circulating concentrations of cardiac enzymes have been used as markers of myocardial damage from ischemia. Serum aspartate aminotransferase, lactate dehydrogenase (LDH), and creatine kinase (CK) are the principal enzymes in clinical use. The enzymes are released after irreversible tissue injury. Because these enzymes are present in many tissues, the specificity is reduced; however, the sensitivity is excellent.

Measurement of isoenzymes of LDH and CK has improved the specificity. The isoenzymes of LDH are composed of four subunits that are different combinations of a heart (H) or muscle (M) type and show different electrophoresis mobilities. LDH_1 is present in heart muscle and is the component released after myocardial infarction. Similarly, CK isoenzymes are dimers of either muscle (M) or brain (B) subunits. CK-MB is found almost exclusively in heart muscle, and increased concentrations are very specific for myocardial injury.

The first enzyme released after acute myocardial infarction is CK, which is increased by 4–5 hours, peaks (two- to tenfold) by 24 hours, and declines over 3–4 days. Aspartate aminotransferase activity is increased by 6–12 hours, peaks at 18–36 hours, and declines over 3–4 days. LDH has the slowest rise, with the initial increase being present by 24–28 hours, peaks occurring within 3–6 days, and values returning to normal by 14 days. Increases in the LDH_1 fraction precede increases in the total LDH and may be present by 8–24 hours. There is some evidence that the enzyme changes in children with myocardial infarction are qualitatively similar to those in adults, but the peak concentrations, especially of CK, may be reduced. In pediatric practice, CK isoenzymes are most frequently used.

Cardiac troponin I and *troponin T* are polypeptide subunits of the myofibrillar regulatory troponin complex. Both are unique myocardial antigens expressed as tissue-specific isoforms and show a high sensitivity and specificity for myocardial injury. They are not found in skeletal muscle during neonatal development or during adulthood, even after acute myocardial injury. The sensitivity of cardiac troponin I and troponin T is similar to that of CK-MB for the diagnosis of acute myocardial infarction. Furthermore, increases in cardiac troponin I and troponin T persist for up to 5–7 days in plasma, which permits flexibility in the timing of blood sampling. Measurement of levels of cardiac troponin I or cardiac troponin T or both is a sensitive and specific method for the diagnosis of perioperative myocardial infarction that avoids the high incidence of false diagnosis associated with the use of CK-MB as a diagnostic marker. With regard to cardiac transplantation a recent study found that increased donor serum cardiac troponin T concentrations measured just before organ retrieval were associated with significant increases in the inotropic requirements immediately after cardiac transplantation, which suggests that some degree of myocardial injury had occurred before organ donation. Increased donor cardiac troponin T values may be a useful predictor of early allograft dysfunction and may influence the decision to use the heart for transplantation.

- At 2–4 hours, electron microscopic changes appear (swelling of mitochondria, endoplasmic reticulum, fragmentation of myofibrils).
- Light-microscopic changes may appear in 4–6 hours but are rarely detectable with certainty before 12–24 hours.
- Coagulative necrosis of the necrotic fibers is recognized by nuclear pyknosis, dark pink staining, and loss of striations in the cytoplasm.

Clinical Features

Ischemic pain is the dominant symptom of myocardial infarction. It is a tightening, retrosternal pain that is not relieved by rest or vasodilators.

- Rarely, myocardial infarction may occur without pain ("silent infarction").
- The onset of pain is sudden and may occur during exercise, excitement, rest, or even sleep.
- Pain is often accompanied by sweating, changes in heart rate (due to autonomic stimulation), and hypotension.
- Fever and neutrophil leukocytosis are common.

The diagnosis of myocardial infarction is made by

- Electrocardiography, which shows elevation of the ST segment, T-wave inversion, and, in transmural infarction, an abnormal Q wave.
- Serum enzyme changes. Myoglobin, troponin I, troponin T, CK-MB isoenzyme, and LDH_1 levels are elevated (Fig. 3).

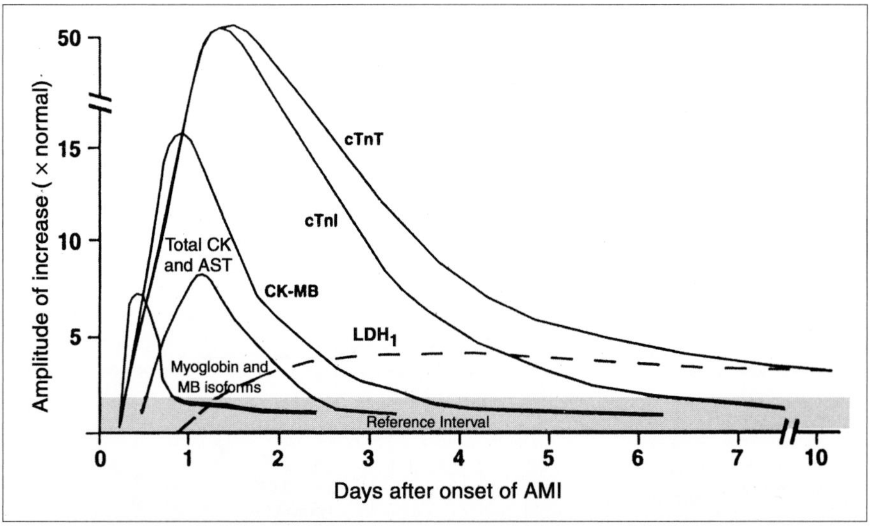

Fig. 3. Serial serum measurements of cardiac markers after acute myocardial infarction (AMI). AST, aspartate aminotransferase; CK-MB, creatine kinase MB isoenzyme; cTnI, cardiac troponin I; cTnT, cardiac troponin T; and LDH_1, lactate dehydrogenase fraction 1.

Diagnosis

Diagnosis of Myocardial Infarction by Seven Enzyme Markers

See Fig. 4 and Table 3.

Interpretation of Markers for Diagnosis of Acute Myocardial Infarction

See Table 4.

Primary Pulmonary Hypertension

Pulmonary arterial hypertension of unknown cause, for which secondary causes have been ruled out. Three pathologic subtypes have been identified: (a) thrombotic (56%), (b) plexogenic (28%), and (c) venoocclusive (16%).

Genetics

Seven percent familial; autosomal dominant with variable expression.

Predominant Sex

Incidence higher in females than in males (3:1)

Signs and Symptoms

- Loud P_2 (>80%)
- Right ventricular lift (>80%)
- Dyspnea (>75%)
- Murmur of tricuspid insufficiency (50–80%)
- Increased jugular venous pressure (50–80%)
- Right ventricular S_4 (50–80%)
- Chest pain (>50%)
- Fatigue (>50%)
- Palpitations (<50%)
- Syncope, dizziness (<50%)
- Cough (<50%)

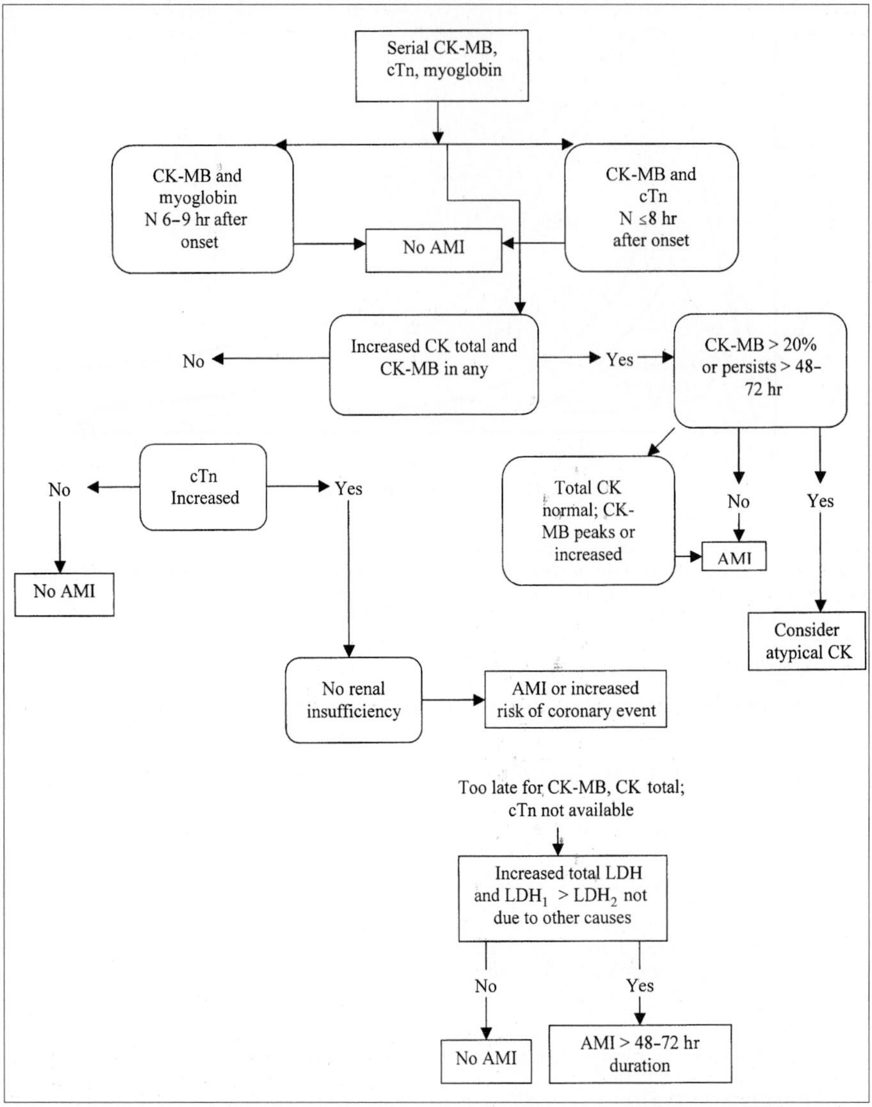

Fig. 4. Diagnosis of myocardial infarction by seven enzyme markers. AMI, acute myocardial infarction; CK, creatine kinase; CK-MB, creatine kinase MB isoenzyme; cTn, cardiac troponin; LDH, lactate dehydrogenase; LDH_1, lactate dehydrogenase fraction 1; LDH_2, lactate dehydrogenase fraction 2; N, negative.

- Raynaud phenomenon (<10%)
- Hepatomegaly (<50%)
- Pulmonic ejection click (<50%)
- Right ventricular S_3 (<50%)
- Murmur of pulmonic insufficiency (<50%)
- Lower extremity edema (<50%)
- Superficial thrombophlebitis (5%)

Table 3. Summary of Marker Levels after Acute Myocardial Infarction

Serum Marker	Earliest Increase (hr)[a]	Peak (hr)[a]	Duration of Increase (hr)[a]	Amplitude of Increase (× normal)	Specificity (%)[b]	Sensitivity at Peak (%)[b]
Troponin T	3–4	10–24	10–14 d		80	>98
Troponin I	4–6	10–24	4–7 d		95	>98
CK total	4–8	24–36	36–48	6–12	57–88	93–100
CK-MD	3–4	15–24	24–36	16	93–100	94–100
$CK\text{-}MB_2/MB_1$	2–4	4–6	16–24		94	95
Myoglobin	1–3	6–9	12–24	10	70	75–95
$CK\text{-}MM_3/MM_1$	6	10	~2			
Myosin light chain	3–8	24–35	10–15			
Electrocardiogram					100	63–84
LDH[c]	10–12	48–72	11	3	88	87
LDH_1[c]	8–12	72–144	8–14		85	40–90
LDH_1/LDH_2[c]	>6		>3		94–99	61–90
AST[d]	6–8	24–48	4–6	5	48–88	89–97
ALD[d]	Usually normal unless liver damage is present (e.g., congestive heart failure)					

ALD, aldolase; AST, aspartate aminotransferase; CK, creatine kinase; CK-MB, creatine kinase MB isoenzyme; LDH, lactate dehydrogenase.

Note: High degree of myocardial perfusion in cardiac surgery or contusion patients may lead to earlier and higher peaks and faster washout, causing shorter duration of increased values. Range of reported values given because different studies used different time periods after onset of symptoms, size of infarct, benchmarks for establishing the diagnosis, patient populations, instrumentation, etc.

[a]Time periods represent average reported values.

[b]Depends on time after onset of acute myocardial infarction (AMI). Sensitivity is lower at earlier or later times after myocardial damage.

[c]Replaced by cardiac troponin for diagnosis of AMI.

[d]Not used for diagnosis of AMI.

Causes

- Unknown; possible pulmonary arteriolar hyperactivity and vasoconstriction; occult thromboembolism; possible autoimmune disorder (high frequency antinuclear antibodies)
- In Europe, reports of primary pulmonary hypertension associated with anorectic agent aminorex fumarate in late 1960s, and with tainted rapeseed oil
- HIV-positive patients may have an increased incidence of primary pulmonary hypertension
- Anorectic agents (fenfluramine hydrochloride and dexfenfluramine hydrochloride)
- Amphetamines

Laboratory Findings

Positive results for antinuclear antibodies (one-third of patients)

Drugs that may alter laboratory results include hydralazine hydrochloride, procainamide hydrochloride, isoniazid, etc.

Other disorders that may alter laboratory results include connective tissue diseases, lupus erythematosus, scleroderma

Pathologic Findings

- Medial hypertrophy and arterial thrombosis are common in all subtypes.
- Plexogenic pulmonary arteriopathy (30–70%): laminar "onion skin" intimal proliferation, focal medial disruption, aneurysmal dilatation.

Table 4. Interpretation of Markers for Diagnosis of Acute Myocardial Infarction

ECG	cTn	CK Total	CK-MB	Myoglobin	Interpretation
+	+	+	+	+	AMI.
+	±	±	±	±	AMI. Confirm with cTn level for risk stratification and to monitor angioplastic/thrombolytic therapy.
–	+	–	–	–	AMI or unstable angina with increased risk of subsequent coronary event.
–	–	–	–	–	AMI or unstable angina. Confirm with serial ECG and serial measurement of CK-MB and cTn.
–	+	±	±	±	AMI or unstable angina.
–	–	–	–	+	Follow up cTn or CK-MB levels to rule out early AMI.
–	–	+	–	–	Not AMI.

+, increased; –, not increased; ±, increased or decreased; AMI, acute myocardial infarction; CK, creatine kinase; CK-MB, creatine kinase MB isoenzyme; cTn, cardiac troponin; ECG, electrocardiogram.

- Microthromboemboli (20–50%).
- Venoocclusive disease (10–15%).

Special Tests

- Electrocardiogram: right ventricular hypertrophy and right-axis deviation.
- Pulmonary function testing: arterial hypoxemia, reduced diffusion capacity, hypoxemia, hypocapnia.
- Ventilation/perfusion scan: must rule out proximal pulmonary artery emboli.
- Exercise test: reduced maximal O_2 consumption, high minute ventilation, low anaerobic threshold, reduced maximal oxygen pulse, increased DO_2A–a. Correlation between severity of disease and results on 6-minute walk test.

Imaging Studies

- Chest radiograph: enlarged central pulmonary arteries with pulmonary arterial branches attenuated. Right ventricular enlargement is a late finding. If there are increased interstitial markings, consider lung parenchymal disease or venoocclusive disease.
- Echo Doppler ultrasonography: right ventricular enlargement and overload; it is important to rule out underlying cardiac disease such as atrial septal defect with secondary pulmonary hypertension or mitral stenosis.
- Ultrasonography, fast computed tomography: sensitivity probably equal to that of pulmonary angiogram with lower contrast dose.

Diagnostic Procedures

- Chest radiograph, pulmonary function tests, arterial blood gas values, and ventilation/perfusion scan should be done.
- Cardiac catheterization: right heart catheterization is necessary to measure pulmonary artery pressures and hemodynamics; rule out underlying cardiac disease and response to vasodilator therapy.
- Pulmonary angiography: should be done if segmental or larger defect on ventilation/perfusion scan. Use caution in cases of pulmonary hypertension, as it can lead to hemodynamic collapse; use low osmolar agents, subselective angiograms.
- Lung biopsy may be performed but is usually not required.

Disorders with Severe Cardiac Manifestations in Infancy[7]

Disorders of lipid transport or metabolism	Systemic carnitine deficiency Carnitine palmityl transferase II deficiency β-Oxidation defects (long-chain acyl dehydrogenase deficiency, long-chain 3-hydroxyacyl coenzyme A dehydrogenase deficiency, multiple acyl coenzyme A dehydrogenase deficiency)

Lysosomal storage disorders	Glycogen storage diseases
	  Acid maltase deficiency (type 2, Pompe disease)
	  Others (rare)
	Mucopolysaccharidosis type IH (Hurler syndrome)
	Mucolipidosis type II (I-cell disease)

Mitochondrial (respiratory chain) disorders	Defects of nuclear DNA
	  Individual respiratory complex deficiencies
	    Histiocytoid (oncocytic) cardiomyopathy (complex III)
	    Autosomal-recessive Leigh syndrome (complex IV)
	  Barth syndrome
	Defects of mitochondrial DNA
	  Kearns-Sayre syndrome
	  Transfer RNA point mutations
	  Maternally inherited Leigh syndrome

Others	Transient cardiomyopathy in infants of diabetic mothers Infantile presentation of autosomal dominant hypertrophic cardiomyopathy

Bibliography

Bayer AS, Bolger AF, Taubert KA, et al. Diagnosis and management of infective endocarditis and its complications. *Circulation* 1998;98:2936–2948.

Brouqui P, Raoult D. Endocarditis due to rare and fastidious bacteria. *Clin Microbiol Rev* 2001;14:177–207.

Frontera JA, Gradon JD. Right-side endocarditis in injection drug users: review of proposed mechanisms of pathogenesis. *Clin Infect Dis* 2000;30:374–379.

Goldenberger D, Kunzli A, Vogt P, et al. Molecular diagnosis of bacterial endocarditis by broad-range PCR amplification and direct sequencing. *J Clin Microbiol* 1997;35:2733–2739.

Manoff SB, Vlahov D, Herskowitz A, et al. Human immunodeficiency virus infection and infective endocarditis among injecting drug users. *Epidemiology* 1996;7:566–570.

Mylonakis E, Calderwood SB. Infective endocarditis in adults. *N Engl J Med* 2001;345:1318–1330.

Patel R, Piper KE, Rouse MS, et al. Frequency of isolation of *Staphylococcus lugdunensis* among staphylococcal isolates causing endocarditis: a 20-year experience. *J Clin Microbiol* 2000;38:4262–4263.

Ribera E, Miro JM, Cortes E, et al. Influence of human immunodeficiency virus 1 infection and degree of immunosuppression in the clinical characteristics and outcome of infective endocarditis in intravenous drug users. *Arch Intern Med* 1998;158:2043–2050.

Strom BL, Abrutyn E, Berlin JA, et al. Risk factors for infective endocarditis: oral hygiene and nondental exposures. *Circulation* 2000;102:2842–2848.

Wallach J. *Interpretation of diagnostic tests*, 7th ed. Philadelphia: Lippincott Williams & Wilkins, 2000.

[7]Gilbert-Barness E, Barness L. *Metabolic diseases: foundations of clinical management, genetics and pathology.* Natick, MA: Eaton Publishing, 2000:687.

8 Pulmonary Function Tests

Evaluation of Pulmonary Function

Peak Expiratory Flow Rate

Maximum flow rate generated during a forced expiratory maneuver. Useful in following the course of asthma and response to therapy.

Predicted average peak expiratory flow rates for normal children are shown in Table 1.

Spirometry

Plots airflow versus time. Measurements are made from a rapid, forceful, and complete expiration from total lung capacity to residual volume (forced vital capacity maneuver).

Forced vital capacity (FVC): Maximum volume of air exhaled from the lungs after a maximum inspiration. FVC <15 mL/kg may be an indication for ventilatory support.

Forced expiratory volume in 1 second: Volume exhaled during the first second of FVC maneuver. Single best measure of airway function.

Forced expiratory flow 25–75: Mean rate of airflow over the middle half of the FVC between 25% and 75% of FVC. Sensitive to small-airway obstruction.

Interpretation of spirometry results is shown in Table 2.

Lung Volume Measurement

Total lung capacity, functional residual capacity, and residual volume cannot be determined by spirometry and require determination by helium dilution or nitrogen washout testing, or body plethysmography.

Interpretation of lung volume measurements is shown in Table 2.

Flow-Volume Curves

Plot of airflow versus lung volume. Useful in characterizing different patterns of airway obstruction.

Maximal Inspiratory and Expiratory Pressures

Obtained by asking patient to inhale/exhale against fixed obstruction. Low pressures suggest neuromuscular problem or submaximal effort. An inspiratory pressure <20–25 cm H_2O (negative inspiratory force) may be an indication for ventilatory support (Fig. 1).

Pulmonary Gas Exchange

Arterial blood gas (ABG) concentrations: Used to assess oxygenation (Pao_2), ventilation, $Paco_2$, and acid-base status (pH and HCO_3^-).

Table 1. Predicted Average Peak Expiratory Flow Rates (PEFR) for Healthy Children

Height (in.)	PEFR (L/min)	Height (in.)	PEFR (L/min)
43	147	56	320
44	160	57	334
45	173	58	347
46	187	59	360
47	200	60	373
48	214	61	387
49	227	62	400
50	240	63	413
51	254	64	427
52	267	65	440
53	280	66	454
54	293	67	467
55	307		

From Polger G, Promedhat V. *Pulmonary function testing in children: techniques and standards*. Philadelphia: WB Saunders, 1971.

Table 2. Interpretation of Spirometry and Lung Volume Readings

	Obstructive Disease (Asthma, Cystic Fibrosis)	Restrictive Disease (Interstitial Fibrosis, Scoliosis, Neuromuscular Cause)
Spirometry		
FVC[a]	Normal or reduced	Reduced
FEV_1[a]	Reduced	Reduced[d]
FEV_1/FVC[b]	Reduced	Normal
FEF_{25-75}	Reduced	Normal or reduced[d]
PEFR[a]	Normal or reduced	Normal or reduced[d]
Lung volumes		
TLC[a]	Normal or increased	Reduced
Rv[a]	Increased	Reduced
RC/TLC[c]	Increased	Unchanged
FRC	Increased	Reduced

FEV, forced expiratory volume; FEV_1, forced expiratory volume in 1 sec; FEF, forced expiratory flow; FRC, functional reserve capacity; FVC, forced vital capacity; PERF, peak expiratory flow rate; RC, residual capacity; Rv, residual volume; TLC, total lung capacity.
[a]Normal range: ± 20% of predicted.
[b]Normal range: >85%.
[c]Normal range: 20 ±10%.
[d]Reduced proportional to FVC.
From Johnson KB. *The Johns Hopkins Hospital—The Harriet Lane handbook*, 13th ed. St. Louis, MO: Mosby, 2000.

Venous blood gas concentrations: Peripheral venous samples are strongly affected by the local circulatory and metabolic environment. Can be used to assess acid-base status. $P{CO_2}$ averages 6–8 mm Hg higher than $Pa{CO_2}$, and pH is slightly lower.

Capillary blood gas concentrations: Correlation with arterial sampling is generally best for pH, moderate for $P{CO_2}$, and worst for $P{O_2}$.

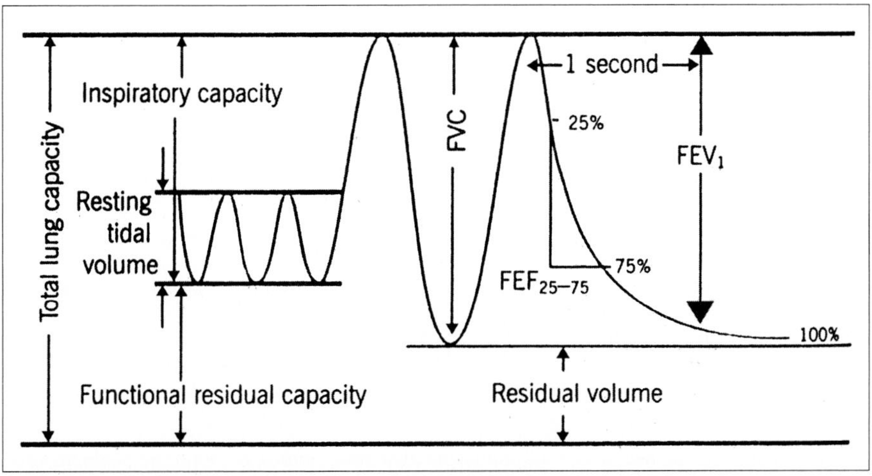

Fig. 1. Graph of normal values for respiratory function studies. FEF_{25-75}, forced expiratory flow over the middle half of the FVC between 25% and 75% of FVC; FEV_1, forced expiratory volume in 1 second; FVC, forced vital capacity.

Normal Mean Arterial Blood Gas Values[1]

	pH	Pa_{O_2} (mm Hg)	Pa_{CO_2} (mm Hg)	HCO_3^- (m Eq/L)
Newborn (birth)	7.26–7.29	60	55	19
Newborn (24 hr)	7.37	70	33	20
Infant (1–24 mo)	7.40	90	34	20
Child (7–19 yr)	7.39	96	37	22
Adult (normal range)	7.35–7.45	90–110	35–45	22–26

Analysis of Acid-Base Disturbances

1. Pure respiratory acidosis (or alkalosis): 10 mm Hg rise (fall) in Pa_{CO_2} results in an average 0.08 fall (rise) in pH.
2. Pure metabolic acidosis (or alkalosis): 10 mEq/L fall (rise) in HCO_3^- results in an average 0.15 fall (rise) in pH.

Expected Compensatory Response

See Table 3.

Pulse Oximetry

Arterial Oxygen Saturation

Noninvasive method of indirectly measuring arterial oxygen saturation (Sa_{O_2}). Uses light absorption characteristics of oxygenated and deoxygenated hemoglobin to estimate O_2 saturation.

Oxyhemoglobin Dissociation Curve

The oxyhemoglobin dissociation curve relates O_2 saturation to Pa_{O_2}. Increased hemoglobin affinity for oxygen (shift to the left) occurs with alkalemia, hypothermia,

[1]Rogers MC. *Textbook of pediatric intensive care*, 2nd ed. Baltimore: Williams & Wilkins, 1992.

Table 3. Calculation of Expected Compensatory Response

Disturbance	Primary Change	pH	Expected Compensatory Response
Acute respiratory acidosis	↑$PaCO_2$	↓pH	↑HCO_3^- by 1 mEq/L for each 10 mm Hg rise in $PaCO_2$
Acute respiratory alkalosis	↓$PaCO_2$	↑pH	↓HCO_3^- by 1–3 mEq/L for each 10 mm Hg fall in $PaCO_2$
Chronic respiratory acidosis	↑$PaCO_2$	↓pH	↑HCO_3^- by 4 mEq/L for each 10 mm Hg rise in $PaCO_2$
Chronic respiratory alkalosis	↓$PaCO_2$	↑pH	↓HCO_3^- by 1–3 mEq/L for each 10 mm Hg fall in $PaCO_2$
Metabolic acidosis	↓HCO_3^-	↓pH	↓$PaCO_2$ by 1.0–1.5 × fall in HCO_3^-
Metabolic alkalosis	↑HCO_3^-	↑pH	↑$PaCO_2$ by 0.25–1.0 × rise in HCO_3^-

hypocapnia, decreased 2,3-diphosphoglycerate, increased fetal hemoglobin, and anemia. Decreased hemoglobin affinity for oxygen (shift to the right) occurs with acidemia, hyperthermia, hypercapnia, and increased 2,3-diphosphoglycerate.

Important Uses of Oximetry

1. Rapid and continuous assessment of oxygenation in acutely ill patients
2. Monitoring of patients requiring oxygen therapy
3. Assessment of oxygen requirements during feeding, sleep, and exercise
4. Home monitoring of physiologic effects of apnea and bradycardia

Capnography

Measures CO_2 concentration of expired gas by infrared spectroscopy or mass spectroscopy. End-tidal CO_2 correlates with $PaCO_2$ (usually within 5 mm Hg of $PaCO_2$ in healthy subjects). Can be used for demonstrating proper placement of endotracheal tube, continuously monitoring CO_2 trends in ventilated patients, and monitoring ventilation during polysomnography.

Diffusing Capacity[2]

Measures gas transfer across alveolar-capillary membrane. Dilute CO is exposed to alveoli during a single breath, and the change in concentration indicates a rate of diffusion (in milliliters per minute per millimeter of mercury). The rate depends on area and permeability of alveolar-capillary membrane and hemoglobin concentration.

Ventilatory Assistance

Ventilator Parameters

1. Peak inspiratory pressure: maximum inspiratory pressure attained during the respiratory cycle
2. Positive end-expiratory pressure: airway pressure maintained between inspiratory and expiratory phases (prevents alveolar collapse during expiration, decreasing work of reinflation and improving gas exchange)
3. Rate (intermittent mandatory ventilation) or frequency (hertz): number of mechanical breaths delivered per minute, or rate of oscillations of high-frequency oscillatory ventilation (HFOV)

[2]Johnson KB. *The Johns Hopkins Hospital—The Harriet Lane handbook,* 13th ed. St. Louis, MO: Mosby, 2000.

4. Inspired oxygen concentration (FIO_2): fraction of oxygen present in inspired gas
5. Inspiratory time: length of time spent in the inspiratory phase of the respiratory cycle
6. Tidal volume: volume of gas delivered during inspiration
7. Power: amplitude of the pressure waveform in HFOV
8. Mean airway pressure: average pressure over entire respiratory cycle

Ventilator Management

Parameters predictive of successful extubation

1. Normal $PaCO_2$.
2. Peak inspiratory pressure generally <14–16 cm H_2O.
3. Positive end-expiratory pressure <2–3 cm H_2O (infants) or <5 cm H_2O (children).
4. Intermittent mandatory ventilation <2–4 breaths per minute (infants); children may be weaned to continuous positive airway pressure.
5. FIO_2 <40% (maintaining PaO_2 >70).
6. Maximum negative inspiratory pressure >20–25 cm H_2O.

Reference Data

1. Minute ventilation (V_E)
   V_E = respiratory rate × tidal volume
   $V_E \times PaCO_2$ = constant (for volume-limited ventilation)
   Normal tidal volume = 10–15 mL/kg
2. Henderson-Hasselbach equation
   $$pH = 6.1 + \log \frac{HCO_3^-}{(0.03 \times PaCO_2)}$$
3. Alveolar gas equation
   $PAO_2 = PIO_2 - (PaCO_2/R)$
   $PIO_2 = FIO_2 \times (PB - 47 \text{ mm Hg})$
   PAO_2 = partial pressure of O_2 in the alveoli
   PIO_2 = partial pressure of inspired O_2 = 150 mm Hg at sea level on room air
   $PACO_2$ = partial pressure of alveolar CO_2 = partial pressure of arterial CO_2 ($PaCO_2$)
   R = respiratory exchange quotient (CO_2 produced ÷ O_2 consumed) = 0.8
   PB = atmospheric pressure = 760 mm Hg at sea level
4. Alveolar-arterial oxygen gradient (A–a gradient)
   A–a gradient = $PAO_2 - PaO_2$.
   Obtain ABG measuring PaO_2 and $PaCO_2$ with patient on 100% FIO_2 for at least 15 minutes.
   Calculate the PAO_2 (see earlier) and then the A–a gradient.
   The larger the gradient, the more serious the respiratory compromise. A normal gradient is 20–65 mm Hg on 100% O_2 or 5–20 mm Hg on room air.
5. Oxygen content (CaO_2)
   O_2 content of sample (mL/dL) = [O_2 capacity × O_2 saturation (as decimal)] + dissolved O_2.
   O_2 capacity = hemoglobulin (g/dL) × 1.34.
   Dissolved O_2 = PO_2 (of sample) × 0.003.
   Hemoglobulin carries more than 99% of O_2 in blood under standard conditions.
6. Arteriovenous O_2 difference ($AVDO_2$)
   $AVDO_2$ = CaO_2 – mixed venous O_2 content.
   Usually done after placing patient on 100% FIO_2 for 15 minutes.
   Obtain ABG and mixed venous blood sample (best obtained from pulmonary artery catheter) and measure O_2 saturation in each sample.
   Calculate arterial and mixed venous oxygen contents and then $AVDO_2$ (normal = 5 mL/100 dL).
   Used in the calculation of O_2 extraction ratio.
7. O_2 extraction ratio
   $$O_2 \text{ extraction} = \left(\frac{AVDO_2}{CaO_2}\right) \times 100.$$

Normal range 28–33%.
Calculate $AVDO_2$ and O_2 contents.
Extraction ratios are indicative of the adequacy of O_2 delivery to tissues, with increasing extraction ratios suggesting that metabolic needs may be outpacing the oxygen content being delivered.

8. Oxygenation index (OI)

$$OI = \frac{[\text{Mean airway pressure}(\text{cm}H_2O) \times FIO_2 \times 100]}{PaO_2}.$$

OI >35 for 5–6 hours is one criterion for initiation of extracorporeal membrane oxygen support.

9. Intrapulmonary shunt fraction (Qs/Qt)

$$\frac{Qs}{Qt} = \frac{(\text{A–a gradient}) \times 0.003}{(AVDO_2) + (\text{A–a gradient})}.$$

Qt, cardiac output; Qs, flow across right-to-left shunt.
Formula assumes blood gas levels obtained on 100% FIO_2.
Represents the mismatch of ventilation and perfusion and is normally <5%.
A rising shunt fraction (usually >15–20%) is indicative of progressive respiratory failure.

Calculation of Alveolar-Arterial Oxygen Gradient[3]

The alveolar-arterial oxygen gradient, or $P(A\text{–}a)O_2$, can be calculated from the ABG results. It is useful in confirming the presence of a shunt.

$P(A\text{–}a)O_2 = PAO_2 - PaO_2$
PAO_2 = the alveolar oxygen tension calculated as shown later
PaO_2 = the arterial oxygen tension measured by ABG determination
PAO_2 can be calculated by the following formula:

$$PAO_2 = (PB - PH_2O)(FIO_2) - \frac{PaCO_2}{R}$$

PB = barometric pressure (760 mm Hg at sea level)
PH_2O = 47 mm Hg
FIO_2 = the fraction of O_2 in inspired gas
$PaCO_2$ = the arterial CO_2 tension measured by ABG determination
R = the respiratory quotient (0.8)

Normal $P(A\text{–}a)O_2$ is 12 mm Hg or less for infants, children, and adolescents.
In pure ventilatory failure, the $P(A\text{–}a)O_2$ remains 12–20 mm Hg. In oxygenation failure, it increases.

Respiratory Rate

See Table 4.

Lymph Node (Scalene) Biopsy

Biopsy of scalene fat pad even without palpable lymph nodes.
May also yield positive results in various granulomatous disease (e.g., tuberculosis, sarcoidosis).

Thoracoscopy and Open Lung Biopsy

Interstitial lung disease, pulmonary and nodules
Diagnosis of pleural malignancy
Accuracy = 96%; sensitivity = 91%; specificity = 100%; negative predictive value = 93%
Diagnosis of pulmonary infection or neoplasm when BAL is not diagnostic

[3]Marshall SA, Ruedy J. *On call: principles and protocols.* Philadelphia: WB Saunders, 1993.

Table 4. Respiratory Function

Mean Respiratory Rate ± 1 Standard Deviation					
Age (yr)	Boys	Girls	Age (yr)	Boys	Girls
0–1	31 ± 8	30 ± 6	9–10	19 ± 2	19 ± 2
1–2	26 ± 4	27 ± 4	10–11	19 ± 2	19 ± 2
2–3	25 ± 4	25 ± 3	11–12	19 ± 3	19 ± 3
3–4	24 ± 3	24 ± 3	12–13	19 ± 3	19 ± 2
4–5	23 ± 2	22 ± 2	13–14	19 ± 2	18 ± 2
5–6	22 ± 2	21 ± 2	14–15	18 ± 2	18 ± 3
6–7	21 ± 3	21 ± 3	15–16	17 ± 3	18 ± 3
7–8	20 ± 3	20 ± 2	17–18	17 ± 2	17 ± 3
8–9	20 ± 2	20 ± 2	17–18	16 ± 3	17 ± 3

Microscopic Examination of Stained Nasal Smear

Large numbers of eosinophils suggest allergy. Does not correlate with blood eosinophilia. Presence of eosinophils and neutrophils suggests chronic allergy with superimposed infection.

Large numbers of neutrophils suggest infection.

Gram stain and culture of pharyngeal exudate may show significant pathogen.

Special Stains

Giemsa Stain of Bronchoalveolar Lavage Specimen

Normal <3% neutrophils, 8–18% lymphocytes, 80–89% alveolar macrophages

Finding of >10% neutrophils: Indicates acute inflammation [e.g., bacterial infection, including *Legionella* infection; acute respiratory distress syndrome (ARDS); drug reaction].

Finding of >1% squamous epithelial cells: Indicates that a positive culture finding may reflect saliva contamination.

Finding of >80% macrophages: Common in pulmonary hemorrhage. Aspergillosis is the only infection associated with significant alveolar hemorrhage, which may also be found in >10% of patients with hematologic malignancies.

Finding of >30% lymphocytes: May indicate hypersensitivity pneumonitis (often up to 50–60% with more cytoplasm and large, irregular nucleus).

Finding of >10% neutrophils and >3% eosinophils: Characteristic of idiopathic pulmonary fibrosis; alveolar macrophages predominate. Lymphocyte percentage may be increased.

Finding of >105 colony-forming bacteria/mL indicates bacterial infection if <1% squamous epithelial cells are present on Giemsa stain.

Gram Stain

Presence of many bacteria suggests bacterial infection if there are <1% squamous epithelial cells, especially if culture shows >104 bacteria/mL.

No bacteria suggests that bacterial infection is unlikely, but *Legionella* should be ruled out with direct fluorescent antibody test if Giemsa stain shows increased neutrophils.

Combined with methenamine silver or Papanicolaou stain, 94% sensitivity for diagnosis of *Pneumocystis* infection; increased to 100% when bronchoalveolar lavage (BAL) is combined with transbronchial biopsy.

Acid-Fast Stain

Positive result may indicate *Mycobacterium tuberculosis* or *Mycobacterium avium-intracellulare* infection.

Toluidine Blue Stain

May show *Pneumocystis carinii* cysts in *Pneumocystis* pneumonia or *Aspergillus* hyphae in immunocompromised host with invasive aspergillosis.

Prussian Blue–Nuclear Red Stain

Strongly positive result indicates severe alveolar hemorrhage; moderately positive findings indicates some hemorrhage; absence of effect indicates infection with corresponding organism.

Direct Fluorescent Antibody Stain

Direct fluorescent antibody stain for *Legionella*, herpes simplex virus 1 and 2 (stains bronchial epithelial cells and macrophages), and cytomegalovirus (CMV; stains mononuclear cells) may indicate infection with corresponding organism.

Papanicolaou Stain

Atypical cytology may be due to cytotoxic drugs, radiation therapy, viral infection (intranuclear inclusions of herpesvirus or CMV), tumor.

Oil Red O Stain

Shows many large intracellular fat droplets in one-third to two-thirds of cells in some patients with fat embolism due to bone fractures but in <3% of patients without embolism.

Respiratory Diseases

Acute Nasopharyngitis

Bacterial: Group A β-hemolytic streptococci cause 10–30% of cases seen by doctors; *Haemophilus influenzae*, *Mycoplasma pneumoniae*, etc. Mere presence of staphylococci, pneumococci, α- and β-hemolytic streptococci (other than groups A, C, and G) in throat cultures does not establish them as cause of pharyngitis and does not warrant antibiotic treatment.

Viral [e.g., Epstein-Barr virus, CMV, adenovirus, respiratory syncytial virus (RSV), herpes simplex virus, coxsackievirus].

M. pneumoniae

Chlamydia pneumoniae

Fungus, allergy, foreign body, trauma, neoplasm.

Idiopathic (no cause is identified in 50% of cases).

Upper Airway Disease

Symptoms and Evaluation

The symptoms of upper airway obstruction are stridor or noisy breathing caused by rapid, turbulent flow through an obstructed or narrowed portion of the airway. Inspiratory stridor is common with lesions above or at the level of the larynx, whereas expiratory stridor is more often seen with lesions below the level of the vocal cords. Other symptoms include a weak or muffled cry, a barking cough, feeding difficulties, retractions, tachypnea, and tachycardia. Hypoventilation with a rising CO_2 is seen before cyanosis.

The most common presentation of upper airway disease is respiratory distress and noisy breathing. Stridor at or near birth is often an indicator of laryngomalacia.

With the widespread availability of *H. influenzae* B vaccines in recent years, the incidence of epiglottitis has dropped dramatically.

The most helpful laboratory evaluation is measurement of arterial blood gases. The patient with respiratory acidosis in this situation is in grave danger. The white blood cell (WBC) count can be helpful, as it is usually more elevated with bacterial infections and has a larger component of polymorphonuclear cells with juvenile forms.

Causes of Upper Airway Obstruction[4]

Congenital Lesions
- Intrinsic lesions
  - Subglottic stenosis
  - Web
  - Cyst
  - Laryngocele
  - Tumor
  - Laryngomalacia
  - Laryngotracheoesophageal cleft
  - Tracheomalacia
  - Tracheoesophageal fistula
- Extrinsic lesions
  - Vascular ring
  - Cystic hygroma
- Birth trauma
- Neurologic lesion
- Craniofacial anomalies
- Metabolic disorders—hypocalcemia

Acquired Lesions
- Infections
  - Retropharyngeal abscess
  - Ludwig angina
  - Laryngotracheobronchitis
  - Epiglottitis
  - Fungal infection
  - Peritonsillar abscess
  - Diphtheria
  - Bacterial tracheitis
- Trauma, internal
  - Postextubation croup
  - Posttracheostomy removal
- Trauma, external
- Thermal or chemical burns
- Foreign-body aspiration
- Systemic disorders
- Internal or external neoplasms
- Neurologic lesions
- Chronic upper airway obstruction
- Hypertrophic tonsils, adenoids
- Tight surgical neck dressing

Acute Sinusitis

Often precipitated by obstruction due to viral upper respiratory tract infection, allergy, foreign body.

Streptococcus pneumoniae and *H. influenzae* cause >50% of cases; also anaerobes, *Staphylococcus aureus, Streptococcus pyogenes* (group A).

Moraxella catarrhalis causes 20% of cases in children.

Viruses cause 10–20% of cases.

Pseudomonas aeruginosa and *H. influenzae* are predominant organisms in cystic fibrosis (CF) patients.

Mucor spp. and *Aspergillus* spp. should be ruled out in patients with diabetes or acute leukemias and in renal transplant recipients.

Anaerobes (e.g., streptococci, *Bacteroides* spp.) are found in 50% of cases of chronic sinusitis.

Needle aspiration of sinus is required for determination of organism. Cultures of nose, throat, and nasopharynx specimens do not correlate well.

Mucosal biopsy may be indicated if aspirate is not diagnostic in unresponsive patient with acute infection.

Pain and tenderness over the sinuses with purulent nasal discharge should present for 3 or more weeks. Bending the body forward may aggravate pain.

Imaging by radiography, computed tomography, or magnetic resonance imaging is associated with many false-positive results as upper respiratory tract infections commonly produce similar imaging abnormalities.

Immotile Cilia Syndrome

See Fig. 2.

Clinical manifestations of immotile cilia syndrome are chronic rhinitis, sinusitis, otitis, bronchitis, bronchiectasis, frontal headaches, and a poor sense of smell. Many patients have nasal polyps. Men are infertile; women suffer reduced fertility. The disorder has an autosomal-recessive mode of inheritance.

Diagnosis is by electron microscopic examination of cilia from a nasopharyngeal biopsy.

[4]Rogers MC, ed. *Textbook of pediatric intensive care.* Baltimore: Williams & Wilkins, 1987.

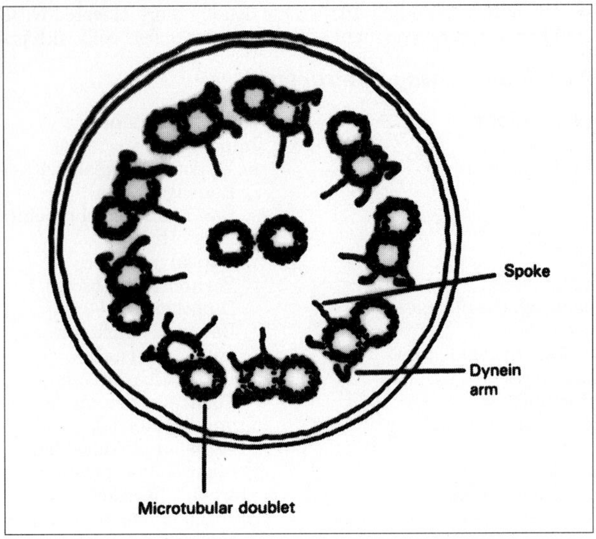

Fig. 2. Diagram of a cilium showing nine peripheral and one central doublet.

Dynein Arms

Absence or shortness or dynein arms is the most common lesion associated with a defect in mucociliary transport.

Radial Spokes

Defective radial spokes may be present.

Central Microtubules

Absence of central microtubules is more frequently an acquired lesion.

Ciliary Membrane

The membrane surrounding the axoneme may play a crucial role in the control of ciliary activity. Membrane alteration is usually excessive membranes.

Croup, Epiglottitis, Laryngotracheitis

Signs and Symptoms

Croup, acute laryngotracheobronchitis, is characterized by a barking cough with an accompanying hoarse voice. Inspiratory stridor and respiratory distress may occur. Signs are usually worse at night, are due to inflammation and edema of the subglottic area, and follow an upper respiratory tract infection. Causes are infections with parainfluenza virus types 1 and 3, and less commonly with adenovirus, influenza viruses A and B, and RSV.

Bacterial tracheitis may follow croup. The patient appears toxic and develops a significant fever. Purulent secretions exude from below the larynx. Usual organisms are *S. aureus* or group B streptococci and, less commonly, *M. catarrhalis*, nontypeable *H. influenzae*, and anaerobic organisms. If untreated, respiratory obstruction occurs. Toxic shock syndrome has been associated with bacterial tracheitis.

Acute epiglottitis causes a toxic appearance in a child with severe respiratory distress and a significant fever. The patient usually sits up with neck extended, may drool, and refuses to speak or speaks with a soft voice. The usual causative organism has been *H. influenzae*, and since the corresponding vaccine has been used, incidence has decreased.

Retropharyngeal abscess may be caused by similar organisms and may cause significant fever and respiratory distress. The posterior pharynx appears swollen.

Angioneurotic edema, an allergic reaction, may cause acute respiratory distress. The offending substance is frequently identifiable. Rash, bronchospasm, and circulatory collapse may occur.

Compression due to hemangioma or lymphangioma or foreign-body aspiration may cause hoarseness, voice abnormalities, and severe respiratory distress.

Diagnosis

Diagnosis of severe respiratory distress is facilitated by radiographic imaging. Radiography of the neck commonly reveals a steeple-like appearance of the supraglottic area. In tracheitis, the tracheal wall appears ragged. With epiglottitis, the epiglottis appears thickened. The retropharyngeal area appears swollen in a lateral neck radiograph. For any of these suspected diagnoses, the condition is a high-risk emergency, and direct visualization may be necessary.

Clinical characteristics differentiating laryngotracheobronchitis from epiglottitis include the following[5]:

Characteristic	Laryngotracheobronchitis	Epiglottitis
Age	6 mo to 3 yr	2–6 yr
Onset	Gradual	Rapid
Cause	Viral	Bacterial
Swelling site	Subglottic	Supraglottic
Symptoms		
Cough/voice	Hoarse cough	No cough; muffled voice
Posture	Any position	Sitting
Mouth	Closed; nasal flaring	Open, chin forward, drooling
Fever	Absent to high	High
Appearance	Often not acutely ill	Anxious; acutely ill
Radiograph	Narrow subglottic area	Swollen epiglottis and supraglottic structures
Palpation of larynx	Nontender	Tender
Recurrence	May recur	Rarely recurs
Seasonal incidence	Winter	None
Common organism	RSV	*H. influenzae*

Lower Airway Disease

Lower airway disease can be divided into disorders of the bronchi and conducting airways and diseases of the alveoli. The two most common diseases of the conducting airways are bronchiolitis and asthma, and there is evidence of overlap between the two processes. Acute respiratory failure after injury to the alveolar capillary unit may occur after a variety of insults. These can include infectious pneumonias, inhalational injuries, sepsis, or shock. Injury to the alveolar capillary unit results in a common group of pathophysiologic findings currently referred to in the literature as ARDS.

Bronchiolitis

Bronchiolitis is an acute inflammatory disease of the lower respiratory tract that results in obstruction of the small airways. It is most commonly seen in infants 1–2 years of age. Viral agents include RSV, parainfluenza, rhinovirus, adenovirus, influenza, and, occasionally, mumps.

Clinically, the infant presents with expiratory wheezing, tachypnea, retractions, and irritability. There is often a low-grade fever, cyanosis, and feeding difficulties. Aus-

[5]Rogers MC, ed. *Textbook of pediatric intensive care*. Baltimore: Williams & Wilkins, 1987.

cultation reveals diffuse wheezing, prolonged expiration, and rales. Younger infants have a significant risk of apnea.

Asthma

A disorder of the tracheobronchial tree characterized by mild to severe obstruction to airflow due to bronchoconstriction precipitated by a variety of stimuli, including allergies, infectious agents, exercise, emotional stress, or certain drugs. Symptoms vary, are generally episodic or paroxysmal, and may be persistent. The clinical hallmark is wheezing, but cough may be the predominant symptom. Commonly misdiagnosed as recurrent pneumonia or chronic bronchitis.

Acute symptoms are characterized by narrowing of large and small airways due to spasm of bronchial smooth muscle, edema and inflammation of the bronchial mucosa, and production of mucus.

Occurs in a setting in which asthma is likely and other conditions such as foreign-body aspiration and CF have been excluded.

Affects 7–19% of children.

Predominant ages are <10 years (50% of cases) and young adulthood (16–40 years), but may occur at any age.

Predominant sex
- Children <10 years, boys affected more than girls
- Puberty, boys and girls affected equally
- Adult onset, women affected more than men

Signs and Symptoms

Variation in pattern of symptoms; paroxysmal, constant, abnormal pulmonary function tests without symptoms

Wheezing

Cough

Periodic symptoms

Prolonged expiration

Hyperresonance

Decreased breath sounds

Nocturnal attacks

Pulsus paradoxus

Cyanosis

Tachycardia

Accessory respiratory muscle use

Flattened diaphragm

Nasal polyp (seen in CF and aspirin sensitivity)

Clubbing is not seen in asthma.

Growth is usually normal.

Causes

Allergic factors
- Air-borne pollens
- Molds
- House dust (mites)
- Animal dander
- Feather pillows

Other factors
- Smoke and other pollutants
- Infections, especially viral
- Aspirin
- Exercise
- Sinusitis
- Gastroesophageal reflux
- Sleep (peak expiratory flow rate lowest at 4 a.m.)
- Current research focuses on inflammatory response (including abnormal release of chemical mediators, eosinophil chemotactic factor, neutrophil chemotactic factor, and leukotrienes, etc.) and muscle relaxants.

Risk Factors

Positive family history

Viral lower respiratory tract infection during infancy

Differential Diagnosis

Foreign-body aspiration (should always be considered), CF, viral respiratory infections (croup, bronchiolitis), epiglottitis, bronchopulmonary aspergillosis, tuberculosis, hyperventilation syndrome, mitral value prolapse, habitual cough, recurrent pulmonary emboli, congestive heart failure, chronic obstructive pulmonary disease, hypersensitivity, pneumonia

Laboratory Tests

Complete blood count (normal)
Nasal eosinophils
Immunoglobulin levels (immunoglobulin E levels elevated in allergic bronchopulmonary aspergillosis)
Immunodeficiency screening
Sweat test in patients with chronic childhood asthma
Arterial blood gas levels in status asthmaticus

Pathologic Findings

Smooth muscle hyperplasia; mucosal edema; thickened basement membrane; inflammatory response; hyperinflated lungs; mucus plugging; increased airway resistance; decreased airflow rates; ventilation-perfusion mismatching. Bronchiectasis is not seen except in association with allergic bronchopulmonary aspergillosis.

Special Tests

Home monitoring of peak flow rates; report if peak flow drops below 70% of baseline
Pulmonary function tests to detect reversible airway obstruction
Allergy testing
Purified protein derivative (tuberculin) yearly
Exercise tolerance testing

Imaging

Chest radiograph (hyperinflation, atelectasis, air leak)

Diagnostic Procedures

Bronchoscopy: rarely indicated.
Spirometry: decreased forced expiratory volume in 1 second.
Chest radiography: do at least one, but not necessary with each exacerbation.

Some Factors That Precipitate Bronchoconstriction in Asthma

Allergy (Mediator Release)

Histamine
Slow-reacting substance of anaphylaxis
Prostaglandins
Thromboxane
Other substances

Autonomic Imbalance

Excessive cholinergic response
Reduced α-adrenergic responsiveness
Nonspecific irritant

Infections

Viral respiratory tract infection

Pharmacologic Agents

α-Adrenergic blockade (propranolol)
Prostaglandin inhibitors (aspirin and nonsteroidal antiinflammatory drugs)

Exercise

Psychogenic

Acute Bronchitis

Viruses (e.g., rhinovirus, coronavirus, adenovirus, influenza) cause most cases.
M. pneumoniae, C. pneumoniae, Bordetella pertussis, Legionella spp.

Chronic Bronchitis

WBC and erythrocyte sedimentation rate normal or increased.
Eosinophil count increased if there is allergic basis or component.
Smears and cultures of sputum and bronchoscopic secretions should be taken.
Laboratory findings due to associated or coexisting diseases (e.g., emphysema, bronchiectasis).

Acute exacerbations are most commonly due to
- Viruses
- *M. pneumoniae*
- *H. influenzae*
- *S. pneumoniae*
- *M. catarrhalis* (*Branhamella catarrhalis*)

Bronchiectasis

WBC usually normal unless pneumonitis is present.
Mild to moderate normocytic normochromic anemia with chronic severe infection.
Sputum abundant and mucopurulent (often contains blood); sweetish smell.
Sputum bacterial smear and cultures should be obtained.
Laboratory findings due to complications (pneumonia, pulmonary hemorrhage, brain abscess, sepsis, cor pulmonale).
Rule out CF of the pancreas and hypogammaglobulinemia or agammaglobulinemia.

Pneumonia Due to Microorganisms

Bacteria

S. pneumoniae: Causes 60–70% of bacterial pneumonia in patients requiring hospitalization. May cause 25% of hospital-acquired cases of pneumonia. Blood culture results positive in 25% of untreated cases during first 3–4 days. Decreasing with vaccination.
Staphylococcus: Causes <1% of all acute bacterial pneumonia with onset outside the hospital but more frequent after outbreaks of influenza; may be secondary to measles, mucoviscidosis, prolonged antibiotic therapy, debilitating diseases (e.g., leukemia, collagen disease). Frequent cause of nosocomial pneumonia. Bacteremia in <20% of patients.
H. influenzae: Important in 6- to 24-month age group; rare in adults except for middle-aged men with chronic lung disease or alcoholism, or both, and patients with immunodeficiency (human immunodeficiency virus infection, multiple myeloma, chronic lymphocytic leukemia). Can mimic pneumococcal pneumonia; may be isolated with *S. pneumoniae*. Decreasing with vaccination.
Gram-negative bacilli (e.g., *Klebsiella pneumoniae*, enterobacteria, *Escherichia coli*, *Proteus mirabilis*, *P. aeruginosa*): Common causes of hospital-acquired pneumonia but unlikely outside the hospital. *K. pneumoniae* causes 1% of primary bacterial pneumonias, most commonly in alcoholic patients and patients with upper lobe pneumonia; tenacious red-brown sputum is typical.
Tubercle bacilli
Legionella pneumophila
M. pneumoniae: Most common in young adult male population (e.g., armed forces camps)
C. pneumoniae, Chlamydia psittaci
Others (e.g., *Streptococcosis*, *Francisella tularensis*, *Yersinia pestis*)

Viruses

Influenza, parainfluenza, adenoviruses, RSV, echovirus, coxsackievirus, reovirus, CMV, viruses of exanthems, herpes simplex virus, hantavirus

Rickettsiae

Coxiella burnetii (Q fever is most common in endemic area); typhus organisms

Fungi

P. carinii, Histoplasma, and *Coccidioides* in particular; *Blastomyces*, *Aspergillus*

Protozoa

Toxoplasma

Microorganisms in Pneumonia Associated with Specific Disorders

Human immunodeficiency virus infection	*S. pneumoniae, H. influenzae, S. aureus*, Gram-negative bacilli, *P. carinii, M. tuberculosis* and *M. avium-intracellulare*, *Toxoplasma gondii*, *Cryptococcus*, *Nocardia*, CMV, *Histoplasma*, *Coccidioides immitis*, *Legionella*, *M. catarrhalis*, *Rhodococcus equi*
Atypical pneumonia	*M. pneumoniae, C. psittaci, C. pneumoniae, Coxiella burnetii, Francisella tularensis,* many viruses

Laboratory Diagnosis

WBC count is frequently normal or slightly increased in nonbacterial pneumonias; considerable increase in WBC count is more common in bacterial pneumonia. In severe bacterial pneumonia, WBC count may be very high or low or normal. Because individual variation is considerable, WBC count has limited value in distinguishing bacterial and nonbacterial pneumonia.

Urine protein, WBCs, hyaline, and granular casts in small amounts are common. Ketones may occur with severe infection. Check for glucose to rule out underlying diabetes mellitus.

Sputum reveals abundant WBCs in bacterial pneumonias. Gram stain shows abundant organisms in bacterial pneumonias (e.g., *Pneumococcus, Staphylococcus*). Culture sputum for appropriate bacteria. Presence of many organisms and WBCs on sputum smear but absence of pathogens on aerobic culture may indicate aspiration pneumonia. Sputum is not appropriate for anaerobic culture.

Blood culture and sputum culture and smear for Gram stain should be performed before antibiotic therapy is started.

Nasopharyngeal aspirate specimens may identify *S. pneumoniae* with few false-positives, but *S. aureus* and Gram-negative bacilli often represent false-positive findings.

In *H. influenzae* pneumonia, sputum culture results are negative in >50% of patients with positive culture results from blood, pleural fluid, or lung tissue, and the organism may be present in the sputum in the absence of disease.

Specimens obtained by transtracheal aspiration (puncture of cricothyroid membrane) generally yield a faster, more accurate diagnosis.

Brush bronchoscopy and BAL have high sensitivity.

Diagnostic lung puncture to determine specific causative agent as a guide to antibiotic therapy may be indicated in critically ill children.

Open lung biopsy is gold standard, with 97% accuracy but 10% complication rate. For pleural effusions that are aspirated, Gram stain and culture should be performed.

Respiratory pathogens isolated from blood, pleural fluid, or transtracheal aspirate (except in patients with chronic bronchitis) or identified by bacterial polysaccharide antigen in urine may be considered the definite causal agent.

Urine testing for capsular antigen from *S. pneumoniae* or type B *H. influenzae* by latex agglutination gives positive results in 90% of bacteremic pneumococcal pneumonias and 40% of nonbacteremic pneumonias. May be particularly useful when antibiotic therapy has already begun.

Acute-phase serum specimen should be stored at onset. If causal diagnosis is not established, a convalescent-phase serum sample should be taken. A 4× increase in antibody titer establishes the causal diagnosis [e.g., *L. pneumophila*, *Chlamydia* spp., respiratory viruses (including influenza and RSV), *M. pneumoniae*].

Lipid Pneumonia

Sputum shows fat-containing macrophages that stain with Sudan. They may be present only intermittently; sputum should be examined more than once.

Opportunistic Pulmonary Infections

See Table 5.

Lung Abscess

Marked increase in sputum; abundant, foul, purulent; may be bloody; contains elastic fibers.

Gram stain is diagnostic; sheets of polymorphonuclear cells with a bewildering variety of organisms.

Bacterial cultures (including tubercle bacilli) show anaerobic as well as aerobic organisms; rule out amebas, parasites.

Cytologic examination for inflammatory cells.

Blood culture may be positive in acute stage.

Increased WBC in acute stages (15,000–30,000/mm^3)

Increased erythrocyte sedimentation rate

Table 5. Opportunistic Pulmonary Infections

Organism	Preferred Specimen	Direct Stain	Antigen or Nucleic Acid	Culture Turnaround Time
Usual bacteria	SP	Gram stain	NA	Routine, 3–4 d
Fungi	BAL	Wet mount	Cryptococcal and histoplasmal antigens	Mycologic media, 6–8 wk
Nocardia spp.	BAL	Modified acid fast	NA	Blood agar, 4–6 wk
Legionella spp.	BAL	DFA	Urine antigen only for serotype 1	Special media, 2–7 d
Mycobacteria spp.	BAL	Acid fast	NA	Mycobacterial media, ≥8 wk
Viruses	BAL, NPS	FAB for specific viruses	FAB for CMV, HSV, VZV	Shell vial 1–2 d; ≥2 wk for traditional
Pneumocystis spp.	BAL, SISP	FAB, Giemsa, toluidine blue O	PCR	Noncultivable
Mycoplasma spp.	BAL	None	PCR[a]	Special media,[b] 7–10 d
Chlamydia spp.	BAL	None	PCR[a]	Cell culture,[b] 3–5 d

BAL, bronchoalveolar lavage, brushings, bronchial biopsy, open lung biopsy, percutaneous needle biopsy; CMV, cytomegalovirus; DFA, direct fluorescent antibody stain; FAB, fluorescent antibody; HSV, herpes simplex virus; NA, not applicable; NPS, nasopharyngeal swab or wash; PCR, polymerase chain reaction; SISP, saline-induced sputum; SP, sputum; VZV, varicella-zoster virus.
[a]Research laboratories only.
[b]Culture is different; not routinely offered by clinical laboratories.
From Shelhamer JH, Gill VJ, Quinn TC, et al. The laboratory evaluation of opportunistic pulmonary infections. *Ann Intern Med* 1996;124:585–599.

Normochromic normocytic anemia in chronic stage
Albuminuria is frequent

Pulmonary Embolism and Infarction

No laboratory test is diagnostic.
Less than 10% of emboli lead to infarction.
Measurement of arterial blood gas levels (obtained when patient is breathing room air) is the most sensitive and specific laboratory test.
Po_2 <80 mm Hg in 88% of cases, but normal Po_2 does not rule out pulmonary embolus. In appropriate clinical setting, Po_2 <88 mm Hg (even with a normal chest radiograph) is indication for lung scans and search for deep vein thromboses. Po_2 >90 mm Hg with a normal chest radiograph suggests a different diagnosis. Normal complete lung scans exclude the diagnosis.
Hypocapnia and slightly elevated pH.
Increased WBC in 50% of patients but is rarely >15,000/mm^3 (whereas in acute bacterial pneumonia is often >20,000/mm^3).
Increased erythrocyte sedimentation rate.
Triad of increased levels of lactate dehydrogenase (LDH) and bilirubin with normal aspartate aminotransferase level is found in only 15% of cases.
Serum enzymes differ from those in acute myocardial infarction.
In 80% of patients, serum LDH levels (due to isoenzymes LDH_2 and LDH_3) increase on first day, peak on second, normal by tenth day.

Serum aspartate aminotransferase level is usually normal or only slightly increased.
Cardiac troponin level not increased.
Serum indirect bilirubin level is increased (as early as fourth day) to 5 mg/dL in 20% of cases.
Pleural effusion may occur.
Measure Leiden factor V, protein S, protein C, antithrombin.
Plasma D-dimer can be measured (using enzyme-linked immunosorbent assay or latex agglutination kits). Tests detect lysis of fibrin clot only, whereas fibrinogen degradation products test detects lysis of both fibrin clot and fibrinogen. At appropriate cutoff level, has >80% sensitivity but only 30% specificity. Negative predicative value >90%; normal test result useful in excluding pulmonary embolism in patients with low pretest probability. Value less than cutoff level (which varies with assay kit) obviates need for pulmonary angiography. Increased in
- Deep venous thrombosis
- Disseminated intravascular coagulation with fibrinolysis
- Renal, liver, or cardiac failure
- Major injury or surgery
- Inflammation (e.g., arthritis, cellulitis), infection (e.g., pneumonia)
- Thrombolytic therapy

Obstructive Emphysema

Laboratory findings due to decreased lung ventilation
Po_2 decreased and Pco_2 increased
Ultimate development of respiratory acidosis
Secondary polycythemia
Cor pulmonale

Pneumothorax

Accumulation of air or gas between the parietal and visceral pleurae.
Spontaneous pneumothorax may be primary or secondary.
Secondary pneumothorax may occur as a complication of an underlying lung disease.
Traumatic pneumothorax may coexist with hemothorax after resuscitation.
In tension pneumothorax, the air in the pleural space is under higher pressure than air in adjacent lung and vascular structures.

Signs and Symptoms

Sudden, sharp chest pain made worse by breathing, coughing, or moving the chest
Asymmetric chest movements
Dyspnea
Cyanosis (sometimes)
Moderate to profound respiratory distress
Tension pneumothorax: weak, rapid pulse, pallor, neck vein distension, anxiety, tracheal deviation
Shock
Circulatory collapse
Diminished breath sounds and voice sounds

Causes

Perforation of the visceral pleura and entry of gas from the lung
Gas generated by microorganisms in an empyema
Penetration of the chest wall, diaphragm, mediastinum, or esophagus
Blunt trauma to thorax

Risk Factors

Trauma (broken rib, ruptured bronchus, perforated esophagus)
Rupture of superficial lung bulla after coughing or blowing a musical instrument

Vigorous or stretching exercises
Flying (high altitude) after loss of pressurization
Diving (ascension or rapid decompression)
Pneumoconioses
Tuberculosis
Pneumonia due to *M. tuberculosis*, *Klebsiella* spp., *S. aureus*
Subpleural *Pneumocystis carinii* pneumonia (in patients with acquired immunodeficiency syndrome patients on *P. carinii* pneumonia prophylaxis via pentamidine aerosol)
Bronchial obstruction
Chronic obstructive pulmonary disease (particularly emphysema)
Neoplasms
Endometriosis (during menstruation)
Rare diseases (Marfan disease, Ehlers-Danlos syndrome)
Rupture of an infected abscess
Lymphangioleiomyomatosis
CF
Cigarette smoking
Intubation ventilation

Laboratory Tests

Arterial blood gas levels in significant pneumothorax
pH <7.35
PO_2 <80 mm Hg (10.6 kPa)
PCO_2 >45 mm Hg (6.0 kPa)

Imaging Studies

Chest radiography
Air without lung markings peripherally, mediastinal shift to contralateral side
Small pneumothorax may be evident only with expiratory or lateral decubitus film

Histiocytosis X

Diagnosis is established by open lung biopsy.
Pulmonary disorder is the major manifestation of this disease; bone involvement in minority of cases with lung disease. Pleural effusion is rare.
BAL specimens show increase in total number of cells; 2–20% Langerhans cells, small numbers of eosinophils, neutrophils, and lymphocytes, and 70% macrophages.
Mild decrease in PO_2, which falls with exercise.

Heiner Syndrome

Anemia, respiratory embarrassment, and splenomegaly in milk-consuming infants. Sputum may contain hemosiderin-laden macrophages. Eosinophilia may be present. Chest radiograph reveals patchy infiltrates.

Goodpasture Syndrome

Alveolar hemorrhage and glomerulonephritis (usually rapidly progressive) associated with antibody against pulmonary alveolar and glomerular basement membranes.
Proteinuria and red blood cells and casts in urine.
Renal function may deteriorate rapidly or renal manifestations may be decreased.
Serum may show antiglomerular basement membrane immunoglobulin G antibodies by enzyme immunoassay. Titer may not correlate with severity of pulmonary or renal disease.
Eosinophilia absent and iron-deficiency anemia more marked than in idiopathic pulmonary hemosiderosis.
Sputum or BAL specimens showing hemosiderin-laden macrophages may be a clue to occult pulmonary hemorrhage.

Renal biopsy specimens may show characteristic linear immunofluorescent deposits of immunoglobulin G and often complement, and focal or diffuse proliferative glomerulonephritis.

Other causes of combined pulmonary hemorrhage and glomerulonephritis are

- Wegener granulomatosis
- Hypersensitivity vasculitis
- Systemic lupus erythematosus
- Polyarteritis nodosa
- Endocarditis
- Mixed cryoglobulinemia
- Allergic angiitis and granulomatosis (Churg-Strauss syndrome)
- Behçet syndrome
- Henoch-Schönlein purpura
- Pulmonary-renal reactions due to drugs (e.g., penicillamine)

Cystic Fibrosis

CF, one of the most common fatal genetic disorders in the United States, is recognized by a classic triad of elevated sweat chloride concentration, pancreatic insufficiency, and chronic pulmonary disease. A defect in a single gene on chromosome 7 encodes a cyclic adenosine monophosphate–regulated chloride channel called the *CF transmembrane conductance regular* (CFTR), which usually resides on the apical membrane of epithelial cells lining the airways, biliary tree, intestines, vas deferens, sweat ducts, and pancreatic ducts.

Deficits in interleukin-10 production, inhibition of the Jak-Stat1 signaling cascade, and other abnormalities have been identified in the airway epithelial cells of CF patients.

In whites, it is estimated to occur in 1 in 2,000 to 1 in 300 live-born infants with equal sex occurrence. A higher incidence is reported in the United Kingdom and Ireland; among blacks the incidence is 1 in 4,000, and among Asians it is 1 in 90,000. One in 27 whites carries a mutant CFTR gene.

Sweat Analysis

A sweat chloride concentration greater than 40 mEq/L (mean + 3 SD of the CF heterozygote carrier group) in the presence of some appropriate clinical manifestation (chronic pulmonary disease, pancreatic insufficiency, or both) or an appropriate family history (sibling or first cousin who has CF) is diagnostic. Typically, sweat production is stimulated by iontophoresis of pilocarpine into the skin. Sweat then is collected on a preweighed filter that is carefully shielded from evaporation or contamination, leached from the filter, and analyzed for chloride by titrimetric analysis. The Wescor system (Wescor Company, Logan, UT), because it is a closed system that requires no fluid transfers, can provide accurate readings with less sweat. If testing is attempted during the first month of life, the infant may not produce an adequate amount of sweat, and the test will not be useful; however, quantitative pilocarpine iontophoresis can be used successfully in infants younger than 6 weeks of age undergoing routine diagnostic evaluations to follow up newborn screening test results positive for CF. CF heterozygote carrier infants with one F508 mutant allele show phenotypic manifestations of CF, including subclinical elevations of sweat chloride. Technical errors, except for errors in dilution of the sample, tend to produce elevated values, so a "positive" result always must be confirmed by a second test. Approximately 5% of patients who have CF exhibit sweat chloride values less than 60 mEq/L. Many physicians suggest age distribution for a positive value (i.e., 60 μg/L before age 20 years, >80 μg/L after age 20 years). There should not be more than a 10-mEq/L difference between the sodium and chloride values. The sweat test is suspect if too great a difference exists.

Diseases that may demonstrate falsely elevated sweat chlorides include the following:

- Untreated adrenal insufficiency
- Ectodermal dysplasia
- Hereditary nephrogenic diabetes insipidus
- Glucose-6 phosphatase deficiency
- Glycogen storage diseases

- Malnutrition
- Hypothyroidism
- Mucopolysaccharidosis
- Fucosidosis
- CF genetic testing

At least 750 CFTR mutations associated with CF are known; the commercially available probes test for only 70. Although these 70 mutations can be used to identify more than 90% of all CF genes, failure to find 2 abnormal genes does not rule out the disease, because in approximately 1% of those with the disease no abnormal gene can be found, and in approximately 18% more, only 1 abnormal gene is identified.

A deletion of phenylalanine at position 508 (ΔF508) accounts for more than 70% of cases of CF and is associated with severe pancreatic insufficiency and pulmonary disease. There is a simplified screening test for heterozygotes with this mutation.

Molecular genotypes are correlated with the severity of pancreatic insufficiency, but not with severity of pulmonary disease. An exception is the 455E CFTR mutant (in which alanine is changed to glutamic acid at position 455), which has been associated with mild lung disease and accounts for 3% of cases of CF in the Netherlands.

It is now possible to detect the common CFTR mutation in 85% to 90% of carriers, and thus population screening is feasible.

Nasal Potential-Difference Measurements

Nasal potential-difference measurements are measurements of the potential difference (voltage) that use as the reference electrode a saline-filled butterfly needle inserted subcutaneously in the forearm, and as the mucosal electrode, a saline-filled polyethylene tube that gently touches the mucosa near the anterior turbinate. The voltage measured correlates with the movement of sodium across cell membranes. Measurements are repeated after mucosal perfusion with amiloride, which blocks the epithelial sodium channel, causing a large drop in potential difference, which is greater in patients with CF (73%) than in normal subjects (53%). Nasal potential-difference measurements may demonstrate abnormal CFTR function more reliably than the sweat test.

Although these measurements may prove more accurate than sweat testing, the lack of commercial equipment and practical difficulties will probably restrict their use.

The immunoreactive trypsinogen test alone is not adequate to screen for CF, and research is needed to develop more accurate and feasible screening methods. It is associated with up to 15% false-negative results.

Diagnostic criteria for CF are shown in the following table:

Presence of one or more characteristic clinical features
OR
Family history of CF
OR
Positive neonatal screening test
AND
Evidence of CFTR abnormality:
Sweat chloride >60 mEq/L
OR
Mutation analysis with two characteristic alleles
OR
Nasal transmembrane potential difference

Involvement in the lung by the CF results in nearly all the mortality from the disease. Three organisms predominate: *H. influenzae*, *S. aureus*, and *P. aeruginosa*. *Haemophilus* and *Staphylococcus* appear and disappear. *Staphylococcus* reaches maximum prevalence of approximately 50% at ages 6 to 17 years and declines thereafter, and *Haemophilus* is most prevalent (approximately 20% to 25% of patients) at ages 2 to 5 years.

Pseudomonas eventually becomes established in the lungs of most CF patients, reaching 80% prevalence by age 18 years. Once established, it is not eradicated despite prolonged intensive antibiotic therapy.

Predominant Signs and Symptoms of Cystic Fibrosis

Common Presentations

Newborns and infants
- Failure to thrive
- Malabsorption
- Meconium ileus

Children
- Failure to thrive
- Malabsorption
- Recurrent nasal polyposis
- Recurrent respiratory disease
- Frequent bulky, foul smelling, pale stools with high fat content
- Vitamin deficiencies (A, D, E, K)

Adolescents and young adults
- Azoospermia
- Malabsorption
- Recurrent sinopulmonary disease

Uncommon Presentations

All age groups
- Biliary cirrhosis and portal hypertension
- Diabetes mellitus
- Edema and hypoproteinemia, hypoprothrombinemia
- Enlarged submaxillary glands
- Gallstones, biliary colic
- Hemoptysis
- Colonic strictures with high-dose enzyme replacement (310,000 U lipase/kg/d)
- Meconium ileus equivalent, intestinal obstruction syndrome
- Meconium peritonitis
- Meconium plug syndrome
- Persistent metabolic alkalosis
- Rectal prolapse
- Recurrent hyponatremia/hypochloremia and heat prostration
- Colonic strictures with high-dose enzyme replacement (710,000 U lipase/kg/d)

Pseudomonas in Cystic Fibrosis

Recovery of mucoid *Pseudomonas* from the lung should prompt diagnostic investigation for CF. Newborn screening by genetic testing provides early diagnosis for CF. The Wisconsin CF Neonatal Screening Project[6] has followed these CK patients at six monthly intervals with serum IgG, IgA, and IgM antibody titers of at least 1:256 to *P. aeruginosa*. This can be assessed by enzyme-linked immunoabsorbent assay using cell lysate, exotoxin A, and elastase as antigens. This has provided early detection of *P. aeruginosa* 6 to 12 months before the organism can be isolated from oropharyngeal cultures and affords the ability for early treatment.

Later in life, some patients acquire *Burkholderia cepacia* infection, which is associated with poorer lung function and poorer prognosis. *B. cepacia* is classified into several groups called *genomavars*, some of which have proven to be especially transmissible ("epidemic strains").

Genetics and Epidemiology

More than 1,000 different mutations have been described in the CF gene. The ΔF508 mutation, in which a phenylalanine residue is deleted at position 508 in this 1480–amino acid protein, is present in approximately 70% of CF alleles in the United States. Approximately 50% of American CF patients are homozygous for the ΔF508 mutation. Some mutations are concentrated in particular ethnic groups, such as the A455 E mutation in Dutch CF patients and the W1282X mutation in Ashkenazi Jewish patients.

Acute Respiratory Distress Syndrome

ARDS is characterized by respiratory distress with hypoxemia, decreased pulmonary compliance, and increased shunt (Qs/Qt) fraction, and radiologic evidence of diffuse pulmonary infiltrates.

There is development of proteinaceous hemorrhagic edema in the interstitium, alveolar wall, and alveolus because of the loss of alveolar capillary membrane integrity. This proteinaceous fluid can coalesce and form hyaline membranes. There is loss of

[6]West SE, Zeng L, Lee BL, et al. Respiratory infections with *Psuedomonas aeruginosa* in children with cystic fibrosis. *JAMA* 2002;287(22):2958–2967.

compliance and reduced lung volumes with severe arterial hypoxemia and a large venous admixture.

The clinical presentation is characterized by hyperventilation and then the gradual onset of respiratory distress. Hypoxemia is profound and unresponsive to delivery of supplemental oxygen by face mask or nasal prongs.

The assessment and care of these children require a plethora of laboratory-based support services. Any injury to the body that causes shock or a systemic inflammatory response can result in ARDS.

Close monitoring of serum electrolyte level, frequent blood gas measurement, and monitoring of other organ functions is essential.

Bedside devices that provide on-line measures of respiratory function, such as pulse oximetry and end tidal CO_2 monitoring, should improve the speed of response to changes in clinical status and may result in lowering the frequency of measurement of arterial blood gases.

Respiratory Diseases in the Newborn

Type II alveolar cells synthesize and secrete pulmonary surfactant, a phospholipid protein mixture that decreases surface tension and prevents alveolar collapse. It is produced in increasing quantities from 32 weeks' gestation. Factors that accelerate lung maturity include maternal hypertensive states, sickle cell disease, narcotic addition, intrauterine fetal growth retardation, and prolonged rupture of membranes.

Respiratory distress syndrome (RDS) occurs in 60% of infants of <30 weeks' gestation who have not received steroids and decreases to 35% for those who have received antenatal steroid treatment. Between 30 and 40 weeks' gestation, that rate is 25% in untreated infants and 10% in those who have received steroid treatment.

Risk increases in infants of mothers with diabetes, those delivered by cesarean section without antecedent labor, those undergoing perinatal asphyxia, second twins, and those born to mothers with a previous infant with respiratory distress syndrome.

Diagnosis

Respiratory distress worsens during the first few hours of life, progresses over 48–72 hours, and subsequently improves. Recovery is accompanied by brisk diuresis. Classically, on chest radiograph, filum lung fields have a reticulogranular pattern that may obscure the heart border.

Hypoxemia

Hypoxemia is evident on arterial blood gas analysis, but increases of carbon dioxide are seen as the disease progresses.

The primary biochemical defect in RDS is a deficiency of pulmonary surfactant. Pulmonary surfactant is composed of 80–90% phospholipid and 10% protein. The phospholipid fraction is the primary surface-tension–lowering component of pulmonary surfactant. Four distinct surfactant-associated proteins have been described. SP-A is the most abundant lipid-associated protein in pulmonary surfactant.

The other major surfactant-associated proteins, B, C, and D, are small hydrophobic molecules.

Congenital surfactant protein B deficiency occurs in infants at full term, presents with severe respiratory distress shortly after birth, and frequently leads to treatment with extracorporeal membrane oxygenation (ECMO). Lung transplant is currently the only available therapy.

Assessment of Fetal Lung Maturity

1. Measurement of lecithin/sphingomyelin ratio. Most common assay used. Sphingomyelin content is constant in amniotic fluid during the first 35 weeks (Fig. 3).
2. Direct assay of the major phospholipid components of surfactant, with phosphatidylglycerol the most common component used.
3. Measurement of surfactant protein A concentration by either enzyme-linked immunosorbent assay or radioimmunoassay techniques is available but not frequently done.

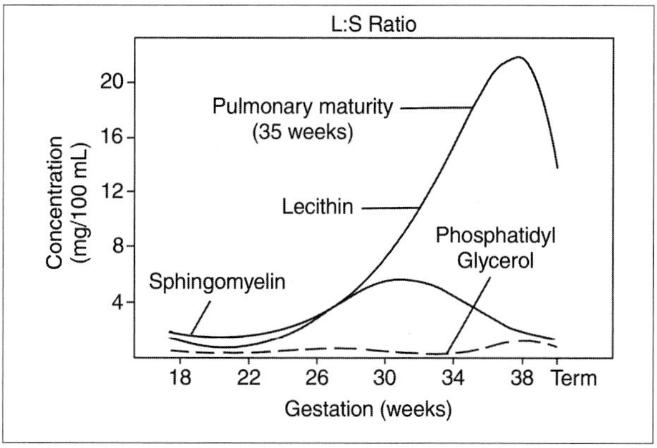

Fig. 3. Levels of sphingomyelin (S), lecithin (L), and phosphatidyl glycerol by gestational age in determination of pulmonary maturity.

Causes of Hyaline Membranes and Bronchopulmonary Dysplasia

Prematurity
Oxygen administration
Patent ductus arteriosus → pulmonary edema
Airway damage (anoxic)
Maternal diabetes (insulin inhibits surfactant by impeding maturation)
Cesarean section (impedes secretion of surfactant from type 2 alveolar cells)
Deficiency of vitamin E and vitamin A

Causes of Surfactant Deficiency

Prematurity
Pulmonary immaturity
Asphyxia
Cesarean section
Aspiration of amniotic fluid and meconium
Birth position as second of twins
Maternal hemorrhage
Congenital deficiency of surfactant protein B

Pulmonary Alveolar Proteinosis (Surfactant B Deficiency)

Rare disease characterized by amorphous, lipid-rich, proteinaceous material in alveoli.
Periodic acid–Schiff-positive material appears in sputum.
Phenolsulfonphthalein dye injected intravenously is excreted in sputum for long periods of time.
BAL fluid contains increased total protein, albumin, phospholipids, and carcinoembryonic antigen.
Antibodies to surfactant protein A (enzyme-linked immunosorbent assay) in sputum and BAL are present.
Serum carcinoembryonic antigen level is increased and correlates with BAL findings. Reflects severity of disease and decreases with response to treatment.
Routine laboratory test findings are nonspecific.
Serum LDH level is increased when protein accumulates in lungs and becomes normal when infiltrate resolves; correlates with serum carcinoembryonic antigen.
Decreased arterial O_2.
Secondary polycythemia may occur.
Diagnosis usually requires open lung biopsy. Electron microscopy shows many lamellar bodies.

Persistent Pulmonary Hypertension of the Newborn

Idiopathic or secondary to conditions leading to increased pulmonary vascular resistance. Most commonly seen in term or postterm infants, infants born via cesarean section, and infants with a history of fetal distress and low Apgar scores. Usually present within 12–24 hours of birth. Accounts for up to 2% of all neonatal intensive care unit admissions.

Physiologic conditions associated with persistent pulmonary hypertension of the newborn:

1. Vasoconstriction secondary to hypoxemia and acidosis (neonatal sepsis)
2. Interstitial pulmonary disease (meconium aspiration syndrome)
3. Hyperviscosity syndrome (polycythemia)

Anatomic Anomalies

Pulmonary hypoplasia either primary or secondary to congenital diaphragmatic hernia or renal agenesis.

Diagnostic Features

Severe hypoxemia (PaO_2 <35–45 mm Hg in 100% O_2) disproportionate to radiologic changes.

Structurally normal heart with right-to-left shunt at foramen ovale or ductus arteriosus; decreased postductal oxygen saturations compared with preductal values. Difference of at least 7–15 mm Hg between preductal and postductal PaO_2 is significant.

Must distinguish from cyanotic heart disease.

Hyperoxia Test

Supplemental oxygen is increased to 100%. Obtain blood gas levels after 20 minutes. Hypoxemia will improve if due to pulmonary parenchymal disease but not if related to persistent pulmonary hypertension of the newborn or cyanotic heart disease.

Conditions Associated with Persistent Pulmonary Hypertension of the Newborn[7]

Prenatal and Perinatal Conditions	Postnatal Conditions
Prolonged maternal aspirin or indomethacin therapy	Neonatal asphyxia
Maternal pregnancy-induced or chronic hypertension	Meconium aspiration syndrome
Maternal intravenous drug use	Sepsis neonatorum
Oligohydramnios	Pulmonary hypoplasia
Placental insufficiency and intrauterine hypoxia	Congenital diaphragmatic hernia
Postmaturity	RDS
Meconium staining of amniotic fluid	Cold stress
Perinatal asphyxia	Hypoglycemia
	Hypocalcemia
	Systemic hypotension
	Myocardial dysfunction
	Polycythemia and hyperviscosity

Apnea of Prematurity

Apnea of prematurity results from developmental immaturity of the respiratory control centers. Apnea is defined as a cessation of respiration that lasts at least 15 seconds. It is frequently accompanied by cyanosis, hypotonia, and bradycardia. The incidence and severity of apnea vary inversely with gestational age.

Laboratory Tests and Blood Gas Monitoring for Neonatal Intensive Care Units

Ideally, blood gas measurements should be done in the neonatal intensive care unit. Blood gas values should be available within 10–15 minutes. Results of emergent studies should be available within 60 minutes, and of routine studies within 4–6 hours.

[7]Soldin SJ, Rifai N, Hicks JM. *Biochemical basis of pediatric disease*, 3rd ed. Washington: American Association for Clinical Chemistry Press, 1998.

Unique problems of premature infants, especially with regard to infection, include the pathogenicity of organisms such as *Staphylococcus epidermidis* that might otherwise be dismissed as contaminants.

Bedside monitoring includes pulse oximetry and, to a lesser extent, transcutaneous Po_2 and Pco_2 monitoring.

Most critically ill newborns require arterial blood gas measurements every 1–2 hours and complete blood count and measurement of electrolyte levels and calcium concentrations every 12–24 hours. Important in the newborn, and especially the preterm infant, are total, direct, and indirect serum bilirubin levels.

Drug monitoring is needed in the neonatal intensive care unit, including monitoring of serum aminoglycoside, vancomycin hydrochloride, caffeine, and theophylline concentrations. When a new drug is started, concentrations need to be monitored daily until therapeutic levels are achieved. Nutritional monitoring must be undertaken if an infant is on hyperalimentation; this includes measurement of levels of serum electrolytes, glucose, phosphorus, magnesium, and triglycerides, and liver function studies. If a coagulopathy is suspected, coagulation profiles must be available, including platelet counts, prothrombin time, partial thromboplastin time, and levels of fibrinogen, D-dimer, and fibrin degradation products.

For infants on ECMO, arterial blood gas levels must be measured often (every 1–2 hours). This frequency can be decreased to every 2–4 hours if an in-line venous saturation monitor is used. The membrane lung blood gases will have an extremely high Po_2 (300–500 torr) due to the efficiency of the membrane lung. Laboratory tests needed every 8–12 hours include hemoglobin level, hematocrit, and levels of calcium, sodium, potassium, chloride, and CO_2. The membrane lung binds platelets, and therefore platelet values should be determined every 8 hours. Platelet counts are kept between 60,000 and 200,000 mm^3. Laboratory tests should include phosphorus level, magnesium level, serum osmolality, blood urea nitrogen level, creatinine level, and total, direct, and indirect bilirubin levels. Infants on ECMO require very little sodium replacement (1–2 mEq/kg/day), high potassium replacement (4–5 mEq/kg/day), and relatively high calcium replacement (40–50 mg of elemental calcium/kg/day).

Prolonged heparinization requires the use of a bedside test to determine activated clotting times. Centers use various systems; the Hemachron (International Technidyne, Edison, NJ) uses only 0.25 mL per sample. Activated clotting times are kept between 180 and 250 seconds depending on the bleeding complications in the patient. When disseminated intravascular coagulation is considered in an ECMO patient, prothrombin time and partial thromboplastin times obtained using the heptasorb method should be available as well as measurements of antithrombin III, fibrin degradation products, fibrinogen, and D-dimer. Plasma free hemoglobin levels are also needed on a daily basis.

Bibliography

Davis PB. Cystic fibrosis. *Pediatr Rev* 2001;22:257–264.

Davis PB, Drumm ML, Konstan MW. State of the art: cystic fibrosis. *Am J Resp Crit Care Med* 1996;154:1229–1256.

Durie PR. Pancreatic aspects of cystic fibrosis and other inherited causes of pancreatic dysfunction. *Med Clin North Am* 2000;84:609–620.

Farrell PM, Koscik RE. Sweat chloride concentrations in infants homozygous or heterozygous for F508 cystic fibrosis. *Pediatrics* 1996;97(4):524–528.

Fiel SB. Cystic fibrosis. *Clin Chest Med* 1998;19:423–567.

Gilbert-Barness E, ed. *Potter's pathology of the fetus and infant.* St. Louis: Mosby–Year Book, 1997.

Gilbert-Barness E, Barness L. *Cystic fibrosis in metabolic diseases: foundations of clinical management, genetics, and pathology.* Natick, MA: Eaton Publishing, 2000.

Hallman M, Bry K. Nitric oxide and lung surfactant. *Semin Perinatal* 1996;20:173–185.

Johnson KB. *The Johns Hopkins Hospital—The Harriet Lane handbook*, 13th ed. St. Louis, MO: Mosby, 2000.

Lewis DA, Noeton JJ. *On call pediatrics,* 2nd ed. Philadelphia: WB Saunders, 2001.

The Neonatal Inhaled Nitric Oxide Study Group. Inhaled nitric oxide in full-term and nearly full-term infants with hypoxic respiratory failure. *N Engl J Med* 1997;336:597–604.

Nogee LM, Garnier G, Dietz HC, et al. A mutation in the surfactant protein B gene responsible for fatal neonatal respiratory disease in multiple kindreds. *J Clin Invest* 1994;93:1860–1863.

2000 Red book—Report of the committee on infectious diseases, 25th ed. American Academy of Pediatrics, 2000.

Roberts JD, Fineman JR, Morin FC, et al. Inhaled nitric acid oxide and persistent pulmonary hypertension of the newborn. *N Engl J Med* 1997;336:605–610.

Schedin U, Norman M, Gustafsson LE, et al. Endogenous nitric oxide in the upper airways of premature and term infants. *Acta Paediatr* 1997;86:1129–1135.

Schidlow DV, Taussig LM, Knowles MR. Cystic Fibrosis Foundation Conference Report on Pulmonary Complications of Cystic Fibrosis. *Pediatr Pulmonol* 1993;15:187–198.

Soldin SJ, Rifai N, Hicks JM. *Biochemical basis of pediatric disease*, 3rd ed. Washington, DC: American Association for Clinical Chemistry Press, 1998.

Taussig LM. *Cystic fibrosis*. New York: Thieme-Stratton, 1984.

Tizzano F, Buchwald M. Cystic fibrosis: beyond the gene to therapy. *J Pediatr* 1992;120:337–343.

Tizzano F, Buchwald M. Recent advances in cystic fibrosis research. *J Pediatr* 1993;122:985–988.

Wallach J. *Interpretation of diagnostic tests*, 7th ed. Philadelphia: Lippincott Williams & Wilkins, 2000.

West SEH, Zeng L, Lee BL, et al. Respiratory infections with *Psuedomonas aeruginosa* in children with cystic fibrosis. *JAMA* 2002;287(22):2958–2967.

9 Gastrointestinal Diseases

Malabsorption and Malnutrition

Malnutrition and failure to grow are frequent consequences of malabsorption, which is one of the presentations of gastrointestinal disease. Other causes of malnutrition include lack of intake of food, lack of specific nutrients (e.g., iron, protein, zinc, etc.), excessive intake of one or a few nutrients as in "imbalanced" diets (e.g., amino acids), hypermetabolic states (e.g., infection, hyperthyroidism, exercise), or excess losses (e.g., diarrhea).

Chronic Malnutrition

Chronic protein-calorie malnutrition can lead to compromise of pancreatic and small bowel function. In developed countries, primary malnutrition is rare, and chronic digestive disorders account for many cases of malnutrition in children. Environmental deprivation is an important cause, as are feeding disorders (improper volume or dilution of formula). Protein-calorie malnutrition appears to contribute to the cycle of protracted diarrhea of infancy, perhaps through impairment of the functional capacity of the bowel, impairment of immune function, or the development of small-bowel bacterial overgrowth. Worldwide, exocrine pancreatic insufficiency is often attributable to malnutrition, not to a primary pancreatic disease.

Patients with kwashiorkor may have severely flattened small intestinal villi; these abnormalities are probably attributable to coexisting infections and infestations. In marasmus, villus structure is relatively well preserved, although microvillus changes and intracellular electron microscopic abnormalities are observed. Chronic malnutrition can lead to impaired immune function; bacterial overgrowth of the upper intestine is seen in malnourished subjects.

Carbohydrates

Breath Hydrogen Test

Hydrogen gas is produced by bacterial fermentation of undigested carbohydrate that reaches the colon. Hydrogen is absorbed into the blood and diffuses into the expired air. A rise in expired hydrogen concentration after oral loading with a particular carbohydrate indicates its malabsorption. In the lactose H_2 breath test, the nondigestible sugar lactulose is ingested. Usually, little H_2 is detectable for approximately 2 hours after the ingestion of lactulose. This represents the time taken for the lactulose to reach the large intestine. If H_2 is detected earlier, this could be due to bacterial contamination of the small intestine or intestinal hurry.

In the glucose H_2 breath test, glucose is ingested. Normally, little H_2 appears, as it is all absorbed before it comes into contact with bacteria. However, H_2 will appear in the breath if there is bacterial contamination of the small intestine or intestinal hurry.

Fast infants for 4–6 hours; fast older children for 12 hours. Give 2 g/kg (max: 50 g) of desired carbohydrate as a 20% solution (10% in infants younger than 6 months). Collect end-expired air in sealed plastic bags by aspirating 5 mL of air after each breath to a total of 20–30 mL via nasal prong attached to a face mask. H_2 is measured by gas chromatography on baseline sample (before carbohydrate load) and on q30-minute samples for 3 hours and is reported in parts per million.

Elevation in H_2 concentration >20 ppm above baseline is considered significant.

Breath hydrogen may be detected in children with gastric ulcers due to metabolism by *Helicobacter pylori*. The child should not be taking antibiotics at the time of the study as colonic bacteria growth may be suppressed.

Measurement of carbohydrate in stool using the Clinitest reagent for reducing substances is simple and can be performed at bedside. This is not an accurate screening test. The test is easily performed by combining ten drops of water with five drops of stool and then adding a Clinitest tablet. The color change can be quantified as trace to 4+ using a color sheet provided by the manufacturer. Only 2+ or higher should raise the possibility of sugar malabsorption. Sucrose is not a reducing sugar and requires hydrolysis with hydrochloric acid before analysis.

Stool pH lower than 5.6 is also suggestive of carbohydrate malabsorption. Stool electrolyte content less than 290 mOsm/L occurs with osmotic diarrhea and may be seen with carbohydrate malabsorption.

Monosaccharide and Disaccharide Absorption

To diagnose malabsorption of a specific carbohydrate by measuring the change in blood glucose after an oral dose of the carbohydrate in question:

- Have the patient fast 4–6 hours prior to test. Give tests carbohydrate (lactose, sucrose, maltose, glucose, galactose) orally or by gastric tube in a dose of 2.0 g/kg as a 10% solution (maximum dose of 50 g). For maltose, the dose is 1.0 g/kg.
- Measure serum glucose prior to carbohydrate dose and 30, 60, 90, and 120 minutes after the dose. Note the number and character of stools. Perform a Clinitest determination for reducing substances on all stools passed during the test and for 8 hours after the test is completed.
- A rise in blood glucose 25 mg/dL over the fasting level within the test period is considered normal. An increase of <20 mg/dL is abnormal and suggests malabsorption of the test carbohydrate.
- Malabsorption also is suggested if during or within 8 hours of test the patient develops diarrhea, stool pH <5.5, >0.5% stool-reducing substances.

Fecal pH and Sugars

There is wide variation in normal fecal pH depending on the diet. pH values of <5 suggest fermentation of unabsorbed sugars to organic acids and gases in the colon. In malabsorption of specific sugars, the stools are usually watery, frothy, and irritant. Clinitest tablets (Ames) are most often used to check fresh feces for reducing substances and will detect sugars such as glucose, lactose, and maltose. Sucrose does not react but can be converted to a reducing sugar by briefly boiling the sample with dilute hydrochloric acid. Identification of any sugars present can be undertaken using thin-layer chromatography and Clinistix (Ames), which will detect glucose only. Normal stool may contain small amounts of reducing substances (up to 0.25%). Values >0.5% are abnormal. False-negatives arise if the offending sugar is completely broken down in the colon.

Fat

A screening test for malabsorption is a microscopic examination of stool for fat. The test can be performed by mixing a small amount of stool with several drops of water or Sudan red stain. Fat droplets separate and can be easily identified, especially with a Sudan stain. The presence of more than six to eight droplets per low-power field is abnormal. Droplets accumulate at the edges of the coverslip. In disorders with pancreatic insufficiency (cystic fibrosis or Shwachman syndrome), the droplets number in the hundreds. Some malabsorption syndromes, such as gluten-sensitive enteropathy, are not always associated with fat in the stool. Serum carotene or vitamin E levels have also been used as a screening test for fat malabsorption.

Quantitative Fecal Fat

Quantitative determination of fecal fat excretion may be used to aid in diagnosis or management of fat malabsorption syndromes.

Patient should be on a normal diet with adequate fat content (35% of diet calories) and caloric intake for 2 days before beginning the test. No meals should be omitted and no medications given during the test period.

Adjust amount of fat administered to the child according to age. Attempt to deliver:
- 25 g/day in infants
- 50 g/day in toddlers
- 100 g/day in school-aged children

Record all foods given to estimate fat intake.

Collect and freeze all stools passed within 72 hours. Determine total fecal fatty acid content. For children with diarrhea or constipation, give carmine red marker (0.6 to 0.9 g) at beginning of test and again 72 hours later. Collect all stools appearing between the marker regardless of time interval.

Interpretation

Normal: Total fecal fatty acid (FA) excretion of <5.0 g fat/24 hour for children >2 years old.

Coefficient of absorption (CA):

$$CA = \frac{\text{g fat ingested} - \text{g fat excreted}}{\text{g fat ingested}} \times 100$$

Normal[1]:

Premature infants	60–75%
Newborn infants	80–85%
10 mo–3 yr	85–95%
>3 yr	95%

Fecal Electrolytes and Osmolality

Diarrhea can be divided into secretory and osmotic types. In osmotic diarrhea, malabsorbed nutrients or poorly absorbed compounds (e.g., laxatives such as lactulose) enter the colon, where the action of bacteria produces osmotically active compounds that retain water in the colon. In secretory diarrhea, the normal handling of electrolytes by the gut is disrupted. Determination of the fecal osmotic gap may help in the investigation of diarrhea, but is not diagnostically useful, presumably because diarrhea is often caused by several mechanisms working together. In secretory diarrhea, the measured osmolality of the stool water is similar to the calculated serum osmolarity [i.e., 2([NA] + [K])mmol/L]. In osmotic diarrhea, the measured osmolality is usually considerably higher than the calculated serum osmolarity (e.g., an osmotic gap of 100 mmol/Kg). For measurement of fecal osmolality, the stool specimen needs to be sufficiently liquid to allow centrifugation and separation of a water supernatant. Specimens should be fresh, as continued degradation of stool constituents by bacteria may increase the measured osmolality.

Fecal Enzymes

Measurement of pancreatic enzymes such as chymotrypsin and trypsin in feces can be used to screen for pancreatic insufficiency. Fecal pancreatic enzymes are reduced in severe pancreatic insufficiency, but these tests are insensitive in mild cases. Fecal chymotrypsin is considered more reliable than trypsin, as it is more resistant to degradation in the gut. Simple photometric assays are available using synthetic substrates such as succinyl-ala-ala-pro-phe-4-nitroanilide. The enzymes are inactivated in the colon. Antibiotic treatment may inhibit bacterial breakdown, leading to falsely normal results. Pancreatic supplements should be stopped 5 days before the test. A test for detecting pancreatic dysfunction is available that involves the measurement of fecal pancreatic elastase. This enzyme is measured immunologi-

[1]Silverman A, Roy CC. *Pediatric clinical gastroenterology.* St. Louis: CV Mosby, 1983:901. Shmerling DH, et al. Fecal fat and nitrogen in healthy children and in children with malabsorption or maldigestion. *Pediatrics* 1970;46:690.

cally, which overcomes the problem of interference of bovine pancreatic extracts in the chymotrypsin assay.

Tests

D-Xylose absorption tests.

D-Xylose is a sugar not metabolized by humans. It is absorbed in the upper small bowel.

It estimates the functional surface area of the duodenojejunal intestinal mucosa by measuring the absorption of an oral dose of D-xylose. Either the elevation in serum concentration or the urinary excretion of D-xylose may be used to quantitate D-xylose absorption. Absorption is independent of bile salts, pancreatic exocrine secretions, and intestinal mucosal disaccharidases. It is unreliable in patients with edema, renal disease, delayed gastric emptying, severe diarrhea, rapid transit time, or small bowel bacterial overgrowth.

Older children are fasted for 8 hours prior to the test; younger infants need fast for only 4–6 hours. Give D-xylose 14.5 g/m^2 BSA (max: 25 g) as a 10% water solution orally or via nasogastric tube. Collect all urine for 5 hours. Ensure adequate urine flow using supplementary oral or intravenous fluid.

The quantity of xylose is measured colorimetrically; 5-hour urinary excretion ≥25% of the administered dose is normal for children over 6 months. Values between 15% and 23% are questionable. Urinary excretion of <15% is abnormal. In infants younger than 6 months, values <10% are abnormal.

Protein

Measurement of stool α_1-antitrypsin levels is helpful in diagnosing protein-losing enteropathy.

Normally none is detectable.

Other Tests

Microbiologic tests, imaging techniques, and endoscopy/biopsy may provide more useful diagnostic information. The best diagnostic test is histologic examination of an intestinal biopsy specimen; flattened villi suggest gluten-sensitive enteropathy (coeliac disease) or tropical sprue. The histologic appearance may suggest Crohn disease or infiltration. Radiologic investigations may be useful in detecting infiltration.

Infections are a common cause of diarrhea and vomiting in children. The stools may contain blood and mucus, and tests for fecal reducing substances may be positive as a result of rapid transit and impaired absorption. Illness may be prolonged by secondary lactose intolerance after damage to the mucosa.

Permeability Tests

Disaccharides (e.g., lactulose) and large molecules (e.g., Cr-EDTA) are generally absorbed minimally. In intestinal disease, however, the gut becomes more permeable to them, probably via a paracellular mechanism, and their absorption increases. This has been used in some intestinal permeability tests, such as the ratios of lactulose/mannitol or ^{51}CrEDTA/^{14}C mannitol absorption in stools. The use of a ratio not only increases the discrimination of the test, because the changes in the urinary excretion of the two test compounds are in opposite directions, but also avoids the problem of abnormal renal function affecting the interpretation.

Intestinal Permeability Tests

Test Substance(s)	Absorption and Excretion In active small bowel Crohn or villous atrophy
Xylose	Decreased
^{51}CrEDTA	Increased
Lactulose	Increased

Mannitol	Decreased
Lactulose/mannitol ratio	Increased
^{51}CrEDTA /^{14}C mannitol	Increased

Gastric Acid Analysis

Determine status of acid secretion in hypergastrinemia patients being treated for gastrinoma.

Determine if patients who have undergone surgery for ulcer disease and who have complications are secreting acid.

Interpretation

1-hour basal acid	
<2 mEq	Normal, gastric ulcer, or carcinoma
2–5 mEq	Normal, gastric or duodenal ulcer
>5 mEq	Duodenal ulcer
>20 mEq	Zollinger-Ellison syndrome (Z-E syndrome)
1 hour after stimulation by pentagastrin	
0 mEq	Achlorhydria, gastritis, gastric carcinoma
1–20 mEq	Normal, gastric ulcer, or carcinoma
20–35 mEq	Duodenal ulcer
35–60 mEq	Duodenal ulcer, high normal, Z-E syndrome
>60 mEq	Z-E syndrome
Ratio of basal acid to post-stimulation outputs	
20%	Normal, gastric ulcer, or carcinoma
20–40%	Gastric or duodenal ulcer
40–60%	Duodenal ulcer, Z-E syndrome
>60%	Z-E syndrome

Hematologic Studies

A hypochromic, microcytic blood smear indicates iron deficiency; a macrocytic smear suggests deficiency and therefore malabsorption of folic acid or vitamin B_{12}. Acanthocyte transformation of erythrocytes occurs in abetalipoproteinemia. A blood smear may also suggest a lymphocyte defect or neutropenia associated with Shwachman-Diamond syndrome.

Imaging Procedures

Used primarily to identify local lesions in the abdomen; these procedures have limited application to the study of children with malabsorption disorders. Plain roentgenograms and barium contrast studies may suggest a site and cause of intestinal stasis. Although flocculation of normal barium and dilated bowel with thickened mucosal folds have been attributed to diffuse malabsorptive lesions such as celiac disease; these abnormalities are nonspecific. Ultrasound can detect alterations in pancreatic function, biliary tree abnormalities, and stones. Retrograde studies of the pancreatic and biliary tree using contrast injection are reserved for rare cases requiring careful delineation of the biliary and pancreatic ducts.

Fecal Occult Blood

Fecal occult blood testing can detect or confirm intestinal bleeding in a variety of conditions and, as in adults, is used in the investigation of unexplained anemia. Blood loss may be intermittent, so testing is usually conducted on three random stool specimens. The commonly used Hemoccult slides (Smith Kline Beecham Corp.) detect the peroxidase activity of heme by the oxidation of guaiac resin to give a blue coloration of the test strips. Ingestion of high doses of vitamin C can produce false-negative results.

Stool Screening Procedures

Fecal leukocytes: The presence of white cells suggests bacterial infection.

Microscopic Examination of Diarrheal Stools for Leukocytes

Primarily polymorphonuclear leukocytes (PMNs)—any number of PMNs found in less than two-thirds of cases:
Shigellosis: 70% have >5 PMNs/oil immersion field.
Salmonellosis: 30% have >5 PMNs/oil immersion field.
Campylobacter infection: 30% have >5 PMNs/oil immersion field.
Rotavirus infection: 11% have >5 PMNs/oil immersion field.
Invasive *Escherichia coli* colitis
Yersinia infection
Ulcerative colitis
Clostridium difficile infection (pseudomembranous colitis)
Primarily mononuclear leukocytes
Typhoid
Leukocytes absent
Cholera
Noninvasive *E. coli* diarrhea
Other bacterial toxins (e.g., *Staphylococcus, Clostridium perfringens*)
Viral diarrheas
Parasitic infestations (e.g., *Giardia lamblia, Entamoeba histolytica, Dientamoeba fragilis*)
Drug effects
pH and reducing substances: To screen for carbohydrate malabsorption and colonic fermentation; stool will be acidic and reducing substances will be present if malabsorption is occurring.
Occult blood (Gastroccult/Hemoccult): Blood present in stool may indicate bacterial infection, inflammation, or protein allergy/intolerance.
Sudan III: To screen for fecal fat malabsorption.
Stool electrolytes and osmotic gap: Stool osmotic gap may be calculated with the formula: $290^{*} - 2 \times [(Na) \times (K)]$
Secretory diarrheas tend to have elevated stool [Na] and a resultant lower osmotic gap (<100 mOsm/L). In malabsorption or viral illness, the stool tends to have decreased [Na] and increased stool osmotic gap (>100 mOsm/L).

*Plasma osmolality of 290 is used because stool osmolarity will increase after stool excretion due to bacterial fermentation, which continues in the sample.

Diagnostic Studies

The results of the history and physical examination and the above stool screening procedures should help to direct further studies including complete white blood cell count, erythrocyte sedimentation rate, electrolytes, radiographic studies, cultures for bacteria, viruses, and parasites, fecal fat collection, breath hydrogen test, sweat chloride tests, and endoscopy with intestinal biopsy.

Tests for Vitamin B_{12} Absorption

In the Schilling test, an injection of 25 mg of vitamin B_{12} is given to saturate body stores. A tracer dose of radioactive vitamin B_{12} with or without intrinsic factor is given by mouth. Urinary excretion is measured over the next 24 hours. With defective absorption, less than 5% of the label appears in the urine. Defective absorption in the absence of intrinsic factor occurs with pernicious anemia. Defective absorption in the presence of intrinsic factor suggests bacterial overgrowth in the bowel and occurs in those after resection of large portions of the ileum.
In juvenile pernicious anemia, intrinsic factor production in the stomach is defective. Vitamin B_{12} malabsorption results, leading to megaloblastic anemia and growth failure. Gastric structure and function are otherwise normal.
Transcobalamin II deficiency is an inherited defect of protein necessary for intestinal transport of vitamin B_{12}. The result is severe megaloblastic anemia, diarrhea, and vomiting.
In Imerslund syndrome, ileal absorption of vitamin B_{12} is defective. Ileal structure and function are otherwise normal. Megaloblastic anemia develops toward the end of the first year. Proteinemia is commonly present.

Urinary and serum methylmalonate elevations are usual in those with vitamin B_{12} deficiency.

Congenital Malabsorption of Folic Acid

A few patients have had folic acid deficiency in infancy as the result of a specific defect in folic acid assimilation. In addition to megaloblastic anemia, they had cerebral degeneration.

Amino Acid Transport Defects

Amino acid uptake into the intestinal mucosa is defective in cystinuria, but these patients have no gastrointestinal symptoms. In Hartnup disease, malabsorption of neutral amino acids including tryptophan leads to ataxia, intellectual deterioration, a pellagra-like skin rash, and, at times, diarrhea. Methionine malabsorption is associated with episodes of diarrhea in fair-complexioned, retarded children whose urine has sweet odor and contains excess β-hydroxybutyric acid. In the blue diaper syndrome, tryptophan absorption is defective.

Gastrin (Serum)

Patient should fast and not take peptic ulcer medication. Serum is separated promptly and frozen.

Test is by immunoassay. It is used in patients with atypical peptic ulcer disease and Z-E syndrome but not with typical peptic ulcer disease. Other causes of elevated gastrinoma include atrophic gastritis and pernicious anemia.

Normal serum level is <100 ng/L. Diagnostic levels are >500 ng/L.

Increased Serum Gastrin with Gastric Acid Normal or Slight Hypersecretion

RA
Diabetes mellitus
Pheochromocytoma
Vitiligo
Chronic renal failure with serum creatinine >3 mg/dL; occurs in 50% of patients
Pyloric obstruction with gastric distention
Short-bowel syndrome due to massive resection or extensive regional enteritis
Incomplete vagotomy

Small-Bowel Biopsy

Small-bowel biopsy identifies diseases of the small-bowel mucosa that are associated with histologic findings, including gluten-sensitive enteropathy, abetalipoproteinemia, lymphangiectasia, congenital microvillus inclusion disease, eosinophilic gastroenteritis, infectious disorders, and Whipple disease (rare in children). The biopsy can be safely performed by upper gastrointestinal endoscopy. At the time of biopsy, in addition to mucosa, it is possible to collect aspirates for examination for *Giardia* or bacterial culture. Mucosal samples can be frozen to assay for disaccharidase activities later. Reduction of a specific enzyme or group of enzymes is consistent with a specific deficiency (e.g., lactase or sucrase-isomaltase deficiency).

Gastroesophageal Reflux Disease

Gastroesophageal reflux disease (GERD) occurs in almost all infants and slowly resolves over the first year of life. Disease is manifested by dysphagia, bronchospasm, cough, failure to thrive, and intermittent apnea. In older children, in addition, heartburn, chest pain, chronic cough, loss of dental enamel, vomiting, and acid hypersecretion may occur. Incidence is increased in developmentally delayed infants and children, those with repaired tracheoesophageal fistula, those with hiatal hernia, and those consuming foods that irritate the esophageal mucosa or medicines that lower the pressure of the lower esophageal sphincter.

Tests include esophageal pH monitoring, esophageal manometry, gastric analysis, chest x-ray for aspiration pneumonia, and fluoroscopic esophagography. Acid pH is found above the lower esophageal sphincter. On fluoroscopy, barium flows from the stomach to the esophagus.

Diarrhea

Diarrhea, a common presentation of gastrointestinal diseases, is the passage of frequent loose watery stools due to a derangement in intestinal water and electrolyte transport or to disturbances in motility.

Food-sensitive enteropathies are commonly seen in infants and may occur at any age.

Intolerance to cow's milk or infant formulas occurs in 0.3–7.0% of infants. No test is specific, but elimination diets or measurement of serum IgE may be helpful. In the older child, in addition, skin or radioallergosorbent assay test (RAST) may be used. Stools may contain blood.

Infectious Diarrhea

Diarrhea may result from infection of the gastrointestinal tract, gastroenteritis (enteral diarrhea) or from infections [e.g., upper respiratory, pneumonia, hepatitis, or urinary infection (parenteral diarrhea)]. Enteral diarrhea may be caused by viruses, bacteria, protozoan, or be antibiotic associated (colitis). Testing is only indicated when diarrhea is severe or persistent. Tests include feces for microscopy culture, and antigen detection and blood culture. If protozoa are suspected, examine feces for ova, cysts, and parasites (q.v.). If dehydration is severe, determine electrolytes and other customary tests for dehydration (q.v.).

Causes for Diarrhea

Acute (course self-limited, lasting <14 days)

Infectious (bacterial, viral, parasitic): Rotavirus, Norwalk agent, adenovirus, *Yersinia*, *Salmonella*, *Shigella*, enterotoxic *E. coli* (0157), *C. difficile*, *Campylobacter jejuni*, *Klebsiella*

Chronic (course lasting >14 days)

Infectious (bacterial, viral, parasitic): Enteroadherent *E. coli*, *Giardia*, amebiasis, cryptosporidium, *C. difficile*, human immunodeficiency virus

Inflammatory: ulcerative colitis, Crohn disease

Malabsorption

Impaired intraluminal digestion: cystic fibrosis, Schwachman syndrome, interrupted enterohepatic circulation (Crohn disease, ileal resection), Johanson-Blizzard syndromes, biliary atresia, impaired bile acid synthesis, bacterial overgrowth

Mucosal malabsorption: celiac disease, combined immune deficiency, hypogammaglobulinemia, IgA deficiency, A-abetalipoproteinemia, food protein sensitivity, intestinal lymphangiectasia, short-bowel syndrome, congenital sucrose-isomaltase deficiency, lactase deficiency

- Allergic
- Malignancy: neuroblastoma, ganglioneuroma
- Intestinal obstruction: Hirschsprung disease, malrotation
- Malnutrition
- Radiation

Secretory (Abnormal Electrolyte Transport) Diarrhea

Increased water and chloride secretion; normal water and sodium absorption may be inhibited.

Causes

Exogenous

Laxatives (e.g., aloe, anthraquinones, bisacodyl, castor oil, dioctyl sodium sulfosuccinate, phenolphthalein, senna)

Drugs

Diuretics (e.g., furosemide, thiazides), asthma drugs (theophylline), thyroid drugs
Cholinergic drugs
Myasthenia gravis (cholinesterase inhibitors)
Cardiac (quinidine) and antihypertensives [angiotensin-converting enzyme (ACE) inhibitors]
Antidepressants (clozapine)
Gout (colchicine)
Toxins (e.g., arsenic, mushrooms, organophosphates, alcohol)
Bacterial toxins (e.g., *S. aureus, E. coli, Vibrio cholerae, Bacillus cereus, C. jejuni, Yersinia enterocolitica, Clostridium botulinum* and *perfringens*)
Endogenous
Hormones

- Serotonin (carcinoid)
- Calcitonin (medullary carcinoma of thyroid)
- Villous adenoma
- Vipoma

Gastric hypersecretion
Z-E syndrome
Systemic mastocytosis
Basophilic leukemia
Short-bowel syndrome
Bile salts (e.g., disease or resection of terminal ileum)
Fatty acids (e.g., disease of small intestine mucosa, pancreatic insufficiency)
Congenital (e.g., congenital chloridorrhea, congenital sodium diarrhea)

Exudative Diarrhea

Active inflammation of bowel mucosa
Inflammation:
Infectious [e.g., *Shigella, Salmonella, Campylobacter, Yersinia, C. difficile*, tuberculosis (TB) organisms, amebas viruses]
Idiopathic (e.g., ulcerative colitis, Crohn disease)
Injury (e.g., radiation)
Ischemia (e.g., mesenteric thrombosis)
Vasculitis
Abscess (e.g., diverticulosis)
Stool contains blood and pus.
Some features of osmotic diarrhea may be present.
20–40% of cases of acute infectious diarrhea remain undiagnosed.

Toddler Diarrhea

Children 1–4 years of age may have loose, occasionally watery stools after each meal. If weight gain is normal or almost normal with no other symptoms, investigation is usually unnecessary. Decreased intake of fruit juices or carbonated liquids may decrease stool frequency. Diarrhea spontaneously resolves.

Inherited Disorders Affecting Gut Function

See Table 1.

Gastrointestinal Causes of Hypoproteinemia

Inflammatory bowel disease
Gluten-sensitive enteropathy
Cystic fibrosis
Shwachman syndrome
Disorders with secondary small-bowel mucosal damage (e.g., infectious disorders)
Intestinal lymphangiectasia (primary or secondary)
Hypertrophic gastropathy
Eosinophilic gastroenteropathy

Table 1. Inherited Disorders Affecting Gut Function (All Are Autosomal Recessive Except As Noted)

Defect	Effects	Symptoms/Signs	Investigations
Marked reduction of brush border lactase activity	Maldigestion of lactose	Neonatal form (rare): diarrhea, vomiting, malnutrition Late-onset form (common): flatulence, abdominal pain, diarrhea	Acid feces containing lactose Reduced lactase activity on intestinal biopsy
Absence or marked reduction of brush border sucrase-isomaltase activity	Maldigestion of sucrose and dextrins	Diarrhea with or without vomiting when sucrose/dextrins introduced into diet	Acid feces containing sucrose Reduced sucrase activity on intestinal biopsy Hydrogen breath test
Reduced activity of brush border trehalase activity	Maldigestion of trehalose (autosomal dominant)	Abdominal pain, diarrhea after consumption of large amount of trehalose	Acid feces containing trehalose Reduced trehalose activity on intestinal biopsy
Defect in Na^+/glucose cotransporter	Malabsorption of glucose and galactose	Severe diarrhea, dehydration Failure to thrive	Acid feces containing glucose and galactose Normal activity of brush border disaccharidases Flat glucose tolerance test, normal xylose tolerance test
Abetalipoproteinemia (defective apo B48 and B100)	Malabsorption of lipids	Steatorrhea, acanthocytosis, ataxia, retinitis pigmentosa	Low serum cholesterol and triglycerides Absent chylomicrons, low-density lipoproteins, very-low-density lipoprotein, and apo B Low VITE acanthocytes
Pancreatic lipase deficiency	Maldigestion of lipids	Gross steatorrhea	Fecal fat Lipase activity in duodenal fluid
Familial chloride diarrhea	Defective reabsorption of chloride from ileum and colon	Severe diarrhea, dehydration	High fecal chloride loss

Acrodermatitis enteropathica	Defective zinc absorption	Diarrhea, failure to thrive, skin lesions	Serum zinc usually low Low serum alkaline phosphatase (Zn dependent) Monitor clinical response to oral zinc
Congenital enteropeptidase deficiency (decreased activation of trypsin and other pancreatic proteases)	Maldigestion of proteins	Diarrhea, vomiting, failure to thrive Edema, adaption occurs; normal diet tolerated later in life	Analysis of duodenal fluid for protease activity ± enteropeptidase in reaction mixture Enteropeptidase activity on intestinal biopsy
Lysinuric protein intolerance	Decreased absorption of lysine, arginine, ornithine	Diarrhea, failure to thrive, vomiting	Raised urine and low plasma lysine, arginine, and ornithine
Defective transport of lysine, arginine, ornithine	Increased loss in urine	Hepatomegaly	Raised blood ammonia and increased orotic acid excretion after a protein load
Glucose-galactose malabsorption	Decreased absorption of disaccharides	Watery diarrhea	Stool reduces substance sugar challenge
Sucrase-isomaltase deficiency	Starch, sucrose intolerance	Watery diarrhea	Eliminate dietary sucrose, starch
Fructose intolerance	Fructose ingestion severe diarrhea, failure to thrive, decreased vitamins A, E	Severe diarrhea, jaundice, hepatomegaly	Liver, fructoaldolase
Chylomicron retention disease	Atherosclerosis	Coronary artery disease, liver disease	Biopsy of enterocytes (absent chylomicrons)

Milk protein sensitivity
Trypsinogen or enterokinase deficiency

Disaccharidase Deficiencies

Clinical Manifestations

Watery osmotic diarrhea with stools with low pH (pH <5.6) contain excess sugar and tend to excoriate the buttocks.

Diagnosis

If the disaccharide involved is a reducing sugar (lactose), the standard Clinitest examination (Bayer Corp., Elkhart, IN) will be 2+ or greater in most cases. Disaccharidase activities can be assayed in mucosal biopsy specimens. Breath hydrogen excretion after an oral sugar load is a useful noninvasive technique for detecting disaccharide intolerance.

Lactose Intolerance

Inability to digest lactose (the primary sugar in milk) into its constituents, glucose and galactose, due to low levels of lactase enzyme in the brush border of the duodenum.

Congenital lactose intolerance—very rare.

Primary lactose intolerance—genetically controlled. Adults in whom a low level of lactase has developed after childhood. Lactose activity develops later in the fetus and intolerance occurs in extremely premature infants. Symptoms are experienced after consumption of milk. Intolerance varies with amount of lactose consumed. Primary lactose intolerance varies according to race: 75–90% of American Indians, blacks, Asians, Mediterraneans, and Jews; less than 5% of descendants of Northern and Central Europeans.

Secondary lactose intolerance—inability to digest lactose caused by any condition injuring the intestinal mucosa (e.g., diarrhea) or a reduction of available mucosal surface (e.g., resection). Especially with rotavirus disease. Also fairly common with giardiasis and ascariasis, inflammatory bowel disease (IBD), abetalipoproteinemia, immunoglobulin, deficiency, sprue, cystic fibrosis, and the acquired immunodeficiency syndrome (AIDS) malabsorptive syndrome. Many lactose-intolerant women regain ability to digest lactose during pregnancy. Duration of the intolerance determined by the nature and course of the primary condition.

50% or more of infants with acute or chronic diarrhea have lactose intolerance, especially with rotavirus disease. Also, fairly common with giardiasis and ascariasis, inflammatory bowel disease, and the AIDS malabsorption syndrome.

Lactose malabsorption—inability to absorb lactose. This does not necessarily parallel lactose intolerance.

Signs and symptoms of lactose intolerance include bloating, cramping, abdominal discomfort, diarrhea or loose stools, flatulence, rumbling (borborygmi).

Only one-third to one-fifth of people with lactose malabsorption will develop symptoms. Degree of symptoms varies with lactose load and with other foods consumed at the same time.

In children—vomiting is common; frothy, acid stools; malnutrition can occur.

Laboratory Tests

Low fecal pH and reducing substances only valid when stools are collected fresh and assayed immediately.

Special Tests

Lactose breath hydrogen test—especially in children
Lactose absorption test—alternative to lactose breath hydrogen test in adults

Diagnostic Procedures

Small-bowel biopsy for assay of lactase activity—may be normal if deficiency is focal or patchy (not readily available and usually not necessary).

Sucrase-Isomaltase Deficiency

The only relatively common congenital deficiency of disaccharidase activities, a combination deficiency of sucrase and isomaltase, is inherited as an autosomal-recessive trait and occurs in about 0.2% of North Americans. Symptoms usually begin when a sucrose or glucose polymer-containing diet is started. Patients may be intolerant of starch, but because isomaltase acts only on the branch points of the starch molecule, isomaltase deficiency itself is relatively asymptomatic. The symptoms are bloating, watery diarrhea, and failure to thrive. Recurrent abdominal pain has not been attributed to sucrose-isomaltose intolerance. Because sucrose is not a reducing sugar, its presence is not detected in the stool by Clinitest unless the specimen is first hydrolyzed with hydrochloric acid. Breath testing usually demonstrates an increased hydrogen gas after sucrose ingestion. Affected patients improve quickly after dietary sucrose is reduced to minimal amounts.

Glucose-Galactose Malabsorption

This is a rare autosomal-recessive congenital disorder of intestinal glucose-galactose absorption.

Watery stools follow the ingestion of glucose, breast milk, or conventional formulas. Most dietary sugars are polysaccharides or disaccharides with glucose or galactose moieties. The patient may be bloated, and, if diarrhea persists, dehydration and acidosis can be severe, resulting in death. The stools are acidic and contain sugar.

Severe diffuse mucosal damage, particularly in a young infant, may also impair the glucose-galactose carrier sufficiently and cause intolerance to these sugars.

Isolated Enzyme Deficiencies

Isolated deficiencies of trypsinogen, enterokinase, lipase, and colipase have been reported. Although enterokinase is a brush border enzyme, deficiency causes pancreatic insufficiency because pancreatic proteins remain inactive. Deficiencies of trypsinogen or enterokinases manifest with failure to thrive, hypoproteinemia, and edema. Isolated amylase deficiency has not been shown to exist as primary, permanent enzyme deficiency. Pancreatic enzyme replacements restore normal digestion function.

Congenital Chloridorrhea

This rare autosomal-recessive condition is characterized by profound watery diarrhea beginning at birth due to ion transport defect in ileum and colon. It is characterized by hypochloremic, hypokalemic acidosis with volume depletion, copious acidic chloride-rich watery diarrhea, and normal intestinal mucosal histology. Maternal hydramnios is almost always present.

It is similar to the rarer autosomal-recessive condition of congenital sodium diarrhea with sodium-rich alkaline stool and systemic acidosis.

Congenital Sodium Diarrhea

A few patients have been described with profuse watery diarrhea from birth. There was maternal polyhydramnios and neonatal abdominal distention; however, unlike chloride diarrhea, this condition was characterized by acidosis and fecal chloride concentration less than sodium concentration.

Primary Hypomagnesemia

This specific defect in magnesium transport causes severe hypomagnesemia and, secondarily, hypocalcemic tetany in infancy. Other aspects of intestinal function are normal. The findings are reversed by large supplements of magnesium, which must be continued indefinitely.

Celiac Disease

Celiac disease is a severe, permanent intolerance of gluten. Presentation is variable. Typically, young children present with diarrhea, vomiting, abdominal distention, malnutrition, steatorrhea, flatulence, abdominal pain, weight loss, and growth failure; clubbing of fingers and edema may occur.

The disease may be insidious in older children, who may present with short stature, anemia, delayed puberty, or a variety of nongastrointestinal complaints. Biochemical tests are of little help in the diagnosis other than to document malabsorption. α-Gliadin antibodies, found in 80–90% of children with untreated celiac disease, provide a useful screening test. Serum titres of antibodies to reticulum and endomysium are increased in untreated disease and are the most specific noninvasive tests. The antibody titer falls on gluten withdrawal and may be normal within 6 months. A rise in titer thereafter is a good indicator of noncompliance. Transglutaminase is the target antigen for antiendomysial antibodies and an ELISA test for antitransglutaminase antibodies has been developed. Other laboratory tests include:

72-hour fecal fat showing >7% fat malabsorption

D-xylose test showing malabsorption of this sugar

Decreased prothrombin time

Decreased serum neutral fats, cholesterol, vitamins E, A, B_{12}, and C, folic acid, serum iron, calcium, and total protein

Pancreatic secretion is decreased as a result of lowered cholecystokinin and secretion.

Upper gastrointestinal series shows flocculation of barium, edema, and flattening of mucosal folds.

As many as 2–5% of first-degree relatives have symptomatic gluten-sensitive enteropathy. The disorder is associated with HLA antigen types DR7, DR3, DQ_W3, and B8. Histologic findings on small intestinal biopsy confirm the diagnosis.

Pathology

Small intestinal mucosa on small-bowel biopsy shows short, flat villi, deepened crypts, and irregular vacuolated surface epithelium with lymphocytes in the epithelial layer. Infections such as rotavirus enteritis, *Giardia lamblia*, or tropical sprue can cause villus flattening and elongated crypts but not the marked abnormalities of enterocytes. Flat mucosa occurs in kwashiorkor but may represent a response to infestation rather than to undernutrition. Tropical sprue can cause a lesion that is indistinguishable from that of celiac disease. Some cases of cow's milk protein or soy protein intolerance are associated with lesions similar to those of celiac disease in children. In immune deficiency, eosinophilic gastroenteritis, and autoimmune enteropathy, villi can be partially shortened. Infants with familial enteropathy have short villi, but the crypt dimensions are normal.

Laboratory findings due to frequently associated diseases (e.g., especially lymphoma of intestine and elsewhere; also dermatitis herpetiformis, insulin-dependent diabetes, selective IgA deficiency, carcinoma of esophagus, small intestine, and breast; possibly IgA nephropathy, ulcerative colitis, thyroid disease, primary biliary cirrhosis, sclerosing cholangitis) may be similar. Diagnosis should be considered in cases of iron-deficiency anemia without demonstrable bleeding, unexplained folate deficiency, or unexplained osteopenic bone disease.

Tropical Sprue

This syndrome is characterized by generalized malabsorption associated with a diffuse lesion of the small intestinal mucosa that occurs only in persons who have lived in or visited certain tropical regions. It occurs in some Caribbean countries (not Jamaica), northern South America, Africa, and parts of Asia. Fever and malaise precede the onset of watery diarrhea. In approximately 1 week, acute features subside and chronic malabsorption, intermittent diarrhea, and anorexia lead eventually to severe malnutrition. Patients have evidence of diffuse malabsorption, including steatorrhea and carbohydrate intolerance. Megaloblastic anemia is the result of folate and vitamin B_{12} deficiencies. Biopsy of the small intestinal mucosa shows villus shortening, increased crypt depth, and an increase in chronic inflammatory cells in the lamina propria.

Gastrointestinal Bleeding

Upper Gastrointestinal Bleeding

Nosebleed
Oral or pharyngeal trauma
Esophagitis or gastritis
Esophageal varices
Mallory-Weiss tear
Peptic ulcer, duodenitis
Swallowed maternal blood (newborn)

Lower Gastrointestinal Bleeding

Anorectal fissure (complication of constipation)
Colitis (ulcerative, ischemic, infectious)
Hemorrhoids
Meckel diverticulum
Intussusception
Hemolytic-uremic syndrome
Crohn disease
Milk protein allergy (infants)

Inflammatory Bowel Disease

IBD is a group of idiopathic chronic disorders and includes Crohn disease and ulcerative colitis (UC). The etiology is poorly understood, and the natural course is characterized by unpredictable exacerbations and remissions. The most common time of onset of IBD is during adolescence and young adulthood but may begin in the first year of life.

In children, there are added problems of poor growth and delayed puberty. An infectious cause should be excluded, followed by radiologic investigations, endoscopy, and biopsy. Assessment of the acute phase response may help distinguish Crohn disease from ulcerative colitis. The response is poor or absent in ulcerative colitis, with acute phase protein concentrations lower than expected for the degree of inflammation. Crohn disease produces a more marked acute phase response. C-reactive protein and α_1-antichymotrypsin provide a useful screen for inflammation in adults and may be used to monitor progress. There is no acute phase response in irritable bowel syndrome.

Ulcerative Colitis

UC is one of a group of inflammatory bowel diseases of unknown etiology characterized by intermittent bouts of inflammation of all or portions of the colon, manifested by recurrences of rectal bleeding, abdominal pain, fever, weight loss, and arthritis.

Laboratory studies include anemia and hypoalbuminemia. Blood antineutrophil cytoplasm antibodies are found in most patients. Endoscopy reveals colitis with no skip areas. X-ray may reveal loss of haustral markings.

Crohn Disease

Children with Crohn disease often appear chronically ill. They commonly have weight loss and are often malnourished. Linear growth retardation frequently precedes clinical presentation. There may be abdominal pain or tenderness that is either diffuse or localized to the right lower quadrant. A tender mass or fullness may be palpable in the right lower quadrant. Large anal skin tags (1–3 cm diameter) or perianal fistulas with purulent drainage are suggestive of Crohn disease. Digital clubbing, arthritis, and skin manifestations such as erythema multiforme may be present.

Findings on colonoscopy may include patchy, nonspecific inflammatory changes (erythema, friability, loss of vascular pattern), aphthous ulcers, linear ulcers, nodularity, and strictures. On biopsy, only nonspecific inflammatory changes may be found.

Some patients with Crohn disease have a mutated NOD_2 gene. Many patients have antisaccharomyces antibodies.

Comparison of Crohn Disease and Ulcerative Colitis

Feature	Crohn Disease	Ulcerative Colitis
Abdominal mass	Common	Not present
Rectal bleeding	Not present	Sometimes
Rectal disease	Occasional	Nearly universal
Ileal involvement	Common	None
Perianal disease	Unusual	Common
Strictures	Common	Unusual
Fistula	Common	Unusual
Discontinuous (skip) lesions	Common	Not present
Transmural involvement	Usual	Less common
Crypt abscesses	Less common	Common
Granulomas	Common	Unusual
Risk for colonic cancer	Slightly increased	Greatly increased
Pyoderma gangrenosum	Less common	Present
Erythema nodosum	Common	Less common
Mouth ulcers	Common	Rare
Cholangitis	Present	Less common

Colitis, Pseudomembranous

Pseudomembranous colitis (PC) is an inflammatory bowel disorder associated with antibiotic use and with mild diarrhea, or it may progress to a severe colitis. Frequently, stool culture is positive for *C. difficile.*

Stool culture is nondiagnostic because some strains are nontoxigenic, and >50% of healthy neonates, 2–5% of healthy adults, and 25% of adults recently treated with antibiotics are carriers. Nontoxigenic strains may be found in 10–20% of hospitalized patients. PCR of stool for toxin A and/or B may be available.

Abdominal x-ray reveals distorted haustral markings and colonic distention.

Computed tomography (CT) scan shows thickened or edematous colonic wall with pericolonic inflammation.

Note: Avoid barium enemas.

Homozygous Hypobetalipoproteinemia

An autosomal-dominant trait. This form is indistinguishable from abetalipoproteinemia. However, the parents of these patients as heterozygotes have reduced plasma low-density lipoprotein (LDL) and apoprotein-β concentrations, unlike the parents of patients with abetalipoproteinemia, who have normal levels.

Abetalipoproteinemia

This autosomal-recessive condition is associated with severe fat malabsorption from birth. Children fail to thrive during the first year of life and their stools are pale, foul smelling, and bulky. The abdomen is distended, and deep tendon reflexes are absent as a result of peripheral neuropathy.

After 10 years of age, intestinal symptoms are less severe, ataxia develops, and a loss of position and vibration senses occurs. In adolescence retinitis pigmentosa develops.

Diagnosis

Diagnosis rests on finding acanthocytes in the peripheral blood and extremely low plasma levels of cholesterol (<50 mg/dL). Chylomicrons and very-low-density lipoproteins are not detectable, and the LDL fraction is virtually absent from the circulation; marked triglyceride accumulation in villus enterocytes occurs in the fasting duodenal mucosa. Usually, steatorrhea occurs in younger patients. Patients have mutations of the microsomal triglyceride transfer protein (MTP) gene resulting in absence of MTP function in the small bowel. This protein is required for normal assembly and secretion of very-low-density lipoproteins and chylomicrons. The neuropathy is the result of vitamin E deficiency.

Hormone-Secreting Tumors

Certain tumors secrete hormones which cause severe diarrhea. Many of these hormones have been identified (Table 2).

Other Malabsorptive Syndromes

Intestinal Lymphangiectasia

This disorder is characterized by dilatation of intestinal lymphatic vessels and leakage of lymph into the intestinal lumen and, at times, the peritoneal cavity. Because absorbed fat is normally transferred from the intestine via the lymphatic vessels, children with this disorder have steatorrhea with protein-losing enteropathy and may have lymphocyte depletion. Manifestations may include any combination of hypoalbuminemia, hypogammaglobulinemia, edema, lymphocytopenia, fat malabsorption, and chylous ascites. Intestinal lymphangiectasia can be primary or can result from abdominal or thoracic surgical damage to lymphatic vessels, chronic right-sided heart failure, constrictive pericarditis, retroperitoneal tumor, or malrotation with lymphatic obstruction. Primary intestinal lymphangiectasia is the result of a congenital abnormality of lymphatic drainage from the intestine and may be associated with abnormalities in lymphatic drainage from other regions of the body. Turner and Noonan syndromes have been associated with intestinal lymphangiectasia.

The diagnosis is suggested by an elevated fecal α_1-antitrypsin level consistent with protein-losing enteropathy. The characteristic radiologic findings of uniform, symmetric thickening of mucosal folds throughout the small intestine are usually present on small-bowel contrast radiographs. The diagnosis is confirmed by the presence of collections of abnormal dilated lacteals with distortion of villi on peroral small bowel biopsy. The disorder may be seen only in the submucosa, thus requiring surgical biopsy of the intestine.

Microvillus Inclusion Disease (Congenital Microvillus Atrophy)

Microvillus inclusion disease is a disorder that presents at birth with intractable, watery diarrhea and severe malabsorption. It appears to be the most common cause of persistent diarrhea that begins in the neonatal period, inherited in an autosomal recessive pattern. The findings on small-bowel biopsy are the key to the diagnosis and include villus atrophy, crypt hypoplasia, and, on electron microscopy, microvillus inclusions in enterocytes and colonocytes. The somatostatin analog octreotide has been used as treatment and may reduce the volume of stool output in some infants. Epidermal growth factor has been used with equivocal results. Infants with this disorder require total parenteral nutrition for survival and may be candidates for bowel transplantation.

Tufting Enteropathy

Tufting enteropathy (intestinal epithelial dysplasia) is a disorder that presents in the first weeks of life with persistent watery diarrhea. Onset of symptoms is not immediately after birth as in microvillus inclusion disease. On small-bowel biopsy, the distinctive feature is that 80–90% of the epithelial surface contains focal epithelial

Table 2. Diarrhea Caused by Hormone-Secreting Tumors

Name	Site	Hormone	Manifestations	Therapy
APUDomas[a]				
VIPoma	Pancreas	VIP	Watery diarrhea, achlorhydria, hypokalemia	Somatostatin Resection
Somatostatinoma	Pancreas	Somatostatin	Massive diarrhea[b]	Resection
Gastrinoma	Pancreas	Gastrin	Peptic ulcer, diarrhea	Cimetidine Tumor resection
Carcinoid	Intestinal argentaffin cells	Serotonin	Diarrhea, crampy abdominal pain, flushing, wheezing, cardiac valve damage	Somatostatin Resection
Mastocytoma	Cutaneous intestine, liver, spleen	Histamine, VIP	Pruritus, flushing, apnea, if VIP is positive, diarrhea	H_1- and H_2-blocking agents cromolyn, steroids Resection if solitary
Medullary carcinoma	Thyroid	Calcitonin, VIP, prostaglandins	Watery diarrhea	Thyroidectomy
Neurogenic				
Ganglioneuroma, ganglioneuroblastoma	Extraadrenal sites and adrenals	Catecholamines, VIP	Massive watery diarrhea	Resection
Pheochromocytoma	Chromaffin cells; abdominal >other sites	Catecholamines, VIP	Hypertension, tachycardia, sweating, anxiety, watery diarrhea[b]	Resection

APUDoma, amine precursor uptake and decarboxylation of amino acids; VIP, vasoactive intestinal polypeptide.
[a]APUDoma cells are neural crest cell derivatives of the gastroenteropancreatic endocrine system.
[b]Reported only in adults.
From Behrman RE, Kliegman RM, Jenson HB, eds. *Nelson textbook of pediatrics,* 16th ed. Philadelphia: WB Saunders Co. 2000, with permission.

"tufts" (teardrop-shaped groups of closely packed enterocytes with apical rounding of the plasma membrane). On electron microscopy of small-bowel epithelium, the major finding is shortening of the microvilli. The intestinal lesion does not respond to removal of dietary antigens or the use of immunosuppressive therapy. This may be a disorder of cell-cell and cell matrix interactions.

Other Chronic Inflammatory Intestinal Disorders

Immune-Inflammatory

Congenital immunodeficiency disorders
Acquired immunodeficiency diseases
Dietary protein enterocolitis
Behçet syndrome
Lymphoid nodular hyperplasia
Eosinophilic gastroenteritis
Graft-versus-host disease

Vascular-Ischemic

Systemic vasculitis [systemic lupus erythematosus (SLE), dermatomyositis]
Henoch-Schönlein purpura
Hemolytic-uremic syndrome

Other

Prestenotic colitis
Diversion colitis
Radiation colitis
Neonatal necrotizing enterocolitis
Typhlitis
Hirschsprung colitis
Intestinal lymphoma
Laxative abuse

Immunodeficiency

Gastrointestinal symptoms are a common manifestation of many immune deficiency states, including AIDS, congenital neutrophil and T- and B-cell immune deficiencies, and conditions of medical immune suppression (cancer and transplantation therapy). The more common congenital disorders associated with bowel disease include severe combined immunodeficiency, agammaglobulinemia, Wiskott-Aldrich syndrome, common variable immunodeficiency disease, and chronic granulomatous disease. Gastrointestinal symptoms of congenital X-linked hypogammaglobulinemia tend to be milder.

Chronic giardiasis and rotavirus infection have been noted to cause malabsorption in children with immune deficiencies. In children with AIDS, other organisms, including opportunistic infections that can interfere with bowel function, include *Cryptosporidium parvum,* cytomegalovirus, *Mycobacterium avium–intracellulare, Isospora belli, Enterocytozoon bieneusi, Candida albicans,* astrovirus, calicivirus, adenovirus, and the usual bacterial enteropathogens.

Autoimmune Enteropathy

Autoimmune enteropathy is a poorly characterized syndrome of chronic diarrhea and malabsorption. If symptoms initially develop after the first 6 months of life, the disorder is likely to be mistaken for gluten enteropathy. Histologic findings in the small bowel include partial or complete villous atrophy, crypt hyperplasia, and an increase in chronic inflammatory cells in the lamina propria. Specific serum anti-enterocyte antibodies may be identified in 50% of patients by indirect immunofluorescent staining of small-bowel mucosa colon and the kidney. Extraintestinal autoimmune disorders are usual and include arthritis, membranous glomerulonephritis, insulin-dependent diabetes, thrombocytopenia, autoimmune hepatitis, hypothyroidism, and hemolytic anemia.

Motility Disturbances

Motility disturbances may alter absorption rates. Decreased small intestine motility may be due to hypothyroidism, diabetes mellitus, or scleroderma. Increased small intestinal motility is found with hyperthyroidism, carcinoid syndrome, and enteral infections. Increased colonic motility is seen in the irritable bowel syndrome.

Constipation

A decreased frequency of stooling associated with painful or difficult passage of hard stool.

Causes of Constipation

- "Functional" idiopathic
- Dietary: low dietary fiber, starvation
- Psychosocial: emotional disturbance, mental retardation
- Anatomic/obstructive: Hirschsprung disease, imperforate/stenotic anus, meconium ileus (cystic fibrosis)
- Endocrine: hypothyroidism
- Drugs: antacids, anticonvulsants, diuretics, lead, opiates, phenothiazines
- Electrolyte abnormalities, hypokalemia, hypocalcemia
- Spinal abnormalities: meningomyelocele, spinal cord injury, spinal tumors
- Distal ileal obstructive syndrome (cystic fibrosis)

"Functional" constipation tends to present with encopresis, recurrent periumbilical pain (60% of patients), enuresis (30% of those with encopresis), large bulky dry stool, abdominal distention, poor appetite, and poor growth.

Hirschsprung Disease

In infancy, the newborn does not pass meconium within 48 hours of birth. Later, child may vomit, develop a distended abdomen, and fail to thrive.

Early recognition of Hirschsprung disease before the onset of enterocolitis is essential in reducing morbidity and mortality.

Diagnosis

Rectum is empty on digital examination. Rectal suction biopsies should be performed no closer than 2 cm to the dentate line to avoid the normal area of hypoganglionosis at the anal verge. The biopsy material should contain an adequate sample of submucosa to evaluate for the presence of ganglion cells. The biopsy specimen can be stained for acetylcholinesterase using a frozen section. Patients with aganglionosis demonstrate a large number of hypertrophied nerve bundles that stain positively for acetylcholinesterase with an absence of ganglion cells.

Distinguishing Features of Hirschsprung Disease and Functional Constipation[2]

Variable	Functional (Acquired)	Hirschsprung Disease
History		
Onset of constipation	After 2 yr of age	At birth
Encopresis	Common	Very rare

[2]Behrman RE, Kliegman RM, Jenson HB, eds. *Nelson textbook of pediatrics,* 16th ed. Philadelphia: WB Saunders Co, 2000.

Failure to thrive	Uncommon	Possible
Enterocolitis	None	Possible
Forced bowel training	Usual	None
Examination		
Abdominal distention	Rare	Common
Poor weight gain	Rare	Common
Anal tone	Normal	Normal
Rectal examination	Stool in ampulla	Ampulla empty
Malnutrition	None	Possible
Anorectal manometry	Distention of the rectum causes relaxation of the internal sphincter	No sphincter relaxation or paradoxical increase in pressure
Rectal biopsy	Normal	No ganglion cells Increased acetylcholinesterase staining
Barium enema	Massive amounts of stool, no transition zone	Transition zone, delayed evacuation (<24 hr)

Encopresis

Encopresis is the regular passage of fecal material into clothes or other inappropriate places by a child older than 4 years of age.

Constipation usually accompanies encopresis (there is a subgroup of children who do not have constipation).

Unrecognized constipation and/or stool retention often precedes the symptom presented to the care provider. Large amount of fecal material is found on abdominal, pelvic, or rectal exam.

Often there is intermittent periumbilical pain and a history of painful bowel movements. Some have had recurrent urinary tract infections. Anal fissure or painful defecation anal stenosis or anterior displacement of the anus may be found.

No test is diagnostic.

Pyloric Stenosis

Pyloric stenosis (PS) is a progressive stenosis of the pyloric canal occurring in infancy due to hypertrophy of the pylorus.

It presents as intermittent, nonbilious, projectile vomiting of increasing frequency and severity. The infant is hungry after vomiting. Abdominal examination reveals palpable tumor (olive) in right upper quadrant.

Early laboratory tests indicate hypochloremic alkalosis with low serum chloride and high bicarbonate. Later tests may indicate acidosis with low bicarbonate and low potassium.

Abdominal ultrasound by experienced radiologist will usually outline the pyloric tumor.

Barium swallow (performed only when diagnosis is not clinically clear) reveals strong gastric contractions and elongated, narrow pyloric canal (string sign).

Bulimia Nervosa

Classified in purging and nonpurging subtypes. Purging often by self-induced vomiting, laxatives, or diuretics. Nonpurging type consists of binges followed by sharply restricted diet and/or vigorous exercise, reported in approximately 2% of females; high among university women. True incidence is not known, as this is a secretive disease.

Signs and Symptoms

- Patients may switch back and forth between purging and nonpurging bulimia and be of average weight or somewhat obese; most are slightly below average weight with frequent fluctuations in weight. Patients deny that there is a problem. They gobble high-calorie foods during binges and are preoccupied with weight control.

- They prefer vigorous exercise, especially running and aerobics, and abuse diet pills, diuretics, laxatives, ipecac, and thyroid medication.
- Diabetic patients often withhold insulin. They collect and hoard food.
- Vomiting (may be effortless).
- They may have abdominal pain, parotid swelling, eroded teeth, and scarred hands or abrasions on back of hands.
- Cardiomyopathy and muscle weakness due to ipecac abuse may occur.

Laboratory Tests

All results may be within normal limits. Check for blood urea nitrogen and electrolytes.

Abdominal Pain/Tenderness

Gastroenteritis
Constipation
Mesenteric adenitis
Urinary tract infection
Inflammatory bowel disease
Pneumonia
Ketoacidosis
Cholecystitis
Renal stones
Testicular torsion
Porphyria
Celiac disease
Irritable bowel syndrome
Appendicitis
Meckel diverticulum
Sickle cell crisis
Ovarian pathology
Inguinal hernia
Pelvic inflammatory disease
Ectopic pregnancy
Peptic ulcer
Gastritis
Drug/toxin ingestion
Pancreatitis

Peptic Ulcers

Gastritis is an inflammation of the gastric mucosa. An ulcer is the disruption of the mucosal lining. Duodenal ulcers are more common than gastric ulcers. Signs and symptoms include abdominal pain, vomiting, and acute and chronic blood loss. Nocturnal pain causes awakening. Pain may be relieved by food, antacids, or antisecretory agents. The cause of most peptic ulcers is *H. pylori* or *H. jejuni* infection (see Chapter 5). Gastritis is commonly caused by corticosteroids, NSAIDs, smoking, or other drugs.

Laboratory tests include: peripheral blood for anemia, fecal blood, and serology or urea breath test for *H. pylori*. Endoscopy with biopsy and culture for *H. pylori* is diagnostic. X-ray after barium meal may be suggestive.

Acute Appendicitis

Acute appendicitis occurs at any age and is an emergency before perforating. In contrast to gastroenteritis and anorexia, pain begins before vomiting. Pain localizes to the right lower quadrant. Rectal examination may elicit tenderness and a mass in the same area.

Tests include moderate leukocytosis, and sometimes pyuria, hematuria, or albuminuria. Imaging may reveal a gas-filled appendix, radiopaque fecalith, or deformed cecum.

CT scan can demonstrate an abnormal appendix.

Ascites in Fetus or Neonate

Nonimmune (occur in 1:3,000 pregnancies)

Cardiovascular abnormalities causing congestive heart failure (e.g., structural, arrhythmias) (40% of cases)

Chromosomal (e.g., Turner and Down syndromes are most common; trisomy 13, 15, 16, 18) (10–15% of cases)

Hematologic disorders (any severe anemia) (10% of cases)

Inherited, e.g.,
- α Thalassemia
- Hemoglobinopathies
- G-6-PD deficiency
- Other RBC enzyme defects

Acquired, e.g.,
- Fetal-maternal hemorrhage
- Twin-to-twin transfusion
- Congenital infection (parvovirus B 19)
- Methemoglobinemia

Congenital defects of chest and abdomen
- Structural, e.g.,
  - Diaphragmatic hernia
  - Cystic adenomatoid malformation of lung
  - Fetal lymphatic dysplasia
  - Midgut volvulus
  - Intestinal malrotation

Peritonitis due to
- Gastrointestinal tract perforation
- Congenital infection [e.g., syphilis, TORCH (*t*oxoplasmosis, *o*ther agents, *r*ubella, *c*ytomegalovirus, *h*erpes simplex) syndrome, hepatitis]
- Meconium peritonitis due to complications of cystic fibrosis

Lymphatic duct obstruction

Biliary atresia

Bile ascites (rare) due to biliary tree perforation caused by congenital stenosis, choledochal cyst or stone
- Intermittent acholic stools, dark urine, fluctuating hyperbilirubinemia.
- Bile-stained ascitic fluid with increased protein (2–4 mg/dL).
- Intravenous administration of iodine 131 (^{131}I)-labeled rose bengal appearing in ascitic fluid makes the diagnosis early before bile staining occurs.

Nonstructural, e.g.,
- Congenital nephrotic syndrome
- Cirrhosis
- Cholestasis
- Hepatic necrosis
- Gastrointestinal tract obstruction

Lower genitourinary (GU) tract obstruction (e.g., usually due to posterior urethral valves, urethral atresia, ureterocele)—most common cause
- Inherited skeletal dysplasias (enlarged liver causing extramedullary hematopoiesis)

Fetal tumors, most often teratomas and neuroblastomas

Vascular placental abnormalities

Genetic metabolic disorders, e.g.,
- Hurler syndrome
- Gaucher disease
- Niemann-Pick disease
- I-cell disease
- Beta-glucuronidase deficiency

Immune (maternal antibodies reacting to fetal antigens, e.g., Rh, C, E, Kell)

Pancreas

Acute Pancreatitis

Causes of acute pancreatitis (Table 1) include trauma, drugs, toxins, ketoacidosis, and others.

Clinical Manifestations

The patient with acute pancreatitis has abdominal pain, persistent vomiting, and fever. The pain is epigastric and steady, often resulting in the child's assuming an antalgic position with hips and knees flexed, sitting upright, or lying on the side, and appears acutely ill. The abdomen may be distended and tender. An abdominal mass may be palpable.

Diagnosis

Acute Pancreatitis

In patients with signs of acute pancreatitis, pancreatitis is highly likely (clinical specificity = 85%) when lipase ≥ 5× upper levels of normal (ULN), if values change significantly with time, and if amylase and lipase changes are concordant. (Lipase should always be determined whenever amylase is determined.) Urinary lipase is not clinically useful. Lipase/amylase ratio >3 (and especially >5) indicates alcoholic rather than nonalcoholic pancreatitis. Acute pancreatitis or organ rejection is highly likely if lipase is ≥5× ULN, but unlikely if <3× ULN.

Serum amylase increase begins in 3–6 hours, rises rapidly within 8 hours in 75% of patients, reaches maximum in 20–30 hours, and may persist for 48–72 hours, with >95% sensitivity during first 12–24 hours. The increase may be ≤40× normal, but the height of the increase and rate of fall do not correlate with the severity of the disease, prognosis, or rate of resolution; however, an increase of >7–10 days suggests an associated cancer of pancreas or pseudocyst, pancreatic ascites, or nonpancreatic cause. Similar high values may occur in obstruction of pancreas (especially when seen more than 2 days after onset of symptoms) or may have normal values, even when dying of acute pancreatitis. May also be normal in patients with relapsing chronic pancreatitis and patients with hypertriglyceridemia (technical interferences with test). Frequently normal in acute alcoholic pancreatitis. Acute abdomen due to gastrointestinal infarction or perforation rather than acute pancreatitis is suggested by only moderate increase in serum amylase and lipase (<3× ULN), with evidence of bacteremia. 10–40% of patients with acute alcoholic intoxication have elevated serum amylase (approximately half of amylases are salivary type); patients often present with abdominal pain, but increased serum amylase is usually <3× ULN.

In healthy persons, 40% of total serum amylase is pancreatic type, and 60% is salivary type.

The serum amylase level is typically elevated in patients with acute pancreatitis for up to 4 days. A variety of other conditions may also cause hyperamylasemia without pancreatitis. Elevation of salivary amylase may mislead the clinician to make the diagnosis of pancreatitis in a child with abdominal pain. Some laboratories can separate amylase isoenzymes into pancreatic and salivary fractions. Serum lipase is more specific than amylase for acute inflammatory pancreatic disease and typically remains elevated 8–14 days longer than serum amylase. Serum lipase may also be elevated in nonpancreatic diseases.

Serum calcium is decreased in severe cases 1–9 days after onset (due to binding to soaps in fat necrosis). The decrease usually occurs after amylase and lipase levels have become normal. Tetany may occur. (Rule out hyperparathyroidism if serum calcium is high or fails to fall with hyperamylasemia of acute pancreatitis.)

Increased urinary amylase tends to reflect serum changes by a time lag of 6–10 hours, but sometimes increased urine levels are higher and of longer duration than serum levels. The 24-hour level may be normal even when some of the 1-hour specimens show increased values. Measurement of amylase levels in hourly samples of urine may be useful. Ratio of amylase clearance to creatinine clearance is increased (>5%), and it decreases tubular reabsorption of amylase (e.g., severe burns, diabetic ketoacidosis, chronic renal insufficiency, multiple myeloma, acute duodenal perforation).

Serum bilirubin may be increased when pancreatitis is of biliary tract origin but is usually normal in alcoholic pancreatitis. Serum alkaline phosphatase, alanine aminotransferase, and aspartate aminotransferase may increase and parallel serum bilirubin rather than amylase, lipase, or calcium levels.

Serum trypsin (by RIA) is increased. High sensitivity makes a normal value useful for excluding acute pancreatitis. But low specificity (increased in a large proportion of patients with hepatobiliary, bowel, and other diseases and renal insufficiency; increased in 13% of patients with chronic pancreatitis and 50% with pancreatic carcinoma) and RIA technology limit use.

WBC is slightly to moderately increased (10,000–20,000/mm^3).

Methemalbumin may be increased in serum and ascites in hemorrhagic (severe) but not edematous (mild) pancreatitis; may distinguish these two conditions but not useful in diagnosis of acute pancreatitis.

Abnormalities that may be present include hemoconcentration (hematocrit increased in severe hemorrhagic pancreatitis), coagulopathy, leukocytosis, hyperglycemia, glucosuria, hypocalcemia, elevated gamma glutamyl transpeptidase, hyperbilirubinemia, hypokalemia, metabolic acidosis, or lactic acidosis.

Pancreatic stimulation tests are rarely performed. A tube is positioned in the duodenum and fluid collected after IV injection of secretin with or without cholecystokinin.

Etiology of Acute Pancreatitis in Children

Infectious
Coxsackie B virus
Epstein-Barr virus
Hepatitis A, B
Influenza A, B
Leptospirosis
Malaria
Measles
Mumps
Mycoplasma
Reye syndrome: varicella, influenza B
Rubeola
Rubella

Altered gastrointestinal tract permeability
Ischemic bowel disease or frank perforation
Esophageal rupture
Perforated or penetrating peptic ulcer
Postoperative upper abdominal surgery, especially partial gastrectomy (up to 2× normal in one-third in patients)
Renal insufficiency often increased

Traumatic
Blunt injury
Burns
Child abuse
Radiation
Surgical trauma
Total body cast

Drug Induced
Aminosalicylic acid
Azathioprine
Corticosteroids
Dexamethasone
Estrogens
Ethacrynic acid
Ethanol
Furosemide
Mercaptopurine
Phenformin
Thiazides
Triamcinolone
Valproic acid

Miscellaneous
α_1-Antitrypsin deficiency
Brain tumor
Cases of intracranial bleeding
Chronic liver disease
Cystic fibrosis
Diabetic ketoacidosis
Dissecting aneurysm
Duplication cyst
Head trauma
Hemochromatosis
Hemolytic uremic syndrome
Hypercalcemia
Hyperlipidemia: types I, IV, V
Hyperparathyroidism
Hypertriglyceridemia
Kawasaki syndrome
Malnutrition
Organic acidemia
Peptic ulcer
Polyarteritis nodosa
Renal failure
Renal transplant
Splenic rupture
Systemic lupus erythematosus
Transplantation: bone marrow, heart, liver, kidney, pancreas
Vasculitis
Venom (spider, scorpion) even without pancreatitis

Obstructive
Ampullary disease
Ascariasis
Biliary tract malformation
Cholelithiasis and choledocholithiasis (stones or sludge)
Clonorchis
Common bile duct obstruction
Endoscopic retrograde cholangiopancreatography complication
Pancreas divisum
Pancreatic ductal abnormalities
Postoperative
Sphincter of Oddi dysfunction
Sphincter of Oddi spasm (e.g., opiates, codeine, methyl/codeine, cholinergics, chlorithiazole)
Tumor

Differential Diagnosis of Hyperamylasemia

Pancreatic Pathology

Acute or chronic pancreatitis
Complications of pancreatitis (pseudocyst, ascites, abscess)
Factitious pancreatitis

Salivary Gland Pathology

Parotitis (mumps, *Staphylococcus aureus*, cytomegalovirus, human immunodeficiency virus, Epstein Barr virus)
Sialadenitis (calculus, radiation)
Eating disorders (anorexia nervosa, bulimia)

Intraabdominal Pathology

Biliary tract disease (cholelithiasis)
Peptic ulcer perforation
Peritonitis
Intestinal obstruction
Appendicitis

Systemic Diseases

Metabolic acidosis (diabetes mellitus, shock)
Renal insufficiently, transplantation
Burns
Pregnancy
Drugs (morphine)
Head injury
Cardiopulmonary bypass

Poor Prognostic Laboratory Findings

On admission
- WBC >16,000/mm^3
- Blood glucose >200 mg/dL
- Serum lactate dehydrogenase >350 U/L
- Serum aspartate aminotransferase >250 U/L

Within 48 hours
- Serum calcium <8.0 mg/dL
- Decrease in Hct >10 points
- Increase in blood urea nitrogen >5 mg/dL
- Arterial Po_2 <60 mm Hg
- Metabolic acidosis with base deficit >4 mEq/L

Mortality
- 1% if three signs are positive
- 15% if three or four signs are positive
- 40% if five or six signs are positive
- 100% if seven or more signs are positive

Degree of amylase elevation has no prognostic significance.

Complications of Pancreatitis

Pseudocyst
Ascites
Abscess
Polyserositis (peritoneal, pleural, pericardial, synovium)
Chronic pancreatitis, in which there is a defect in pancreatic exocrine function leading to malabsorption, is not associated with leakage of pancreatic enzymes into blood. Repeated bouts of acute pancreatitis will lead to development of chronic pancreatitis.

Chronic Pancreatitis

Cholecystokinin-secretin test measures the effect of IV administration of cholecystokinin and secretin on volume, bicarbonate concentration, and amylase output of duodenal contents and increase in serum lipase and amylase. This is the most sensitive and reliable test for chronic pancreatitis. Some abnormality occurs in >85% of patients with chronic pancreatitis. Amylase output is the most frequent abnormality.

Normal duodenal contents:

- Volume: 95–235 mL/hr
- Bicarbonate concentration: 75–120 mEq/L
- Amylase output: 87,000–267,000 mg

Serum amylase and lipase increase after administration of cholecystokinin and secretin in ~20% of patients with chronic pancreatitis. They are more often abnormal when duodenal contents are normal. Normally, serum lipase and amylase do not rise above normal limits.

Fasting serum amylase and lipase are increased in 10% of patients with chronic pancreatitis.

Laboratory findings due to malabsorption (occurs when >90% of exocrine function is lost) and steatorrhea.

- Bentiromide test is usually abnormal with moderate to severe pancreatic insufficiency.
- Schilling test may show mild malabsorption of vitamin B_{12}.
- Xylose tolerance test and small-bowel biopsy are not usually done but are normal.

Chemical analysis of fecal fate demonstrates steatorrhea. It is more sensitive than tests using triolein ^{131}I.

Triolein ^{131}I testing is abnormal in one-third of patients with chronic pancreatitis.

Starch tolerance test is abnormal in 25% of patients with chronic pancreatitis.

Laboratory findings due to chronic pancreatitis:

- Alcoholism in 60–70%
- Idiopathic in 30–40%
- Obstruction of pancreatic duct (e.g., trauma, pseudocyst, pancreas divisum, cancer, or obstruction of duct or ampulla)
- Other causes occasionally [e.g., cystic fibrosis, primary hyperparathyroidism, heredity, protein caloric malnutrition, miscellaneous (Z-E syndrome), Shwachman syndrome, α_1-antitrypsin deficiency, trypsinogen deficiency, enterokinase deficiency, hemochromatosis, parenteral hyperalimentation]
- Radioactive selenium scanning of pancreas yields variable findings in different clinics

CT, ultrasonography, and endoscopic retrograde cholangio-pancreatography (ERCP) are most accurate for diagnosing and staging chronic pancreatitis.

Serum lipid, calcium, and phosphorus levels should be determined. Stools are evaluated for Ascaris, and a sweat test is performed. Plain abdominal films are evaluated for the presence of pancreatic calcifications. Abdominal ultrasound or CT scanning is performed to detect the presence of a pseudocyst. The biliary tract is evaluated for the presence of stones.

ERCP is a technique that can be used to define the anatomy of the gland and should be performed as part of the evaluation of any child with idiopathic, nonresolving, or recurrent pancreatitis and in patients with a pseudocyst before surgery. In these cases, ERCP may detect a previously undiagnosed anatomic defect.

A hereditary form of chronic pancreatitis is transmitted as an autosomal-dominant trait with symptoms beginning in the first decade. The gene for this disorder has been cloned and mapped to the long arm of chromosome 7.

Macroamylasemia

Serum amylase persistently increased (often 1–4× normal) without apparent cause.

Serum lipase is normal. Normal pancreatic to salivary amylase ratio.

Urine amylase normal or low.

Amylase-creatinine clearance ratio <1% with normal renal function is very useful for this diagnosis; should make the clinician suspect this diagnosis.

Diagnosis

Macroamylase is identified in serum by special gel filtration or ultracentrifugation technique.

May be found in ~1% of randomly selected patients with 2.5% of persons with increased serum amylase. Same findings may also occur in patients with normal-molecular-weight hyperamylasemia in which excess amylase in principally salivary gland isoamylase types 2 and 3.

When associated with pancreatic disease, serum lipase may be elevated.

Decreased Serum Amylase

Extensive marked destruction of pancreas (e.g., acute fulminant pancreatitis, advanced chronic pancreatitis, advanced cystic fibrosis). Decreased levels are clinically significant only in occasional cases of fulminant pancreatitis.

Severe liver damage (e.g., hepatitis, poisoning, toxemia of pregnancy, severe thyrotoxicosis, severe burns).

Methodologic interference by drugs (e.g., citrate and oxalate decrease activity by binding calcium ions).

Amylase-creatinine clearance ratio = (urine amylase concentration ÷ serum amylase concentration) × (serum concentration ÷ urine concentration) × 100.

Normal: 1–5%.

Macroamylasemia: <1%; very useful for this diagnosis (high serum amylase).

Acute pancreatitis: >5%.

Diabetic glucose tolerance test results in 65% of patients with chronic pancreatitis and frank diabetes in >10% of patients with chronic relapsing pancreatitis. When glucose tolerance test is normal in the presence of steatorrhea, the cause should be sought elsewhere than in the pancreas.

Pancreolauryl Test

This test for normal pancreatic enzyme secretions is designated for use in adults but can be used in children. Fluorescein dilaurate is ingested and, in the absence of pancreatic disease, is digested by pancreatic lipase to release fluorescein, which is absorbed into the bloodstream and ultimately excreted into urine. Thus, low excretion of fluorescein may be the result of abnormal digestion, abnormal absorption, or abnormal renal function. To compensate for the latter two, fluorescein alone is taken on another day. The urinary excretion of fluorescein after taking fluorescein dilaurate is compared to that after taking fluorescein. A normal result is greater than 30%. The BT-PABA (N-benzoyl-1-tyrosylpara-amino-benzoic acid) test is similar. In this test, PABA is released by the action of chymotrypsin and is measured in urine. To compensate for renal function, the test is repeated with unconjugated PABA.

Pseudocyst of Pancreas

Serum direct bilirubin is increased (>2 mg/dL) in 10% of patients.

Serum alkaline phosphatase is increased in 10% of patients.

Fasting blood sugar is increased in <10% of patients.

Duodenal contents after secretin-pancreozymin stimulation usually show decreased bicarbonate content (<70 meq/L) but normal volume and normal content of amylase, lipase, and trypsin.

Findings of pancreatic cyst aspiration:

- High fluid viscosity and CEA indicate mucinous differentiation and exclude pseudocyst, serous cystadenoma, other nonmucinous cysts or cystic tumors.
- Increased CA 72-4, CA 15-3, and tissue polypeptide antigen are markers of malignancy; if all are low, pseudocyst or serous cystadenoma is most likely.
- CA 125 is increased in serous cystadenoma.
- Pancreatic enzymes, leukocyte esterase, and NB/70K are increased in pseudocysts.
- Cytologic examination.

Shwachman Syndrome

This is an autosomal-recessive syndrome (1:20,000 births), consisting of pancreatic insufficiency; neutropenia, which may be intermittent; neutrophil chemotaxis defects; metaphyseal dysostosis; failure to thrive; and short stature. Patients present in infancy with poor growth and greasy, foul-smelling stools that are characteristic of malabsorption. These children can be readily differentiated from those with cystic fibrosis by their normal sweat chloride levels, lack of the cystic fibrosis gene, characteristic metaphyseal lesions, and fatty pancreas on CT examination.

Recurrent pyogenic infections (otitis media, pneumonia, osteomyelitis, dermatitis, sepsis) are common and are a frequent cause of death. Thrombocytopenia is found in 70% of patients and anemia in 50%. Pathologically, the pancreatic acini are replaced by fat with little fibrosis. Islet cells and ducts are normal. The fatty pancreas has a characteristic hypodense appearance on CT and magnetic resonance scans.

Pearson Syndrome

This is a sporadic mitochondrial DNA mutation affecting oxidative phosphorylation that manifests in infants with severe macrocytic anemia and variable thrombocytopenia. The bone marrow demonstrates vacuoles in erythroid and myeloid precursors as well as ringed sideroblasts. In addition to severe bone marrow failure, pancreatic insufficiency contributes to growth failure.

Other Syndromes Associated with Pancreatic Insufficiency

Johanson-Blizzard syndrome is characterized by pancreatic insufficiency, deafness, low birth weight, microcephaly, midline ectodermal scalp defects, psychomotor retardation, hypothyroidism, dwarfism, absent permanent teeth, and aplasia of the alae nasae. Congenital pancreatic hypoplasia, congenital rubella, and other syndromes (Alagille) are other causes of pancreatic insufficiency.

Cystic Fibrosis

Cystic fibrosis (discussed in more detail in Chapter 8) is the most common lethal genetic disease. It is due to abnormalities of the CFTR gene and is the most common cause of malabsorption among white American children. By the end of the first year of life, 90% of children with cystic fibrosis have pancreatic insufficiency, leading to malnutrition. Signs and symptoms in the newborn include meconium ileus, diarrhea, failure to thrive, and jaundice; later, chronic obstructive pulmonary disease, liver failure, and diabetes mellitus occur.

Transport of chloride is defective, and exocrine pancreatic ducts are obstructed. Diagnostic tests include measurement of intestinal and stool trypsin, sweat chloride (sweat test), newborn serum trypsin, and determination of CFTR gene.

Bibliography

Barr RG, Watkins JB, Perman JA. Mucosal function and breath hydrogen excretion: comparative studies in the clinical evaluation of children with nonspecific abdominal complaints. *Pediatrics* 1981;68:526.

Behrman RE, Kliegman RM, Jenson HB, eds. *Nelson textbook of pediatrics,* 16th ed. Philadelphia: WB Saunders Co., 2000.

Branski D, Lerner A, Lebenthal E. Chronic diarrhea and malabsorption. *Pediatr Clin North Am* 1996;43:307.

Cosgrove M, Al-Atia RF, Jenkins HR. The epidemiology of pediatric inflammatory bowel disease. *Arch Dis Child* 1996;74:460.

Dieterich W, Laag E, Schöpper H, et al. Autoantibodies to tissue transglutamine as predictors of celiac disease. *Gastroenterology* 1998;115:1317.

Dundas SA, Dutton J, Skipworth P. Reliability of rectal biopsy in distinguishing between chronic inflammatory bowel disease and acute self-limiting colitis. *Histopathology* 1997;31:60.

Gilbert-Barness E, ed. *Potter's pathology of the fetus and infant*. St. Louis: Mosby–Year Book, 1997.

Goulet OJ, Revillon Y, Jan D, et al. Neonatal short bowel syndrome. *J Pediatr* 1991;119:18.

Hyams JS, Davis P, Grancher K, et. al. Clinical outcome of ulcerative proctitis in children. *J Pediatr* 1996;129:81.

Kleinman RE, Klish W, Lebethal E, et al. Role of juice carbohydrate malabsorption in chronic nonspecific diarrhea in children. *J Pediatr* 1992;120:825.

Leonberg BL, Chuang E, Eicher P, et al. Long-term growth and development in children after home parenteral nutrition. *J Pediatr* 1998;132.

Mack DR, Forstner GG, Wilchanski M, et al. Shwachman syndrome: pancreatic dysfunction and variable phenotypic expression. *Gastroenterology* 1996;111:1593.

Mäki M, Collin P. Celiac disease. *Lancet* 1997;349:1755.

Mergener K, Baillie J. Chronic pancreatitis. *Lancet* 1997;350:1379.

Montes R, Perman JA. *Semin Pediatr Gastroenterol Nutr* 1991;2:2.

Murphy MS, Eastham EJ, Nelson R, et al. Noninvasive assessment of intraluminal lipolysis using a CO_2 breath test. *Arch Dis Child* 1990;65:574.

Pavli P, Cavanaugh J, Grimm M. Inflammatory bowel disease: Germs or genes? *Lancet* 1996;347:1198.

Perman JA, Barr RG, Watkins JB. Sucrose malabsorption in children: noninvasive diagnosis by interval breath hydrogen determination. *J Pediatr* 1978;93:17.

Proujansky R, Fawcett PT, Gibney KM, et al. Examination of antineutrophil cytoplasmic antibodies in childhood inflammatory bowel disease. *J Pediatr Gastronenterol Nutr* 1993;17:193.

Report to working group of European society of pediatric gastroenterology and nutrition: revised criteria for diagnosis of celiac disease. *Arch Dis Child* 1990;65:909.

Riddlesherger MM. Evaluation of the gastrointestinal tract in the child: CT, MRI, and isotopic studies. *Pediatr Clin North Am* 1988;35:281.

Rossi TM, Tjota A. Serologic indicators of celiac disease. *J Pediatr Gastronenterol Nutr* 1998;26:205.

Sartor RB. Cytokines in intestinal inflammation: Pathophysiological and clinical considerations. *Gastroenterology* 1994;106:533.

Volta U, De Franceschi L, Lari F, et al. Celiac disease hidden by cryptogenic hypertransaminasemia. *Lancet* 1998;352:26.

Wallach J. *Interpretation of diagnostic tests*, 7th ed. Philadelphia: Lippincott Williams & Wilkins, 2000.

Weizman Z. An update on diseases of the pancreas in children. *Curr Opinion* 1997;9:484.

Whitecomb DC, Gorry MC, Preston RA, et al. Hereditary pancreatitis is caused by a mutation in the cationic trypsinogen gene. *Nat Genet* 1996;14:141.

10 Liver Disease

Tests for Evaluation of Liver Function

Biochemical Investigation of Prolonged Jaundice

See Fig. 1 and Table 1.

Standard Indicators Measured to Assess Liver Function

Blood

Bilirubin (total and direct or conjugated)
Alanine aminotransferase (ALT)
Albumin
Calcium
Sodium
Creatinine
Lactate
β-Hydroxybutyrate
Thyroid hormones (check that neonatal screening tests have been performed)
Galactose-1-phosphate uridyltransferase (qualitative screen)
Prothrombin time
Alkaline phosphatase (ALP)
γ-Glutamyltransferase
Cholesterol
Phosphate
Potassium
Fasting glucose
Free fatty acids
Qualitative amino acids
α_1-Antitrypsin
Glucose-6-phosphate dehydrogenase (if in high-risk group, check that screening has been performed)
Partial thromboplastin time

Urine

Amino acids
Sugars
Organic acids
If plasma amino acid tests show an increased tyrosine or methionine level, second-line tests are
  Plasma α-fetoprotein level
  Urinary succinylacetone level
If the baby is acutely ill, consider
  Measurement of ammonia and orotic acid levels to test for urea cycle defects and urgent investigations for fatty acid oxidation and glycogen storage disorders.
In patients with persistent cholestasis of unknown cause, disorders of bile acid synthesis, Zellweger syndrome, cystic fibrosis, and Niemann-Pick disease type C should also be considered.

Indications for Liver Function Tests

Tests of liver function are indicated in patients with suspected

1. Impaired biliary secretion
2. Hepatocellular damage
3. Synthetic dysfunction

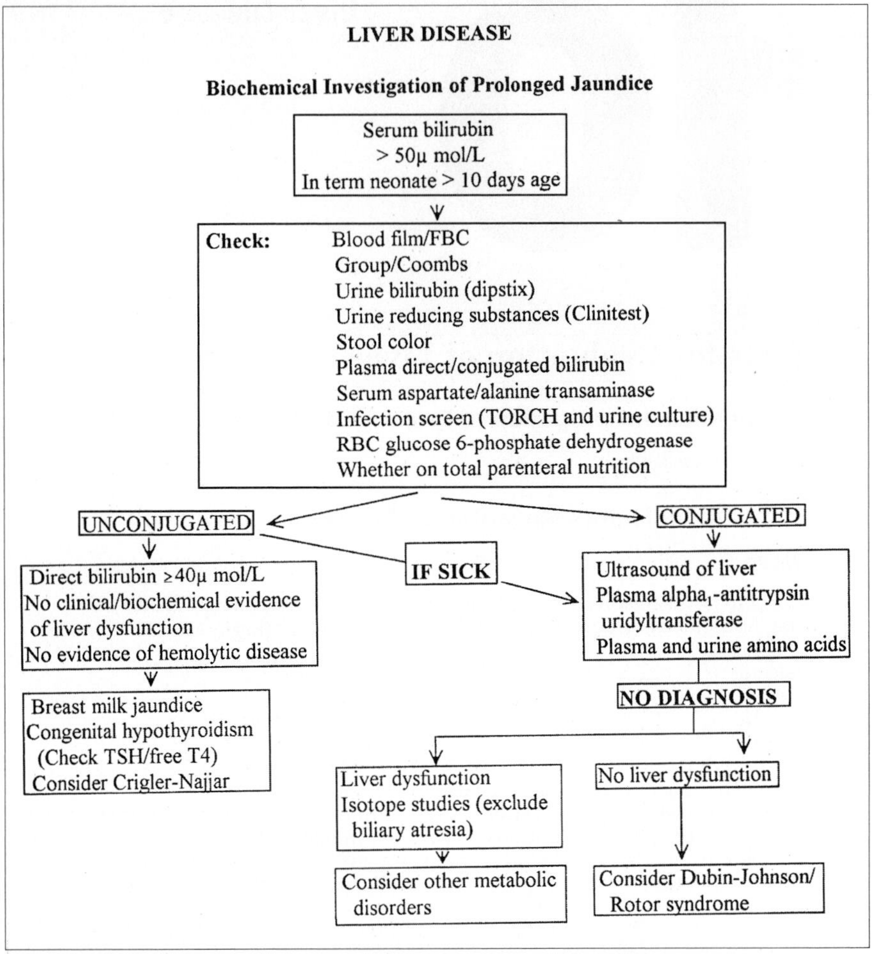

Fig. 1. Algorithm for biochemical investigation of prolonged jaundice. FBC, full blood count; RBC, red blood cells; T_4, thyroxine; TORCH, toxoplasmosis, other infections, rubella, cytomegalovirus infection, and herpes simplex; TSH, thyroid-stimulating hormone.

Evaluation of Liver Function Test Results

See Table 2.

Albumin

Serum albumin level is low in liver disease but is also nonspecifically low in a number of other disorders. It behaves as a negative acute-phase reactant. Thus, its synthesis is reduced, whereas the synthesis of positive acute-phase reactants such as α_1-antitrypsin is increased.

Bilirubin

Free bilirubin is unconjugated bilirubin that is not bound to albumin.

Laboratory methods for measuring bilirubin level are usually based on the method of Jendrassik and Grof, which relies on a chemical reaction between bilirubin and a

Table 1. Causes of Jaundice in the Newborn

Disorder	Type of Jaundice	Supporting Information	Further Investigation
Breast-feeding	U	Jaundice spontaneously resolves if breast-feeding halted. No clinical or biochemical evidence of liver dysfunction.	—
Infection	C/U	Improves with treatment.	Infection screen Urine culture
Rhesus/ABO isoimmunization	C	History of early hemolytic jaundice.	—
TPN	C	History of TPN.	None if resolves after TPN has been discontinued
Biliary atresia	C	Pale stools.	Liver ultrasonography, diisopropyl iminodiacetic acid scan
α_1-Antitrypsin deficiency	C	—	Plasma α_1-antitrypsin level
Hypothyroidism	U	Clinical signs.	Thyroid-stimulating hormone, free thyroxine levels
Alagille syndrome	C	Characteristic facies congenital abnormalities.	Hypoplasia or reduced intrahepatic bile ducts on liver biopsy
Galactosemia	C	Cataracts. Urinary reducing substances positive. Hypoglycemia, abnormal clotting.	Erythrocyte galactose-1-phosphate uridyltransferase level
Tyrosinemia type I	C	Serum amino acids increased. Aminoacidemia. Hepatocellular disease. Increased serum α-fetoprotein.	Plasma amino acid levels (tyrosine and methionine) Urine succinylacetone level
Zellweger syndrome	C	Hypotonia. Dysmorphic features. Neurologic dysfunction.	Plasma levels of very-long-chain fatty acids
Glucose-6-phosphate dehydrogenase deficiency	U	Usually presents early. Family history of occurrence due to drugs. Mediterranean, Asian, or African ethnicity.	Erythrocyte glucose-6-phosphate dehydrogenase level
Crigler-Najjar syndrome types I and II	U	No liver dysfunction.	Glucuronide levels in bile Glucuronyl transferase level in liver
Cystic fibrosis	C	Meconium ileus may occur.	Plasma/blood spot immunoreactive trypsin Sweat Na and Cl levels

C, conjugated hyperbilirubinemia; TPN, total parenteral nutrition; U, unconjugated hyperbilirubinemia.

Table 2. Evaluation of Liver Function Test Results

Enzyme	Source	Increased	Decreased	Comments
AST/ALT	Liver Heart Skeletal muscle Pancreas RBCs Kidney	Hepatocellular injury Rhabdomyolysis Muscular dystrophy Hemolysis Liver cancer	Vitamin B_6 deficiency Uremia	ALT more specific than AST AST >ALT in hemolysis AST/ALT >2 in 90% of adults
Alkaline phosphatase	Liver Osteoblasts Small intestine Kidney Placenta	Hepatocellular injury Bone growth, disease, trauma Pregnancy Familial	Low phosphate levels Wilson disease Zinc deficiency Hypothyroidism Pernicious anemia	Highest in cholestatic conditions Must be differentiated from bone source
GGT	Bile ducts Renal tubules Pancreas Small intestine Brain	Cholestasis Newborn period Induced by drugs	Estrogen therapy Artificially low in hyperbilirubinemia	Not found in bone Increased in 90% of primary liver disease Biliary obstruction Intrahepatic cholestasis Induced by alcohol Specific for hepatobiliary disease in nonpregnant patient
5'-NT	Liver cell membrane Intestine Brain Heart Pancreas	Cholestasis		Specific for hepatobiliary disease in nonpregnant patient
Ammonia	Bowel Bacteria Protein metabolism	Hepatic disease secondary to urea cycle dysfunction Hemodialysis Valproic acid use Urea cycle enzyme deficiency Organic acidemia and carnitine deficiency		Converted to urea in liver

ALT, alanine aminotransferase; AST, aspartate aminotransferase; GGT, γ-glutamyl transpeptidase; 5'-NT, 5'-nucleotidase; RBC, red blood cell.
From The Johns Hopkins Hospital, Siberry G, Iannone R. *Harriet Lane handbook*, 15th ed. St. Louis: Mosby, 2000.

diazotizing reagent that produces a colored product. Methods for the measurement of total bilirubin level include use of an accelerator (e.g., caffeine), which ensures that all bilirubin species react.

No methods in common use specifically measure indirect bilirubin. Conjugated bilirubin is reported as "direct," unconjugated as "indirect." Bilirubin is reported as total and direct; unconjugated is the calculated difference.

Impaired biliary secretion (obstructive jaundice) causes elevated levels of conjugated bilirubin; hepatocellular damage causes elevated levels of both conjugated and unconjugated bilirubin and alteration of liver enzymes; and synthetic dysfunction causes no consistent hyperbilirubinemia but lack of specific proteins, such as albumin and prothrombin. Hemolysis is followed by an increase in unconjugated bilirubin and a decrease in serum haptoglobin, the hemoglobin-binding protein.

In most forms of liver disease, the ability to secrete conjugated bilirubin into bile is impaired and a conjugated-fraction hyperbilirubinemia results. The ability of the liver to take up and conjugate bilirubin may also be impaired; thus, accompanying unconjugated-fraction hyperbilirubinemia may occur. Because conjugated bilirubin is filtered at the glomerulus, urine bilirubin level is increased, the amount of bilirubin reaching the gut is decreased, the production of urobilinogen decreases, and urine urobilinogen level is low.

Clotting Factor

Synthesis of, for example, prothrombin and other vitamin K–dependent proteins is deficient in liver disease.

Lactate Dehydrogenase

Lactate dehydrogenase is not generally used as a marker of liver damage. It is present in the liver cytoplasm, and its level is increased in conditions in which ALT level is increased. The liver contains the lactate dehydrogenase-5 isoenzyme and is not measured in the specific lactate dehydrogenase isoenzyme-1 assays used for the detection of myocardial infarction.

Immunoglobulins

Immunoglobulin (Ig) levels can be increased in chronic liver disease. The increase is predominately in IgG in autoimmune liver disease, whereas IgM levels are raised in viral hepatitis.

Markers of Enzyme Induction and Release

Markers of enzyme induction and release, such as ALP, γ-glutamyl transpeptidase (GGT), and 5'-nucleotidase, are membrane-bound enzymes in the hepatocyte. They are not soluble and do not leak out of the cell when the plasma membrane is damaged; therefore, they are not good markers of hepatocellular damage. Increases in serum of the activity of soluble forms of these enzymes often accompany cholestasis. 5'-Nucleotidase is a relatively liver-specific enzyme, but its measurement in serum is not routinely performed, having been superseded by measurement of GGT. Although GGT is found in tissues other than the liver, including the kidney, the liver is usually the source of significant increases in serum GGT. An elevated serum GGT level is a sensitive indicator of liver disease in which induction (by anticonvulsants or alcohol) can be excluded.

Because ALP is found in tissues other than liver, an increase in its serum activity is not specific for liver disorders. Increase occurs most notably in bone disease. In bone disease, the increase is of a different isoenzyme than that which increases in liver disease. The different isoenzymes of ALP can be distinguished by a variety of techniques, including electrophoresis. Alternatively, the bone isoenzyme can be measured specifically using an immunologic assay.

ALP levels in neonates, particularly in premature neonates, are up to five times the upper limit of the normal reference range for adults. Older infants (from age 6 months) and prepubertal children have ALPs two to three times the upper limit of normal. The growth spurt occurring at puberty increases the reference range to five times the upper limit of normal for adults. In the absence of disease, the serum activity of the liver isoenzyme remains fairly constant.

Long-term administration of anticonvulsant drugs induces increased serum levels of GGT.

Markers of Hepatocellular Damage

Irrespective of the cause of hepatic damage, when any individual cell is irreversibly damaged, its plasma membrane loses its integrity, which allows its soluble cytoplasmic contents to leak out and enter the bloodstream. Severe damage is associated with the leaking of the contents of intracellular organelles such as mitochondria. In theory, any of a number of the soluble components of the hepatocyte cytoplasm could be used as a marker of hepatocyte damage. A marker with a very short half-life is useful for detecting recent and continuing liver disease, whereas one with a longer half-life is useful in excluding liver disease.

Transferases

α-Glutathione S-Transferase

α-Glutathione S-transferase is a cytoplasmic enzyme that is largely liver specific. It is the most sensitive indicator of hepatocellular damage. It is slow and expensive to measure, however, and the test is not readily available. The enzyme has a very *short* half-life (<1 hour) and is excellent for detecting recent-onset liver disease.

Aspartate Aminotransferase and Alanine Aminotransferase

The transferases are the most commonly used markers of hepatocellular damage. Hepatocytes contain both aspartate aminotransferase (AST) and ALT. ALT is not present to any great extent in tissues other than liver, so it is a more specific marker of liver disease. Within the liver, it exhibits a periportal to perivenous gradient, and within the cell it is located exclusively in the cytoplasm. It has a plasma half-life of approximately 47 ± 10 hours.

AST is present in liver, cardiac muscle, and skeletal muscle. There are both cytoplasmic and mitochondrial forms of the enzyme. The cytoplasmic form of the enzyme exhibits a periportal to perivenous gradient, but the mitochondrial enzyme is uniformly distributed. It has a plasma half-life of 17 ± 5 hours.

Other Markers of Liver Disease

In extremely severe liver disease, urea and glucose levels may be low and ammonia levels may be high, but these are poor indicators of liver function. Any child who is encephalopathic due to liver disease has elevated serum ammonia levels. Measurement of ammonia is useful in the investigation of Reye syndrome and in the investigation of suspected inborn errors of metabolism.

Typical Changes in Liver Function Indicators in Different Disease States

	Bilirubin	Alkaline Phosphatase	Alanine Aminotransferase
Hemolysis	↑	N	N
Obstructive liver disease	↑	↑	N
Hepatocellular liver disease	↑	N/↑	↑

↑, increased; N, normal.

Liver Disorders

α-Fetoprotein Elevation

Elevated levels of α-fetoprotein in serum are found in primary hepatoma, during the first 12 months of life, and in tyrosinemia.

Levels of α-fetoprotein may be elevated in patients with germ cell tumors.

Cirrhosis

Cirrhosis is the end result of hepatic cell necrosis from a variety of injurious agents. Although the active phase of liver disease is manifested by abnormal liver function test results or hyperbilirubinemia and decrease in synthesis of essential proteins, in the final phase only abnormalities of prothrombin time and partial thromboplastin time and decreased albumin levels are present. In the precirrhotic phase, the liver may be large on physical examination, and larger than the spleen. As the disease progresses, the liver scars and becomes small.

Causes of cirrhosis in the infant include the following:

- Biliary obstruction
  - Extrahepatic biliary atresia
  - Choledochal cyst
  - Tyrosinemia
- Cholestatic disease
  - Familial cholestatic syndromes
  - Paucity of intrahepatic bile ducts
  - Sclerosing cholangitis
- Infection
  - Neonatal hepatitis
  - Other viral infections
- Vascular disease
  - Venoocclusive disease
  - Congestive cardiac failure
- Miscellaneous
  - Total parenteral nutrition
  - Malnutrition
  - Histiocytosis X
  - Drugs, toxins
  - Idiopathic disease
- Metabolic disorders
  - Galactosemia
  - Fructosemia
  - Glycogen storage disease type 4
  - α_1-Antitrypsin deficiency
  - Gaucher disease
  - Niemann-Pick disease
  - Wolman disease
  - Cholesterol ester storage disease
  - Mucopolysaccharidoses
  - Wilson disease
  - Neonatal hemochromatosis
  - Argininosuccinic aciduria
  - Peroxisomal disorders
  - Fatty acid oxidation disorders
  - Mitochondrial abnormalities
- Hereditary syndromes
  - Indian childhood cirrhosis
  - Congenital hepatic fibrosis
  - Progressive neuronal degeneration (Alpers disease)

Cholestasis

Causes include

- α_1-Antitrypsin deficiency
- Inborn errors of bile acid synthesis
- Drug effects
- Total parental nutrition
- Progressive familial intrahepatic cholestasis (Byler disease)
- Cystic fibrosis
- Hyper- or hypothyroidism
- Idiopathic hypopituitarism
- Hemophagocytic lymphohistiocytosis
- Neonatal hemochromatosis
- Galactosemia
- Fructosemia
- Tyrosinemia type I
- Niemann-Pick disease types B and C
- Glycogen storage disease, type 4
- Wolman disease
- Gaucher disease
- Generalized peroxisomal disorders

Cholestasis with Ductal Paucity

Syndromic

Caused by Alagille syndrome

Nonsyndromic

Causes include
- Ductopenic allograft rejection

Familial Intrahepatic Cholestatic Syndromes

Causes include
- Byler syndrome (progressive intrahepatic cholestasis)
- Norwegian cholestasis (Aagenaes syndrome)
- North American Indian cholestasis
- Greenland Eskimo cholestasis
- Benign recurrent intrahepatic cholestasis

Obstructive Cholestasis

Causes include
- Biliary atresia
- Congenital bile duct anomalies (choledochal cyst)
- Cholelithiasis
- Primary sclerosing cholangitis
- Infectious cholangitis
- Cholangitis associated with Langerhans-cell histiocytosis

Drugs That May Affect the Liver

Drugs that produce predictable hepatotoxicity include cytotoxins, salicylate, acetaminophen (paracetamol), and ferrous sulfate. Liver function test results show a cholestatic, hepatitic, or mixed pattern.

Drugs and chemicals that may cause abnormal liver function test results include the following:

Class	Example(s)
Steroid drugs	Oral contraceptives
Antibiotics	Sulfonamides, penicillin, tetracycline hydrochloride
Anticonvulsants	Carbamazepine, phenytoin
Anesthetics	Halothane
Analgesics	Salicylate, acetaminophen
Cytotoxics	Cyclophosphamide, 6-mercaptopurine
Antitubercular drugs	Rifampicin, isoniazid
Solvents	Toluene
Others	Cocaine, alcohol

Hepatitis

Neonatal Hepatitis

Table 3 lists infections causing neonatal hepatitis.

Viral Hepatitis

Hepatitis C virus (HCV) has been identified in approximately 90% of patients diagnosed as having non-A, non-B hepatitis. Incubation period is 2–26 weeks. Infection frequently occurs after percutaneous exposure to blood, such as during intravenous drug use or blood product administration. Signs and symptoms are similar to those of other types of viral hepatitis. Assays include detection of IgG antibodies against the virus.

Hepatitis E, like hepatitis A, is transmitted by enteric contamination. Incubation period is 30–40 days, and the disorder is clinically similar to hepatitis A. Diagnosis is by detection of IgG and IgM antibodies to the virus.

Screening for Hepatitis Viruses

There are two main modalities of testing for the hepatitis viruses and several subclasses within each. The two main modalities are

Table 3. Infections Causing Neonatal Hepatitis

	Time of Presentation	Diagnostic Test(s)
Transplacental		
Rubella	Day 1	Maternal and infant rubella IgM levels
CMV infection	Day 1	Maternal and infant CMV IgM levels
Toxoplasmosis	Day 1	Maternal and infant toxoplasmosis IgM level
Syphilis	Day 1	Mother seropositive, infant titer high or rising
Perinatally acquired		
Herpes simplex	First week	Isolation from vesicles or swab specimens
CMV infection	Late	CMV-specific IgM level or culture
Hepatitis A	Late	Serologic testing
Hepatitis B	Any	Serologic testing
Coxsackievirus infection	Any	Coxsackievirus B antibody level
		Viral culture (stool and throat swabs specimens)

CMV, cytomegalovirus; Ig, immunoglobulin.

1. Tests that detect the presence of host-generated antibodies against the particular hepatitis viral antigens
2. Tests that detect nucleic acids themselves (known collectively as *direct detection methods*)

Serologic Testing

Examples of assays used to test for the hepatitis group viruses are the Ortho 3.0 (Ortho-Clinical Diagnostics, Raritan, NJ) and Abbott HCV 2.0 HCV enzyme immunoassay (Abbott Labs, Abbott Park, IL).

The Ortho-Clinical 3.0 and the Abbott 2.0 assays are qualitative enzyme-linked immunosorbent assays (ELISAs) for the detection of antibody to HCV in human serum or plasma.

The Abbott HCV 2.0 (enzyme immunoassay) method also detects the antibodies to proteins expressed by the virus. The Abbott 2.0 kit has been widely used for initial screening. It is relatively inexpensive, but the assay results require further confirmation with more sensitive and specific tests.

Kits for the detection of hepatitis B virus (HBV) surface antigen are also manufactured by both Abbott and Ortho-Clinical. Two tests by Abbott Laboratories measure HBV surface antigen (AUSAB enzyme immunoassay) and HBV core antigen (CORZYME recombinant enzyme assay). These assays can detect antibodies to HBV surface antigen in the presence of other hepatitis markers and other viral antibodies and antigens.

Two other widely used HBV assays developed by Ortho-Clinical Diagnostics are the VITROS system tests for HBsAg and anti-HBs.

Nucleic Acid Amplification–Based Testing Techniques

Nucleic acid amplification–based testing techniques coupled with the extremely sensitive DNA detection method of Southern blotting identifies early infection. An individual may be infectious, but the organism may not be detectable by traditional serologic assays. The period before serologic tests yield positive results is estimated to be approximately 14 days from infection for human immunodeficiency virus infection and from 40 to 80 days from infection for HCV infection. The use of nucleic acid testing to screen blood products is expected to reduce the risk of HCV infection from 1:100,000 (current risk per unit transfused) to between 1:500,000 and 1:1,000,000.

Pooling Algorithms for Mass Screening

For testing to be economically feasible, pool testing or screening of many samples with a single test is suggested.

One pooling method combines equal amounts of 512 antibody-negative plasma samples into one master pool for testing. If the master pool is negative for the target markers, then all 512 samples are released. If, however, the master pool test yields

Table 4. Serologic Markers of Viral Hepatitis

Stage of Infection	HAV	HBV	HCV	HDV	HEV
Acute disease	Anti-HAV IgM	HBcAb IgM	Anti-HCV	HDAg	Anti-HEV[a]
Chronic disease	NA	HBsAg	Anti-HCV	Anti-HDV	NA
Infectious state	HAV RNA[b]	HBeAg, HBsAg, HBV DNA[c]	Anti-HCV, HCV RNA	Anti-HDV, HDV RNA[b]	HEV RNA[b]
Recovery	None	HBeAb, HBsAb	None	None	None
Carrier state	NA	HBsAg	None	Anti-HDV, HDAg	NA
Immunity screen	Anti-HAV, total (includes anti-HAV IgG)	HBsAb, total HBcAb	None	None	Anti-HEV[a]

HAV, hepatitis A virus; HBcAb, hepatitis B core antigen; HBeAb, hepatitis Be antigen; HBsAb, hepatitis B surface antigen; HBV, hepatitis B virus; HCV, hepatitis C virus; HDAg, hepatitis D antigen; HDV, hepatitis D virus; HEV, hepatitis E virus; Ig, immunoglobulin; NA, not available.
[a]Not available in United States.
[b]Only available in research laboratories.
[c]Only available for investigational use.

positive results for one or more markers, subpools of the same samples are tested further to identify the suspect individual donations.

Coupling of the newer nucleic acid amplification–based tests with serologic testing has resulted in a reduction in posttransfusion hepatitis and the incidence of hepatitis cases among persons who use plasma-derived products.

HEPTIMAX

A new test for HCV is the ultrasensitive quantitative test HEPTIMAX (Quest Diagnostics, Inc.). The test detects levels of HCV through an innovative application of transcription-mediated amplification technology. The HEPTIMAX test is capable of detecting immune-level quantities of HCV.

Serologic Markers of Viral Hepatitis

See Table 4 and Figs. 2 and 3.

Hepatitis B

Serologic Marker	Significance
HBsAg (HBV surface antigen)	Acute or chronic infection
Anti-HBs (antibody to HBsAg)	Immunity (due to viral clearance)
HBeAg (HBV e antigen)	Active viral replication
Anti-HBe (antibody to HBeAg)	Asymptomatic carrier
IgM anti-HBc (IgM antibody to core antigen)	Acute HBV infection
Anti-HBc (IgG and IgM antibody to core antigen)	Present or past HBV infection
HBV DNA [quantitation of DNA by polymerase chain reaction (PCR)]	Active viral replication

Hepatitis D

Serologic Marker	Significance
HDAg [hepatitis D virus (HDV) antigen]	Acute infection
anti-HDV IgM (IgM antibody to HDAg)	Acute or chronic HDV
anti-HDV IgA (IgA antibody to HDAg)	Superinfection or chronic HDV
HDV RNA (quantitation of RNA by PCR)	Acute or chronic HDV

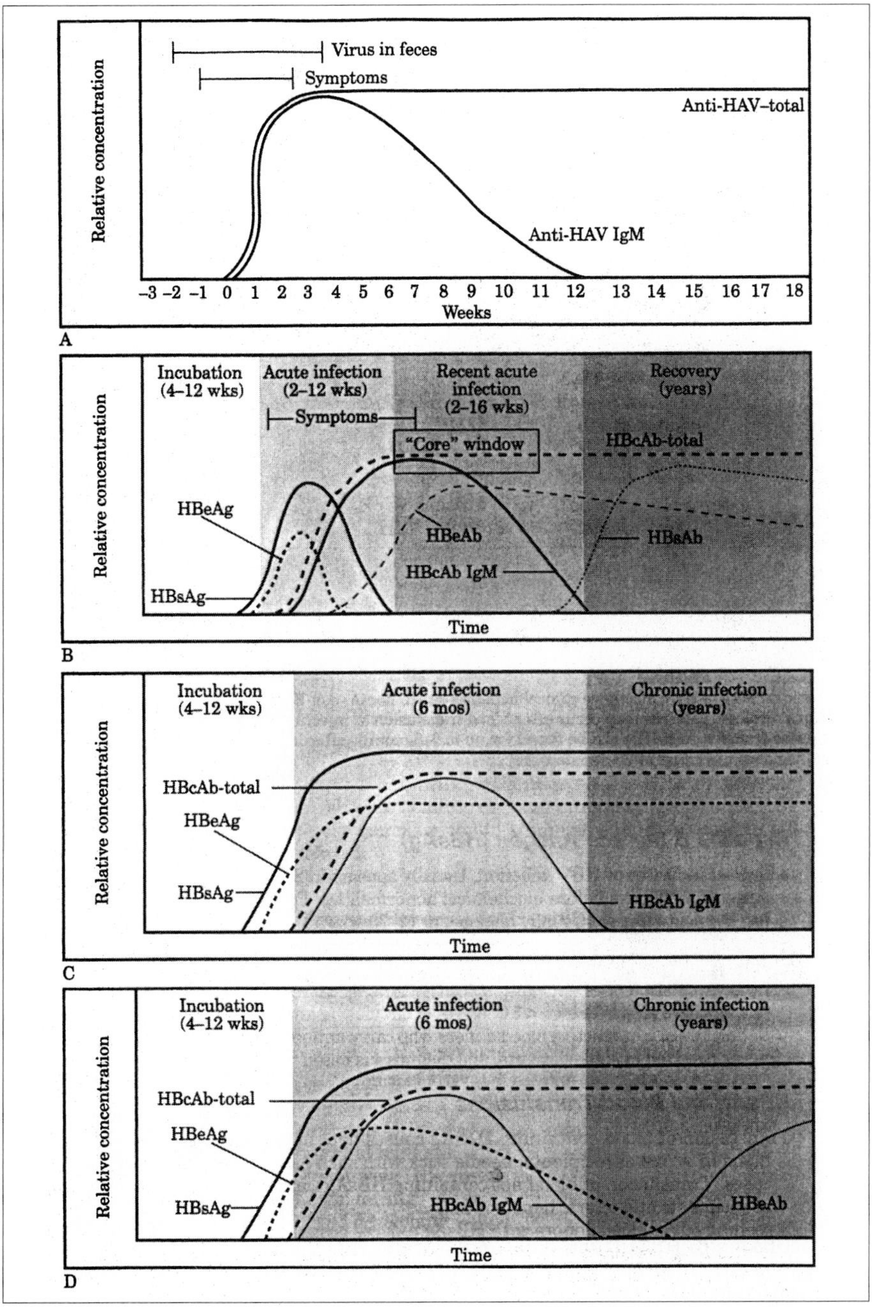

Fig. 2. Hepatitis serologic profiles. **A:** Antibody response to hepatitis A virus (HAV). **B:** Hepatitis B core window identification. **C:** Hepatitis B chronic carrier profile, no seroconversion. **D:** Hepatitis B chronic carrier profile, late seroconversion. HBcAg, hepatitis B core antigen; HBeAg, hepatitis Be antigen; HBsAg, hepatitis B surface antigen; IgM, immunoglobulin M. (Reproduced with permission from Hepatitis Information Center, Abbott Laboratories, Abbott Park, IL.)

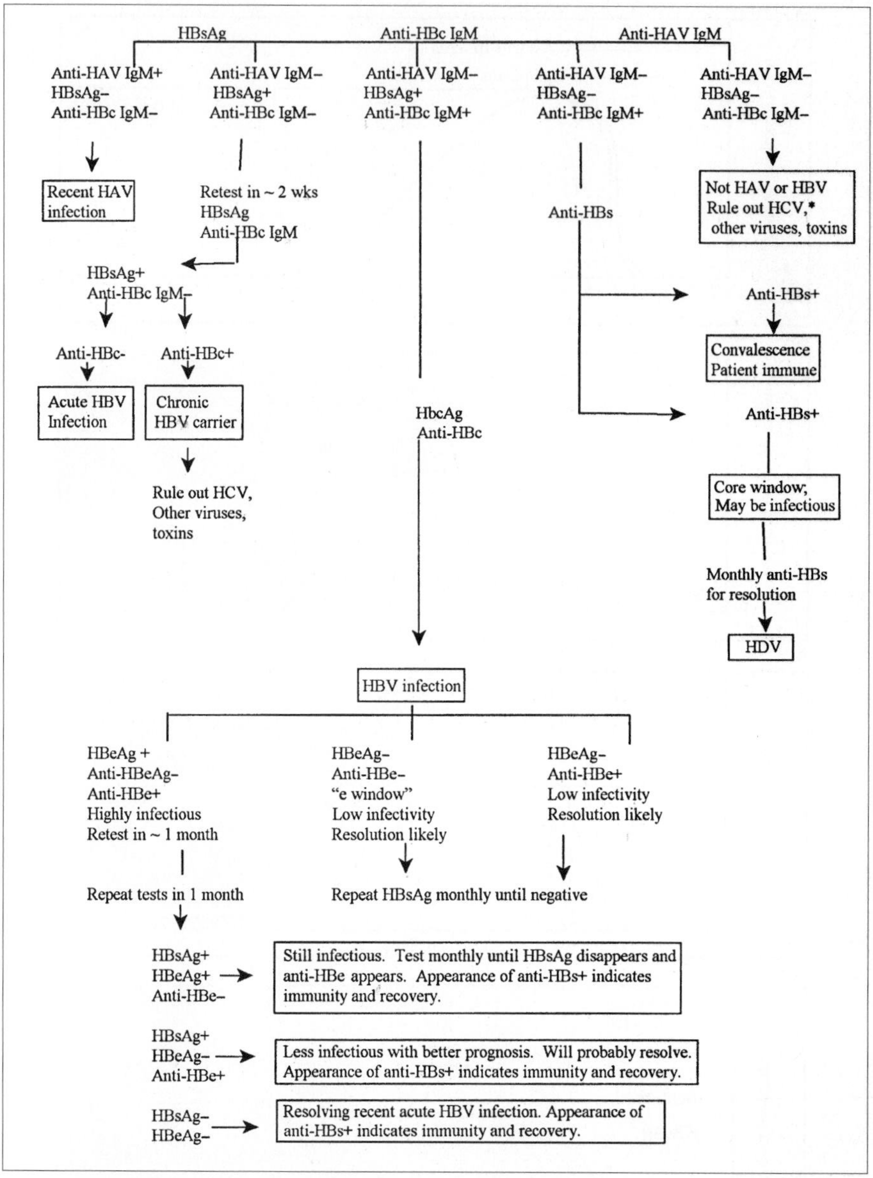

Fig. 3. Algorithm for diagnosis of hepatitis. *Do anti–hepatitis C virus (HCV). Anti-HAV, antibodies to hepatitis A virus (HAV); anti-HBc, antibodies to hepatitis B core antigen; anti-HBs, antibodies to HBsAg; anti-HBe, antibodies to HBeAg; HBeAg, hepatitis Be antigen; HBsAg, hepatitis B surface antigen; HBV, hepatitis B virus; HDV, hepatitis D virus; IgM, immunoglobulin M.

Hyperbilirubinemia, Neonatal

Diagnosis

The evaluation of serum bilirubin concentrations in newborn infants by means of a percentile-based normogram can predict the risk of hyperbilirubinemia. In one study, infants who had serum bilirubin concentrations in the high-risk category (>95th percentile) 18–72 hours after birth had a 40% probability of subsequent moderately severe hyperbilirubinemia (serum bilirubin concentration of >17 mg/dL), whereas infants with concentrations placing them in the low-risk category (<40th percentile) had a probability of zero. Meaningful follow-up data after hospital discharge were available for only 2,976 of 13,003 eligible infants. Nonetheless, normograms can identify infants who are at risk for severe hyperbilirubinemia.

Transcutaneous Measurement of Bilirubin

Newer noninvasive transcutaneous devices use multiwavelength spectral reflectance. In 897 newborn infants from various racial and ethnic groups, the serum bilirubin concentration ranged from 2 to 28 mg/dL (34–479 μmol/L), and the results of transcutaneous measurements of bilirubin correlated well with the serum concentrations ($r^2 = 0.88$).

Measurement of Carbon Monoxide to Evaluate Bilirubin Production

Hemolysis and bruising increase the production of bilirubin. Although the degree of jaundice and the rate of production of bilirubin are not always correlated because the rate of elimination of bilirubin varies among infants, early identification of infants in whom large amounts of bilirubin are produced is important. Carbon monoxide and bilirubin are produced in equimolar amounts when heme is degraded; measurements of carbon monoxide in exhaled air can be used as an index of bilirubin production. Exhaled carbon monoxide can be measured reproducibly.

Typical Changes in Levels of Bilirubin and Its Metabolites in Hyperbilirubinemias of Different Causes

See Table 5.

Conjugated-Fraction Hyperbilirubinemia

The presence of conjugated-fraction hyperbilirubinemia in the neonate is always pathologic and arises from a variety of causes.

Table 5. Typical Changes in Bilirubin and Its Metabolites in Hyperbilirubinemias Due to Different Causes

	Serum		Urine	
	Total Bilirubin	Conjugated Bilirubin	Bilirubin	Urobilinogen
Hemolysis	↑	N	N	↑
Physiologic hyperbilirubinemia	↑	N	↑	N
Liver disease	↑	↑	↑	N/↓
Gilbert disease	↑	N	N	N/↓
Crigler-Najjar syndrome	↑	N	N	N/↓

↑, increased; ↓, decreased; N, normal.

Causes of Neonatal Hyperbilirubinemia

Unconjugated	Conjugated
Physiologic (transient, appears days 1–2, resolves by days 7–10 in term babies)	Cholestasis/liver disease
Severe bruising	Parental nutrition
Breast-milk jaundice	Pyloric stenosis
Hemolysis	Cystic fibrosis
Blood group incompatibility	Infection
Inherited disorders of bilirubin conjugation	Inherited disorders
Hypothyroidism	Congenital abnormalities of the biliary tree
Rare endocrine disorders	Drugs

Risk Factors for Neonatal Hyperbilirubinemia

Maternal Factors

- Race or ethnic group
  - Native American
  - Asian
  - Greek Islander
- Complications during pregnancy
  - ABO incompatibility
  - Rh incompatibility
  - Diabetes mellitus
- Use of oxytocin in hypotonic solutions during labor
- Breast-feeding*

*Breast milk contains a competitive inhibitor of hepatic uridine diphosphate glucuronosyltransferase (late-onset breast-milk jaundice).

Perinatal Factors

- Birth trauma
  - Ecchymoses
  - Cephalhematoma
- Infection
  - Viral
  - Bacterial
  - Protozoal

Neonatal Factors

- Prematurity
- Genetic factors
- Familial disorders of conjugation
  - Crigler-Najjar syndrome types I and II
  - Gilbert syndrome
- Other enzymatic defects causing hemolysis
  - Pyruvate kinase deficiency
  - Hexokinase deficiency
  - Glucose-6-phosphate dehydrogenase deficiency
  - Congenital erythropoietic porphyria
- Erythrocyte structural defects causing hemolysis
  - Elliptocytosis
  - Spherocytosis
- Polycythemia causing hemolysis
- Drugs
  - Chloramphenicol
  - Benzyl alcohol
  - Streptomycin sulfate
  - Sulfisoxazole
- Low intake of breast milk (early-onset breast-milk jaundice)

Hyperphosphatasemia, Benign Transient (Idiopathic Hyperphosphatasemia of Infancy)

Transient marked increases in serum ALP levels are not uncommon in children. These increases are apparently benign, with no clinical or biochemical evidence of liver or bone disease, and typically occur in children <5 years of age.

Electrophoresis shows a diffuse band corresponding to the bone isoenzyme and a second band, intermediate in mobility to the main liver band and "biliary" ALP. Results of inhibitor, heat, neuraminidase, sialidase, and lectin treatment are consistent with the second band's being a liver isoenzyme with increased sialylation. The increased sialic acid content of the liver isoenzyme may slow the hepatic clearance. The etiology is uncertain, and induction by viral infection has been proposed. Enzyme activity usually falls to normal within 4 months.

Hypothyroidism

Hypothyroidism is usually associated with prolonged jaundice. This is identified in neonatal screening programs or investigated by measurement of serum free thyroxine and thyroid-stimulating hormone levels. Typically, the thyroid-stimulating hormone level is increased, with values >100 mU/L.

Jaundice

Breast-Milk Jaundice Syndrome

A small proportion (approximately 2.5%) of breast-fed babies develop a prolonged unconjugated-fraction hyperbilirubinemia at 10–21 days, known as *breast-milk jaundice syndrome*. Bilirubin values may be as high as 300 µmol/L (17.5 mg/dL). The jaundice resolves if breast-milk consumption is discontinued for a few days, and it is usually possible to restart breast-feeding without recurrence of jaundice or with only mild hyperbilirubinemia.

Breast-feeding jaundice, in contrast to breast-milk jaundice, occurs in the first few days of life. Bilirubin is mainly conjugated, and the increase is probably due to inadequate volume of intake.

Hemolysis

The appearance of jaundice within the first 48 hours of life may be due to hemolysis. In developed countries, blood-group incompatibilities between the mother and child are now rare due to the use of anti-D Ig (RhoGAM, Rh Ig) to prevent sensitization to the D antigen. ABO and other rare blood group incompatibilities can also produce hemolytic disease. If the mother's blood group is Rh negative, maternal anti-D titer is monitored to detect sensitization. In cases of sensitization, amniotic fluid indirect bilirubin level should be determined. A number of inherited abnormalities of the red cell may also present in this way, including spherocytosis, glucose-6-phosphate dehydrogenase deficiency, pyruvate kinase deficiency, and red cell membrane defects.

At the birth of a sensitized infant, cord blood hemoglobin level should be measured and bilirubin and antiglobulin levels determined on infant red cells (direct Coomb test). Sensitized infants may not be visibly jaundiced at birth.

Infections

Infection is the most common cause of nonphysiologic jaundice in infants in the first month of life. Many viral and bacterial infections cause hepatitis in the neonate. Investigation requires bacterial culture of blood and urine and viral serologic testing. Serum IgM level is raised in intrauterine infection; for healthy infants at the age of 2 weeks, the range is 0.05–0.2 g/L.

Cultures or DNA tests for toxoplasmosis, rubella, cytomegalovirus infection, herpes simplex infection, viral hepatitis, echovirus infection, and syphilis (TORCHES) are performed, in addition to tests for the more common organisms.

Neonatal Jaundice

In full-term infants, jaundice appearing before 2 days or persisting or appearing after 10 days requires further investigation. Estimation of total bilirubin and direct bilirubin levels is useful despite technical problems with the measurement of the latter fraction. Elevated levels of unconjugated, lipid-soluble bilirubin are toxic to the brain, causing kernicterus. Presence of bilirubin in urine on dipstick testing is a sensitive indicator of elevated conjugated bilirubin levels. Twenty-five percent or more of conjugated bilirubin in bilirubinemia suggests liver disease.

Obstructive Jaundice

The main causes of extrahepatic biliary obstruction in the neonate are biliary atresia and choledochal cyst. Biochemical tests show a predominantly conjugated-fraction hyperbilirubinemia with increase of liver enzymes. Diagnosis relies on ultrasonography, technetium scan, biopsy, and, ultimately, laparotomy.

Physiologic Jaundice

Physiologic jaundice occurs in at least 50% of normal babies. Development of the bilirubin-conjugating enzyme is delayed, and unconjugated bilirubinemia results. The jaundice becomes apparent after 1–2 days and usually fades by 7–10 days. These babies are well and thriving. In bottle-fed babies, serum bilirubin values are usually <200 μmol/L (11.7 mg/dL); in breast-fed babies, values are slightly higher. Higher values may occur in premature infants; values peak later, and increases may persist for up to 14 days. Several factors have been implicated, such as liver immaturity, increased bilirubin load from reduced red cell survival, reabsorption of bilirubin from the gut, bruising at birth, dehydration, and infection.

Liver Failure, Neonatal: Differential Diagnosis

See Table 6.

Endocrine Disorders

A number of rare endocrine abnormalities, including hypopituitarism, diabetes insipidus, hypoadrenalism, and hypoparathyroidism, may also present with jaundice in the neonatal period.

Parenteral Nutrition

Prolonged parenteral nutrition may cause cholestatic liver disease in some neonates. This complication is more common in sick, premature infants than in full-term infants.

Inherited Disorders

Several inherited disorders present with conjugated-fraction hyperbilirubinemia in the neonate. See the following section on Metabolic Diseases Causing Liver Disorders. See also Chapter 17, Metabolic and Hereditary Diseases.

Metabolic Diseases Causing Liver Disorders

(See also Chapter 17, Metabolic and Hereditary Diseases.)

A wide range of inborn errors of metabolism are associated with liver damage. Conditions include urea cycle disorders, defects in fatty acid oxidation and mitochondrial oxidative phosphorylation, amino acid disorders, and glycogen storage diseases. Many of the disorders that present acutely in neonates occur as late-onset forms in children.

Examples of inherited disorders that may present with neonatal jaundice are the following:

Galactosemia
Hereditary fructose intolerance
Cystic fibrosis
Niemann-Pick disease type C
Byler disease
Tyrosinemia type I
Zellweger syndrome
α_1-Antitrypsin deficiency
Defects in bile acid synthesis

Table 6. Differential Diagnosis in Neonatal Liver Failure

Disease Category	Disease	Diagnostic Tests
Metabolic	Galactosemia	Levels of reducing substances in urine
		Red blood cell galactose-1-phosphate uridyltransferase level
	Tyrosinemia	Plasma quantitative amino acid levels
		Urine succinylacetone level
		α-Fetoprotein level
	Neonatal hemochromatosis	Salivary gland or liver biopsy
		Hypersaturation of transferrin with decreased absolute transferrin concentrations
		Appropriate pattern of hepatic and extrahepatic siderosis on magnetic resonance imaging
	Δ^4-3-oxosteroid 5β-reductase deficiency	Urinary bile acid analysis by fast-atom-bombardment mass spectroscopy
	Hereditary fructose intolerance	Liver aldolase activity
		Allele-specific oligonucleotide analysis of peripheral genomic DNA
	α_1-Antitrypsin deficiency	Quantitative serum α_1-antitrypsin level
		Protease inhibitor typing
	Zellweger syndrome	Plasma levels of very long plasma fatty acids
	Niemann-Pick disease type C	Skin biopsy for fibroblast culture
		Studies of cholesterol esterification and accumulation
	Glycogen storage disease type 4	Skin biopsy for branching enzyme assay in cultured fibroblasts
		Liver biopsy
Infectious	Parvovirus B19	IgM level
		Blood PCR
	Echovirus 9	Culture from pharynx or blood
		PCR
	Coxsackievirus	Culture from urine or blood
		PCR
	Adenovirus	IgM level
		Culture from urine or blood
	Cytomegalovirus	Buffy-coat antigen level
		IgM level

(continued)

Table 6. (continued)

Disease Category	Disease	Diagnostic Tests
	Herpes simplex virus	Culture from nasopharynx or rectal swab specimen
		Buffy-coat PCR
	Hepatitis A virus	IgM level
	Hepatitis B virus	HBsAg level
		PCR
	Hepatitis C virus	PCR
	Rubella	IgM level
		Culture from urine or nasopharynx
	Syphilis	Venereal Disease Research Laboratories or rapid plasma reagin test
	Toxoplasma	DS-IgM EIA or ISAGA
	Human herpes virus 6	Blood PCR
Other	Hemophagocytic lymphohistiocytosis	Identification of hemophagocytic histiocytosis in liver and bone marrow
	Mitochondrial cytopathy	Presence of lactic acidosis
		Muscle or liver biopsy for analysis of respiratory chain enzyme function
	Neonatal lupus erythematosus	Maternal anti-Ro/SS-A and anti-La/SS-B antibodies
	Hepatic neuroblastoma	Ultrasonography or computed tomography
		Biopsy of mass
	Budd-Chiari syndrome	Doppler ultrasonography

DS-IgM EIA, double sandwich IgM enzyme immunoassay; HBsAb, hepatitis B surface antigen; Ig, immunoglobulin; ISAGA, IgM immunosorbent agglutination assay; PCR, polymerase chain reaction.
From Murray KF, Kowdley KV. Neonatal hemochromatosis. *Pediatrics* 2001;108(4):960–964.

α_1-Antitrypsin Deficiency

Characteristics

Deficiency of α_1-antitrypsin is an inherited condition that may account for up to 40% of cases of neonatal hepatitis. α_1-Antitrypsin is a plasma glycoprotein synthesized by the liver. It has a molecular weight of 52 kd, which permits entry into tissue spaces. It is a member of the serpin family (serine protease inhibitors) and functions in the inhibition of neutrophil elastase. Elastase has the highest affinity for elastin, which is found in the lungs.

α_1-Antitrypsin is encoded by a single gene on chromosome band 14q32:1. The alleles are inherited codominantly. More than 75 variants are now known. For the most common variants, letters have been assigned according to their electrophoresis mobility: F (fast), M (medium), S (slow), and Z (very slow). The heterozygous state occurs in 10–15% of the general population and is associated with α_1-antitrypsin levels that are 60% of normal; the homozygous state occurs in 1 in 2,000 and is accompanied by serum levels that are 1% of normal.

The most common phenotype is protease inhibitor M (Pi M). α_1-Antitrypsin deficiency is associated with emphysema as a result of increased proteolytic damage to the lungs. In some phenotypes (Pi Z, M_{MALTON}, M_{DUARTE}), α_1-antitrypsin accumulates in the hepatocyte.

Approximately 15% of individuals with the ZZ phenotype present with neonatal hepatitis, or, more rarely, hemorrhagic disease. Biochemical abnormalities include increased levels of bilirubin, aminotransferases, and ALP. Clinically and biochemically, the presentation may be indistinguishable from that of biliary atresia. Other patients with the Z phenotype may present later in childhood or adulthood with chronic liver disease and no reliable history of neonatal illness. Of infants with neonatal hepatitis, approximately 30% progress to cirrhosis and death by age 20 years, approximately 5% of these in the first year. By age 10, approximately 45% have clinical or biochemical evidence of liver disease. Liver disease resolves in the remainder. Pulmonary disease is more characteristic in later childhood and adulthood.

Quantitation of α_1-antitrypsin uses immunochemical methods and Pi phenotyping by isoelectric focusing or polyacrylamide gel. Isoenzyme quantitation or DNA analysis is confirmatory.

α_1-Antitrypsin values may be low in hepatic necrosis and in protein-losing states. Absence of an α_1-antitrypsin band is obvious on routine serum electrophoresis, but phenotyping should be undertaken using isoelectric focusing, in conjunction with immunofixation. Family studies are required to confirm the ZZ genotype. PCR methods can be used for prenatal diagnosis.

Although all ZZ individuals accumulate α_1-antitrypsin in hepatocytes, 20–40% develop clinically significant liver disease. Deficiency of α_1-antitrypsin (ZZ genotype) may present with liver disease in the older child.

Prenatal Diagnosis of α_1-Antitrypsin Deficiency by DNA Testing

Alleles of the α_1-antitrypsin gene are as follows:

	Serum α_1-Antitrypsin	α_1-Antitrypsin Function	Phenotype
Normal	Normal (150–350 mg/dL)	Normal	Pi MM
Deficiency severe	<50 mg/dL	Normal	Pi ZZ (>95% of cases) Pi Sz (rare) Pi SS (rare) Pi MZ (rare)
Null	Undetectable		Pi null-null (very rare) Pi Z-null (very rare)
Dysfunctional	Normal	Abnormal	

Z alleles are rare in Asians and blacks.
Threshold protection level for emphysema = 80 mg/dL.

Crigler-Najjar Syndrome

Crigler-Najjar syndrome is an inherited deficiency of the hepatic conjugating enzyme.

In the rare type I Crigler-Najjar syndrome, whose mode of inheritance is autosomal recessive, the enzyme is completely absent. This leads to severe unconjugated-fraction hyperbilirubinemia [bilirubin >340 μmol/L (>20 mg/dL)], which is recognized within a few days of birth. Without intensive treatment, death from the neurologic sequelae of kernicterus invariably occurs by 18 months of age. With continuous phototherapy with or without plasmapheresis, however, patients can survive longer. The only hope of cure is liver transplantation.

In type II Crigler-Najjar syndrome, a partial deficiency of the enzyme leads to a less severe unconjugated-fraction hyperbilirubinemia [bilirubin 100–340 μmol/L (6–20 mg/dL)]. Treatment with phenobarbitone induces the conjugating enzyme and reduces the serum bilirubin concentration and thus the jaundice.

Cystic Fibrosis

Liver complications are common in cystic fibrosis. Fatty filtration of the liver is usually found on liver biopsy, and 5–10% of adolescents have cirrhosis.

Infants with cystic fibrosis may rarely present with neonatal hepatitis.

Dubin-Johnson Syndrome

Dubin-Johnson syndrome is predominantly a conjugated-fraction hyperbilirubinemia with approximately 60% of the total bilirubin being direct reacting. Jaundice is recognized by puberty in half of the cases and by age 20 years in two-thirds. Bilirubin is usually <90 μmol/L (5 mg/dL) but can be up to 400 μmol/L (23 mg/dL). It is generally a benign disorder and is inherited as an autosomal-recessive trait. Bilirubin is taken up and conjugated normally by the liver, but conjugated bilirubin fails to be excreted into bile. Thus, bilirubin is retained in the liver and regurgitated into blood. A characteristic finding on the bromosulfophthalein test, in which bromosulfophthalein disappears normally from blood by 45 minutes but reappears at approximately 90 minutes, is pathognomonic for the syndrome. The disorder is associated with a highly pigmented liver, presumably due to the accumulation of bilirubin metabolites. An abnormality of coproporphyrin excretion is also present. Although the total urine coproporphyrin excretion is normal, 80–90% is in the form of coproporphyrin 1, whereas the usual proportion of this form is 25%.

Galactosemia

Galactosemia is caused by a deficiency of galactose-1-phosphate uridyltransferase required for the conversion of galactose (derived from lactose in milk) to glucose. Galactose-1-phosphate accumulates. High concentrations of galactose result in the production of potentially toxic compounds such as galactitol, involved in the formation of cataracts, and galactonate. A finding of galactose in the urine should prompt withdrawal of lactose from the diet and subsequent assessment of liver marker levels. Liver and renal dysfunction give rise to a generalized aminoaciduria. Diagnosis is based on the measurement of galactose-1-phosphate uridyltransferase activity in red cells.

Gilbert Syndrome

Gilbert syndrome is a mild unconjugated-fraction hyperbilirubinemia that affects approximately 70% of the population. The condition is benign and the hyperbilirubinemia usually presents between the ages of 10 and 30 years. Although the condition is present at birth, bilirubin concentrations rarely exceed approximately 100 μmol/L (6 mg/dL). The bilirubin concentration is increased by fasting and reduced by phenobarbitone administration, which induces the hepatic conjugating enzyme. AST, ALT, ALP, and GGT levels (liver function test results) are normal. Once all hematologic and hepatic causes of hyperbilirubinemia have been eliminated, Gilbert syndrome is the likely diagnosis.

Lysosomal Storage Disorders

Lysosomal storage disorders may cause hepatomegaly, splenomegaly, or both, with a range of other effects such as coarse facies, skeletal changes, and eye problems. Central nervous system involvement usually predominates. Investigation of lysosomal storage diseases relies heavily on clinical suspicion, as the diagnosis may require examination of bone marrow for storage cells and measurement of specific white cell enzyme levels.

Rotor Syndrome

Rotor syndrome, like Dubin-Johnson syndrome, is a disease of a benign conjugated-fraction hyperbilirubinemia and has many other similar features, including mode of inheritance, age at recognition, and degree of hyperbilirubinemia. The liver is not pigmented, however, and response to the bromosulfophthalein test, as in other hepatobiliary disorders, is a reduction in clearance and no regurgitation. Urinary excretion of coproporphyrin is increased, with 60% being coproporphyrin 1, a proportion similar to that in other hepatobiliary disorders.

Tyrosinemia Type I

In tyrosinemia type I, a deficiency of fumarylacetoacetase is found. The accumulating fumarylacetoacetate is converted to succinylacetoacetate and a "cabbage-like" odor is present. Diagnosis requires the demonstration of succinylacetone excretion in the urine together with fumarylacetoacetase deficiency in fibroblasts or lymphocytes.

Zellweger Syndrome

Zellweger syndrome is the classic example of a peroxisomal disorder. Typically, affected babies present with dysmorphic features, hypotonia, and abnormal liver function test results. Diagnosis involves the measurement of compounds metabolized or synthesized in peroxisomes, such as plasma very-long-chain fatty acids.

Reye Syndrome

Characteristics

Reye syndrome is an acute noninflammatory encephalopathy with liver dysfunction. It can occur at any age but is seen most often in childhood. The mortality rate is high, and many survivors suffer permanent brain damage. Typically, vomiting and altered consciousness develop in a child who appears to be recovering from a common viral illness such as influenza or chickenpox. The patient is not usually jaundiced, and there are no clinical signs of liver disease. Approximately 30% of children have seizures. There may be spontaneous recovery or progression to coma and brain death. Death in Reye syndrome is a result of marked cerebral edema. There is fatty infiltration of the liver and other organs, including muscle. The liver has a characteristic appearance on biopsy. Electron microscopy shows abnormalities in mitochondrial structure, and many of the biochemical changes are consistent with generalized mitochondrial dysfunction. Liver aminotransferase levels are elevated, with increased serum ammonia level and hypoglycemia. Prothrombin time is prolonged. Creatine kinase level is increased. In survivors, the mitochondria recover, and liver function test results return to normal. Uncontrolled lipolysis and reduced β-oxidation result in high concentrations of free fatty acids, which are converted to dicarboxylic acids and excreted in the urine.

The diagnosis of classical Reye syndrome is reserved for cases in which there is no obvious cause of the cerebral edema and liver dysfunction. Other causes of coma with abnormalities of liver function test results, such as severe infections and prolonged hypoxia, should be ruled out.

Drugs and toxins have been implicated in the development of Reye syndrome–like illnesses. Much attention has focused on salicylate, and the general use of aspirin by children <12 years of age is contraindicated.

Inborn Errors of Metabolism Presenting with a Reye Syndrome–Like Illness

Ornithine transcarbamylase deficiency
Carbamyl phosphate synthetase deficiency
Late-onset citrullinemia
Glutaric aciduria type 2
Biotinidase deficiency
Isovaleric acidemia

Medium-chain acyl–coenzyme A (CoA) dehydrogenase deficiency
Primary carnitine deficiency
Long-chain acyl–CoA dehydrogenase deficiency
Carnitine palmitoyltransferase deficiency
3-Hydroxy, 3-methylglutaryl–CoA lyase deficiency
Methylmalonic aciduria
Ethylmalonic adipic aciduria
Fructose-1,6-diphosphatase deficiency
Propionic acidemia
α_1-Antitrypsin deficiency
Pyruvate dehydrogenase deficiency

Stenosis, Pyloric

Infants with pyloric stenosis may be jaundiced due to increased levels of conjugated bilirubin. Dehydration may be part of the cause, and pyloric hypertrophy may partially obstruct the common bile duct.

Thromboembolism, Hepatic

Although there are many causes of thromboembolism related to liver disease, the majority of liver-related thromboembolisms occur secondary to liver transplantation in the postoperative period. Most frequently, thromboembolisms are limited to the transplanted vessels and include portal vein thrombosis (PVT).

Thrombosis

Hepatic Artery Thrombosis

Hepatic artery thrombosis (HAT) is a serious event that has a slightly delayed presentation, occurring approximately 1–2 weeks after transplantation. Dermatan sulfate, a circulating proteoglycan with anticoagulant activities, is present before and during the first days postoperatively.

The clinical course of HAT is usually fulminant but can be indolent with a late onset. The clinical presentation can include fulminant liver failure, biliary complications, and biliary sepsis.

Testing with pulsed Doppler ultrasonography combined with real-time ultrasonography of the liver parenchyma is commonly used to detect HAT; it has a sensitivity of approximately 70%. Because both false-positive and false-negative results may occur, angiography is usually required to confirm the diagnosis of HAT. Angiography has also been reported to give false-positive results as determined by autopsy findings. The extremely low flow that occurs in the hepatic arteries of small children contributes to the diagnostic difficulty. Computed tomography of the liver may be of aid in equivocal cases. Spiral computed tomography has been shown to be both sensitive and specific for the detection of HAT in adults.

Hepatic Vein Thrombosis

Hepatic vein thrombosis or Budd-Chiari syndrome is rare in children. It may be secondary to inferior vena cava obstruction, protein C deficiency, paroxysmal nocturnal hemoglobinuria, and congenital membranous malformation of the inferior vena cava.

Hepatic venoocclusive disease of the liver is seen after high-dose cytoreductive therapy before bone marrow failure.

Symptoms of hepatic vein thrombosis include abdominal pain, abdominal distention, and symptoms and laboratory signs of liver failure.

Portal Vein Thrombosis

In newborns, PVT most commonly occurs secondary to umbilical vein catheterization, with or without infection. The causes of PVTs in older children include liver transplantation, intraabdominal sepsis, splenectomy, sickle cell anemia, and the presence of antiphospholipid antibodies. In approximately 50% of children, an underlying cause is not identified. In contrast to adults, in whom PVT is most frequently secondary to cirrhosis, liver function is usually normal in children with PVT.

Clinical Presentation

PVT may present acutely as an acute abdomen, especially in adolescents. More commonly, PVT presents with symptoms reflecting a chronic obstruction including gastrointestinal bleeding and asymptomatic splenomegaly. If gastrointestinal bleeding occurs, it is usually recurrent.

Diagnosis

Radiographic tests to detect PVT include ultrasonography, magnetic resonance imaging, angiography, and computed tomographic scans.

Variceal hemorrhagic complications are an important clinical consequence of portal hypertension secondary to PVT. Less commonly, portal hypertension may be associated with fatal pulmonary hypertension.

Liver Disease in Older Children

Autoimmune Chronic Active Hepatitis

The presentation of autoimmune chronic active hepatitis varies from acute hepatitis to cirrhosis. Raised aminotransferase levels, hyperbilirubinemia, and often a low albumin level are present; IgG level is usually >16 g/L, and IgM level may be increased. Non–organ-specific autoantibodies are present.

Viral Hepatitis

Both acute and chronic hepatitis in childhood are most commonly caused by viral infections. Acute infections include those due to the hepatotrophic viruses [hepatitis A, B, C, D (hepatitis B dependent), and E] and those due to many other viruses, such as cytomegalovirus and Epstein-Barr virus (infectious mononucleosis). There may be hepatic involvement in numerous childhood viral illnesses, such as measles and adenovirus infections. The patient may have no symptoms of liver involvement, and it may be detected only by raised levels of aminotransferases on liver function tests. Hepatitis B, C, and D can progress to chronic infection.

The child with *hepatitis A* is almost always asymptomatic. Aminotransferase levels typically are increased up to 4 days before the development of jaundice, although bilirubin is detectable in the urine at this stage. Aminotransferase levels usually peak within 1 week at 1,000–5,000 IU. Bilirubin is usually at a level of <350 μmol/L (<20.5 mg/dL) and is predominantly conjugated. Increased aminotransferase levels may persist for several months. The diagnosis of hepatitis A infection is confirmed by detection of anti–hepatitis A virus IgM antibody.

Symptomatic *hepatitis B* follows an incubation period of 45–100 days, with jaundice and elevated aminotransferase levels. Papular acrodermatitis (Gianotti-Crosti syndrome) and glomerulonephritis may occur. Presence of hepatitis B surface antigen indicates acute or chronic infection.

Hepatitis D virus is a defective virus that infects only in the presence of hepatitis B. Incubation is 2 weeks to 4 months. Signs and symptoms are similar to those of hepatitis B but more severe than those of hepatitis B alone.

Wilson Disease

Wilson disease is an inherited disorder of copper metabolism. Inheritance is autosomal recessive with an incidence of 1 in 30,000. The gene has been mapped to chromosome band 13q14:3 and encodes for a copper-transporting adenosine triphosphatase, similar to the protein affected in Menkes syndrome. In Wilson disease, excretion of copper into the bile is defective, and usually serum concentrations of the copper-containing protein ceruloplasmin are reduced. Copper accumulates in the liver and, once the hepatic storage capacity is overwhelmed, it affects other tissues, including the brain and kidneys. Without treatment, the condition is fatal. Clinical presentation of Wilson disease is variable. It should be suspected in any child >5 years of age with unexplained liver disease or hemolytic anemia, and in older children with undiagnosed neurologic abnormalities.

Diagnosis relies on biochemical tests and careful examination of the eyes for evidence of copper deposition (Kayser-Fleischer rings). Ceruloplasmin level is below the reference range (0.2–0.6 g/L) in approximately 80% of patients but may be normal or increased with inflammation. Levels of this protein may also be low in protein-losing states and fulminant hepatic failure from other causes. Estrogens (from pregnancy and oral contraceptive use) increase the serum concentrations. Values in neonates are low (0.08–0.23 g/L in infants <4 months), which hampers diagnosis in siblings of affected children. Up to 20% of heterozygotes have low serum ceruloplasmin concentrations.

Baseline urine copper excretion is increased in the majority of cases. Urine copper excretion is generally >64 µg/24 hours (>1.0 µmol/24 hours). Liver copper values are increased, with concentrations in excess of 250 µg/g dry weight (the normal range is 15–50 µg/g). Heterozygotes have intermediate values. Urine copper excretion is assessed before and after administration of chelating agents. In Wilson disease, urine copper excretion is >1.6 mg/24 hours (25 µmol/24 hours) after administration of 1 g of penicillamine (with 500 mg given before the start of the collection and a second dose 12 hours later).

DNA methods that use flanking microsatellite markers can be used in family studies. Direct mutation analysis is difficult, as there are a large number of mutations and most patients are compound heterozygotes.

Other Causes of Liver Disease in Older Children

Reye syndrome
Hyperphosphatasemia
Drugs

Bibliography

Cacciola I, Pollicino T, Squadrito G, et al. Occult hepatitis B virus infection in patients with chronic hepatitis C liver disease. *N Engl J Med* 1999;341:22–26.

Czaja AJ. The variant forms of autoimmune hepatitis. *Ann Intern Med* 1996;125:588–598.

Gilbert-Barness E, Barness LA. *Metabolic diseases: foundations of clinical management, genetics and pathology.* Natick, MA: Eaton Publishing, 2000.

Lemon SM. Type A viral hepatitis: epidemiology, diagnosis, and prevention. *Clin Chem* 1997;43:1494–1499.

Masuko K, Mitsui T, Iwano K, et al. Infection with hepatitis GB virus C in patients on maintenance hemodialysis. *N Engl J Med* 1996;334:1485–1490.

Press RD, Flora K, Gross C, et al. Hepatic iron overload: direct HFE (HLA-H) mutation analysis vs quantitative iron assays for the diagnosis of hereditary hemochromatosis. *Am J Clin Pathol* 1998;109:577–584.

Ranson JHC. Etiological and prognostic factors in human acute pancreatitis: a review. *Am J Gastroenterol* 1982;77:633–638.

Sheth SG, Gordon FD, Chopra S. Nonalcoholic steatohepatitis. *Ann Intern Med* 1997;126:137–145.

Soldin SJ, Rifai N, Hicks JW. *Biochemical basis of pediatric disease*, 3rd ed. Washington, DC: AACC Press, 1998.

Stremmel W, Meyerrose KW, Niederau C, et al. Wilson disease: clinical presentation, treatment and survival. *Ann Intern Med* 1991;115:720–726.

Tietz NW, Shuey DF. Lipase in serum—the elusive enzyme: an overview. *Clin Chem* 1993;39:746–756.

Wallach J. *Interpretation of diagnostic tests*, 7th ed. Philadelphia: Lippincott Williams & Wilkins, 2000.

11 Hematologic Disorders

Hematologic Indices

Normal Blood Levels

The following normal values are compiled from published literature:

Bilirubin	
Total	
<1 day	<5.8 mg/dL
1–2 days	<8.2 mg/dL
3–5 days	<11.7 mg/dL
>1 mo	<1.0 mg/dL
Direct	
1 mo to adult	<0.6 mg/dL
Bleeding time	<9 min
D-Dimer	Any positive test result is significant
Erythrocyte sedimentation rate (ESR)	
Newborn (0–48 hr)	0–4 mm/hr
Child	4–20 mm/hr
Adult male	0–10 mm/hr
Adult female	0–20 mm/hr
Ferritin	
Child	7–144 µg/L
Adult male	30–265 µg/L
Adult female	10–110 µg/L
Fibrin degradation products	
Titer of 1:25	Borderline positive
Titer of 1:50	Positive
Fibrinogen	200–400 mg/dL
Folate [red blood cells (RBCs)]	150–450 µg/mL
Free erythrocyte protoporphyrin (FEP)	<3 µg/g hemoglobin <50 µg/dL whole blood <130 µg/dL packed RBCs
Haptoglobin	40–180 mg/dL
Hemoglobin A_{1C}	3.0–7.7% of total hemoglobin
Hemopexin	
Premature	2–26 mg/dL
Newborn	8–42 mg/dL
1–12 yr	40–70 mg/dL
>12 yr	50–100 mg/dL
Iron	
Newborn	110–270 µg/dL
4–10 mo	30–70 µg/dL
3–10 yr	53–119 µg/dL
Adult	72–186 µg/dL
Partial thromboplastin time, activated	
Preterm	70 sec

Full term	45–65 sec
Child/adult	30–45 sec
Prothrombin time	
Preterm	17 (range, 12–21) sec
Full term	16 (range, 13–20) sec
Child/adult	13 (range, 12–14) sec
Red blood count	
Term infant, cord blood	4.0–6.0 × 10^{12}/L
3 mo	3.2–4.8 × 10^{12}/L
1 year	3.6–5.2 × 10^{12}/L
3–6 yr	4.1–5.5 × 10^{12}/L
10–12 yr	4.0–5.4 × 10^{12}/L
Adult female	3.8–5.8 × 10^{12}/L
Adult male	4.5–6.5 × 10^{12}/L
Red cell distribution width (RDW)	11.5–14.5 × 10^{12}/L (no subnormal values reported)

High in iron deficiency, hemoglobin H (HbH) disease, S β thalassemia, fragmentation of RBCs, hemoglobinopathy traits (AC); some patients with anemia of chronic disease, glucose-6-phosphate dehydrogenase (G-6-PD) deficiency.

5 mL blood in ethylenediaminetetraacetic acid (EDTA) tube; 2 mL blood in special pediatric EDTA tube

Method: Part of full blood count on many automated instruments.

The RDW may assist in the classification of anemia, in association with the blood film and the other RBC indices [mean corpuscular volume (MCV), mean corpuscular hemoglobin (MCH), and mean corpuscular hemoglobin concentration (MCHC)].

Transferrin	
Newborn	130–275 mg/dL
Adult	220–400 mg/dL
Vitamin B_{12}	211–785 pg/mL

Blood Volume

Age	Total Blood Volume (mL/kg)
Premature infants	90–105
Term newborns	78–86
>1 mo	78
>1 yr	74–82
Adult	68–88

Age-Specific Values for Standard Hematologic Indices

Table 1 shows value for hemoglobin, hematocrit (Hct), and other hematologic indices by age.

Table 2 provides red cell values on the first postnatal day for infants of ≥24 weeks' gestational age.

Table 3 gives the proportion of different categories of white blood cells (WBCs) by age.

Hematologic Values in Preterm Infants (Compared with Term Infants)

Red Blood Cell Parameters

Lower hemoglobin and Hct levels at birth

Higher MCV, reticulocyte percentage, and number of nucleated RBCs at birth

Shorter RBC survival time (35–50 days versus 60–80 days for term infant)

More rapid and more pronounced physiologic anemia; nadir at 1–2 months

White Blood Cell Parameters

WBC count 30–50% lower at birth

Table 1. Age-Specific Hematologic Indices

Age	Hgb (g%), Mean[a] (–2 SD)	Hct (%), Mean (–2 SD)	MCV (fL), Mean (–2 SD)	MCHC (g% RBC), Mean (–2 SD)	Retic (%)	WBC/mm³ × 1,000, Mean (±2 SD)	Platelets (10³/mm³), Mean (±2 SD)	Nucleated RBCs/mm³
26–30 wk gestation[b]	13.4 (11)	41.5 (34.9)	118.2 (106.7)	37.9 (30.6)	—	4.4 (2.7)	254 (180–327)	
28 wk	14.5	45	120	31.0	(5–10)	—	275	
32 wk	15.0	47	118	32.0	(3–10)	—	290	
Term[a] (cord)	16.5 (13.5)	51 (42)	108 (98)	33.0 (30.0)	(3–7)	18.1 (9–30)	290	500
1–3 days	18.5 (14.5)	56 (45)	108 (95)	33.0 (29.0)	(1.8–4.6)	18.9 (9.4–34.0)	192	200
2 wk	16.6 (13.4)	53 (41)	105 (88)	31.4 (28.1)	—	11.4 (5–20)	252	0
1 mo	13.9 (10.7)	44 (33)	101 (91)	31.8 (28.1)	(0.1–1.7)	10.8 (4.0–19.5)	—	
2 mo	11.2 (9.4)	35 (28)	95 (84)	31.8 (28.3)	—	—	—	
6 mo	12.6 (11.1)	36 (31)	76 (68)	35.0 (32.7)	(0.7–2.3)	11.9 (6.0–17.5)	—	
6 mo–2 yr	12.0 (10.5)	36 (33)	78 (70)	33.0 (30.0)	—	10.6 (6–17)	(150–350)	
2–6 yr	12.5 (11.5)	37 (34)	81 (75)	34.0 (31.0)	(0.5–1.0)	8.5 (5.0–15.5)	(150–350)	
6–12 yr	13.5 (11.5)	40 (35)	86 (77)	34.0 (31.0)	(0.5–1.0)	8.1 (4.5–13.5)	(150–350)	
12–18 yr								
Male	14.5 (13)	43 (36)	88 (78)	34.0 (31.0)	(0.5–1.0)	7.8 (4.5–13.5)	(150–350)	
Female	14.0 (12)	41 (37)	90 (78)	34.0 (31.0)	(0.5–1.0)	7.8 (4.5–13.5)	(150–350)	
Adult								
Male	15.5 (13.5)	47 (41)	90 (80)	34.0 (31.0)	(0.8–2.5)	7.4 (4.5–11.0)	(150–350)	
Female	14.0 (12)	41 (36)	90 (80)	34.0 (31.0)	(0.8–4.1)	7.4 (4.5–11.0)	(150–350)	

Hct, hematocrit; Hb, hemoglobin; MCHC, mean corpuscular hemoglobin concentration; MCV, mean corpuscular volume; RBC, red blood cells; retic, reticulocytes; SD, standard deviation; WBC, white blood cell count.

[a]Under 1 mo, capillary Hb exceeds venous: 1 hr, 3.6-g% difference; 5 days, 2.2-g% difference; 3 wks, 1.1-g% difference.

[b]Values are from fetal samplings.

Adapted from Forestier F, Daffos F, Galacteros F, et al. *Pediatr Res* 1986;20:342–346; Oski FA, Naiman JL. *Hematological problems in the newborn infant.* Philadelphia: WB Saunders, 1982; Nathan D, Oski FA. *Hematology of infancy and childhood.* Philadelphia: WB Saunders, 1993; Metoth Y, Zaizov R, Varsano I. *Acta Paediatr Scand* 1971;60:317–23; and Wintrobe MM. *Clinical hematology.* Philadelphia: Lea & Febiger, 1981.

Table 2. Red Cell Values on the First Postnatal Day by Gestational Age

	Gestational Age (wk)							
	24–25 (n = 7)	26–27 (n = 11)	28–29 (n = 7)	30–31 (n=35)	32–33 (n = 23)	34–35 (n = 23)	36–37 (n = 20)	Term (n = 19)
RBC ($\times 10^{12}$/L)	4.65 ± 0.43	4.73 ± 0.45	4.62 ± 0.75	4.79 ± 0.74	5.0 ± 0.76	5.09 ± 0.5	5.27 ± 0.68	5.14 ± 0.7
Hemoglobin	19.4 ± 1.5	19.0 ± 2.5	19.3 ± 1.8	19.1 ± 2.2	18.5 ± 2.0	19.6 ± 2.1	19.2 ± 1.7	19.3 ± 2.2
Hematocrit	0.63 ± 0.04	0.62 ± 0.08	0.60 ± 0.07	0.60 ± 0.08	0.60 ± 0.08	0.61 ± 0.07	0.64 ± 0.07	0.61 ± 0.074
MCV (fL)	135.0 ± 0.2	132.0 ± 14.4	131.0 ± 13.5	127.0 ± 12.7	123.0 ± 15.7	122.0 ± 10.0	121.0 ± 12.5	119.0 ± 9.4
Reticulocytes	6.0 ± 0.5	9.6 ± 3.2	7.5 ± 2.5	5.8 ± 2.0	5.0 ± 1.9	3.9 ± 1.6	4.2 ± 1.8	3.2 ± 1.4
Weight (g)	725 ± 185	993 ± 194	1,174 ± 128	1,450 ± 232	1,816 ± 192	1,957 ± 291	2,450 ± 213	2,550 ± 220

Values are mean ± 1 standard deviation. Counts performed on heel-prick blood.
MCV, mean corpuscular volume; RBC, red blood cells.
Reproduced from Wallach J. *Interpretation of diagnostic tests*. 7th ed. Philadelphia: Lippincott Williams & Wilkins, 2000.

Table 3. Age-Specific White Cell Differential

	Total Leukocytes		Neutrophils[a]			Lymphocytes			Monocytes		Eosinophils	
Age	Mean	Range	Mean	Range	%	Mean	Range	%	Mean	%	Mean	%
Birth	—[b]	—	4.0	2.0–6.0	—	4.2	2.0–7.3	—	0.6	—	0.1	—
12 hr	—	—	11.0	7.8–14.5	—	4.2	2.0–7.3	—	0.6	—	0.1	—
24 hr	—	—	9.0	7.0–12.0	—	4.2	2.0–7.3	—	0.6	—	0.1	—
1–4 wk	—	—	3.6	1.8–5.4	—	5.6	2.9–9.1	—	0.7	—	0.2	—
6 mo	11.9	6.0–17.5	3.8	1.0–8.5	32	7.3	4.0–13.5	61	0.6	5	0.3	3
1 yr	11.4	6.0–17.5	3.5	1.5–8.5	31	7.0	4.0–10.5	61	0.6	5	0.3	3
2 yr	10.6	6.0–17.0	3.5	1.5–8.5	33	6.3	3.0–9.5	59	0.5	5	0.3	3
4 yr	9.1	5.5–15.5	3.8	1.5–8.5	42	4.5	2.0–8.0	50	0.5	5	0.3	3
6 yr	8.5	5.0–14.5	4.3	1.5–8.0	51	3.5	1.5–7.0	42	0.4	5	0.2	3
8 yr	8.3	4.5–13.5	4.4	1.5–8.0	53	3.3	1.5–6.8	39	0.4	4	0.2	2
10 yr	8.1	4.5–13.5	4.4	1.8–8.0	54	3.1	1.5–6.5	38	0.4	4	0.2	2
16 yr	7.8	4.5–13.0	4.4	1.8–8.0	57	2.8	1.2–5.2	35	0.4	5	0.2	3
21 yr	7.4	4.5–11.0	4.4	1.8–7.7	59	2.5	1.0–4.8	34	0.3	4	0.2	3

Number of leukocytes is in thousands per cubic millimeter; ranges are estimates of 95% confidence limits, and percentages refer to differential counts.
[a]Neutrophils include band cells at all ages and a small number of metamyelocytes and myelocytes in the first few days of life.
[b]Insufficient data for a reliable estimate.
Reproduced with permission from Dallman PR. Developmental changes in number. In: Rudolph AM, ed. *Pediatrics,* 18th ed. Norwalk, CT: Appleton & Lange, 1987:1061. Data on infants under the age of 1 month are derived from Manroe BL, Weinberg AG, Rosenfeld CR, et al. *J Pediatr* 1979;95:89–98; and Weinberg AG, Rosenfeld CR, Manroe BL, et al. *J Pediatr* 1985;106:462–466. Other values are from Albritton EC, ed. *Standard value in blood.* Philadelphia: WB Saunders, 1952.

Hematologic Procedures and Tests

Procedures for Hematologic Studies

Microhematocrit

1. Fill standard microhematocrit tube with blood and seal one end with clay. Centrifuge (12,000 g) for 5 minutes.
2. Falsely high Hcts caused by increased plasma trapping occur with short centrifugation time and in disorders with decreased red cell deformability.

Wright Staining Technique

1. Place air-dried blood smears, film side up, on staining rack.
2. Cover smear with undiluted Wright stain and leave for 2–3 minutes.
3. Add equal volume of distilled water and blow gently on the surface until a greenish metallic sheen appears. Leave diluted stain on smear for 2–6 minutes.
4. Without disturbing the slide, flood with water and wash until stained smear is pinkish red. Blot dry.

Hematologic Indices

1. MCV: Average RBC volume. Usually measured directly by electronic counters. Expressed in femtoliters (fL, 10^{-15} L).

$$MCV = \frac{Hct(\%) \times 10}{\text{RBC count (millions/mm}^3)}$$

2. MCH: Average quantity of hemoglobin per red cell expressed in picograms (pg, 10^{-12} g).

$$MCH = \frac{Hb(g\%) \times 10}{\text{RBC count (millions/mm}^3)}$$

3. MCHC: Grams of hemoglobin per 100 mL packed cells. High value in congenital spherocytic hemolytic anemia and hemoglobulin SC (sickle cell) disease; may be low in iron deficiency.

$$MCHC = \frac{Hb(g\%) \times 100}{Hct(\%)}$$

4. RDW: Statistical description of heterogeneity of red cell size. Increases with anisocytosis, reticulocytosis, iron deficiency. Increased in newborns. Normal in thalassemia minor.

$$\text{RDW} = \frac{(\text{Standard deviation of MCV} \times 100)}{\text{MCV}}$$

Reticulocyte Count

1. Mix equal amounts of new methylene blue or brilliant cresyl blue with whole blood. After 10–20 minutes, prepare thin smears.
2. Count the number of reticulocytes (cells containing reticulum or blue granules) per 100 red cells and report as percentage of RBCs.

Platelet Estimation

Use Wright-stained blood smear to approximate platelet count. Always examine periphery of smear or coverslip, as platelet clumps may be deposited there. For rough approximation, one platelet per oil-immersion field corresponds to 10,000–15,000 platelets/mm^3. Platelet clumps usually indicate >100,000 platelets/mm^3.

Erythrocyte Sedimentation Rate

Should be determined within 1 hour after obtaining blood.

Collect venous blood in EDTA- or oxalate-containing tube.

Place 1 mL in a Wintrobe tube, using a long Pasteur pipette. Fill carefully from the bottom of the tube; do not shake tube or allow air bubbles to form in the column of blood. Place the tube vertically.

Read depth of fall of RBC column at the end of 60 minutes.

Anemia, tilting of column, warming, or shaking may artificially increase the ESR. Hypo- or afibrinogenemia, old or cold blood, excessive anticoagulant, sickle cell anemia, congestive heart failure, polycythemia, trichinosis, and pertussis may decrease the ESR. ESR is elevated in newborns with infections or with ABO hemolysis.

Cold Agglutinins: Rapid Screening Test

(See also Anemia, Hemolytic, Autoimmune.)

1. Collect four or five drops of blood in 60 × 7 mm Wasserman tube containing approximately 0.2 mL of 3.8 sodium EDTA.
2. Cap tube and place in ice water bath for 30–60 seconds.
3. Tilt tube and observe blood as it runs down wall of tube.
4. Definite floccular agglutination (seen with unaided eye), which disappears on warming to 37°C, is considered a positive (3–4+) test. A control sample is useful for interpretation.
5. Positive test result frequently correlates with cold agglutinin titer of >1:64. Seventy-five percent to 85% of patients with atypical pneumonia and a positive test result develop serologic evidence of mycoplasma pneumonia infection.

Serum Complement Measurement

Serum complement is measured spectrophotometrically by lysis of 50% of an RBC suspension in 1 hour. This is achieved by 50–100 U of complement in most laboratories, but normal ranges must be determined for each laboratory.

Serum complement is decreased in cold autoimmune hemolytic anemia (AIHA) due to complement binding by antibodies. Levels also may be decreased in warm AIHA when complement is fixed to the cell membrane. Lytic complement tests are not easily performed and often require the services of reference laboratories.

Automated Complete Blood Cell Count

Routine analyses provided by hematology analyzers and automated instruments

- RBCs
- Hemoglobin
- Hct
- MCV
- MCH
- RDW
- WBCs
- White blood cell differential
- Platelets
- Mean platelet volume

Blood Cell Analysis

Mean Corpuscular Volume

The MCV is decreased in severe iron-deficiency anemia and thalassemias. The MCV may be increased in many of the sideroblastic anemias, although microcytosis is more common in the hereditary types. The reticulocyte count may be modestly decreased, normal, or modestly increased. Indices are often normal in patients with hemoglobin levels >10 g/dL (>100 g/L). RBC number in thalassemias is not proportional to the low hemoglobin level or degree of microcytosis. Iron-deficiency anemia usually shows concordant decrease in RBC number, hemoglobin levels, and MCV; it may also be associated with mild thrombocytosis.

Peripheral Blood Smear Morphology

Hypochromia and microcytosis are present in severe iron-deficiency anemia but may be lacking in patients with less severe iron depletion. Sideroblastic anemias usually have notable anisocytosis and poikilocytosis in addition to hypochromia. Occasionally, dysplastic features may be noted in WBCs in idiopathic cases. Target cells and basophilic stippling are usually prominent in the thalassemias.

Bone Marrow Examination

Bone marrow examination usually is not required for the diagnosis of iron-deficiency anemia or thalassemia but is important in documenting a sideroblastic anemia. The only specific bone marrow findings in microcytic anemias are decreased or absent stainable storage iron in iron-deficiency anemia, increased reticuloendothelial iron with decreased sideroblastic iron in anemia of chronic diseases (ACD), and the presence of ringed sideroblasts in sideroblastic anemias. Iron stores are often increased in thalassemias.

Special Hematologic Stains

Special stains are on peripheral blood or bone marrow aspirate (BMA).

Stain	Use
Wright-Giemsa	Routine cytomorphology
Leukocyte alkaline phosphatase	Suspected myeloproliferative process [e.g., chronic myelogenous leukemia (CML)]
Tartrate-resistant acid phosphatase	Suspected hairy cell leukemia
Iron stain (Prussian blue)	Detection and quantitation of iron deposits
Myeloperoxidase	Detection and quantitation of myeloblasts
Sudan black B	Detection and quantitation of myeloblasts
Periodic acid–Schiff (PAS)	Identification of blasts
Specific esterase (chloroacetate esterase)	Identification and quantitation of myeloblasts, granulocytes, percentage of granulocytic precursors
Nonspecific esterase (α-naphthyl acetate esterase)	Identification and quantitation of monoblasts, monocytes, percentage of monocytic precursors
Combined esterase (specific and nonspecific)	Differentiation of acute monoblastic, acute myelomonocytic, and acute myelogenous leukemia
RBC inclusions	
Microcytes with stippling	Thalassemia; lead or heavy metal poisoning
Cabot rings	Occasionally seen in severe hemolytic anemias and pernicious anemia
Howell-Jolly bodies (dark purple spherical bodies) (Color Fig. 1A,B)	Megaloblastic anemia; thalassemia; hyposplenism; postsplenectomy state
Pappenheimer bodies (siderotic granules; purple coccoid granules at periphery) (Color Fig. 1C)	Anemias with defect of incorporating iron into hemoglobin (e.g., sideroblastic anemia, thalassemia, lead poisoning, pyridoxine-unresponsive and pyridoxine-responsive anemias)
	Iron overload
Heinz bodies (precipitates of denatured hemoglobin) (Color Fig. 1D)	Congenital G-6-PD deficiency
	Hemolytic anemias induced by drugs (e.g., dapsone, phenacetin)
	Unstable hemoglobin disorders after splenectomy

Evaluation of Red Blood Cell Production and Breakdown

Phases of Life Cycle	Laboratory Tests or Findings
Bone marrow production	Reticulocyte count, bone marrow cellularity, iron 59 uptake
RBC circulation	Hemoglobin/Hct, chromium 51 (^{51}Cr) RBC survival studies
RBC sequestration	^{51}Cr RBC sequestration
RBC breakdown	Hemoglobinemia; increased serum levels of haptoglobin, bilirubin, lactate dehydrogenase, methemalbumin; increased bone marrow iron
Excretion	Hemosiderinuria, hemoglobinuria

Evaluation of Iron Levels

Serum Iron Quantitation and Measurement of Total Iron-Binding Capacity

Procedure

Serum iron is freed from transferrin by acidification of the serum and is reduced to the ferrous form. After the protein has been precipitated, the iron in the filtrate is detected spectrophotometrically after reaction with a chromogen such as bathophenanthroline sulfonate. Total iron-binding capacity (TIBC) is measured by adding iron to the serum and then removing excess unbound iron by magnesium carbonate absorption. The bound iron is then released from transferrin and reduced, and its concentration is measured as in the serum iron test. The TIBC also can be determined by measuring transferrin with immunodiffusion.

Interpretation

The normal range of values is as follows:

1. Serum iron concentration: 60–180 μg/dL (12.7–35.9 μmol/L)
2. TIBC: 250–410 μg/dL (45.2–77.7 μmol/L)
3. Percent saturation: 20–50%

The serum iron level and percent saturation are low in both iron-deficiency anemia and ACD. The value for percent saturation is often reduced to <16% in iron-deficiency anemia and is frequently >16% in ACD. The TIBC is uniformly increased in severe uncomplicated iron-deficiency anemia and is decreased or normal in microcytic ACD. In mild iron-deficiency anemia, both the serum iron concentration and TIBC may be normal. Serum iron concentration is increased in the sideroblastic anemias and in some cases of thalassemia.

Serum iron concentrations show wide diurnal variations, with highest levels in the morning. Thus, specimens should be collected in the morning, and oral iron therapy should be withdrawn 24 hours before the blood sample is drawn. Iron dextran administration causes plasma iron levels to be elevated for several weeks. A normal plasma iron level and iron-binding capacity do not rule out the diagnosis of iron deficiency when the hemoglobulin level of the blood is >9 g/dL.

Serum Ferritin Quantitation

Principle

Ferritin is a storage complex of the protein apoferritin and iron. The largest quantities of ferritin are found in the liver and reticuloendothelial cells. Ordinarily, serum ferritin concentration reflects the amount of stored iron.

Procedure

Reliable estimation of serum ferritin levels is achieved with a sensitive radioimmune method using a sandwich technique. Ferritin is removed from the serum by solid-phase antiferritin antibodies, and radioactively labeled antiferritin antibodies are then permitted to bind to the removed ferritin.

Interpretation

The normal concentration of serum ferritin varies from 10 to 500 ng/mL. In iron-deficiency anemia, serum ferritin level is diminished. Elevated ferritin levels are common in iron overload state, including sideroblastic anemia, neonatal iron storage disease, and hemochromatosis. Serum ferritin levels are also elevated in patients with inflammatory diseases and in patients with Gaucher disease.

Serum Soluble Transferrin Receptor Assay

The transferrin receptor is a transmembrane protein that transfers iron from plasma transferrin into the cell. Most transferrin receptors are found in the cell membrane, but a truncated form of the tissue receptor that is complexed with transferrin is found in soluble form in the serum. Transferrin receptor levels reflect iron status, with receptor synthesis being rapidly induced by decreased iron levels.

Serum transferrin receptors are assayed with a sandwich enzyme immunoassay that uses a polyclonal antibody against the serum transferrin receptor protein. Commercially available kits can detect the protein in ranges from 0.85 to 20 mg/L.

Levels of serum soluble transferrin receptors >3.1 mg/L have been used as an indicator of iron deficiency.

Elevated serum soluble transferrin receptor levels have been noted, irrespective of patient iron status, in patients with hematologic malignancies or conditions with increased effective or ineffective hematopoiesis (i.e., hemolytic anemias, hemoglobinopathies, or deficiencies of vitamin B_{12} or folate). Normal ranges for pediatric patients are not well established.

Free Erythrocyte Protoporphyrin Measurement

FEP levels are elevated in patients with anemias associated with failure of iron incorporation into heme.

Whole anticoagulated blood is collected. There is also a spot test for blood specimens collected on filter paper.

FEP is extracted from RBCs with ethyl acetate and acetic acid, and is quantitated fluorometrically.

FEP is normally <100 μg/dL packed RBCs. Elevated levels are seen in patients with iron deficiency, erythropoietic protoporphyria, chronic disease states associated with decreased transferrin saturation, and acquired idiopathic sideroblastic anemia. Marked elevation of FEP level is seen in patients with sideroblastic anemia secondary to lead intoxication, with FEP values >300 μg/dL packed RBCs. In patients with microcytic anemias associated with abnormal globin synthesis rather than abnormal heme synthesis (such as thalassemia minor), FEP levels are normal.

Hemoglobin Electrophoresis

(See also Hemoglobinopathies.)

Cellulose acetate electrophoresis separates hemoglobin variants based on molecular charge. Hemoglobins are reported in order of relative abundance; for example, sickle cell trait is ASA_2, sickle cell disease is SFA_2, β thalassemia is elevated A_2.

Bone Marrow Examination

Bone Marrow Aspiration

Smear
- Romanowsky stain
- Cytochemical stain
- Immunocytochemical stain
- Image analysis
- *In situ* hybridization

Cell suspension
- Flow cytometry
- Cytogenetics
- DNA-RNA extractions

Bone Marrow Biopsy

Imprints
- Romanowsky stain
- Immunocytochemical analysis
- Cytochemical analysis

Sections
- Hematoxylin and eosin stain
- Giemsa stain
- Iron analysis
- Immunocytochemical analysis

In young infants, hematopoiesis occupies 80% to 100% of the marrow spaces. Erythrocytes grow in islands in the center of the medullary cavity. The more immature forms of the granulocytic series grow in proximity to the bone trabeculae or close to small arteries. Megakaryocytes develop in proximity to the central capillaries of the marrow spaces.

Stainable Bone Marrow Iron

Principle

Normoblasts that contain one or more particles of stainable iron are called *sideroblasts*. Iron is stored as ferritin (iron complexed to the apoferritin protein) and hemosiderin (iron-protein complexes with a high iron content and denatured ferritin aggregates).

Hemosiderin is the stainable form of storage iron that appears blue when treated with an acid potassium ferricyanide solution used in the Prussian blue reaction.

Specimens

Sectioned BMA fragments (clot section) or particle smears are used for the assessment of reticuloendothelial iron, but BMA films must be used to detect sideroblasts.

Note: Iron staining may be decreased in decalcified sections due to leaching out of iron during the decalcification process.

The BMA is stained with Prussian blue.

Hemosiderin granules are seen in reticuloendothelial cells in every third or fourth oil-immersion field. With reduced iron stores, either no or only a few hemosiderin granules are seen in the entire preparation. With increased iron stores, hemosiderin granules are seen in every oil-immersion field, often deposited in clumps. Increased iron is generally present in the marrow of patients with anemia who are not iron deficient. Decreased bone marrow sideroblasts are seen in iron-deficiency anemia, after acute blood loss when reticuloendothelial stores have not yet been depleted, and in ACD. Sideroblastic anemia is characterized by the presence of ring sideroblasts, normoblasts that contain iron granules that surround at least two-thirds of the nuclear circumference.

Indications for Bone Marrow Examination

Abnormalities in blood counts or peripheral blood smears
- Unexplained cytopenias
- Unexplained leukocytosis or abnormal WBCs
- Teardrop cells or leukoerythroblastosis
- Rouleaux
- No or low reticulocyte response to anemia

Evaluation of systemic disease
- Unexplained splenomegaly, hepatomegaly, lymphadenopathy
- Tumor staging (solid tumors, lymphomas)
- Monitoring of chemotherapy effect
- Fever of unknown origin (with bone marrow cultures)
- Evaluation of trabecular bone in metabolic disease (undecalcified bone should be used)

Osmotic Fragility Test

The osmotic fragility test indirectly measures the presence of spherocytes. A cell that is spherocytic in the resting state has less membrane redundancy than a normal biconcave cell, so less water can enter before cellular rupture occurs.

Blood freshly drawn into heparin or EDTA is used. Samples older than 48 hours may show an artefactual shift toward increased fragility.

The tests should be carried out on freshly drawn blood and, if necessary, on blood that has been incubated at 37°C for 24 hours. Osmotic fragility tests on incubated samples are more sensitive for detecting low levels of hemolysis. This may be useful when hereditary spherocytosis is suspected clinically but the levels of hemolysis seen with fresh blood are within normal ranges. However, the increase in sensitivity for detection of osmotic fragility is offset by a loss of specificity in the incubated-sample test.

Increased osmotic fragility is an essential diagnostic feature of hereditary spherocytosis. In mild forms of the disease, however, it is not uncommon to find only a minimal increase in osmotic fragility on freshly drawn blood. Results of osmotic fragility tests on incubated blood are almost always abnormal in such cases. Decreases in hemolysis or decreased osmotic fragility are seen in thalassemia, iron deficiency, and other conditions in which there is an increase in the ratio of surface area to volume for the RBC.

Special Diagnostic Procedures

Evaluation of Anemia

Anemia is defined by age-specific norms. Common general screening studies include
1. Complete blood cell count (CBC) with differential and reticulocyte count.
2. Blood smear to examine morphology of cells, indices, and size distribution.

3. Urinalysis for bilirubin, blood, protein, glucose. Also perform microscopic examination.
4. Stool test for occult blood.
5. Serum bilirubin, blood urea nitrogen, creatinine levels.
6. Coombs test.

After a clinical history is taken and physical examination and screening tests are performed, the evaluation of hypochromic anemias may include

1. Estimation of serum iron levels and total iron-binding capacity, ferritin, or serum transferrin receptor levels. These measurements reflect iron stores and help to distinguish iron deficiency from other causes of microcytic, hypochromic anemia.
2. Tests to diagnose sickle hemoglobin: Any substance that reduces oxygen tension will cause red cells containing HbS (sickle cell hemoglobin) to sickle. Positive results on a sickle preparation are found in the sickle cell hemoglobinopathies (SS, SC, S thal, and others), as well as in sickle trait (AS); 8% of black children have positive results on sickle preparation. All positive test results should be confirmed with hemoglobin electrophoresis.
   Sulfite solution—sickle preparation: Mix one or two drops of 2% sodium metabisulfite or sodium hyposulfite on a slide with one drop of blood; apply coverslip. Read preparation at 30 minutes and again at 3 hours. Positive test result: presence of sickled cells.
   Sickledex (solubility test using dithionate reduction of HbS): Used in many commercial and hospital diagnostic laboratories.
3. Iron trial: Adequate iron therapy should result in reticulocytosis peaking 7–10 days into therapy. A significant increase in hemoglobin concentration should be evident after 3–4 weeks of therapy.
4. FEP measurement.
5. Hemoglobin electrophoresis (cellulose acetate electrophoresis or isoelectric focusing).
6. Examination of aspirated bone marrow for stainable iron, the most direct assessment of iron stores. Associated dysplasia or demonstration of ringed sideroblasts may reflect a sideroblastic anemia.
7. Specific red cell enzyme tests (e.g., G-6-PD, pyruvate kinase).
8. Assays for indicators of hemolysis
   Haptoglobin: binds free hemoglobin (see also Anemia, Hemolytic). Decreased with intravascular and extravascular hemolysis and hepatocellular disease. Falsely normal or increased levels may occur in association with inflammation, infection, or malignancy.
   Hemopexin: binds free heme groups. Decreased with intravascular hemolysis, renal disease, and hepatocellular disease. Hemopexin levels usually not increased with inflammation, infection, or malignancy.
9. Cytogenetic analysis to document a myelodysplastic syndrome, which shows cytogenetic abnormalities in up to 80% of affected patients. Cytogenetic abnormalities associated with myelodysplasia include complex chromosomal defects, monosomy 7, deletion of 5q, and trisomy 8.
10. Determination of globin chain synthetic ratios, which is often the only means of making a positive diagnosis of mild forms of thalassemias.

Diagnostic Procedures for Leukemia, Lymphomas, and Pediatric Malignant Tumors

Flow cytometry, molecular diagnostics, fluorescent *in situ* hybridization (FISH), and conventional chromosome metaphase spread analysis are the most commonly used adjunctive studies in the diagnosis of hematopoietic tumors. These techniques often provide diagnostic information beyond that seen with routine light microscopy. Although they are useful and often necessary, these techniques are not required for the diagnosis of many common hematopoietic disorders. Many of these specialized tests are relatively expensive and should be used judiciously.

Flow Cytometry

Flow cytometry is a rapid and reliable technique for immunophenotyping of hematopoietic cells. Flow cytometry has a broad range of uses in the evaluation of hemato-

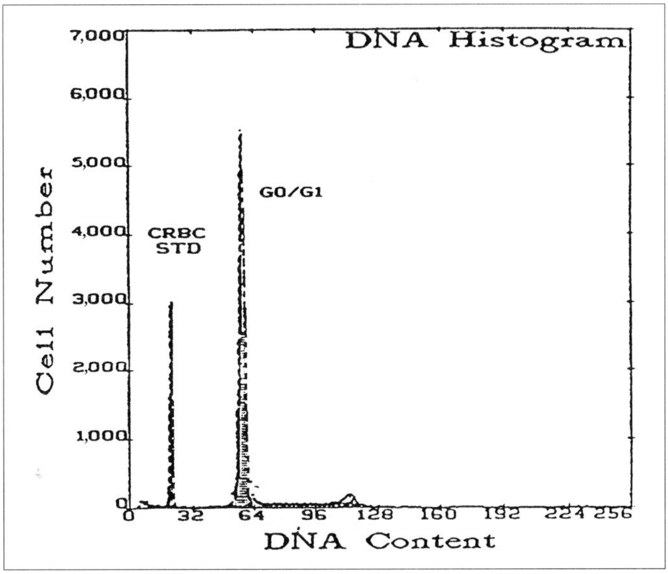

Fig. 2. A typical histogram of a diploid nephroblastoma includes three peaks: chicken red blood cell standard (CRBC STD), G_0/G_1 diploid peak, and small G_2/M peak, which has twice the DNA content of the G_0/G_1 peak. Diploid cells: DNA index = 1.00; percent of total = 100.0%; G_2 phase = 0.5%; S phase = 15.1%; G_0/G_1 coefficient of variation = 2.3%. (Reproduced with permission from Marshall T, Rutledge JC. Flow cytometry DNA applications in pediatric tumor pathology. *Perspect Pediatr Pathol* 2001;23:55.)

poietic processes. One of the most common is immunophenotyping of peripheral blood, lymph node, and bone marrow samples to establish the diagnosis of leukemia or lymphoma, detect clonality, and identify lineage. Flow cytometry has many other uses, including determining CD4/CD8 ratios and absolute counts, establishing the presence of congenital immunodeficiencies, and determining the ploidy and S phase of tumors.

In flow cytometry, cells are passed singly in a fluid stream through a beam of light. The light source is typically a laser, and as the cells pass through the laser beam, photons of light are emitted and scattered. These photons are separated and collected by forward and side light-scatter detectors. The detected light signal is converted into a digital signal with the aid of photomultipliers. The digital signal generated by each cell is proportional to its light emission and is plotted on a histogram. One of the most important requirements of flow cytometry is the passage of single cells through the light source. This is achieved by forcing an isotonic (sheath) fluid through a cylindrical nozzle to create a laminar flow. The sample, also suspended in isotonic fluid, is introduced simultaneously into the nozzle. The differential pressure under which the sample and the sheath fluid are forced into the nozzle results in the hydrodynamic focusing of the cells in the center of the fluid stream, so that they pass singly through the light source.

Mature lymphocytes, which are relatively small cells with round nuclei and little cytoplasmic granulation, exhibit low forward and low side light scatter. In contrast, granulocytes, which are larger in size with abundant cytoplasmic granulation, exhibit increased forward and increased side light scatter. Flow cytometry allows identification of lymphocytic, monocytic, and granulocytic cell populations. Abnormal cell populations also can be detected by their aberrant light scatter patterns (Figs. 2–5).

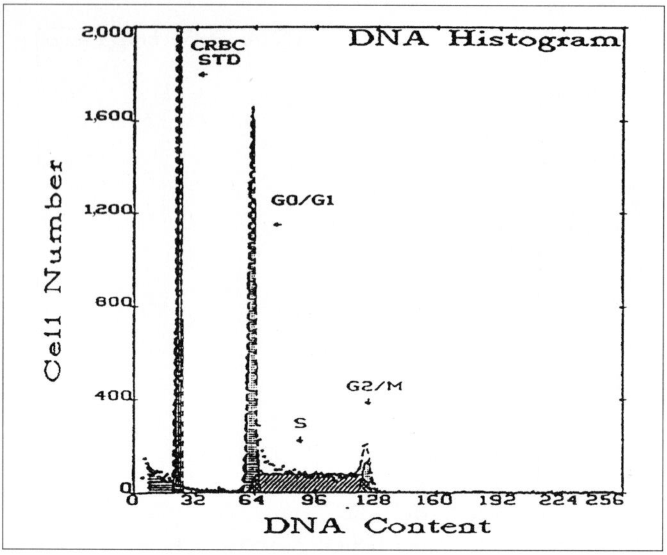

Fig. 3. Histogram of a diploid Burkitt lymphoma. Compared to Fig. 2, the S phase is enormous at 42%, which correlates with the rapid turnover of this tumor. Diploid cells: DNA index = 1.00; percent of total = 100.9%; G_2 phase = 6.2%; S phase = 42.4%; G_0/G_1 coefficient of variation = 2.3%. CRBC STD, chicken red blood cell standard. (Reproduced with permission from Marshall T, Rutledge JC. Flow cytometry DNA applications in pediatric tumor pathology. *Perspect Pediatr Pathol* 2001;23:55.)

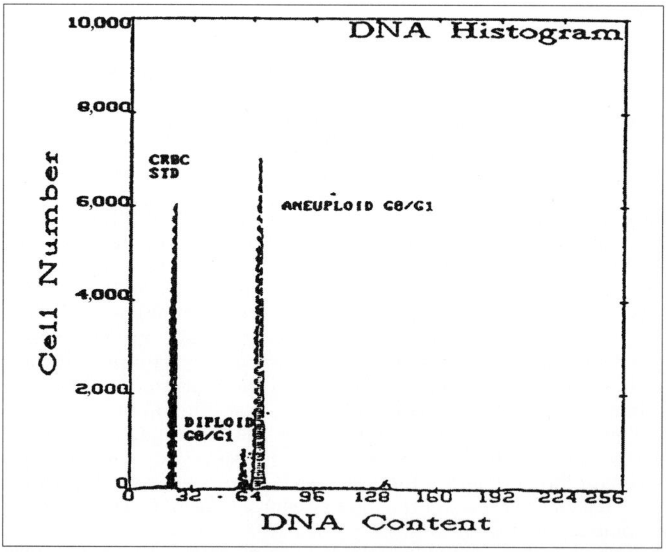

Fig. 4. A small diploid peak (normal cells) is dwarfed by a large aneuploid peak in this specimen from a patient with acute lymphoblastic leukemia (ALL). The S phase of 10% is typical of ALL. The DNA index is only 1.13, which makes this a near-diploid aneuploid peak. Diploid cells: DNA index = 1.00; percent of total = 8.9%; G_0/G_1 coefficient of variation = 1.6%. Aneuploid cells: DNA index = 1.13; percent of total = 91.1%; G_2 phase = 0%; S phase = 10.3%; average S phase = 9.4%; G_0/G_1 coefficient of variation = 1.6%. CRBC STD, chicken red blood cell standard. (Reproduced with permission from Marshall T, Rutledge JC. Flow cytometry DNA applications in pediatric tumor pathology. *Perspect Pediatr Pathol* 2001;23:55.)

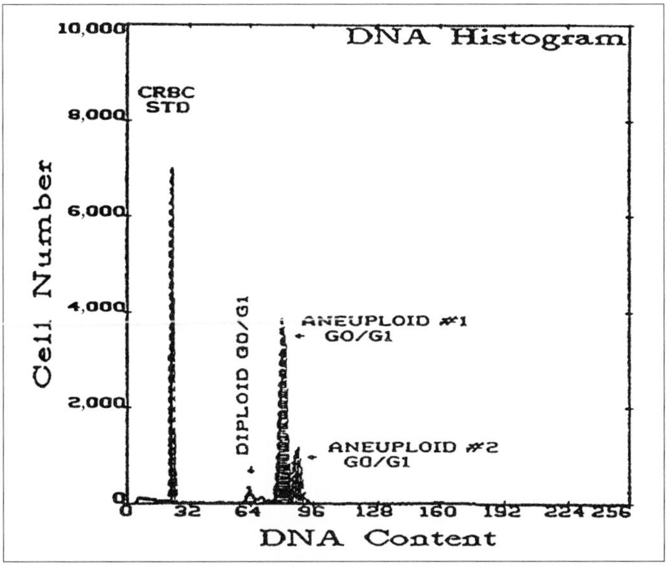

Fig. 5. A neuroblastoma shows two aneuploid peaks. Because of the overlap, the S and G_2 phases could not be determined. Diploid cells: DNA index = 1.00; percent of total = 6.4%; G_0/G_1 coefficient of variation = 2.2%. Aneuploid cells No. 1: DNA index = 1.2; percent of total = 71.0%; average S phase = 3.8%; percent of total = 22.6%; average aneuploid S phase = 1.8%; G_0/G_1 coefficient of variation = 1.9%. CRBC STD, chicken red blood cell standard. (Reproduced with permission from Marshall T, Rutledge JC. Flow cytometry DNA applications in pediatric tumor pathology. *Perspect Pediatr Pathol* 2001;23:55.)

In addition to the intrinsic light-scattering properties of hematopoietic cells, flow cytometry uses numerous fluorochrome-conjugated antibodies that can tag individual cells to further delineate their antigenic profile. The most widely used fluorochromes are fluorescein isothiocyanate and phycoerythrin. When hematopoietic cells are mixed and incubated with these fluorochrome-conjugated antibodies, the antibodies bind to those cells that express the corresponding antigen on their surface.

Fresh peripheral blood or BMA samples anticoagulated with heparin (green top tube), acid citrate dextrose (yellow top tube), or EDTA (lavender top tube) are acceptable. Heparin is the preferred anticoagulant, but only heparin sodium—not heparin lithium—should be used. Lymph node or other tissue samples should be submitted fresh (not fixed) in transport medium or an isotonic salt solution. If a BMA specimen cannot be obtained, a fresh bone marrow core biopsy sample may be submitted. Body fluids such as pleural and peritoneal fluids can be submitted fresh but should be anticoagulated if they are contaminated with blood. Specimens in heparin lithium and fixatives such as formalin, B5, Bouin fixative, and alcohol solutions are unacceptable for analysis.

Specimens should be kept at ambient temperature and analyzed within 24 hours of collection. Frozen specimens are unacceptable.

Approximately 5 mL of peripheral blood (depending on WBC count), 1–2 mL of bone marrow, and 500 mg of lymph node or other tissue are minimum requirements for adequate analysis.

Most laboratories have standard panels of antibodies they use for specific disease processes or groups of disease processes such as acute leukemias, chronic leukemias, or lymphomas. As preliminary results are obtained on a specific case, additional antibodies may need to be added to further characterize the hematologic process. Many lymphomas and leukemias have specific, characteristic antigen expression patterns that aid in their diagnosis.

Southern Blot Hybridization

Southern blot hybridization allows the identification of clonal B-cell and T-cell populations through the detection of antigen receptor gene rearrangements. Certain chromosomal translocations also can be identified.

The B-cell antigen receptor proteins, or immunoglobulins, are composed of two subunits. These include an immunoglobulin heavy chain (IgH) and a light chain (IgL). The light chains can be either κ or λ type, but not both. Two identical heavy-chain subunits combine with two identical light-chain subunits to form an intact immunoglobulin molecule. The gene for the IgH is located on the long arm of chromosome 14, and the genes for κ– and λ–light chains are located on the short arm of chromosome 2 and the long arm of chromosome 22, respectively.

The intact T-cell receptor is a heterodimer composed of two different subunits. The subunits comprise four possible types, including α, β, γ, or δ. The α subunits combine only with β subunits, γ subunits combine only with δ subunits, and vice versa. Therefore, the T-cell receptor located on the cell membrane is either an α/β or a γ/δ heterodimer. The majority of T cells contain an α/β heterodimer on their cell membranes. The gene that codes for the α and δ subunits is located on the long arm of chromosome 14. Those that code for the β and γ subunits are located on the long and short arms of chromosome 7, respectively.

Five to 7 mL of whole blood, 1–2 mL of bone marrow, or 2 mm^3 of tissue is required. Fresh whole blood (anticoagulated with EDTA or heparin sodium), bone marrow, body fluid, or unfixed tissue samples are acceptable for Southern blot hybridization. As an anticoagulant, EDTA is preferred over heparin. Whole blood, bone marrow, and tissue samples frozen at –20°C or –70°C are acceptable as long as any associated RBCs are lysed before freezing. If samples will not be analyzed within 24 hours, they should be refrigerated (at 2–8°C) or frozen. Refrigerated blood and bone marrow samples may be stored for up to 1 week. Frozen blood, bone marrow, and tissue samples can be stored at –20°C or –70°C for 2 weeks or 1–2 years, respectively, before analysis.

Polymerase Chain Reaction Testing

Polymerase chain reaction (PCR) is an *in vitro* method of amplifying specific segments of DNA using enzymes. It is a highly sensitive technique with the potential to detect a single copy of DNA within a specimen.

In hematopathology, this procedure is primarily used to detect chromosomal translocations as well as B-cell and T-cell antigen receptor gene rearrangements. The detection of DNA sequences that span a translocation site, such as t(15;17) seen in acute myelogenous leukemia (AML) type M_3 or t(14;18) associated with follicular lymphoma, provide diagnostic and prognostic information regarding a specific neoplastic process. Negative PCR results are often followed by Southern blot hybridization analysis because the latter is more sensitive.

For PCR studies, sample types similar to those recommended for Southern blot hybridization are generally acceptable. EDTA is the preferred anticoagulant; heparin should not be used. Although fresh unfixed samples are preferred, tissue samples fixed in formalin are acceptable. Mercury-based fixatives such as B5 should not be used. Refrigerated blood and bone marrow samples may be stored for approximately 1 week as long as the RBCs have been removed or the WBC component has been isolated. Frozen samples may be stored at –20° or –70°C for up to 1 year after removal of the RBCs. Fresh tissue samples should be snap-frozen in liquid nitrogen and can be stored at –70°C for 1–2 years.

Approximately 1 mL of blood, 0.5 mL of bone marrow, or 0.5 mm^3 of tissue is required.

PCR is a highly sensitive and efficient process. It is important to have stringent PCR amplification procedures and conditions in place to prevent contamination of the product and ensure amplification. Intact DNA is a requirement for the process. As with Southern blot hybridization, detection of a clonally rearranged band by PCR does not definitively indicate malignancy. Such bands have been detected in reactive processes such as chronic gastritis and autoimmune disorders. In addition, it is important to interpret the result and its significance in combination with the morphology and clinical history. Occasionally, very small populations of minimal residual disease are detected by PCR, but they have little or unknown clinical significance and do not predict relapse.

Cytogenetic Analysis

Cytogenetic analysis has become an integral part of the workup and diagnosis of many hematopoietic disorders. It is particularly important in the evaluation and classification of leukemias, lymphomas, and myelodysplastic and myeloproliferative syndromes. Traditional cytogenetic analysis, or karyotyping, evaluates chromosome metaphase preparations to detect structural and numeric abnormalities. Such abnormalities are detected in >50% of patients with acute leukemias. Specific chromosomal abnormalities have been associated with a number of disorders, including t(15;17) with acute promyelocytic leukemia, t(14;18) with follicular lymphoma, and inversion of chromosome 16 in AML M_4 with eosinophilia.

Although cytogenetic analysis is often valuable and frequently essential in diagnosing hematopoietic neoplasms, the need for viable tumor cells and the relatively long turnaround time are major disadvantages. Often a morphologic impression must be rendered before the cytogenetic results are available. More recent techniques such as FISH, particularly interphase FISH analysis, have allowed specific cytogenetic questions to be answered more quickly.

Conventional Chromosome Metaphase Spread Analysis

Chromosome metaphase spread analysis is used to detect structural and numeric chromosomal abnormalities. The mechanism by which cytogenetic alterations induce disease often involves the activation or inactivation of specific oncogenes. Many hematopoietic tumors exhibit chromosomal abnormalities such as translocations, deletions, and inversions, and can be identified by the characteristic size and staining patterns of the long and short arms of individual chromosomes. Although these chromosomal alterations occasionally are nonspecific, they are frequently characteristic for specific disorders. New or additional chromosome abnormalities are commonly associated with disease progression.

Two to 3 mL of fresh bone marrow or peripheral blood anticoagulated with sodium heparin is necessary. A bone marrow sample is preferable if available, but peripheral blood is acceptable. The specimen should be kept at ambient temperature and transported to the cytogenetics laboratory within 24 hours. Frozen samples exposed to extreme temperatures are unacceptable.

Metaphase spread analysis requires a specimen containing viable cells capable of mitotic division. Because these samples must be grown in culture, they must be acquired under sterile conditions.

Fluorescent *In Situ* Hybridization

FISH is used to detect numeric and structural chromosomal abnormalities within intact cells or metaphase spreads. It is particularly useful in the detection of specific chromosomal translocations.

FISH takes advantage of the double-stranded and complementary-sequence arrangement of DNA. Fluorescently labeled probes consisting of single-stranded DNA sequences can bind complementary denatured DNA segments to identify specific chromosomes or gene sequences in intact cells. Depending on the formation sought, different types of probes are used. The fluorescent reporting molecule can be directly attached to the DNA sequence or can be attached to an antibody that detects the DNA sequence through an indirect reporter system. Centromeric, telomeric, and repeat-sequence probes are commonly used to identify chromosomes and detect the loss or gain of a particular chromosome (numeric abnormalities). Unique-sequence probes such as cosmid and yeast artificial chromosome probes are used to locate a specific DNA sequence. Unique-sequence probes are useful in the identification of chromosomal translocations.

Bone marrow and peripheral blood samples anticoagulated with heparin sodium are both acceptable, but bone marrow samples are preferred to whole-blood samples. Samples should be transported to the laboratory at ambient temperature within 24 hours. Formalin-fixed tissue samples are acceptable for interphase FISH analysis. Neither Bouin solution nor B5 should be used. For metaphase FISH analysis, only viable cell samples are acceptable.

The signal detected depends on the probe and fluorescent dye used. A positive signal is detected as a single colored dot observed under the fluorescence microscope. Two colors, red and green, are distinct in cells lacking the translocation, and the fusion color (signal) appears in those with a translocation. If the translocation is present, a single third fusion colored dot or signal is detected. If

Table 4. Hematologic Parameters of Frequent Causes of Anemia

	Iron Deficiency	β Thalassemia Trait	Chronic Inflammation	Lead Poisoning	Sickle Disease
Reticulocyte count	Low	Low	Normal	Low	
RDW	↑	↓	Normal	↓	
Ferritin	↓	Normal to ↑	Normal	↓ to normal	
FEP	↑	Normal	↑	↑	
Iron	↓	Normal	↓	↓ to normal	↑
TIBC	↑	Normal	↓		
Electrophoresis	Normal	↑ HbA_2 or F	Normal	Normal	HbSS
ESR	Normal	Normal	↑	Normal	Low
Smear	Hypochromic, target cells	Normochromic, microcytic	Varies	Basophilic stippling	Sickle

↑, increased; ↓, decreased; ESR, erythrocyte sedimentation rate; F, fetal hemoglobin; FEP, free erythrocyte protoporphyrin; HbA_2, hemoglobin A_2; HbSS, hemoglobin SS; RDW, red cell distribution width; TIBC, total iron-binding capacity.

numeric probes are used, the number of signals detected per cell equals the number of the particular chromosome present. Chromosome losses or gains can be detected in this manner.

Interphase FISH analysis is significantly quicker than traditional G-banding metaphase analysis because the cells do not need to be grown in culture. It has the disadvantage of not allowing the entire chromosomal pattern to be analyzed, so that some useful information is potentially missed.

Anemias and Other Erythrocyte Disorders

Aciduria, Hereditary Orotic

Hereditary orotic aciduria is a rare inborn error of *de novo* pyrimidine synthesis characterized by megaloblastic anemia unresponsive to treatment with vitamin B_{12} or folic acid and increased urinary excretion of orotic acid accompanied by macroscopic crystalluria, which may result in obstructive nephropathy. Inheritance is autosomal recessive. Delayed development of motor and cognitive skills is apparent in the majority of cases. Other clinical features include sparse hair, poor nail growth, immune dysfunction, cardiac malformations, strabismus, and malabsorption.

Diagnosis

Red cell hypochromia (despite adequate iron stores), megaloblastic anemia, orotic aciduria, and positive results on a specific enzyme assay are common features.

Anemia

Hematologic Parameters of Frequent Causes of Anemia

See Table 4.

Classification of Anemias

Anemias can be classified by red cell size as follows:

MCV	Size	Type of Anemia
Low	<75 fL	Microcytic
Normal	75–95 fL	Normocytic
High	>95 fL	Macrocytic

Table 5 shows a categorization of various types of anemia.

Anemia, Aplastic

Aplastic anemia is an anemia in which the bone marrow fails to produce adequate numbers of peripheral blood elements. The usual course is insidious. Pure red cell aplasia is a related syndrome that is caused by a selective failure of the production of erythroid elements.

Causes of aplastic anemia include idiopathic disease (approximately 50% of the cases), injury to pluripotential stem cells, destruction of pluripotential stem cells, immunologic injury, toxic exposure (e.g., exposure to benzene or inorganic arsenic; infectious hepatitis; radiation exposure; use of certain drugs, especially antibiotics, anticonvulsants, gold), pregnancy (rare), and inherited condition (constitutional anemia).

Table 5. Classification of Anemia

Reticulocyte Count	Microcytic Anemia	Normocytic Anemia	Macrocytic Anemia
Low	Iron deficiency Lead poisoning Chronic disease Aluminum toxicity Copper deficiency Protein malnutrition Pyridoxine deficiency	Chronic deficiency RBC aplasia (TEC, infection, drug induced) Malignancy Juvenile rheumatoid Arthritis Endocrinopathies Renal failure	Folate deficiency Vitamin B_{12} deficiency Aplastic anemia Congenital bone marrow dysfunction (Diamond-Blackfan or Fanconi syndrome) Drug induced Trisomy 21 Hypothyroidism
Normal	Thalassemia trait Sideroblastic anemia	Acute bleeding Hypersplenism Dyserythropoietic anemia II	—
High	Thalassemia syndromes Hemoglobin C disorders	Antibody-mediated hemolysis Hypersplenism Microangiopathy (HUS, TTP, DIC, Kasabach-Merritt syndrome) Membranopathies (spherocytosis, elliptocytosis) Enzyme disorders (G-6-PD, pyruvate kinase deficiencies) Hemoglobinopathies	Dyserythropoietic anemia I, III Active hemolysis

DIC, disseminated intravascular coagulation; G-6-PD, glucose-6-phosphate dehydrogenase; TEC, transient erythroblastopenia of childhood; HUS, hemolytic-uremic syndrome; RBC, red blood cell; TTP, thrombotic thrombocytopenic purpura.

Risk factors that predispose to aplastic anemia are viral illness, toxin exposure, and tumors of the thymus (red cell aplasia).

Laboratory Findings

Pancytopenia
Leukopenia
Thrombocytopenia
Decreased reticulocytes
Normal TIBC
Hematuria
Increased fetal hemoglobin (Fanconi anemia)
Molecular determination of abnormal gene (Fanconi anemia)

Anemia
Neutropenia
Increased bleeding time
Increased serum iron level secondary to transfusion
Borderline-high MCV >104 fL
Abnormal liver function test results (hepatitis)
Increased chromosomal breaks under specialized conditions (constitutional anemia)

Constitutional (Fanconi) anemias are associated with congenital anomalies. Signs and symptoms are dyspnea, ecchymoses, petechiae, fatigue, fever, hemorrhage, menorrhagia, occult blood in stool, melena, epistaxis, pallor, palpitations, progressive weakness, retinal flame hemorrhages, systolic ejection murmur, and weight loss. Constitutional symptoms include short stature, microcephaly, radius and thumb anomalies, renal anomalies, hypospadias, and hyperpigmentation.

Pathologic Findings

In the normochromic forms RBC bone marrow shows
- Increased iron stores
- Decreased cellularity (<10%)
- Decreased megakaryocytes
- Decreased myelocytes
- Decreased erythroid precursors

Diagnostic Tests

Diagnostic tests for Fanconi anemia include assay for chromosome breakage (constitutional anemia) and measurement of fetal hemoglobin level.

Types

- Primary (50% of cases)
- Secondary (50% of cases)
- Large granular lymphocytosis, T-cell type
- Drug related
  - Chloramphenicol
  - Phenylbutazone
  - Anticonvulsants
  - Sulfonamides
  - Gold
  - Chemotherapy agents
- Toxin induced
  - Benzene
  - Insecticides
  - Solvents
- Infection related
  - Hepatitis
  - Epstein-Barr virus (EBV) infection
  - Influenza
  - Other infections
- Due to other conditions and exposures
  - Radiation exposure
  - Immune disorders
  - Paroxysmal nocturnal hemoglobinuria

Chronic lymphocytic leukemia
Other neoplasms
Pearson syndrome
Thymoma

Pearson syndrome is a fatal disorder that involves the hematopoietic system, exocrine pancreas, liver, and kidney. Hematologic findings include pancytopenia with RBC macrocytosis. Examination of BMA reveals vacuolization of myeloid and erythroid precursors as well as ringed sideroblasts. The syndrome is classified among the mitochondrial cytopathies. Phenotypic variations of "classic" Pearson syndrome have been proposed on the basis of different mitochondrial DNA deletions.

Another congenital bone-marrow–failure syndrome in which hematologic complications rarely occur in the first 2 years of life includes dyskeratosis congenita.

Anemia, Congenital Dyserythropoietic

Laboratory Findings

Laboratory findings in congenital dyserythropoietic anemia (CDA) include macrocytic anemia in types I and III and normocytic anemia in type II. Morphologic findings in the peripheral blood smears show anisocytosis, poikilocytosis, basophilic stippling, and a disproportionally low reticulocyte count with respect to the degree of anemia. Associated with all types of CDA are transferrin saturation and increased plasma iron level. Both are indicators of dyserythropoiesis.

The bone marrow shows erythroid hyperplasia with a low myeloid/erythroid (M/E) ratio in all types. Although cytologic changes vary with each type, all types share the morphologic aberration associated with premature destruction of the developing erythroblasts: dyserythropoiesis. Vacuolated macrophages and siderocytes are present in all types.

In the bone marrow of patients with CDA type I, the RBC abnormalities are limited to the late erythroid forms (polychromatophilic and orthochromatic erythroblasts) without change in the pronormoblasts. The maturation of the erythrocytes is megaloblastoid and asynchronous. A low percentage of the erythroblasts are binucleated (less than 10%), and others have chromatin bridges connecting both nuclei. Defective hemoglobinization of some erythroblasts is also seen.

The most extensive biochemical studies in CDA, on HEMPAS (*h*ereditary *e*rythroblastic *m*ultinuclearity associated with *p*ositive *a*cidified *s*erum) or type II CDA, demonstrate that the major enzymatic defect can be linked to an aberrant glycosylation of transferrin.

In the bone marrow of patients with CDA type II, nuclear abnormalities are seen in all erythroblasts (Color Fig. 6). The percentage of morphologically aberrant erythroblasts is up to 50%. The erythroblasts can be binucleated, multinucleated, or multilobulated with chromatin bridges. In some cases, macrophages contain inclusions that are positive for the PAS. These macrophages are present in association with the abnormal erythroblasts. Electron microscopy shows a linear structure around the periphery of the erythroblasts running parallel to the cell membrane. This change is not pathognomonic of type II, however, as it is seen in other dyserythropoietic states with the exception of type I.

The most useful laboratory test for the diagnosis of CDA type II is the acidified serum test. In a normal subject a large percentage of red cells are lysed in the presence of acidified serum from that person. In CDA, the patient's serum does not lyse its own cells. This is in contrast to paroxysmal nocturnal hemoglobinuria in which the patient's acidified serum lyses its own cells.

In the bone marrow of patients with CDA type III, there are large numbers of multinucleated erythroblasts (containing up to eight nuclei) and some giant mononucleated erythroblasts.

The morphologic findings by light microscopy and electron microscopy are not limited to CDAs but can be seen in, for example, thalassemias, aplastic anemia, erythroleukemia, and postchemotherapy states. It is the proportion of these changes in the bone marrow that is striking in the CDAs.

Table 6 shows peripheral blood and bone marrow findings in patients with congenital dyserythropoietic anemias.

Table 6. Peripheral Blood and Bone Marrow Findings in Patients with Congenital Dyserythropoietic Anemia

	CDA I	CDA II[a]	CDA III
Blood			
RBC size	Macrocytic	Normocytic	Normocytic to macrocytic
RBC morphology	Anisopoikilocytosis	Anisopoikilocytosis	Anisopoikilocytosis
Anemia	Mild to moderate	Mild to severe	Mild
Bone marrow			
Erythroid hyperplasia	Prominent	Prominent	Prominent
Erythroid morphology	Megaloblastic; internuclear chromatin bridging, nuclear budding; occasional binucleate forms	Normoblastic; bi- or multinucleated normoblasts; nuclear karyorrhexis	Megaloblastic; "gigantoblasts" (up to 12 nuclei); nuclear karyorrhexis
Other laboratory results			
Acidified serum test	– (rarely +)	+	–
Sugar water test	– (rarely +)	–	–
Agglutination by anti-t and anti-I	Slight	+	+ (variable)

+, present; –, absent; CDA, congenital dyserythropoietic anemia; RBC, red blood cells.
[a]A designation of HEMPAS [hereditary erythroblastic multinuclearity with positive acidified serum (test)] is sometimes applied to patients with CDA II.
From Kjeldsberg C, et al. *Practical diagnosis of hematologic disorders,* 3rd ed. Chicago: American Society of Clinical Pathologists Press, 2000.

Anemia, Hemolytic

See Table 7.

Diagnostic Tests

Examination of Blood

Normochromic normocytic anemia, which may be hemolytic, is evidenced by polychromasia, macrocytosis, and the presence of microspherocytes, nucleated RBCs, or RBC agglutination. Anemia may be severe (hemoglobin level <3 g/dL) with normochromic normocytic indices. There is variable reticulocytosis, but the reticulocyte count is usually increased. In acute hemolysis, a nonspecific stress granulocytosis with a left shift may be present. The leukocytosis can reach leukemoid proportions [$>50 \times 10^3/mm^3$ ($>50 \times 10^9/L$)]. Schistocytes (fragmented RBCs) are present in disseminated intravascular coagulation, hemolytic-uremic syndrome, and thrombotic thrombocytopenic purpura (Color Fig. 7B). Bone marrow examination usually is not required. If performed, it demonstrates a hypercellular marrow. Prolonged severe hemolysis may result in relative deficiencies of folic acid or vitamin B_{12}, which causes superimposed megaloblastic maturation. Occasionally, bone marrow examination may reveal an underlying lymphoproliferative disorder associated with autoantibody production.

Hemoglobinopathy Evaluation

A comprehensive method is used to identify the presence of abnormal or atypical hemoglobins in whole blood. If an abnormal hemoglobin variant is detected by high-pressure liquid chromatography, additional techniques are used to identify the variant hemoglobin or hemoglobins. These techniques may include dithionite

Table 7. Hemolytic Anemias

Hereditary disorders	
Membrane defects	Hereditary spherocytosis, hereditary elliptocytosis, stomatocytosis, hereditary xerocytosis, pyropoikilocytosis, Macleod syndrome, Rh deficiency syndrome, other rare membrane disorders
Enzyme defects	G-6-PD deficiency, pyruvate kinase, deficiency, glutathione pathway deficiency, deficiencies of the pentose pathway
Hemoglobin defects	Amino acid substitutions: hemoglobin S, hemoglobin C, etc.; decreased production: thalassemia
Acquired or extrinsic disorders	
Infection, trauma	Bacterial: *Clostridium perfringens* infection
	Protozoal: malaria
	Viral: *Mycoplasma* infection, infectious mononucleosis
	Physiochemical damage: burns, oxidative and nonoxidative
	Mechanical damage: heart valve prosthesis (aortic), ulcerative colitis, hemolytic-uremic syndrome, TTP, DIC
Antibody	Alloantibody: incompatible transfusion, fetal-maternal blood group incompatibility
	Autoantibody: idiopathic, secondary to malignant lymphomas, collagen vascular diseases, viral infections, secondary to drugs
Other	Paroxysmal nocturnal hemoglobinuria

DIC, disseminated intravascular coagulation; G-6-PD, glucose-6-phosphate dehydrogenase; TTP, thrombotic thrombocytopenic purpura.

solubility testing, alkaline and acid electrophoresis, isopropanol and heat stability studies, and isoelectric focusing.

Serum Haptoglobin Quantitation

Haptoglobin is decreased or absent in hemolysis, liver failure, and rare genetic variants. A low serum haptoglobin level indicates that hemolysis may be present if liver function is normal.

Normal values are usually 40–80 mg/dL (0.4–0.8 g/L). With active hemolysis, values of <10 mg/dL (<0.1 g/L) are seen. In cold-type autoimmune hemolytic anemia (AIHA) secondary to viral or *Mycoplasma* pneumonia, haptoglobin may be increased as an acute-reactant protein, which obscures expected decreases with hemolysis.

Ham Test for Acid Hemolysis

A Ham test is performed to exclude paroxysmal nocturnal hemoglobinuria, which is caused by an acquired clonal defect of the RBC membrane rather than an antibody-mediated process. Whenever antibody hemolysis is suspected, paroxysmal nocturnal hemoglobinuria should be considered and excluded.

False-positive hemolysis results are seen if the acidified sera contains a cold agglutinin. True-positive results occur only with human (not guinea pig) complement. The acid hemolysis test can be confirmed with sucrose lysis.

Nonenzymatic Disorders Associated with Hemolytic Anemia

Runner's Anemia

A careful history taking is critically important for recognition of runner's anemia, which is due to plasma volume expansion, with hemolysis from the pounding of feet on pavement, and hemoglobinuria. Gastrointestinal blood loss may also contribute to anemia in long-distance runners. Runner's anemia should be considered when, amidst a constellation of signs and symptoms, mild anemia is well tolerated by an avid runner.

Red Cell Membrane Defects

Diagnostic Tests for Red Blood Cell Membrane Defects

Tests include CBC, microscopic examination of the peripheral blood smear, Coombs test, measurement of serum haptoglobin level, osmotic fragility test, and determination of bilirubin level. The RBC indices reflect the degree of anemia, which is in most cases a hemoglobin level of <10 g/dL, with low MCV and high MCHC. The reticulocyte count is elevated, RDW is above normal, the Coombs test result is negative, and osmotic fragility is increased. The direct bilirubin level is above normal.

Plasma hemoglobin is increased (hemoglobinemia). If the amount of free hemoglobin cannot be metabolized by the liver, hemoglobin is excreted by the kidney (hemoglobinuria). Because of RBC destruction, lactate dehydrogenase is released, and its level in the serum increases. The BMA shows RBC hyperplasia with a striking increase in pronormoblasts. The M/E ratio is decreased and the storage of iron is increased.

When an RBC membrane defect is suspected, the diagnosis may be facilitated by examination of blood smears of both parents, because in most such defects the pattern of inheritance is dominant.

Spherocytosis and Elliptocytosis

Spherocytosis and elliptocytosis are hereditary erythrocyte membrane defects. Abnormalities in these proteins may lead to premature hemolysis, as in hereditary spherocytosis, or may have little effect on RBC life span, as in most cases of hereditary elliptocytosis.

Hereditary spherocytosis in the most common type of hereditary hemolytic anemia among individuals of northern European origin, but it occurs in all races throughout the world. It is seen in approximately 1 in 5,000 individuals in the United States. The inheritance is autosomal dominant. In this disease, a primary defect in membrane stability is caused by a quantitative decrease in the amount of spectrin or, more rarely, by formation of an abnormal spectrin that does not interact with other proteins within the RBC skeleton. Spherocytes are less flexible than normal RBCs, which leads to retention within the spleen. This causes accelerated loss of cellular membrane to form the characteristic spherocytes and premature cellular destruction.

Clinical Findings

The more severe forms of the disease are diagnosed in early childhood. Clinical manifestations usually are first noted in children or adolescents. Typical complaints include mild jaundice and nonspecific manifestations of anemia, such as weakness. Because of an increased bilirubin turnover, patients with this condition have a high incidence of pigment gallstones. Usually, patients can maintain nearly normal hemoglobin levels owing to increased RBC production by the bone marrow. Infection or other stress may lead to acute episodes due to increased splenic activity (hemolytic crisis) or decreased bone marrow production (aplastic crisis). The most consistently positive physical finding is splenomegaly, which may be marked. Variable degrees of jaundice and scleral icterus are frequently seen. The most consistent and therapeutically important feature of hereditary spherocytosis is the clinical cure of hemolytic anemia by splenectomy. RBC life span after this procedure is restored to normal or near normal.

Peripheral Smear Findings in Hereditary Spherocytosis and Elliptocytosis

Hemoglobin levels in patients with hereditary spherocytosis and hemolytic elliptocytosis frequently range between 9 and 12 g/dL (90 and 120 g/L); the MCV is usually in the normal range but may be elevated in the presence of prominent reticulocytosis. The MCHC in hereditary spherocytosis is characteristically elevated to levels as high as 37 g/dL (370 g/L) [normal, 26–34 g/dL (260–340 g/L)], due to membrane loss without loss of cellular hemoglobin. The reticulocyte count usually ranges between 5% and 15% (0.05 and 0.15).

Spherocytes on the peripheral blood film appear as densely staining RBCs that are slightly smaller than normal with an absence of central pallor (Color Fig. 8A). The increased intensity of staining is partially caused by increased cellular thickness due to the spherical shape and the increased MCHC. In the mild forms of the disease, spherocytes may not be present in large numbers.

Prominent macrocytosis and polychromasia may be present in association with very high reticulocyte count.

Hereditary elliptocytosis is a heterogeneous group of disorders characterized by the presence of elliptocytes in the peripheral blood smear (Color Fig. 8B). These represent RBCs that have failed to regain their normal biconcave shape following passage through the microcirculation. A wide variety of RBC membrane skeletal defects have been associated with hereditary elliptocytosis, including dysfunctional spectrin molecules, decreased spectrin content, and band 4.1 defects or deficiency. Unlike patients with hereditary spherocytosis, 90% of patients with hereditary elliptocytosis do not experience clinically significant hemolysis. Hereditary elliptocytosis is usually inherited as an autosomal-dominant trait.

Diagnostic Tests for Spherocytosis and Elliptocytosis

1. Hematologic evaluation, with attention to RBC morphologic characteristics, MCHC, and the reticulocyte count
2. Osmotic fragility test
3. Direct antiglobulin test to rule out AIHA as a cause for spherocytosis

Elliptocytes are readily identified on the stained blood film. Because this generally represents a benign anomaly, hereditary elliptocytosis should be considered the cause of anemia only when evidence for hemolysis, such as an elevated reticulocyte count, is found.

Hereditary elliptocytosis may present either as a primary morphologic disorder with little or no hemolysis or, much more rarely, with a moderately severe hemolytic anemia. Patients with the usual form of hereditary elliptocytosis have no anemia or splenomegaly. Patients with the hemolytic forms of the disease, composing approximately 10% of cases, may have splenomegaly and often show spherocytes and fragmented RBCs, in addition to elliptocytes, in the peripheral blood smear. Elliptocytosis is diagnosed when most or all of the cells on the smear have an oval shape with a long diameter that is two or more times the short diameter.

Bone Marrow Examination

The bone marrow characteristically shows normoblastic erythroid hyperplasia when significant hemolysis occurs. During aplastic crises, erythroid precursors are diminished and evidence of viral infection, such as parvovirus B19, may be seen.

Erythroenzymopathies Associated with Hereditary Hemolytic Anemia

The human genes encoding all known enzymes, other than P5'N, central to red cell metabolism have been cloned. Apart from a few examples due to mutations that result in premature termination of translation, or aberrant messenger RNA splicing and adenosine deaminase overproduction, in which the basic defect that up-regulates transcription appears to lie outside the structural gene, the majority of erythroenzymopathies are caused by missense mutations.

Missense mutations that destabilize intersubunit contact or alter the conformation of the active site are generally associated with markedly diminished enzyme activity and correspondingly more severe clinical expression.

The following mutations are seen in enzymopathies associated with hereditary hemolytic anemia:

Enzyme	Acronym	Locus
Glucose-6-phosphate dehydrogenase	G-6P-D	Xq28
Pyruvate kinase	PK-L/R	1q21
Phosphofructokinase	PFK-M	1cen-q32
Glucosephosphate isomerase	GP1	19q13.1
Glutathione synthetase	GSHS	20q11.2
Triosephosphate isomerase	TPI	12p13
Phosphoglycerate kinase	PGK1	Xq13
Hexokinase	HK1	10q22
Aldolase	ALD-A	16q22-q24
Adenylate kinase	AK1	9q34.1

Glucose-6-Phosphate Dehydrogenase Deficiency

Deficiency of G-6-PD enzyme is the most prevalent inborn metabolic disorder of RBCs, affecting more than 400 million people worldwide, and is an important cause of inheritable hemolytic anemia.

Deficiency of G-6-PD results from the inheritance of an abnormal G-6-PD enzyme gene located on the X chromosome. More than 100 different mutations have been described. Two isotypes of G-6-PD, termed *A* and *B*, can be distinguished by electrophoretic mobility. The B isoform is the most common type of enzyme found in all population groups. The G-6-PD A isoform migrates more rapidly on electrophoretic

Table 8. Clinical Features of Variants of Glucose-6-Phosphate Dehydrogenase Deficiency

Clinical Feature	G-6-PD A$^-$	G-6-PD^{MED}, G-6-PD^{IOWA}	G-6-PD^{CANTON}
Drug-induced hemolysis	Moderate	Moderate	Moderate
Infection-induced hemolysis	Common	Common	Common
Favism	Not seen	Common	Not usually seen
Neonatal icterus	Rare	Observed	Observed
Hereditary nonspherocytic hemolytic anemia	Not seen	Occasionally	Not seen
Degree of hemolysis	Moderate	Severe	Moderate
Chronic hemolysis	Not seen	Not seen	Not seen

G-6-PD, glucose-6-phosphate dehydrogenase.

gels than does the normal B enzyme. It has similar enzymatic activity to the B isoform, however, and is not associated with disease. Up to 11% of U.S. black men have a G-6-PD variant (G-6-PD A$^-$) that has the same electrophoretic mobility as G-6-PD A but is unstable, which results in enzyme loss and ultimate enzyme deficiency as the RBC ages. Thus, older circulating RBCs from individuals with this variant may contain only 5–15% of the normal amount of enzymatic activity. Mediterranean (G-6-PD^{MED}) is found frequently in Sicilians, Greeks, Sephardic Jews, and Arabs. Several other variants, such as G-6-PD^{CANTON} and G-6-PD^{MAHIDOL}, are common in Asian populations. The population distribution of G-6-PD deficiency reflects its probable origins in tropical and subtropical areas and possible conferring of increased resistance to malarial infection.

G-6-PD deficiency may occur in heterozygous females. The wild-type G-6-PD allele may render the enzyme activity of a red cell lysate normal. Cytochemical staining with tetrazolium, which is capable of detecting minor populations of *Gd* red cells, may be helpful.

Clinical Findings

G-6-PD deficiency usually manifests as an episode of acute hemolysis after infection or ingestion of an oxidant drug in an otherwise apparently healthy person. Hemolysis begins acutely in the case of infection or within 1 to 3 days, leading to plasma hemoglobinemia (pink to brown plasma), hemoglobinuria (dark or black urine), and jaundice. Rarely, patients may have a clinical picture of chronic hemolysis or be asymptomatic.

Heinz bodies are seen in unstained or supravital preparations of RBCs that are not seen in Giemsa- or Wright-stained smears. Testing for G-6-PD deficiency should not be performed until several days after hemolytic crisis and reticulocytosis have resolved. Several screening tests have been developed, including the fluorescent spot test, the methemoglobin reduction test, and the ascorbate-cyanide test. All have been standardized by a World Health Organization (WHO) scientific group.

Clinical features of variants of glucose-6-phosphate dehydrogenase deficiency are summarized in Table 8.

Hemolytic Crisis

In G-6-PD A$^-$ deficiency, the hemolytic anemia is usually self-limited because the young RBCs produced in response to hemolysis have nearly normal G-6-PD levels and are relatively resistant to hemolysis. In contrast, other types of G-6-PD deficiency, such as G-6-PD^{MED} (in which there are decreased levels of the enzyme in all RBCs), may cause severe hemolysis that requires transfusion therapy. Other stresses that may precipitate acute hemolytic anemia in people who are severely G-6-PD deficient are the neonatal state and exposure to fava beans.

Exposure to the following agents is commonly associated with hemolysis in G-6-PD deficiency:

- Antimalarial agents
  - Primaquine
  - Quinacrine
- Sulfonamides

Sulfanilamide
Salicylazosulfapyridine
Sulfacetamide sodium
Other antibacterial agents
Nitrofurantoin
Nitrofurazone
Para-aminosalicylic acid
Nalidixic acid
Acetanilid
Sulfones
Diaminodiphenyl sulfone
Thiazolsulfone
Miscellaneous agents
Dimercaprol
Naphthalene (mothballs)
Methylene blue
Trinitrotoluene (TNT)

Pyruvate Kinase Deficiency

Various RBC enzymatic defects produce hemolytic anemias characterized by a lack of spherocytes and few distinguishing features on the blood film. The most common glycolytic enzyme defect causing hemolytic anemia is pyruvate kinase deficiency, although it is a rare disorder.

A congenital hemolytic anemia occurs in homozygotes for the autosomal-recessive gene. Concentration of 2,3-diphosphoglycerate is increased and adenosine triphosphate generation is impaired, which allows potassium leakage from the RBC. Jaundice and anemia may occur in the neonatal period; kernicterus has been reported. Macrocytosis, polychromatophilia, and increased reticulocytes characterize the peripheral blood smear; diagnosis depends on marked reduction of pyruvate kinase activity in the RBCs.

Disorders of Glutathione Metabolism

Three defects of glutathione metabolism associated with decreased red cell glutathione have been implicated in hemolytic anemia; glutathione reductase, glutamylcysteine synthetase, and glutathione synthetase deficiencies.

Two phenotypes are recognized: In the red cell type of glutathione deficiency, there is mild hemolytic anemia that may be exacerbated by oxidant stress; glutathione deficiency may also result in a multisystem disorder characterized by hemolysis, metabolic acidosis, neurologic abnormalities, neutropenia, and susceptibility to bacterial infection.

Diagnosis

Urinary excretion of 5-oxoproline is markedly elevated. Enzyme analysis is required to definitively diagnose these conditions.

Chronic nonspherocytic hemolytic anemias of varying severity have been associated with deficiencies of other enzymes in the glycolytic pathway, including hexokinase, glucose phosphate isomerase, and aldolase, which are inherited as autosomal-recessive disorders. Phosphofructokinase deficiency occurs primarily in Ashkenazi Jews in the United States and results in hemolysis associated with a myopathy of glycogen storage disease type 7.

Diphosphoglycerate Mutase Deficiency

Diphosphoglycerate mutase (DPGM) acts in the Rapoport-Luebering shunt to regulate the metabolism of 2,3-diphosphoglycerate (DPG). Its main catalytic function is the conversion of 1,3-DPG to 2,3-DPG. In addition, DPGM possesses phosphatase activity that is responsible for the conversion of 2,3-DPG to 3-phosphoglycerate and functions, albeit at low efficiency, as a monophosphoglycerate mutase. Human DPGM activity is confined to red cells. The 2,3-DPG is the most abundant glucolytic intermediate and serves to lower the affinity of hemoglobin for oxygen, thereby shifting the oxygen dissociation curve to the right.

Disorders of Erythrocyte Nucleotide Metabolism

Several disorders of erythrocyte nucleotide metabolism associated with hemolytic anemia have been described. By comparison with disorders of glycolysis, the mechanism by which they mediate premature red cell destruction is poorly understood.

Adenylate Kinase Deficiency

Three isoenzymes of adenylate kinase have been identified. Adenylate kinase 1 is found in red cells, muscle, and brain in cases of hemolytic anemia. Elevation of red cell adenosine triphosphate concentration has been observed in the majority of cases.

Pyrimidine 5'-Nucleotidase Deficiency

Pyrimidine 5'-nucleotidase exists as two isoenzymes, P5'N or uridine monophosphate hydrolase 1 and 2, which have different substrate specificities and are encoded by separate structural loci. Hemolytic anemia is the result of deficiency in P5'N-1 (uridine monophosphate hydrolase 1). Deficiency of P5'N is associated with hemolytic anemia of mild to moderate severity, which may worsen during infection or pregnancy.

There is accumulation in the red cell of pyrimidine phosphates and their derivatives, particularly the phosphodiesters cytosine diphosphate–choline and cytosine diphosphate–ethanolamine. This forms the basis of a screening test to establish the diagnosis. Normally, adenosine phosphates account for at least 97% of cellular nucleotides. In P5'N deficiency the presence in red cell perchloric acid extracts of significant concentrations of pyrimidine compounds shifts the ultraviolet absorption spectrum from the normal peak at 257 nm to a peak of 265–270 nm. The diagnosis may be confirmed by specific enzyme assay. A conspicuous feature of P5'N deficiency is basophilic stippling (ribonucleoprotein aggregates), which may be visible in up to 5% of red cells. Blood collected in EDTA must be examined fresh, because after 3 hours stippling is no longer discernible. Alternatively, a stained blood film may be prepared from heparinized blood. The activity of P5'N is increased in young red cells. When corrected for reticulocytosis, the enzyme activity in homozygous P5'N deficiency is generally approximately 5% of that in normal red cells. Typically, heterozygotes exhibit 50% P5'N activity, although overlapping of values with those of normal subjects renders carrier detection difficult in some.

Acquired P5'N deficiency is seen in lead poisoning and underlies the mechanism of lead-induced hemolytic anemia. Patients with severe acute lead toxicity have enzyme levels comparable to those found in homozygous deficiency states.

Overproduction of Adenosine Deaminase

Clinically, overproduction of adenosine deaminase (ADA) is characterized by a well-compensated hemolytic anemia showing dominant inheritance. Red cell ADA levels are increased up to 100-fold, reflecting up-regulation of transcription of the ADA gene. This phenomenon appears specific to red cells, because ADA levels in other cells are normal.

Congenital Methemoglobinemia Due to Deficiency of Cytochrome b_5 Reductase

In steady-state levels, methemoglobin normally comprises <1% of total hemoglobin. The principal pathway by which functional hemoglobin is restored involves the transfer of electrons from nicotinamide adenine dinucleotide (reduced form) to methemoglobin mediated by cytochrome b_5. A defect in this pathway underlies hereditary methemoglobinemia. Homozygous deficiency of cytochrome b_5 reductase classically results in a benign clinical disorder characterized by congenital cyanosis. Most affected children are otherwise asymptomatic, even in the face of methemoglobin levels of up to 50%. Transient cyanosis may occur spontaneously in heterozygotes for cytochrome b_5 reductase deficiency in the neonatal period and after exposure to oxidizing compounds in later childhood. Cytochrome b_5 reductase must be distinguished from other causes of cyanosis at birth, including cardiac or pulmonary disease and toxic methemoglobinemia, to which newborns and infants, whose physiologic red cell cytochrome b_5 reductase activity is approximately 50% that of adult levels, are particularly susceptible. Conjunctival cyanosis, a cardinal sign of hereditary methemoglobinemia, is usually absent in hypoxemia due to cyanotic cardiac or respiratory disease. Drugs and toxins that can induce methemoglobin formation include nitrites, sulfonamides, dapsone, metoclopramide, doxorubicin hydrochloride, vitamin K analogs, antimalarial agents, benzocaine, and aniline dyes.

Deficiency of cytochrome b_5 reductase is limited to the red cells in the majority of cases. In contrast to this form, in which affected individuals are "more blue than sick," a severe lethal disorder (type II) results from deficiency of cytochrome b_5 reductase in all somatic cells. Generalized cytochrome b_5 reductase deficiency is characterized by failure to thrive, mental retardation, and neurologic abnormalities, including microcephaly, opisthotonos, athetoid movements, and hypertonia, which lead to early death. A third form of cytochrome b_5 reductase deficiency (type III) without neurologic involvement has been described in which there is enzyme deficiency in red cells, platelets, and leukocytes but not in other cells.

Diagnosis

Diagnosis of cytochrome b_5 reductase deficiency is based on the demonstration of methemoglobin in the absorption spectrum of hemolysate. This disappears on the addition of cyanide, which distinguishes enzymopathic methemoglobinemia from cases due to an M hemoglobin. The diagnosis is confirmed by evidence of reduced enzyme activity in red cells alone (type I) or in addition to leukocytes and platelets (type II or III).

Hereditary Pyropoikilocytosis

Hereditary pyropoikilocytosis (HPP) is a rare autosomal-recessive hereditary hemolytic anemia. Most of the children affected are black. HPP most commonly presents in infancy with a previous clinical history of jaundice and anemia during the newborn period. The severity of the anemia usually requires some medical intervention such as exchange transfusion or phototherapy.

Laboratory Findings

Laboratory findings include a low MCV and an increase in osmotic fragility. Blood smears show bizarre spiculated and budding RBCs. Micropoikilocytoses, microspherocytosis, elliptocytes, red-cell fragments, and nucleated red cells are also seen.

The diagnosis of HPP is confirmed by analyzing the spectrin using two-dimensional isoelectric focusing polyacrylamide gel electrophoresis, which demonstrates the structural abnormality in the I-domain of the spectrin.

HPP erythrocytes exhibit thermal instability and fragmentation at 45–46°C, in contrast with normal erythrocytes, which fragment at 49°C.

Anemia, Hemolytic, Autoimmune

AIHA is caused by the presence of antibodies against a person's own RBC antigens, which leads to premature lysis resulting in shortened RBC life span. It can appear at any age, including infancy, but is frequent in older age groups. There are two major categories of AIHA. Antibodies that are most active at 37°C give rise to warm-type AIHA and those that are most active at 4°C produce cold-type AIHA.

Warm-type AIHA is the most common, making up approximately 70% of AIHA cases. It is associated with IgG autoantibodies in approximately 90% of cases. Antibodies coat the RBC, which leads to increased recognition and subsequent interaction with splenic macrophages, and thus enhances phagocytosis of the RBC membrane. This results in formation of spherocytes and shortened RBC survival by extravascular hemolysis. The RBC is heavily coated with IgG; complement also binds to the cell membrane. The presence of C3 on the cell surface markedly enhances macrophage-binding efficiency and increases reticuloendothelial-mediated destruction in the liver and spleen.

Cold-type AIHA is caused primarily by IgM autoantibodies called "cold agglutinins." They tend to agglutinate RBCs at low temperatures (optimally at <16°C, but also at temperatures between 25°C and 31°C). Because macrophages have no receptors for this complement, the cell escapes hemolysis in the spleen. This effect is seen in ^{51}Cr survival studies when an initial episode of abrupt cell destruction is followed by a slower second phase, in which cell survival times may approach normal.

AIHA may be either primary (idiopathic) or secondary. The primary type usually develops in older individuals with no evidence of underlying disease and constituting 30–60% of patients with AIHA. The remaining cases are secondary to an underlying disease, drug use, or infection.

Cold-type AIHA may present as an acute onset of anemia. It may occur after an infection such as *Mycoplasma* pneumonia, infectious mononucleosis, or cytomegalovirus (CMV) infection, or it may be found in association with a lymphoproliferative malignancy. The anemia may range from mild to severe, and intravascular hemolysis may occur. Alternatively, cold-type AIHA may have an insidious onset, with minimal symptoms until severe anemia develops. Cold-type AIHA usually is not associated with jaundice or splenomegaly despite marked anemia.

Most people have low, clinically insignificant, or physiologic titers of cold agglutinins (≤1:32) that bind to RBCs only at temperatures well below those found even in exposed extremities. When increased production of the IgM leads to higher titers (≥1:256), the temperature of cellular agglutination rises to approximately 37°C, which results in complement fixation and a positive result on a direct antiglobulin (Coombs) test. Cold-type AIHA is often subdivided into three clinically distinct disease categories: acute postinfectious, chronic idiopathic, and cold agglutinin disease. Acute postinfectious cold-type AIHA (titers of 1:128 to 1:8,000) is usually seen in younger patients and has an acute, often self-limited course; it follows mycoplasmal pneumonia, CMV infection, or EBV infection. Titers of ≥1:256 are observed in cold-type AIHA in elderly women. In chronic cold agglutinin disease, titers may be ≥1:50,000, particularly in diseases associated with a lymphoproliferative process. *Warm-type AIHA* is of abrupt onset, with jaundice and splenomegaly, and anemia may be severe.

Paroxysmal cold hemoglobinuria (PCH) is clinically closely related to cold-type AIHA. It is due to acquisition of an IgG antibody called the Donath-Landsteiner hemolysin. This antibody has a characteristic biphasic mode of action, first adsorbing to RBCs at low temperatures and then causing intravascular hemolysis and hemoglobinuria as the temperature rises to 37°C. It is important to diagnose PCH because it is usually self-limited and treated by keeping the patient warm.

Laboratory Findings

Laboratory Parameters	**Warm Type**	**Cold Type**
Usual immunoglobulin type	IgG	IgM
Direct antibody test	2+–4+	2+–4+
Monospecific sera		
Anti-IgG only	1+	0
Anti-IgG+ anti-C1	1+	0
Anti-C1 only	Rare	1+
Complement activation	Little or none	Yes
Serum complement levels	Normal or decreased	Decreased
Osmotic fragility	Increased	Normal
Peripheral blood findings	Spherocytes, nucleated RBCs	RBC agglutination

Clinical Findings

Clinical Findings	**Warm Type (70%)**	**Cold Type (30%)**
Onset	Abrupt	Insidious
Jaundice	Usually present	Often absent
Splenomegaly	Present	Absent
Age	All ages	All ages
Sex	Slightly more females	Females predominate
Origin of autoantibody		
Idiopathic	50–60%	30–40%
Drug induced	25–30%	1–5%
Lymphoproliferative disorder	10–15%	15–20%
Viral or mycoplasma	0%	25–35%
Other (inflammatory diseases, other malignancies)	5–10%	5–10%

Diagnostic Tests

Donath-Landsteiner Test

The Donath-Landsteiner test facilitates diagnosis of PCH, allowing it to be distinguished from cold-type AIHA. PCH is usually a self-limited disease and is treated conservatively by keeping the patient warm.

The Donath-Landsteiner hemolysin is a complement-dependent IgG antibody that agglutinates cells at 4°C and lyses them at warmer temperatures (usually 37°C).

Table 9. Diseases Associated with Autoimmune Hemolytic Anemia

	Antibody Specificity	
Disease	Warm Antibody	Cold Antibody
Inflammatory disease		
SLE, rheumatoid arthritis, ulcerative colitis	Anti-Rh, LW, Wright	Anti-I, anti-i
Infection		
Mycoplasma	NA	Anti-I
Epstein-Barr virus	NA	Anti-i
Clostridium, Escherichia coli	Anti-T	NA
AIDS	Variable	Anti-I
Drugs		
Methyldopa	Anti-Rh	NA
Quinidine penicillin	Anti-Rh	NA
Malignancy		
Chronic lymphocytic leukemia	Anti-Rh, LW, Wright	Anti-I
Non-Hodgkin lymphoma	Anti-u, En	Anti-I
Hodgkin disease	Anti-Rh	Anti-I
Carcinoma (ovary, thymus, gastrointestinal)	Variable	NA

AIDS, acquired immunodeficiency syndrome; NA, not applicable; SLE, systemic lupus erythematosus.

Other hemolysins may react at a single temperature, 48°C or 37°C, but are not biphasic. The Donath-Landsteiner hemolysin does not lyse cells with reverse incubations of 37°C to 4°C. Warm antibodies are IgG, whereas cold antibodies are IgM.

Presence of a biphasic hemolysin is diagnostic of PCH. PCH often occurs after a viral infection but can also be seen with congenital syphilis, so follow-up serologic testing should be performed. Pathologic findings with BMA include hyperplasia and increased marrow hemosiderin levels.

Antibody Titers for *Mycoplasma* and Viruses

Measurement of antibodies to *Mycoplasma* and viruses requires acute- and convalescent-phase serum samples obtained 7 to 10 days apart to show a rise in titer of antibody for specific organisms.

The tests are usually performed at county or state reference laboratories. The agent suspected should be specified. The most common etiologic agents of interest are *Mycoplasma* and, less frequently, EBV or CMV.

A three-dilution rise in titer is required for the test to aid diagnosis because previous exposure to these viruses is fairly common. IgM antibody suggests recent infection.

Disorders Associated with Autoimmune Hemolytic Anemia

See Table 9.

Anemia, Hypochromic

Causes of hypochromic anemia include

- Disorders of iron metabolism
  - Iron deficiency, inadequate intake, malabsorption
  - Growth spurt
  - Chronic infections or inflammatory states
  - Blood loss, menses
  - Neoplasia
- Disorders of heme synthesis: sideroblastic anemias
  - Hereditary (X-linked or autosomal)
  - Acquired idiopathic causes (myelodysplasia)
  - Toxin induced (lead, drugs, alcohol)

Disorders of globin synthesis: thalassemic syndromes
- α Thalassemia
- β Thalassemia

Anemia, Hypochromic Microcytic

Decreased hemoglobin synthesis results in a hypochromic microcytic anemia. Such a decrease may occur due to deficiencies in either heme or globin chain synthesis. This synthetic defect may arise due to insufficient amounts of iron, abnormal iron metabolism and heme synthesis (due to acquired or hereditary sideroblastic disorders), or secondary to hereditary abnormalities in globin synthesis (such as the thalassemias).

Causes

Iron Deficiency

Iron deficiency is the most common cause of anemia. In infants and children, a negative iron balance usually occurs because the dietary intake of iron is inadequate to meet the requirements for growth. It takes 3 months of iron deficiency to produce an abnormal RBC count. The anemia is hypochromic microcytic (Color Fig. 9).

Reticulocytes are the first cells produced in circulation and reflect iron levels within 72 hours of the time a blood specimen is drawn. They are very early markers of iron deficiency, indicating it before a child is anemic.

A normal range for reticulocyte hemoglobin content (RHc) is 25.6–29.6. Iron-deficiency anemia results in an RHc level of 19.2 ± 2.04.

If the RHc level is <24, the likelihood is 50% that a child has iron-deficiency anemia.

If the RHc level is >29, there is no chance that the child is iron deficient.

Renal dialysis patients have slightly different values, with an RHc level <26 predicting iron deficiency with 100% sensitivity and 80% specificity.

Interpretation of the results of iron studies is shown in Table 10.

Anemia of Chronic Disease

ACD is often normochromic and normocytic but also may present as a hypochromic microcytic anemia.

Sideroblastic Anemias

Sideroblastic anemias are characterized by abnormal iron metabolism within the RBC itself. In these disorders, iron sequestered in the developing RBC mitochondria distorts the mitochondria and is unavailable for heme synthesis. Iron stains show a characteristic pattern of iron around the nucleus, forming a ringed sideroblast. Sideroblastic anemias may be hereditary (either X-linked or autosomal), idiopathic (usually as part of a myelodysplastic disorder), or secondary to a toxic insult (drugs, lead, or alcohol). Hereditary sideroblastic anemias are extremely rare in comparison with acquired forms.

Table 10. Interpretation of the Results of Iron Studies

	Iron	Iron-Binding Capacity	Transferrin Saturation	Ferritin	Trial of Oral Iron
Iron deficiency	Decreased	Increased	Decreased	Decreased	Hemoglobin normalizes
Iron deficiency + acute-phase response	Decreased	Normal or decreased	Normal or decreased	"Normal" <100 μg/L	Partial response
Acute-phase response	Decreased	Decreased	Decreased	Increased	No response
Iron overload	Increased	Normal or decreased	Increased	Increased	Not appropriate

Hereditary Disorders of Globin Synthesis

Hereditary disorders of globin synthesis, or thalassemic syndromes, are common in Asian, Mediterranean, and black populations.

Lead poisoning

Lead intoxication leads to microcytic anemia, and hematologic findings may resemble those of thalassemia. Nonhematologic manifestations of lead intoxication, however, particularly neurologic complications, often dominate. The spectrum of clinical presentations of lead intoxication ranges from abdominal pain, vomiting, malaise, and behavioral changes to acute encephalopathy with rapid progression to coma and death.

Diagnostic Tests

Hypochromic and microcytic anemia and basophilic stippling of erythrocytes on peripheral blood smears are noted early in lead-poisoned infants and children. Basophilic stippling is a result of the inhibition of the RBC enzyme 5-pyrimidine nucleotidase, which normally removes nucleotide chains from the RBC after its nucleus has been extruded. In lead poisoning, these chains persist, and the nucleotide remnants stain blue on a regular Wright stain, causing a stippling of the RBC.

Lead interferes with porphyrin synthesis and prevents iron incorporation into porphyrin III, which impairs iron use as well as globin synthesis.

Lead intoxication and iron deficiency may coexist. Both lead poisoning and iron deficiency cause FEP to accumulate in the blood and levels are elevated in both conditions, although extremely high levels are seen more commonly in lead intoxication. Further testing, such as the determination of blood lead level, is necessary to ascertain the cause of elevated FEP. When lead intoxication is suspected, a whole-blood lead level should be obtained.

Clinical Findings

Severe anemia is associated with pallor, weakness, dizziness, palpitations, and even dyspnea. Some patients with iron deficiency may have cheilitis or spooning of the nails (koilonychia). Food cravings for ice, clay (pica), dirt, starch, or pickles also are common.

Laboratory Findings

Pertinent laboratory findings in microcytic hypochromic anemia are shown in Table 11.

Tests helpful in distinguishing anemia of chronic disease from iron deficiency are shown in Table 12.

Anemia, Megaloblastic

Megaloblastic anemia occurs when the coenzyme forms of folate or vitamin B_{12} or both are deficient.

Vitamin B_{12} circulates in the peripheral blood bound to various proteins. Except in infants, total body stores of vitamin B_{12} are abundant and are sufficient for adequate supply for 2 to 5 years. Folate is very heat labile and is destroyed readily in the cooking process.

Except in infants, total body stores of folate are moderate and are sufficient to maintain normal cellular proliferation for 3–5 months. Because of the relatively short time that folate stores meet host needs, the incidence of folate deficiency secondary to inadequate intake is substantially greater than that of vitamin B_{12} deficiency.

Clinical Findings

Patients with megaloblastic anemia characteristically present with moderate to severe fatigue and malaise of several months' duration. Their skin may be lemon yellow because of the combined effects of moderately increased bilirubin level and the marked pallor of the underlying anemia. Because the defective DNA synthesis affects all proliferating cells, such patients experience atrophy of the mucosal surfaces of the

Table 11. Pertinent Findings in Microcytic Hypochromic Anemia

Cause of Anemia	RBC Number	Red Cell Distribution Width	Anisopoikilocytosis	Basophilic Stippling	Serum Iron	Bone Marrow Iron	Total Iron-Binding Capacity	% Saturation	Soluble Serum Transferrin Receptor
Iron deficiency	Decreased	Increased	Yes	No	$\downarrow$	$\downarrow$	$\uparrow$	$\uparrow$	High
Thalassemia minor	Normal or increased	Normal	No	Yes	$\uparrow$	$\uparrow$	$\downarrow$	$\uparrow$	Variable
Sideroblastic anemias									
Hereditary	Decreased	Variable	Variable	Yes	$\uparrow$	Increased ringed sideroblasts	$\downarrow$	$\uparrow$	Variable
Acquired	Decreased	Dimorphic population	Yes	Yes	$\uparrow$	Increased ringed sideroblasts	$\downarrow$	$\uparrow$	
Chronic disease	Decreased	Variable	Variable	No	$\downarrow$	Decreased in siderocytes; increased in RE cells	$\downarrow$	$\downarrow$	Normal

$\uparrow$, increased; $\downarrow$, decreased; RBC, red blood cell; RE, reticuloendothelial.

Table 12. Tests Helpful in Distinguishing Anemia of Chronic Disease from Iron Deficiency

Test	Anemia of Chronic Disease	Iron Deficiency
Red blood cell size	Normocytic to slightly microcytic	Microcytic
Red blood cell hemoglobin	Normochromic to hypochromic	Hypochromic
Serum iron level	Decreased	Decreased
Total iron-binding capacity	Decreased	Increased
Transferrin saturation	Decreased	Decreased
Serum ferritin level	Normal to slightly increased	Decreased
Marrow iron stains		
Reticuloendothelial	Increased	Absent
Sideroblastic	Decreased	Absent

tongue, gastrointestinal tract, and vagina. This can cause pain in the mouth and vagina, and can lead to secondary malabsorption in the gastrointestinal tract.

Although the neurologic manifestations of pernicious anemia have been well described, patients with folate deficiency also may rarely develop neuropsychiatric disorders, including irritability, forgetfulness, sleepiness, and depression. Occasionally, patients with folate deficiency manifest peripheral neuropathy similar to that described in patients with vitamin B_{12} deficiency.

Morphologic and Histologic Findings

Peripheral Blood Smear Morphology in Megaloblastic Anemia

The peripheral blood smear characteristically contains numerous oval macrocytes as well as schistocytes of various sizes, broken erythrocytes, and spherocytes (Color Fig. 10).

RBC fragmentation occurs because of the increased fragility of large erythrocytes, which probably are damaged during their passage through the spleen.

Basophilic stippling and Howell-Jolly bodies also have been seen in RBCs.

When the Hct value drops below 20%, nucleated RBCs may be found in the blood.

Hypersegmentation of mature neutrophils is a characteristic feature that appears very early in the development of megaloblastic anemia. Hypersegmentation can be manifested by cells with six or more nuclear lobes or by an elevation in the mean neutrophil lobe count.

Blood Cell Measurements

A moderate to severe normochromic macrocytic anemia with MCVs ranging from 100 to 150 μm^3; the MCHC is normal. The RDW is markedly elevated in megaloblastic anemia because of extreme anisocytosis. Circulating macrocytes are often disrupted, producing minute RBC fragments. The reticulocyte count is very low; in severe cases, the neutrophil and platelet counts also are decreased.

Bone Marrow Examination

The bone marrow is hypercellular with erythroid and granulocytic hyperplasia. Mitotic activity is abundant. The proliferating erythroid and myeloid cell lines show megaloblastic changes. The nuclei are large with finely dispersed chromatin, whereas the cytoplasm is more mature with effective hemoglobinization. The myeloid abnormalities are giant bands, metamyelocytes, and nuclear hypersegmentation of mature granulocytes (Color Fig. 10B). Large megakaryocytes may also be present.

Characteristics of Vitamin B_{12} and Folate

Table 13 describes the characteristics of vitamin B_{12} and folate.

Table 14 and Figure 11 describe the physiology and metabolism of vitamin B_{12} and folate.

Table 13. Characteristics of Vitamin B_{12} and Folate

	Vitamin B_{12}	Folate
Origin	Synthesized exclusively by bacteria	Synthesized by plants and microorganisms
Dietary source	Meat, fish, dairy products (heat stable)	Vegetables (especially green leafy) and fruits (heat labile)
Parent compound	Cyanocobalamin	Pteroylglutamic acid
Recommended daily allowance (μg)		
Infants	0.3	25–35
Children	0.7–1.4	50–100
Adults	2.0	400
Pregnant women	2.2	800
Lactating women	2.6	400
Normal blood levels	150–1,000 pg/mL	>3.7 ng/mL (red blood cells: 130–640 ng/mL)
Normal total stores[a] (major storage site)	3,000–5,000 mg (liver)	20–70 mg (liver)
Storage duration on deficient diet	2–5 yr	3–5 mo

[a]Total stores are much smaller in infants.

Table 14. Physiologic Characteristics of Vitamin B_{12} and Folate

	Vitamin B_{12}	Folate
Physiology of absorption	Vitamin B_{12} released from food by gastric acid, gastric enzymes, and small-bowel enzymes→free vitamin B_{12} bound to R binders primarily; some also binds to intrinsic factor (IF)→pancreatic enzymes degrade R binder–B_{12} complexes→released B_{12} is then bound to IF.	Polyglutamate deconjugated by conjugase enzymes in bile and small-bowel lumen.
Site of absorption	Vitamin B_{12}–IF complex adheres to receptors on brush border of ileum (pH- and calcium-dependent process).	Deconjugated folate absorbed in jejunum.
Physiology of circulation	30% of vitamin B_{12} binds to transcobalamin II (TCII), which delivers it to liver, bone marrow, and other sites; 70% of vitamin B_{12} binds to TCI, TCIII, and R binders, which deliver it exclusively to liver.	Folate circulates unbound in blood as 5-methyl tetrahydrofolate (THF).
Entry into cells	TCII–B_{12} attaches to specific membrane receptors. Vitamin B_{12} transferred across plasma membrane (TCII degraded in this process).	Vitamin B_{12} necessary for folate (THF form) to pass across plasma membranes and be retained in cell.
Function	Two active forms, methylcobalamin and 5-deoxyadenosyl cobalamin, which facilitate formation of methionine and succinate, respectively.	THF essential for all one-carbon transfer reactions in mammalian cells. THF required for both purine and pyrimidine synthesis.

	Vitamin B_{12}	Folate
Biologically active form(s)	Coenzyme B_{12} (5-deoxyadenosyl cobalamin) and methylcobalamin	5-methyl THF
Reactions requiring vitamin B_{12} and/or folate cofactors	I. Homocysteine $\xrightarrow{\text{methylcobalamin}}$ Methionine; 5-methyl THF → THF Failure in this pathway results in megaloblastosis; reaction also important in central nervous system methylation, and for incorporation of folate into cells II. Methylmalonate $\xrightarrow{\text{Coenzyme } B_{12}}$ Succinate Failure of this reaction not involved in neurologic disease or megaloblastosis	I. Required for both purine and pyrimidine synthesis II. Rate-limiting step in DNA synthesis (pyrimidine synthesis) dUMP → dTMP; THF → DHF III. Required for methionine synthesis (See I, vitamin B_{12}) IV. Folate also essential in amino acid synthesis

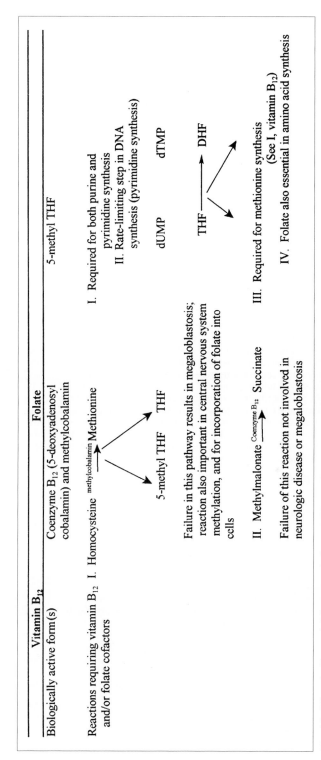

Fig. 11. Vitamin B_{12} and folate metabolism. DHF, dihydrofolic acid; dTMP, deoxythymidine monophosphate; dUMP, deoxyuridine monophosphate; THF, tetrahydrofolate.

Mechanisms of vitamin B_{12} deficiency include the following:

	Example	**Condition/Disorder**
Inadequate intake	Dietary deficiency	Strict vegetarianism
Increased requirement	Growth, development	Pregnancy, lactation
Defective absorption	Decreased intrinsic factor	Pernicious anemia, congenital intrinsic factor deficiency
	Decreased pancreatic enzymes	Pancreatitis
	Lack of calcium or abnormal pH	Zollinger-Ellison syndrome
	Defective ileal mucosa	Sprue, regional enteritis, surgical resection
	Parasitic or bacterial overgrowth	Tapeworm, blind loop
	Drug interference with absorption	Alcoholism, colchicine treatment, para-amino salicylic acid treatment
Defective transport	Decreased transcobalamin II level	Congenital deficiency of transcobalamin II (rare)
Disorders of metabolism	Suppression of inhibition of metabolic enzymes	Nitrous oxide administration, enzyme deficiencies
		Inborn errors of metabolism (rare)

The most commonly encountered cause of defective absorption of B_{12} is decreased intrinsic factor in patients with pernicious anemia. Intrinsic factor is secreted by gastric parietal cells stimulated by gastrin and histamine. The antibodies directed against intrinsic factor and parietal cells commonly detected in patients with pernicious anemia may cause the decreased level of intrinsic factor.

Dietary deficiency of folate is common in those with chronic alcoholism, in drug abusers, and in patients in low socioeconomic groups who consume inadequate diets. Excessive cooking destroys folate. Increased folate is required by infants, pregnant and lactating women, and patients with either malignancies or chronic hemolytic anemias. Premature infants have very low folate stores and are highly susceptible to folate deficiency. In individuals requiring anticonvulsant medications, the rate of folate metabolism is increased.

Diagnostic Tests

Serum vitamin B_{12}, serum folate, and RBC folate levels are measured. Levels found in megaloblastic anemia are given in Table 15.

Other laboratory tests for diagnosis of megaloblastic anemia are shown in Table 16.

Table 15. Serum Vitamin B_{12}, Serum Folate, and Red Blood Cell Folate Levels in Megaloblastic Anemia

Disorder	Serum Vitamin B_{12}	Serum Folate[a]	RBC Folate
Vitamin B_{12} deficiency	Decreased, <100 pg/mL (<74 pmol/L)	Normal or increased	Decreased
Folate deficiency	Normal or mildly decreased	Decreased	Decreased
Deficiency of both vitamin B_{12} and folate	Decreased	Decreased	Decreased

RBC, red blood cell.
[a]Fluctuates with changes in dietary folate.

Table 16. Laboratory Tests for Diagnosis of Megaloblastic Anemia

Test	Specimen	Procedure	Interpretation	Notes and Precautions
Vitamin B_{12}	Serum	Competitive protein-binding assay.	Decreased in PA and other anemias secondary to vitamin B_{12} deficiency; possible moderate decrease in patient with severe folate deficiency.	Low values common in HIV-1 infected patients; may not reflect true deficiency.
Folate	Serum	Competitive protein-binding assay.	Decreased in anemias due to folate deficiency; normal or increased in PA.	False-normal results in some patients with concurrent severe iron deficiency. Levels fluctuate with diet. Falsely elevated level with hemolyzed specimen.
RBC folate	Lysed RBCs	Similar to serum folate assay except lysed erythrocytes are used.	Because RBCs are metabolically inactive, RBC folate level reflects patient's folate status at the time these cells are formed; decreased level in folate and vitamin B_{12} deficiency.	Because vitamin B_{12} is required for folate to enter cell, level is decreased in either B_{12} or folate deficiency or in combined deficiency.
LDH	Serum/heparinized plasma	LDH catalyzes oxidation of lactate to pyruvate with reduction of NAD to NADH. Absorbance of NADH measured.	Markedly elevated LDH in megaloblastic anemia due to intramedullary destruction of cells.	Hemolysis falsely elevates results.
Iron, IBC	Serum/heparinized plasma	—	Increased serum iron, storage iron, and IBC in megaloblastic anemias due to increased iron use in erythropoiesis.	—
IF antibodies	Serum	Competitive protein-binding assay.	Present in 50% of patients with PA.	Very specific for PA, present in only 70% of patients.
Parietal cell antibodies	Serum	Immunofluorescent test using sections of mouse stomach and appropriate control tissues.	Fluorescence of parietal cells in stomach sections (with negative controls) indicates patient has parietal cell antibodies.	Sensitive for PA (positive in 90% of patients) but also found in other disorders.

(continued)

Table 16. (continued)

Test	Specimen	Procedure	Interpretation	Notes and Precautions
Indirect bilirubin	Serum	—	Mildly increased in megaloblastic anemia due to hemolysis of some abnormal RBCs and intramedullary destruction.	—
Gastrin	Serum	Competitive protein-binding assay.	Markedly increased in PA.	Specialized referral test.
Methylmalonate	Serum/plasma/urine	Gas chromatography–mass spectrometry or high-pressure liquid chromatography.	Increased in vitamin B_{12} deficiency; normal in folate deficiency.	Highly sensitive and specific; useful in early detection of vitamin B_{12} deficiency.
Total homocysteine	Serum/plasma/urine	Gas chromatography–mass spectrometry or high-pressure liquid chromatography.	Increased in both vitamin B_{12} and folate deficiency; also increased in some patients with inborn errors of metabolism.	Highly sensitive; useful in early detection of deficiency.
Orotic acid	Urine	Gas chromatography–mass spectrometry or high-pressure liquid chromatography.	Crystalluric.	Non-B_{12}, folate responsive.

HIV-1, human immunodeficiency virus 1; IBC, iron-binding capacity; IF, intrinsic factor; LDH, lactate dehydrogenase; NAD, nicotinamide adenine dinucleotide; NADH, reduced form of nicotinamide adenine dinucleotide; PA, pernicious anemia; RBC, red blood cell.

Serum Folate Quantitation

Serum folate is currently measured using a competitive protein-binding assay analogous to that used for vitamin B_{12}. Using current methodologies, these two assays can be performed simultaneously. The amount of labeled folate that binds to folate-binding proteins is inversely proportional to the amount of the patient's folate.

Decreased serum folate levels are detected in patients with megaloblastic anemia secondary to folate deficiency, whereas normal or increased levels of serum folate are found in patients with pernicious anemia.

Because serum folate level shows significant fluctuation with diet, a patient can have a normal serum folate level and actually be folate deficient. Folate deficiency also can be masked by a concurrent, more severe iron deficiency in which the serum and RBC folate levels may be normal. Hemolyzed blood samples elevate serum folate levels because of the large amounts of folate normally present in erythrocytes.

Red Blood Cell Folate Quantitation

RBC folate is measured by ion capture assay analogous to that used for measuring serum folate using whole blood. RBCs are lysed with ascorbic acid. Vitamin B_{12} cofactor is necessary for folate to enter and be retained within RBCs; therefore, decreased RBC folate is found in patients with either folate or vitamin B_{12} deficiency.

Serum Vitamin B_{12} Quantitation

Most laboratories currently use a competitive protein-binding assay for the determination of serum B_{12} levels. In this assay, a patient's vitamin B_{12} competes with fluorescently labeled B_{12} for a fixed number of binding sites on a solid matrix. The amount of labeled B_{12} that binds is inversely proportional to the patient's vitamin B_{12} levels. Decreased vitamin B_{12} levels are seen in patients with pernicious anemia and all other types of megaloblastic anemia caused by vitamin B_{12} deficiency. In patients with pernicious anemia and coexisting disease (such as iron deficiency, liver disease, hemoglobinopathy, or myeloproliferative disorders), the vitamin B_{12} level may be normal or even increased. Falsely low levels may be seen in patients with severe folate deficiency, pregnant women, women taking oral contraceptives, and patients with transcobalamin deficiency. Serum vitamin B_{12} levels are often low in patients infected with human immunodeficiency virus (HIV) 1, although only a small proportion of these patients appear to have a true deficiency.

Schilling Test

The first part of the Schilling test measures only the patient's ability to absorb vitamin B_{12}. Intrinsic factor and vitamin B_{12} are given to the patient in the second part of the test. The third part uses antibiotics to destroy bacteria and is designed to detect intestinal bacterial overgrowth disorders. The patient ingests radiolabeled vitamin B_{12}, and then an injection of a loading dose of unlabeled vitamin B_{12} is given. A 24-hour urine sample is collected and the amount of radioactivity in this sample is measured. In patients with pernicious anemia, the urinary excretion of labeled vitamin B_{12} is normal only when intrinsic factor is administered. The patient must have normal renal function and normal intestinal mucosa for the test results to be valid. Some patients who cannot absorb dietary vitamin B_{12} are able to absorb the crystalline vitamin B_{12} that is used, so that a false-normal result occurs.

Ancillary Tests

Several other laboratory tests, including measurements of levels of serum lactate dehydrogenase, bilirubin, serum and storage iron, intrinsic factor antibodies, and parietal cell antibodies, and gastrin test and deoxyuridine suppression test can be useful in evaluating patients with megaloblastic anemia. Excess of metabolites such as methylmalonic acid and total homocysteine may be diagnostic.

Most patients with pernicious anemia have parietal cell and intrinsic factor antibodies.

Gastrin Test

Gastrin stimulates parietal cells to secrete intrinsic factor and hydrochloric acid; typically, serum gastrin levels are markedly elevated in patients with pernicious anemia. Some parietal cell antibodies may be directed against the gastrin receptor, which explains the failure of parietal cells to respond to gastrin. The achlorhydria in gastric juices is secondary to the failure of parietal cells to produce hydrochloric acid; achlorhydria is a further stimulus for gastrin secretion.

Deoxyuridine Suppression Test

The deoxyuridine suppression test is for intranuclear vitamin B_{12} and folate levels and is based on studies of thymidine synthesis. This test of cultured blood lymphocytes or bone marrow cells distinguishes the primary and salvage pathways used in thymidine synthesis. It assesses both vitamin B_{12} and folate levels, because cofactors of both vitamins are required in the primary metabolic pathway of thymidine synthesis. The salvage pathway is favored when a deficiency of either vitamin exists. If nucleated blood cells are deficient in either vitamin B_{12} or folate, the salvage pathway is favored, which results in increased incorporation of radioactively labeled material into cell nuclei. With the addition of the deficient vitamin, the metabolic pathway reverts back to the primary synthetic pathway, and the radioactivity within the nucleus decreases. This test is useful in selected patients when other test results fail to confirm a vitamin B_{12} or folate deficiency.

Anemia, Normocytic

The normocytic normochromic anemias with low reticulocyte counts develop because of failed RBC production. The differential diagnosis of this group of anemias includes pure red cell aplasia, dyserythropoietic anemia, renal disease, infection, and drug-related aplasia. When low-reticulocyte, normocytic, normochromic anemia occurs in the presence of a decrease in WBCs and platelets, the diagnosis includes leukemia, aplastic anemia, and tumor infiltration of the marrow.

Aplasia, Red Cell

Clinical and laboratory features of various types of red cell aplasia are summarized in Table 17.

Congenital Red Blood Cell Aplasia

Diamond-Blackfan anemia (also known as *hypoplastic anemia*, *erythrogenesis imperfecta*, *congenital nonregenerative anemia*, *congenital pure red cell aplasia*, and *constitutional red cell aplasia*) is a constitutional disorder of erythropoiesis in which erythroid progenitors fail to follow the course of differentiation of the erythrocytic series toward reticulocytes. The anemia is present at birth or soon after, and in most cases the diagnosis is established before 6 months of age. Of the cases reported, 25% are associated with malformations of the bones and heart or other physical abnormalities.

Laboratory Findings

Laboratory findings in Diamond-Blackfan anemia include high MCV (>95 fL), normal RDW, and reticulocytopenia. The characteristics of all these hematologic values persist through the patient's life. The RBCs in the blood smear (peripheral blood) are macrocytic (Color Fig. 12). They have an abnormal concentration of fetal hemoglobin (HbF) and increased expression of i antigen, as well as fetal levels of RBC hexose monophosphate shunt and glycolytic enzymes, all characteristic of the fetal RBC. Increased erythrocyte adenosine deaminase levels have been reported in 90% of patients with Diamond-Blackfan anemia; however, their clinical significance is not yet clear. Quantitative changes in the WBC and platelet counts are absent or minimal.

BMA and bone marrow biopsy (BMB) specimen are cellular with a selective deficiency of the erythroid series. In the bone marrow, large pronormoblasts are sometimes present and even increased in numbers, but late normoblasts are absent. Myelopoiesis and thrombopoiesis are normal. Because of the age of the patient when the diagnosis is established, the lymphocyte count in the BMA is usually high.

Transitory Erythroblastopenia of Childhood

Transitory erythroblastopenia of childhood is the most common acquired RBC aplasia in infancy. Transitory erythroblastopenia of childhood usually presents in a previously healthy child between 6 months and 4 years of age with a recent onset of marked anemia. It is often associated with a recent viral infection and is followed by spontaneous recovery. An increase in the prevalence of transitory erythroblastopenia of childhood has been reported in the United States and other countries.

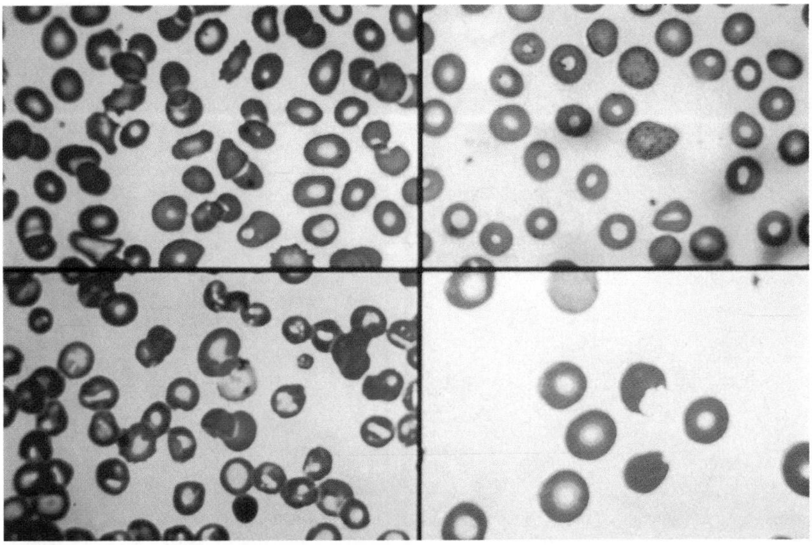

A B C D

Color Fig. 1. **A:** Howell-Jolly bodies—round granules representing nuclear remnants occurring in asplenia, after splenectomy, in congenital dyserythropoietic anemia (CDA), and in megaloblastic anemias. **B:** Basophilic stippling—punctate granules, representing ribosomal material occurring in lead toxicity, CDA hemoglobinopathies, and pyrimidine 5'-nucleotidase deficiency. **C:** Pappenheimer bodies—threadlike granules of variable size that stain positively for iron with Prussian blue; observed in liver disease, CDA, megaloblastic anemias, and hemoglobinopathies. **D:** "Bite" cell from a patient with glucose-6-phosphate dehydrogenase deficiency showing membrane defects from extrusion of Heinz bodies. **A–D:** Wright stain, 1,000×.

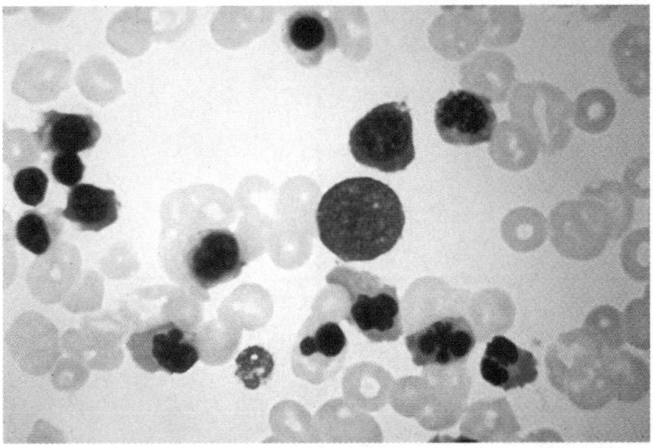

Color Fig. 6. Bone marrow specimen demonstrating erythroid precursors with multinuclearity in HEMPAS (hereditary multinuclearity with positive acid serum). (Wright stain, 1,000×.)

A 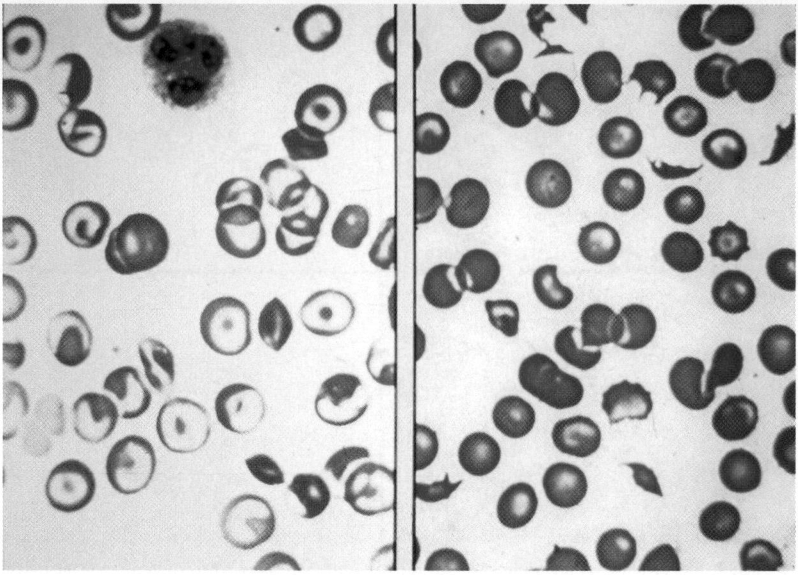 B

Color Fig. 7. A: Target cells with abnormal hemoglobin distribution, observed in hemoglobinopathies (hemoglobin C and hemoglobin S hemoglobinopathies, and thalassemia). **B:** Schistocytes (fragmented red blood cells) in a patient with hemolytic-uremic syndrome. Causes of schistocytic hemolysis include acute renal allograft rejection, mechanical damage secondary to prosthetic heart valve, hypertensive angiopathy, preeclampsia and eclampsia, thrombotic thrombocytopenic purpura, hemolytic-uremic syndrome, disseminated intravascular coagulation, and vasculitides. **A, B:** Wright stain, 1,000×.

A B
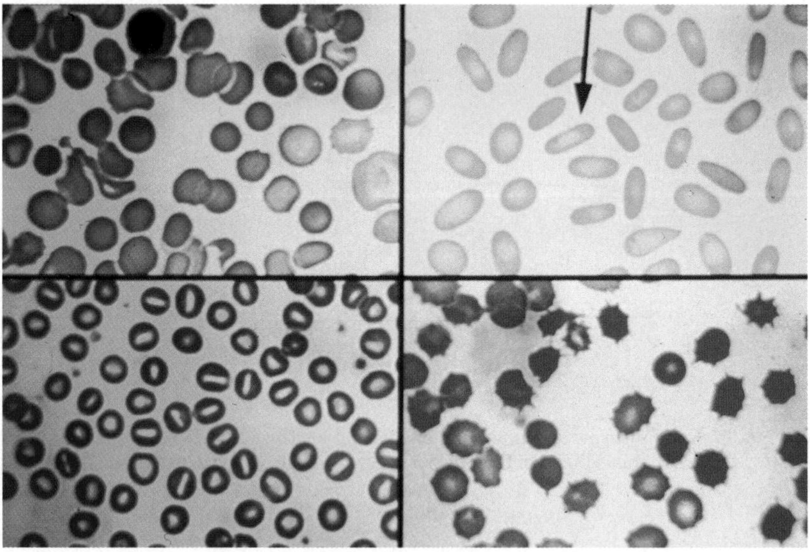
C D

Color Fig. 8. A: Spherocytes—round red blood cells without central pallor, frequently microcytic; observed in ABO incompatibility, burns, congenital hereditary spherocytosis, autoimmune hemolytic anemia. **B:** Elliptocytes—elongated or oval cells; normally up to 10% found in normal smear; observed in iron deficiency, thalassemia, and hereditary elliptocytosis (ovalocytosis). **C:** Stomatocytes—cells with slitlike central pallor; observed in Rh_0 disease. **D:** Acanthocytes (spur cells)—3–12 spicules of unequal length; observed in liver disease, abetalipoproteinemia, Macleod phenotype, pyruvate kinase deficiency, asplenia, and vitamin E deficiency. **A–D:** Wright stain, 1,000×.

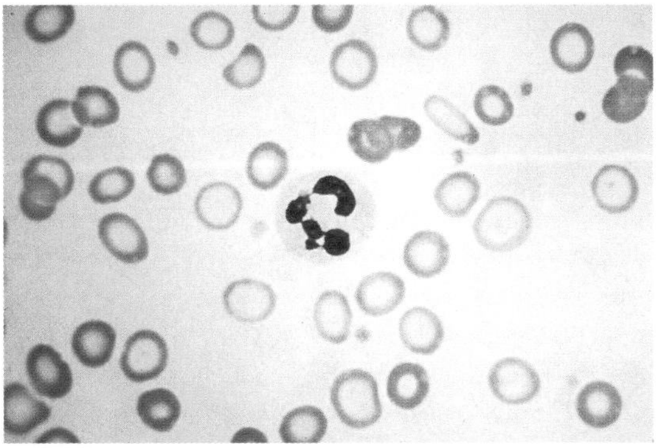

Color Fig. 9. Blood smear from a child with severe iron-deficiency anemia showing microcytosis, anisocytosis, hypochromia, and elongated elliptocytes (Wright stain, 1,000×). Bone marrow findings include mild erythroid hyperplasia, small normoblasts with uneven hemoglobinization, and absent iron stores.

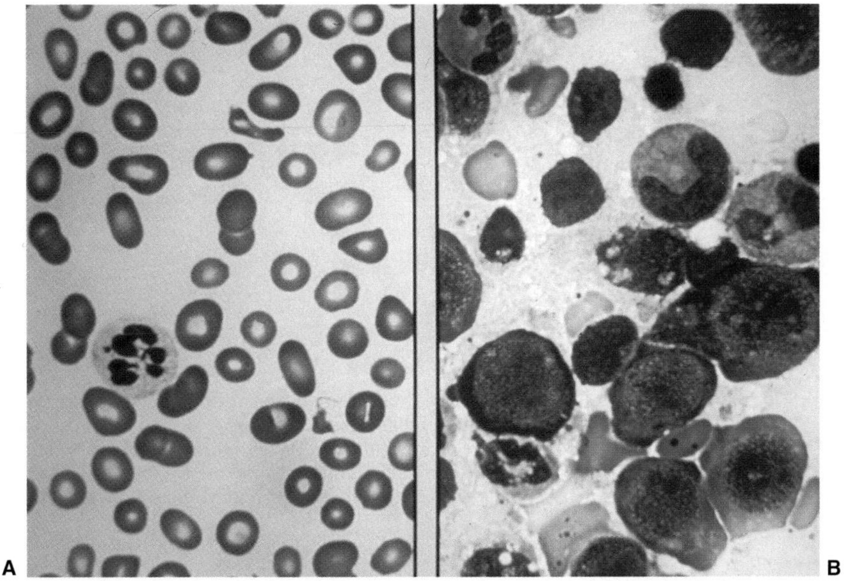

Color Fig. 10. **A:** Peripheral blood smear from a child with megaloblastic anemia secondary to folate deficiency. The erythrocytes show anisocytosis, macrocytosis, and ovalocytosis. A hypersegmented neutrophil with six lobes is present, which is one of the most sensitive indicators of megaloblastic anemia. **B:** Bone marrow specimen from a child with folate deficiency. Orthochromic megaloblasts are characterized by enlarged nuclei and mature cytoplasm with abundant hemoglobin. Giant band forms are typical of megaloblastic change of the myeloid series. **A, B:** Wright stain, 1,000×.

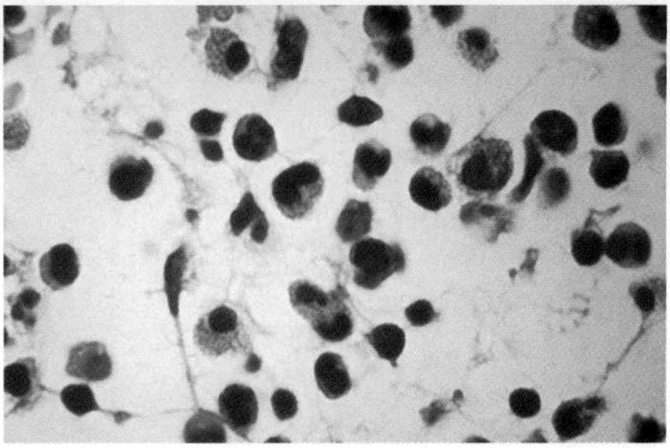

Color Fig. 12. Bone marrow sample with complete absence of erythroid precursors in patient with Diamond-Blackfan syndrome (Wright stain, 1,000×). The disorder is characterized by a normochromic macrocytic anemia, reticulocytopenia, and normocellular bone marrow with red cell aplasia (may exhibit red cell hypoplasia or, rarely, hyperplasia). Diamond-Blackfan syndrome is differentiated from transient erythroblastopenia of childhood by reticulocytopenia, elevated fetal hemoglobin levels during all phases of disease, and elevated deaminase levels.

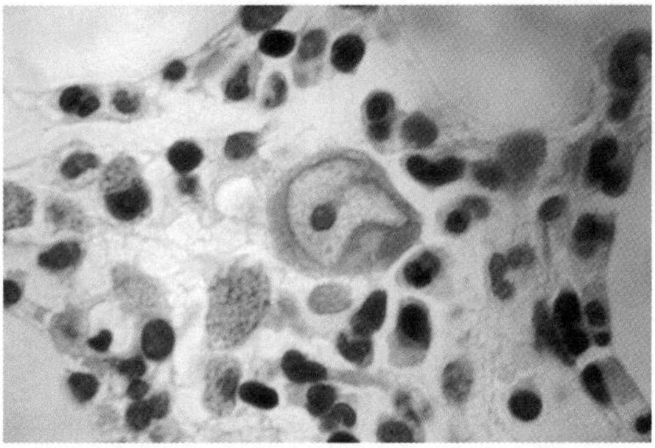

Color Fig. 13. Megaloblastoid erythroid precursors with inclusion-like nuclei in parvovirus infection in patient with acquired immunodeficiency syndrome (AIDS) (Wright stain, 1,000×). The loss of erythroid precursors (transient aplastic crisis) may occur in sickle cell disease, thalassemia, Chédiak-Higashi syndrome, and enzyme deficiency. Patients may develop varying degrees of neutropenia, thrombocytopenia, or pancytopenia. Infection leads to chronic red cell aplasia in AIDS.

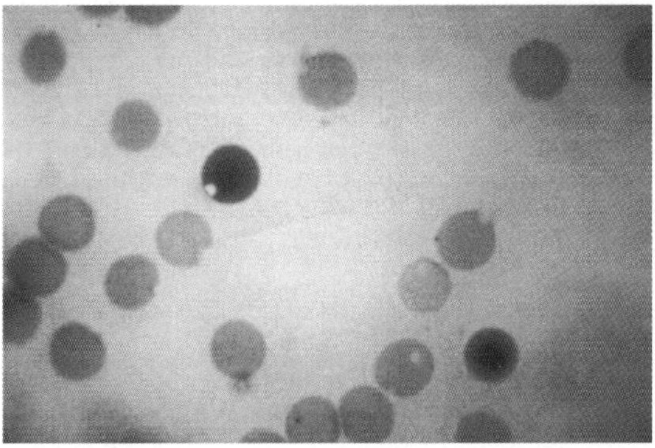

Color Fig. 14. Betke-Kleihauer test specimen exhibiting fetal cells in maternal circulation (percentage of bleed calculated by multiplying percentage of fetal cells ×50 (1,000×).

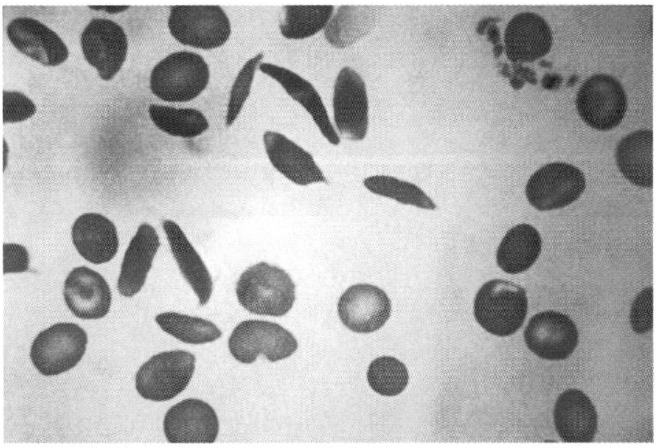

Color Fig. 15. Peripheral blood smear from an infant with homozygous hemoglobin S sickle cell crisis. Typical findings include normocytic normochromic anemia (average, 7.5 g/dL) beginning in late infancy; presence of variable numbers of sickled cells, target cells, and ovalocytes; and polychromasia. Thrombocytosis and Howell-Jolly bodies may be seen if there is functional asplenia (Wright stain, 1,000×).

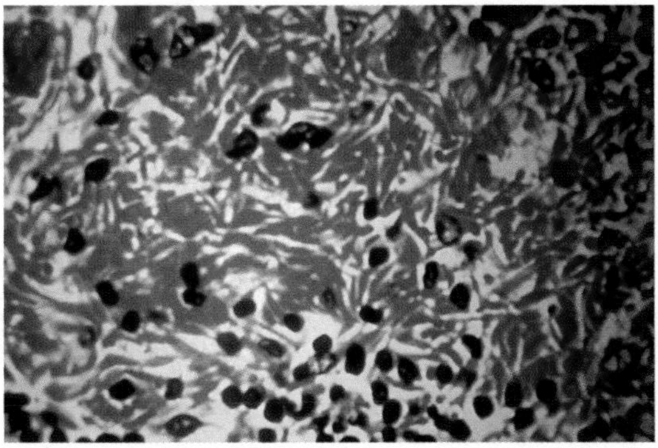

Color Fig. 16. Section of spleen from a young child with sickle cell anemia displaying engorged sinuses packed with irreversibly sickled red cells. In later life, repeated splenic infarcts lead to "autosplenectomy" (hematoxylin and eosin stain, 400×).

A,B

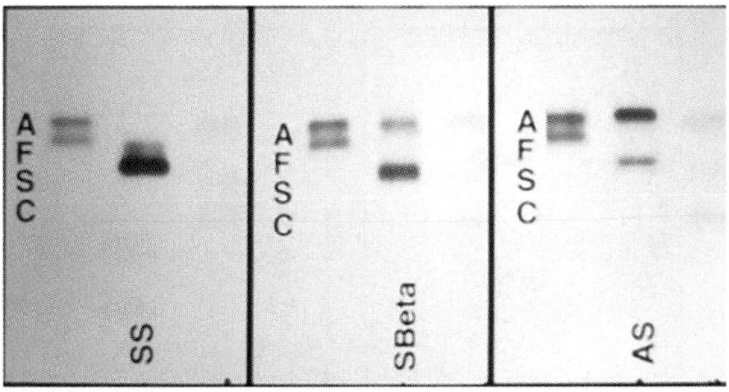

C

Color Fig. 17. Hemoglobin electrophoresis on cellulose acetate at pH 8.5. **A:** Homozygosity for hemoglobin S (HbS) in a 7-month-old girl (HbS 70%). **B:** Sickle/β^+ (SBeta) thalassemia in a 2 year old (HbS 61%). **C:** Sickle cell trait (AS) in an 18-month-old boy (HbS 38%). AFSC, control containing hemoglobins A, F, S, and C; SS, sickle cell anemia.

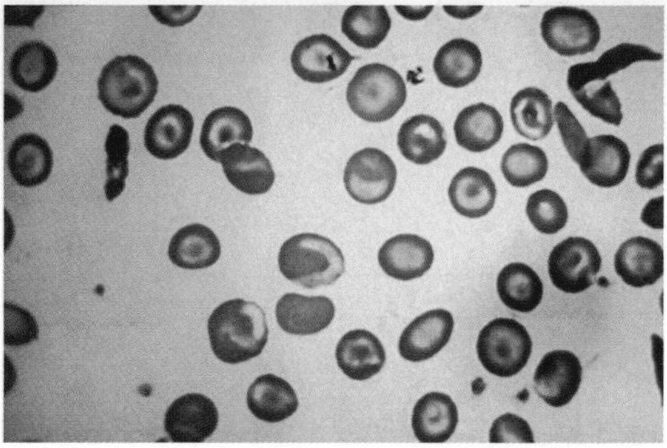

Color Fig. 18. Peripheral blood smear from a patient with sickle cell disease. Characteristic changes include target cells, polychromasia, and irregular elongated crystals (Wright stain, 1,000×).

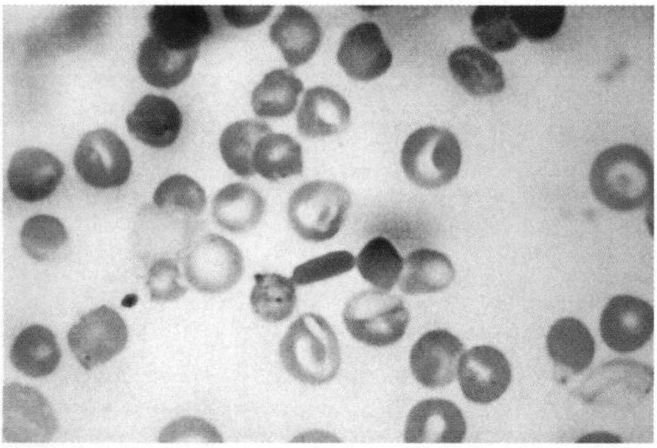

Color Fig. 19. Peripheral smear from patient with hemoglobin C (HbC) disease showing numerous target cells and occasional microspherocytes and an HbC crystal in a patient after splenectomy. Formation of crystals can be accentuated by incubation of the red cells in 3% NaCl solution (Wright stain, 1,000×). Hematologic findings in HbC disease include mild to moderate anemia, large numbers of target cells, minor population of microspherocytes, mild reticulocytosis, and occasional HbC hexagonal crystals in erythrocytes.

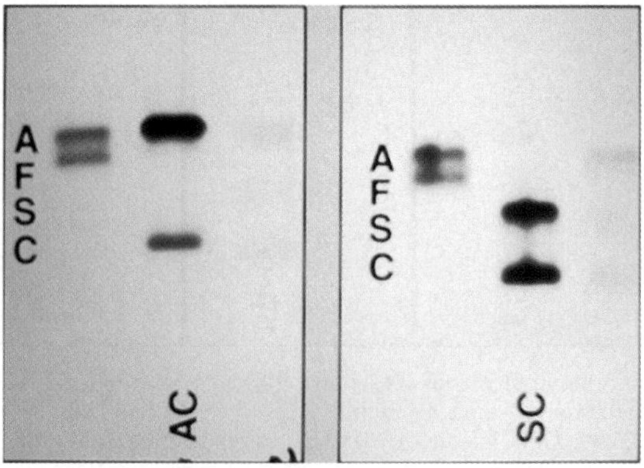

A B

Color Fig. 20. Hemoglobin electrophoresis on cellulose acetate pH 8.5. **A:** Hemoglobin C trait [65% hemoglobin A, 35% hemoglobin C (AC)]. **B:** Sickle cell–hemoglobin C disease [52% hemoglobin S, 48% hemoglobin C (SC)]. AFSC, control containing hemoglobins A, F, S, and C.

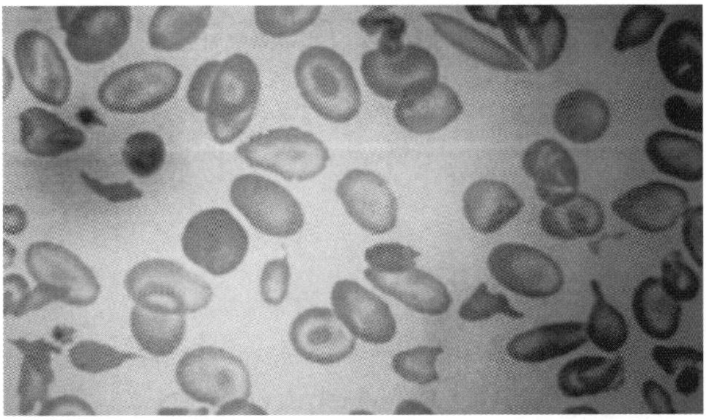

Color Fig. 21. Peripheral blood from a patient with β thalassemia major exhibiting anisocytosis, marked hypochromia, numerous target cells, and basophilic stippling (Wright stain, 1,000×).

A

B

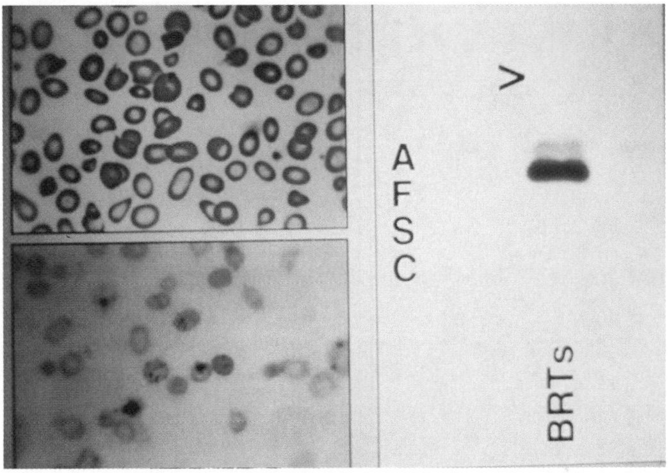

C

Color Fig. 22. A: Blood smear from a patient with hemoglobin H (HbH) disease. Red cells are characterized by marked anisocytosis, microcytosis, occasional target cells, and polychromia (Wright stain, 1,000×). **B:** Blood smear from a patient with HbH disease stained with brilliant cresyl blue demonstrating numerous punctate Heinz bodies (1,000×). **C:** Hemoglobin electrophoresis performed at an alkaline pH showing a faint band of hemoglobin Bart (BRTs) (*arrow*) migrating anodal to hemoglobin A in an infant with HbH disease. AFSC, control containing hemoglobins A, F, S, and C.

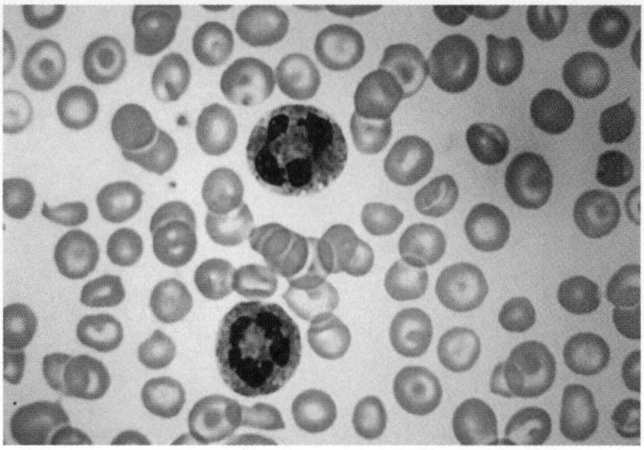

Color Fig. 24. Blood smear from a patient with β thalassemia minor showing microcytosis and occasional target cells (Wright stain, 1,000×).

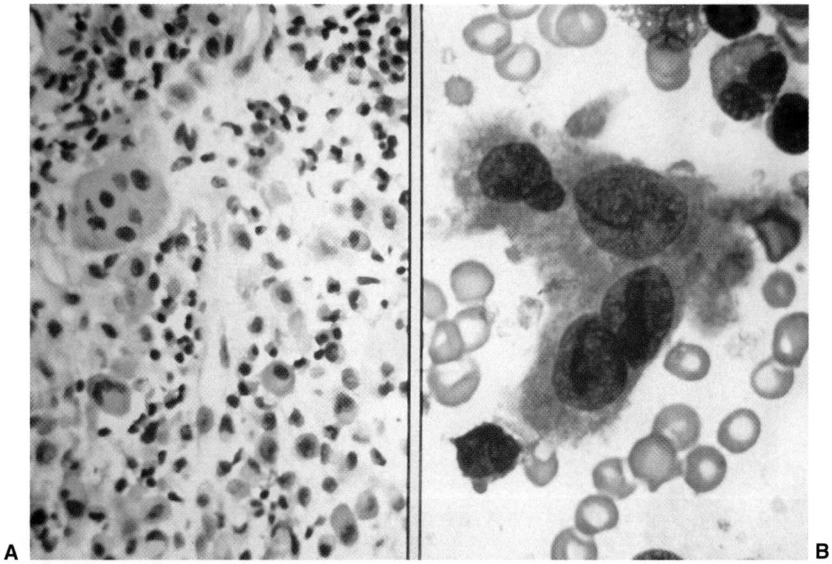

Color Fig. 25. A: Lymph node specimen from a patient with Langerhans cell histiocytosis demonstrating eosinophils and multinucleated giant cells. Lesions tend to be sinusoidal (hematoxylin and eosin stain, 400×). **B:** Bone marrow aspirate with cells exhibiting typical groove (folded nuclei) (Wright stain, 1,000×). The lymph nodes exhibit histiocytic aggregates, with necrosis, eosinophilia, and multinucleated giant cells. Immunohistochemical assays yield positive results for S-100, vimentin, LN-2, and LN-3, and negative results for leukocyte common antigen.

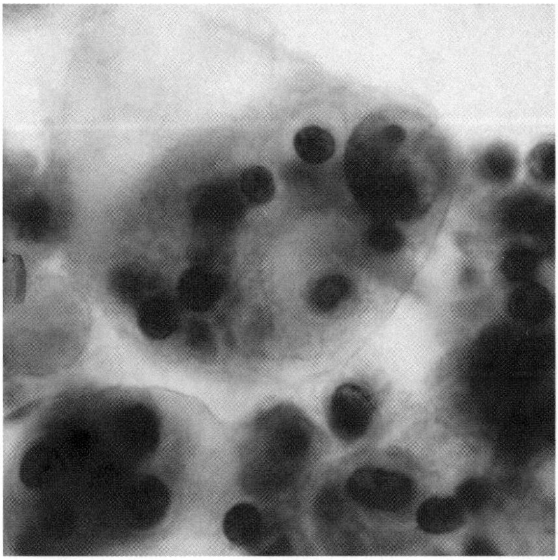

Color Fig. 26. Rosai-Dorfman massive lymphadenopathy with sinus histiocytes (Rosai-Dorfman disease) from lymph node biopsy (hematoxylin and eosin stain, 400×).

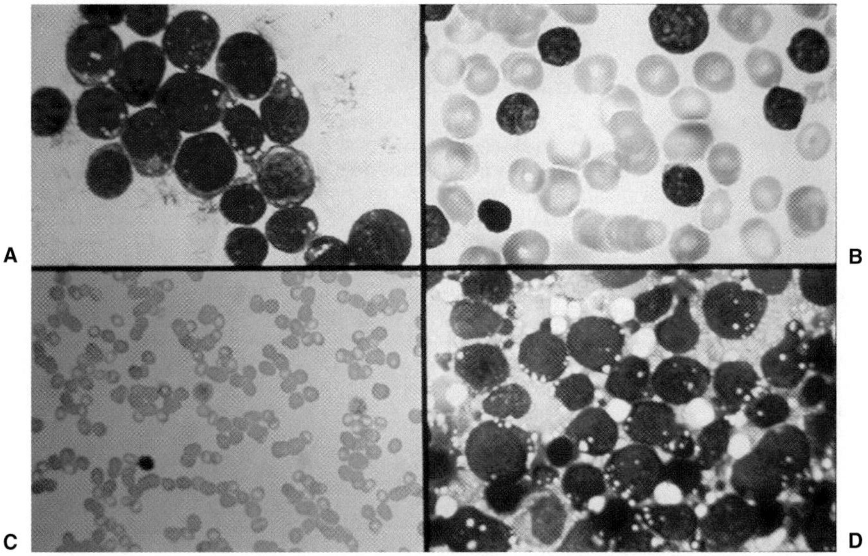

Color Fig. 27. Morphology in French-American-British (FAB) classification of acute lymphoblastic leukemia (ALL). **A:** Bone marrow aspirate smear of patient with ALL L_1 showing monotonous small lymphoblasts with scant cytoplasm and inconspicuous nucleoli. Peripheral blood findings usually include anemia, thrombocytopenia, and a leukocytosis [up to 50,000/mL white blood cells (WBCs)]. Leukopenia or normal WBC counts may be seen (Wright stain, 1,000×). **B:** Smear from patient with FAB category L_2 disease with lymphoblasts characterized by heterogeneity, nuclear folds, nucleoli, and more abundant cytoplasm than in L_1 (Wright stain, 1,000×). **C:** Bone marrow aspirate from patient with FAB category L_3 disease showing the characteristic morphology of blasts. The blasts display large round nuclei, a fine chromatin pattern, nucleoli, and abundant cytoplasm with vacuoles (Wright stain, 400×). **D:** Smear from patient with ALL L_1 with immunohistochemical staining directed against terminal deoxynucleotidyl transferase (TdT) (1,000×). TdT expression is usually seen in precursor B- and T-cell ALL.

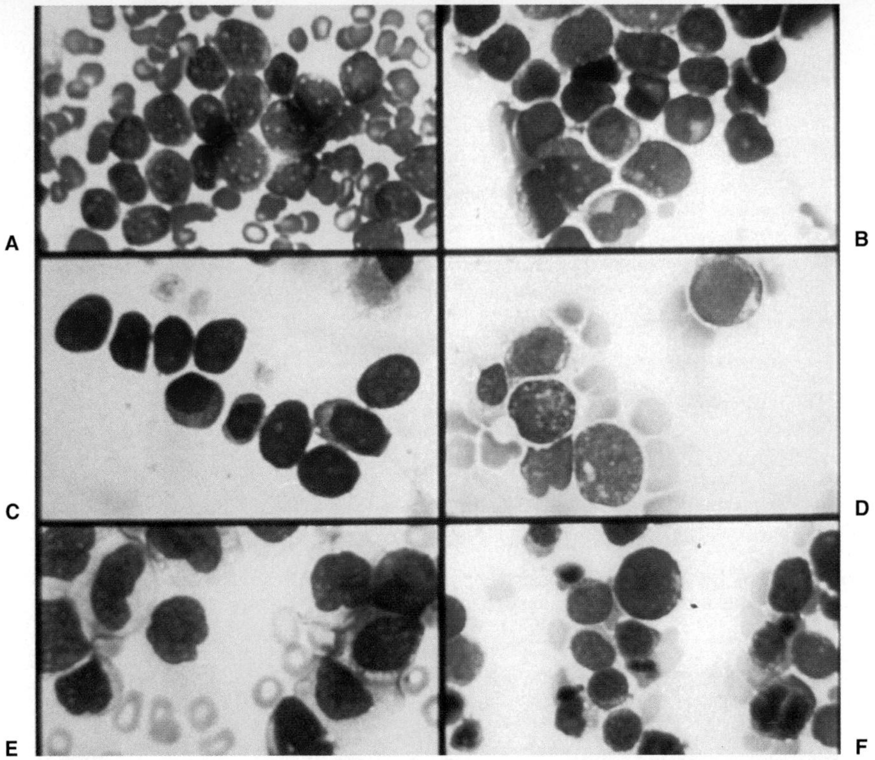

Color Fig. 29. **A:** Bone marrow smear from a patient with acute myelogenous leukemia (AML) type M_1 (French-American-British classification). The myeloblasts show little evidence of maturation. In some cases, distinguishing AML M_1 from acute lymphoblastic leukemia type L_2 by morphology and cytochemistry is very difficult. In these cases, immunophenotypic analysis is usually definitive. **B:** Bone marrow smear from a patient with AML type M_2. Maturation in more than 10% of the tumor cells as evidenced by primary and secondary granulation of the cytoplasm. **C:** Bone marrow smear from a patient with AML type M_3. The leukemic cells contain numerous primary granules and Auer rods. **D:** Bone marrow aspirate from a patient with acute myelomonocytic leukemia with eosinophilia (AML M_4 E). Smear shows atypical dysplastic eosinophils with granules. **E:** Bone marrow smear from a patient with AML type M_5 B. **F:** Bone marrow smear from a patient with erythroleukemia (AML M_6). Myeloblasts are admixed with dysplastic erythroid precursors. **A–F:** Wright stain, 1,000×.

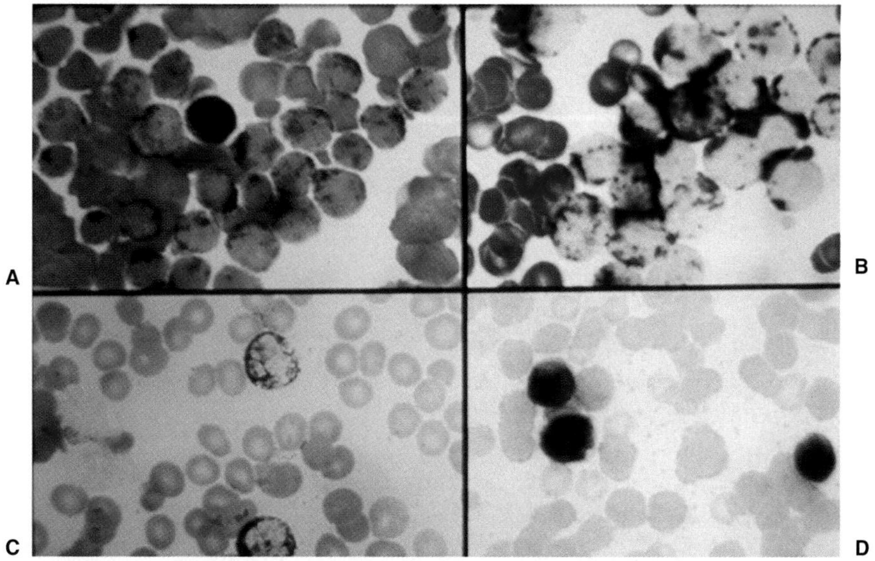

Color Fig. 30. A, B: Bone marrow smears from a patient with acute myelogenous leukemia type M_2 (French-American-British classification) stained with myeloperoxidase stain **(A)** and Sudan black B stain **(B)**. Cytochemical reaction is identified in many of the blasts (1,000×). **C, D:** Bone marrow smears from a patient with acute myelogenous leukemia type M_4 stained with chloroacetate esterase **(C)** and nonspecific esterase **(D)**. Positive staining for both enzymes is consistent with acute myelomonocytic leukemia. **A–D:** 1,000×.

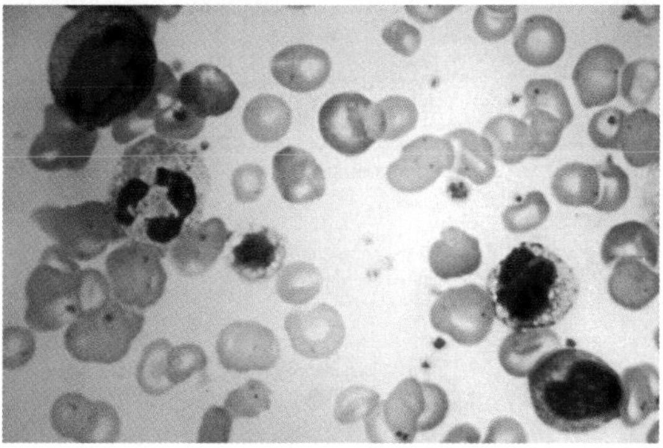

Color Fig. 32. Peripheral blood smear from a child with chronic myelomonocytic leukemia, adult type. Peripheral smear is characterized by leukocytosis, left shift, and basophilia (Wright stain, 1,000×).

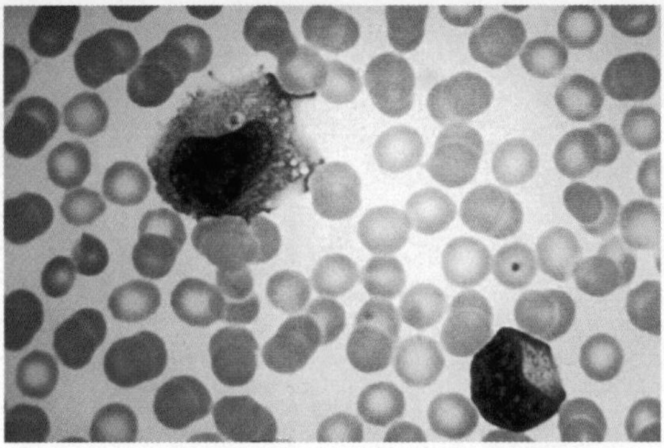

Color Fig. 33. Peripheral blood smear from a patient with infectious mononucleosis demonstrating atypical lymphocytes (Wright stain, 1,000×).

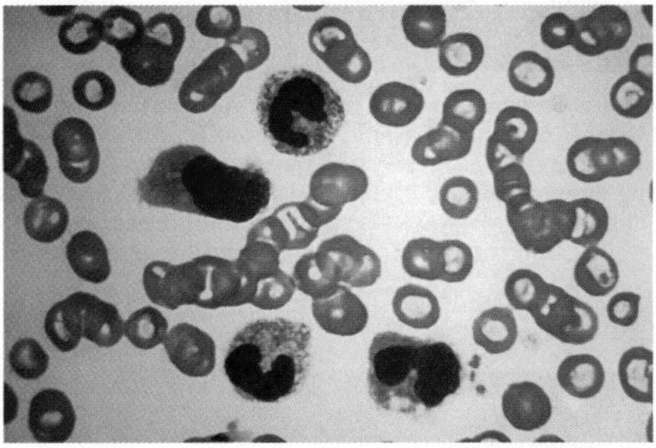

Color Fig. 34. Toxic granules (Döhle bodies)—heavy azurophilic (primary) granules in cytoplasm of neutrophils in a child with meningitis. The granules are present in cases of infection or severe burns and after radiation exposure (Wright stain, 1,000×).

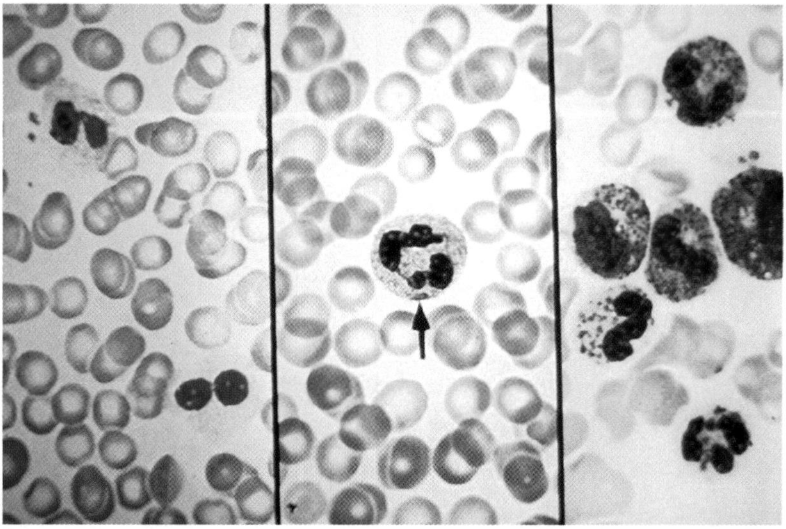

A,B C

Color Fig. 35. **A:** Pelger-Huët anomaly; autosomal-dominant inheritance; heterozygotes have bilobed neutrophil nuclei, homozygotes have monolobed nuclei. The neutrophils have normal function. Pseudo–Pelger-Huët cells may be seen in myeloproliferative disorders, myxedema, influenza, aplastic anemia, and metastatic tumor, and after sulfonamide therapy. **B:** Döhle bodies represented by a bluish inclusion in periphery of cytoplasm of neutrophils in a patient with burn. **C:** Alder-Reilly anomaly; large metachromatic granules are identified in neutrophils, lymphocytes, monocytes, and plasma cells of patients with mucopolysaccharide storage disease. **A–C:** Wright stain, 1,000×.

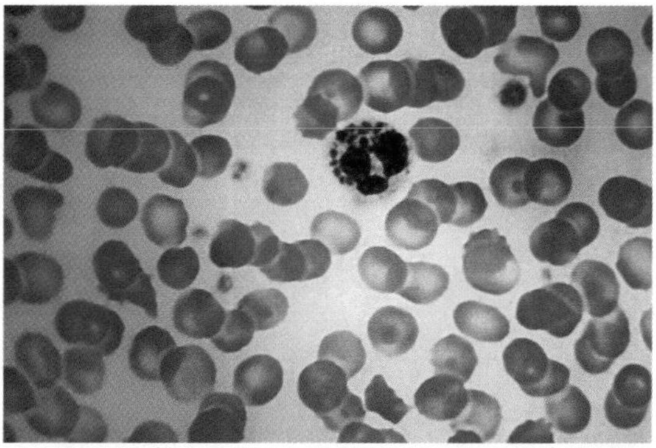

Color Fig. 36. Peripheral blood smear from a patient with Chédiak-Higashi syndrome. The neutrophil shows striking giant granules representing coalesced specific and primary granules. This autosomal-recessive disease results in incomplete degranulation on stimulation and poor chemotaxis. Clinical findings include partial oculocutaneous albinism, gingivitis, neuropathies, and hepatosplenomegaly (Wright stain, 1,000×).

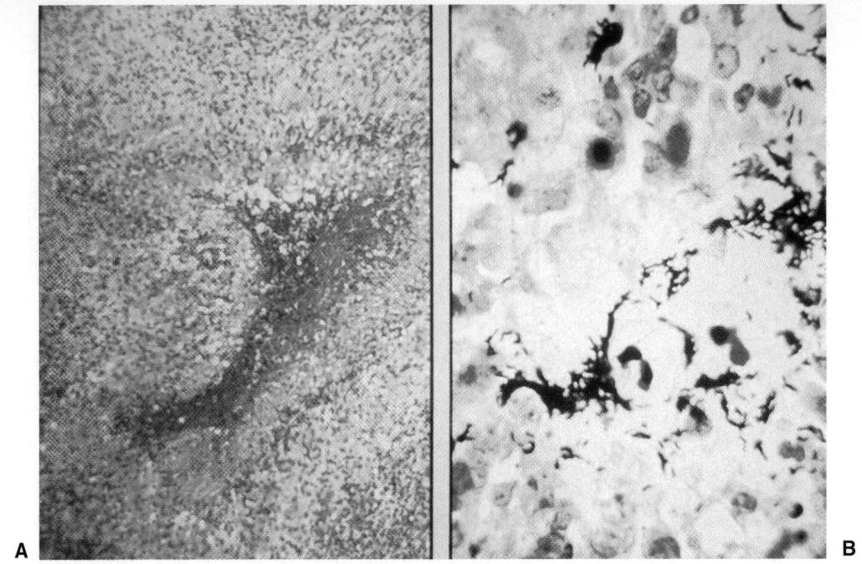

Color Fig. 37. **A:** Necrotizing granulomas and abscesses in lymph node specimen from a patient with cat-scratch disease (hematoxylin and eosin stain, 100×). **B:** Specimen stained with Warthin-Starry stain exhibiting wavy organisms of cat-scratch disease (1,000×). The disease is benign and self-limiting. Clinical findings include papular eruption after scratch by cat and regional lymphadenopathy persisting up to months. Histopathologic findings include lymph nodes demonstrating necrotizing, suppurative granulomatous process with multinucleated giant cells and stellate abscesses; polymerase chain reaction studies and immunofluorescent testing reveal the offending organism, *Bartonella henselae*, identified in tissue as wavy bacilli on Warthin-Starry stain.

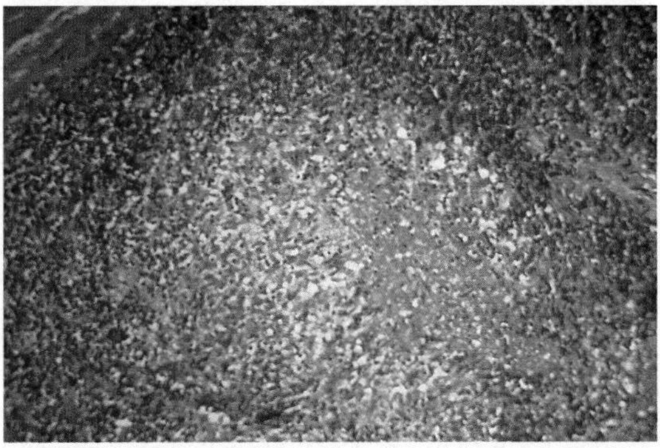

Color Fig. 38. Lymph node specimen from a patient with Kikuchi-Fujimoto disease demonstrating necrotic zone with prominent karyorrhectic debris, absent neutrophils, and occasional immunoblasts; may be indistinguishable from systemic lupus erythematosus (hematoxylin and eosin stain, 400×). Clinical findings include adenopathy, fever and chills, sweats, nausea and vomiting, pain in chest or right lower quadrant, myalgia or arthralgia, and rash; the disorder shows a higher incidence among young women; resolution occurs in 1–4 months.

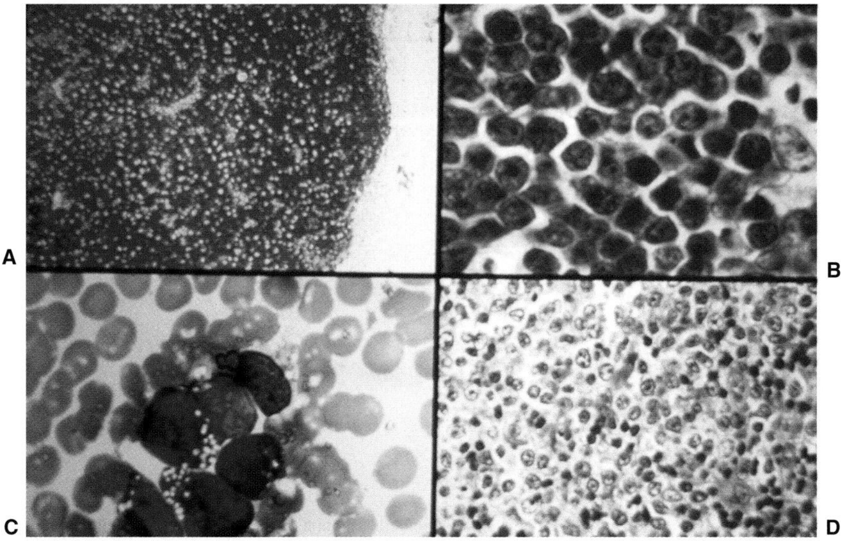

Color Fig. 40. A: Omental mass from a young boy with small noncleaved cell lymphoma (SNCL), Burkitt type. Low-power appearance is a "starry sky" pattern caused by evenly distributed tingible-body macrophages (hematoxylin and eosin stain, 100×). **B:** High-power section from the same patient exhibiting round uniform nuclei, prominent nucleoli, amphophilic cytoplasm, and a high mitotic rate (hematoxylin and eosin stain, 400×). **C:** Wright-stained touch imprint showing tumor cells with deeply basophilic vacuolated cytoplasm (1,000×). **D:** SNCL, non-Burkitt type. The tumor cells show more variability in nuclear shape and more prominent nucleoli (hematoxylin and eosin stain, 400×).

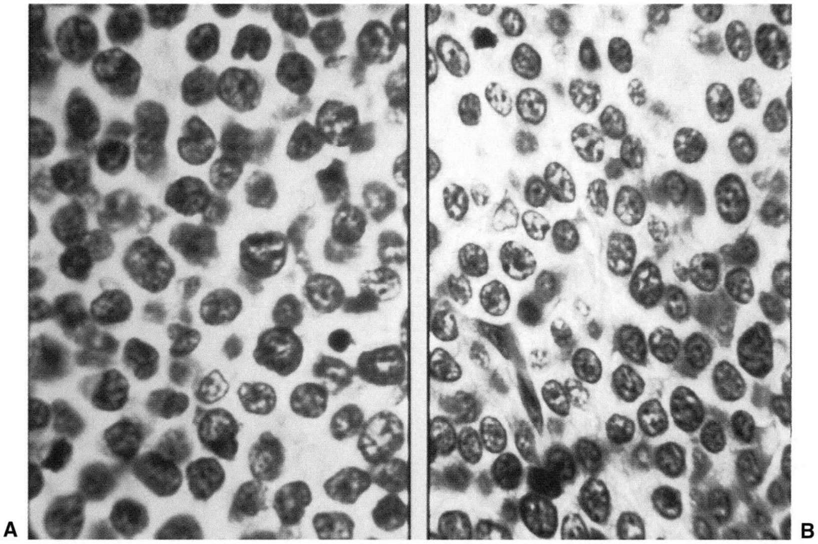

Color Fig. 41. A: Mediastinal mass from a patient with lymphoblastic lymphoma. The convoluted nuclei, fine chromatin pattern, and inconspicuous nucleoli are typical. **B:** Mass from a different patient with nonconvoluted histologic pattern. Histopathologic characteristics of lymphoblastic lymphoma includes a diffuse pattern with occasional "starry sky" appearance; uniform small round cells or variably sized cells with convoluted nuclei; fine chromatin pattern; inconspicuous nucleoli; very high mitotic rate; and invasion of pericapsular tissue and vessel walls. Tumors test positive for T-cell markers (UCHL-1). **A, B:** Hematoxylin and eosin stain, 1,000×.

Table 17. Red Cell Aplasia

Type	Clinical Features	Blood	Bone Marrow
Constitutional aplastic anemia			
Fanconi anemia	Autosomal-recessive disease with associated bone, skin, and renal abnormalities Mental retardation Underlying DNA repair defect	Thrombocytopenia is typically initial abnormality. Pancytopenia develops by midchildhood. Decreasing reticulocytes.	Initially normocellular/hypercellular with variable megaloblastic changes. Eventual aplasia. Substantial late development of myelodysplasia or acute myelogenous leukemia.
Dyskeratosis	X-linked recessive disorder with skin, nail, and mucosal abnormalities Mental retardation Likely DNA repair defect	Gradual development of pancytopenia. Decreased reticulocytes.	Initially normocellular/hypercellular; eventual aplasia in one-half of patients. Reports of late development of acute myelogenous leukemia.
Shwachman-Diamond syndrome	Autosomal recessive; associated bone abnormalities in some patients	Neutropenia predominates. One-fourth of cases progress to pancytopenia. Decreased reticulocytes.	Initial abnormalities are granulocytic. Eventual in one-fourth of patients. Some patients develop acute myelogenous leukemia.
Constitutional red cell aplasia			
Diamond-Blackfan anemia	Onset of anemia at birth or early infancy Several genetic types Short stature, hypertelorism, retardation Likely intrinsic progenitor cell defect	Macrocytic anemia with decreased reticulocytes.	Only rare erythroblasts. Other lineages unremarkable. Increased hematogones.
Acquired aplastic anemia	Onset at any age Most cases idiopathic Other cases linked to infections, toxin, drugs, radiation, immune disorders	Pancytopenia. Normal morphology. Decreased reticulocytes.	Panhypoplasia. Variable lymphoid infiltrates.

(continued)

Table 17. (continued)

Type	Clinical Features	Blood	Bone Marrow
Acquired red cell aplasia			
Transient erythroblastopenia of childhood	Patient usually >1 year old	Normocytic, normochromic anemia. Decreased reticulocytes.	Only rare erythroblasts evident. Other lineages unremarkable. Variable lymphocytosis.
Parvovirus-induced red cell aplasia	Any age Typically, either underlying constitutional anemia or immunodeficiency	Variable red blood cell morphology depending on underlying chronic anemia. Decreased reticulocytes.	Only erythroblasts evident; these cells may contain intranuclear inclusions ("lantern cells").[a] Other lineages usually unremarkable. Infection transient in immunocompetent, sustained in immunocompromised patients.
Acquired sustained pure red cell aplasia	Adolescence through adulthood Both idiopathic and secondary types	Normocytic, normochromic anemia. Decreased reticulocytes.	Only rare erythroblasts evident. Other lineages unremarkable.

[a]Unusual features such as increased erythroblasts and intact erythroid maturation noted in occasional cases.

Laboratory Findings

Decreased hemoglobin and Hct with normochromic and normocytic anemia (MCV of 80–95 fL) occurs with a variable degree of reticulocytopenia. If the reticulocyte count is determined at the beginning of the recovery phase, however, it may be high. The WBC count is normal or slightly low. Mild to moderate increases in platelet counts are commonly seen.

BMA is often performed to exclude malignancy. The cellular composition of the aspirated material may be quite variable with a large myeloid/erythroid (M/E) ratio. It may exhibit erythroblastopenia with normal maturation of the myeloid and megakaryocytic series. The lymphocyte counts are often high, and lymphocytes appear morphologically mature. "Lymphoid-like" cells are slightly more numerous and are intermixed with the hematopoietic cells. An alternative finding on BMA corresponds to the maturation arrest of the erythrocytic series and is characterized by a large number of pronormoblasts. Even more unusual is the finding of hyperplasia of the erythrocytic series.

BMB specimens are usually cellular with a selective decrease of the erythrocytic series; occasionally, small, ill-defined granulomas can be seen. The diversity of the laboratory findings described in the peripheral blood and bone marrow should be correlated with the clinical stage of the disease at the time that those laboratory studies are performed.

Red Blood Cell Aplasia Associated with Parvovirus Infection

Infection by human parvovirus B19 (HPVB19) in the nonimmunocompromised child has a subclinical course. Infection in children with hereditary hemolytic anemias and congenital or acquired immunodeficiencies often has a severe clinical course with worsening of the anemia, preceded by an infectious syndrome that can be life threatening. HPVB19 infection is the etiologic agent of the aplastic crisis seen in children with hereditary hemolytic diseases. Furthermore, HPVB19 infection can provide the first clue in the diagnosis of hereditary hemolytic anemias in children with compensated anemia.

Laboratory Findings

In a child with hereditary hemolytic anemia, a sudden drop in hemoglobin concentration is combined with reticulocytopenia relative to the hemoglobin concentration. Occasionally, the anemia is associated with thrombocytopenia or pancytopenia; these hematologic associations are seen in immunodeficient children. The peripheral blood smear exhibits marked anisopoikilocytosis and atypical lymphocytes.

In HPVB19 infection, the BMA smear is characterized by giant pronormoblasts with a decrease in late normoblasts if the BMA is done in the early stages of the infection (Color Fig. 13). Viral inclusions are not readily identified on the smears; they may sometimes be recognized in the late erythroid forms, but not in the giant pronormoblasts with the Wright-Giemsa stain. Viral inclusion can be distinguished from nuclear debris by recognizing the gray-pink cytoplasmic rim of the normoblast and the dark purple or lilac inclusions surrounding a lucent central area. These are so-called lantern cells.

The BMB is cellular with a large M/E ratio due to the decrease in the number of late erythroid cells. Large pronormoblasts with a purple-blue cytoplasm and a round nucleus with prominent nucleoli are seen in the hematoxylin and eosin–stained sections. The nucleus of an infected RBC contains an eosinophilic inclusion surrounded by a halo due to the condensation of the nuclear chromatin around the nuclear membrane. A characteristic finding is the absence of an inflammatory reaction in the marrow. The definitive diagnosis can be made in the BMA by immunocytochemical methods with a monoclonal antibody to the capsid protein of HPVB19, or alternatively by a highly sensitive PCR assay. Further proof of recent infection by the virus can be obtained by measuring serum titers of a specific B19 IgM antibody, which is generally detected within 3 days of clinical symptoms; titers start declining after the first month.

If the patient is immunosuppressed, the infection may persist, becoming chronic as a result of the inadequate antibody response. Patients may have more extensive marrow damage with severe pancytopenia.

Other viruses that commonly infect immunosuppressed patients can produce intranuclear inclusions in the cells of the bone marrow; however, HPVB19 produces its cytopathic effect only in erythroid cells. This effect is the hallmark of HPVB19 infection but is not associated with CMV or herpes infection. In addition, the necrotic effect produced by herpes virus is absent, and the cytomegaly and cytoplasmic inclusions seen in CMV infection are also absent in HPV19 infection. Immunohistochemical stains are available for the identification of herpes and CMV if necessary.

Hepatitis and EBV infections have been linked to aplastic anemia. Many drug treatments and some toxic exposures have been associated with acquired aplastic anemia.

Clinical Findings

Patients with hypoplastic or aplastic anemia may present with weakness, fatigue, or tachycardia. If pancytopenia is present, additional findings can include petechiae and purpura secondary to thrombocytopenia, as well as fever from neutropenia-associated infections.

Diagnostic Tests

Infants and young children should be evaluated for the other manifestations of hereditary hypoplastic disorders, including physical and radiographic defects and family history.

Hemolytic Disease of the Newborn

Hemolytic disease of the newborn (HDN; also known as *erythroblastosis fetalis*) develops owing to the transfer across the placenta of specific maternal antibodies against RBC antigens of the fetus. When severe, anemia can result in extramedullary hematopoiesis, secondary organ dysfunction, heart failure, hydrops, and death. The term *erythroblastosis* refers to the presence of immature erythrocytes in the peripheral blood from accelerated hematopoiesis. It occurs when the fetus inherits a paternal blood group antigen lacking in the mother. The RhD antigen is most frequently implicated. Only IgG is capable of crossing the placenta, and the degree of hemolysis is dependent on the amount of the antibody as well as the binding avidity of the IgG subtype. Evidence suggests that clinically significant hemolysis correlates with subtype IgG3, whereas IgG1 is not associated with hemolysis.

Maternal sensitization to fetal RBC antigens is primarily due to fetal-maternal hemorrhage during pregnancy or, more commonly, at the time of delivery, when the largest volume of blood exchange may occur. The two major types of fetal-maternal incompatibility are ABO group incompatibility and Rh incompatibility. Approximately 9% of pregnancies involve an Rh-negative mother and an Rh-positive fetus.

Antibodies against ABO-incompatible blood antigens are very common but usually do not cause severe hemolytic disease. This arises in a mother of blood group O with a fetus who is blood group A, B, or AB. It may occur during any pregnancy, even the first, because it is postulated that in addition to RBCs, secreted A or B substance may cross the placenta to induce maternal production of an IgG isotype of anti-A or anti-B in addition to the IgM anti-A and anti-B IgG antibodies normally present. The IgG antibody then crosses the placenta, attaching to the fetal RBCs. Antibody avidity is usually poor, so hemolytic disease is slow to appear and usually becomes apparent 3 to 4 days after delivery.

Rh_0 (anti-D) incompatibility usually appears after the first pregnancy as a result of fetal-maternal transfer of Rh-positive blood during pregnancy or delivery. It is much less common with the current use of prophylactic anti-Rh immune globulin. Occasionally, other antibodies are involved in fetal-maternal incompatibility. The mechanism is the same as that for anti-D.

In severe Rh-mediated hemolysis (25% of patients), RBC destruction occurs *in utero*. This leads to severe anemia with high-output congestive heart failure and anasarca (hydrops fetalis). Mild disease (50% of patients) may present as a mild hemolytic anemia requiring no therapy, whereas patients with moderate disease (25%) have significant anemia and severe jaundice and are at risk for development of kernicterus. Jaundice is not seen until after birth, when placental transport of bilirubin is lost, the neonatal liver assumes bilirubin metabolism, and the infant's skin is exposed to light. The immature infant liver is initially unable to conjugate bilirubin rapidly enough in the face of hemolysis, which leads to high levels of indirect bilirubin and jaundice. The indirect bilirubin is also deposited in the lenticulostriate nucleus of the brain (kernicterus), which may cause mental retardation, motor spasticity, deafness, and death.

Signs and Symptoms

Pallor	Respiratory distress
Hepatomegaly	Splenomegaly
Ascites	Hypotension, shock
Edema, anasarca, hydrops	Jaundice of newborn
Purpura, bleeding problems	Fetal death *in utero*

Maternal isoimmunization to other blood group antigens (Kell, Duffy, Kidd, M, S, Diego, etc.) is unusual but may cause serious disease.

After prior transfusion with incompatible blood in any Rh-positive pregnancy in an Rh-negative woman who has not received prophylactic immunotherapy (Rh immune globulin), the risk of Rh sensitization is up to 16% during or after a term pregnancy, approximately 3% with spontaneous abortion, and 5–6% with surgical abortion. Sensitization by exposure to fetal blood can also occur with ectopic pregnancy, amniocentesis, chorionic villus sampling, placental trauma or manipulation, and abruptio placentae. Prophylaxis with Rh immune globulin greatly reduces but does not totally eliminate the risk.

Other Clinical and Laboratory Findings

Findings	**ABO**	**Rh_0**
Clinical		
Pregnancy associated with disease	Any, including the first	After the first pregnancy
Clinical severity	Unpredictable	Most severe with each antigen-positive pregnancy
Prenatal evaluation	None needed	Sequential anti-Rh_0 titers, amniocentesis
Onset of jaundice	3–4 d after delivery	Intrauterine or immediately after delivery
Treatment (options listed by increasing severity of hemolysis)	None; phototherapy or rarely exchange therapy	None; early delivery, phototherapy, exchange transfusion, or intrauterine transfusion
Laboratory		
Direct Coombs test	± to 1+	2+ to 4+
Fetal blood group	A, B, or AB	Rh_0 positive
Antibody causing hemolysis	Anti-A or anti-B	Anti-Rh_0 (anti-D)
Maternal blood group	O, A, B	Rh_0 or D^u negative
Maternal antibody screening	Negative	Positive
Peripheral blood (newborn)	Microspherocytes	Not diagnostic

Diagnostic Tests

Prenatal studies may anticipate clinical disease in the newborn and may direct prenatal or postnatal management. These studies include sequential titrations of anti-D levels in the mother's serum and amniocentesis to determine levels of intrauterine hemolysis.

Studies include

1. Identification of anemia in fetus or newborn.
2. Determination of maternal blood group and antibody screening (indirect Coombs test in maternal blood).
3. Determination of blood group of newborn.

4. Direct antiglobulin test of newborn RBCs and RBC eluates (Coombs test). Prior administration of Rh_0 (D) immune globulin may lead to weakly (false) positive results on indirect Coombs test in mother and direct Coombs test in infant.
5. Examination of a peripheral blood smear from the infant or cord blood for microspherocytes, reticulocytes, and nucleated RBCs.
6. Serial serum bilirubin tests (hyperbilirubinemia, indirect bilirubin), if serologic evidence is present for HDN.
7. Identification of thrombocytopenia.
8. Tests of father's and mother's blood if serologic evidence of HDN is not present, yet the newborn is experiencing hemolysis of undetermined cause and the direct antiglobulin test result is positive. Such testing is expected to exclude unusual incompatibilities between paternal antigens expressed by the child and maternal antibodies.
9. Neutralization studies. Although such studies can be performed to classify the maternal antibody as IgG or IgM, knowledge of which helps to estimate likelihood of placental passage, they are rarely necessary or clinically helpful.

Blood Group Testing

Standard typing procedures that detect direct agglutination of RBCs by anti-A, anti-B, and anti-D antibodies are used. All Rh_0-negative cells also are tested for D^u, the partial or gene-suppressed D^u antigen.

In ABO hemolytic disease, mother's blood is usually group O (i.e., negative for A or B antigens), and the infant's blood is group A, B, or AB. Disease also may arise in a group A infant. In Rh hemolytic disease, the mother is Rh negative, and the infant is Rh positive. Where the serologic possibility of both ABO and Rh disease is possible (i.e., O-negative mother with an A- or B-positive child), hemolytic disease is more likely caused by ABO incompatibility, because the major blood group incompatibility has usually lysed Rh-incompatible cells throughout the pregnancy. Mothers who are Rh positive are not excluded from having infants with hemolytic disease, because they may be negative for minor antigens in the complex (such as C or E) and their offspring may be positive.

Direct Antiglobulin (Coombs) Test

A clinically significant direct antiglobulin test result is positive (1–4+) with broad-spectrum reagents. Monospecific reagents identify the adsorbed globulin type. In warm-type AIHA, monospecfic reagents for IgG or IgG and complement give positive results. Monospecific reagents in cold-type AIHA show only complement, because IgM antibody quickly separates from RBCs collected at 37°C. C3d is believed to be a clinically significant fraction in AIHA, because it indicates prior absorption of C3 to the RBC membrane. Very weak complement reactions (±) are not significant, but weak anti-IgG reactions may occasionally be clinically important.

Very rarely, AIHA is present without a positive direct antiglobulin test result, so that ultrasensitive methods or radioisotopic analysis are required to detect antibody molecules on the RBCs. These test are not generally available and must be done by a specific reference laboratory.

An indirect Coombs test, or its modifications, depicts serum antibody binding to RBCs after incubation of test cells with the patient's serum. This is followed by washing and addition of direct antibody reagents to detect cell-bound complement or immunoglobulin. Enzymatic treatment of cells (by ficain, papain, bromelain, or trypsin) may increase the detection of very low levels of antibody. Alternatively, direct agglutination of saline-suspended cells also depicts serum RBC antibodies. If screening tests show positive results, the antibody is identified.

The patient's serum and RBC mixtures are tested at 37°C and 4°C. In addition to panels of reagent RBCs, the patient's own cells and specimens of cord blood are included. The presence of agglutination or hemolysis is significant and is graded 0 to 4+.

Warm autoantibodies agglutinate test cells strongly at 37°C with no increase at 4°C by indirect antiglobulin tests and enzyme techniques. These are usually an IgG subtype.

Cold autoantibodies are usually IgM and show strong reactivity at 4°C and weaker reactivity at 37°C. Sometimes, this differential reactivity is more apparent with diluted serum, in saline-washed suspensions, or in enzyme-treated cells.

Maternal Antibody Screening and Identification

Maternal serum is screened for antibody, usually early in pregnancy and sporadically thereafter, to detect the presence of IgG or IgM antibodies. Antibody levels are assessed to determine fetal risk, and, if necessary, the father's RBC antigens are tested as a predictive measure of fetal expression.

Common RBC antibodies found in pregnant women are anti-Le^a and anti-Le^b. These antibodies do not produce neonatal disease because they are IgM and cannot cross the placenta, and all infants are Le^a and anti-Le^b negative. Thus, some antibodies are more significant for the mother in a postpartum hemorrhage than for the infant with HDN.

The current practice of administering Rh immune globulin at 28 weeks of gestation to prevent possible sensitization by the fetus results in a spuriously positive result on maternal antibody screening due to a weak anti-D (titer of <1:4). Unlike antibody produced as a consequence of true maternal sensitization, these antibodies do not give a "crisp" pattern of identification.

Acid Elution (Betke-Kleihauer) Test for Detection of Fetal-Maternal Hemorrhage

Fetal-maternal hemorrhage of even small numbers of Rh-positive fetal RBCs may sensitize an Rh-negative mother, unless she is adequately immunized postpartum with Rh immune globulin. Doses are standardized to compensate for fetal hemorrhage volume of 15 mL of packed RBCs or less. Intrapartum Rh immune globulin is administered at 20–28 weeks of gestation, but Kleihauer-stained peripheral smears usually are not useful at this time because the number of potentially positive cells is minimal. (See also Chapter 3.)

Fetal hemoglobin is resistant to acid elution, whereas adult hemoglobin is not. This resistance is the basis of the acid elution (Betke-Kleihauer) test. A maternal peripheral smear is treated with dilute acid buffer for 10 minutes and then stained. The maternal erythrocyte adult hemoglobulin is leached into the buffer, which leaves RBC ghosts, whereas the fetal RBCs remain as dense red erythrocytes (Color Fig. 14).

Very thin peripheral blood smears fixed in 80% alcohol are prepared from maternal blood collected in EDTA.

Dried smears are placed in McIlvaine buffer (pH 3.2) for 10 minutes, then washed in distilled water. The smear is then stained with erythrosin and counterstained with hematoxylin. Two thousand cells are counted, and the percentage of densely staining cells with fetal hemoglobin (presumably fetal in origin) is calculated. The percentage can be converted to milliliters by a nomogram, and 300 mg of Rh immune globulin is administered intramuscularly for each 15 mL of packed RBCs calculated. Control smears should be made from cord blood specimens (positive) mixed 1:10 with adult blood (negative), because questionably positive cells are sometimes seen even with the negative control. Test kits are available, so small laboratories may perform this test.

Flow cytometric tests to detect fetal cells, using staining for HbF in permeabilized RBCs, allow detection of a very small number of fetal cells within a sample. It is the best test now available in terms of ease, accuracy, and reproducibility.

Amniocentesis for measurement of amniotic fluid bilirubin level is helpful in estimating the rate of RBC destruction and expected degree of fetal anemia. The procedure is done when maternal Rh antibody has been identified and has a significant titer >1:16 to 1:23 by indirect antiglobulin techniques. The first procedure is usually performed at 16–18 weeks of gestation. At least two sequential tests are performed to determine whether the differential absorption is increasing or decreasing. Specimens are obtained every 1–2 weeks or, in borderline cases, every few days. If significant hemolysis is suspected based on increased levels of amniotic fluid bilirubin, fetal blood sampling or intrauterine transfusion may be required. False elevations in absorbance are seen when hemoglobin or meconium contaminate the specimen.

Intrauterine transfusion has a success rate of approximately 85% unless hydrops is present, in which case the success rate is less than 25%.

Other Special Tests

Test for elevated amniotic fluid bilirubin levels (change in optical density at 450 nm)

Paternal blood typing, which may exclude risk to pregnancy

Imaging

Ultrasonography can demonstrate hepatomegaly, abdominal enlargement, ascites, or signs of hydrops. Doppler flow studies of fetus are experimental in assessing degree of anemia. Fetus may be severely affected without hydrops; ultrasonography is poor at predicting need for intervention.

Since the RhD gene has been cloned to chromosome 1, its DNA sequence can be amplified by PCR. A noninvasive procedure to determine fetal RhD from maternal blood with PCR technology is possible.

Macrocytosis

Causes include the following:

- Normal neonatal state
- Megaloblastic anemia
- Down syndrome
- Hyperthyroidism
- Diamond-Blackfan syndrome
- Pearson syndrome
- Chronic hemolytic states
- Cytotoxic drug effects
- Congenital dyserythropoietic anemia
- Hereditary orotic aciduria
- Lesch-Nyhan syndrome
- Copper deficiency
- Goat-milk anemia

Hemoglobinopathies

Human hemoglobin variants generally result from a point mutation of the DNA that leads to a single amino acid substitution of one of the globin chains.

During the first weeks of intrauterine life, oxygen is carried by the embryonic hemoglobins Gower-1 ($\zeta_2\ \varepsilon_2$), Gower-2 ($\alpha_2\ \varepsilon_2$), and Portland ($\zeta_2\ \delta_2$). After the eighth gestational week, HbF ($\alpha_2\ \delta_2$) is the predominant hemoglobin. At about the time of birth, hemoglobin production is gradually shifted to hemoglobin A ($\alpha_2\ \beta_2$).

Fetal Hemoglobin, Increased

Fifty percent of patients with β thalassemia minor have high levels of HbF; even higher levels are found in virtually all patients with β thalassemia major. In sickle cell disease, HbF >30% protects the cell from sickling; therefore, even infants homozygous for hemoglobin S (HbS, sickle cell hemoglobin) have few problems before age 3 months.

Persistence of HbF is seen in

- Nonhereditary refractory normoblastic anemia (one-third of patients).
- Pernicious anemia (50% of untreated patients); increases after treatment and then gradually decreases. Minimal elevation occurs in 5% of patients with other types of megaloblastic anemia.
- Some cases of leukemia, especially juvenile myeloid leukemia with HbF of 30–60%, absence of the Philadelphia chromosome.
- Multiple myeloma.
- Molar pregnancy.
- Chromosome abnormalities (e.g., trisomy 13, 21).
- Acquired aplastic anemia (due to drugs, toxic chemicals, or infections, or idiopathic); level returns to normal only after complete remission. Better prognosis in patients with higher initial level.
- Some chronic viral infections (e.g., CMV, EBV).

Hemochromatosis

Hemochromatosis is a hereditary disorder in which the small intestine absorbs excessive iron. Because the body lacks a way to excrete iron, the excess is stored in glands and muscle, such as the liver, pancreas, and heart. Over the years, the involved organs begin to fail.

The genetic form is an autosomal-recessive mutation in the HFE gene, associated with HLA-A3, HLA-B14, and HLA-B7.

Heterozygote frequency is 1 in 10.

Although this disorder is present from birth, symptoms usually present in the fifth and sixth decades.

Signs and Symptoms

Weakness (83%)
Arthralgia (43%)
Amenorrhea (22%)
Neurologic symptoms (6%)
Increased skin pigmentation (75%)
Splenomegaly (13%)
Jaundice (10%)
Ascites (6%)
Hypoalbuminemia
Hepatic tenderness
  Increased serum glutamic-oxaloacetic transaminase
  Decreased lactic dehydrogenase
Abdominal pain (58%)
Loss of libido or potency (38%)
Decreased follicle-stimulating hormone, testosterone
Dyspnea on exertion (15%)
Hepatomegaly (83%)
Loss of body hair (20%)
Peripheral edema (12%)
Gynecomastia (8%)
Testicular atrophy
Diabetes mellitus symptoms
Hemosiderinuria

Causes

The mechanism for increased iron absorption in the face of excessive iron stores is unknown. Iron metabolism appears normal in this disease except for a higher level of circulating iron.

Iron overload may be due to thalassemia, sideroblastic anemia, liver disease, excess iron intake, long-term transfusion.

Some variables influence the age of onset and severity of symptoms. Vitamin supplements may contain large amounts of iron as well as vitamin C, which enhances iron absorption. Alcohol increases the absorption of iron (by as much as 41%) in patients with symptomatic disease.

Loss of blood, such as blood loss in women because of menstruation and pregnancy, delays the onset of symptoms.

Diagnostic Evaluation

Iron Tests

Transferrin saturation [(serum iron concentration ÷ TIBC) × 100] >70% is virtually diagnostic of iron overload; levels of ≥45% warrant further evaluation.

Serum ferritin levels >300 μg/L for men and postmenopausal women and >200 μg/L for premenopausal women are suggestive of the disorder.

Pathologic Findings in Organs

Increased hepatic parenchymal iron stores; hepatic fibrosis and cirrhosis with hepatomegaly; pancreatic enlargement; excess hemosiderin in liver, pancreas, myocardium, thyroid, parathyroid, joints, skin; cardiomegaly; joint deposition of iron

Special Tests

After the diagnosis is established, oral glucose tolerance test to rule out diabetes and echocardiogram to rule out cardiomyopathy should be considered.

Imaging Studies

Computed tomographic (CT) scan, magnetic resonance imaging, and magnetic susceptibility measurement are being studied for measuring body iron.

Other Diagnostic Procedures

Examination of liver biopsy specimen for stainable iron is the standard for diagnosis. Presence or absence of cirrhosis can also be ascertained.

DNA PCR testing for HFE gene mutations C282Y and H63D, which are present in 85–90% of patients, is used.

Sickle Cell Anemia

Sickle cell anemia is a chronic hemoglobinopathy transmitted genetically, marked by moderately severe chronic hemolytic anemia, periodic acute painful episodes, and increased susceptibility to intercurrent infections, especially with *Streptococcus pneumoniae*. The heterozygous condition (HbA/HbS) is called *sickle cell trait* and is usually asymptomatic, with no anemia.

Sickle cell anemia is autosomal recessive due to homozygous presence of a variant hemoglobin, HbS, or sickle hemoglobin. Approximately 1 in 500 black Americans and 1 in 1,000 Hispanics have sickle cell anemia; 9% of black Americans have sickle cell trait.

Causes

HbS is produced by substitution of valine for glutamic acid in the sixth amino acid position of the β chains of the hemoglobin molecule. When deoxygenated HbS polymerizes, it forms long rods that change RBC from biconcave to sickle shaped (Color Fig. 15).

At the cellular level, sickled RBCs are inflexible, odd shaped, and rigid and cause increased blood viscosity, stasis, and mechanical obstruction of small arterioles and capillaries, which leads to distal ischemia. Sickled cells become sequestered in the sinusoids of the spleen (Color Fig. 16). Sickle RBCs are also more fragile than normal, which leads to hemolytic destruction in blood and the reticuloendothelial system.

Signs and Symptoms

Sickle cell anemia is often asymptomatic in the early months of life; after 6 months of age, the earliest symptoms are pallor and symmetric, painful swelling of the hands and feet (hand-foot syndrome). Chronic hemolytic anemia develops. Symptoms include painful crisis involving bones, joints, abdomen, back, and viscera. These crises account for 90% of all hospital admissions of patients with sickle cell anemia. Mild scleral icterus; increased susceptibility to infections, especially pneumococcal sepsis and staphylococcal or *Salmonella* infections; osteomyelitis; functional asplenia; and delayed physical and sexual maturation, especially in boys, are common. Many multisystem complications may occur, particularly in later childhood and adolescence, especially episodes of acute chest syndrome (which presents a clinical picture consistent with pneumonia or infection).

A variety of crises and infections occur. The bases may be as follows:

1. Vasoocclusive ("painful crisis"): most common; pain results from tissue necrosis secondary to vascular occlusion and tissue hypoxia. Progressive organ failure and acute tissue damage result from repeated vasoocclusive episodes.
2. Aplastic crisis: temporary suppression of RBC production of bone marrow by severe infection.
3. Hyperthermolytic crisis: accelerated hemolysis; increased RBC fragility and shortened life span.
4. Sequestration crisis: splenic sequestration of blood (only in infants and young children).

Patients with sickle cell anemia have susceptibility to infection with impaired or absent splenic function and a defect in the alternate pathway of complement activation.

Risk factors in sickle cell anemia include

1. Vasoocclusive crisis: hypoxia, dehydration, infection, fever, acidosis, cold, anesthesia, strenuous physical exercise, smoking
2. Aplastic crisis: severe infections, human parvovirus B19 infection, folic acid deficiency
3. Hyperhemolytic crisis: acute bacterial infections and exposure to oxidant drugs

Diagnosis

The diagnosis of hemoglobinopathies is by electrophoretic analysis of hemoglobin (Color Fig. 17A–C): isoelectric focusing, electrophoresis in cellulose acetate at alkaline pH and agar gel at acid pH, and electrophoresis of separated globin chains.

Prenatal diagnosis by means of molecular tests with probes for the common mutations is possible.

In addition to the well-recognized HbA of normal adult erythrocytes, HbF of the normal fetus, and HbS of sickle cell anemia, many other abnormal hemoglobins have been discovered by electrophoresis. Hemoglobulins that have been recognized in addition to these are designated C, D, E, G, H, I, J, and K. Disorders in which combinations of abnormalities have been seen include sickle cell anemia with HbC (Color Fig. 18), HbD, HbE, and HbG; thalassemia with HbS, HbC, HbE, and HbG; spherocytosis with HbS; and elliptocytosis with hemoglobinopathy.

Hb electrophoresis: HbS predominates, variable amount of HbF, no HbA. (In sickle cell trait, both HbS and HbA are present.)

Screening tests: Sodium metabisulfite reduction test; Sickledex test.

Anemia: Hemoglobin level of approximately 8 g/dL (1.24 mmol/L); RBC indices usually normal but MCV >75 μm^3 (75 fL). Reticulocytosis of 10–20%, leukocytosis, bands normal in absence of infection, and thrombocytosis are typical. Peripheral smear shows few sickled RBCs, polychromasia, and nucleated RBCs. The peripheral smear in HbC disease shows numerous target cells and occasional microspherocytes (Color Fig. 19) and HbC crystals after splenectomy. The smear in HbC trait (Color Fig. 20A) contains 65% HbA and 35% HbC, whereas in HbSC disease (Color Fig. 20B), it contains approximately 52% HbS and 48% HbC. Target cells are seen in thalassemia, HbC disease, and HbS disease (Color Fig. 7A). Serum bilirubin level is mildly elevated [2–4 mg/dL (34–68 μmol/L)]; fecal and urinary urobilinogen levels are high. ESR is low, serum lactate dehydrogenase level is elevated, and haptoglobin is absent or present at very low levels.

If HbF, HbS, and HbA are present in a newborn, the differential diagnosis includes sickle cell trait or HbS/β^+ thalassemia. Repeat studies at 1 year of age may clarify the diagnosis.

Prenatal diagnosis can be accomplished using recombinant DNA techniques. Cells from the amniotic fluid can be tested for the aberrant gene at 16–20 weeks' gestation or chorionic villi can be sampled as early as 8–12 weeks.

Thalassemia Syndromes

The thalassemias are a heterogenous group of inherited disorders, all characterized by a failure to synthesize one of the two globin chains (α or β) of HbA. The α globin chain gene resides on chromosome 16, and the β gene chain resides on chromosome 11.

The thalassemias can be classified clinically according to the degree of clinical severity, genetically according to their abnormal globin synthesis, or at the molecular level according to their particular gene mutation. Classification of the thalassemias is also complicated by the high frequency with which other structural hemoglobin abnormalities are associated with thalassemia, such as the presence of HbS, HbC, and HbE.

Two main clinical forms of α thalassemia are due to α globin chain deficiency. The first is one for which there is no production of α chain owing to the deletion of both chain genes in both alleles of chromosome 16. This form of α thalassemia is incompatible with life and produces fetal death associated with hydrops fetalis syndrome (Bart disease). The second is characterized by a reduced production of α globin due to deletion of three of four α chain genes. In this form (HbH disease), the anemia is moderate to severe. Examination of the peripheral blood smear shows, in addition to target cells, the inclusion of rod-shaped bodies in the RBCs. These bodies represent precipitates of HbH. Individuals who lack two α globin genes have thalassemia trait, and those who lack one α globin gene are silent carriers.

Thalassemia major (Cooley anemia), thalassemia intermedia, and thalassemia minor are due to a deficiency of the β chain of hemoglobin. The characteristic laboratory finding is mild hypochromic microcytic anemia. The β thalassemia trait is clinically silent and is diagnosed when a peripheral blood smear is examined for other causes. Laboratory findings in thalassemia minor include hypochromic microcytic anemia (hemoglobin levels of 9–10 g/dL and MCV <75 fL) and elevated RDW. The peripheral blood smear shows anisopoikilocytosis. Target cells (Color Fig. 21), in which the cell surface is increased in disproportion to its volume, are the characteristic RBC form. Resistance to falciparum malarial infections on the part of carriers of thalassemia genes may have been a selective force for their survival.

Clinical and hematologic features of the principal forms of thalassemia are summarized in Table 18.

α Thalassemia

Four α globin genes are present in normal individuals, and four distinct forms of α thalassemia have been identified corresponding to deletions of one, two, three, or all four of these genes.

Deletion of a single α globin gene produces the silent carrier α thalassemia phenotype. No hematologic abnormality is usually evident, except for mild microcytosis. Approximately 25% of black Americans have this form of α thalassemia.

Individuals lacking two α globin genes exhibit the features of α thalassemia trait, with mild microcytic anemia. In affected newborns, small quantities of hemoglobin Bart (γ_4) can be identified by hemoglobin electrophoresis. Beyond approximately 1 month of age, hemoglobin Bart is no longer detectable, and the levels of HbA_2 are increased.

Deletion of three of the four α globin genes is associated with a thalassemia intermedia–like syndrome: HbH syndrome. Microcytic anemia in this condition is accompanied by abnormal RBC morphology (Color Fig. 22A), with prominent intracellular inclusions present in the RBCs after supravital intracellular staining (Color Fig. 22B). HbH (β_4) is highly unstable; it can be readily identified by electrophoresis (Color Fig. 22C), but unless special measures are taken to prevent its precipitation during sample preparation, it may escape detection.

The most severe form of α thalassemia, resulting from deletion of all of the α globin genes, is accompanied by a total absence of α chain synthesis. Because HbF, HbA, and HbA_2 all contain α chains, none of these hemoglobins is produced.

β^0 Thalassemia

Homozygous β^0 thalassemia usually becomes symptomatic as a hemolytic anemia during the second 6 months of life. Blood transfusions are necessary in these patients to prevent profound weakness and cardiac decompensation. Without transfusion, life expectancy is no more than a few years. In untreated cases or in those receiving infrequent transfusions, hypertrophy of erythropoietic tissue occurs in medullary and extramedullary locations. The spleen and liver are enlarged by extramedullary hematopoiesis and hemosiderosis and cause mechanical discomfort and secondary hypersplenism. The bones become thin, and pathologic fractures may occur. Expansion of the marrow of the face and skull produces characteristic facies. Radiographs of the skull show a characteristic hair-on-end appearance (Fig. 23). Pallor, hemosiderosis, and jaundice produce a greenish-brown complexion. Growth is impaired in older children; puberty is delayed or absent because of secondary endocrine abnormalities. Diabetes mellitus resulting from pancreatic siderosis may occur. Cardiac complications, including intractable arrhythmias and chronic congestive failure caused by myocardia sclerosis, have been common terminal events. Bone marrow transplantation is effective.

Large numbers of nucleated RBCs circulate, especially after splenectomy. The hemoglobin level falls progressively to lower than 5 g/dL unless transfusions are given. The conjugated serum bilirubin level is elevated. The serum iron level is high, with saturation of the transferrin and very high levels of HbF in the RBCs. Dipyrrolic compounds render the urine dark brown, especially after splenectomy.

The homozygous expression of milder (β^+) thalassemia genes produces a Cooley anemia–like syndrome of lesser severity (thalassemia intermedia). Skeletal deformities and hepatosplenomegaly develop in these patients, but their hemoglobin levels are usually maintained at 6–8 g/dL without transfusion. Nevertheless, they may develop severe hemosiderosis, attributable to their greatly increased gastrointestinal iron absorption.

Several structurally abnormal hemoglobins produce β thalassemia–like hematologic changes and, when present in combination with a gene for β thalassemia, result in a thalassemia intermedia syndrome. Among these are the hemoglobin Lepore variants, which are composed of chains in combination with hybrid δβ fusion globin chains. The Lepore hemoglobins are identified by electrophoresis, in which they exhibit HbS-like mobility.

Most forms of heterozygous β thalassemia are associated with mild anemia. The hemoglobin concentrations typically average 2–3 g/dL lower than age-related normal

Table 18. Clinical and Hematologic Features of the Principal Forms of Thalassemia[a]

Type of Thalassemia	Globin Genotype	Hematologic Features	Clinical Expression	Hemoglobin (Hb) Findings
β Thalassemias				
β^0 Homozygous	β^0/β^0	Severe anemia; normoblastemia	Cooley anemia	HbF >90% No HbA HbA2 increased
β^+ Homozygous	β^+/β^+	Anisocytosis, poikilocytosis; moderately severe anemia	Thalassemia intermedia	HbA: 20–40% HbF: 60–80%
β^0 Heterozygous	β/β^0	Microcytosis, hypochromia, mild to moderate anemia	May have splenomegaly jaundice	Increased HbA2 and HbF
β^+ Heterozygous	β/β^-	Microcytosis, hypochromia, mild anemia	Normal	Increased HbA2 and HbF
β Silent carrier, heterozygous	β/β^-	Normal	Normal	Normal
δβ Heterozygous	$\delta\beta/(\delta\beta)^0$	Microcytosis, hypochromia, mild anemia	Usually normal	HbF: 5–20% HbA2: normal or low
γδβ Heterozygous	$\gamma\delta\beta/(\gamma\delta\beta)^0$	Newborn: microcytosis, hemolytic anemia, normoblastemia Adult: similar to heterozygous δβ	Newborn: hemolytic disease with splenomegaly Adult: similar to heterozygous δβ	Normal
α Thalassemias				
α Silent carrier	–,α/α, α	Mild microcytosis or normal	Normal	Normal
α Trait	–,α/–, α or –,–/α, α	Microcytosis, hypochromia, mild anemia	Usually normal	Newborn: Hb Bart (γ4), 5–10% Child or adult: normal
HbH disease	–,α/–,–	Microcytosis, inclusion bodies by supravital staining; moderately severe anemia	Thalassemia intermedia	Newborn: Hb Bart (γ4), 20–30% Child or adult: HbH, 4–20% (γ4)
α-Hydrops fetalis	–,–/–,–	Anisocytosis, poikilocytosis; severe anemia	Hydrops fetalis, usually stillborn or neonatal death	Hb Bart (γ4), 80–90%; no HbA or HbF

[a]From Behrman RE, Kliegman RM, Jenson HB. *Nelson textbook of pediatrics,* 16th ed. Philadelphia: WB Saunders, 2000.

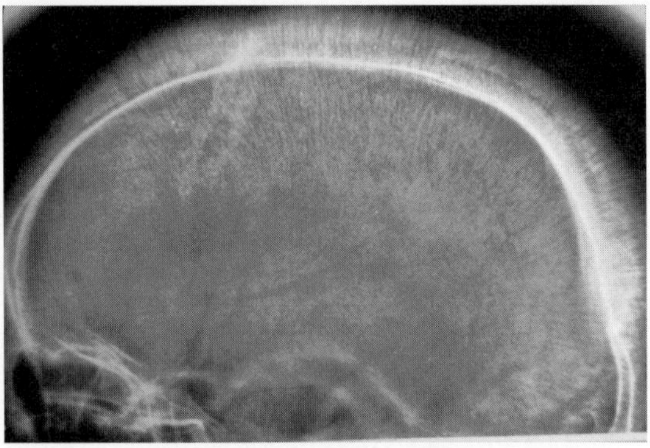

Fig. 23. Skull radiograph of a child with thalassemia major showing typical "hair-on-end" appearance due to an expanded erythron.

values. The RBCs are hypochromic and microcytic, with poikilocytosis, ovalocytosis, and, often, basophilic stippling. Target cells may be present (Color Fig. 24). The MCV is low, averaging 65 fL, and the MCH values are also low (<26 pg). Overt signs of hemolysis are usually absent. The serum iron level is normal or elevated.

More than 90% of persons with thalassemia trait have diagnostic elevations of HbA_2 of 3.4–7.0%. Approximately 50% of these individuals also have slight elevations of HbF, approximately 2–6%. In a small number of otherwise typical cases, normal levels of HbA_2 with HbF levels ranging from 5% to 15% are found, representing the $\delta\beta$ type of thalassemia. The silent carrier form of thalassemia produces no demonstrable abnormality in heterozygous individuals, but the gene for this condition, when inherited with a gene for β^0 thalassemia, results in a thalassemia intermedia syndrome.

A deletion defect that involves the γ, δ, and β globin genes produces a clinical picture similar to that of thalassemia trait. In the newborn period, however, this defect is accompanied by significant hemolytic disease with microcytosis, normoblastemia, and splenomegaly. The hemolytic process is self-limited, but supportive transfusions may be required.

If MCV and MCH values are found to be in the range associated with the carrier states for thalassemia, HbA_2 level should be determined. It is elevated in the majority of cases of β thalassemia. If the HbA_2 level is normal and a carrier state is expected, it is essential to refer the patient to a center that can analyze for the α globin genes. It is important to distinguish between the homozygous state for α^+ thalassemia ($-\alpha/-\alpha$) and the heterozygous state for α^0 thalassemia ($--/\alpha\alpha$); in the former, the patient is not at risk for having offspring homozygous for α^0 thalassemia with its attendant obstetric risks. In those rare cases in which the blood picture resembles that of heterozygous β thalassemia but the HbA_2 level is normal and the α globin genes are intact, the differential diagnosis lies between a nondeletion form of thalassemia and a normal HbA_2 form of β thalassemia. These conditions must be distinguished by globin chain synthesis analysis and further DNA studies. Hemoglobin electrophoresis in these cases may exclude a coexisting structural hemoglobin variant.

Leukemias and Other Leukocyte Disorders

Table 19 shows the distribution of white blood cell types by age group.

Basophilia

Basophils generally account for <2% of WBCs, and the absolute basophil count is characteristically $<0.1 \times 10^3/mm^3$.

Table 19. Distribution of White Blood Cell Types by Age Group

	Neonates	1–3 yr	4–7 yr	8–12 yr	Adult
Neutrophils	4.5–12.0	1.5–7.0	1.6–9.0	1.4–7.5	2.0–7.5
Eosinophils	<2.0	0.1–0.5	0.1–1.4	0.04–0.75	0.6–2.4
Basophils	<0.1	<0.1	<0.2	<0.2	<0.1
Monocytes	0.2–1.6	0.1–1.5	0.06–1.0	0.06–0.8	0.2–0.8
Lymphocytes	2.2–7.0	2.2–5.5	2.0–5.0	1.4–3.8	1.5–4.0

Basophilia is defined as an absolute basophil count $>0.2 \times 10^3/mm^3$. Conditions occasionally associated with reactive basophilia include allergic disorders such as ulcerative colitis and rheumatoid arthritis; chronic renal disease; and infections, including influenza, chickenpox, and, historically, smallpox. The absolute basophil count may be modestly increased after radiation exposure.

Basophils are recognized in the peripheral blood and bone marrow by their distinctive secondary granule, which is large and deeply basophilic, and often obscures the segmented nucleus. These secondary granules contain numerous proteins that include heparin, histamine, eosinophil chemotactic factor, arylsulfatase A, slow-reacting substance of anaphylaxis, and other substances.

Basophils are closely related to tissue mast cells. Both basophils and mast cells function in immediate hypersensitivity reactions via granule release. Basophil degranulation occurs in response to the binding of IgE antibodies to Fc receptors on the cell membrane.

Causes

Allergic or hypersensitivity reactions
Inflammatory disorders (collagen vascular disease)
Endocrinopathy
Renal disease
Rare infections
Irradiation
Rare carcinomas
Medications (estrogen, antithyroid agents)

Eosinophilia

Eosinophilia is defined as an absolute eosinophil count $>0.6 \times 10^3/mm^3$. The most common causes are drug treatments, allergies, or parasitic infections. An eosinophilia-myalgia syndrome secondary to L-tryptophan ingestion and therapy with pharmacologic doses of recombinant human interleukins are associated with a brisk, reactive eosinophilia.

Tumor-associated blood eosinophilia is generally associated with more advanced disease and unsatisfactory prognosis. In these patients, the sustained blood eosinophilia with subsequent degranulation can result in tissue damage, which further compromises the overall debilitated condition of the patient.

Eosinophil production is influenced by the synergistic action of interleukin-1, interleukin-3, and interleukin-5 produced in the bone marrow microenvironment. These interleukins, most notably interleukin-5, stimulate production of eosinophils. These mature eosinophils characteristically have bilobed nuclei and contain abundant large, refractile eosinophilic granules.

Eosinophil recruitment into tissue is mediated by chemokines such as eotaxin. Eosinophils demonstrate two main functions: (a) modulation of immediate hypersensitivity reactions and (b) destruction of parasites. Secondary granules contain major basic protein, peroxidase, arylsulfatase, histamine oxidase, and eosinophil cationic protein. The surface membranes of eosinophils express Fc receptors for IgE, IgG, and certain complement components.

A sustained peripheral blood eosinophilia can result in endothelial and endomyocardial damage from intravascular degranulation of these cells. The potent cytolytic enzymes contained within eosinophil secondary granules damage endothelial cells throughout the body. As a consequence, either thrombosis or endomyocardial fibrosis may result.

Causes of Reactive Eosinophilia

Allergic and hypersensitivity reactions
Drug allergies
Cytokine therapy (recombinant human interleukins)
Cutaneous disorders
Connective tissue diseases, collagen vascular diseases
Parasitic infections
Neoplasms (carcinoma, lymphoma, Hodgkin disease, acute lymphoblastic leukemia)
Immunodeficiency disorders
Sarcoidosis
Recovery from streptococcal and some other infections

Findings in Peripheral Blood

Eosinophils have a diurnal variation; levels are highest in the morning and decrease in the afternoon.

Hypersegmented (trilobed), hypogranular, degranulated, or vacuolated eosinophils are especially prominent in chronic and myeloproliferative disorders formerly termed *idiopathic hypereosinophilic syndromes.*

Diagnostic Tests

Bone Marrow Examination

Bone marrow examination generally is not required in patients with straightforward reactive eosinophilia unless indicated for other reasons such as tumor staging. However, both bone marrow examination and cytogenetic studies are valuable in patients with a possible myeloproliferative disorder or other neoplasm in which the eosinophils are likely to be part of a clonal process.

Additional Tests

If a parasitic infection is suspected, both stool examination for ova and parasites and serologic tests for parasites may be warranted.

The FISH technique can be applied to smear preparations in which eosinophil identification is readily apparent, whereas assessment of eosinophil clonality by either molecular or cytogenetic techniques requires a purified eosinophil population.

Measurement of serum interleukin-5 levels may be useful in selected patients with presumed secondary eosinophilia.

Although nonspecific, the determination of serum IgE levels may be useful.

Nasal eosinophilia is common in allergic rhinitis, and abundant eosinophils in sputum may be evident in patients with Löffler pneumonia. Charcot-Leyden crystals may be present.

Serologic tests for collagen vascular disorders may be helpful.

Granulocytic Disorders of Abnormal Morphology, Hereditary

See Table 20.

Histiocytosis

Classification of Histiocytic Syndromes[1]

Class I: Langerhans cell histiocytosis (LCH)

Class II: histiocytosis of mononuclear phagocytic system other than LCH (infection-associated hemophagocytic syndrome, familial hemophagocytic lymphohistiocytosis)

[1]Writing Group of the Histiocytic Society. Histiocytosis syndromes in children. *Lancet* 1987;1:208–209.

Table 20. Hereditary Granulocytic Disorders of Abnormal Morphology

Disorder	Granulocyte Feature	Other Blood, Bone Marrow Abnormalities	Inheritance	Other Findings
Pelger-Huët anomaly	Bilobed or nonsegmented neutrophil nuclei; cytoplasm normal	No other lineage abnormalities No functional abnormalities	Autosomal dominant	No associated findings
May-Hegglin anomaly	Large blue cytoplasmic inclusions resembling giant Döhle bodies	Thrombocytopenia Enlarged platelets Variable neutropenia Inclusions also in eosinophils, basophils, and monocytes	Autosomal dominant	Many patients are asymptomatic
Chédiak-Higashi syndrome	Giant cytoplasmic granules	Neutropenia, thrombocytopenia All granulated cells and even lymphocytes/natural killer cells affected Represents fused lysosomes Functional defects of neutrophils Some patients develop infection, usually Epstein-Barr virus–associated hemophagocytic syndrome (accelerated phase) or Epstein-Barr virus–induced lymphoproliferative disorders	Autosomal recessive	Partial oculocutaneous albinism Frequent pyogenic infections Both neutrophil function defects and immunodeficiency from decreased natural killer cell function Mild bleeding tendency Progressive peripheral neuropathy
Alder-Reilly anomaly	Intense azurophilic granulation of neutrophil cytoplasm	Eosinophils and basophils contain large basophilic granules Vacuolated/abnormally granulated lymphocytes in some cases	Autosomal recessive	Associated with several different types of genetic mucopolysaccharide disorders
Specific granule deficiency	Absence of secondary granules in cytoplasm, imparting a pale appearance; also nuclear hyposegmentation	Abnormal granules (subset) in platelets and eosinophils	Autosomal recessive	Recurrent infections

(continued)

Table 20. (continued)

Disorder	Granulocyte Feature	Other Blood, Bone Marrow Abnormalities	Inheritance	Other Findings
Myelokathexis	Shape abnormalities; pyknotic nuclei; hypersegmentation	Striking bone marrow abnormalities affecting granulopoiesis Neutropenia; intramedullary death of granulocytes Functional defects of neutrophils and monocytes	Not well characterized	Growth retardation Skeletal abnormalities
Hereditary hypersegmentation of neutrophils	Increased mean nuclear lobe index	No other abnormalities	Autosomal dominant	No associated findings
Hereditary giant neutrophils	Enlarged overall neutrophil size with hypersegmentation	Only a subset of neutrophils affected Other lineages unremarkable	Autosomal dominant	No associated findings

Class III: malignant histiocytic disorder (acute monocytic leukemia, malignant histocytosis, histocytic leukemia)

Class I (Langerhans Cell Histiocytosis)

Histiocytoses are a complex and protean group of disorders that can affect almost any organ. Bone marrow involvement in a histiocytic proliferation is usually better detected in BMA than in BMB specimens, because cytoplasmic detail and phagocytic material are better recognized in BMA samples.

Langerhans cell histiocytosis (class I) is a group of disorders previously referred to as *histiocytosis X*, *Letterer-Siwe disease*, *Hand-Schüller-Christian disease*, or *eosinophilic granuloma*. LCH is a proliferative disorder of histiocytes in which the consistent pathologic finding is the Langerhans cells, dendritic cells that originate in the bone marrow mononuclear phagocytic system.

The diagnosis of LCH is suggested by a constellation of clinical symptoms, of which the infiltration of bone and skin are dominant features. LCH can present clinically as a generalized or focal disorder. In young children, the most common clinical presentation is the generalized form, in which histologic examination is required for diagnosis.

Histiocytes have light pink eosinophilic cytoplasm, with an oval or elongated grooved nucleus, fine chromatin, and a small nucleolus. The inflammatory reaction includes multinucleated giant cells, lymphocytes, plasma cells, and eosinophils; sometimes, there are areas of necrosis and macrophages with cytoplasmic debris.

The diagnosis is confirmed by immunohistochemical stains (Color Fig. 25A, B) In the BMA specimen, histiocytes appear isolated or in small groups, intermixed among the hematopoietic cells. The best cytochemical stains are acid phosphatase, which strongly stains the cytoplasm of the histiocytes, and α-naphthol-acetate esterase (ANAE). The acid phosphatase activity is inhibited by tartrate, but if abundant phagocytic material is present, tartrate-resistant coarse granules may persist. Strong diffuse cytoplasmic reaction is also obtained with the ANAE stain, inhibited by sodium fluoride. The recognition of histiocytes generally does not require cytochemical analysis. Monoclonal antibodies of choice are S-100 protein and CD1a. Use of CD1 assay is limited to examination of smears or frozen sections, or flow-cytometric studies. CD68, a macrophage-associated antigen usually confined to the Golgi area, is present in a large proportion of LCH cases. At the ultrastructural level, the Langerhans cells are identified by the presence of racquet-shaped Birbeck granules, the organelles that define this entity.

Thrombocytopenia and sometimes neutropenia are present.

Class II Histiocytosis

Class II comprises a group of lesions in which there is an accumulation of phagocytic histiocytes (not Langerhans cells) and lymphocytes. Infection-associated hemophagocytic syndrome (IAHS) and familial hemophagocytic lymphohistiocytosis are the primary members of class II histiocytic syndromes. Also included in class II are sinus histiocytosis with massive lymphadenopathy (Rosai-Dorfman disease) (Color Fig. 26) and other histiocytic syndromes.

Infection-Associated Hemophagocytic Syndrome

IAHS is a clinicopathologic disorder characterized by a generalized proliferation of histocytes. Risdall and colleagues in 1979 proposed that it was related to viral infections in an immunocompromised patient; other infections produce a similar picture in immunocompromised and nonimmunocompromised patients.

Laboratory findings include anemia with reticulocytopenia associated with granulocytopenia or pancytopenia, and monocytes with phagocytosis and vacuolization on a peripheral blood smear.

BMA is particularly useful for morphologic identification of hemophagocytic histiocytes. In most cases, the BMA specimen yields hypocellular spicules. The proportion of hemophagocytic histiocytes observed in the BMA sample can range from sparse to numerous. The erythroid and granulocytic series are decreased with preservation of the megakaryocytes, which sometimes may be prominent. A rare event is a decrease of RBC precursors with maturation arrest of the myeloid series. Lymphocytes and plasma cells are intermixed with histiocytes in the hypocellular spicules. The histiocytes are morphologically benign. Phagocytosis of all hematopoietic cells can be observed, but the phagocytosis of multiple mature and nucleated RBCs is notable. Macrophages with hemosiderin in their cytoplasm are abundant.

In infancy, IAHS is usually a self-limited disorder; if associated with immunodeficiency, it may be fatal.

Familial Hemophagocytic Lymphohistiocytosis

Familial hemophagocytic lymphohistiocytosis is an autosomal-recessive systemic disorder. The clinical presentation is characterized by fever, hepatosplenomegaly, and pancytopenia. Distinguishing the disorder from IAHS in a young child is difficult and sometimes impossible in the absence of a family history.

Laboratory findings in the active phase of the disease include anemia and thrombocytopenia or pancytopenia associated with hypertriglyceridemia, hypofibrinogenemia, and cerebrospinal fluid pleocytosis.

The BMA specimen is usually cellular or hypercellular. Erythrophagocytosis by bland histiocytosis is striking. Hemophagocytic histiocytes are required for the diagnosis. Cytochemical stains are consistent with the histiocytic origin of the phagocytic cells; acid phosphatase and ANAE stains give positive results. During infection a BMA specimen in familial hemophagocytic lymphohistiocytosis may be indistinguishable from that in IAHS.

Class III

Class III disorders include acute monocytic leukemia [French-American-British (FAB) classification M_5], malignant histiocytosis, and true histiocytic lymphoma.

Monoclonal antibody evaluation, immunohistochemical analysis, and molecular biologic analysis indicate that true malignant histiocytic disorders are rare. What was called *malignant histiocytosis* for the first 80 years of the twentieth century is now classified as *Ki-1 positive (large-cell anaplastic) lymphoma*, which presents in children as a systemic disorder with lymphadenopathy and frequent extranodal involvement of skin, liver, and spleen. The immunophenotype and genotype are crucial to the identification of children with the disorder. They express CD30 (Ki-1 antigen) and epithelial membrane antigen. The expression of other antigens such as common leukocyte antigen (CD45) is variable. Most cases express a T-cell phenotype and lack expression of CD68, a macrophage marker. The immunophenotype may not always reveal lymphocytic lineage, and genomic studies are necessary to demonstrate T- or B-cell clonal rearrangement. The cytogenetic abnormality described in Ki-1 positive lymphoma is t(2:5).

The current practice of administering Rh immune globulin at 28 weeks of gestation to prevent possible sensitization by the fetus results in a spurious positive maternal antibody screening result due to a weak anti-D (titer of <1:4). Unlike antibody produced as a consequence of true maternal sensitization, these antibodies do not give a "crisp" pattern of identification.

Leukemia

The FAB classification of the leukemias is based on the morphology, immunology, and cytogenetic findings, and characterizes these disorders in a precise manner.

The FAB morphologic classification of acute lymphoblastic leukemias (ALLs) is shown in Table 21.

Procedures for Diagnosis of Leukemia

CBC
Peripheral blood smear examination
BMA and trephine biopsy
Appropriate cytochemical studies on blood and bone marrow specimens
Immunophenotyping of leukemic blasts by flow cytometry or immunohistochemical analysis
Bone marrow cytogenetic studies
Molecular studies as indicated

Table 21. French-American-British Morphologic Classification of Acute Lymphoblastic Leukemias

Cytologic Features	L_1	L_2	L_3
Cell size	Small cells predominate	Large, heterogeneous in size	Medium to large and homogenous
Amount of cytoplasm	Scant	Variable; often moderately abundant	Moderately abundant
Nucleoli	Not visible, or small and inconspicuous	One or more present, often large	One or more present, often prominent
Nuclear shape	Regular; occasional clefting or indentation	Irregular; clefting and indentation common	Regular; oval to round
Nuclear chromatin	Homogeneous in any one case	Variable; heterogeneous in any one case	Finely stippled and homogeneous
Basophilia of cytoplasm	Variable; usually moderate	Variable; occasionally intense	Intensely basophilic
Cytoplasmic vacuolation	Variable	Variable	Prominent

From Kjeldsberg C, Elenitoba-Johnson K, Foucar K, et al. *Practical diagnosis of hematologic disorders,* 3rd ed. Chicago: American Society of Clinical Pathologists Press, 2000:447.

Cerebrospinal fluid examination

Radiographic studies for assessment of extramedullary disease as indicated

Other biochemical and microbiologic studies as indicated

Automated instruments that combine flow cytometry with cytochemical analysis may provide a preliminary characterization of acute leukemia. The peripheral blood smear often shows anisopoikilocytosis of RBCs and blasts. Sometimes, lymphocytes with atypical forms represent the larger number of WBCs. Lymphoblast morphology in the peripheral blood is variable, and cytologic findings may not always match the morphologic observation of BMA smears.

The FAB classification of any leukemia requires a well-spread bone marrow smear. Electron micrographic studies are rarely required, since lineage can often be established by flow-cytometric studies.

Cytochemical stains are used in the diagnosis of leukemias. ANAE reaction is positive in some cases of ALL of B-cell lineage with numerous fine granules. In T-cell lineage leukemias, the stain gives strongly positive results with a single dot pattern in the Golgi apparatus. Sodium fluoride does not inhibit the reaction. The use of acid phosphatase, like ANAE, gives positive results in some ALLs of B-cell lineage. In such cases, the pattern is characterized by numerous fine and coarse granules.

The FAB classification defines those categories of ALL referred to as L_1, L_2, and L_3. Of the immunocytochemical stains applied in the diagnosis of ALL, TdT (terminal deoxynucleotidyl transferase) is one of the most useful. TdT is a DNA polymerase found in the nucleus of a small proportion of normal bone marrow cells and in the cortical lymphocytes of the thymus. It is present in the majority of L_1 and L_2 lymphoblasts of ALLs of both precursor B- and T-cell lineage, but absent in L_3 ALLs. By the use of anti-TdT monoclonal antibodies, the presence of TdT can be demonstrated on smears by immunofluorescence or the immunoperoxidase technique and by flow cytometry in cell suspensions. The presence of nuclear TdT is not specific for ALL; TdT is occasionally present in some myeloid leukemias, particularly monocytic leukemias, and a large number of TdT-positive cells (Color Fig. 27D) may be seen in the bone marrow of children after chemotherapy without leukemic involvement, and in other disorders.

BMB specimens in ALL with L_1 or L_2 morphology usually show hypercellularity and an almost complete replacement of hematopoietic cells by a monotonous lymphoblast population (Color Fig. 27A, B). The cytoplasm of the lymphoblast is sparse;

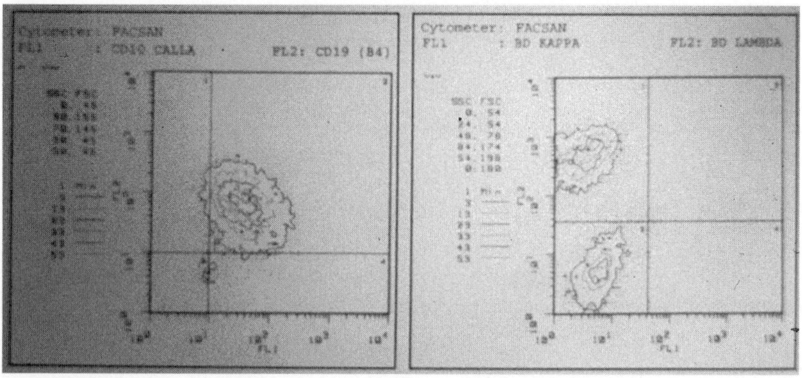

A B

Fig. 28. A: Results of flow cytometry of peripheral blood from a 3-year-old boy with acute lymphoblastic leukemia (ALL). The leukemic cells show positivity for the pan–B cell marker CD19 and CD10 (CALLA). **B:** Results of flow cytometry of bone marrow specimen of a patient with B-cell ALL demonstrating monoclonal λ surface immunoglobulin.

the nucleus can be round, indented, or folded, with a dispersed chromatin and nucleoli that are inconspicuous or small. Rarely in ALL the marrow is hypocellular with foci of leukemic involvement.

The L_3 blast is present in approximately 5% of cases of ALL. Morphologically and immunologically, it is identical to the Burkitt lymphoma cell. The L_3 cell (Color Fig. 27C) is approximately twice the size of a lymphocyte. The nucleus is round and is surrounded by a rim of deeply basophilic cytoplasm that usually contains vacuoles. On air-dried preparations, nucleoli are generally seen. Macrophages with debris in their cytoplasm are often present. Whenever this type of leukemia is diagnosed, a careful search for an extramedullary mass should be undertaken to rule out the possibility of a Burkitt lymphoma in the leukemic phase. L_3 ALL is strongly associated with the cytogenetic translocation of t(8:14).

A mature B-cell phenotype (Burkitt) is found in $\leq$5% of ALL cases. Surface immunoglobulin expression and light chain restriction are present, as this is the definition of a mature B cell. CD19, CD20, and CD22 will also usually be present. Presence of CD10 is variable. CD34 and TdT are absent. Mature B-cell ALL is commonly associated with, but not restricted to, L_3 morphology and t(8:14).

Techniques for ALL immunophenotyping include flow cytometry (Fig. 28A) with panels of monoclonal antibodies (Fig. 28B) and immunocytochemical stains on smears.

The most common immunophenotype in infantile ALL is HLA-DR/CD19 positive. CD10 is found less frequently in infants than in older children.

T-cell lineage ALL is rare in infancy. Most of the cases studied by flow cytometry are $CD7^+$. Of the other T-cell surface markers, CD1, CD3, and CD8 are highly specific but are found in fewer cases. If flow-cytometric studies are not conclusive for T-cell ALL, immunocytochemical analysis can be performed on BMA smears. Of the markers available, cytoplasmic CD3 is the most sensitive.

In childhood ALLs, there is often aberrant expression of one or more myeloid antigens: CD33, CD13, CD15, and CD14. This aberrant expression may be seen in up to 30–50% of precursor-B ALLs and 25–30% of T-cell ALLs.

A chromosomal aberration in infancy is t(4;11)(q21;q23). This karyotype is associated with hyperleukocytosis $>100 \times 10^9$/L.

The structural anomalies in ALL are predominately rearrangements or translocations. Of these, the most common is rearrangements of TEL-AML1 at 12p13, which occurs in approximately 25% of precursor B-cell childhood ALL. Molecular analysis demonstrates that this rearrangement is usually part of t(12;21) in which TEL is fused to AML1 at 21q22.

Translocation t(9;22)(q34;q11) is also found in 30% of adult ALL but only 5% of childhood ALL. This (9;22) translocation of ALL is karyotypically indistinguishable from that seen in CML, but the molecular lesions are different. In ALL, a 190-kd fusion protein (p190) is produced, whereas in CML the fusion protein is a 210-kd molecule (p210). The difference is due to the location of the BCR breakpoint. In AML, the breakpoint is in the major breakpoint cluster region (M-bcr); in ALL, it is in a locus that is referred to as the *minor breakpoint region* (M-bcr).

Also seen in ALL is the t(8;14)(q24;q32) and its variant t(2;8)(p12;q24) and t(8;22)(q24;q11). The translocation fuses c-MYC at 8q24 with one of the immunoglobulin gene sequences on chromosomes 2, 14, and 22, which leads to c-MYC dysregulation. This anomaly is strongly associated with L_3 (Burkitt) morphology; however, t(8;14) and variants have been reported in cases lacking the mature B-cell phenotype.

Translocation (1;19)(q23;p13) occurs in approximately 25% of precursor B-cell childhood ALL but <3% of adult ALL. The usual translocation fuses E2A at 19p13 with PBXI at 1q23. ALL with t(1;19) is associated with a distinctive precursor B-cell phenotype showing expression of CD10, CD19, CD22, TdT, HLA-DR, and rarely CD15 but not CD20, CD34, or myeloid-associated antigens.

A newer WHO classification of tumors of hematopoietic and lymphoid malignancies was introduced recently. While the FAB classification attempted and achieved, in part, a standardized classification of hematopoietic malignancies, the hope of the newer WHO classification is to go beyond the morphologic classification by continuously incorporating new changes into the FAB classifications of acute leukemias and myelodysplastic-myeloproliferative syndromes affecting pediatric patients. These include

1. Replacing the L_1 and L_2 ALL with the immunologic classifications of precursor-B and precursor-T lymphoblastic leukemia
2. Moving L_3 ALL into Burkitt lymphoma
3. Lowering the blast count from 30% to 20% for the diagnosis of AML and eliminating refractory anemia with excess blasts in transformation
4. Subdividing refractory anemia with excess blasts into two types based on blast percentages
5. Recognizing distinct cytogenetic-molecular AML subtypes
6. Recognizing AML with multilineage dysplasia and therapy-related AML as distinct leukemias
7. Establishing criteria for juvenile myelomonocytic leukemia and atypical chronic myeloid leukemia lacking the Philadelphia chromosome

The transcriptional control genes altered in leukemia are shown in Table 22.

Leukemia, Acute Lymphoblastic

ALL is the most frequent childhood neoplasm. The clinical presentation is characterized by fever, pallor, and bleeding in the form of petechiae or large hemorrhages. On physical examination, hepatosplenomegaly, lymphadenopathy, and bone tenderness are common.

Laboratory Findings and Prognostic Indicators

Laboratory findings include anemia, neutropenia, and thrombocytopenia. Thirty percent of children with ALL, however, may have normal or high platelet counts. The WBC count is variable. The initial WBC count is classified into one of three categories for prognosis of survival. Patients with a WBC count $<10 \times 10^9$/L have the most favorable prognosis; those with a WBC count of $>50 \times 10^9$/L have an unfavorable prognosis; those with a WBC count of $>10 \times 10^9$/L but $<50 \times 10^9$/L have an intermediate prognosis.

Prognostic indicators in ALL are listed in Table 23.

Immunophenotypes and Antigen Expression Patterns in Acute Lymphoblastic Leukemia

T-cell lineage immunophenotypes in ALL are shown in Table 24.

B-cell lineage immunophenotypes in ALL are shown in Table 25.

Common antigen expression patterns in ALL are shown in Table 26.

Table 22. Altered Transcriptional Control Genes in Leukemia

	Cytogenetics	Genes
Acute lymphoblastic leukemia		
B-cell ALL-Burkitts	t(8;14)(q24;q32)	MYC
	t(2;8)(p12;q24)	MYC
	T(8;22)(q24;q11)	MYC
Pre–B cell ALL	t(17;19)(q22;p13)	E2A-HLF
	t(1;19)(q23;p13)	E2A-PBX1
	t(4;11)(q21;q23)	MLL-AF4
	t(9;22)(q34;q11)	BCR-ABL
	t(12;21)(p13;q22)	TEL-AML1
T-cell ALL	t(8;14)(q24;q11)	MYC-IGH
	t(7;19)(q35;p13)	LYL1
	t(1;14)(p32;q11)	TAL1 (SCL)
	t(7;9)(q35;q34)	TAL2
	t(11;14)(p15;q11)	LMO1(RBTN1)
	t(11;14)(p13;q11)	LMO2(RBTN2)
	t(7;11)(q35;p13)	LMO2(RBTN2)
	t(10;14)(q24;q11)	HOX11
	t(7;10)(q35;q24)	HOX11
	t(9;22)(q34;q11)	BCR-ABL
Myeloid leukemias		
AML, granulocytic	t(8;21)(q22;q22)	AML1-ETO
	t(9;22)(q34;q11)	BCR-ABL
Myelodysplasia	t(3;21)(q26;q22)	AML-EAP
CML, blast crisis	t(3;21)(q26;q22)	AML-EV11
	t(9;22)(q34;q11)	BCR-ABL
AML, undifferentiated	t(3;v)(q26;v)	EV11
	t(9;22)(q34;q11)	BCR-ABL
AML, myelomonocytic	inv(16)(p13;q22)	CBFbeta-MYH11
AML, monocytic	t(9;11)(p21;q23)	MLL-AF9
AML, promyelocytic	t(15;17)(q21;q21)	PML-RARalpha
	t(11;17)(q23;q21)	PLZF-RARalpha
	t(5;17)(q32;q12)	NPM-RARalpha
AML, undifferentiated	t(16;21)(p11;q22)	FUS-ERG
	t(12;22)(p12;q12)	TEL-MN1
Mixed-lineage leukemias		
Pre–B cell ALL	t(4;11)(q21;q23)	MLL-AF4
AML (monocytic)	t(9;11)(p21;q23)	MLL-AF9
ALL/AML	t(11;19)(q23;p13.3)	MLL-ENL
AML	t(11;19)(q23;p13.1)	MLL-ELL
	t(1;11)(q21;q23)	MLL-AF1Q
	t(1;11)(p32;q23)	MLL-AFIP
	t(6;11)(q27;q23)	MLL-AF6
	t(10;11)(p12;q23)	MLL-AF10
	t(11;17)(q23;q21)	MLL-AF17
	t(X;11)(q13;q23)	MLL-ARX1

ALL, acute lymphocytic leukemia; AML, acute myelogenous leukemia; CML, chronic myelogenous leukemia.

Table 23. Prognostic Indicators in Acute Lymphoblastic Leukemia

	Favorable	Less Favorable
Clinical		
Age	2–10 yr	<2 yr, >10 yr
Sex	Female	Male
Race	White	Black
WBC count	$<10 \times 10^3/mm^3$ ($<10 \times 10^9/L$)	$>50 \times 10^3/mm^3$ ($>50 \times 10^9/L$)
Rapidity of cytoreduction	Bone marrow free of disease by day 14	Residual disease at day 14
Relapse	No relapse	Relapse
Morphologic	L_1	?L_2, ?L_3
Immunophenotypic	$CD10^+$ precursor B cell	$CD\text{-}10^-$ precursor B-cell, precursor T-cell ALL, ?B-cell ALL (SIg)
Cytogenetic	Hyperdiploidy >50 t(12;21)	Translocation [especially t(9;22) t(4;11)] and t(1,19) near haploidy, near tetraploidy, del 17p

ALL, acute lymphoblastic leukemia; SIg, surface immunoglobulin; WBC, white blood cell.
From Brunning RD, McKenna RW. Tumors of the bone marrow. Acute lymphoblastic leukemias. In: *Atlas of tumor pathology,* 3rd Series, Fascicle 9. Washington: Armed Forces Institute of Pathology, 1994:100–142.

Table 24. T-Cell Lineage Immunophenotype in Acute Lymphoblastic Leukemia

	CD7	CD3	CD2	CD1	CD4	CD8	CD10
Early (immature thymocyte)	+	+ (cytoplasmic)	+				–
Intermediate (common thymocyte)	+	+ (cytoplasmic surface)	+	+	+	+	+
Mature (medullary thymocyte)	+	+ (surface)	+		±	+	–

+, present; –, absent; ±, sometimes present.

Table 25. B-Cell Lineage Immunophenotype in Acute Lymphoblastic Leukemia

	HLA-DR	CD19	CD10	CD20	CIg	SIg
Early precursor	+	+	–	–	–	–
Early pre-pre–B cell	+	+	+	±	–	–
Pre–B cell	+	+	+	+	+	–
B cell	–	+	–	±	±	+

+, present; –, absent; ±, sometimes present; CIg, intracytoplasmic immunoglobulin; SIg, surface immunoglobulin.

Table 26. Common Antigen Expression Patterns of Acute Lymphoblastic Leukemias

	CD1	CD2	CD3	CD4	CD5	CD7	CD8	CD10	CD19	CD20	CD22	CD24	CD34	TdT	DR	SIg
B cell																
B-precursor ALL								+/–	+	–/+	–	+	+	+	+	–
Pre-B ALL								+	+	+/–	–/+	+	+	+/–	+	–
B-ALL								+/–	+	+	+	+	–	–	+	+
T-cell																
T-ALL	+	+	+ (C)	+	+	+	+	+/–					–/+	+	–/+	

+, present; –, absent; +/–, often present; –/+, occasionally present; ALL, acute lymphoblastic leukemia; C, usually cytoplasmic; SIg, surface immunoglobulin.

Table 27. Common Cytogenetic Findings in Acute Leukemias, Chronic Leukemias, and Myelodysplastic-Myeloproliferative Syndromes

Condition	Clinical Findings
Acute myelogenous leukemias	
M_0	No consistent finding
M_1	No consistent finding
M_2	t(8;21)(q2;q22)
M_3	t(15;17)(q22;q12–21)
M_4	inv(3)(q21;q26)
M_4E	inv(16)(p13;q22)/t(16;16)
M_5	t(9;11)(p22;q23)
M_6	No consistent finding
M_7	t(1;22)(p13;q13)
ALLs	
Precursor B-cell ALL	t(9;22)(q34;q11)
Precursor T-cell ALL	t(1;19)(q23;p13)
B-cell ALL	t(8;14)(q24;q32), also t(2;8) and t(8;22)
T-cell ALL	t(11;14)(p13;q11), t(10;14)(q24;q11)
Chronic leukemia	
Hairy cell leukemia	+14, –6q
B-cell CLL	+12, –13, +14(q32)
B-cell PLL	t(11;14)(q13;q32)
T-cell PLL	t/del 14q11
T-cell CLL	inv(14)(q11;q52)
Others	
CML	t(9;22)(q34;q11)
MDS	–5, –7, –12p, –20p
5q-syndrome	–5q

ALL, acute lymphoblastic leukemia; CLL, chronic lymphocytic leukemia; CML, chromic myelogenous leukemia; MDS, myelodysplastic syndrome; PLL, prolymphocytic leukemia.
From Kjeldsberg C, Elenitoba-Johnson K, Foucar K, et al. *Practical diagnosis of hematologic disorders,* 3rd ed. Chicago: American Society of Clinical Pathologists Press, 2000.

Common cytogenetic findings associated with acute leukemias, chronic leukemias, and myelodysplastic-myeloproliferative syndromes are shown in Table 27.

Leukemia, Acute Myelogenous

AML presents with an initial high WBC count and leukemic extramedullary involvement. The frequency of leukemia in children with constitutional chromosomal abnormalities, for example, Down syndrome and Klinefelter syndrome, is high.

AML is the most common type of leukemia in early infancy; ALL is the most common in childhood. Like ALL, AML comprises a heterogeneous morphologic group of malignancies.

Conspicuous morphologic markers of AML are azurophilic linear structures known as *Auer rods*, which may be seen in M_2, M_3, and M_4 leukemia subtypes but are not necessarily present in all cases of AML. Some AML subtypes may occur in infants or young children; acute monocytic leukemia (M_5) and acute megakaryocytic leukemia (M_7) are the most frequent types seen in this age group.

Laboratory Findings

The classification of AML is shown in Table 28.

Laboratory findings in the peripheral blood of AML include anemia and thrombocytopenia. The leukocyte count has a wide range; in infancy, it is frequently markedly

Table 28. Classification of Acute Myelogenous Leukemia

	AML Type	Bone Marrow Findings[a]
M_0	Minimal differentiation	>30% blasts[b] <3% blasts MPO/SBB positive >20% blasts reactive for myeloid-associated antigens Negative for lymphocyte antigens
M_1/M_2	No differentiation	>30% blasts[b] >3% blasts MPO/SBB positive <10% promyelocytes and more mature granulocytes >30% myeloblasts and abnormal[a] Hypergranular promyelocytes
M_3	Promyelocytic leukemia	Intense MPO/SBB positivity Blasts and promyelocytes with multiple Auer rods (faggot cells) t(15;17) chromosomal abnormality
M_4	Myelomonocytic leukemia	>30% myeloblasts, monoblasts, and promonocytes[b] >20% granulocytic cells >20% monocytic cells Monocytosis ≥5 × 10^9/L
M_5	Monocytic leukemia	>30% myeloblasts, monoblasts, and promonocytes[b]
	A	>80% monocytic cells with >80% monoblasts
	B	>30% myeloblasts, monoblasts, and promonocytes[a] >80% monocytic cells with <80% monoblasts Predominance of promonocytes
M_6	Erythroleukemia	>50% erythroblasts >30% of nonerythroid cells are myeloblasts[a]
M_7	Megakaryocytic leukemia	>30% blasts[b] >50% megakaryocytic cells (megakaryoblasts, promegakaryocytes, and megakaryocytes) by immunologic markers or ultrastructural study

AML, acute myelogenous leukemia; MPO, myeloperoxidase; SBB, Sudan black B.
[a]Percentages are of bone marrow nucleated cells.
[b]The new World Health Organization classification lowers the blast count from 30% to 20% for AML. The classification "refractory anemia with excess blasts in transformation" (RAEBIT) has been eliminated.
Modified from Knowles DM. *Neoplastic hematopathologic.* Baltimore: Williams & Wilkins, 1992.

increased (>100 × 10^9/L). The percentage of blasts in the peripheral blood smear is variable but is usually high in infancy. Other cytomorphologic abnormalities in the granulocytes include abnormalities in the cytoplasmic granules of polymorphonuclear leukocytes, pseudo–Pelger-Huët forms, and multiple chromatin appendages in the polymorphonuclear leukocyte nuclei.

The BMA specimen obtained from infants with AML is usually cellular. The percentage of blasts is variable, but for diagnosis, blasts should represent ≥30% of the nucleated marrow cells. The FAB classification defines the blast category by their morphologic and cytochemical characteristics in accordance with their differentiation. Cytochemical stains are useful for the classification of AMLs. Myeloperoxidase is the best single marker for M_0 through M_4 FAB subtypes. It can be demonstrated in M_1 through M_4 leukemias by routine cytochemical procedures or by the use of antimyeloperoxidase monoclonal antibodies on smear or flow cytometry when the results of routine cytochemical staining are negative.

Cytogenetic studies show chromosomal rearrangements in most AMLs. Despite the variability of karyotype profiles described in AMLs, certain changes are distinctively nonrandom. Some of the abnormalities are associated with specific morphologic AML FAB subtypes and may be associated with other structural chromosomal abnormalities. The most frequent change in karyotype of infantile AML involves chromosome 11.

AML M_0 blasts stained with Romanovsky stains have a moderate amount of light blue cytoplasm, a round nucleus with dispersed chromatin, two or more nucleoli, and peripheral condensation of the chromatin around the nucleoli. Routine cytochemical stains for myeloperoxidase and Sudan black yield negative results. In certain cases, immunocytochemistry can detect myeloperoxidase in the blasts, but in others myeloperoxidase is demonstrated only as scattered granules in the blasts by electron microscopy. By flow cytometry, >20% of the blasts express HLA-DR, CD13, or CD33 (or some combination), and often CD34.

AML M_1 blasts have a moderate amount of light blue cytoplasm and may contain a few granules or a single Auer rod (Color Fig. 29A). The presence of Auer rods is sufficient to establish the diagnosis, but in most cases they are absent. The diagnosis should be confirmed by stain for myeloperoxidase or by Sudan black, the cytochemical stains of choice. Three percent or more of the blasts should show positive results for the diagnosis of AML. By flow cytometry, in a large proportion of cases, >20% of the blasts express HLA-DR, CD33, and CD13. The expression of CD34 is not uniform. Common cytogenetic abnormalities associated with AML M_1 are monosomy 7 and trisomy 8.

AML M_2 blasts may show a large range of morphologic variations of the cytoplasm and the nucleus; the hallmark is the presence of multiple azurophilic granules occasionally clumped in the cytoplasm (Color Fig. 29B). One or two cytoplasmic Auer rods are frequently seen. Cytochemical stains are used to confirm the positivity of the azurophilic granules for myeloperoxidase (Color Fig. 30A) and Sudan black reactivity (Color Fig. 30B). By flow cytometry, >20% of the blasts express HLA-DR, CD13, and CD33. The expression of CD34 and other myelomonocytic surface markers such as CD11 and CD14 is not uniform. Translocation (8;21) is a cytogenetic aberration frequently associated with M_2 AML. This translocation often expresses CD19 and CD56 on the surface in addition to the characteristic myeloid surface markers. This chromosomal translocation results in the formation of the AML1-ETO fusion gene. This may interfere with transcription at a large number of genes involved in myelopoiesis and lymphopoiesis.

AML M_3, acute promyelocytic leukemia (APL) (Color Fig. 29C), is a distinctive form of AML and occurs in 3–10% of childhood AML; it is often associated with disseminated intravascular coagulation. Hypofibrinogenemia is of clinical significance for management. Patients with APL typically present with low WBC counts, peripheral blood cytopenias, and coagulopathy. APL is characterized by the t(15;17)(q24;q22) abnormality, which results in the fusion of the retinoic acid receptor-α gene (RAR) with the PML gene (15q24). The RAR gene product is a nuclear transcription factor that becomes active on binding its naturally occurring ligand, retinoic acid (vitamin A) and heterodimerizing with a second retinoic acid receptor family protein (RXR). This retinoic acid receptor pathway appears to be required for the normal differentiation of myeloid cells. The chimeric PML-RAR gene is present in essentially all cases of APL and produces a hybrid PML-RAR protein. The administration of pharmacologic doses of all-*trans* retinoic acid (not *cis* retinoic), however, has been shown to induce terminal myeloid maturation in APL and has been used as a highly successful model for cytodifferentiative therapy in AML. Overall, the outcome for patients with APL is substantially better than that for the group of pediatric AML patients as a whole, and the eradication of detectable disease at the molecular level has emerged as a significant prognostic factor. The peripheral blood smear exhibits findings consistent with microangiopathic hemolytic anemia. Two morphologic variants of APL are included under the M_3 group of the FAB classification: hypergranular and microgranular, or hypogranular variants (vM_3). Peripheral blood leukopenia is often associated with the hypergranular variant.

Promyelocytes with multiple coarse azurophilic granules in their cytoplasm and large numbers of Auer rods, called *faggot cells*, are present in the peripheral blood and BMA specimens of patients with the classic form of APL. Small promyelocytes with a basophilic cytoplasm and heavy granulation are often seen in BMA samples of patients with this variant.

The hypogranular and microgranular variant of APL is characterized by promyelocytes with small or scanty azurophilic granules. Multiple Auer rods are found much less often in the peripheral blood but may be observed on BMA smears. Promyelocytes with a bilobated nucleus (dumbbell shaped) and fine azurophilic granules are commonly seen in the APL vM_3. Sometimes the differentiation of these promyelocytes from abnormal monocytes may be difficult and should be based on cytochemical stains and immunologic surface markers.

Cytochemical stains are similar in both morphologic variants of APL; myeloperoxidase, Sudan black, and chloroacetate esterase strongly stain the granules and Auer rods of the promyelocytes. On occasion, the Auer rod profiles appear like a negative long crystal outlined by dense staining. ANAE may show a weak positivity in some APLs in contrast to monocytic leukemia, in which strongly positive results to ANAE and sensitivity to sodium fluoride are seen. By flow cytometry, >80% of the promyelocytes are HLA-DR negative, CD13 positive or CD33 positive, or both. The combined cytochemical and flow-cytometric data are useful in the differential diagnosis of microgranular APL from acute monocytic leukemia.

Association exists between the clinicopathologic picture of any variant of APL and the chromosomal translocation (15;17) and other chromosomal abnormalities.

AML M_4 (Color Fig. 29D) is characterized by a simultaneous clonal proliferation of blasts from the granulocytic and monocytic series. There are cytomorphologic variations in the blasts in peripheral blood and in BMA specimens. The blasts are intermixed with larger blasts with abundant gray-blue cytoplasm that in some cases have a fine azurophilic cytoplasmic granulation and may contain Auer rods. The nuclear shape is variable. It may be round, oval, or lobulated or indented. The chromatin has a fine network appearance. Light blue nucleoli are present and often multiple.

The diagnosis of AML M_4 requires that ≥20% of the blasts have monocytic differentiation, which is demonstrated by a strong positive stain with chloroacetate (Color Fig. 30C) and nonspecific esterase (Color Fig. 30D) sensitive to sodium fluoride.

A variant of M_4 AML in which >3% of the eosinophils are counted in the BMA differential is included as AML M_4 Eo in the FAB classification. In this subtype, no consistent association with peripheral blood eosinophilia exists. In the BMA sample, the eosinophils not only are increased but also are morphologically abnormal. The cytoplasm contains dark (basophilic) granules in addition to the normal eosinophilic granules. The nuclei of the immature eosinophils may be similar to the nuclei of the monocytes. Cytochemically, these eosinophils stain positively with PAS and chloroacetate esterase in contrast to normal eosinophils.

Cytogenetic aberrations associated with FAB category M_4 involve chromosomes 4, 6, and 11. The specific karyotype associated with M_4 is inv 16.

AML M_5 (Color Fig. 29E) is uncommon in infancy. Of the two variants described in the FAB classification, acute monoblastic leukemias (M_5A) and acute monocytic leukemia (M_5B), M_5B is the more frequent form in infancy. The blasts in M_5A are characterized by abundant cytoplasm, sometimes with azurophilic granules or vacuoles. The nucleus is large and of variable shape. Nucleoli are prominent. The cytoplasm stains strongly with ANAE, and the stain is sensitive to sodium fluoride. The intensity of the stain is not uniform in all blasts. Myeloperoxidase stain and Sudan black stain are negative. The fine granules stain positively with PAS. Weakly positive results with TdT stain can be observed in a large number of blasts in monoblastic leukemias. By flow cytometry, a large percentage of blasts are positive for HLA-DR, CD11, CD13, CD15, CD14, and CD34.

Rearrangement in the long arm of chromosome 11, t(9;11) is the most frequent cytogenetic abnormality associated with M_5 AML.

AML M_6 (erythroleukemia) (Color Fig. 29F) is extremely rare in infancy. It has been reported in Down syndrome. The diagnosis of true erythroid leukemia is complicated by the frequency with which myeloblast levels progressively increase during the course of the disease. The diagnosis depends on the presence of 30–50% erythroblasts, in addition to morphologic abnormalities of the erythroblasts. M_6 erythroblasts in BMA samples are usually large, with a deep blue cytoplasm that may contain vacuoles. Nuclear abnormalities are diverse. The nucleus may be single or multiple. Megaloblastic changes are observed and dyserythropoiesis is striking. Myeloblasts are present and associated with dysgranulopoiesis. In the peripheral blood, the RBC precursors are observed at different stages of maturation. Numerous basophilic reticulocytes are also common. PAS is the cytochemical stain of

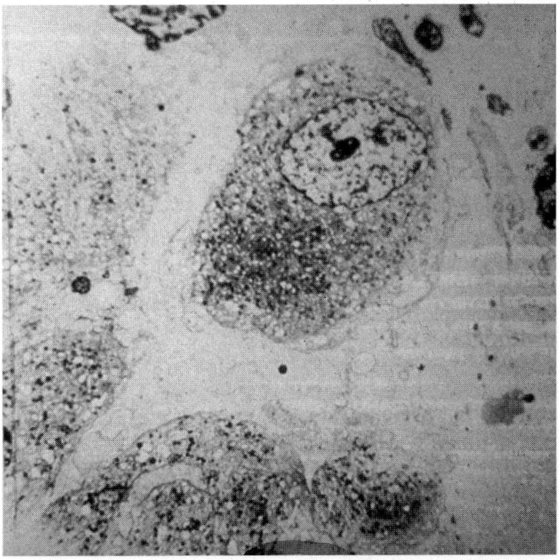

Fig. 31. Electron micrograph showing megakaryoblasts in a case of acute megakaryocytic leukemia.

choice. Large globular or granular blocks showing PAS positivity are present in the erythroblasts. By flow cytometry, assays for glycophorin A (GPA) give positive results. Other monoclonal and polyclonal antibodies can be used to study a leukemia morphologically suspicious for M_6 but negative for glycophorin A. Anticarbonic anhydrase I and spectrin have been recommended in such cases.

AML M_7 (acute megakaryoblastic leukemia) (AMKL) is rare among the acute leukemias, comprising 10% of AMLs. It is characterized by trisomy 21, inversions or translocations of chromosomes 3, t(9;22), t(1;22) in infants. The FAB classification includes this leukemia under the subtype 7. It is more common in children <3 years of age, with a high incidence in infants with Down syndrome. It is also seen in Klinefelter syndrome (XXY syndrome).

Children with Down syndrome and AMKL often have episodes of hematologic abnormalities, of which the most frequent is thrombocytopenia, with spontaneous recovery; they often present before 1 year of age with marked organomegaly.

Laboratory findings include anemia in almost all cases, thrombocytopenia (not always present), and large platelets or megakaryocyte fragments or both. The percentage of blasts is variable in the peripheral blood, but a diagnosis of AMKL based on cell morphology alone is difficult to establish. Blasts from AMKL can be misclassified as atypical lymphocytes in the peripheral blood. A BMA sample is difficult to obtain, and a "dry tap" is frequent. The marrow is usually partially replaced by blast cells that show marked morphologic variations of nucleus and cytoplasm. The blasts may be small, similar to lymphoblasts, or very large (>20 μm) with round nucleus and prominent nucleolus as seen by electromicroscopy (Fig. 31). The cytoplasm is light blue, with or without fine azurophilic granules, and with single or multiple blebs. The nucleus may be small and round, reminiscent of a lymphoblast, or large or irregular, with binucleated or multinucleated bizarre forms, or both, that are intermixed. Clustering of blasts may give the appearance of metastatic tumor.

Monoclonal antibodies useful in the diagnosis of AMKL are CD61, CD41, CD33, and HLA-DR. HLA-DR is seen in the early stages of megakaryocytic differentiation, while cytoplasmic CD41 is seen in the late stages. CD33 is seen in the intermediate forms and those that have acquired CD61. Flow cytometry might yield a low percentage of positive monoclonal antibodies, owing to the clumping of the megakaryoblasts.

Table 29. Antigen Expression in Acute Myelogenous Leukemia

	Type of Acute Myelogenous Leukemia				
Antigen	M_0, M_1, M_2	M_3	M_4, M_5	M_6	M_7
CD13	+	+	+	+	+/–
CD33	+	+	+	+	+/–
HLA-DR	+	–/+	+	–/+	+/–
CD64	–/+	+/–	+	–	–
CD14	–/+	–	+	–	–
CD36	–/+	–	+	+	+
CD71	+/–	+/–	+/–	+	+/–
Glycophorin A	–	–	–	+/–	–
CD41 and CD61	–	–	–	–	+

+, present; –, absent; +/–, often present; –/+, occasionally present.

The most frequent cytogenetic abnormalities associated with AMKL in children without Down syndrome are t(1:22) and aberrations of chromosome 21. Numerical and structural abnormalities in the cytogenetic analysis are less common in children with Down syndrome and AMKL, than in those without Down syndrome.

The new WHO classification has defined two types of refractory anemia with excess blasts based on the percentage of blasts:

Type 1	5% blasts in the marrow <5% blasts in the blood
Type 2	10–19% blasts in the marrow 5–19% blasts in the blood and <10% blasts in the bone marrow <20% blasts with Auer rods

Antigen expression in AML is summarized in Table 29.

Cytochemical and immunocytochemical findings for AML are shown in Table 30.

Table 30. Cytochemistry and Immunocytochemistry in Acute Leukemia

Reaction	Primary Normal Cells Manifesting Reaction	Major Diagnostic Use
Myeloperoxidase	Neutrophil series, eosinophils (cyanide resistant), monocytes ±	Myeloid leukemia without maturation (M_1), myeloid leukemia with maturation (M_2), microgranular promyelocytic leukemia (M_3)
Sudan black B	Neutrophil series, monocytes ±	M_1, M_2, microgranular M_3
Chloroacetate esterase	Neutrophil series	M_1, M_2, microgranular M_3, granulocytic sarcomas
Nonspecific esterase (α-naphthyl acetate esterase)	Monocytes (inhibited by sodium fluoride)	Myelomonocytic leukemia (M_4); monocytic leukemia, poorly differentiated (M_5A); monocytic leukemia, differentiated (M_5A)
Periodic acid–Schiff		Erythroleukemia (M_6), acute lymphoblastic leukemias
Terminal deoxynucleotidyl transferase	T- and B-lymphocyte precursors	Acute lymphoblastic leukemias

Common cytogenetic findings associated with acute leukemias, chronic leukemias, and myelodysplastic-myeloproliferative syndromes are shown in Table 27.

Prognostic Implications of Chromosome Findings in Acute Myelogenous Leukemia

Prognostic Group	Chromosome Findings
Favorable	inv(16) or t(16;16)
	t(8;21)
	Single miscellaneous defects
Intermediate	t(15;17)
	+8
	t(9;1) (children)
	Normal
Unfavorable	–7 or 5, del 7q
	t(11q23)
	inv(3q)
	Complex abnormalities

Leukemia, Chronic Myeloid (Chronic Myelomonocytic Leukemia), Juvenile

CML is uncommon in infancy and childhood. Two forms of the disease have been described. One is similar to the adult type and is seen in children >5 years of age. The other form, originally described as Philadelphia chromosome–negative CML or juvenile chronic myeloid leukemia, is a panmyelopathy now classified as a myeloproliferative disorder and a variant of chronic myelomonocytic leukemia. This differs from the CML seen in older children and adults in its clinical, morphologic, cytogenetic, and molecular features. It often presents clinically in infancy with a distinct eczematous facial rash, lymphadenopathy, hepatomegaly, and marked splenomegaly.

Clinical Features and Hematologic Findings[2]

	Juvenile-type CML <5 yr	Adult CML >5 yr
Lymphadenopathy	Common	Uncommon
Skin lesions	Common	Unusual
Bacterial infections	Common	Unusual
WBC count >100,000/mL	Unusual	Common
Hemoglobin level >12 g/dL	Common	Variable
Platelets	Decreased	Usually increased
Monocytosis	Common	Unusual
Circulating pronormoblasts	Common	Unusual
HbF increased	Common	Unusual
Philadelphia chromosome	Absent	>90%
bcr-abl fusion gene	Absent	Present
Leukocyte alkaline phosphatase decreased	Variable	Common
Median survival	1–2 yr	4–5 yr
Blastic phase	Unusual	Common

Other Laboratory Findings

Laboratory findings in chronic myelomonocytic leukemia include normochromic normocytic anemia, leukocytosis ($<100 \times 10^9$/L), and thrombocytopenia. The peripheral blood smear (Color Fig. 32) demonstrates circulating pronormoblasts or normoblasts or both, immature granulocytes, and prominent monocytosis. Basophilia may be present. The number of RBCs with i antigen and the level of serum and urinary muramidase are also increased. Score on the granulocyte leukocyte

[2]From Nathan DG, Oski FA. *Hematology of infancy and childhood*. Philadelphia: WB Saunders, 1993.

alkaline phosphatase test, a test commonly used in the differential diagnosis of adult CML, is low but may be normal.

The BMA specimen is hypercellular with preservation or slight elevation of the M/E ratio. The erythrocytic series is dyserythropoietic with multinucleated forms. Monocytes are increased. Megakaryocytes are normal or decreased. The percentage of blasts is low, <30% if transformation to AML has not occurred.

The BMB specimen is hypercellular, with trilineage maturation and an increase in reticulin. The bone marrow karyotype at diagnosis lacks the Philadelphia chromosome and can be normal. No specific abnormalities of the karyotype are associated with chronic myelomonocytic leukemia in infants. New clones may emerge if transformation to AML takes place, and frequently monosomy 7 develops. At the molecular level, no bcr rearrangement occurs such as characterizes the adult type of CML.

Leukemia, Congenital

The term *congenital leukemia* is usually applied to those cases diagnosed at birth but is sometimes used for cases developing shortly after birth or in the first few months of life.

The diagnostic signs of acute leukemias in older children, such as leukocytosis with an increase in the number of blasts in the peripheral blood associated with an increase in blasts in the bone marrow of >30%, are not valid for the diagnosis of acute leukemia in the neonate. *Leukemoid reactions*, which are characterized by high WBC counts, with an increase in the number of immature WBCs, should be distinguished from leukemia. One cause of the leukemoid reaction is fetal infection produced by rubella, CMV infection, herpes simplex, toxoplasmosis, and bacterial infections. In HDN, increased numbers of immature WBCs are associated with the presence of nucleated RBCs, RBC fragments, teardrops, target cells, and often large platelets on blood smears. Cytogenetic studies should be performed to rule out Down syndrome if other causes for leukemoid reaction are absent.

Cutaneous-specific leukemic infiltrates occur in up to 50% of cases of congenital leukemia, and the infant may have a "blueberry muffin" appearance. A skin biopsy specimen from the lesion shows a dense infiltration of the dermis and subcutaneous tissue by large, pleomorphic mononuclear cells.

Leukocytosis

Common causes of leukocytosis of nonmalignant origin in infancy include the following:

Condition	Type
Bacterial infections, except pertussis	Neutrophilic
Allergy	Eosinophilic
Urticaria	Basophilic, eosinophilic
Neutropenia or agranulocytosis	Monocytic
Recovery phase from acute infection	Monocytic, eosinophilic
Malaria	Monocytic
Congenital syphilis	Monocytic
Rickettsial infections	Monocytic
Tuberculosis	Monocytic
Parasitic infestation	Eosinophilic
Immunodeficiencies	Eosinophilic
Drug reactions	Eosinophilic
Tissue injury	Neutrophilic
Inflammation	Neutrophilic
Asplenia	Neutrophilic
Asphyxia	Neutrophilic
Hypoxia	Neutrophilic

Milk precipitin disease	Eosinophilic
Eosinophilic gastroenteritis	Eosinophilic
Systemic mastocytosis	Eosinophilic
Hereditary eosinophilia	Eosinophilic
Viral infections	Neutrophilic, monocytic, lymphocytic

Lymphocytopenia

In children <16 years, absolute lymphocyte counts are higher than in adults. The lower reference value is approximately $2.0 \times 10^3/mm^3$. Approximately 80% of circulating lymphocytes in the blood are $CD3^+$ T lymphocytes, and approximately two-thirds of cases of T lymphocytopenia have a decrease in the absolute number of T lymphocytes and of $CD4^+$ T lymphocytes in particular.

Severe combined immunodeficiency disease is characterized by profound defects in cellular and humoral immunity with prominent lymphocytopenia. The common form is X-linked and is a mutation of the γ chain of the interleukin-2 receptor. Other cases of severe combined immunodeficiency disease result from autosomal-recessive inheritance, commonly deficiencies of the purine-degradation enzymes adenine deaminase and nucleoside phosphorylase.

Infants with DiGeorge syndrome usually exhibit profound lymphocytopenia. Aplasia of the thymus and the parathyroid gland results from a defect in embryogenesis of the third and fourth pharyngeal pouches. The T-cell areas of all tissues, including lymph nodes and spleen, are depleted.

Wiskott-Aldrich syndrome, an X-linked recessive disease characterized by eczematoid dermatitis, thrombocytopenia, and recurrent opportunistic infections, is associated with lymphocytopenia.

The signs and symptoms of patients with lymphocytopenia are those characteristic of the underlying disease process.

Diagnostic Tests

CBC with differential and platelet count.

BMA and BMB may be indicated if the reason for the lymphocytopenia is unclear or to confirm a suspected diagnosis.

Quantitative immunoglobulin determination.

Immunophenotypic analysis of peripheral blood lymphocytes by flow cytometry.

Ancillary tests such as skin tests to evaluate cellular immunity.

Other tests dependent on the clinical setting to determine the underlying cause. These include tests for HIV, antinuclear antibodies (systemic lupus erythematosus), and lymph node biopsy (sarcoidosis).

Cultures for patients suspected of having infection.

In adults, the lymphocyte count is $<1.0 \times 10^3/mm^3$. In children, it is $<2.0 \times 10^3/mm^3$. Granulocytopenia may be present. Normochromic normocytic anemia is present in many of the diseases associated with lymphocytopenia.

Immunophenotypic Analysis of Peripheral Blood Lymphocytes by Flow Cytometry

Labeled monoclonal antibodies bind to T cells, B cells, their subsets, and other hematopoietic cells. Labeled cells can then be enumerated with flow cytometry.

In flow cytometry, a fluid system delivers the cell sample past an excitation light beam in a single-file stream. The scattered light and any fluorescence emitted from this interaction (from dyes used to stain specific cell molecules) are collected and converted to electrical signals. These then can be analyzed to give quantitative information about specific cell characteristics.

Sixty percent to 80% of circulating lymphocytes are T cells, 10–20% are B cells, and 5–10% are natural killer cells. The T-cell population consists of helper T cells ($CD4^+$) and suppressor T cells ($CD8^+$); the helper T cells outnumber the suppressor T cells 2 to 1.

The normal ranges of bone marrow lymphocytes and immunophenotype in infants as measured by flow cytometry are shown in Table 31.

Table 31. Normal Ranges of Bone Marrow Lymphocytes and Immunophenotype[a] in Infants Aged 7 Days to 24 Months

	%
Lymphocytes	8–50
CD19	9–56
CD10	8–72
CD7	12–69
CD4	7–32
CD8	1–28
Kappa	7–28
Lambda	3–22

[a]Flow cytometry: lymphoid region gated. Values were obtained from bone marrow donors and patients without hematologic disease.

Laboratory Findings

Bone Marrow

Bone marrow findings depend on the underlying disorder and recent therapeutic approaches. In some congenital immunodeficiency states, lymphocyte numbers are decreased.

Quantitation of Immunoglobulins

Immunoglobulin production is altered when there is a defect in the B-cell population alone or when a combined defect involving B and T lymphocytes exists. Defects in antibody production also can result from severe defects in T-lymphocyte function, because in humans, all antigens seem to be T-lymphocyte dependent.

Causes of Lymphocytopenia

Autoimmune Disorders

The lymphocytopenia seen in autoimmune disorders such as systemic lupus erythematosus is likely mediated by autoantibodies.

Systemic Diseases

Lymphocytopenia is associated with severe burns, protein-losing enteropathies, severe congestive heart failure, thoracic duct injury, and other primary diseases of the gut or intestinal lymphatics. The lymphocytopenia of renal insufficiency and sarcoidosis may be secondary to defective T-lymphocyte proliferative responses.

Iatrogenic Factors

Radiotherapy induces lymphocytopenia. Helper T lymphocytes are more sensitive than are suppressor T cells; the helper/suppressor ratio can be decreased for months after exposure to radiation. Chemotherapeutic agents, such as alkylating agents, can cause profound lymphocytopenia that may persist for years. Lymphocytopenia in response to corticoid therapy usually resolves after discontinuance of the drugs. Lymphocytopenia often is associated with anesthesia and surgical stress and is secondary to redistribution, perhaps related to endogenous steroid release. In thoracic duct damage, lymphocytes are lost from the body.

Idiopathic Factors

A syndrome of isolated $CD4^+$ T-cell depletion in the absence of evidence for a retroviral infection has been identified. The cause of this condition is unknown.

Nutritional Deficiencies

Nutritional deficiencies are associated with lymphocytopenia. Protein-calorie malnutrition is a common cause of lymphocytopenia worldwide. The lymphocytopenia probably is due to decreased production or synthesis and is characterized by decreased numbers of circulating $CD4^+$ T cells and increased numbers of $CD8^+$ T cells.

Infectious Diseases

Lymphocytopenia is prominent in acquired immunodeficiency syndrome (AIDS) and is due to selective loss of the $CD4^+$ T lymphocytes. The lymphocytopenia in AIDS is

Table 32. Reference Intervals for Lymphocyte Subsets by Age Group

	Age Group					
	Neonate	Infant	1–3 yr	3–6 yr	7–17 yr	Adult
Total lymphocytes	2.2–7.0	2.5–6.5	2.2–5.5	2.0–5.0	1.4–3.8	1.5–4.0
CD3	2.4–3.7	1.7–3.6	1.8–3.0	1.8–3.0	1.4–2.0	0.6–2.4
CD4 (T4)	1.5–2.4	1.7–2.8	1.0–1.8	1.0–1.8	0.7–1.1	0.5–1.4
CD8 (T8)	1.2–2.0	0.8–1.2	0.8–1.5	0.8–1.5	0.6–0.9	0.2–0.7
CD19	0.7–1.5	0.5–1.5	0.7–1.3	0.7–1.3	0.3–0.5	0.04–0.5
CD16	0.8–1.8	0.3–0.7	0.2–0.6	0.2–0.6	0.2–0.3	0.2–0.4
CD4/CD8 ratio	1.2–6.2	—	—	1.0–3.2	—	—

Values represent cell count × 10^9/L.

secondary to a direct cytopathic effect of the HIV. The host immune response also may contribute to the progressive loss of T lymphocytes.

Other viral or bacterial infections also are associated with lymphocytopenia.

Lymphocytosis

Reference ranges for lymphocyte subsets by age group are shown in Table 32.

Lymphocytosis usually represents a specific response to an underlying disorder or condition. The most common cause is infectious mononucleosis (IM) caused by EBV infection. In CMV infection, the clinical and peripheral blood picture is similar to that in EBV IM. Lymphocytosis is also seen in viral hepatitis, childhood viral infections, drug reactions, infectious lymphocytosis, transient stress lymphocytosis, pertussis, and persistent polyclonal B-cell lymphocytosis associated with cigarette smoking. The route of transmission of EBV seems to be intimate contact with saliva from a previously infected person. EBV infects B lymphocytes in the oropharynx, which then disseminate the virus throughout the reticuloendothelial system, provoking an intense immunologic response responsible for the immunopathology and symptoms of EBV IM. The majority of the reactive lymphocytes in the blood during the acute infection are T lymphocytes of the cytotoxic-suppressor (CD8) phenotype. IM is characterized by the production of heterophil antibody and EBV-specific antibodies, including those directed against viral capsid antigen (VCA), early antigen (EA), and Epstein-Barr nuclear antigen (EBNA). The humoral response seems to be important for preventing recurrent infections. IM typically occurs between the ages of 10 and 25 years. Characteristic symptoms include sore throat, fever, headache, malaise, nausea, and anorexia. Lymphadenopathy, usually cervical, is almost always present. More than 50% of patients have splenomegaly, and mild hepatitis may be present. Acute EBV infections are common in early childhood but often are asymptomatic or characterized by clinical symptoms not recognized as IM.

Diagnostic Tests

CBC with leukocyte differential

Morphologic examination of the peripheral blood smear

Testing for IM heterophil antibody

Hemoglobin and Hct measurements usually are normal in IM. Mild hemolysis occasionally is present, but clinically significant anemia is uncommon. When anemia is present, it is usually an autoimmune hemolytic anemia caused by RBC autoantibodies. RBC autoantibodies with anti-N and anti-I specificities have been described in IM. An absolute lymphocytosis >4.0 × 10^3/mm^3 usually is present. The total leukocyte count is increased and ranges from 10 to 30 × 10^3/mm^3; counts exceeding this range are rare. The leukocytosis begins approximately 1 week after the onset of symptoms, peaks during the second or third week, and persists for 2–8 weeks. A mild to moderate neutropenia often is present. Rarely, agranulocytosis may complicate IM. Mild thrombocytopenia is present in approximately one-third of patients with IM; severe thrombocytopenia is rare. The neutropenia and thrombocytopenia apparently are secondary to an immune mechanism.

Hematologic Tests

Peripheral Blood Smear

Lymphocytes have a characteristic morphologic appearance (Downey cells) (Color Fig. 33). They usually are large with abundant blue cytoplasm and coarse but dispersed chromatin. Nucleoli are absent or indistinct. Peripheral or radiating basophilia of the cytoplasm often is present, and scattered azurophilic granules may be noted. Immunoblasts observed frequently are medium to large lymphocytes with moderate amounts of basophilic cytoplasm, round to oval nuclei with a coarsely reticular chromatin pattern, and visible nucleoli. In some cases, reactive lymphocytes are small with minimal basophilic cytoplasm, condensed chromatin, and indented or lobulated nuclei. This type of cell is uncommon in IM but may be prominent in some patients, especially young children. Circulating plasma cells often are present in small numbers.

The erythrocytes in blood smears from patients with IM usually are normochromic and normocytic, but spherocytes and increased polychromasia may be apparent if an AIHA is present. The platelets have normal morphologic features, but the number may be slightly decreased.

Peripheral blood shows

- Fifty percent mononuclear cells (lymphocytes and monocytes) in blood smear
- At least ten reactive lymphocytes per 100 leukocytes
- Marked lymphocyte heterogeneity

Serologic Profile

Table 33 shows the serologic profile in EBV IM.

Heterophil Antibody Assay

Heterophil antibodies are produced in EBV IM. They appear within the first 2 weeks of illness and usually are undetectable 3–6 months after the acute illness.

The IM heterophil antibody is of the IgM class and reacts with beef, sheep, and horse erythrocytes; it does not react with guinea pig kidney tissue. This characteristic separates the IM heterophil antibody from cross-reacting Forssman-type antibodies.

Most clinical laboratories use one of the several commercially available rapid tests or "monospot" tests to detect heterophil antibodies. Test results are positive in more than 96% of the teenagers and young adults with IM. False-positive results occur but are uncommon.

A small percentage of teenagers and young adults with EBV IM do not produce heterophil antibodies. These cases represent heterophil-negative IM. The incidence of heterophil negativity is much higher in infants and young children. Approximately 75% of children with IM from 2 to 4 years of age and fewer than 25% of children with IM <2 years produce heterophil antibodies. When the heterophil antibody cannot be detected, EBV-specific serologic tests can be used to confirm the diagnosis of EBV IM.

Table 33. Serologic Profile in Infectious Mononucleosis (Epstein-Barr Virus Infection)

Antibody	Acute (0–3 mo)	Recent (3–12 mo)	Past (>12 mo)
Heterophil	Positive	Negative	Negative
EBV specific			
VCA IgM	Positive	Negative	Negative
VCA IgG	Positive	Positive	Positive
EA	Positive or negative	Positive or negative	Negative
EBNA	Negative	Positive	Positive

EA, early antigen; EBNA, Epstein-Barr nuclear antigen; EBV, Epstein-Barr virus; Ig, immunoglobulin; Negative, no detectable antibody; Positive, detectable antibody; VCA, viral capsid antigen.

Epstein-Barr Virus–Specific Serologic Tests

Almost all patients develop antibodies of the IgG and IgM types to VCA early in the course of the disease. The IgM anti-VCA titers diminish rapidly during convalescence, and VCA is usually undetectable at 12 weeks, whereas positive IgG anti-VCA titers persist for life. Antibody to EA (anti-EA) appears during the acute phase of the disease and then declines. Antibodies to EBNA do not appear until symptoms have resolved and then persist indefinitely.

Assays for EBV-specific antibodies are usually done with indirect immunofluorescence microscopy. Enzyme-linked immunosorbent assays, Western blot analysis, and other immunoassays are also available.

An acute primary infection is characterized by the following: (a) the presence of IgM anti-VCA, (b) high titers of IgG anti-VCA, (c) detection of anti-EA, and (d) the absence of anti-EBNA. The presence of IgG anti-VCA and anti-EBNA with absence of IgM anti-VCA indicates a remote infection.

Bone Marrow Examination

A bone marrow examination is not indicated to diagnose IM.

Lymphocytosis, Infectious

Infectious lymphocytosis is a benign illness of young children that is presumably of viral origin. The patients often are asymptomatic, but fever, abdominal pain, or diarrhea may be present. Organomegaly does not occur. The symptoms resolve within a few days. Leukocyte counts in infectious lymphocytosis range from 35.0 to $100.0 \times 10^3/mm^3$. The predominant lymphocyte has been reported to be a T cell or natural killer cell, but increased numbers of B lymphocytes have been observed. The lymphocytes appear morphologically mature, and eosinophilia may be present in the later stages of the disease. The lymphocytosis may persist for several weeks.

Table 34 shows the differential diagnosis and tests in infectious lymphocytosis.

Lymphocytosis, Transient Stress

The lymphocytes in transient stress lymphocytosis consist of mature or mildly reactive-appearing lymphocytes. Large granular lymphocytes occasionally are prominent in these patients. The lymphocytosis resolves quickly, often within a few hours, and is followed by a neutrophilia. The lymphocytosis represents an expansion of the normal lymphocyte population and is thought to be secondary to epinephrine release.

Monocytosis

Monocytes circulate briefly in the peripheral blood and migrate to tissues, where they mature into a variety of cells composing the monocyte/histiocyte/immune cell system. Monocytes generally compose only 2–9% of WBCs, with an absolute count of $0.1–0.9 \times 10^3/mm^3$.

Monocytosis is defined as an absolute monocyte count $>1.0 \times 10^3/mm^3$ in adults and $1.2 \times 10^3/mm^3$ in neonates.

Peripheral Blood Smear Morphology

Reactive monocytes characteristically exhibit cytoplasm that is frequently vacuolated. Cytoplasmic granulation also may be prominent.

Causes

Chronic infections, tuberculosis, listeriosis, syphilis
Hodgkin disease
Recovery from agranulocytosis
Collagen vascular diseases
Gastrointestinal disorders (immune mediated)
Non-Hodgkin lymphomas
Sarcoidosis
Multiple myeloma

Table 34. Differential Diagnosis and Tests in Lymphocytosis

Disease	Test	Interpretation
EBV-IM	Heterophil test	Positive results in association with characteristic blood smear morphologic features indicate EBV-IM.
	EBV-specific serologic tests	IgM and IgG antibodies to viral capsid antigens indicate acute infection.
Cytomegalovirus	Antigenemia assay	Positive results indicate acute infection.
	Serologic test for antibody using EIA or other method	Change from negative to positive result or fourfold or greater rise in titer in paired serum samples indicates acute infection.
Toxoplasmosis	Serologic tests by EIA for *Toxoplasma gondii*–specific antibodies	Elevated *Toxoplasma gondii*–specific IgM and IgG antibody levels indicate acute infection.
Adenovirus	Culture	Positive results in acute infection.
Acute HIV infection	Test for HIV-specific antibody by EIA with confirmation of positive results (e.g., by Western blot)	Positive results indicate infection with HIV.
Human herpesvirus 6	Virus isolation by culture or detection of viral DNA	Detection of virus or DNA indicates acute infection.
Hepatitis A, B, C	Serologic tests by EIA	Hepatitis A–specific IgM is present in acute infection.
		Presence of hepatitis B surface antigen in absence of antibody indicates acute infection.
		Antibody to hepatitis C virus present in acute infection.
Rubella	Serologic test for antibody using EIA or other method	Rise in antibody titers in paired serum samples or presence of rubella virus–specific IgM indicates acute infection.
Bordetella pertussis	Culture of nasal swab; direct fluorescent antibody staining procedure for clinical specimens or cultures	Identification of bacteria indicates acute infection.

EBV, Epstein-Barr virus; EIA, enzyme immunoassay; HIV, human immunodeficiency virus; Ig, immunoglobulin; IM, infectious mononucleosis.

Hemolytic anemia
Chronic neutropenia
Rare carcinomas
Splenectomy
Immune thrombocytopenic purpura

Myelodysplastic Syndromes

Monosomy 7

The myelodysplastic syndrome that occurs in association with bone marrow monosomy 7 in infants has characteristic clinical features that distinguish it from acute leukemia associated with monosomy 7 in older children and adults. A wide range is seen in the age of presentation during childhood; the median age is 10 months. Most infants with monosomy 7 are boys. The usual clinical presentation includes marked hepatosplenomegaly and recurrent respiratory and skin infections.

Laboratory Findings

Laboratory findings in patients with monosomy 7 are macrocytic anemia (MCV >95 fL), leukocytosis or leukopenia, and thrombocytopenia. The thrombocytopenia may or may not be persistent after the treatment of the infection. HbF level is normal or slightly elevated, and abnormal neutrophil functions are reported. The peripheral blood smear reveals macrocytic RBCs and often nucleated RBCs. The granulocytic and monocytic cells show abnormal cytoplasmic granulation, and either hypogranular or hypergranular forms are seen. Partial degranulation of the eosinophils is often noted. Nuclear abnormalities include pseudo–Pelger-Huët anomaly.

The BMA specimen is cellular with or without excess of blasts. Dysplastic changes are seen in the erythrocytic, granulocytic, and megakaryocytic lines. Small mononuclear megakaryocytes may be difficult to identify, and immunocytochemical analysis with CD61 may be necessary for their recognition. The BMB specimen is hypercellular. A striking feature is the morphologic variability in the distribution of megakaryocytes; they can form large clusters or appear small and mononuclear (micromegakaryocytes) or both. Monosomy 7 is limited to the hematopoietic cells. The number of metaphase cells lacking one chromosome in the karyotype varies.

Hematologic Findings in Myelodysplastic Syndromes

Blood

- Anemia
- Anisopoikilocytosis
  - Oval macrocytes
  - Hypochromatic cells
  - Dimorphic populations
- Decreased polychromatophilic cells
- Basophilic stippling
- Nucleated RBCs
- Vacuolated RBCs
- Howell-Jolly bodies
- Neutropenia
- Neutrophilia (rare)
- Immature granulocytes
- Hypogranularity
- Nuclear hyposegmentation (pseudo–Pelger-Huët change)
- Nuclear "sticks"
- Hypersegmentation (occasionally)
- Hypercondensed chromatin
- Circulating myeloblasts (<5%)
- Thrombocytopenia
- Large platelets
- Hypogranular platelets
- Vacuolated platelets
- Abnormal platelet granules
- Micromegakaryoctyes

Bone Marrow

- Dyserythropoiesis
  - Erythroid hyperplasia (occasionally hypoplasia)
  - Nuclear-cytoplasm asynchrony
  - Megaloblastic chromatin
  - Karyorrhexis
  - Multinuclearity
  - Internuclear bridging
  - Nuclear fragments
  - Ringed sideroblasts
  - PAS-positive erythroblasts
- Dysgranulopoiesis
  - Increased myeloblasts and immature granulocytes
  - Abnormally localized immature precursors
  - Maturation defects
    - Hypogranularity
    - Abnormal granules
    - Abnormal nuclei
  - Myeloperoxidase-deficient neutrophils
  - Increased monocytes
  - Increased basophils
- Dysmegakaryopoiesis
  - Increased or decreased megakaryocytes
  - Clusters of megakaryocytes
  - Micromegakaryocytes
  - Monolobation or hypolobation
  - Odd-numbered nuclei
  - Multiple widely separated nuclei
  - Hypogranulation

Cytogenetic Findings in Myelodysplastic Syndromes

Common cytogenetic findings associated with myelodysplastic-myeloproliferative syndromes, acute leukemias, and chronic leukemias are shown in Table 27.

Myeloproliferative Syndromes

Chronic

Table 35 summarizes the differential characteristics of chronic myeloproliferative syndromes.

Table 35. Differential Characteristics of Chronic Myeloproliferative Syndromes

Variable	Myeloproliferative with Myeloid Metaplasia	Essential Thrombocythemia	Chronic Myelogenous Leukemia (Adult)	Polycythemia Vera
Hemoglobulin	Decreased	Normal or decreased	Decreased	Normal or increased
Leukocyte count	Usually $<30 \times 10^3/mm^3$ ($<30 \times 10^9/L$)	Usually $<20 \times 10^3/mm^3$ ($<20 \times 10^9/L$)	Usually $<50 \times 10^3/mm^3$ ($<50 \times 10^9/L$)	Usually $<20 \times 10^3/mm^3$ ($<20 \times 10^9/L$)
Differential count	Moderate number of immature granulocytes	Usually normal	Many immature granulocytes	Usually normal
Eosinophilia and/or basophilia	Usually present	May be present	Present	May be present
RBC morphology	Anisocytosis and teardrop poikilocytosis	Normal or hypochromic, microcytic	Usually normal	Normal or hypochromic, microcytic
Nucleated RBCs	Common	Rare	Rare	Rare
Platelet count	Normal, increased, or decreased	Increased	Normal, increased, or decreased	Normal or increased
Bone marrow	Hypercellular with increasing fibrosis	Hypercellular with megakaryocytosis	Marked myeloid hyperplasia	Hypercellular with decreased iron stores
LAP	Variable, usually increased	Usually normal	Decreased	Usually increased
Ph^1	Absent	Absent	Present	Absent
ber-abl rearrangement	Absent	Absent	Present	Absent
Splenomegaly	Marked	Absent or mild	Moderate	Absent or mild

LAP, leukocyte alkaline phosphatase; Ph^1, Philadelphia chromosome; RBC, red blood cell.

Transient

Transient myeloproliferative syndrome is a rare syndrome with the clinical and hematologic characteristics of acute leukemia in the peripheral blood; it usually resolves spontaneously. Synonyms for this syndrome include transitory abnormal myelopoiesis, transient myelodysplasia, transient leukemia, and transient myelodysplastic disorder. The most common association is trisomy 21, or chromosome 21 mosaicism in a phenotypically normal neonate. Rarely, the disorder occurs in a cytogenetically normal child. Hepatosplenomegaly is the common clinical denominator of all patients with transient myelodysplastic disorder.

Laboratory findings include anemia, thrombocytopenia, and leukocytosis, as high as 100×10^9/L with up to 80% blasts. Immunophenotypes are heterogeneous. The blast population is myeloid, megakaryocytic, erythroid, lymphoid, or mixed, and the proportion varies from case to case. In sharp contrast with peripheral blood, the BMA specimen often has a lower percentage of blasts, usually <30%—a useful criterion for distinction from acute leukemia.

The course of transient myelodysplastic disorder is variable. Usually, there is spontaneous recovery within the first month of life, but some patients are at high risk for a malignant hematologic disease.

Neutropenia

In normal adults, the range for absolute neutrophil count is 1.5–$7.0 \times 10^3/mm^3$. In neonates and infants, the lower limit is approximately $2.5 \times 10^3/mm^3$, whereas the lower limit of normal for children and adults is $1.5 \times 10^3/mm^3$. Approximately one-fourth of healthy black children and adults demonstrate an absolute neutrophil count that ranges from 1.0 to $1.5 \times 10^3/mm^3$.

Neonates may develop neutropenia from maternal factors such as hypertension, drug treatments given to the mother during late gestation, and maternal antibodies that cross the placenta and attack fetal granulocytes. A variety of distinct constitutional neutropenic disorders may manifest during the neonatal period and include rare hereditary disorders. Severe sustained neutropenia characterizes Kostmann syndrome and Chédiak-Higashi syndrome, whereas patients with cyclic neutropenia exhibit episodic loss of neutrophils followed by a rebound recovery. As with neonates, infection is a common cause of neutropenia in older children. Because of the variety of underlying causes, patients with neutropenia have diverse clinical manifestations.

Causes

Neonate	Infections
	Maternal hypertension or drug treatment
	Maternal antibody production (e.g., in systemic lupus erythematosus)
	Constitutional disorders such as cyclic neutropenia
	Infantile genetic agranulocytosis
	Kostmann syndrome
	Chédiak-Higashi syndrome
	Phenotypic abnormalities
Infant/child	Infections
	Autoimmune neutropenia
	Neoplasms replacing bone marrow
	Idiosyncratic drug reactions
	Myeloablative therapies
	Constitutional neutropenic disorders
	Megaloblastic anemias, adult-type pernicious anemia
	Copper deficiency (rare)
	Hypersplenism
	Metabolic disease (e.g., aminoacidemia, organic acidemia)
	Aleukemic leukemia
	Aplastic anemia
	Idiopathic

Constitutional disorders associated with neutropenia include the following:

Disorder	Age of Onset	Type of Defect
Cyclic neutropenia	Early infancy	Proliferation
Kostmann syndrome	Birth/early infancy	Proliferation
Shwachman-Diamond syndrome	Birth/early infancy	Proliferation
Immunodeficiency disorders, reticular dysgenesis	Early infancy	Proliferation
Chédiak-Higashi syndrome	Early infancy	Maturation
Myelokathexis	Early infancy	Maturation
Fanconi anemia	Infancy/childhood/ adulthood (rare)	Proliferation
Dyskeratosis congenita	Infancy	Proliferation

Bone Marrow Findings in Nonneoplastic Neutropenic Disorders

Disorder or Condition	Comments
Aplastic anemia	All lineages absent or reduced (proliferation defect).
Radiotherapy, chemotherapy (proliferation defect)	All lineages suppressed or absent.
Myelophthisis (proliferative effect)	Bone marrow replaced by infiltrative disorder.
Drug-induced neutropenia (proliferation or survival defect)	Variable; most cases exhibit almost complete granulocytic aplasia with occasional blasts and promyelocytes. Other cases characterized by granulocytic hyperplasia with a decrease in mature forms (e.g., drug-induced immune destruction).
Immune-mediated neutropenia (survival or proliferation defect)	Generally granulocytic hyperplasia with decreased mature neutrophils is found, although immune mechanisms also responsible for suppressing granulocyte and other lineages. Prominent ingestion of neutrophils by macrophages possible. Immune aberrations may be primary or secondary to neoplastic or nonneoplastic disorders.
Vitamin B_{12} or folate deficiency (maturation defect)	Markedly hypercellular bone marrow with pronounced megaloblastic changes; intramedullary cell death.
Infection-associated neutropenia (proliferation or survival defect)	Variable bone marrow morphology; some infections (especially viral) suppress progenitor cells, inducing hypoplasia. Other infections cause decreased neutrophil survival, and bone marrow shows granulocytic hyperplasia.

Disorders Associated with Neutropenia

Immune Neutropenia

The immune neutropenias are classified as isoimmune and autoimmune. In both cases, neutrophil-specific antigens have been identified. Isoimmune neutropenia in the newborn presents with infection in the first 2 weeks of life. No specific clinical finding, except mucocutaneous infection, is associated with autoimmune neutropenia.

Laboratory findings in isoimmune neutropenia include normal or decreased WBC count associated with monocytosis and eosinophilia. The BMA specimen shows myeloid hyperplasia with a decrease in the mature forms of the granulocytic series. Shortly after birth, neutrophil antibodies are detected in the serum of both mother and child. The mechanism of isoimmune neutropenia is secondary to the transfer of maternal antibodies from mother to fetus.

Alloimmune Neonatal Neutropenia

In alloimmune neonatal neutropenia, a granulocytic analog of HDN, the mother produces antibodies against granulocyte antigens that she lacks but that the fetus has inherited from the father. Granulocyte-specific IgG antibodies formed by the mother can cross the placenta and cause fetal neutropenia. Although protected *in utero* by the sterile environment, affected neonates may develop mild to severe infections during the first days of life. An absolute neutrophil count is often required to define this disorder, as the total leukocyte count may be normal in these infants. Unlike red cell fetal-maternal incompatibilities, alloimmune neonatal neutropenia does occur during first pregnancies. Circulating antibodies may be detected in the mother, and sometimes in the infant, with granulocyte agglutination or granulocyte immunofluorescence assays. Absorption of circulating antibody by infant granulocytes, however, may reduce circulating antibody to an undetectable level in the neonate. Antibodies to NA1, NA2, NB1, MB2, and Mart have been reported to cause this condition, as well as antibodies reactive against granulocytes without specificity for unknown antigens. Testing the maternal serum against the paternal granulocytes may be necessary to detect antibody to a low-frequency antigen. Typing of the parents' granulocytes is useful in cases in which a granulocyte antibody is undetectable in maternal serum and may indicate the probability of future offspring's being affected.

Autoimmune Neutropenia

In primary autoimmune neutropenia in children and adults, antibodies to NA1, NA2, and NB1 have been implicated, as well as antibodies reactive against granulocytes but without specificity for known antigens. Circulating antibodies have been detected in indirect testing using granulocyte agglutination, granulocyte immunofluorescence, and the monoclonal antibody immobilization to granulocyte antigen assay. In cases in which adequate numbers of the patient's granulocytes can be isolated, direct granulocyte immunofluorescence testing may detect bound antibody when levels of circulating antibody are too low to be reactive in indirect testing.

Testing the patient's own granulocytes and serum may be useful in differentiating auto- and alloimmune antibodies.

Secondary autoimmune neutropenia due to granulocyte antibodies is associated with Felty syndrome, systemic lupus erythematosus, and thyroid disease. The relationship of chronic idiopathic neutropenias to immune neutropenias is not known. Many of the patients with idiopathic neutropenias do not have detectable granulocyte antibodies. However, the maturation arrest in the myeloid series of the bone marrow that is often seen is similar to that in patients with known immune neutropenias such as alloimmune neonatal neutropenia and autoimmune neutropenia.

Transfusion Reactions

In transfusion reactions, a general association may be seen between the occurrence of febrile reactions and the presence of granulocyte antibodies detected by leukoagglutination. This is a relatively nonspecific technique using cell suspensions containing leukocytes of all types, as well as platelets. With the development of more sophisticated leukocyte antibody methods, the specificity of these antibodies may be more precisely defined. Granulocyte agglutination and HLA antibody screening may be informative in determining the cause of some transfusion reactions.

Acute Lung Injury

Transfusion-related acute lung injury (TRALI) is recognized as a life-threatening complication of blood-component transfusion therapy. It is the third most frequent cause of transfusion-related death after ABO incompatibility and bacterial contamination. TRALI is a well-characterized clinical constellation of symptoms including dyspnea, hypotension, and fever. The chest radiograph shows bilateral pulmonary infiltrates without evidence of cardiac compromise of fluid overload. Symptoms typically begin 1–2 hours after transfusion and are fully manifest within 1–6 hours. Products typically implicated are whole blood, packed RBCs, fresh frown plasma, cryoprecipitate, and platelets (concentrates or apheresis). The cause of TRALI may be related to the presence of anti-HLA or antigranulocyte antibodies, or both, in the plasma of donors. One or both of these antibody types have been found in 89% of TRALI cases. Recent information suggests that HLA class II antibodies may also be implicated in cases of TRALI.

Diagnostic Tests

In the neutrophil antibody screen, granulocyte (neutrophil)-specific antibodies are detected by testing against a panel of granulocyte-typed donor cells in the granulocyte agglutination and granulocyte immunofluorescence assays.

HLA (panel-reactive antibody) antibody screen (multiwell enzyme-linked immunosorbent assay) is first performed. If the screen is positive, the HLA (panel-reactive antibody) antibody identification can be performed.

The monoclonal antibody immobilization to granulocyte antigen assay may be performed to differentiate between HLA and granulocyte-specific antibodies, if the HLA class I antibody screen is positive.

The Neutrophil Serology Laboratory is the designated reference laboratory for the American National Red Cross Blood Services. Testing is offered to Red Cross affiliates and other institutions. Inquiries regarding these services may be directed to the Neutrophil Serology Laboratory at (612) 291–6797.

Cyclic Neutropenia

Cyclic neutropenia is a disorder of neutrophils with an autosomal-dominant mode of inheritance characterized by a periodic decline in the number of neutrophils in the peripheral blood, with intervening periods of normal neutrophil counts. Considered a benign disorder, it is usually diagnosed after the newborn period during infancy. The clinical symptoms of the neutropenic cycle are infections; the severity of the infection depends on the degree of the neutropenia.

Laboratory Findings

Regular oscillations of the neutrophil counts occur every 19–23 days. The decrease in the number of neutrophils in each cycle may be associated with normal neutrophilic counts or neutropenia associated with monocytosis. The BMA findings that accompany the decrease of neutrophils in peripheral blood may vary. The BMA specimen may be hypocellular or show an arrest of maturation in the granulocytic series at the myelocyte stage with an increase of monocytes and plasma cells.

Kostmann Syndrome

Kostmann syndrome, or severe congenital neutropenia, is a disorder of neutrophils inherited in an autosomal-recessive manner that is characterized by infections starting during the first month of life. Laboratory findings include severe neutropenia, with a granulocyte count $<0.5 \times 10^9$/L, associated with monocytosis and moderate eosinophilia. BMA examination shows a decrease in mature forms of the neutrophils, with blockage of the maturation at the promyelocyte or myelocytic stage with or without vacuolization of the immature myeloid cells.

Shwachman-Diamond Syndrome

Shwachman-Diamond syndrome is chronic hypoplastic neutropenia with pancreatic insufficiency.

Neutrophilia

Neutrophilia, often exceeding 30×10^3/mm^3 (30×10^9/L), is typical at birth. Shortly after birth, the absolute neutrophil count decreases, and lymphocytes predominate by 2 weeks of age. The normal range for absolute neutrophil count in infants is $2.5–7.0 \times 10^3$/mm^3, whereas the normal range for children and adults is $1.5–7.0 \times 10^3$/mm^3.

Beyond the neonatal period, neutrophilia is defined as an absolute neutrophil count $>10 \times 10^3$/mm^3. Constitutional neutrophilia is rare and is generally linked to neutrophil migration defects.

Pronounced toxic changes with toxic granules in the neutrophils (Color Fig. 34), a limited left shift, and normal absolute basophil count indicate a reactive neutrophilia.

Causes

Infections

- Primarily bacterial infections
- Less common in viral, mycobacterial, leptospiral, or toxoplasmal infections
- Hantavirus pulmonary syndrome

Drugs, hormones
- Excess colony-stimulating factor (therapeutic administration, colony-stimulating factor–producing tumors)
- Epinephrine (therapeutic administration or endogenous production)
- Corticosteroids (therapeutic administration or endogenous production)
- Poisons, toxins, venoms, lithium

Tissue necrosis
- Burns, trauma, infarct
- Acute gout

Inflammatory disorders
- Collagen vascular disorders
- Other autoimmune disorders

Metabolic
- Ketoacidosis
- Uremia
- Eclampsia

Constitutional (rare)
- Hereditary neutrophilia
- Familial cold urticaria
- Leukocyte adhesion deficiency

Miscellaneous
- Stress, severe exercise
- Pregnancy
- Smoking
- Acute hemorrhage, hemolysis
- Splenectomy

Neutrophils, Hereditary Cytologic Variants

Nuclear abnormalities of neutrophils include the Pelger-Huët anomaly, hereditary hypersegmentation of the neutrophils, and hereditary giant neutrophils. These disorders have an autosomal-dominant inheritance pattern, and none has clinical significance. The diagnosis of these congenital nuclear anomalies can be made by examining the peripheral blood of both parents. Acquired forms of these nuclear morphologic abnormalities, however, are associated with various hematologic disorders.

The Pelger-Huët anomaly is characterized by a failure in nuclear segmentation; most of the neutrophils have two segments or are unsegmented (Color Fig. 35A) and should be differentiated from eosinophils. Acquired Pelger-Huët anomaly is associated with AML, myeloproliferative disorders, hypothyroidism, infections, and use of sulfonamide medications. Eosinophils have a bilobated nucleus and eosinophilic granules in their cytoplasm.

Hereditary hypersegmentation of the neutrophils is characterized by an increased number of segments of the neutrophils, up to nine to ten from the normal three to five. When acquired, this abnormality is associated with vitamins B_{12} and folic acid deficiency.

Hereditary giant neutrophils are characterized by an increase in neutrophil diameter and in the number of segments of each neutrophil. These changes are seen in a small percentage of the neutrophils.

In Alder-Reilly anomaly, an autosomal-recessive disorder, the neutrophil granules are larger and stain lavender or blue (Color Fig. 35C). Similar cytoplasmic abnormalities of the granulocytes may be seen in mucopolysaccharidoses.

Döhle bodies may be seen in the neutrophils of patients with infectious diseases and burns (Color Fig. 35B). In Chédiak-Higashi syndrome, leukocytes contain giant cytoplasmic granules (Color Fig. 36).

Investigation

Investigation entails the taking of a detailed history for evidence of recurrent infections, findings suggestive of a constitutional disorder, symptoms of a current infection, and symptoms of an underlying immunologic disorder or occult neoplasm.

Investigation for drug therapy, toxin, or alcohol exposure.
Physical examination for possible splenomegaly, evidence of occult infection, or evidence of neoplasm.
CBC with differential. Serial CBCs may be necessary to document either a cyclic pattern or neutrophil recovery in patients with transient neutropenia.
Morphologic review of blood smear for evidence of hematopoietic neoplasms, infection-related changes, megaloblastic features, and features of constitutional disorders such as Chédiak-Higashi syndrome.
Evaluation of other hematopoietic lineages for morphologic or numeric abnormalities.
Laboratory workup for possible infection, if clinically suspected.
In selected patients, laboratory assessment of immune status, tests for collagen vascular disorders, or serologic studies for viral infections.
Various radiographic studies in selected patients, including those with suspected constitutional neutropenic disorders, to assess for constitutional bony defects, evidence of neoplasm, or evidence of infection.
Bone marrow examination. This is generally required in adult patients with new-onset neutropenia. Likewise, bone marrow evaluation is necessary in children with suspected neoplasms, aplasia, and selected infections. Many children, however, develop transient neutropenia after presumed viral infections. In these children, who are otherwise healthy and have only isolated neutropenia, a "watch-and-wait" approach is often taken. A bone marrow examination is unlikely to be considered in these children unless spontaneous neutrophil recovery is not evident within 1–2 months.

Other Tests

Numerous ancillary tests may be warranted in selected neutropenic patients, including tests for folate and vitamin B_{12} levels, tests for collagen vascular disease, assessment of immune status, granulocyte antibody studies, cytogenetic studies, serologic tests for infectious agents, neutrophil survival studies, and determination of copper levels.

Posttransplantation Lymphoproliferative Disorder

Posttransplantation lymphoproliferative disorders (PTLDs) may arise in the asymptomatic patient incidental to other clinical or radiographic findings, and they may be localized to systemic involvement. An unexplained infectious syndrome in a transplant patient should raise the suspicion of a PTLD. PTLD can present as early as <1 month to as late as several years after transplantation. In general, PTLD is remarkable for having a short posttransplantation time of onset. The time of onset is shorter in patients treated with cyclosporine and tacrolimus than in those in the precyclosporine era. In a large series, 47% of cases occurred within 6 months, 62% within 1 year, and 90% within 5 years after transplantation. PTLDs that are not associated with EBV tend to arise at a later time than those that are not associated with the virus. PTLDs of T-cell origin are uncommon and may also arise later in the posttransplantation course.
The clinical presentation of PTLD is heterogeneous but may be

1. An IM-like syndrome with or without generalized lymphadenopathy
2. One or more extranodal tumors
3. A fulminant and disseminated presentation with sepsis

A mononucleosis syndrome may occur early after transplantation, particularly in association with a primary EBV infection.
A PTLD that occurs later is more likely to be circumscribed anatomically and to be associated with a more gradual clinical course. Extranodal disease with visceral involvement is common with gastrointestinal, pulmonary, or central nervous system symptoms. Lymphadenopathy is generally painless, and atypical lymphocytes may or may not be present in the peripheral blood.
Most patients with PTLD present with at least one tumor. Approximately two-thirds of these tumors are extranodal, and approximately one-third are nodal. The allograft may be involved.

Lymphadenopathy, Lymphomas, and Other Pediatric Tumors

Lymphadenopathy

Causes of lymphadenopathy include the following[3]:

- Infection
  - Viral infection
  - IM*
  - CMV infection*
  - HIV infection†
  - Postvaccinal lymphadenitis‡
- Bacterial
  - Staphylococcal infection*
  - Streptococcal infection*
  - Tuberculosis*
  - Cat-scratch disease‡ (Color Fig. 37A, B)
  - Syphilis*
  - Chancroid‡
  - Chlamydial infection*
  - Lymphogranuloma venereum‡
- Protozoal
  - Toxoplasmosis*
- Fungal
  - Cryptococcal infection*
  - Histoplasmosis*
  - Coccidioidomycosis*
- Autoimmune disorders
  - Sjögren syndrome‡
  - Rheumatoid arthritis*
- Iatrogenic causes
  - Drug hypersensitivity (phenytoin, phenylbutazone, methyldopa, meprobamate, hydralazine hydrochloride)*
  - Serum sickness*
  - Silicone exposure
- Malignancy
  - Hodgkin lymphoma*
  - Non-Hodgkin lymphoma*
  - Acute and chronic leukemia*
  - Metastatic cancer*
- Other disorders
  - Castleman disease* (giant lymph node hyperplasia)
  - Kikuchi-Fujimoto lymphadenitis‡ (Color Fig. 38)
  - Sarcoidosis*
  - Dermatopathic lymphadenopathy‡
  - Histiocytosis X*
  - Sinus histiocytosis with massive lymphadenopathy*
  - Abnormal immune response*

*Localized or generalized lymphadenopathy.
†Generalized lymphadenopathy.
‡Localized lymphadenopathy.

[3]Kjeldsberg C, Elenitoba-Johnson K, Foucar K, et al. *Practical diagnosis of hematologic disorders*, 3rd ed. Chicago: American Society of Clinical Pathologists Press, 2000:347.

Table 36. Clinical Features of Common Pediatric Lymphomas

Clinical Features	Diagnosis	Comment
Mediastinum		
Child or teenager, male, rapid growth	Lymphoblastic (convoluted) T lymphoma	May have respiratory failure, pleural or pericardial effusion, superior vena caval syndrome, rapid response to steroids
Teenager or young adult, female, rapid growth	Large B-cell lymphoma	May have compression symptoms
Teenager or young adult, female, slow growth	Hodgkin disease, nodular sclerosing type	May have superior vena caval obstruction, tracheal compression, parasternal mass
Abdomen, gastrointestinal tract, ovary		
Child or young adult, rapid growth	Small transformed (noncleaved) lymphoma, Burkitt type	Nonendemic form
Nodes, cervical or axillary		
Child or teenager, slow growth	Hodgkin disease, lymphocyte-predominant type	
Child or teenager, rapid growth	Anaplastic large-cell lymphoma, $CD30^+$	May present with small-cell variant with clinical features suggesting infection
Bone		
Child, rapid growth	Small transformed (noncleaved) lymphoma, Burkitt type	Endemic form

Modified from Collins RD, Swerdlow SA. *Pediatric hematopathology.* New York: Churchill Livingstone, 2001.

Lymphoma

Lymphomas are generally classified into two main histologic types: Hodgkin lymphoma and non-Hodgkin lymphoma (NHL). Hodgkin lymphoma is extremely rare in children <3 years of age. NHL is frequently associated with leukemia or immunodeficiency disease. Blast cells in peripheral blood and bone marrow make the differentiation of lymphoma from ALL difficult. Lymph node biopsy is required for the diagnosis of lymphomas.

NHL in childhood is virtually limited to three histologic types:

1. Lymphoblastic lymphoma: 30–35% small noncleaved cell (undifferentiated)
2. Burkitt and non-Burkitt types: 40–50%
3. Large-cell lymphoma: 15–20%

Clinical and Genetic Features of Pediatric Lymphomas

Table 36 lists the clinical features of common pediatric lymphomas.

Table 37 gives the cell of origin, major genotypic and karyotypic abnormalities, and EBV association in the major types of pediatric lymphoma.

Table 38 shows common cytogenetic findings in various types of malignant lymphoma.

Processing of Lymph Node Biopsy Specimens

See Figure 39.

Table 37. Cell of Origin, Major Genotypic and Karyotypic Abnormalities, and Epstein-Barr Virus (EBV) Association in Major Types of Pediatric Lymphomas

Diagnosis	Cell Type and Other Important Cellular Constituents	Major Genotypic or Karyotypic Abnormalities	EBV Association
Burkitt lymphoma	B cell similar to those in follicular center or transformed memory-type B cell	MYC rearrangement from 8q24 immunoglobulin heavy chain (14q32) or, less often, to κ (2p11) or λ (22q11); MYC mutations	Endemic: almost all EBV positive Sporadic: 10–40% EBV positive
T-lymphoblastic lymphoma[a]	Thymic type I lymphoblast	Translocations involving T-cell receptor (α, β, γ, or δ chains on 14q11, 7q32, 14q11, or 7p15, respectively) and protooncogenes (mostly transcription factors)	None
Anaplastic large-cell (Ki-1 antigen positive) lymphoma	Cytotoxic T cell; less often, "null" (indeterminate) cell	t(2;5)(P23;P35) involving nucleophosmin gene (5) and anaplastic lymphoma kinase gene (2) with NPM/ALK fusion product ("p80")	Usually none
HD, nodular lymphocyte predominance	Follicular center B cell ("L and H" Reed-Sternberg variants)	No consistent abnormality in these clonal B cells	None
HD, nodular sclerosis and mixed cellularity types	Reed-Sternberg cells in some cases resemble follicular center cells but do not show immunoglobulin gene expression; some cases of T-cell origin; others undefined Reactive cellular elements that, like Reed-Sternberg cells, are important in cytokine secretion	No consistent abnormality but typically aneuploid	>50% EBV positive, with highest proportion in children <10 years old

HD, Hodgkin disease.
From Collins RD, Swerdlow SH. *Pediatric hematopathology.* New York: Churchill Livingstone, 2001.

Table 38. Common Cytogenetic Findings in Malignant Lymphomas

SLL	–14(q2–24), t(11;18)(q21;q21), –6q
FL	t(14;18)(q32;q21)
MCL	t(11;14)(q13;q32)
MZL	+3, t(11;18)
DLBL	t(3;14)(q27;q32), t(3;22)(q27;q11)
LPL	No consistent finding
ALCL	t(2;5)(p23;q35)
Burkitt	t(8;14)(q24;q32), t(2;8)(p12;q24), t(8;22)(q24;q11)
MF	–6q, +14
ATLL	–6q, –14q
MM	1q abnormalities

ALCL, anaplastic large-cell lymphoma; ATLL, adult T-cell lymphoma/leukemia; Burkitt, Burkitt lymphoma; DLBL, diffuse large-B-cell lymphoma; FL, follicular lymphoma; LPL, lymphoplasmacytic lymphoma; MCL, mantle cell lymphoma; MF, mycosis fungoides; MM, multiple myeloma; MZL, marginal zone lymphoma; SLL, small lymphocytic lymphoma.
From Kjeldsberg C, Elenitoba-Johnson K, Foucar K, et al. *Practical diagnosis of hematologic disorders*, 3rd ed. Chicago, IL: American Society of Clinical Pathologists Press, 2000.

Lymphoma, Burkitt

Pathology and Pathogenesis

EBV infection has a major role in the pathogenesis of Burkitt lymphoma. The EBV genome is present in tumor cells in 95% of endemic cases in equatorial Africa compared to 20% of sporadic cases in the United States. How EBV contributes to the pathogenesis of Burkitt lymphoma remains unclear. Preexisting immunodeficiency (congenital or acquired) also predisposes to the development of NHL.

Burkitt lymphoma and non-Burkitt small noncleaved lymphoma may be nodal and extranodal. They usually arise in the abdomen and the cervical region. Burkitt lym-

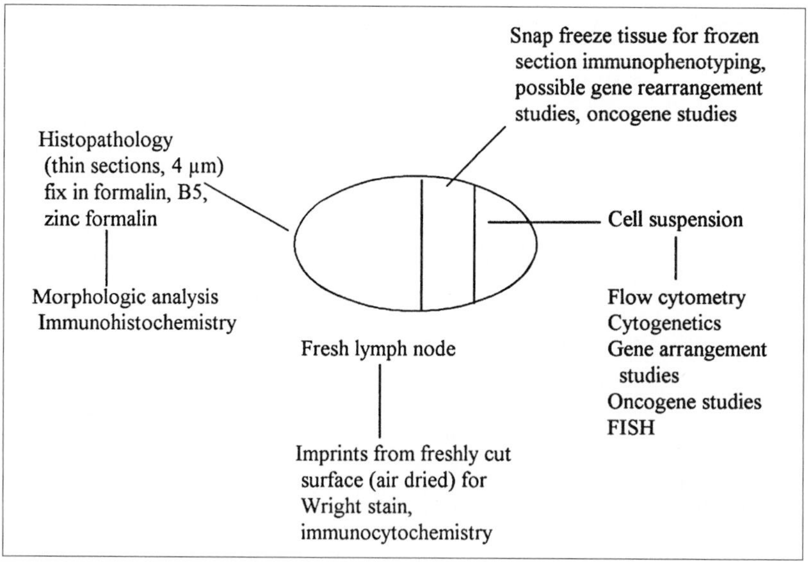

Fig. 39. Scheme for processing lymph node biopsy specimens. FISH, fluorescent *in situ* hybridization.

Table 39. Cytogenetic Findings in Diffuse B-Cell Lymphoma

	Cytogenetics	Gene
Large cell	t(3;14)(q27;q32)	BCL6
	t(3;4)(q27;p11)	BCL6
Anaplastic	t(2;5)(p23;q35)	NPM-ALK
	t(10;14)(q24;q32)	LYT10
B-cell CLL	t(14;19)(p32;p13)	BCL3
B-cell lymphoma	t(10;14)(q24;q32)	LYT10
Lymphoplasmacytoid B-cell lymphoma	t(9;14)(p13;q32)	PAX5

CLL, chronic lymphocytic leukemia.

phoma is the most common type of lymphoma in tropical Africa but occurs sporadically worldwide. The African form frequently affects the jaw and may result from stimulation of the immune system by EBV. Cytogenic rearrangements include t(8;14)(q24;q32)—90% of cases; and t(8;22)(q24;q11) and t(2;8)(q13;q24) and t(2;8)(q13;q24)—10% of cases. These rearrangements translocate the C-*myc* oncogene from the long arm of chromosome 8 to the immunoglobulin heavy-chain locus on chromosome 14 or to light-chain loci on chromosomes 2 and 22.

Non-African Burkitt lymphoma usually presents as an intraabdominal mass arising from Peyer patches in the ileocecal region or from mesenteric lymph nodes. Intussusception or intestinal obstruction may occur. Involvement of ovaries, kidney, and retroperitoneum is not uncommon. Bone marrow involvement is associated with central nervous system disease and short survival.

Diagnosis

Histologically, monotonous, intermediate-sized cells usually involve the paracortical (T-cell) areas of the lymph node. The cytoplasm is moderate and the nucleus round with prominent nucleoli. Histiocytes with abundant cytoplasmic and nuclear debris are intermixed with the neoplastic cells, which gives the "starry sky" appearance (Color Fig. 40). The main morphologic difference between B-cell–derived Burkitt lymphoma and non-Burkitt lymphoma is the variability in the size and shape of the nucleus of the cells in non-Burkitt lymphoma. The revised European-American classification for non-Burkitt lymphoma is "High-grade B-cell lymphoma, Burkitt-like."

Lymphoma, Diffuse B-cell

See Table 39.

Lymphoma, Hodgkin

Hodgkin lymphoma (Hodgkin disease) accounts for approximately 5% of cancers in children and adolescents <15 years old in the United States. The possible role of EBV is supported by serologic studies. It predominantly affects patients <10 years old at diagnosis, with roughly equal gender incidence in adolescence. Preexisting immunodeficiency, either congenital or acquired, increases the risk of developing Hodgkin disease.

Differential Diagnosis of Hodgkin Lymphoma[4]

- Nodular lymphocyte predominance
  - Progressive transformation of germinal centers
  - Nodular paracortical hyperplasia

[4]Kjeldsberg C, Elenitoba-Johnson K, Foucar K, et al. *Practical diagnosis of hematologic disorders*, 3rd ed. Chicago: American Society of Clinical Pathologists Press, 2000:347.

Lymphocyte-rich classic Hodgkin lymphoma
T-cell/histiocyte-rich large-B-cell lymphoma
Small lymphocytic lymphoma/classic lymphocytic lymphoma
Follicular hyperplasia
Follicular lymphoma

Lymphocyte-rich classic Hodgkin disease
Nodular lymphocyte predominance Hodgkin disease
Follicular lymphoma
Mantle cell lymphoma
Reactive hyperplasia

Nodular sclerosis Hodgkin disease
Anaplastic large-cell lymphoma
Peripheral T-cell lymphoma
Primary mediastinal (thymic) large-B-cell lymphoma
Mediastinal seminoma (germinoma)
Metastatic neoplasms (e.g., carcinoma, melanoma)
Necrotizing granulomatous lymphadenitis (e.g., cat-scratch disease)

Mixed cellularity
T-cell/histiocyte-rich large-B-cell lymphoma
Peripheral T-cell lymphoma
Anaplastic large-cell lymphoma
IM
Angioimmunoblastic lymphadenopathy

Lymphocyte depletion Hodgkin disease
Nodular sclerosis, syncytial type
Anaplastic large-cell lymphoma
Large-cell non-Hodgkin lymphoma

Diagnostic Tests

Pathologic Findings

The Reed-Sternberg cell, a large (15- to 45-μ in diameter) cell with multiple or multilobulated nuclei is considered the hallmark of Hodgkin disease, although similar cells are seen in IM, NHL, and other conditions. The cellular origin of the Reed-Sternberg cell remains in dispute. An infiltrate of apparently normal lymphocytes, plasma cells, and eosinophils surround the Reed-Sternberg cell and vary with the histologic subtype. Other features that distinguish the histologic subtypes include various degrees of fibrosis and the presence of collagen bands and necrosis. The four major histologic subtypes are

1. Lymphocyte predominant
2. Nodular sclerosing
3. Mixed cellularity
4. Lymphocyte depleted

Historically, prognosis is linked to histologic subtype, with lymphocyte predominant disease having the most favorable prognosis and lymphocyte depleted the least favorable.

Hodgkin disease appears to arise in lymphoid tissue and spreads to adjacent lymph node areas. Hematogenous spread occurs, which leads to involvement of the liver, spleen, bone, bone marrow, or brain, and is usually associated with systemic symptoms. Levels of various cytokines have been shown to be elevated in patients' sera or are produced by cultured cell lines or Hodgkin disease tissue. They may well be responsible for the systemic symptoms of fever and night sweats (interleukin-1 or interleukin-2) and weight loss (tissue necrosis factor).

Various degrees of cellular immune impairment can be identified in the majority of patients newly diagnosed with Hodgkin disease. The severity of the immune defect varies with the extent of disease and persists even after successful curative therapy.

Painless, firm, cervical or supraclavicular adenopathy is the most common presenting sign. Inguinal or axillary adenopathy sites are uncommon areas of presentation. An anterior mediastinal mass is often present and disappears quickly with therapy. Depending on the extent and location of nodal and extranodal disease, patients might present with symptoms and signs of airway obstruction, pleural or pericardial effusion, hepatocellular dysfunction, or bone marrow infiltration (anemia, neutropenia, or thrombocytopenia). Nephrotic syndrome is a rare complication.

Because of the impaired cellular immunity, concomitant tuberculous or fungal infections may complicate Hodgkin disease and predispose to complications during immunosuppressive therapy. Varicella-zoster infections occur at some time during the course of the disease in approximately 30% of cases.

Biopsy Findings

Excisional biopsy is preferred over needle biopsy to ensure that adequate tissue is obtained, both for light microscopy and for appropriate immunocytochemical studies, culture, and cytogenetic analysis if routine studies fail to provide a firm diagnosis. Hodgkin disease is rarely diagnosed with certainty on frozen-section samples. Ideally, a portion of the biopsy specimen should be frozen and stored to allow for other studies.

Staging

Once the diagnosis of Hodgkin disease is established, extent of disease (i.e., stage) should be determined.

Cotswald Modification of the Ann Arbor Staging Classification for Hodgkin Disease[5]

Stage I	Involvement of a single lymph node region (I) or a single extralymphatic organ or site (IE)
Stage II	Involvement of two or more lymph node regions on the same side of the diaphragm (II) or localized involvement of an extralymphatic organ or site (IIE)
Stage III	Involvement of lymph node regions on both sides of the diaphragm (III) or localized involvement of an extralymphatic organ or site (IIIE) or spleen (IIIS) or both (IIISE)
III_1	With or without involvement of splenic hilar, celiac, or portal nodes
III_2	With involvement of paraaortic, iliac, or mesenteric nodes
Stage IV	Diffuse or disseminated involvement of one or more extralymphatic organs with or without lymph node involvement
A	No symptoms
B	Fever, drenching sweats, weight loss, pruritus
X	Bulky disease: More than one-third the width of the mediastinum >10 cm maximal dimension of nodal mass
E	Involvement of a single extranodal site, contiguous or proximal to a known nodal site

Staging Procedures in Hodgkin Disease[6]

Required procedures

- Clinical history and physical examination
- Lymph node biopsy, BMB
- Radiologic studies: chest radiograph; CT scan of chest and whole abdomen, including the pelvis; lymphangiography
- Laboratory tests: CBC; serum alkaline phosphatase and lactate dehydrogenase levels; liver and renal function tests, including uric acid level and urinalysis; ESRz
- Bilateral iliac crest BMB

Ancillary studies (when clinically indicated)

- Skeletal radiographic examination
- Gallium whole-body scanning
- Laparotomy to include splenectomy, liver biopsy, and intraabdominal lymph node biopsy (celiac, porta hepatis, mesenteric, paraaortic, iliac nodes), if information is likely to affect therapy

[5]Lister TA, Crowther D, Sutcliffe SB, et al. Report of a committee convened to discuss the evaluation and staging of patients with Hodgkin disease: Cotswald meeting. *J Clin Oncol* 1989;7(11):1630–1636.

[6]Kjeldsberg C, Elenitoba-Johnson K, Foucar K, et al. *Practical diagnosis of hematologic disorders*, 3rd ed. Chicago: American Society of Clinical Pathologists Press, 2000:347.

Lymphoma, Large-Cell

Large-cell lymphomas are a heterogeneous group that includes Ki-1 positive lymphoma. Large-cell lymphoma may involve peripheral lymph nodes, nasopharynx, gastrointestinal tract, mediastinum, lungs, bone, gonads, skin, and soft tissue.

Diagnosis

The cells have large nuclei and less cytoplasm than reactive histocytes. Large-cell lymphoma can be divided into large cleaved, large noncleaved, and immunoblastic subtypes. The large noncleaved types have round or oval vesicular nuclei with two or three prominent basophilic nucleoli. The large cleaved form has scant cytoplasm, coarsely clumped chromatin, and indistinct cytoplasm. The immunoblastic form has round or oval nuclei with one or several large, central nucleoli. No significant difference in the clinical course of large-cell lymphoma correlates with the histologic subtype.

Fifty percent to 60% of large-cell lymphomas are of B-cell origin. The Ki-1 antigen (CD30) may be present in large-cell lymphoma, and this form has a helper T-cell phenotype and is characterized by peripheral lymph node and skin involvement.

Lymphoma, Lymphoblastic

Lymphoblastic lymphoma cells are usually derived from T-cell precursors. Clinically, children present with massive leukocytosis, an anterior mediastinal mass, massive generalized lymphadenopathy, and organomegaly with frequent dissemination to the bone marrow, gonads, and central nervous system. Gingival hyperplasia or priapism may be associated with very high peripheral WBC counts.

Diagnosis

Morphologically, lymphoblastic lymphoma is characterized by a diffuse nodal involvement. The malignant cells have scanty cytoplasm, and the nucleus is convoluted (Color Fig. 41A) or nonconvoluted (Color Fig. 41B) with rare nucleoli. Lymphoblastic lymphoma has a diffuse monotonous pattern but usually demonstrates a selective involvement of the paracortical (T-cell) areas of the lymph node. Eighty percent of the lymphomas are T cell and are reactive for the T-cell marker UCHL-1.

Chromosomal translocation involving protooncogenes (e.g., tel, rhomb2, rhombi, hox11, ly11, myc, lck) and T-cell receptor genes on chromosomes 7 or 14 results in activation of the protooncogene, which contributes to malignant transformation in some cases of lymphoblastic lymphoma.

Lymphoma, Non-Hodgkin

NHL results from malignant clonal proliferation of lymphocytes of T-cell, B-cell, or indeterminate cell origin. NHL occurs with an annual incidence of 9.1 in 1 million white children and 46 in 1 million black children <15 years of age in the United States. In equatorial Africa, 50% of childhood cancers are lymphoma. Unlike in Hodgkin disease, the incidence of NHL increases steadily throughout life. In some situations there is overlap with ALL. Patients with lymphoblastic NHL and those with >25% lymphoblasts in the bone marrow are arbitrarily classified and treated as if they had ALL, whereas patients with B-cell ALL are treated similarly to patients with Burkitt lymphoma even if no extramedullary disease is present.

Classification

Classification of Non-Hodgkin Lymphoma in Children

Type	Incidence	Cell Type
Lymphoblastic	30–35%	80% T cell
Burkitt	40–45%	Mostly B cell, IgM
Small-cell non-Burkitt	5%	Mostly B cell
Large-cell anaplastic	15%	B cell; rarely T cell

Classification of T-Cell and B-Cell Pediatric Lymphomas

Type	Presenting Sites
T-cell lymphomas	
Lymphoblastic (convoluted)	Thymus or anterior mediastinum
Anaplastic large-cell, CD 30 positive, small-cell variant	Nodes (cervical, axillary, and skin)
Natural killer–like T cell	Hepatosplenic (intestinal?)
Mycosis fungoides	Skin
B-cell lymphomas	
Large transformed (noncleaved) cell	Nodes, anterior mediastinum
Small transformed (noncleaved), Burkitt type	Ileum, elsewhere in abdomen, gonads, bone
Follicular center cell, nodular, small cleaved	Nodes, superficial
Immunoblastic lymphoma	Nodes, soft tissue
Lymphoblastic	Mediastinum (?), skin

Staging

Pretreatment Studies for Staging Pediatric Non-Hodgkin Lymphoma

CBC
Serum levels of electrolytes, uric acid, lactate dehydrogenase, creatinine, calcium, phosphorus
Liver function tests
Chest radiograph and chest CT scan if radiograph is abnormal
Abdominal and pelvic ultrasonography or CT scan or both
Gallium scan, bone scan, or both
Bilateral BMA and BMB
Spinal fluid cytologic examination

Staging System for Non-Hodgkin Lymphoma in Childhood[7]

Stage I	A single tumor (extranodal) or single anatomic area (nodal), with the exclusion of mediastinum or abdomen
Stage II	A single tumor (extranodal) with regional node involvement Two or more nodal areas on the same side of the diaphragm Two single (extranodal) tumors with or without regional node involvement on the same side of the diaphragm A primary gastrointestinal tract tumor, usually in the ileocecal area, with or without involvement of the associated mesenteric nodes only, which must be grossly (>90%) resected
Stage III	Two single tumors (extranodal) on opposite sides of the diaphragm Two or more nodal areas above and below the diaphragm Any primary intrathoracic tumor (mediastinal, pleural, thymic) Any extensive primary intraabdominal disease
Stage IV	Any of the above, with initial involvement of central nervous system, bone marrow, or both at time of diagnosis

Features of Pediatric Non-Hodgkin Lymphoma

Table 40 shows the morphologic, cytochemical, and immunotypic features of pediatric non-Hodgkin lymphoma.

NHL Tumors, Pediatric

Table 41 lists antibodies commonly used in the immunophenotyping of pediatric non-Hodgkin lymphoma.

Immunohistochemical Staining Patterns of Pediatric Tumors

See Table 42.

[7]Murphy SB. Classification, staging and end results treatment of childhood non-Hodgkin lymphomas: dissimilarities from lymphomas in adults. *Semin Oncol* 1980;7:332–339.

Table 40. Comparison of Morphologic, Cytochemical, and Immunotypic Features of Childhood Non-Hodgkin Lymphoma

	Type of Lymphoma			
Detection Method	Lymphoblastic	Burkitt (Small Noncleaved)	Small Noncleaved Non-Burkitt (High-Grade B-Cell Burkitt-Like)	Large Cell ("Histiocytic")
Imprint cytology, Wright stain	FAB L_1 or FAB L_2 blasts	FAB L_3 blasts	FAB L_3 blasts	Variable, large transformed lymphocytes
Nuclear size	Smaller than macrophage nucleus	Approximates macrophage nucleus; nuclear monotony	Approximates macrophage nucleus; nuclear variability	Larger than macrophage nucleus
Nuclear chromatin	Delicate	Coarsely reticulated	Coarsely reticulated	Clumped, vesicular
Nucleoli	Small, inconspicuous	Prominent	Prominent	Variable, often prominent
Mitotic index	High	High	High	Variable
Cytoplasm	Scant	Moderate	Moderate	Moderate to abundant
Cytoplasmic vacuoles	Inconspicuous	Prominent	Prominent	Inconspicuous
Periodic acid–Schiff stain	Occasionally positive	Negative	Negative	Occasionally positive
Methyl green pyronine stain	Negative or focal positive	Strongly positive	Strongly positive	Variable, usually positive
Terminal deoxynucleotidyl transferase	Positive	Negative	Negative	Negative
Immunologic markers	Immature T cell, precursor	Mature B surface IgM (CD19, 20, 22, 79)$^+$, CD10$^+$, CD5$^-$, CD23$^-$	Usually B (CD19, 20, 22, 79a)$^+$; may be non-B, non-T; rarely T; CD5$^-$, usually CD10$^-$	Usually B; Ki-1 antigen positive non-B; non-T
Cytogenic translocation	t(1:19), t(10:14), t(11:14), t(1:14)	t(8:14), t(8:22), t(2:8)	t(8:14), t(8:22), t(2:8)	t(14:18), t(8:14); in anaplastic large cell

FAB, French-American-British classification of acute lymphoblastic leukemia.
Adapted from Perkins SL, Segal GH, Kjeldsberg CR. Classification of non-Hodgkin lymphoma in children. *Semin Diagn Pathol* 1995;12:303–313. From Gilbert-Barness E, ed. *Potter's pathology of the fetus and infant.* St. Louis: Mosby–Year Book, 1997.

Table 41. Commonly Used Antibodies in Immunophenotyping of Pediatric Non-Hodgkin Lymphoma

Antibody	Application	Use
B cell		
CD19	F	B cells, all stage of development
CD20	P, F	Mature B cells, does not detect precursor B cells or plasma cells
CD22	F	Mature B cells
CD79a	P	B cells, all stages of development
κ/λ	P, F	Cell surface expression in mature B cells, used to detect monoclonal populations
T cell		
CD1a	P, F	Immature T cells, histocytes
CD2	F	Pan T-cell marker
CD3	P, F	Pan T-cell marker
CD4	P, F	Marks T helper cells
CD5	P, F	Pan T-cell marker; coexpressed on some B-cell lymphomas
CD7	F	Pan T-cell markers
CD8	P, F	Marks T suppressor cells
CD43	P	T-cell marker, will also mark myeloid cells, plasma cells, and some B-cell lymphomas
CD45RO	P	T-cell marker
Others		
CD10 (CALLA)	P, F	Common lymphoblastic leukemia antigen; seen in precursor B and T cells, in follicular center cells, and in Burkitt lymphoma
CD30	P, F	Activation antigen associated with anaplastic large-cell lymphomas
CD45	P, F	Common leukocyte antigen; may be decreased in precursor B and T cells or absent in some immunoblastic large-cell lymphomas
TdT	P, F	Terminal deoxytidyltransferase; marker of precursor T and B cells
ALK	P	Detects fusion protein of t(2;5) or inv(2) seen in anaplastic large-cell lymphomas
p80	P	Detects fusion protein of t(2;5) seen in anaplastic large-cell lymphomas

F, flow or frozen tissue; P, paraffin.

Bone Marrow Metastases and Childhood Malignant Tumors

Of the nonhematologic malignancies of childhood, neuroblastoma and rhabdomyosarcoma are the most frequent metastatic neoplasms to the bone marrow.

BMB specimens show

- Marrow without abnormal architecture, infiltrate, or fibrous stoma, although it may be very hypocellular
- Marrow with similar features but with a pathologic increase in reticulin
- Marrow with distorted architecture, increased fibrous stroma, and abnormal although not frankly malignant mononuclear cells
- Marrow with an obvious infiltrate of malignant cells

Osteoblasts positive for neural cell adhesion molecule (NCAM) may be present. Neural cell adhesion molecule has also been found to be expressed by Ewing's tumor,

Table 42. Immunohistochemical Staining Patterns of Pediatric Tumors

	Antibody								
Tumor	Vimentin	Desmin, Actin	Keratin	NSE	Neurofilament	S-100 Protein	LCA, B- and T-Cell Markers	NB84	013 (HBA 71 MIC2)
Small round cell									
Malignant lymphoma	+/–	–	–	–	–	–	+	–	–
Ewing's sarcoma and extraosseous Ewing's sarcoma	+	–	+/–	–	–	–	–	+/–	+
Desmoplastic small round cell tumor	+	+	+	+	–	–	–	–	–
PPNET	+	–	+/–	+	–	–	–	–	–
Neuroblastoma	+	–	–	+	+/–	+/–	–	+	–
Rhabdomyosarcoma	+	+	–	–	–	–	–	–	–
Nephroblastoma (Wilms tumor)	+	–	+	–	–	–	–	–	–
Others									
Chondroblastoma	+	–	–	–	–	+	–	–	–
Pheochromocytoma	–	–	–	+	+	+	–	–	–
Osteogenic sarcoma	+	–	–	–	–	–	–	–	–

+, present; –, absent; +/–, often present; –/+, occasionally present; NSE, neuron-specific enolase; PPNET, peripheral primitive neuroectodermal tumor.

peripheral neuroectodermal tumor, rhabdomyosarcoma, medulloblastoma, retinoblastoma, and pinealoblastoma. Neurone-specific enolase is also expressed by most of the neural-origin tumors.

The tyrosine hydroxylase gene is thought to be specific for neuroblastoma; very small numbers of putative neuroblasts can be detected in aspirated bone marrow. Some molecular techniques such as FISH can be applied directly to BMA specimens to detect chromosomal or genetic features of neuroblasts that are known to be of prognostic significance: Amplification of N-*myc*, deletions of chromosome 1p, and hyperdiploidy can be demonstrated in intact tumor cells on bone marrow smears.

Bibliography

Al-Mulla ZS, Christensen RD. Neutropenia in the neonate. *Clin Perinatol* 1995;2:711–739.

Alter BP. Arms and the man or hands and the child: congenital anomalies and hematologic syndromes. *J Pediatr Hematol Oncol* 1997;19:287–291.

Association for Molecular Pathology. Recommendations for in-house development and operation of molecular diagnostic tests. *Am J Clin Pathol* 1999;111:449–463.

Bagby GC. Leukopenia and leukocytosis. In: Goldman L, Bennett JC, eds. *Cecil textbook of medicine*, 21st ed. Philadelphia: WB Saunders, 2000:919–933.

Baranger L, Bauchel A, Leverger G, et al. Monosomy-7 in childhood hemopoietic disorders. *Leukemia* 1990;4:345.

Bennett JM, Catovsky D, Danie MT, et al. Criteria for the diagnosis of acute leukemia of megakaryocyte lineage (M7). A report of the French-American-British Cooperative Group. *Ann Intern Med* 1985;103:460.

Beutler E. Hereditary and acquired sideroblastic anemias. In: Beutler E, Coller BS, Kipps TJ, et al., eds. *Williams hematology*, 5th ed. New York: McGraw-Hill, 1995:747–751.

Bitter MA, Franklin WA, Larson RA, et al. Morphology in ki-1 (CD30)-positive lymphoma is correlated with clinical features and the presence of a unique chromosomal abnormality (2;5)(p23;q35). *Am J Surg Pathol* 1990;14:305.

Bitter MA, LeBeau MM, Larson RA, et al. A morphologic and cytochemical study of acute myelomonocytic leukemia with abnormal marrow eosinophils associated with Inv (16)(pp13q22). *Am J Clin Pathol* 1984;81:73.

Bonilla FA, Rosen FS, Geha RS. Primary immunodeficiency diseases. In: Nathan DG, Orkin SH, eds. *Nathan and Oski's hematology of infancy and childhood*. Philadelphia: WB Saunders, 1998:1023–1050.

Bowman J. Assays to predict the clinical significance of blood group antibodies. *Semin Perinatol* 1998;5:412–416.

Bowman JM. Alloimmune hemolytic disease of the fetus and newborn. In: Lee GR, Foerster J, Lukens JN, et al., eds. *Wintrobe's clinical hematology*, 10th ed. Baltimore, MD: Williams & Wilkins, 1999:1210–1232.

Brigden EA, Graydon C. Eosinophilia detected by automated blood cell counting in ambulatory North American outpatients: incidence and clinical significance. *Arch Pathol Lab Med* 1997;121:963–967.

Bucceri V, Shetty V, Yoshida N, et al. The role of an antimyeloperoxidase antibody in the diagnosis and classification of acute leukaemia: a comparison with light and electron microscopy cytochemistry. *Br J Haematol* 1992;80:62–68.

Bux J, Behrens G, Jaeger G, et al. Diagnosis and clinical course of autoimmune neutropenia in infancy: analysis of 240 cases. *Blood* 1998;91:181–186.

Cartwright GE. *Diagnostic laboratory hematology*, 4th ed. New York: Grune & Stratton, 1968.

Castelino DJ, McNair P, Kay TWH. Lymphocytopenia in a hospital population: what does it signify? *Aust N Z Med* 1997;27:170–174.

Cerezo L, Shuster JJ, Pulen J, et al. Laboratory correlates and prognostic significance of granular acute lymphoblastic leukemia in children. A Pediatric Oncology Group Study. *Am J Clin Pathol* 1991;95:526–531.

Chadburn A, Chen JM, Hsu DT, et al. The morphologic and molecular genetic categories of posttransplantation lymphoproliferative disorders are clinically relevant. *Cancer* 1998;82:1978–1987.

Chan JKC, Ng CS, Hui PK, et al. Anaplastic large cell Ki-l lymphoma. Delineation of two morphological types. *Histopathology* 1989;15:11–34.

Chessels JM, Swansbury GJ, Reeves B, et al. Cytogenetics and prognosis in childhood lymphoblastic leukaemia: results of MRC UKALL X. *Br J Haematol* 1997;99:93–100.

Chott A, Kaserer L, Augustin I, et al. Ki-l positive large cell lymphoma. A clinicopathological study of 41 cases. *Am J Surg Pathol* 1990;14:439–448.

Christensen RD, Anstall HB, Rothstein G. Review: deficiencies in the neutrophil system of newborn infants and the use of leukocyte transfusions in the treatment of neonatal sepsis. *J Clin Apheresis* 1982;1:33–41.

Claas FH. Immune mechanisms leading to drug-induced blood dyscrasias. *Eur J Haematol Suppl* 1996;60:64–68.

Coleman WB, Tsongalis GJ. *Molecular diagnostics for the clinical laboratorian.* Totowa, NJ: Humana Press, 1997.

Cordero L, Cuadrado R, Hall CB, et al. Primary atypical pneumonia: an epidemic caused by *Mycoplasma pneumoniae*. *J Pediatr* 1967;71(1):1–12.

Corey SJ, Locker J, Oliveri DR, et al. A non-classical translocation involving 17q12 retinoic acid receptor alpha in acute promyelocytic leukemia with atypical features. *Leukemia* 1994;8:1350–1353.

Cunningham FG, MacDonald PC, Gant NF, eds. *Williams' obstetrics*, 19th ed. Norwalk, CT: Appleton & Lange, 1993.

Cynober T, Mohandes N, Tchernia G. Red cell abnormalities in hereditary spherocytosis: relevance to understanding of the variable expression of clinical severity. *J Lab Clin Med* 1996;128:259–269.

Dauwerse JG, Kievits T, Beverstock GC, et al. Rapid detection of the chromosome 16 inversion in acute nonlymphocytic leukemia, subtype M4: regional localization of the breakpoint in the 16p. *Cytogenet Cell Genet* 1990;53:126–128.

Davis BH, Olsen S, Biglow NC, et al. Detection of fetal red cells in fetomaternal hemorrhage using a fetal hemoglobin monoclonal antibody by flow cytometry. *Transfusion* 1998;38:749–756.

De Andres B, Rakasz E, Hagen M, et al. Lack of Fc-epsilon receptors on murine eosinophils: implications for the functional significance of elevated IgE and eosinophils in parasitic infections. *Blood* 1997;89:3826–3836.

Dehner LP. Ki-l lymphoma. *Pediatr Pathol* 1991;11:183–189.

Delaunay J. Genetics disorders of the red cell membranes. *FEBS Lett* 1995:369:34–37.

Dierlamm J, Stul M, Vranckx H, et al. FISH and related techniques in the diagnosis of lymphoma. *Cancer Surv* 1997;30:3–20.

Dorfman RF, Berry GJ. Kikuchi's histiocytic necrotizing lymphadenitis: an analysis of 108 cases, with emphasis on differential diagnosis. *Semin Diagn Pathol* 1988;5:329–345.

Duerbeck NB, Seeds JW. Rhesus immunization in pregnancy: a review. *Obstet Gynecol Surv* 1993;48(12):801–810.

Duguid JK. ACP Broadsheet No. 150, March 1997. Antenatal serologic testing and preventing of hemolytic disease of the newborn. *J Clin Pathol* 1997;50:193–196.

Eber SW, Armburst R, Schroter W. Variable clinical severity of hereditary spherocytosis: relation to erythrocytic spectrin concentration, osmotic fragility, and autohemolysis. *J Pediatr* 1990;117:409–416.

Eldinbany MM, Totonchi KF, Joseph NJ, et al. Usefulness of certain red blood cell indices in diagnosing and differentiating thalassemia trait from iron deficiency anemia. *Am J Pathol* 1999;111:676–682.

Enokihara H, Kajitani H, Nagashima S, et al. Interleukin 5 activity in sera from patients with eosinophilia. *Br J Haematol* 1990;75:458–462.

Faderl S, Kantarjian HM, Talpaz M, et al. Clinical significance of cytogenetic abnormalities in adult acute lymphoblastic leukemia. *Blood* 1998;91:3995–4019.

Fan H, Gulley M, Gascoyne R, et al. Molecular methods for detecting t(11;14) translocations in mantle-cell lymphomas. *Diagn Mol Pathol* 1998;7:209–214.

Favara BE. Histiocytosis syndromes: classification, diagnostic features, and current concepts. Leuk Lymphoma 1990;2:141.

Favara BE, Jaffe R. The histopathology of Langerhans' cell histiocytosis. *Br J Cancer Suppl* 1994;23:S17–S23.

Foucar K. Constitutional and reactive myeloid disorders. In: Foucar K, ed. *Bone marrow pathology,* 2nd ed. Chicago: American Society of Clinical Pathologists Press, 2000.

Foucar K, Duncan MH, Smith KJ. Practical approach to the investigation of neutropenia. *Clin Lab Med* 1993;13:879–894.

Foucar KM. Reactive lymphoid proliferations in blood and bone marrow. In: Foucar K, ed. *Bone marrow pathology,* 2nd ed. Chicago: American Society of Clinical Pathologists Press, 2000.

Frizzera G, Wu CD, Inghirami G. The usefulness of immunophenotypic and genotypic studies in the diagnosis and classification of hematopoietic and lymphoid neoplasms. *Am J Clin Pathol* 1999;111[Suppl 1]:S13–S39.

Fukai K, Ishii M, Kadoya A, et al. Chédiak Higashi syndrome. *J Dermatol* 1993;20:231–237.

Gassmann W, Loffler J, Thiel E, et al. Morphological and cytochemical findings in 150 cases of T-lineage acute lymphoblastic leukaemia in adults. *Br J Haematol* 1997;97:372–382.

Gersen SL, Keagle MB. *The principles of clinical cytogenetics.* Totowa, NJ: Humana Press, 1999.

Gilbert-Barness E. *Potter's pathology of the fetus and infant.* St. Louis: Mosby–Year Book, 1997.

Good RE, Anderson V. Immunodeficiency disorders. In: Gilbert-Barness E, ed. *Potter's pathology of the fetus and infant.* St. Louis: Mosby–Year Book, 1997.

Green R, Miller JW. Folate deficiency beyond megaloblastic anemia: hyperhomocysteinemia and other manifestations of dysfunctional folate status. *Semin Hematol* 1999;36:47–64.

Griffin JP. Rapid screening for cold agglutinins in pneumonia. *Ann Intern Med* 1969;70:701–705.

Guohui Lu, Altman AJ, Benn PA. Review of the cytogenetic changes in acute megakaryoblastic leukemia: one disease or several? *Cancer Genet Cytogenet* 1993;67:81–89.

Guyatt GH, Oxman AD, Ali M, et al. Laboratory diagnosis of iron deficiency anemia. *J Gen Intern Med* 1992;7:145–153.

Hadley AG. In vitro assays to predict the severity of hemolytic disease of the newborn. *Transfus Med Rev* 1995;9:302–313.

Hage C, William CHL, Favara BE, Isaacson PG. Langerhans' cell histiocytosis (histiocytosis X): immunophenotype and growth fraction. *Hum Pathol* 1993;24:840–845.

Hann IM, Gibson BES, Letsky EA, eds. *Fetal and neonatal haematology.* London: Bailliere-Tindall, 1991.

Harris N, Jaffe E, Stein H, et al. A revised European-American classification of lymphoid neoplasms: a proposal from the International Lymphoma Study Group. *Blood* 1994;84:1361–1392.

Harris NL, Jaffe ES, Diebold J, et al. The World Health Organization classification of hematological malignancies: report of the Clinical Advisory Committee meeting, Arlie House, Virginia, November 1997. *Mod Pathol* 2000;13:193–207.

Hartwell EA. Use of Rh globulin: ASCP practice parameters. American Society of Clinical Pathologists. *Am J Clin Pathol* 1998:110:281–292.

Hashimoto C. Autoimmune hemolytic anemia. *Clin Rev Allergy Immunol* 1998;16:285–295.

Hassoun H, Palek J. Hereditary spherocytosis: a review of the clinical and molecular aspects of the disease. *Blood Rev* 1996;10:129–147.

Haurie C, Dale DC, Mackey MC. Cyclical neutropenia and other periodic hematological disorders: a review of mechanisms and mathematical models. *Blood* 1998;92:2629–2640.

Hayhoe FGH, Flemans RJ. *Color atlas of hematological cytology,* 3rd ed. St. Louis, MO: Mosby–Year Book, 1992.

Henry K, Symmers W St C. *Thymus, lymph nodes, spleen and lymphatics,* 3rd ed. Edinburgh: Churchill Livingstone, 1992. *Systemic pathology*; vol 7.

Henter JI, Elinder G, Ost A. FHL Study Group of the Histocyte Society: diagnostic guidelines for hemophagocytic lymphohistiocytosis. *Semin Oncol* 1991;19:29–33.

Hickey SM, Strasburger VC. What every pediatrician should know about infectious mononucleosis in adolescents. *Pediatr Clin North Am* 1997;44:1541–1556.

Homans AC, Barker BE, Forman EN, et al. Immunophenotypic characteristics of cerebral spinal fluid cells in children with acute lymphoblastic leukemia at diagnosis. *Blood.* 1990;76:1807–1811.

Hoxie JA. Hematologic manifestations of HIV infection. In: Hoffman R, Benz EJ Jr, Shattel SJ et al., eds. *Hematology: basic principles and practice*, 3rd ed. New York: Churchill Livingstone, 2000:2430–2457.

Hurwitz CA, Raimondi SC, Head D, et al. Distinctive immunophenotypic features of t(8;21)(q22;q22) acute myeloblastic leukemia in children. *Blood* 1992;80:3182–3188.

Iselius L, Jacobs P, Morton N. Leukemia and transient leukaemia in Down syndrome. *Hum Genet* 1990;85:477485.

Jaffe ES. Histiocytosis in lymph nodes. *Semin Diagn Pathol* 1988;5:376–390.

Jennings CD, Foon KA. Recent advances in flow cytometry: application to the diagnosis of hematologic malignancy. *Blood* 1997;90:2863–2892.

Jurco S, Starling K, Hawkins EP. Malignant histiocytosis in childhood. *Hum Pathol* 1983;14:1059–1065.

Kamb ML, Murphy JJ, Jones JL, et al. Eosinophilia-myalgia syndrome in L-tryptophan-exposed patients. *JAMA* 1992;267:77–82.

Kaneko Y, Shikano T, Maseki N, et al. Clinical characteristics of infant acute leukemia with or without 11q23 translocations. *Leukemia* 1988;2:672–676.

Kelleher JF, Carbone TV. Monosomy 7 in an infant with neurofibromatosis. *Am J Pediatr Hematol Oncol* 1991;13:338–341.

Keren DF, Hanson CA, Hurtubise GJ. *Flow cytometry and clinical diagnosis*. Chicago: American Society of Clinical Pathologists Press, 1994.

Kersey JH. Fifty years of studies of the biology and therapy of childhood leukemia. *Blood* 1997;90:4243–4251.

Kipps TJ. Lymphocytosis and lymphocytopenia. In: Beutler E, Lichtman MA, Coller BS, et al, eds. *Williams hematology*, 5th ed. New York: McGraw-Hill, 1995:963–968.

Kjeldsberg C, Elenitoba-Johnson K, Foucar K, et al. *Practical diagnosis of hematologic disorders*, 3rd ed. Chicago: American Society of Clinical Pathologists Press, 2000.

Kjeldsberg CR. The lymph nodes and spleen. In: Stocker JT, Dehner LP, eds. *Pediatric pathology.* Philadelphia: JB Lippincott Co, 1992.

Knowles DM. *Neoplastic hematopathology.* Baltimore, MD: Williams & Wilkins, 1992.

Koc S, Harris JW. Sideroblastic anemias: variations on imprecision in diagnostic criteria, proposal for an extended classification of sideroblastic anemias. *Am J Hematol* 1998;57:1–6.

Koike T, Enokihara H, Arimura H, et al. Serum concentrations of IL-5, GM-CSF, and IL-3 and the production by lymphocytes in various eosinophilia. *Am J Hematol* 1995;50:98–102.

Kotylo PK, Fineberg NS, Freeman KS, et al. Reference ranges for lymphocyte subsets in pediatric patients. *Am J Clin Pathol* 1993;100:111–115.

Kubic VL, Kubic PT, Brunning RD. The morphologic and immunophenotypic assessment of the lymphocytosis accompanying *Bordetella pertussis* infection. *Am J Clin Pathol* 1990;95:809–815.

Lewis SM, Frisch B. Congenital dyserythropoietic anaemias: electron microscopy. In: *Congenital disorders of the erythropoiesis*. CIBA Foundation, Symposium 37, 1975;17:203.

Lilleyman JS. Congenital monocytic leukaemia. *Clin Lab Haematol* 1980;2:243–245.

Malatack J, Blatt J, Penchansky L. Pediatric hematology and oncology. In: Zitelli B, Davis HW, eds. *Atlas of pediatric physical diagnosis*. Philadelphia: JB Lippincott Co, 1992.

Malone M. The histiocytoses of childhood. *Histopathology* 1991;19:105–119.

Marshall T, Rutledge JC. Flow cytometry DNA applications in pediatric tumor pathology. *Perspect Pediatr Pathol* 2001;23:55.

Mast AE, Blinder MA, Gronowski AM, et al. Clinical utility of the soluble transferrin receptor and comparison with serum ferritin in several populations. *Clin Chem* 1998;44:45–51.

Mazzulli T, Drew LW, Yen-Lieberman B, et al. Multicenter comparison of the digene hybrid capture CMV DNA assay (version 2.0), the pp65 antigenemia assay, and cell culture for detection of cytomegalovirus viremia. *J Clin Microbiol* 1999:37;958–963.

Merenstein GB, Gardner SL. *Handbook of neonatal intensive care*, 3rd ed. St. Louis, MO: Mosby, 1993.
Min KW, Read JA, Welch DF, et al. Morphologically variable bacilli of cat scratch disease are identified by immunocytochemical labeling antibodies to *Rochalimaea henselae*. *Am J Clin Pathol* 1994;101:607–610.
Minervini MI, Swerdlow SH, Nalesnik MA. Polymorphism and T-cell infiltration in posttransplant lymphoproliferative disorders. *Transplant Proc* 1999:31:1270.
Mirro J, Zipf TF, Pui CH, et al. Acute mixed lineage leukemia clinicopathologic correlations and prognostic significance. *Blood* 1985;66:1115–1123.
Mollison PL, Cutbush M. Hemolytic disease of the newborn due to fetal maternal ABO incompatibility. *Prog hematol* 1959;2:153.
Mossafa H, Malaure M, Maynadie M, et al. Persistent polyclonal lymphocytosis with binucleated lymphocytes: a study of 25 cases. *Br J Haematol* 1999;104:486–493.
Muffay JC, Rossmann SN, Chintagumpala M. Pathological case of the month, Gilbert-Barness, E (ed.): sinus histiocytosis with massive lymphadenopathy (Rosai-Dorfman disease). *Arch Pediatr Adolesc Med* 1995;149:57–58.
Nathan DG, Oski FA. *Hematology of infancy and childhood*, 4th ed. Philadelphia: WB Saunders, 1993.
Nelson BP, Nalesnik MA, Bahler DW, et al. Epstein-Barr virus negative post-transplant lymphoproliferative disorders: a distinct entity? *Am J Surg Pathol* 2000;242:375–385.
North M, Dallalio G, Donath AS, et al. Serum transferrin receptor levels in patients undergoing evaluation of iron stores: correlation with other parameters, and observed versus predicted results. *Clin Lab Haematol* 1997;19:93–97.
Oski FA. *Principles and practice of pediatrics,* 2nd ed. Philadelphia: JB Lippincott Co, 1994.
Palek J, Jarolim P. Hereditary spherocytosis, elliptocytosis and related disorders. In: Beutler E, Coller BS, Kipps TJ, et al., eds. *Williams hematology,* 5th ed. New York: McGraw-Hill, 1995:536–556.
Palframan RT, Collins PD, Williams TJ, et al. Eotaxin induces a rapid release of eosinophils and their progenitors from the bone marrow. *Blood* 1998;91:2240–2248.
Penchansky L, Kaplan SS, Krause JR. Multiple lineage reactivity in childhood leukemia. *Pediatr Pathol* 1990;10:217–229.
Penchansky L, Kjeldsberg C, et al. *Practical diagnosis of hematologic disorders*, 3rd ed. American Society of Clinical Pathologists Press, 2000.
Penchansky L, Krause JR. Acute leukemia following a malignant teratoma in a child with Klinefelter's syndrome. Secondary leukemia. Review of the literature. *Cancer* 1982;50:684–689.
Penchansky L, Krause JR. Flow cytochemical study of acute leukemia of childhood with the Technicon H-1. *Lab Med* 1991;22:184.
Penchansky L, Pirrotta V, Kaplan SS. Flow cytometric study of the expression of neutral endopeptidase (CD10/CALLA) on the surface of newborn granulocytes. *Mod Pathol* 1993;6:414–418.
Penchansky L, Taylor SR, Krause JR. Three infants with acute megakaryoblastic leukemia stimulating metastatic tumor. *Cancer* 1989;64:1366–1371.
Penchansky L, Willman MR, Gartner JC, Wenger SL. Spontaneous remission of infantile acute nonlymphocytic leukemia for 11 years in a child with normal karyotype. *Cancer* 1993;71:1928–1930.
Peterson L, Foucar K. Granulocytosis and granulocytopenia. In: Bick RL, ed. *Hematology: clinical and laboratory practice*. St. Louis, MO: Mosby, 1993:1137–1154.
Peterson L, Hrisinko MA. Benign lymphocytosis and reactive neutrophilia: laboratory features provide diagnostic clues. *Clin Lab Med* 1993;13:863–877.
Praghakaran K, Wise B, Chen A, et al. Rational management of post-transplant lymphoproliferative disorder in pediatric recipients. *J Pediatr Surg* 1999;34:112–115.
Pui CH. Childhood leukemias. *N Engl J Med* 1995;332:1618–1630.
Pui CH, Behm FG, Crist WM. Clinical and biologic relevance of immunologic marker studies in childhood acute lymphoblastic leukemia. *Blood* 1993;82:343–362.
Pui CH, Frankel LS, Carroll AJ, et al. Clinical characteristics and treatment outcome of childhood acute lymphoblastic leukemia with the t(4;11)(q21;q23): a collaborative study of 40 cases. *Blood* 1991;77:440–447.

Remacha AF, Cadafalch J. Cobalamin deficiency in patients infected with the human immunodeficiency virus. *Semin Hematol* 1999;36;75–87.
Resnik KS, Brod BB. Leukemia cutis in congenital leukemia—analysis and review of the world literature with report of an additional case. *Arch Dermatol* 1993;129:1301–1306.
Risdall RS, McKenna RW, Newbit ME, et al. Virus associated with hemophagocytic syndrome. *Cancer* 1979;44:993–1002.
Robison LL. Down syndrome and leukemia. *Leukemia* 1992;6[Suppl 1]:5–7.
Roizen NJ, Amarose AP. Hematological abnormalities in children with Down syndrome. *Am J Med Genet* 1993;46:510–512.
Rosai J, Dorfman R. Sinus histiocytosis with massive lymphadenopathy. *Cancer* 1972;30:1174–1188.
Rosen FS, Cooper MD, Wedgwood RJP. The primary immunodeficiencies. *N Engl J Med* 1995;333:431–440.
Rosenblatt DS, Whitehead VM. Cobalamin and folate deficiency: acquired and hereditary disorders in children. *Semin Hematol* 1999:36:19–34.
Rowley JD. Recurring chromosome abnormalities in leukemia and lymphoma. *Semin Hematol* 1990;27:122–136.
Scott JR, et al., eds. *Danforth's obstetrics and gynecology*, 7th ed. Philadelphia: JB Lippincott Co, 1994.
Shannon KM, Turham AG, Chang SS, et al. Familial bone marrow monosomy 7. Evidence that the predisposing locus is not on the long arm of chromosome 7. *J Clin Invest* 1989;84:984–989.
Shannon KM, Watterson J, Johnson P, et al. Monosomy 7 myeloproliferative disease in children with neurofibromatosis. Type 1: epidemiology and molecular analysis. *Blood* 1992;79:1311–1318.
Shimizu H, Sawada K, Katano N, et al. Intramedullary neutrophil phagocytosis by histiocytes in autoimmune neutropenia of infancy. *Acta Haematol* 1990;84:201–203.
Shurtleff SA, Buijs A, Behm FG, et al. TEL/AML 1 fusion resulting from a cryptic t(12;21) is the most common genetic lesion in pediatric ALL and defines a subgroup of patients with an excellent prognosis. *Leukemia* 1995;9:1985–1989.
Sievers EL, Dale DC. Non-malignant neutropenia. *Blood Rev* 1996;10:95–100.
Siimes MA, Addiego JE Jr, Dallman PR. Ferritin in serum: diagnosis of iron deficiency and iron overload in infants and children. *Blood* 1974;43:581.
Smith KL, Johnson W. Classification of chronic myelocytic leukemia in children. *Cancer* 1974;34:670–679.
Smith PS. Congenital coagulation protein deficiencies in the perinatal period. *Semin Perinatol* 1990;14:384–392.
Sokol RJ, Booker DJ, Stamps R. ACP Broadsheet No 145. Investigations of patients with autoimmune hemolytic anemia and provision of blood for transfusion. *J Clin Pathol* 1995:48:602–610.
Stansfeld AG, d'Ardenne AJ. *Lymph node biopsy interpretation.* Edinburgh: Churchill Livingstone, 1992.
Steeper TA, Horwitz CA, Hanson M, et al. Heterophil-negative mononucleosis-like illnesses not resulting from Epstein-Barr virus or cytomegalovirus. *Am J Clin Pathol* 1990;93:776–783.
Stewart M. Hemostasis and thrombosis. In: Coleman RW, Hirsh J, Marder VV, et al., eds. *Bleeding in newborn and pediatric patients*. Philadelphia: JB Lippincott Co, 1987:943.
Stockman JA III, Pochedly C, eds. *Development and neonatal hematology.* New York: Raven Press, 1988. Pediatric Hematology/Oncology Series.
Strickler JG, Fedeli F, Horwitz CA, et al. Infectious mononucleosis in lymphoid tissue. *Arch Pathol Lab Med* 1994;117:269–278.
Teggatz JR, Parkin J, Peterson L. Transient atypical lymphocytosis in patients with emergency medical condition. *Arch Pathol Lab Med* 1987;111:712–714.
Telen MJ, Rao N. Recent advances in immunohematology. *Curr Opin Hematol* 1994;1:143–150.
Thomas AT. Autoimmune hemolytic anemias. In: Lee GR, Foerster J, Lukens JN, et al., eds. *Wintrobe's clinical hematology*, 10th ed. Baltimore: Williams & Wilkins, 1999:1233–1263.

Toh BH, van Driel IR, Gleeson PA. Pernicious anemia. *N Engl J Med* 1997;337:1441–1448.

Toren A, Mandel M, Amariglio N, et al. Lack of bcr rearrangement in juvenile chronic myeloid leukemia. *Med Pediatr Oncol* 1991;19:493–495.

Tsang WYW, Chan JKC, Ng CS. Kikuchi's lymphadenitis: a morphologic analysis of 75 cases with special reference to unusual features. *Am J Surg Pathol* 1994;18:219–231.

Uckun FM, Sather HN, Gaynon PS, et al. Clinical features and treatment outcome of children with myeloid antigen positive acute lymphoblastic leukemia: a report from the Children's Cancer Group. *Blood* 1997;90:28–35.

Uckum FM, Sensel MG, Sun L, et al. Biology and treatment of childhood T-lineage acute lymphoblastic leukemia. *Blood* 1998;91:735–746.

Welte K, Zeidler DC, Reiter A, et al. Differential effects of granulocyte-macrophage colony-stimulating factor and granulocyte colony-stimulating factor in children with severe congenital neutropenia. *Blood* 1990;75:1056–1063.

Wickramasinghe SN. The wide spectrum and unresolved issues of megaloblastic anemia. *Semin Hematol* 1999;36:3–18.

Wickramasinghe SN, Matthews JH. Deoxyuridine suppression: biochemical basis and diagnostic applications. *Blood Rev* 1988;2:168–177.

World Health Organization classification of tumors, pathology and genetics. Tumors of the haematopoietic and lymphoid tissues. Lyon, France: International Agency for Research on Cancer Press, 2001.

Worwood M. The laboratory assessment of iron status—an update. *Clin Chim Acta* 1997;259:3–23.

Writing Group of the Histocytic Society. Histocytosis syndromes in children. *Lancet* 1987;1:208–209.

Zittoun J, Zittoun R. Modern clinical testing strategies in cobalamin and folate deficiency. *Semin Hematol* 1999;36:35–46.

Zupanska B. Assays to predict the clinical significance of blood group antibodies. *Curr Opin Hematol* 1998;5:412–416.

12 Coagulation Disorders

Irwin L. Browarsky[1]

Tests of Coagulation

Clotting Evaluation

Evaluation of clotting requires a good history and physical examination, and review of a peripheral blood smear for red blood cell fragmentation, giant or other platelet abnormalities, platelet numbers, and white blood cell (WBC) inclusions or nuclear abnormalities. Platelet counts, activated partial thromboplastin time, prothrombin time (PT), and thrombin time are the first-line studies for evaluating bleeding disorders. Normal clotting depends on adequate platelet number and function as well as adequacy of plasma factors, including those responsible for contact activation, thrombin generation, and fibrinolysis.

Prothrombin Time

The PT is carried out by adding extrinsic factor to the patient's plasma. Plasma is anticoagulated with citrate. After the plasma samples are mixed, the time of appearance of the first fibrin strand is the PT. The PT measures clotting factors in the extrinsic clotting cascade. Normal PT requires the presence of factors VII, X, V, II, and fibrinogen. It may be prolonged with decreased liver synthetic capacity, decreased vitamin K absorption, warfarin sodium therapy, presence of inhibitors, or inadequate sample volume (or high hematocrit), and in specimens obtained from heparin-containing lines. PT is only minimally altered with usual therapeutic doses of heparin sodium.

Activated Partial Thromboplastin Time

Activated partial thromboplastin time (aPTT) measures the intrinsic clotting system; it requires the presence of factors XII, X, XI, IX, VIII, V, and II and fibrinogen and is prolonged in the presence of inhibitors. The determination is similar to that of PT, with kaolin (traditionally) and partial thromboplastin added to the patient's plasma. The end point is the same as for PT.

Thrombin Time

To measure thrombin time, thrombin is added to the patient's plasma and the time for fibrin formation is observed. Thrombin time is abnormal with decreased fibrinogen, abnormality of fibrinogen structure, and in the presence of inhibitors to thrombin, such as heparin.

[1]This chapter written by Dr. Irwin L. Browarsky, Clinical Associate Professor, University of South Florida; Medical Laboratory Director, Tampa General Hospital, Tampa, Florida.

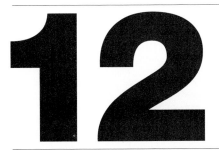

Table 1. Laboratory Tests for Common Bleeding Disorders

Disorder	PT	aPTT	Platelet Count	Platelet Function
von Willebrand disease	Normal	Normal or prolonged	Normal	Normal or abnormal
Hemophilia A or B	Normal	Usually prolonged	Normal	Normal
Thrombocytopenia	Normal	Normal	Decreased	Test not usually indicated
Vitamin K deficiency	Prolonged	Normal or prolonged	Normal	Normal

aPTT, activated partial thromboplastin time; PT, prothrombin time.

Laboratory Test Results in Common Bleeding Disorders

Table 1 shows the results of laboratory tests of coagulation in several common bleeding disorders.

Table 2 summarizes the results for aPTT and PT in inherited deficiencies of clotting factors.

Table 3 outlines the use of aPTT and PT tests in screening for inherited bleeding disorders.

Hemorrhagic Disorders of Platelets

Platelets

Platelets are the smallest anucleated circulating elements of the blood. They are fragments of the bone marrow megakaryocytes. They play a primary role in hemostasis by interacting with blood vessels and coagulation proteins to prevent *in vivo* bleeding. A platelet count $<150 \times 10^9$/L or $>450 \times 10^9$/L should be considered abnormal in a newborn or infant. Normal range for mean platelet volume is 7.5–10.0 fL. Large platelets or degranulated platelets are not counted by automated instruments; their presence may give rise to a falsely low platelet count, and platelets should be examined microscopically to rule out pseudothrombocytopenia. A blood smear

Table 2. Activated Partial Thromboplastin Time and Prothrombin Time in Inherited Deficiencies of Clotting Factors

Disorder	aPTT	PT
Deficiency of HMWK, prekallikrein, factors XII, XI, IX, VIII	Increased	Normal
Deficiency of factors V, X, prothrombin; hypofibrinogenemia	Increased	Increased
Factor VII deficiency	Normal	Increased
Dysfibrinogenemia	Increased or normal	Increased or normal
Factor XIII deficiency	Normal	Normal
α-Antiplasmin	Normal	Normal

aPTT, activated partial thromboplastin time; HMWK, high-molecular-weight kininogen; PT, prothrombin time.

Table 3. Use of Activated Partial Thromboplastin Time and Prothrombin Time Tests in Screening for Inherited Bleeding Disorders

aPTT	PT	Further Testing
Normal	Normal	Platelet function studies, vWF studies, factor XIII screen, α_2-antiplasmin study
Increased	Normal	Factor VIII:c assay; if normal, assay for factor IX, then factor XI; if factor VIII is low, assay for vWF:Ag and ristocetin cofactor activity; exclude inhibitor, heparin
Increased	Increased	Thrombin time; if normal, assays for factors V and X and prothrombin; if thrombin time prolonged, fibrinogen assay by functional and antigenic methods; exclude heparin
Normal	Increased	Factor VII assay

aPTT, activated partial thromboplastin time; PT, prothrombin time; VIII:c, factor VIII coagulant activity; vWF, von Willebrand factor; vWF:Ag, vWF antigen.

review will also exclude platelet agglutination due to cold agglutinins, or satellitosis induced by adherence of platelets to WBCs.

Platelet Counts

The flow cytometric method for platelet counting is rapid and simple, and generates reproducible results. Such testing can be set up easily by any laboratory with a fluorescent flow cytometer. Use of flow cytometry improves the accuracy of platelet counting, particularly in thrombocytopenic samples. Unlike impedance analyzers, the method not only distinguishes large platelets from red blood cells but also discriminates platelets from nonfluorescent platelet-like particles.

Platelet Function

Platelet defects manifest as mucocutaneous hemorrhage, the severity of which is determined by the specific defect and the percent reduction of the platelet protein. Patients with the hereditary thrombocytopenias usually have 50,000–100,000 platelets/mL and are typically asymptomatic unless function is also impaired.

Platelet function has traditionally been assessed by measuring bleeding time. Because of the difficulty of reproducibility, especially in children, there have been numerous attempts to devise other measures of testing platelet function. One of these methods is the PFA, which essentially provides a qualitative measure of platelet aggregation. Using epinephrine, it adequately separates intrinsic platelet dysfunction from an abnormality secondary to drug interaction.

Table 4 lists various abnormalities of platelet function.

A specific and sensitive method to analyze platelet function is the thromboelastograph (TEG), which uses curves to determine the part of the clotting system that is abnormal.

The TEG measures the kinetic changes in a sample of whole blood as the sample clots, retracts, and lyses. The parameters measured by the TEG are

- Reaction time: the period from the time that the blood is placed in the instrument until the initial fibrin formation is detected.
  - The reaction time is prolonged by anticoagulants and shortened by hypercoagulable states.
  - Normal reference range: 4–6 minutes.
  - Measure of speed to reach a certain level of clot strength.
  - Normal reference range: 0–4 minutes.
- α: Measures kinetics of fibrin buildup and cross linking, that is, speed of clot strengthening.
  - α is decreased with use of anticoagulants that affect fibrinogen and platelet function.

Table 4. Abnormalities of Platelet Function

Disease	Inheritance	Adhesion[a]	Collagen[b]	ADP[b]	Ristocetin[b]	Other Functions
Congenital						
Bernard-Soulier disease	AR	↓	N	N	↓	Giant platelets
Glanzmann thrombasthenia	AR	N	↓	↓	N	Absent clot retraction
Storage pool disease	Variable	N	↓	↓	N	Absent dense bodies
von Willebrand disease	AD	↓	N	N	↓	Corrected by factor VIII/vWF
Acquired						
Aspirin use	—	N	↓	↓	N	Decreased cyclooxygenase
Uremia	—	↓	↓	↓	N	Pathogenesis not known
Myeloproliferative diseases	—	↓	↓	↓	N	Pathogenesis not known

↓, decreased; ADP, adenosine diphosphate; AD, autosomal dominant; AR, autosomal recessive; N, normal; vWF, von Willebrand factor.
[a]Tests of adhesiveness are difficult to standardize.
[b]Aggregation induced by collagen, ADP, or ristocetin *in vitro*. Other inducers of aggregation include arachidonic acid and epinephrine; the normal range is 60–100% of control.
From Wallach J. *Interpretation of diagnostic tests,* 7th ed. Philadelphia: Lippincott Williams & Wilkins, 2000.

    - Normal reference range: 55–62 degrees.
- Maximum amplitude: Direct function of maximum dynamic properties of fibrin and platelet bonding. Maximum amplitude represents the ultimate strength of fibrin clot.
    - Maximum amplitude is affected by platelet numbers and platelet function, and to a lesser degree by fibrinogen.
    - Normal reference range: 45–53 minutes.

The TEG therefore measures the kinetics of clot formation, clot dissolution, and clot quality.

For routine preoperative and postoperative testing, a TEG baseline is performed. The turnaround time is approximately 1 hour from the time the specimen is received in the laboratory.

Causes of Thrombocytopenia

In the premature infant
- Respiratory distress syndrome
- Meconium aspiration
- Persistent pulmonary hypertension
- Necrotizing enterocolitis
- Hyperbilirubinemia
- Polycythemia
- Phototherapy

In the full-term newborn
- Erythroblastosis fetalis
- Preeclampsia

- Drug effects
- Immune thrombocytopenia
- Inherited metabolic disorders
  - Methylmalonic acidemia
  - Ketotic glycinemia
  - Holocarboxylase synthetase deficiency
  - Isovaleric acidemia

Platelet Abnormalities That Cause Bleeding[2]

- Thrombocytopenia
  - Decreased production in the bone marrow
    - Aplastic anemia: due to any of numerous causes, including idiopathic
    - Radiation
    - Marrow infiltration by leukemia, metastatic neoplasms, infections
    - Vitamin B_{12} and folate deficiency
    - Hereditary autosomal-dominant form: Wiskott-Aldrich syndrome, May-Hegglin anomaly
  - Pooling (sequestration) of platelets in an enlarged spleen
  - Increased peripheral destruction of platelets
  - Immune mechanisms
    - Idiopathic thrombocytopenic purpura
    - Systemic lupus erythematosus
    - Drug-induced thrombocytopenia (gold salts, quinine, sulfonamides)
    - Neonatal thrombocytopenia: transfer of maternal immunoglobulin G antibodies with activity against fetal platelets
    - Posttransfusion: due to alloantibodies to platelet antigen $P1^{A1}$ (rare but severe)
  - Hypersplenism
  - Increased platelet consumption
  - Disseminated intravascular coagulation
  - Thrombotic thrombocytopenic purpura
  - Hemolytic-uremic syndrome
  - Valve prosthesis, artificial vascular grafts
  - Dilution of platelets: massive transfusions
- Qualitative platelet disorders (abnormal function)
  - Congenital
    - Defects of adhesion: Bernard-Soulier disease
    - Defects of aggregation: thrombasthenia (Glanzmann disease)
    - Abnormal granule release: storage pool disease
    - Wiskott-Aldrich syndrome
    - von Willebrand disease
    - Albinism
  - Acquired
    - Uremia
    - Dysproteinemias
    - Chronic liver disease, especially alcoholic
    - Drug-induced: aspirin, phenylbutazone
    - Myeloproliferative diseases
    - Vascular disorders: many diseases producing vascular damage also affect platelet function

Evaluation of Platelet Disorders

See Fig. 1.

Hereditary Thrombocytopenias and Thrombocytopathies

See Table 5.

[2]Wallach J. *Interpretation of diagnostic tests*, 7th ed. Philadelphia: Lippincott Williams & Wilkins, 2000.

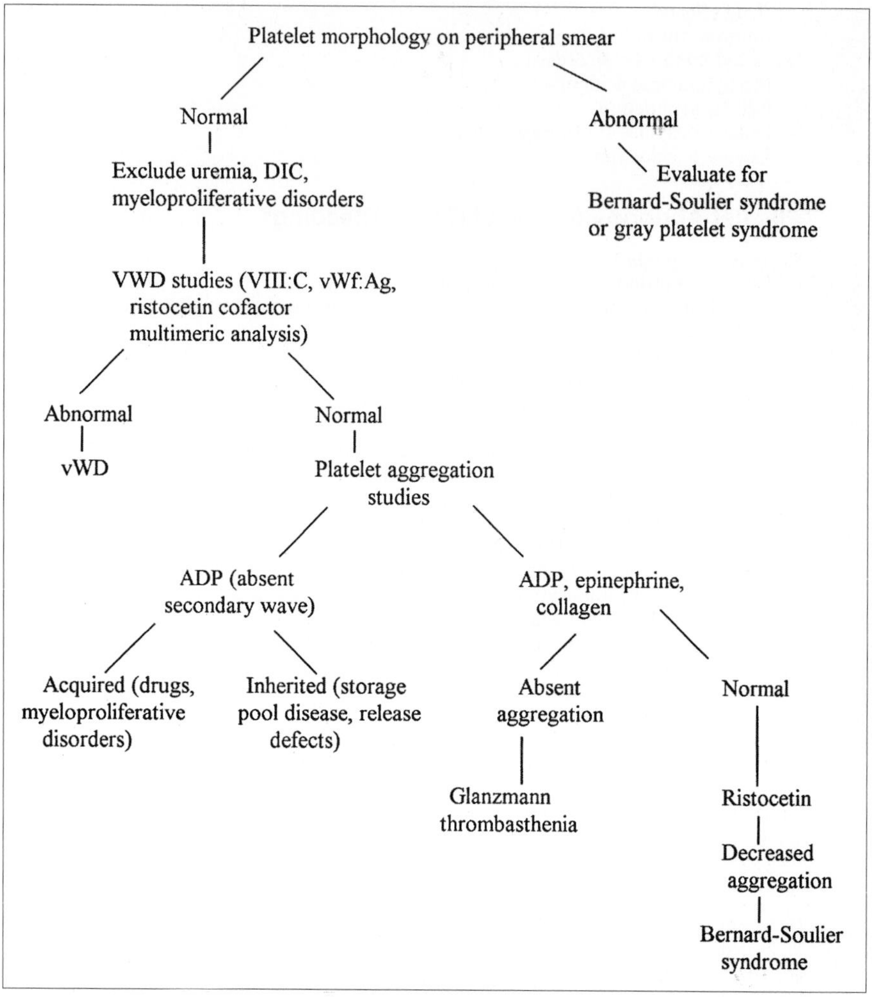

Fig. 1. Evaluation of platelet disorders. ADP, adenosine diphosphate; DIC, disseminated intravascular coagulation; VIII:c, factor VIII coagulant activity; vWD, von Willebrand disease.

Bernard-Soulier Syndrome

Bernard-Soulier syndrome is a rare bleeding disorder with an autosomal-recessive pattern of inheritance. The clinical onset of the disorder at an early age is characterized by mucocutaneous bleeding disproportionate to the degree of thrombocytopenia.

Laboratory Findings

Morphologic and functional platelet abnormalities are found. Platelet counts are normal or moderately decreased. In the peripheral blood smear the platelets are large, up to 30 μm in diameter. The platelet granules are localized in the center of the cell. In the bone marrow aspirate megakaryocytes are normal by light microscopy; on electron microscopy most of the platelets are large and spherical, rather than of the normal discoid shape. Functionally, both platelet adhesion and agglutination are abnormal with prolonged bleeding time and abnormal prothrombin consumption. The platelets show an abnormal aggrega-

Table 5. Hereditary Thrombocytopathies

Disorder	Plt Counts	Morphologic/ Functional Abnormality	Molecular Abnormality	Megakaryocyte or Plt Morphology	Inheritance Pattern	Clinical Findings
Bernard-Soulier disease	N/low	Giant plt/ adhesion	Cell membrane decreased GP Ib, factors V and IX	Multinucleated vacuolated megakaryocytes Dense granules on EM	AR	Hemorrhage
Willebrand platelet syndrome	Low	Giant plt/ adhesion	Cell membrane increased GP Ib	N	AD	Hemorrhage
Storage pool disease	N	N small plt/ granular secretion	Dense body	Decreased dense granules on EM	AD AD	Associated with other hematologic abnormalities Chédiak-Higashi syndrome Wiskott-Aldrich syndrome TAR syndrome
Gray platelets syndrome	Low	Gray stain/ adhesion Large plt	α Granules, qualitative and quantitative	Lack of α granules on EM Myelofibrosis	AR	Hemorrhage
Glanzmann disease	N	N/aggregation	PGP IIb/IIIa	PGP	AR	Hemorrhage
Morehead disease	Low	Giant plt	?	?	AD	
May-Hegglin anomaly	Low	Giant plt Basophilic inclusions Granulocytes	Maturation defect	N	AD	Purpura
Wiskott-Aldrich syndrome	Low	Small plt/ secretion	GT	?	XL	Purpura

AD, autosomal dominant; AR, autosomal recessive; EM, electron microscopy; GP, glycoprotein; GT, glycotransferase; N, normal; PGP, platelet glycoprotein; plt, platelets; TAR, thrombocytopenia absent radii; XL, sex linked.

tion response to ristocetin and normal aggregation response to adenosine diphosphatase, epinephrine, and collagen.

Deficiency of monoclonal antibodies to glycoprotein Ib in the platelets of patients with Bernard-Soulier syndrome facilitates the diagnosis. Radioimmunoassay of glycoprotein Ib in whole blood, or smear immunocytochemical staining with anti–glycoprotein Ib, can be applied to demonstrate the deficiency.

Other Platelet Disorders

Special laboratory tests are required for the diagnosis of other congenital giant platelet syndromes such as May-Hegglin anomaly, gray platelet syndrome, Epstein or Fletchner variants of Alport syndrome, and Mediterranean "macrothrombocytopenia."

Rare causes of thrombocytopenia in the newborn are Kasabach-Merritt syndrome, Wiskott-Aldrich syndrome, amegakaryocytic thrombocytopenia, and a group of hereditary thrombocytopenias associated with inclusions in the leukocytes.

Kasabach-Merritt syndrome is characterized by giant hemangiomas associated with thrombocytopenia. However, large size is not a prerequisite for the syndrome. Large single or multiple hemangiomas are present at birth. The syndrome is characterized by anemia, thrombocytopenia, and coagulation studies consistent with disseminated intravascular coagulation (DIC). The bleeding is due to sludging of blood in the hemangioma, which results in a consumption coagulopathy.

Wiskott-Aldrich syndrome is an X-linked recessive disorder characterized by a triad of immunodeficiency of the cellular and humoral arms of the immune system, eczema, and thrombocytopenia. The defect is expressed primarily by cells derived from the bone marrow. The abnormality is due to an aberrant biosynthesis of X-linked oligosaccharides with abnormal expression of two glycotransferases: platelet membrane glycoprotein and lymphocytic sialophorin (CD43).

Laboratory abnormalities include a decrease in the number and size of the platelets. The number of megakaryocytes appears normal. The most consistent defect is the absence of low circulating levels of i blood group antigens.

Amegakaryocytic thrombocytopenia is a rare heritable disorder. Inheritance is X-linked or autosomal recessive. Low platelet counts can be detected early in life. Bone marrow abnormalities are limited to the megakaryocytic lineage, with a decrease or absence of megakaryocytes.

Chédiak-Higashi syndrome is an autosomal-recessive disorder characterized by oculocutaneous albinism, recurrent infections, large basophilic inclusions in WBCs and macrophages, and decreased platelet survival, associated with decreased aggregation to epinephrine and collagen.

TAR (*t*hrombocytopenia and *a*bsent *r*adius) syndrome is an autosomal disorder that manifests as diminished aggregation of the platelets and thrombocytopenia, with absent radii at birth.

Wiskott-Aldrich syndrome, TAR syndrome, Hermansky-Pudlak syndrome, and Chédiak-Higashi syndrome are among the inherited storage pool defects.

Glanzmann thrombasthenia is an inherited autosomal-recessive condition in which a fibrinogen receptor, glycoprotein IIb-IIIa, is deficient. Heterozygotes are usually asymptomatic. Patients may manifest easy bruising and mucocutaneous hemorrhage. Intraarticular bleeds are unusual. The condition diminishes with age. Platelet aggregation does not respond to usual agents, that is, collagen and epinephrine.

In addition to drugs with variable effects on platelets (inhibition of cyclooxygenase, membrane binding of glycoprotein IIb-IIIa, etc.), many other causes of platelet dysfunction are known, such as uremia, glycogen storage disease, agammaglobulinemia, autoimmune disorders, dysproteinemias, and infections.

Drugs That Affect Platelet Function

Anesthetics
- Cocaine (local)
- Procaine (local)
- Volatile general anesthetics

Antibiotics
- Ampicillin

- Carbenicillin indanyl sodium
- Gentamicin sulfate
- Penicillin G
- Ticarcillin disodium

Anticoagulants
- Dextran
- Heparin sodium

Antiinflammatory agents and analgesics
- Aspirin
- Colchicine
- Ibuprofen (Motrin)
- Indomethacin (Indocin)
- Naproxen (Naprosyn)
- Phenylbutazone (Butazolidin)
- Sulfinpyrazone (Anturane)

Sympathetic blocking agents
- Phenoxybenzamine hydrochloride (Dibenzyline)
- Propranolol hydrochloride (Inderal)

Other drugs
- Abciximab
- Antihistamines (diphenhydramine hydrochloride)
- Clofibrate
- Dipyridamole (Persantine)
- Furosemide (Lasix)
- Glyceryl guaiacolate ether (cough suppressant)
- Hydroxychloroquine sulfate
- Nicotinic acid
- Nitrofurantoin (Furadantin)
- Papaverine hydrochloride (Myobid)
- Quinidine
- Sodium nitroprusside
- Theophylline
- Phenothiazines
- Tricyclic antidepressants: imipramine pamoate (Tofranil), amitriptyline hydrochloride (Triavil, Elavil)
- Verapamil hydrochloride

Miscellaneous substances
- Ethanol
- Hashish compounds

Heparin-Induced Thrombocytopenia

Heparin therapy may induce thrombocytopenia with or without arterial or venous thrombosis. This occurs in two forms: type I, in which there is a slight drop in platelet count, no evidence of antibody formation, and spontaneous remission; and type II, in which there is a marked drop in platelet count to <50% of pretreatment values, vascular thrombosis, correction after heparin withdrawal, and presence of detectable antibodies. The thrombocytopenia is related to reticuloendothelial clearance of the platelet factor 4–heparin complexes. This process occurs in approximately 7 days, which leaves free antibody circulating. Thrombosis occurs in approximately 20% of patients with heparin-induced thrombocytopenia and occurs much more commonly in sick patients in whom there is tissue damage. Even heparin in indwelling lines may precipitate the syndrome.

There are a variety of ways in the clinical laboratory to confirm the impression of heparin-induced thrombocytopenia, such as activation assays and antibody assays. When combined, these procedures result in 100% sensitivity. The enzyme-linked immunosorbent assay is a qualitative immunoassay for detecting *antibodies* reactive with platelet factor 4 when complexed with polyanionic compounds. This test is sensitive but not as specific as flow cytometry, which detects an *activation marker* on platelets, annexin v. A positive result on flow cytometry is a value 2.2% greater than the control.

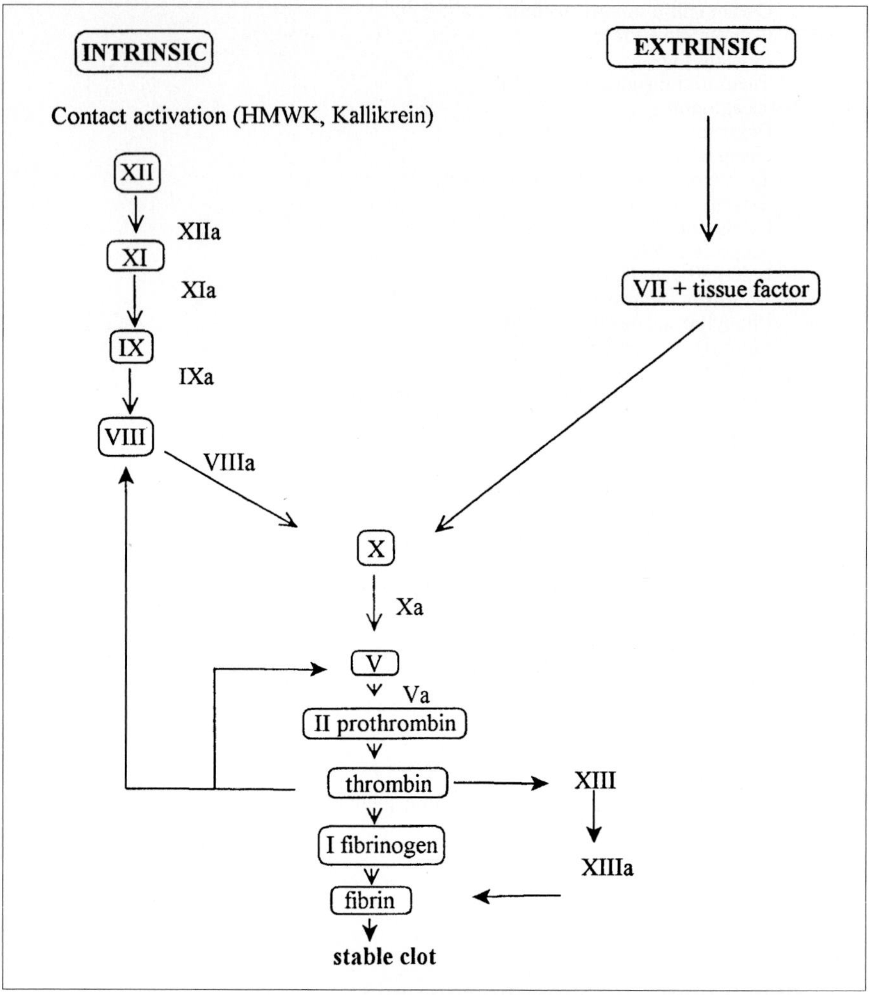

Fig. 2. Coagulation cascade. a (after factor number), activated form; HMWK, high-molecular-weight kininogen.

Coagulation Protein Disorders

Coagulation Cascade

See Figs. 2 and 3.

Bleeding Disorders of Newborn Infants

Table 6 lists bleeding disorders of newborn infants.
Table 7 shows coagulation values by age.
Table 8 shows reference values for the inhibitors of coagulation in healthy children aged 1–16 years compared with adults.

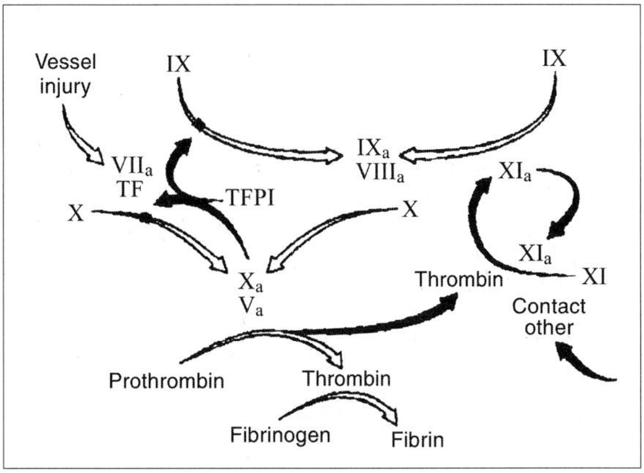

Fig. 3. Current view of coagulation cascade. Revised theory suggests that tissue factor (TF) rather than contact factors initiates cascade. Activated factor VII (VIIa) and TF activates factors X and XI. Activated factor X (Xa) binds tissue factor pathway inhibitor (TFPI), which inactivates factor X. TFPI also feeds back on VIIa/TF to block factor X activation. Factor Xa is also produced by activation of IX and activated factor VIII (VIIIa). a after factor number indicates activated form. [Reproduced with permission from Luchtman-Jones L, Broze GJ Jr. The current status of coagulation. *Ann Med* 1995;27(1):47–52.]

Table 6. Bleeding Disorders of Newborn Infants

Category	Condition	Frequency	Bleeding
Platelet disorders	Congenital thrombocytopenia		
	Neonatal alloimmune thrombocytopenia	Common	Usually
	Thrombocytopenia secondary to uteroplacental factors	Common	Occasionally
	Fanconi syndrome		
	Down syndrome with transient myeloproliferation syndrome		
	Platelet function disorders: Glanzmann thrombasthenia, Bernard-Soulier syndrome		
	Platelet storage pool diseases		
	TAR syndrome (thrombocytopenia absent radius)		
Coagulation protein disorders	Factor VIII deficiency (hemophilia A) and factor IX deficiency (hemophilia B)	Rare	Usually
	Factor XIII deficiency		
	Vitamin K deficiency	Common	Usually
Combinations of platelet and coagulation protein abnormalities	Disseminated intravascular coagulation caused by sepsis, necrotizing enterocolitis, or another condition	Common	Often
Disorders of vascular integrity	Intraventricular hemorrhage in preterm infants	Common	Usually
	Hemangiomas and Kasabach-Merritt syndrome	Rare	Often

Table 7. Age-Specific Coagulation Values

Coagulation Test	Preterm Infant 30–36 Wk, Day 1 of Life	Term Infant, Day 1 of Life	1–5 Yr	6–10 Yr	11–16 Yr	Adult
PT (sec)	15.4 (14.6–16.9)	13.0 (10.1–15.9)	11 (10.6–11.4)	11.2 (10.2–12.0)	11.2 (10.2–12.0)	12 (11.0–14.0)
aPTT (sec)	108 (80–168)	42.9 (31.3–54.3)	30 (24–36)	31 (26–36)	32 (26–37)	33 (27–40)
Fibrinogen (g/L)	2.43 (1.50–3.73)	2.83 (1.67–3.09)	2.76 (1.70–4.05)	2.79 (1.57–4.0)	3.0 (1.54–4.48)	2.78 (1.56–4.0)
Thrombin time (sec)	14 (11–17)	12 (10–16)	—	—	—	—
Factor II (U/mL)	0.45 (0.20–0.77)	0.48 (0.26–0.70)	0.94 (0.71–1.16)	0.88 (0.67–1.07)	0.83 (0.61–1.04)	1.08 (0.70–1.46)
Factor V (U/mL)	0.88 (0.41–1.44)	0.72 (0.43–1.08)	1.03 (0.79–1.27)	0.90 (0.63–1.16)	0.77 (0.55–0.99)	1.06 (0.62–1.50)
Factor VII (U/mL)	0.67 (0.21–1.13)	0.66 (0.28–1.04)	0.82 (0.55–1.16)	0.85 (0.52–1.20)	0.83 (0.58–1.15)	1.05 (0.67–1.43)
Factor VIII procoagulant (U/mL)	1.11 (0.50–2.13)	1.00 (0.50–1.78)	0.90 (0.59–1.42)	0.95 (0.58–1.32)	0.92 (0.53–1.31)	0.99 (0.50–1.49)
vWF (U/mL)	1.36 (0.78–2.10)	1.53 (0.50–2.87)	0.82 (0.47–1.04)	0.95 (0.44–1.44)	1.00 (0.46–1.53)	0.92 (0.50–1.58)
Factor IX (U/mL)	0.35 (0.19–0.65)	0.53 (0.15–0.91)	0.73 (0.47–1.04)	0.75 (0.63–0.89)	0.87 (0.59–1.22)	1.09 (0.55–1.63)
Factor X (U/mL)	0.41 (0.11–0.71)	0.40 (0.12–0.68)	0.88 (0.58–1.16)	0.75 (0.55–1.01)	0.79 (0.50–1.17)	1.06 (0.70–1.52)
Factor XI (U/mL)	0.30 (0.08–0.52)	0.38 (0.10–0.66)	0.97 (0.56–1.50)	0.86 (0.52–1.20)	0.74 (0.50–0.97)	0.97 (0.67–1.27)
Factor XII (U/mL)	0.38 (0.10–0.66)	0.53 (0.13–0.93)	0.93 (0.64–1.29)	0.92 (0.60–1.40)	0.81 (0.34–1.37)	1.08 (0.52–1.64)
PK (U/mL)	0.33 (0.09–0.57)	0.37 (0.18–0.69)	0.95 (0.65–1.30)	0.99 (0.66–1.31)	0.99 (0.53–1.45)	1.12 (0.62–1.62)
HMWK (U/mL)	0.49 (0.09–0.89)	0.54 (0.06–1.02)	0.98 (0.64–1.32)	0.93 (0.60–1.30)	0.91 (0.63–1.19)	0.92 (0.50–1.36)
Factor XIIIa (U/mL)	0.70 (0.32–1.08)	0.79 (0.27–1.31)	1.08 (0.72–1.43)	1.09 (0.65–1.51)	0.99 (0.57–1.40)	1.05 (0.55–1.55)
Factor XIIIx (U/mL)	0.81 (0.35–1.27)	0.76 (0.30–1.22)	1.13 (0.69–1.56)	1.16 (0.77–1.54)	1.02 (0.60–1.43)	0.97 (0.57–1.37)
D-Dimer	—	—	—	—	—	Positive titer = 1:8
FDPs	—	—	—	—	—	Borderline titer = 1:25 Positive titer = 1:50
Coagulation inhibitors						
ATIII (μg/mL)	380 (140–620)	630 (390–970)	1,110 (820–1,390)	1,110 (900–1,310)	1,050 (770–1,320)	1,000 (740–1,260)
α_2-M (U/mL)	1.10 (0.56–1.82)	1.39 (0.95–1.83)	1.69 (1.14–2.23)	1.69 (1.28–2.09)	1.56 (0.98–2.12)	0.86 (0.52–1.20)
C_1-Inh (U/mL)	0.65 (0.31–0.99)	0.72 (0.36–1.08)	1.35 (0.85–1.83)	1.14 (0.88–1.54)	1.03 (0.68–1.50)	1.0 (0.71–1.31)

α_2-AT (U/mL)	0.90 (0.36–1.44)	0.93 (0.49–1.37)	0.93 (0.39–1.47)	1.00 (0.69–1.30)	1.01 (0.65–1.37)	0.93 (0.55–1.30)
Protein C (U/mL)	0.28 (0.12–0.44)	0.35 (0.17–0.53)	0.66 (0.40–0.92)	0.69 (0.45–0.93)	0.83 (0.55–1.11)	0.96 (0.64–1.28)
Protein S total (U/mL)	0.26 (0.14–0.38)	0.36 (0.12–0.60)	0.86 (0.54–1.18)	0.78 (0.41–1.14)	0.72 (0.52–0.92)	0.81 (0.60–1.13)
Fibrinolytic system						
Plasminogen (U/mL)	1.70 (1.12–2.48)	1.95 (±0.35)	0.98 (0.78–1.18)	0.92 (0.75–1.08)	0.86 (0.68–1.03)	0.99 (0.7–1.22)
TPA (ng/mL)	—	—	2.15 (1.0–4.5)	2.42 (1.0–5.0)	2.16 (1.0–4.0)	4.90 (1.40–8.40)
α_2-AP (U/mL)	0.78 (0.4–1.16)	0.85 (±0.15)	10.5 (0.93–1.17)	0.99 (0.89–1.10)	0.98 (0.78–1.18)	1.02 (0.68–1.36)
PAI (U/mL)	—	—	5.42 (1.0–10.0)	6.79 (2.0–12.0)	6.07 (2.0–10.0)	3.50 (0–11.0)

Age-specific RBC/iron indicators

RBC Iron Indicator	Term Neonate	Infant (1–12 mo)	Child	Adolescent	Adult
Erythrocyte sedimentation rate (mm/hr)	0–4	—	4–20	—	0–20 female 0–10 male
Ferritin (ng/mL)	25–200	200–600 (1 mo)	7–140 (6 mo–15 yr)	7–140 (6 mo–15 yr)	10–120 female
		50–200 (2–5 mo)			20–250 male
Folate (serum) (ng/mL)	150–200	75–1,000	>160	>160	140–628
Free erythrocyte protoporphyrin	30–70 µmol/mol heme; <30 µg/dL whole blood	30–70 µmol/mol heme; <30 µg/dL whole blood	30–70 µmol/mol heme; <30 µg/dL whole blood	30–70 µmol/mol heme; <30 µg/dL whole blood	30–70 µmol/mol heme; <30 µg/dL whole blood
Haptoglobin (mg/dL)	5–50	25–185	25–185	25–185	25–185
Hemoglobin A_{1C} (% hemoglobin)	5.0–7.5	5.0–7.5	5.0–7.5	5.0–7.5	5.0–7.5
	77 ± 7 (1 d) 77 ± 6 (5 d) 70 ± 7 (3 wk)	53 ± 11 (6–9 wk) 23 ± 16 (3–4 mo) 5 ± 2 (6 mo) 1.6 ± 1 (8–11 mo)	<2	<2	<2
Hemopexin (mg/dL)	18% of maternal concentration	—	—	—	50–115 >75 pregnant women
Iron (µg/dL)	100–250	40–100	50–120	—	50–170 female 65–175 male

(continued)

Table 7. (continued)

RBC Iron Indicator	Term Neonate	Infant (1–12 mo)	Child	Adolescent	Adult
Methemoglobin (% Hb)	0–1.5%	0–1.5%	0–1.5%	0–1.5%	0–0.15%
TIBC (μg/dL)	150–250	200–400	250–500	300–600	250–425
Transferrin (mg/dL)	130–275	200–360	200–360	220–400	220–400
Vitamin B_{12} (pg/mL)	160–1,300	200–900	200–900	130–800	200–835

α_2-AP, α_2-antiplasmin; α_2-AT, α_2-antitrypsin; α_2-M, α_2-macroglobulin; aPTT, activated thromboplastin time; ATIII, antithrombin III; C_1-Inh, C_1 inhibitor; factor XIIIa, activated factor XIII; FDP, fibrin degradation products; HMWK, high-molecular-weight kininogen; INR, international normalized ratio; PAI, plasminogen activator inhibitor; PK, prekallikrein; PT, prothrombin time; RBC, red blood cell; TIBC, total iron-binding capacity; TPA, tissue plasminogen activator; vWF, von Willebrand factor.
From The Johns Hopkins Hospital, Siberry G, Iannone R. *Harriett Lane handbook*, 15th ed. St. Louis, MO: Mosby, 2000:327–329.

Table 8. Reference Values for Inhibitors of Coagulation in Healthy Children Compared with Adults

	Age			
	1–5 Yr	6–10 Yr	11–16 Yr	Adult
Coagulation Inhibitor	Mean (Boundary)	Mean (Boundary)	Mean (Boundary)	Mean (Boundary)
ATIII	1.11 (0.82–1.39)	1.11 (0.90–1.31)	1.05 (0.77–1.32)	1.0 (0.74–1.26)
α_2-M	1.69 (1.14–2.23)[a]	1.68 (1.28–2.09)[a]	1.56 (0.98–2.12)[a]	0.86 (0.52–1.20)
C_1-Inh	1.35 (0.85–1.83)[a]	1.14 (0.88–1.54)	1.03 (0.68–1.50)	1.0 (0.71–1.31)
α_1-AT	0.93 (0.39–1.47)	1.00 (0.69–1.30)	1.01 (0.65–1.37)	0.93 (0.55–1.30)
HCII	0.88 (0.48–1.28)[a]	0.86 (0.40–1.32)[a]	0.91 (0.53–1.29)[a]	1.08 (0.66–1.26)
Protein C	0.66 (0.40–0.92)[a]	0.69 (0.45–0.93)[a]	0.83 (0.55–1.11)[a]	0.96 (0.64–1.28)
Protein S				
Total	0.86 (0.54–1.18)	0.78 (0.41–1.14)	0.72 (0.52–0.92)	0.81 (0.60–1.13)
Free	0.45 (0.21–0.69)	0.42 (0.22–0.62)	0.38 (0.26–0.55)	0.45 (0.27–0.61)

α_1-AT, α_1-antitrypsin; α-M, α_2-macroglobulin; ATIII, antithrombin III; C_1-Inh, C_1 inhibitor; HCII, heparin cofactor II.
All values are expressed in U/mL, where for all factors pooled plasma contains 10 U/mL, with the exception of free protein S, which contains a mean of 0.4 U/mL. All values are given as a mean, followed by the lower and upper boundary encompassing 95% of the population. Between 20 and 30 samples were assayed for each value for each age group. Some measurements were skewed due to a disproportionate number of high values. The lower limits, which exclude the lower 2.5% of the population, are given.
[a]Values are significantly different from those of adults.
Reproduced from Andrew M, Vegh P, Johnston M, et al. Maturation of the hematopoietic system during childhood. *Blood* 1988;80:1998–2000.

Coagulation parameters for normal newborns, preterm infants, and older children are as follows:

	Term	**Preterm**	**Children**
aPTT (sec)	25–45	35–50	25–40
PT	12–17	14–22	12–14
Thrombin time (sec)	12–16	14–18	12–14
Platelet count (× 10^9/L)	150–400	150–400	150–400
Assays			
Factor I, fibrinogen (mg/dL)	150–300	150–300	175–450
Factor II, prothrombin (U/dL)	23–74	21–54	60–150
Factor V, proaccelerin (U/dL)	50–150	50–150	50–150
Factor VII, proconvertin (U/dL)	20–70	20–45	50–150
Factor VIII, antihemophilic (U/dL)	50–250	50–180	50–150
Factor IX, plasma thromboplastin (U/dL)	20–60	10–25	50–150
Factor X, Stuart factor (U/dL)	20–55	10–45	50–150
Factor XI, plasma thromboplastin antecedent (U/dL)	15–70	5–20	70–120
Factor XII, Hageman factor (U/dL)	25–70	15–45	70–120
Factor XIII (a) (U/dL)	>24	>24	>24
Factor XIII (g) (U/dL)	—	35–120	55–130
Prekallikrein (U/dL)	Reduced	Reduced	60–160
Plasminogen (U/dL)	100–350	110–250	250–400
High-molecular-weight kininogen	Reduced	Reduced	—

Fig. 4 presents an algorithm for evaluation of coagulation studies in neonates.

Bleeding in the Newborn

It was recognized centuries ago that bleeding problems in the neonatal period existed when the circumcision of the fourth son of a woman whose three other sons had

I Platelets decreased
PT increased
aPTT increased
↓
DIC (especially if sick infant, i.e., sepsis)

II Platelets normal
PT increased
aPTT increased
↓
Administer vitamin K

Bleeding continues	Bleeding stops
↓	↓
• Liver disease • Congenital fibrinogen deficiency • Factor V, X deficiency • Inhibitors	Vitamin K deficiency

III Platelets normal
PT normal
aPTT increased
↓
- Hemophilia A, B
- Factor XI deficiency
- von Willebrand disease
- Heparin or other inhibitors

IV Platelets normal
PT increased
aPTT normal
↓
- Factor VII deficiency
- Factor II deficiency

V Platelets normal
PT normal
aPTT normal
↓
- Factor XIII deficiency
- Platelet dysfunction
- von Willebrand disease
- α_2-Antiplasmin deficiency
- Dysfibrinogenemia

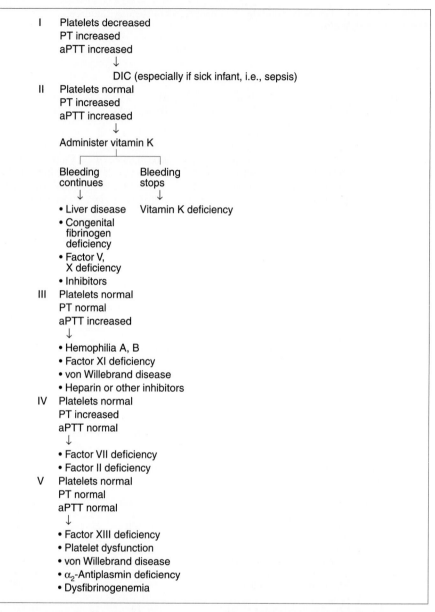

Fig. 4. Evaluation of coagulation studies in neonates. aPTT, activated thromboplastin time; DIC, disseminated intravascular coagulation; GIT, gastrointestinal tract; ITP, idiopathic thrombocytopenic purpura; PT, prothrombin time; SLE, systemic lupus erythematosus; SUBQ, subcutaneous; TAR, thrombocytopenia absent radius. Other causes of neonatal thrombocytopenia include giant hemangiomas, impaired production of megakaryocytes (i.e., TAR and Wiskott-Aldrich syndromes), congenital leukemia, cyanotic heart disease, and metabolic disorders. In relatively well infants, the causes of thrombocytopenia are maternal drug ingestion and immune factors. (continued)

VI Platelets decreased
PT normal
aPTT normal
↓
Maternal platelet count

- Low ↓
  - • ITP
  - • SLE
  - • Drugs
- Normal ↓ Previously affected neonate
  - Yes
  - No
    - Abnormal examination
      - Yes ↓
        - • TAR syndrome
        - • Fanconi syndrome
        - • Trisomy 13, 18
        - • Metabolic causes
        - • Leukemia
        - • Letterer-Siwe disease
      - No ↓
        - Drugs
        - Thrombosis

VII Summary

- • GIT, bleed, day 1—ingested maternal blood (Apt test)
- • Circumcision or SUBQ hematoma—factor deficiency
- • Umbilical cord hemorrhage:
  - Vitamin K deficiency
  - Factor XIII deficiency
  - Fibrinogen abnormality
- • Bleed day 2–3—vitamin K deficiency
- • Petechiae or generalized oozing—platelet problem
- • Oozing in sick patient:
  - DIC
  - Liver disease
- • Intracranial hemorrhage:
  - Trauma
  - Hereditary factor deficiencies
  - Platelet deficiency (or dysfunction)
  - Connective tissue disorder
  - Infections
  - Vascular malformations

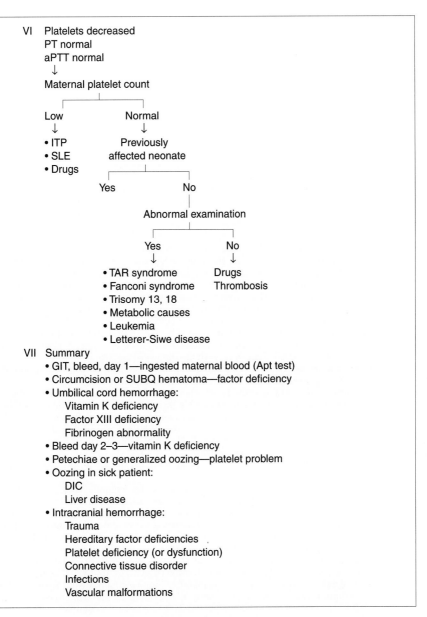

Fig. 4. (continued)

died from bleeding after circumcision was delayed. The neonate's ability to undergo normal clotting is complicated not just by congenital abnormalities but by physiological mechanisms as well. Levels of liver-dependent factors (vitamin K–dependent factors II, VII, IX, X) and factor V, plus contact factors (high-molecular-weight kininogen, Fletcher factor, factor XI, and factor XII) are usually low at birth, which prolongs both PT and aPTT. Infants usually manifest normal values of these factors by 6 months. Levels of normally occurring inhibitors [antithrombin

III (ATIII), protein C, protein S] are also diminished at birth, which balance the tendency to bleed.

Bleeding in newborns may manifest as oozing from the umbilicus, cephalohematomas, gastrointestinal bleeding, bleeding after circumcision, oozing from peripheral venipuncture sites, and bleeding into the skin. Sometimes sick newborns can bleed from mucous membranes, the urinary bladder, and sites of invasive procedures. Cerebral hemorrhage and hemarthrosis are rare as a manifestation of congenital factor deficiencies.

Laboratory Evaluation

Appropriate screening studies for infants with bleeding include examination of the peripheral blood smear, a complete blood count with platelet count, PT, aPTT, and fibrinogen level. (See Tables 1–6.)

After the first 3 days of life, new-onset thrombocytopenia in a newborn usually occurs in a sick infant, with sepsis or necrotizing enterocolitis and DIC, or is associated with thrombosis accompanying an indwelling arterial or venous catheter. Trisomy 13 and 18 are also associated with thrombocytopenia. Neonatal alloimmune thrombocytopenia (NAIT) is a relatively common condition. It may be severe and can lead to death, but it is diagnosable and treatable.

NAIT arises from an incompatibility between antigens on the surface of the platelets the baby inherits from the father and antigens on the surface of the mother's platelets. During pregnancy, with the inevitable mixing of maternal and fetal blood (even without procedures such as amniocentesis or chorionic villous sampling), the mother becomes sensitized to the foreign fetal platelet antigen and forms immunoglobulin G antibodies that cross the placenta and destroy the baby's platelets.

NAIT often presents as diffuse petechiae or mucosal surface bleeding in an otherwise healthy baby. The platelet count can be <10,000/μL to 20,000/μL. Because intracranial hemorrhage may occur around the time of birth or in the first few days of life, a head ultrasonographic examination is indicated when NAIT is suspected. Babies with platelet counts of <20,000/μL or those with bleeding need treatment.

A platelet count between 50,000/μL and 150,000/μL merits careful observation. Platelet counts generally rise slowly toward a normal level.

The diagnosis of NAIT is established when it is shown that the platelet antigens of the mother and father are incompatible and that immunoglobulin G antibody in the mother's serum reacts with the antigen on the father's platelets. In whites, incompatibility in human platelet alloantigen HPA-1 (formerly called $P1^{A2}$) is by far the most common cause of NAIT. National referral laboratories are best for assessment of other incompatibilities.

In women at particular risk for NAIT, screening in pregnancy for this disorder may be recommended.

Thrombocytopenia secondary to maternal factors, for example, connective tissue disorders, is relatively common. Maternal idiopathic thrombocytopenic purpura, whether active (mother has a low platelet count) or previously treated with splenectomy (mother's platelet count has normalized but she still produces antiplatelet antibodies that cross the placenta), is one such factor. True maternal idiopathic thrombocytopenic purpura, if not present before pregnancy, can be difficult to distinguish from gestational incidental thrombocytopenia, in which the mother's platelet count is mildly decreased to between 75,000/μL and 120,000/μL.

Maternal factors associated with neonatal thrombocytopenia that are unrelated to the immune system include preeclampsia or eclampsia, maternal hypertension, the HELLP syndrome (*h*emolysis, *e*levated *l*iver enzymes, *l*ow *p*latelets), drug-induced thrombocytopenia, and diabetes mellitus. A baby with intrauterine growth retardation is at risk. In these babies, the thrombocytopenia usually is moderate or mild, and in the absence of other risks for bleeding, resolves spontaneously in 7–14 days.

Bone marrow evaluation is indicated only if thrombocytopenia persists longer than 3 weeks after birth.

Coagulopathies Associated with Liver Disease

Coagulopathies in babies with liver disease manifest as prolonged PT and low plasma concentrations of many coagulation factors, such as factor V, the vitamin K–dependent factors, and fibrinogen. Causes of neonatal liver disease include inherited disorders, hypoxic damage, viral infections, shock, hydrops, and complications of total parenteral nutrition.

Hemorrhagic Disease of the Newborn

Physiologic deficiencies of the newborn are related to vitamin K–dependent clotting factors and occur in the first few days of life. These factors (II, VII, IX, X) require conversion of their inactive precursors, produced by the liver, by carboxylation of glutamyl residues, a vitamin K–dependent step. The levels of factors II, VII, IX, and X are approximately 50% of normal in umbilical cord blood and decline rapidly to reach a nadir at 48–72 hours of life. In 0.25–0.5% of infants the decline is so extreme that severe hemorrhage may result. Thereafter, the levels of these factors slowly increase but remain in the range of low adult levels for several weeks. The increase results from absorption of vitamin K from the diet. Breast milk has low levels of vitamin K, and symptomatic hemorrhagic disease of the newborn is more common in breast-fed than in formula-fed infants unless vitamin K prophylaxis is given.

Three forms of hemorrhagic disease of the newborn may occur:

1. The classic form presents on days 2–5 with gastrointestinal bleeding, ecchymoses, central nervous system hemorrhage, and oozing from venipunctures.
2. On day 1, a serious bleeding episode may occur, particularly if the mother has taken anticonvulsant drugs, warfarin, rifampin, or isoniazid, which interfere with vitamin K stores in the infant.
3. A late form, seen in breast-fed infants, is usually associated with a variety of disorders that compromise the supply of vitamin K, including cystic fibrosis, diarrhea, α_1-antitrypsin deficiency, hepatitis, and celiac disease.

Predisposing factors are lack of intestinal flora and hepatic immaturity. Earlier feeding (4–8 hours) leads to higher prothrombin values. A single parenteral dose of vitamin K, 0.5 mg, or 1–2 mg orally corrects the bleeding. Prophylactic vitamin K should be given at birth.

Laboratory Studies

Accurate testing of blood in the neonate requires that the blood specimens have adequate anticoagulant proportions and be uncontaminated with tissue thromboplastins or "jelly" from cord collections.

Vitamin K Effects

Mechanisms of Disturbed Vitamin K Effects in the Embryonic Period

Mechanism	**Disorder**
Malabsorption/malnutrition in maternal celiac disease	Vitamin K deficiency, embryopathy
Embryonic enzyme deficiency of vitamin K epoxide reductase	Pseudo–warfarin embryopathy
Pharmacologic inhibition by coumarin derivatives	Warfarin embryopathy

Vitamin K–Dependent Reactions

Activation of	**In**
Coagulation factors II, VII, IX, and X	Liver
Coagulation inhibitor proteins C and S	Liver
Protein Z	Liver
Osteocalcin ([bone 4-carboxyglutamic acid (Gla) protein]	Bone
Matrix Gla protein	Bone
Plaque Gla protein	?
Renal Gla protein(s)	Kidneys

Vitamin K Effects and Their Inhibition

See Fig. 5.

Laboratory Diagnosis

Factor VII and protein C have the shortest half-life of the vitamin K–dependent proteins. Factor VII is therefore the first of the procoagulants to become deficient, which results in an isolated prolongation of the PT. Levels of factors II, IX, and X

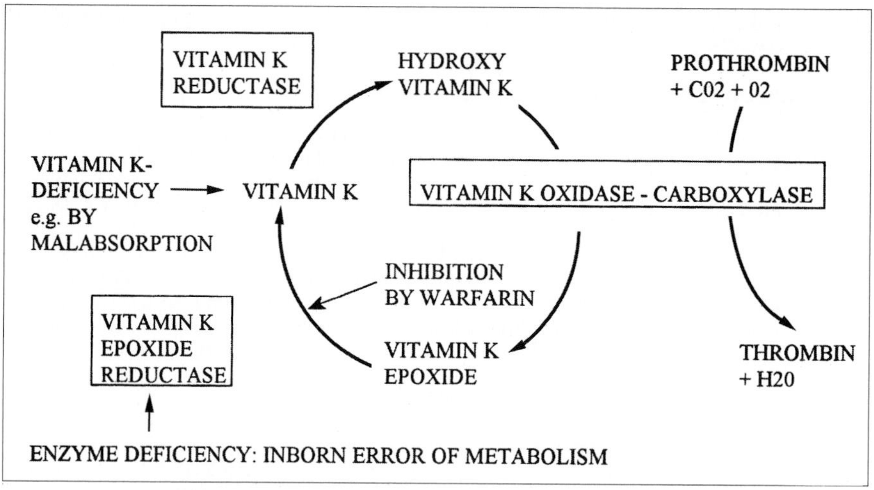

Fig. 5. Vitamin K effects and examples for their inhibition.

then decline, which prolongs the aPTT. Both the PT and aPTT are corrected by a 1:1 mix with normal plasma. Specific factor assays may help distinguish isolated vitamin K deficiency from congenital factor deficiency, liver disease, or DIC. Measurement of decarboxy-prothrombin (protein induced by vitamin K absence), which is increased in vitamin K deficiency, is a more specific test. An additional useful test is the *Echis* prothrombin assay, which measures both carboxylated and decarboxylated forms of prothrombin by comparing factor II activity in a calcium-dependent system to that in a calcium-independent system. A factor II/Echis II ratio of ≤ 0.80 indicates vitamin K deficiency. Vitamin K can be directly quantified. Normal serum levels in adults are around 0.5 ng/mL. Vitamin K assays, however, are too time consuming and expensive for routine diagnostic use.

Despite the sophistication of a number of assays for diagnosing vitamin K deficiency, only the PT is known to correlate with the risk of bleeding. The diagnosis of isolated vitamin K deficiency can be confirmed if administration of a therapeutic dose of vitamin K is followed by a fall in the PT, which can occur in as short a period as 30 minutes if the vitamin is given intravenously. Vitamin K deficiency can complicate other coagulopathies.

Laboratory evaluation for suspected vitamin K deficiency reveals a prolonged PT and deficiencies in factors II, VII, IX, and X; platelet count and fibrinogen levels are normal. Measurements of vitamin K levels do not help make the diagnosis because the levels are physiologically decreased in the newborn.

Congenital Clotting Factor Deficiencies

Physiologic deficiencies of clotting factors are manifest in neonates as deficiencies of vitamin K–dependent factors and contact factors. Levels of factor V, factor VIII, and fibrinogen are usually normal in the neonate. As levels of protein C, S, antithrombin II, and plasminogen are also reduced, a relative balance in the coagulation system is maintained.

Contact factor deficiencies are more typically associated with long aPTT and a predisposition to thrombosis. This is the case with deficiencies of Fletcher factor, Fitzgerald factor, and factor XII. Fletcher factor deficiency can be suspected when increased contact activation (incubation for 10 minutes versus the usual 5) normalizes the aPTT.

Factor XI deficiency accounts for a long aPTT but is responsible for mild bleeding tendencies unrelated to the level of factor XI. Easy bruising, epistaxis, menorrhagia, and bleeding after procedures are common signs. Hemarthroses are unusual. Liver and megakaryocytes are sites of production of factor XI. Factor XI deficiency is an autosomally inherited trait and its activity and antigen are reduced correspondingly. There are 15 known mutations responsible for factor XI deficiency. The most commonly occurring, type II and type III, are due to specific amino acid substitutions and occur in Ashkenazi Jews. Noonan syndrome (dysmorphic facies, short stature, congenital heart disease, easy bruising) may be associated with a partial factor XI deficiency. The lack of correlation of factor level and clinical manifestations is related to a variety of associated defects, most common of which is a qualitative or quantitative platelet factor XI abnormality. This may account for bleeding tendencies. Diagnosis of factor XI deficiency is confirmed by measurement of factor XI activity in the absence of an inhibitor. Performing this test on fresh plasma is recommended, as a relative increase in activity may be seen in a frozen sample. Bleeding time may also be increased, although other disorders should also be excluded in this circumstance.

Common Pathway Factor Deficiencies

Common pathway deficiencies are rare.

Fibrinogen (Factor I) Deficiency

Fibrinogen in the normal newborn is quantitatively normal, but there is usually a prolonged thrombin clotting time (TCT) as a result of slow polymerization of fibrin. Afibrinogenemia, an autosomal-recessive defect, is associated with severe bleeding, including hemarthroses, umbilical cord hemorrhage, menorrhagia, and splenic rupture. Laboratory studies reveal no clotting in the aPTT, PT, or TCT. Fibrinogen deficiency, an autosomal-recessive trait, may be congenital and is usually not associated with significant symptoms, except after surgical or traumatic events. These patients have long PT, aPTT, TCT, and bleeding times.

Hypofibrinogenemia probably represents the heterozygous state of *afibrinogenemia*. Hypofibrinogenemia produces milder forms of bleeding, such as postsurgical bleeding, recurrent abortion, and menorrhagia. The aPTT is usually normal with a slightly prolonged TCT.

Dysfibrinogenemia is due to an amino acid substitution, and each type is named after the city in which the defect was originally noted. Bleeding may be from mucous membranes, may occur after surgery or trauma, and may be associated with poor wound healing. Umbilical cord hemorrhage should raise the possibility of either a fibrinogen abnormality or factor XIII deficiency. Predisposition to thrombosis may also exist. The diagnosis is based on a finding of long TCT with normal antigenic (immunologic) assay.

Factor II Deficiency

Factor II deficiency is inherited as an autosomal-recessive trait and may be associated with a qualitative or quantitative defect. Activation of factor II by prothrombinase results in cleavage of factor Xa to produce fragment 1.2 and prothrombin 2. A deficiency or aberrant prothrombin molecule may result in epistaxis, menorrhagia, or postoperative bleeding.

Factor V Deficiency

Factor V deficiency may be an autosomal-dominant or autosomal-recessive trait. Bleeding in factor V deficiency is very variable and is dependent on levels of factor V (homozygous or heterozygous states), presence or absence of abnormal protein, and the platelet content of factor V. These should be evaluated with PT, aPTT, and a platelet function study. Patients may manifest mild or moderate bleeding phenomena, that is, postoperative or posttraumatic hemorrhage, intracranial hemorrhage in the newborn, deep hematoma, or hemarthroses. Heterozygotes usually do not bleed, as their factor V levels are >40%.

Factor X Deficiency

Factor X deficiency is an autosomal-recessive trait associated with a prolongation of PT, aPTT, and Russell viper venom time, and a normal bleeding time. Patients may present with mucous membrane and skin hemorrhages, exaggerated postoperative bleeding, hemarthroses, or posttraumatic or intracerebral hemorrhage. Umbilical stump bleeding is especially prominent. Spontaneous hyphema has been reported.

Factor VII Deficiency

Factor VII defects are autosomal-recessive traits that may present as umbilical stump bleeds in the newborn or as hemorrhage from mucous membranes later in life. Postoperative and posttraumatic bleeds may be life-threatening. Heterozygotes may have PTs that are only seconds long, are rarely symptomatic, and rarely bleed. Laboratory diagnosis is made by findings of a long PT, normal aPTT, normal Russell viper venom time, and decreased factor VII levels. Factor VII deficiency has been associated with Gilbert disease and Dubin-Johnson syndrome.

Factor XIII Deficiency (Fibrin-Stabilizing Factor Deficiency)

Factor XIII is responsible for clot stabilization and cross linking of the fibrin polymer; deficiency results in reduced clot stability. Deficiency of factor XIII is an autosomal-recessive trait; onset is most often in infancy with bleeding after separation of the umbilical cord stump. Gastrointestinal, intracranial, and intraarticular hemorrhages, and poor wound healing are common clinical manifestations. Routine coagulation studies are normal. The diagnosis may be suspected by the finding of an abnormal solubility of the clot in 5 mol/L urea solution.

Factor VIII and Factor IX Deficiencies (Hemophilia)

Hemophilia A and hemophilia B are hereditary bleeding disorders that result from defects in the factor VIII gene (FVIII) and factor IX gene (FIX), respectively. The genes lead to decreased or absent circulating levels of functional factor VIII or factor IX, which results in excessive and prolonged bleeding. Hemophilia A is the more common form and accounts for 80–85% of cases, whereas hemophilia B accounts for 15–20%. The prevalence of hemophilia A is 1 in 10,000 males, whereas that of hemophilia B is approximately 1 in 50,000 males. Hemophilia has a worldwide distribution and affects all racial groups. The severity of the disease is usually correlated with the degree of factor VIII or factor IX deficiency.

Severe disease occurs when the level is <2% and is associated with the highest incidence of anti–factor VIII antibodies; such severe disease accounts for 5–10% of cases. Moderate disease is found with a 2–5% factor level, and mild disease occurs with levels of 5–25%.

Hemophilia A and B are clinically indistinguishable. Both affect males almost exclusively, and both are characterized by bleeding into joints and soft tissue. The genes for factor VIII and factor IX are on the long arm of the X chromosome, in band Xq28 and band Xq27, respectively.

Deletions, insertions, inversions, and missense mutations have been identified in patients with hemophilia. As many as 50% of patients with severe hemophilia A have an inversion involving intron 21. There is a significant rate of spontaneous mutation in this large gene, because as many as 30% of patients have no family history of hemophilia.

Approximately one-third of cases of hemophilia newly diagnosed in infants result from a spontaneous mutation.

Diagnosis of Hemophilia

Because factors VIII and IX do not cross the placenta, prenatal diagnosis is possible with a cord blood collection using direct determination of the factor levels or DNA probes. Chorionic villus sampling at 9–12 weeks may be performed.

Bleeding may occur in the newborn period, manifested by intraventricular hemorrhage or after circumcision, although the latter is rare. Bleeding during the first year of life is uncommon unless the infant is exposed to trauma or surgery. Bleeding into joints, soft tissue, muscle, or tongue occurs in later childhood when the child begins to walk. Gastrointestinal tract hemorrhage may occur and may be associated with peptic ulcer disease.

Laboratory diagnosis is made when aPTT is prolonged after the patient's plasma is mixed with normal pooled plasma. Low levels of factor VIII clotting activity (factor VIII:c), normal PT, normal levels of von Willebrand factor antigen (vWF:Ag), and normal bleeding time are identified. Antibodies to VIII:c should be evaluated in patients with severe disease and particularly in patients who fail to respond to treatment. Carrier detection and prenatal diagnosis can be performed by restriction fragment length polymorphism (RFLP) analysis of the affected family.

It is now possible to trace the defective allele in some families by examining the inheritance of RFLPs linked to the factor VIII gene and allele-specific oligonucleotide hybridization. Previously, prenatal diagnosis required sampling of fetal blood for coagulant activity. Now, in families with an identifiable RFLP linked to the gene or a known mutation, precise diagnosis is possible early in pregnancy with either chorionic villus biopsy or amniocentesis.

Female carriers of hemophilia, who are heterozygotes, occasionally have factor VIII levels far below 50% due to random inactivation of normal X chromosomes. These symptomatic carriers may bleed excessively with major surgery or with menses. Rarely, true female hemophiliacs arise from consanguinity within hemophilia families or from concomitant Turner's syndrome (monosomy X or monosomy X mosaicism) in a carrier female.

von Willebrand Disease (Vascular Hemophilia)

von Willebrand factor (vWF), an autosomally inherited factor, is a large multimeric glycoprotein that is synthesized in megakaryocytes and endothelial cells. It is stored in specific cellular storage granules, the Weibel-Palade bodies (endothelial cells), and the α granule of platelets. Its major functions are acting as a carrier protein for factor VIII and binding glycoprotein Ib on platelets, which initiates platelet adhesion to damaged vessel walls.

Clinically, patients with vWF deficiency manifest mild to severe hemorrhage, typically from mucocutaneous sites, gastrointestinal tract, central nervous system, or endometrium. The severity of symptoms is usually related to homozygosity or heterozygosity for the von Willebrand gene. Patients with the defect may be asymptomatic as well.

Nosebleeds, bleeding from the gums and tongue, prolonged oozing from cuts, purpura, petechiae, and increased bleeding after trauma or surgery are the initial manifestations. Easy bruisability may be seen in childhood. Excessive bleeding during menses may give the first clue.

The most frequently encountered type of von Willebrand disease (vWD) is referred to as type I. Multimeric analysis reveals all polymeric forms of vWF, but the intensity of the bands is decreased with a reduction of vWF:Ag and vWF activity. The bleeding time is usually prolonged. Asymptomatic or mild forms of this type of vWD are frequently found, in which the level of vWF falls between 40% and 60%; in these patients, the bleeding time is usually normal.

Another type is referred to as type IIA. In this form, there is a qualitative defect of vWF, although the amount of protein synthesized may be normal. The defect appears to be a failure to form intermediate and large multimers, which is revealed on multimeric analysis or on crossed immunoelectrophoresis. The bleeding time is usually prolonged, and the factor VIII level is decreased or normal.

Other types of vWD appear to be less common. In type IIB, patients may not respond to desmopressin (1-desamino-9-D-arginine vasopressin).

Patients with type III vWD have a severe bleeding disorder resembling hemophilia A. These patients have very low levels of factor VIII:c, vWF:Ag, and ristocetin cofactor activity. The laboratory features of vWD are summarized.

Clinical manifestations and laboratory findings in vWD vary over time and include prolonged bleeding time, long aPTT, decreased levels of vWF:Ag, and decreased levels of factor VIII. Other initial studies include assays of ristocetin cofactor and VWF multimers. The aPTT is relatively insensitive in evaluating vWD, and a normal value should not preclude further testing. It should be noted that patients with blood group O typically have a lower normal range of vWF antigen. Use of vWF ristocetin cofactor levels appears best for following response to therapy. The PFA used by many laboratories to screen for platelet function abnormalities may provide an abnormal result when vWF normalizes and a normal PFA finding after treatment (in acquired vWF diseases) when the level of vWF is diminished.

Acquired vWD may occur as an autoimmune event in patients with hypothyroidism, in patients with congenital heart defects, and with those with various tumors, including Wilms tumor.

Table 9. Variants of von Willebrand Disease

Test	Type I	Type IIA	Type IIB	PT-vWD	Type III
vWF:Ag	↓	↓	±↓	±↓	Absent
R:Co (vWF)	↓	↓↓↓	±↓	±↓	Absent
RIPA	±↓	↓↓	Normal	Normal	Absent
RIPA-LD	Absent	Absent	Increased	Increased	Absent
Frequency	70–80%	10–12%	3–5%	0–1%	1–3%

↓, mildly decreased; ↓↓, decreased; ↓↓↓, greatly decreased; ±↓, sometimes decreased; PT-vWD, pseudo–von Willebrand disease; R:Co, ristocetin cofactor activity; RIPA, ristocetin-induced platelet aggregation; RIPA-LD, ristocetin-induced platelet aggregation to low doses of ristocetin; vWF, von Willebrand factor; vWF:Ag, von Willebrand factor antigen.
Adapted from Montgomery RR, Scott JP. Hemostasis: diseases of the fluid phase. In: Nathan DG, Oski F, eds. *Hematology of infancy and childhood,* 4th ed. Vol II. Philadelphia: WB Saunders, 1993.

Table 10. Differences between von Willebrand Disease and Hemophilia A

Characteristic	von Willebrand disease	Hemophilia A
Inheritance	Autosomal dominant	Sex-linked recessive
Hemarthroses or joint damage	Rare	Present in most severe cases
Clinical severity	Usually mild and rarely dangerous or crippling	Mild to severe
Bleeding time	May be prolonged	Normal if test performed correctly
Factor VIII:c level	Usually 6–50%	0–35%
vWF antigen	<50%	>50%
Ristocetin cofactor activity	Abnormal	Normal

Factor VIII:c, factor VIII coagulant activity; vWF, von Willebrand factor.

Variants of von Willebrand Disease

See Table 9.

Distinctions between von Willebrand Disease and Hemophilia

See Table 10.

Thrombotic Disorders

Disseminated Intravascular Coagulation

DIC is a complex disorder due to widespread activation of the clotting mechanism. DIC is a microvascular process that may be precipitated by infection, neoplasms, intravascular hemolysis, vascular disorders, thrombosis, snakebite, massive tissue injury, trauma, hypoxia, shock, acidosis, hypothermia, amniotic fluid aspiration, liver disease, infant and adult respiratory distress syndrome, purpura fulminans, or thermal injury.

In DIC there is generation of fibrin in the blood and consumption of procoagulants and platelets, essentially conversion of plasma to serum.

Signs and symptoms include epistaxis, gingival bleeding, mucosal bleeding, hemoptysis, hematemesis, metrorrhagia, cough, dyspnea, confusion, disorientation, melena, hematuria, oliguria, fever, petechiae, purpura, ecchymosis, hemorrhagic necrosis, localized rales, tachypnea, pleural friction rub, retinal hemorrhage, anuria, thrombosis, stupor, peripheral cyanosis, disseminated fibrin in capillaries, and fibrin thrombi in large vessels.

Important risk factors for DIC include pregnancy, prostatic surgery, head injury, inflammatory state, abruptio placentae, and large hemangiomas.

Diagnostic studies show the following:

Thrombocytopenia	Increased partial thromboplastin time
Decreased fibrinogen levels	Positive result on D-dimer assay
Schistocytosis	Increased prothrombin time
Increased thrombin time	Increased levels of fibrin degradation products
Decreased ATIII levels	Increased bleeding time
Anemia	Leukocytosis
Increased lactate dehydrogenase level	Increased blood urea nitrogen
Decreased level of factor V	Decreased or increased level of factor VIII
Decreased level of factor X	Decreased level of factor XIII
Hemoglobinemia	Hematuria

Testing should consist of serial studies, every 4–6 hours, of aPTT, fibrinogen level, platelet count, and D-dimer level, and review of peripheral smear. Serial evaluation is important, because at the onset, results of some studies may actually be elevated.

Disorders Associated with Disseminated Intravascular Coagulation

- Infectious diseases
  - Gram-positive bacteremia
  - Disseminated fungal infections
  - Rickettsial infections
  - Gram-negative bacteremia
  - Meningococcal sepsis
  - Severe viremias (e.g., hemorrhagic fevers)
  - Neonatal and intrauterine infections
  - Plasmodium falciparum malaria
- Liver diseases
  - Cirrhosis of the liver
  - Massive liver cell necrosis
- Malignant diseases
  - Acute promyelocytic leukemia
  - Metastatic carcinoma, mainly adenocarcinoma
- Obstetric disorders
  - Amniotic fluid embolism
  - Retained dead fetus
  - Abruptio placentae
- Miscellaneous disorders
  - Heat stroke
  - Severe shock
  - Small vessel vasculitides
  - Massive trauma
  - Burns
  - Snakebite (Russell viper)
  - Surgery with extracorporeal circulation
  - Intravascular hemolysis

Chronic localized DIC is uncommon in the pediatric age group and is almost exclusively documented in association with giant hemangiomas (Kasabach-Merritt syndrome). The Kasabach-Merritt syndrome was initially described in 1940 and has its peak incidence in early infancy. The condition can, however, present later in childhood, and although the diagnosis is usually obvious, occult hemangiomas do occur (e.g., in spleen and retroperitoneum) and may exist undetected in the presence of a significant coagulopathy. A rare syndrome of *neonatal purpura fulminans* with DIC is caused by homozygous or compound heterozygous deficiencies of protein C or protein S. Affected infants often manifest blindness and retinal hemorrhage in addition to cerebral infarcts and renal vein thrombosis. Neonates presenting with extensive, multiple, or unusual thrombi are likely to carry two or more thrombophilia traits or acquired coagulopathies resulting from transplacentally acquired antiphospholipid antibodies.

The prevalence of thrombosis increases with puberty and rises steadily thereafter. Cumulatively, the rate of thrombosis is 5–10% over a lifetime.

Thrombocytosis

Essential Thrombocytosis[3]

Peripheral blood findings are as follows:

Red blood cells	Hemoglobin level <13 g/dL or normal red cell mass
WBCs	Usually normal
Platelets	Increased to >600,000 platelets/μL Large platelets with hypogranular forms
Other	Platelet aggregation abnormalities Variable qualitative platelet defects May have prolonged bleeding time
Marrow	Hypercellular marrow with megakaryocytic hyperplasia, megakaryocytic clustering Variable to absent reticulum fibrosis Normal iron stores
Cytogenetics	Usual normal karyotype

Neoplastic Thrombocytosis

Causes of neoplastic thrombocytosis in children include the following[4]:

Myeloproliferative disorders
Lymphoma
Hepatoblastoma
Neuroblastoma

Reactive Thrombocytosis

General Causes

Iron deficiency
Neoplasm
Congenital heart disease (cyanotic)
Trauma
Infection
Parenteral nutrition
Vitamin K deficiency
Asplenia
Hemorrhage
Maternal polydrug use
Down syndrome
Polycythemia
Acute lymphoblastic leukemia

Causes in Children[5]

Trauma, surgery, fracture, hemorrhage
Inflammatory diseases: collagen vascular disease, inflammatory bowel disease, sarcoid
Infections: viral, bacterial
Nutritional: iron deficiency, vitamin B_{12} or folate deficiency
Drug use: corticosteroids
Splenectomy

[3]Collins RD, Swerdlow SH. *Pediatric hematopathology.* Churchill Livingstone, 2001.
[4]Chan KW, Kaikov Y, Wadsworth LD. Thrombocytosis in childhood: a survey of 94 patients. *Pediatrics* 1989;84:1064–1067.
[5]Chan KW, Kaikov Y, Wadsworth LD. Thrombocytosis in childhood: a survey of 94 patients. *Pediatrics* 1989;84:1064–1067.

Thrombophilia and Thrombosis in the Infant and Child

Thrombophilia is a term indicating a genetic predisposition to form excessive blood clots or thrombi.

Thrombosis in infants and children is characterized by a predilection for large vessels and an increased incidence of arterial lesions. Thrombi often occur in later life. Thrombophilia may predispose to vascular disease. Thrombosis in the young is multifactorial, and the coexistence of multiple thrombophilic genes in symptomatic children is common. Thrombophilic children typically develop thrombi in a setting of other predisposing medical conditions and provoking factors. Thrombophilia may be suggested by the occurrence of thrombi in unusual locations or without other apparent provocation.

Thromboses occur more frequently during the perinatal period than during any other period of childhood. The incidence of thrombosis in the newborn infant has been estimated at 5 in 100,000. Thromboses may occur prenatally and usually present clinically within the first 48 hours of life. The cerebral arteries and veins, renal veins, aorta, and vena cava are most commonly affected. Hematuria, thrombocytopenia, and hypertension form a classic clinical triad in neonatal renal vein thrombosis. Neonatal stroke generally manifests with seizures within the first 24 hours of life. The level of consciousness may be normal or depressed. Infants and children beyond the neonatal period suffer arterial and venous stroke at the rate of 2 in 100,000. One-third of children with stroke test positive for anticardiolipin antibodies. Massive aortic thromboses present with absent pulses in the lower extremities, upper extremity hypertension, and cardiovascular collapse. Renal vein thrombosis presents with a flank mass that may be palpable in the delivery room or in the nursery.

Testing after the acute event is best accomplished with noncoagulant-based studies, such as DNA-based polymerase chain reaction testing and homocysteine measurement. The coagulant levels may be spuriously elevated or lowered when patients are on anticoagulant agents or in the presence of acute-phase reactions. Testing 3–6 months after cessation of anticoagulant therapy, if possible, results in more accurate results.

Thrombosis, Deep Vein

Development of single or multiple blood clots within the deep veins of the extremities or pelvis is usually accompanied by inflammation of the vessel wall. The major clinical consequence is embolization, usually to the lung.

Many cases are completely asymptomatic and are diagnosed retrospectively after embolization. Signs include limb pain or swelling, leg pain on dorsiflexion of the foot (Homans sign), palpable tender cord in affected limb, warmth or redness of the skin over the area of thrombosis, fever, nontender swelling of collateral superficial veins, massive edema with cyanosis and ischemia (phlegmasia cerulea dolens).

Causes of deep vein thrombosis include venous stasis, injury to vessel wall, and abnormalities of coagulation. Clinical risk factors are trauma, especially long bone fractures or crush injuries; surgery, particularly hip and knee surgery; prolonged immobility; pregnancy, especially the puerperium; cancers; use of indwelling central venous catheters; use of birth-control drugs; exposure to extremely high altitude (>14,000 feet). Other risk factors are deficiencies of protein C, protein S, ATIII, and all endogenous anticoagulants; presence of antiphospholipid antibodies; nephrotic syndrome; polycythemia vera; homocystinuria; *Campylobacter jejuni* bacteremia; and mutation of factor V (factor V Leiden).

Causes of Thrombosis in Children

Physiologic Characteristics of Neonatal Coagulation That Predispose to Thrombosis

Increased Primary Hemostasis

Increased concentration and size of vWF multimers
Increased hematocrit and viscosity

Increased Thrombin Generation

Increased concentration of factor VIII

Increased tissue factor expression on monocytes and endothelial cells

Decreased Thrombin Regulation

Decreased levels of coagulation inhibitors antithrombin, protein C, and protein S

Decreased Fibrinolysis

Decreased concentration of plasminogen

Fetal plasminogen with reduced and delayed activation

Decreased tissue plasminogen activator (TPA) level

Increased levels of α_2-antiplasmin and plasminogen activator inhibitor 1 (PAI-1)

Genetic Causes of Thrombophilia in Children

Disorders involving excessive primary hemostasis result in platelet clumping and clearance but usually manifest with bleeding rather than thrombosis.

Trait	Frequency of Occurrence
Congenital hemolytic-uremic syndrome/thrombotic thrombocytopenia purpura	
Caused by deficient vWF-cleaving metalloproteinase	Rare
Caused by vascular endothelial cyclooxygenase deficiency	Rare
Platelet glycoprotein Ib mutations resulting in increased platelet/von Willebrand factor interactions (platelet or pseudo–von Willebrand disease)	Rare
Excessive thrombin generation	
Elevated factor VIII level	11% of whites
Factor V G1691A mutation	3–8% of whites
Prothrombin G20210A mutation	1–2% of whites
Deficient thrombin regulation	
Antithrombin deficiency	1 in 5,000
Protein C deficiency	1 in 500
Protein S deficiency	Unknown
Deficient fibrinolysis	
Dysfibrinogenemia	Rare
Plasminogen deficiency	Rare
Multiple effects	
Cystathionine synthase deficiency	Rare
Sickle cell anemia	1 in 400 blacks
β Thalassemia	Population dependent

Acquired Causes Predisposing to Thrombosis in Children

Indwelling vascular catheter

Vascular damage

Trauma

Surgery

Infection, inflammation

Vascular malformation, malignancy, chemotherapy

Cardiac disease

Prosthetic cardiac valves

Systemic lupus erythematosus

Rheumatoid arthritis

Crohn disease

Ulcerative disease

Sickle cell anemia and other hemoglobinopathies

Renal disease

Diabetes mellitus

Use of oral contraceptive agents

Polycythemia, hyperviscosity

Essential thrombocythemia

Hemolytic-uremic syndrome, thrombotic thrombocytopenia purpura

Heparin-associated thrombocytopenia and thrombosis syndrome

Splenectomy (e.g., sideroblastic anemia)

Excessive Thrombin Generation
Presence of lupus anticoagulant with or without anticardiolipin antibody
Increased tissue factor expression with infection, inflammation, malignancy
Deficient Thrombin Regulation
Acquired antithrombin deficiency with nephrotic syndrome
Decreased synthesis of hepatic proteins (e.g., chemotherapy with L-asparaginase)
DIC
Acquired antibodies to coagulation-regulatory proteins
Multiple Defects
Hyperhomocysteinemia
Dietary deficiencies of folate, vitamin B_6, or vitamin B_{12}
Inactivity
Smoking
Coffee drinking
Primary antiphospholipid antibody syndrome

Disorders Associated with Thrombophilia

Antithrombin III Deficiency

ATIII, a glycoprotein that is synthesized in the liver and endothelial cells, forms an inactive complex by binding irreversibly with thrombin. The normal functional level is 75–125%. It inactivates activated factors XII, XI, IX, X, and possibly VII, particularly in the presence of heparin, with which it complexes on a lysine site. Levels <50% are associated with a substantial risk of thrombosis. The disorder is an autosomal trait with variable penetrance and may present in the pediatric population. Altered activity may or may not be associated with reduced antigen levels. A variety of stress-induced clinical settings may predispose to thromboses, especially in leg or mesenteric veins, and result in pulmonary embolism. An isolated case of myocardial infarction has been reported in a newborn with congenital ATIII deficiency.

Increased ATIII levels may be observed in patients on warfarin sodium (Coumadin) or various other drugs such as oral contraceptives, and in patients with congenital factor deficiencies (i.e., of factors V, VIII, IX). Acquired ATIII deficiency may be observed in liver disease, neoplastic syndrome, burns, sepsis, DIC, postoperative state, and enteropathies.

Protein C and Protein S Deficiency

Protein C is a vitamin K–dependent protein, activated by thrombin and mediated via thrombomodulin on endothelial cells. Protein C is a serine protease that inactivates PAI-I, VIIIa, and Va in the presence of a cofactor protein S. The deficiency is inherited as an autosomal-dominant disorder with variable penetrance. Thromboses at an early age, recurrent thromboses, and thromboses at unusual sites should raise suspicions of protein C deficiency. Neonatal purpura fulminans, warfarin-induced necrosis, and recurrent deep vein thromboses are the usual syndromes. Type I protein S deficiency is characterized by a concordant decrease in protein antigen and activity. Type II disease shows normal total and free protein S compartments with a decrease in protein S clotting activity. Type III protein S deficiency is characterized by a normal total protein S with a decrease in both free protein S and protein S clotting activity. Decreased levels of free protein S correlate best with thrombotic risk. Protein S levels are affected by hormone status. Clinically, protein S deficiency manifests similarly to protein C deficiency in severity. The newborn infant has a mean plasma level of total protein S antigen of only 0.20 U/mL, which is related to a low C4 binding protein. Almost all neonatal protein S is functional. A qualitative assay using synthetic chromogen substrate may detect functional deficiency. The test is of limited value in patients on oral anticoagulants. Activated protein C (APC) sensitivity is determined by measuring the ratio of aPTT with and without activated protein C.

Activated Protein C Resistance

APC resistance is the most common predisposition to unexplained deep vein thrombosis, arising in 50% of families with a history of thrombophilia. There appears to be a strong association between APC resistance and a single point mutation in factor V (factor V Leiden). An additional mutation in the factor V gene is FVR506Q, factor V Cambridge. Resistance to protein C is detected when the ratio of aPTT with and without APC is <2.1 (modified coenzyme A test). The molecular defect results from a G to A transition in position 1691 of the factor V gene and can be detected by polymerase chain reaction amplification and DNA sequencing, which detects only levels <20%. Prevalence of carriers of the mutation is 3–4%. Protein C is very much influenced by protein S. Heparin in test plasma can be overcome by using Hepzyme.

Factor V G1691A shows some hormonal interaction and increases the risk of thrombosis, especially stroke, in adolescents in association with the use of oral contraceptive agents or pregnancy, and during the perinatal period. Maternal factor V G1691A may cause thrombus formation in the maternal or fetal placental circulation or both. Elevated levels of factors XI, IX, and VII have also been associated with factor V Leiden.

The mutation in prothrombin G20210A, found in 1–2% of the white population, is the second most common cause of thrombophilia. Prothrombin G20210A has been associated with venous and arterial thrombosis including central nervous system lesions in infants, children, and adolescents. Prothrombin levels may be elevated to 115–130%, and prothrombin fragment 1+2 and thrombin-antithrombin complexes suggest the enhancement of thrombin generation. This abnormality has been observed in patients with other mutations predisposing to thrombosis, especially presence of factor V Leiden.

APC resistance may also be acquired, such as in patients with lupus anticoagulants and in pregnancy, oral contraception use, and acute-phase reactions.

Protein such as thrombomodulin and tissue factor pathway inhibitor that are normally associated with cell surfaces or other compartments may be genetically altered but are difficult to study. Gene sequencing has been performed to detect abnormalities of these proteins, but gene mutations are not always synonymous with protein deficiencies.

Other Genetic Disorders Associated with Thrombophilia

Other rare genetic fibrinolytic defects have been associated with thrombophilia. Decreases in the amount or activity of plasminogen as well as some dysfibrinogenemias have been associated with deficiencies in fibrinolysis. Whether *TPA* deficiency or elevated levels of PAI-1 predispose to familial thrombosis is being studied.

The metabolic disease *homocystinuria*, caused by decreased activity of the enzyme cystathionine synthase is associated with a 50% incidence of early-onset arterial and venous thrombosis as well as premature atherosclerotic vascular disease. Other enzyme deficiencies in the metabolism of homocysteine also result in increased vascular disease. The most common genetic defect of homocysteine metabolism is caused by a thermolabile variant of the methyltetrahydrofolate reductase gene (MTHFR C677T), which is found in a homozygous form in 10% of the population.

Hemoglobinopathies including sickle cell anemia and β thalassemia are associated with a genetic predisposition to thrombosis related to multiple effects, including endothelial cell damage by abnormal red cells as well as acquired protein S deficiency. In addition, congenitally abnormal red cells found in sideroblastic anemia cause recurrent venous thrombosis and pulmonary emboli in affected individuals after splenectomy.

Acquired Disorders Predisposing to Thrombosis

The most common acquired disorders predisposing to thrombosis in children and adolescents are caused by antiphospholipid antibodies, both the lupus anticoagulant and anticardiolipin antibodies. The anticardiolipin antibody is detected using an enzyme-linked immunosorbent assay. Both of these autoantibodies can be of immunoglobulin G, immunoglobulin M, or immunoglobulin A specificity, although immunoglobulin G antibodies are most reliably correlated with clinical pathology.

Lupus anticoagulants occur as true autoantibodies in approximately 40% of children with systemic lupus erythematosus and occasionally in children with juvenile rheumatoid arthritis, ulcerative colitis, Crohn disease, and other collagen vascular diseases. It may be associated with second-trimester spontaneous abortion.

The *antiphospholipid antibody syndrome* often presents in adolescents. This clinical syndrome is characterized by presence of the lupus anticoagulant or anticardiolipin antibody along with other autoantibodies, most often directed against blood cells, including platelets, red blood cells, and WBCs. Antithyroid antibodies are also common. Presence of the lupus anticoagulant is associated with a high rate of venous thrombosis and primary pulmonary thrombi or pulmonary emboli. Anticardiolipin antibodies are found in one-third of children with stroke. In adult women, anticardiolipin antibodies are most commonly found in a clinical constellation including thrombocytopenia, migraine headache, stroke, and recurrent fetal wastage. A few case reports have described familial variants of the antiphospholipid antibody syndrome with lupus anticoagulants.

Measurement of lupus anticoagulant profiles typically requires at least two screening procedures. This may include kaolin clotting time, aPTT, or dilute Russell viper venom time (DRVVT). A positive screen result requires a more specific procedure, such as Staclot LA (Diagnostica Stago, Asnieres-sur-Seine, France) in the presence of a long aPTT or Viperquick LA-Check (Organon Teknika Corporation, Durham, North Carolina) (lupus anticoagulant check) in the presence of an abnormal lupus anticoagulant test result (DRVVT). It should be noted that anticardiolipin antibodies may be positive in up to 25% of the patients who have negative results on studies for the anticoagulants.

Autoantibodies causing acquired deficiencies of protein S, protein C, or antithrombin with or without evidence of a concomitant lupus anticoagulant occasionally are present in children.

Acquired deficiencies of coagulation-regulatory proteins and thrombosis occur in DIC as well as disorders affecting hepatic protein synthesis, such as chemotherapy with L-asparaginase for acute leukemia. *Nephrosis* is associated with urinary losses of antithrombin along with other proteins. An acquired increase in homocysteine secondary to deficiencies of folic acid, vitamin B_6, or vitamin B_{12} is a more common cause of hyperhomocysteinemia than are genetic mutations. There are many lifestyle choices that increase the risk for hyperhomocysteinemia, including smoking, excessive caffeine intake, poor diet, and inactivity.

Prevalence of Inherited Thrombotic Disorders

ATIII deficiency	1–4 %
Protein C deficiency	5–6 %
Protein S deficiency	5–6 %
APC resistance	20–60%

Mechanisms by Which Inherited Thrombotic Disorders Result in Thrombosis[6]

Disorder	Mechanism
Factor V Leiden	Failure of APC to inactivate factor Va due to a highly conserved point mutation
Protein C deficiency	Failure to generate APC; failure to inactivate factors Va and VIIIa
Protein S deficiency	Failure of APC to inactivate factors Va and VIIIa
ATIII deficiency	Failure to inhibit thrombin, factor Xa, and activated factors
Homocysteinemia	Endothelial cell cytotoxicity and perturbation of vascular hemostatic mechanisms
Elevated factor VIII levels	Unknown
Elevated factor IX levels	Unknown
Elevated factor XI levels	Sustained thrombin generation and protection of fibrin from proteolysis
Prothrombin mutation	Elevated plasma prothrombin levels
Dysfibrinogenemia	Abnormal fibrin that resist fibrinolysis
Plasminogen deficiency	Failure to generate plasmin
TPA deficiency	Failure to activate plasminogen
Excess PAI-1 activity	Neutralization of TPA
Thrombomodulin deficiency	Failure to generate APC

[6]Florell SR, Rodgers GM. Inherited thrombotic disorders: an update. *Am J Hematol* 1997;54:53–60.

Table 11. Thrombosis Risks Associated with Various Hypercoagulability Disorders

Site of Thrombosis	Hyperhomo-cysteinemia	Resistance to Activated Protein C	Deficiency of Protein S	Deficiency of Protein C or Antithrombin
Superficial vein thrombosis	–	+	+	–
Subclavian vein thrombosis	+	–	–	–
Proximal deep vein thrombosis, idiopathic distal deep vein thrombosis, or pulmonary embolism	+++	+++	++	++
Distal deep vein thrombosis due to surgery or immobilization	+	+	+	–

–, no increased risk; +, increased risk; ++, strongly increased risk; +++, very strongly increased risk.
From Sole FJ. *N Engl J Med* 2001;345:697,698–699.

Risk Factors for Thrombosis

Table 11 indicates the risk for various thrombotic events associated with various hypercoagulability disorders.

Laboratory Tests for Thrombophilia in Children[7]

Recommended Tests

See Fig. 6.

Level I: Basic evaluation for all children with thrombosis
- Complete blood count with hematocrit, WBC count, differential, and platelet count
- Antithrombin activity
- Protein C activity
- Protein S, free or activity
- Factor VIII activity
- Factor V A1691G gene test or functional activated protein C resistance assay (or both)
- Prothrombin G20210A gene test
- Homocysteine level
- Lupus anticoagulant test
- Anticardiolipin antibody test
- Sickle cell and thalassemia screen or hemoglobin electrophoresis

Level II: Extended evaluation for children with normal level I values and recurrent thrombosis, a positive family history for thrombosis, or severe thrombosis
- Euglobulin clot lysis time
- Plasminogen activity
- Dysfibrinogenemia evaluation: fibrinogen activity, antigen level, thrombin time, reptilase time, level of fibrin degradation products; consider crossed immunoelectrophoresis
- Test for paroxysmal nocturnal hemoglobinuria (sucrose hemolysis)
- If not previously performed:
  - Functional activated protein C resistance (modified assay)
  - Hemoglobin electrophoresis
  - Erythrocyte sedimentation rate, C-reactive protein level

Level III (currently under investigation)
- Lipoprotein(a) level
- Factor XII deficiency
- Factor XI level
- Factor IX level
- Factor VIII level

[7]Manco-Johnson MJ, Nuss R. Thrombophilia in the infant and child. *Adv Pediatr* 2001;48:363–384.

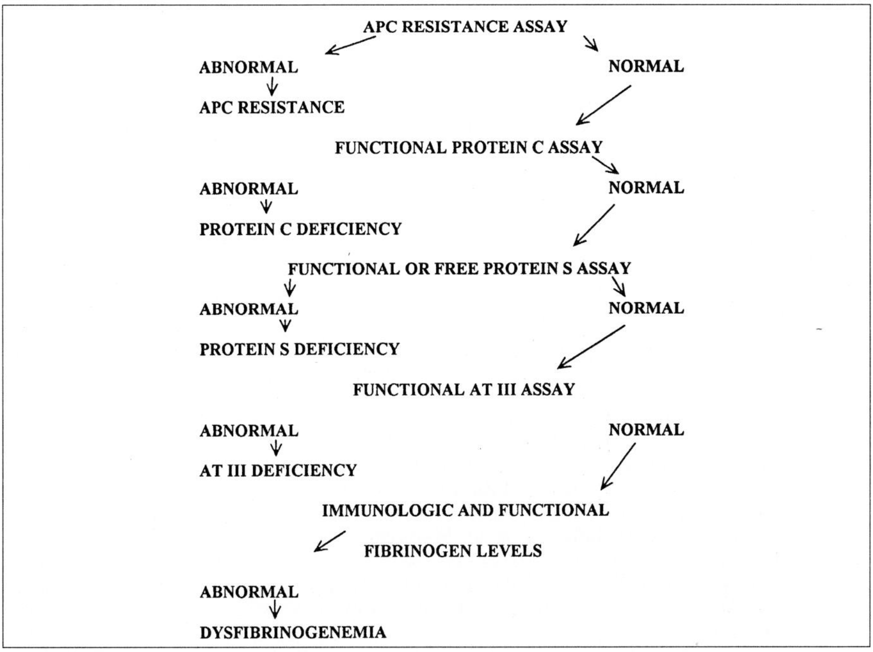

Fig. 6. Venous thromboembolism. APC, activated protein C; ATIII, antithrombin III.

von Willebrand factor level; presence of larger-molecular-weight multimers
Spontaneous platelet aggregation
Platelet receptor polymorphisms
Heparin cofactor II activity deficiency
PAI level
TPA level
Tissue factor pathway inhibitor level
Thrombomodulin level
MTHFR gene test

Precautions and Comments

1. Testing of blood drawn before anticoagulant therapy may lead to spurious results, due to increased levels of factors associated with acute-phase reactions, such as fibrinogen.
2. Testing of blood drawn after anticoagulant therapy may result in falsely low results, such as low levels of protein C in patients taking warfarin.
3. Staclot study (for lupus anticoagulant) can be performed on a heparinized sample.
4. APC resistance manifests interference from both heparin and warfarin as well as in the presence of factor deficiencies or lupus anticoagulants.
5. ATIII level is reduced by heparin. Chromogenic study results are not influenced by heparin (assay, factor Xa).
6. Protein C and protein S demonstrate interference from heparin and warfarin; protein C or protein S may be evaluated by comparison of protein C or protein S, antigens to factor II or X (normal ratio, 1:1); chromogenic study results reliable while patient is taking heparin.

Bibliography

Aysola A, Manack L. Check Sample 8. Chicago: American Society of Clinical Pathologists, 1999.

Baglin TP. Heparin-induced thrombocytopenia thrombosis (HIT/T) syndrome. *J Clin Pathol* 2001;54:272–274.

Baker R, Thomy J, Van Bockxmeer F. Diagnosis of activated protein C resistance (factor V Leiden). *Lancet* 1994;344:1162.
Balasa VV, Gruppo RA, Glueck CJ, et al. The relationship of mutations in the MTHFR, prothrombin, and PAI-1 genes to plasma levels of homocysteine, prothrombin and PAI-1 in children and adults. *Thromb Haemost* 1999;81:739–744.
Bertina RM. Factor V Leiden and other coagulation factor mutations affecting thrombotic risk. *Clin Chem* 1997;43:1678–1683.
Bianco A, Bonduel M, Penalva L, et al. Deep vein thrombosis in a 13-year-old boy with hereditary protein S deficiency and a review of the pediatric literature. *Am J Hematol* 1994;45:330–334.
Bick R. *Disorders of thrombosis and hemostasis*. Chicago: American Society of Clinical Pathologists Press, 1992.
Bollhalder M, Mura C, Landr O, et al. LightCycler PCR assay for simultaneous detection of the H63D and S65C mutations in the HFE hemochromatosis gene based on opposite melting temperature shifts. *Clin Chem* 1999;45:2275–2278.
Brandt R. Diagnosing heparin-induced thrombocytopenia. *CAP Today* 2000;14(5):40, 44, 48, 50–52.
Burrows RF, Kelton JG. Fetal thrombocytopenia and its relation to maternal thrombocytopenia. *N Engl J Med* 1993;329(20):1463–1466.
Butler TJ, Sodoma LJ, Doski JJ, et al. Heparin-associated thrombocytopenias and thrombosis as the cause of a fatal thrombus on extracorporeal membrane oxygenation. *J Pediatr Surg* 1997;32:768–771.
Castle V, Andrew M, Kelton J, et al. Frequency and mechanism of neonatal thrombocytopenia. *J Pediatr* 1986;108:749–755.
Chong BH, Burgess J, Ismail F. The clinical usefulness of the platelet aggregation test for the diagnosis of heparin-induced thrombocytopenia. *Thromb Haemost* 1993;69:344–350.
Coleman R, Hirsh J, et al. *Hemostasis and thrombosis*. Philadelphia: Lippincott Williams and Wilkins, 2001.
Deally C, Hancock BJ, Giddins N, et al. Primary antiphospholipid syndrome: a cause of catastrophic shunt thrombosis in the newborn. *J Cardiovasc Surg (Torino)* 1999;40:261–264.
deRonde H, Bertina RM. Laboratory diagnosis of APC-resistance: a critical evaluation of the test and the development of diagnostic criteria. *Thromb Haemost* 1994;72(6):880–886.
DeVeber F, Monagle P, Chan A, et al. Prothrombotic disorders in infants and children with cerebral thromboembolism. *Arch Neurol* 1998;55:1539–1543.
Ehrenforth S, Junker R, Koch H-G, et al., for the Childhood Thrombophilia Study Group. Multicentre evaluation of combined prothrombotic defects associated with thrombophilia in childhood. *Eur J Pediatr* 1999;158[Suppl 3]:S97–S104.
el-Kalia S, Menon NS. Neonatal congenital factor X deficiency. *Pediatr Hematol Oncol* 1991;8:347–354.
Forbes CD, Madhok R. Genetic disorders of blood coagulation: clinical presentation and management. In: Ratnoff OD, Forbes CD, eds. *Disorders of hemostasis*. Philadelphia: WB Saunders, 1991:423.
Fujita I, Takahashi Y, Sakaguchi T, et al. Congenital factor VII abnormality discovered in an infant at a routine checkup. *Am J Pediatr Hematol Oncol* 1991;13:47–48.
Gill JC, Endres-Brooks J, Bauer PJ, et al. The effects of ABO blood group on the diagnosis of von Willebrand disease. *Blood* 1987;69(6):1691–1695.
Goodnight J, Scott H, Hathaway WE. *Disorders of hemostasis and thrombosis*. New York: McGraw-Hill, 2001:115–124;154–161.
Gorbe E, Nagy B, Varadi V, et al. Mutation in the factor V gene associated with inferior vena cava thrombosis in newborns. *Clin Genet* 1999;55:65–66.
Greinacher A, Mueller-Eckhardt C. Hereditary types of thrombocytopenia with giant platelets and inclusion bodies in the leukocytes. *Blut* 1990;60:53–60.
Harenberg J, Wang LC, Hoffmann U, et al. Laboratory diagnosis of heparin-induced thrombosis, type II, after clearance of platelet factor IV/heparin complex. *J Lab Clin Med* 2001;137:408–413.
Harenburg J, Wang L, Hoffmann U, et al. Improved laboratory confirmation of heparin-induced thrombocytopenia type II. *Am J Clin Pathol* 2001;115:432–438.

Harrison P, Ault KA, Chapman S, et al. An interlaboratory study of a candidate reference method of platelet counting. *Am J Clin Pathol* 2001;115:448–459.
Harum LH, Hon AH, Kato GI, et al. Homozygous factor V mutation as a genetic cause of perinatal thrombosis and cerebral palsy. *Devel Med Child Neurol* 1999;41:777–780.
Heijer MD, Koster R, Blom HJ, et al. Hyperhomocysteinemia as a risk factor for deep-vein thrombosis. *N Engl J Med* 1996;334:759–762.
Hirsh J, Anand SS, Halperin JL, et al. Guide to anticoagulant therapy. *Circulation* 2001;103:3003–3004.
Hong JJ, Kwaan HC. Hereditary defects in fibrinolysis associated with thrombosis. *Semin Thromb Hemost* 1999;25:321–331.
Hourdille P, Pico M, Jandrot-Perrus M, et al. Studies on the megakaryocytes of a patient with Bernard-Soulier syndrome. *Br J Haematol* 1990;76:521–530.
Isenhart CE, Brandt JT. Platelet aggregation studies for the diagnosis of heparin-induced thrombocytopenia. *Am J Clin Pathol* 1993;99:324–330.
Isselbacher KJ, et al., eds. *Harrison's principles of internal medicine*, 13th ed. New York: McGraw-Hill, 1994.
Jy W, Mao WW, Horstman LL, et al. Flow cytometric assay of platelet activation marker selectin (CD62P) distinguishes heparin-induced thrombocytopenia (HIT) from HIT with thrombosis (HITT). *Thromb Haemost* 1999;82:1255–1259.
Kaplan C, Morel-Kopp MC, Kroll H, et al. HPA-5b(Bra) neonatal alloimmune thrombocytopenia: clinical and immunological analysis of 39 cases. *Br J Haematol* 1990;78(3):425–429.
Kitchens CS. Factor XI: a review of its biochemistry and deficiency. *Semin Thromb Hemost* 1991;17:55–72.
Kosch A, Junker R, Kurnik K, et al. Prothrombotic risk factors in children with spontaneous venous thrombosis and their asymptomatic parents. *Thromb Res* 2000;9:531–537.
Kraaijenhagen Ra, in't Anker PS, Koopman MMW, et al. High plasma concentration of factor VIIIc is a major risk factor for venous thromboembolism. *Thromb Haemost* 2000;83:5–9.
Kraus FT, Scheen VI. Fetal thrombotic vasculopathy in the placenta: cerebral thrombi and infarcts, coagulopathies, and cerebral palsy. *Hum Pathol* 1999;30: 659–669.
Kyrle PA, Minar E, Hirschl M, et al. High plasma levels of factor VIII and the risk of recurrent venous thromboembolism. *New Engl J Med* 2000;343:457–462.
Ljung R, Petrini P, Milsson IM. Diagnostic symptoms of severe and moderate haemophilia A and B. A survey of 140 cases. *Acta Paediatr Scand* 1990;79:196–200.
Luchtman-Jones L, Broze GJ Jr. The current status of coagulation. *Ann Med* 1995;27(1):47–52.
Lusher J, Warrier I. Hemophilia A. *Hematol Oncol Clin North Am* 1992;6:1021–1033.
MacDonald PD, Gibson BE, Brownlie J, et al. Protein C activity in severely ill newborns with congenital heart disease. *J Perinat Med* 1992;20:421–427.
Makris M, Leach M, Beauchamp NJ, et al. Genetic analysis, phenotype diagnosis and risk of venous thrombosis in families with inherited deficiencies of protein S. *Blood* 2000;15:1935–1941.
Mammen EF. Factor IX abnormalities. *Semin Thromb Hemost* 1983;9:28.
Mammen EF. Factor XI deficiency. *Semin Thromb Hemost* 1983;9:34.
Manco-Johnson MJ. Disorders of hemostasis in childhood: risk factors for venous thromboembolism. *Thromb Haemost* 1997;78(1):710–714.
Manco-Johnson MJ, Abshire TC, Jacobson LJ, et al. Severe neonatal protein C deficiency; prevalence and thrombotic risk. *J Pediatr* 1991;119:793–798.
Mangasser-Stephan K, Tag C, Reiser A, et al. Rapid genotyping of hemochromatosis gene mutations on the LightCycler with fluorescent hybridization probes. *Clin Chem* 1999;45:1875–1878.
McGann MA, Triplett DA. Interpretation of antithrombin III activity. *Lab Med* 1982;13:742–748.
Meijers JC, Tekelenburg WL, Bouma BN, et al. High levels of coagulation factor XI as a risk factor for venous thrombosis. *N Engl J Med* 2000;342:696–701.
Merchant RH, Agarwal BR, Currimbhoy Z, et al. Congenital factor XIII deficiency. *Indian Pediatr* 1992;29:831–836.

Miletick JP. Thrombophilia as a multigenic disorder. *Semin Thromb Hemost* 1998;24[Suppl 1]:13–20.

Montgomery RR, Scott JP. Hemostasis: diseases of the fluid phase. In: Nathan DG, Oski F, eds. *Hematology of infancy and childhood*, 4th ed. Vol II. Philadelphia: WB Saunders, 1993.

Neal WR, Taylor DT, Cederbaum AI, et al. Another genetic variant of haemophilia B: haemophilia B-Leyden. *Scand J Haematol* 1970;7:82–90.

Nowak-Göttl U, Junker R, Harmeier M, et al. Increased lipoprotein (a) is an important risk factor for venous thromboembolism in childhood. *Circulation* 1999; 100(7):743–748.

Nowak-Göttl U, Sträter R, Heinecke A, et al. Lipoprotein (a) and genetic polymorphisms of clotting factor V, prothrombin, and methylenetetrahydrofolate reductase are risk factors of spontaneous ischemic stroke in childhood. *Blood* 1999;94:3678–3682.

Nurden AT, Caen JP. An abnormal platelet glycoprotein pattern in three cases of Glanzmann's thromboasthenia. *Br J Haematol* 1974;28:253–260.

Nuss R, Hays T, Chudgar U, et al. Antiphospholipid antibodies and coagulation regulatory protein abnormalities in children with pulmonary emboli. *J Pediatr Hematol Oncol* 1997;19(3):202–207.

Öhlin A-K, Norlund K, Marlar MR. Thrombomodulin gene variations and thromboembolic disease. *Thromb Haemost* 1997;78:396–400.

Peacocke M, Siminovitch KA. Wiskott-Aldrich syndrome: new molecular and biochemical insights. *J Am Acad Dermatol* 1992;27:507–519.

Phillips M, Meadows CA, Huang MY, et al. Simultaneous detection of C282Y and H63D hemochromatosis mutations by dual-color probes. *Mol Diagn* 2000;5:107–116.

Press RD. Hereditary hemochromatosis: impact of molecular and iron-based testing on the diagnosis, treatment, and prevention of a common, chronic disease. *Arch Pathol Lab Med* 1999;123:1053–1059.

Ranze O, Ranze P, Magnai HN, et al. Heparin-induced thrombocytopenia in paediatric patients—a review of the literature and a new case treated with danaparoid sodium. *Eur J Pediatr* 1999;158[Suppl 3]:S130–S133.

Roberts HR, Grizzle JE, McLester WD. Genetic variants of hemophilia B: detection by means of a specific inhibitor. *J Clin Invest* 1968;47:360.

Rosenburg R, Bauer K. Thrombosis in inherited deficiencies of antithrombin, Protein C and Protein S. *Hum Pathol* 1987;18:253–267.

Rosendaal FR. Risk factors for venous thrombosis. *Thromb Haemost* 1999;82(2):610–619.

Rosendaal FR. Thrombosis in the young: epidemiology and risk factors. A focus on venous thrombosis. *Thromb Haemost* 1997;78(1):1–6.

Ruggeri Z, Zimmermann T. von Willebrand factor and von Willebrand disease. *Blood* 1987;70:895–904.

Schobess R, Junker R, Auberger K, et al. Factor V G1691 A and prothrombin G20210 A in childhood spontaneous venous thrombosis—evidence of an age-dependent thrombotic onset in carriers of factor V G1691 A and prothrombin G20210 A mutation. *Eur J Pediatr* 1999;158[Suppl 3]:S105–S108.

Schwartz KA. Platelet antibody: review of detection methods. *Am J Hematol* 1988;29:106–114.

Sifontes MT, Nuss R, Hunger SP, et al. Activated protein C resistance and the factor V Leiden mutation in children with thrombosis. *Am J Hematol* 1998;57:29–32.

Sills RH, Marlar RA, Montgomery RR, et al. The clinical spectrum of heterozygous protein C deficiency. *J Pediatr* 1984;105:409–413.

Smith P. Congenital coagulation protein deficiencies in the perinatal period. *Semin Perinatol* 1990;14:384–392.

Stites DP, Stobo JD, Wells JV, eds. *Basic and clinical immunology*, 8th ed. New York: Appleton & Lange, 1994.

Tomer A. A sensitive and specific functional flow cytometric assay for the diagnosis of heparin-induced thrombocytopenia. *Br J Haematol* 2001;98:648–656.

Van Hylckama VA, van der Linden IK, Bertina RM, et al. High levels of factor IX increase the risk of venous thrombosis. *Blood* 2000;95:3678–3682.

Von Ahsen N, Schutz E, Armstrong VW, et al. Rapid detection of prothrombotic mutations of prothrombin (G20210A), factor V (G1691A), and methylene-tetrahydrofolate reductase (C677T) by real-time fluorescence PCR with the LightCycler. *Clin Chem* 1999;45:694–696.

Warketin TE, Kelton JG. Heparin-induced thrombocytopenia. In: Coller BS, ed. *Progress in hemostasis and thrombosis*. Philadelphia: WB Saunders, 1991:1–34.

Weiss A, Gollin JI, Kaplan AP. Fletcher factor deficiency. *J Clin Invest* 1974;53:622–633.

Zeerleder S, Scholesser M, Redondo M, et al. Reevaluation of the incidence of thromboembolic complications in congenital factor XIII deficiency. *Thromb Haemost* 1999;82:1240–1246.

Zimmermann T, Ruggeri Z. von Willebrand disease. *Hum Pathol* 1987;18:140–152.

13 Musculoskeletal and Joint Diseases

Laboratory Studies

Synovial Fluid: Normal Values

Volume	1.0–3.5 mL
pH	Parallels serum
Appearance	Clear, pale yellow, or straw-colored; viscous, does not clot
Fibrin clot	0
Mucin clot	Good
White blood cells (WBCs)	<200/mm^3 (even in presence of leukocytosis in blood)
Neutrophils	<25%
Crystals	
Free	0
Intracellular	0
Fasting uric acid, bilirubin	Approximately the same as in the serum
Total protein	25–30% of serum protein Mean = 1.8 g/dL Abnormal if >2.5 g/dL; inflammation is moderately severe if >4.5 g/dL
Glucose	<10 mg/dL lower than serum level of simultaneously drawn blood
Culture	No growth

Laboratory Tests for Joint Diseases

Hematologic Tests

Acute-phase reactants, for example, erythrocyte sedimentation rate, C-reactive protein level

Anti–*Borrelia burgdorferi* antibodies

Anticardiolipin antigens

Anticytoplasmic antigens

Examination of Synovial Fluid

The fluid obtained at aspiration of a joint should be examined as follows:

- Gram stain
- WBC count and differential
- Glucose test
- Aerobic and anaerobic culture
- Mycobacterial culture
- Acid-fast staining
- Gonococcal culture (in sexually active individuals)

Appearance of the fluid: Sepsis in joints usually results in cloudy or purulent fluid. WBC counts in the fluid are generally >50,000/mm^3, with predominance of neutrophils; the glucose level may be low. Exceptions to these generalizations are common.

In the sexually active adolescent, throat, rectal, and cervical or urethral cultures should also be obtained before starting antibiotic therapy to further evaluate the possibility of gonococcal infection. The organism is more often cultured from these sites than from the synovial fluid.

A bone scan may be helpful in distinguishing osteomyelitis from septic arthritis; the duration of antibiotic therapy is longer for osteomyelitis.

Serum Enzymes in Muscle Diseases

See Table 1.

Measurement of creatinine kinase (CK) level is the test of choice. It is more specific and sensitive than measurement of aspartate aminotransferase and lactate dehydrogenase levels, and more discriminating than measurement of aldolase level, but aspartate aminotransferase is more significantly associated with inflammatory myopathy and its measurement is more useful in these cases.

Increased In

Polymyositis
Muscular dystrophy
Myotonic dystrophy
Some metabolic disorders
Malignant hyperthermia
Prolonged exercise; peak 24 hours after extreme exercise (e.g., marathon); smaller increases in well-conditioned athletes

Normal In

Scleroderma
Acrosclerosis
Discoid lupus erythematosus
Muscle atrophy of neurologic origin (e.g., old poliomyelitis, polyneuritis)
Hyperthyroid myopathy

Decreased In

Rheumatoid arthritis (in approximately two-thirds of patients)

Creatine Kinase Isoenzyme with Muscle and Brain Subunits

The following conditions or disorders may cause increased serum levels of the isoenzyme of creatine kinase with muscle and brain subunits (CK-MB):

Use of ceratin drugs [e.g., alcohol, cocaine, halothane [(malignant hyperthermia), ipecac]
Dermatomyositis polymyositis
Muscular dystrophy [Duchenne muscular dystrophy (DMD), Becker muscular dystrophy (BMD)]
Exercise myopathy (slight to significant increases)
Familial hypokalemia periodic paralysis
Endocrine disorders (e.g., hypoparathyroidism, acromegaly; hypothyroidism rarely increases CK-MB levels)
Rhabdomyolysis
Infections
- Viral (e.g., human immunodeficiency virus, Epstein-Barr virus, influenza virus, picornaviruses, coxsackievirus, echovirus, adenoviruses)
- Bacterial (e.g., *Staphylococcus, Streptococcus, Clostridium, Borrelia*)
- Fungal
- Parasitic (e.g., *Trichinella, Toxoplasma, Schistosoma, Taenia*)

Skeletal muscle trauma

Joint Disorders

Arthritis, Associated with Ulcerative Colitis or Regional Enteritis

Rheumatoid arthritis, ankylosing spondylitis (in $\leq 20\%$ of patients with Crohn disease), or acute synovitis (monarticular or polyarticular) may be present.

Table 1. Serum Enzyme Levels in Muscle Diseases

	Muscular Dystrophy							
	Duchenne		Limb-Girdle		Facioscapulohumeral Dystrophy		Myotonic Dystrophy	Polymyositis
Enzyme	Frequency (%)	Amplitude	Frequency (%)	Amplitude	Frequency (%)	Amplitude	Frequency (%)	Frequency (%)
CK	>95	65	75	25	80	5	50	70
ALD	90	9	25	3	30	2	20	75
AST	90	4	25	2	25	1.5	15	25
LD	90	4	15	1.5	10	1	10	25

ALD, aldolase; AST, aspartate aminotransferase; CK, creatine kinase; LD, lactate dehydrogenase.
Frequency is the average percentage of patients with an increased serum enzyme level when blood is taken at the optimal time. Amplitude is the average number of times the normal level by which serum level is increased.
From Wallach J. *Interpretation of diagnostic tests*, 7th ed. Philadelphia: Lippincott Williams & Wilkins, 2000.

Joint fluid is sterile with regard to both bacteriologic and microscopic findings.
Synovial biopsy findings are similar to those in rheumatoid arthritis.
Abnormal laboratory results (e.g., increased erythrocyte sedimentation rate, WBC count, platelets) are related to activity of bowel disease.
Absent rheumatoid factor and antinuclear antibodies.

Arthritis, Septic

Septic arthritis is characterized by involvement of a single large joint, most commonly the knee, hip, or wrist.
The affected joint is swollen and painful.
Diagnosis depends on examination of joint fluid or examination of a synovial biopsy specimen, which shows caseous granulomas and acid-fast bacilli.

Relative Frequency of Pathogens in Septic Arthritis According to Age

Neonate	1 mo–2 yr	2–5 yr	>5 yr
Staphylococcus aureus	*Haemophilus influenzae*	*S. aureus*	*S. aureus*
Group B streptococci	Group A streptococci	Group A streptococci	Group A streptococci
Gram-negative enteric pathogens	*S. pneumoniae*	*H. influenzae* type B	*Neisseria gonorrhoeae*
	N. meningitidis	*N. meningitidis*	*Pseudomonas aeruginosa*
	P. aeruginosa	*S. pneumoniae*	
	Salmonella species		

Differential Diagnosis of Arthritis

A joint aspirate is often the most rapid and accurate way to establish a diagnosis in a child with arthritis.

Diagnostic Test	Juvenile Rheumatoid Arthritis	Septic Arthritis	Traumatic Arthritis
Appearance	Clear to opalescent	Cloudy or turbid	Clear to blood-tinged
Mucin clot (add a few drops of joint aspirate to a beaker containing 10–20 mL of 5% acetic acid; let stand for 1 min, then shake)	Good to poor	Poor (clot flakes and shreds)	Good (remains a firm and rope-like mass)
White cell count	15,000–25,000/mm³ (50–90% neutrophils)	50,000–100,000/mm³ (90% neutrophils)	<5,000/mm³ (20–50% neutrophils)
Blood glucose/joint fluid glucose difference	10–25 mg/100mL	>50 mg/100 mL	<10 mg/100 mL

Synovial Fluid, Findings in Diseases of Joints

Disease	Findings
Pyogenic arthritis	Purulent fluid exudate; large numbers of neutrophils; culture results positive for bacteria
Tubercular arthritis	Fluid exudate (high protein content and specific gravity); neutrophils and mononuclear cells; culture results positive for *Mycobacterium*
Rheumatoid arthritis	Clear fluid, high protein content; inflammatory cells; neutrophils and mononuclear cells; increased immunoglobulins and complement, rheumatoid factor present in many cases

Osteoarthrosis	Clear fluid, high protein content; no inflammatory cells
Gout	Urate crystals
Chondrocalcinosis (pseudogout)	Calcium pyrophosphate crystals

Table 2 presents synovial fluid findings in various diseases of the joints.
Table 3 lists birefringent materials in synovial fluid.

Muscle Disorders

Differential Diagnosis of Some Muscle Diseases

See Table 4.

Dystrophy, Muscular

Muscular dystrophies are inherited, progressive diseases of muscle with a wide range of clinical expression.
Table 5 lists the most common forms of muscular dystrophy.

Incidence

DMD: 1 per 3,000 male births

Causes

X-linked: DMD and the milder allelic form, BMD, are associated in two-thirds of patients with deletion of a gene at Xp21.2 for production of dystrophin; patients with Emery-Dreifuss muscular dystrophy have an abnormal Xq28 fascioscapulohumeral gene mapped to 4q35.
Dystrophin is the largest human gene that has been isolated, with a 14-base RNA transcript and 2,500 kilobases of genomic DNA spanning 70 exons. The huge size of the gene explains the high mutation rate, with dystrophin presenting a large target for mutational events.

Clinical Features of Duchenne and Becker Muscular Dystrophies

Normal motor milestones until child begins to walk
Clumsiness—frequent falls, toe walking, waddling gait
Weakness—inability to jump or climb stairs, weak neck flexors, Gower sign, lumbar lordosis
Pseudohypertrophy of calf muscles and contractures of heel cords
Kyphosis and scoliosis
Progressive decline in vital capacity
Facial weakness—inability to completely close eyes or whistle, pouting expression with transverse smile
Shoulder and proximal arm weakness: inability to do push-ups, horizontal clavicles, exaggerated biceps muscles ("Popeye" arms), winging of the scapula
Retinal vascular abnormalities in most patients
Toe walking
Contractures of neck, biceps, Achilles tendons—even without significant weakness
Cardiac conduction abnormalities with risk of sudden death
Leg pain, which may be an early complaint

Laboratory Tests

Creatine kinase level:
- Marked elevation in DMD
- Moderate elevation in BMD, FSH
- Normal in congenital muscular dystrophy, late in DMD

Table 2. Synovial Fluid Findings in Various Diseases of Joints

Property	Noninflammatory[a]	Hemorrhagic[b]	Acute Inflammatory[c]	Septic		
Volume	↑	↑	↑	↑		
Appearance	Clear, straw colored	Bloody or xanthochromic	Turbid yellow	Turbid yellow		
Viscosity	High	Variable	↓	↓		
Fibrin clot	Usually 0	Usually 0	+	+		
Mucin clot[d]	Good	Variable	Fair to poor	Poor		
			RF	TB arthritis	Gonorrheal arthritis	Septic arthritis[e,f]
WBC (no/mm³)[g]	<5,000	<10,000	300–100,000	2,500–105,000	1,500–108,000	15,600–213,000
Neutrophils (%)	<25	<50	8–98	29–96	2–96	75–100
Blood/synovia[h] glucose difference (mg/dL)[i]	<10	<25	0–88	0–108	0–97	40–122
Culture[j]	Negative	Negative	Negative	57	26	71

↑, increased; ↓, decreased; +, positive; RF, rheumatoid factor; TB, tuberculosis; WBC, white blood cell count.
[a]For example, degenerative joint disease, traumatic arthritis, some cases of pigmented villonodular synovitis.
[b]For example, tumor, hemophilia, neuroarthropathy, trauma, some cases of pigmented villonodular synovitis.
[c]For example, rheumatoid arthritis, Reiter syndrome, acute gouty arthritis, acute pseudogout, systemic lupus erythematosus.
[d]Mucin clot test adds little additional information to WBC count.
[e]For example, pneumococcal.
[f]In purulent arthropathy of undetermined cause, very high level of synovial fluid lactate (>2,000 mg/dL) indicates a nongonococcal septic arthritis (Gram-negative bacilli, Gram-positive cocci, fungi). Lactate level is <100 mg/dL in gonococcal infection, gout, rheumatoid arthritis, osteoarthritis, trauma.
[g]Use saline instead of acetic acid, which clumps the joint fluid.
[h]Glucose concentration may give spurious results unless obtained after prolonged fasting, and differences between joint and blood samples may not be significant unless >50 mg/dL.
[i]Joint tap should be performed, preferably after the patient has been fasting for >4 hr, and a blood glucose determination should be performed simultaneously.
[j]Material should be cultured aerobically and anaerobically. Culture for tubercle bacilli should be performed.
From Wallach J. *Interpretation of diagnostic tests,* 7th ed. Philadelphia: Lippincott Williams & Wilkins, 2000.

Table 3. Birefringent Materials in Synovial Fluid

Material	Usual Shape, Size	Birefringence	Cause	Location Within or Out of PMNs, Macrophages
Crystals				
Monosodium urate	Needle, rod, parallel edges	Strong; –	Gout	Within or out
Calcium pyrophosphate dihydrate	8–10 μm long rhomboid; may be rod, diamond, square, needle; <10 μm long	Weak; +	Pseudogout	Only within
Calcium oxalate	Bipyramidal	Strong; 0	Long-term renal dialysis	Within or out
Hydroxyapatite, other basic calcium phosphates	Aggregates only; small (1 μm)	Weak; 0	Degenerating, calcifying joint	
Cholesterol	Flat, plate, corner notch; may be needle; often >100 μm			
Cartilage, collagen	Irregular, rodlike	Strong; +		
Steroids			Injection into joint	
Betamethasone acetate	Rods; blunt ends, 10–20 μm	Strong; –		
Cortisone acetate	Large rods	Strong; +		
Methyl prednisone acetate	Small, pleomorphic, tend to clump	Strong; 0		
Prednisone tebutate	Small, pleomorphic, branched, irregular	Strong; +		
Triamcinolone acetonide	Small, pleomorphic fragments; tend to clump	Strong; 0		
Triamcinolone hexacetonide	Large rods, blunt ends, 15–60 μm	Strong; 0		
Anticoagulants			Injection into joint	
EDTA (dry)	Small, amorphous	Weak		
Lithium heparin (not sodium)	May resemble pseudogout	Weak; +		
Other materials				
Debris	Small, irregular; nonparallel, edges	Variable		
Fat (cholesterol esters)	Globules	Strong; Maltese cross		
Starch granules	Round; size varies	Strong; Maltese cross		

+, positive birefringence; –, negative birefringence; 0, no axis. EDTA, ethylenediaminetetraacetic acid; PMN, polymorphonuclear cell.
Crystals are best seen in fresh, wet-mount preparations examined with polarizing light. Hydroxyapatite complexes (diagnostic of apatite disease) and basic calcium phosphate complexes can be identified only by electron microscopy and mass spectroscopy; most cases are suspected clinically but never confirmed.
From Judkins SW, Cornbleet PJ. Synovial fluid crystal analysis. *Lab Med* 1997;28:774.

Table 4. Laboratory Findings in Differential Diagnosis of Some Muscle Diseases

Disease	Complete Blood Cell Count	ESR	Thyroid Function Test Results	Percentage of Patients with Increase in Various Serum Enzyme Levels	Muscle Biopsy Findings	Comments
Myasthenia gravis	N	N	N	N	Lymphorrhages	Cancer of lung should always be ruled out; high frequency of associated diabetes mellitus, especially in older patients
Polymyositis	Total eosinophil count frequently increased	Moderately to markedly increased; occasionally N	N	CK in 65%; levels may vary greatly and become N with steroid therapy; marked increase may occur in children LD in 25%, AST in 25%	Necrosis of muscle with phagocytosis of muscle fibers; infiltration of inflammatory cells Serum α_2- and γ-globulins	Associated cancer in $\leq 17\%$ of cases (especially lung; also breast)
Muscular dystrophy	N	N	N	In active phase, CK in 50%, LD in 10%, AST in 15%	Various degenerative changes in muscle; late muscle atrophy; no cellular infiltration	

AST, aspartate aminotransferase; CK, creatine kinase; ESR, erythrocyte sedimentation rate; LD, lactate dehydrogenase; N, normal.

Table 5. Most Common Forms of Muscular Dystrophies

Type	Frequency	Inheritance	Severity	Age at Onset	Distribution of First Involved Muscles
Duchenne (pseudo-hypertrophic)	Common	XR	Severe, fatal	0–12 yr	Pelvis, legs
Becker	Rare	XR	Mild	10–70 yr	Pelvis, legs
Facioscapulo-humeral	Relatively common	AD	Mild	10–20 yr	Face, shoulders
Emery-Dreifuss (scapulo-humeral)	Rare	XL	Mild	10–20 yr	Shoulders
Limb-girdle	Rare	AR	Moderate	Variable	Pelvis, shoulders
Distal	Very rare	AD	Variable	Adulthood	Hands, feet
Myotonic	Relatively common	AD	Variable, slow progression	Usually adulthood	Face, tongue extremities

AD, autosomal dominant; AR, autosomal recessive; XL, X-linked; XR, X-linked recessive.

Pathologic Findings on Muscle Biopsy Specimens

DMD: fiber splitting, necrosis, regeneration with interspersed fibrosis
FSH: highest yield in supraspinatus muscle with occasional degenerating fibers and small angulated fibers with inflammatory cells
Emery-Dreifuss muscular dystrophy: type I fiber atrophy

Diagnostic Tests

At this time, two methods are used for testing for DMD and BMD (more appropriately called *dystrophinopathies*). In the first, *dystrophin is examined by Western blotting* (immunoblotting) on samples of skeletal, cardiac, or smooth muscle using sheep antidystrophin and immunoperoxidase-conjugated rabbit anti–sheep immunoglobulin G followed by peroxidase development. Myosin staining is used as a control. DMD patients show no immunoreactive dystrophin, whereas BMD patients demonstrate either a decreased amount of dystrophin or a dystrophin molecule of larger or smaller size than normal, or both. Despite the accuracy and sensitivity of the Western blot method, it cannot detect the carrier condition in many carrier females. Direct immunohistochemistry of muscle biopsy specimens in carrier females shows mosaic dystrophin staining after the pattern of random inactivation of the X chromosome containing the normal and abnormal dystrophin alleles.

DNA-based detection of dystrophin gene mutations can be performed using Southern blotting with complementary DNA probes. The use of multiple restriction enzyme–probe combinations allows detection of the approximately 65% of DMD and BMD patients who have gene deletions or duplications. The clustering of dystrophin gene mutations has led to the development of a rapid multiplex polymerase chain reaction assay. Using two mixtures of polymerase chain reaction primers that simultaneously amplify nine exons each, 98% of deletions or duplications detectable by Southern blotting can be identified by polymerase chain reaction. The major advantages of this latter methodology are its speed (1–2 days compared to 1–2 weeks) and small sample requirement (0.5 mL blood versus 20 mL).

Other Diagnostic Procedures

Muscle biopsy of moderately weak muscle (vastus lateralis, triceps).
Dystrophin level in muscle biopsy specimen. In DMD, dystrophin content is <3% of normal; in BMD, dystrophin content is <20% of normal.

DMD and BMD: Dystrophin studies in chorionic villus sample and amniocytes; analysis of fetal red blood cells in maternal blood; preimplantation diagnosis.

Prenatal Diagnosis

For detection of DMD and BMD in families with history of disease or for screening.

Serum CK level is always increased in affected children [5–100 × upper limit of normal (ULN) of adults] to peak by 2 years of age; level then begins to fall as disease becomes manifest. Persistent normal CK levels virtually rule out this diagnosis. Testing should be begun at 2–3 months of age. (Note: Normal children have very high CK levels during first few days, which fall to three times the ULN by fourth day and drop to two to three times the adult level during the first month of life; levels remain higher than adult levels during first 2 years.) Neonatal screening tests that give positive results with whole blood should be confirmed with serum. CK level is more than three times the ULN for age in all boys with DMD and more than twice the ULN in those with BMD. Sex-linked dystrophy is virtually the only cause of high values in normal neonates. High values persist in patients with dystrophy but not in those with false-positive results. Neonatal screening of girls has been discontinued. Prenatal screening at 18–20 weeks of gestation by placental aspiration of fetal blood has been abandoned due to false-negative and false-positive results.

Dystrophy, Myotonic (Steinert Disease)

Myotonic dystrophy is characterized not by muscle weakness but by failure of relaxation of muscle after voluntary contraction (myotonia).

Incidence of myotonic dystrophy is 1 per 10,000 births.

Clinical Features

Onset in late childhood, usually
Facial weakness—open, triangular mouth and droopy eyelids
Sustained muscle contraction with percussion of thenar eminence
Weakness in distal limbs
Mental retardation
High forehead with receding hairline
Cataracts, gonadal dysfunction, cardiac conduction defects and arrhythmias
Abnormal insulin metabolism (diabetes)
Hypothyroidism, addisonian crisis
Difficulty in letting go (myotonia) after handshake
Neonatal form: hypotonia, respiratory distress, hip dislocations; mother usually affected

Risk Factors

Affected parent; autosomal dominant. Myotonic dystrophy more severe if mother is affected parent. The myotonic dystrophy gene has been mapped to chromosome band 19q13.

Special Tests

Electromyography—high-frequency repetitive waxing and waning discharges ("dive-bomber" effect)
Electrocardiography

Imaging

Brain magnetic resonance imaging in congenital myotonic dystrophy shows diffuse white-matter changes resembling leukodystrophy.

Hyperthermia, Malignant

Malignant hyperthermia may occur with most congenital myopathies and occurs with exposure to general anesthetics in susceptible children. Patients develop high fever, rigid muscles, acidosis, rhabdomyolysis, and myoglobinuria.

Myopathy, Congenital and Acquired

The more common types of myopathy are the following:

Disease	Histologic Characteristic
Central core disease	Amorphous central core in myofibrils with absence of myofilaments.
Nemaline myopathy	Elongated crystalline rods composed of tropomyosin present beneath sarcolemma; show periodicity on electron microscope.
Centronuclear myopathy	Nuclei occupy the central port of the myofibril, which lacks myofilaments.
Secondary congenital myopathies	Myopathy is a feature of some forms of glycogen storage disease and certain disorders of lipid metabolism (e.g., carnitine deficiency).
Toxins	Organophosphate exposure, botulism, tick paralysis, eosinophilia myalgia (follows tryptophan ingestion).
Acquired myopathies	Endocrine diseases: thyrotoxicosis, corticosteroid excess (Cushing syndrome, exogenous steroid administration), acromegaly, osteomalacia (hypocalcemia); familial periodic paralysis (potassium deficiency or excess); malignant neoplasms (paraneoplastic syndrome).

Myopathy, Lipid

See Table 6.

Myopathy, Metabolic

See Chapter 17, Metabolic and Hereditary Diseases.
Glycogen storage diseases.
Mitochondrial myopathies (frequently encephalomyopathy). See Tables 7 and 8.

Myositis (Inflammation of Muscle)

Causes

- Infectious diseases
  - Bacterial (pyomyositis)
    - Local infection with pyogenic bacteria usually secondary to trauma, intramuscular injection; staphylococci common
    - Bacteremic myositis, for example, in infective endocarditis, typhoid fever, leptospirosis
    - Gas gangrene (clostridial infection)
  - Viral
    - Coxsackievirus (Bornholm disease); affects mainly chest wall muscles
    - Influenza
    - Many other viruses
  - Parasitic
    - *Trichinella spiralis* (trichinosis)
    - *Toxoplasma gondii*
    - *Taenia solium* (cysticercosis)
    - *Trypanosoma cruzi* (Chagas disease)
  - Exotoxic
    - Diphtheria
- Immune diseases
  - Polymyositis, dermatomyositis. In polymyositis, inflammation of muscles is the dominant clinical manifestation.
  - Other autoimmune diseases: systemic lupus erythematosus, progressive systemic sclerosis
  - Sarcoidosis
  - Myasthenia gravis: associated with anti–striated muscle antibody in serum
- High-dosage radiation (most commonly in treatment of cancer)

Table 6. Lipid Myopathies: Clinical Associations

Deficiency	Onset	Signs and Symptoms
CPT I	Infancy	Hypoglycemia
CPT II	Infancy	Hypoglycemia, hepatomegaly, hypotonia, seizures, cardiomyopathy
	Young adulthood	Myalgia, rhabdomyolysis, myoglobulinuria
Carnitine		
Systemic	Infancy	Hypoketotic hypoglycemia, Reye-LS, lipid myopathy
	Infancy	Dilated cardiomyopathy,[a] nonketotic HG, weakness, vomiting, developmental delay
	Childhood	Progressive cardiomyopathy, lipid myopathy
Myopathic (rare)	Variable	Progressive lipid myopathy
Acyl–coenzyme A dehydrogenases (CADs)		
SCAD (short chain)	Infancy	Nausea, vomiting, FTT, microcephaly, nonketotic HG, hepatomegaly
	Adulthood	Progressive lipid myopathy, CD
MCAD (medium chain)	Infancy	Reye-LS, sudden death (SIDS)
	Later	Lipid myopathy, CD
LCAD (long chain)	Infancy	Cardiomyopathy, Reye-LS, sudden death
	Later	Myopathy, myoglobinuria, CD, hypoglycemia
3-Hydroxyacyl–coenzyme A dehydrogenase	Infancy	Reye-LS, myopathy, cardiomyopathy, neuropathy, SIDS
Glutaric acidemia type II (multiple CAD deficiency)		
ETF, ETF-QO	Neonatal period	Congenital anomalies, hypotonia, hypoglycemia, metabolic acidosis, CD, early death
	Infancy	Similar to that in neonates but without congenital anomalies, longer survival (months), rapidly progressive cardiomyopathy
	Adulthood	Hypoglycemia, myopathy, secondary CD
Coenzyme Q10	Childhood	Lipid myopathy, CNS dysfunctions, seizures, myoglobinuria

CD, secondary carnitine deficiency; CNS, central nervous system; CPT, carnitine palmityl transferase; ETF, electron transfer flavoprotein; ETF-QO, electron transfer flavoprotein ubiquinone oxidoreductase; FTT, failure to thrive; HG, hypoglycemia; Reye-LS, Reye's-like syndrome; SIDS, sudden infant death syndrome.
[a]Treatable with oral carnitine.

Ischemia

Myositis ossificans

- Rare disease of unknown etiology
- Characterized by bone formation in the involved muscle
- Presents as a hard mass in the muscle that may be mistaken for a neoplasm

Systemic infections: With systemic infection, extreme elevations in the levels of muscle enzymes (creatinine phosphokinase, aldolase) may occur. This process is self-limited and usually resolves within a few days. Viral illnesses, Rocky Mountain spotted fever, and leptospirosis may cause similar increase in muscle enzyme levels.

Clinical and Laboratory Findings

Muscle biopsy findings are definitive; also for dermatomyositis and inclusion-body myositis.

Table 7. Syndromic Multisystem Mitochondrial Diseases

Acronym	Meaning	Pattern of Inheritance
KSS	Kearns-Sayre syndrome (PEO, pigmentary retinopathy, heart block)	Sporadic
MELAS	Mitochondrial encephalomyopathy, lactic acidosis, strokelike episodes	Maternal
MERRF	Myoclonus epilepsy with ragged-red fibers	Maternal
NARP	Neuropathy, ataxia, retinitis pigmentosa	Maternal
LHON	Leber hereditary optic neuropathy	Maternal
MNGIE	Mitochondrial neurogastrointestinal encephalomyopathy	AR

AR, autosomal recessive; PEO, progressive external ophthalmoplegia.

Table 8. Infantile Forms of Mitochondrial Disease

Condition	Defect of	Clinical Features
Leigh syndrome (SNE)		LA, H, FTT, CNS
Three major forms:	Complex IV (COX) AR	
	PDC (E1 α) XR	
	ATPase 6 maternal	
Alpers syndrome (PSP)	Complex I, COX, Krebs cycle, PDC	CNS, L
Fumarase	Krebs cycle	H, FTT, CNS
Fatal multisystem disease	Complex I, II	LA, H, CRF
Pearson marrow/pancreas syndrome	Complex I	SA/EPD
Myopathy, LA, RRF	Complex II	CNS, H
Encephalomyopathy	Complex III	LA, H, CNS
Histiocytoid cardiomyopathy	Complex III	Fatal CM
Benign myopathy (reversible)	Complex IV (COX)	RI, LA, H, W
Depletion mtDNA	Complex IV (COX)	H, W, L
ATP-synthetase deficiency	Complex V	LA, CM

AR, autosomal recessive; ATPase, adenosine triphosphatase; CM, cardiomyopathy; CNS, variety of CNS-associated symptoms including seizures, progressive degeneration, visual and hearing defects, myoclonic epilepsy, coma; COX, cytochrome oxidase; CRF, cardiorespiratory failure; FTT, failure to thrive; H, hypotonia; L, liver abnormalities; LA, lactic acidosis; mtDNA, mitochondrial DNA; PDC, pyruvate decarboxylase complex, among most common causes of lactic acidosis with progressive cerebral dysfunction in infancy; PSP, progressive sclerosing poliodystrophy; RI, respiratory insufficiency; RRF, ragged-red fibers; SA/EPD, refractory sideroblastic anemia, exocrine pancreatic dysfunction; SNE, subacute necrotizing encephalopathy; SR, spontaneous recovery of enzymatic activity; W, weakness; XR, X-linked recessive.

Total eosinophil count is frequently increased. WBC count may be increased in fulminant disease.

Mild anemia may occur.

Erythrocyte sedimentation rate is moderately to markedly increased; may be normal; not clinically useful.

Thyroid function test results are normal.

Urine shows a moderate increase in creatine and a decrease in creatinine. Myoglobinuria occurs occasionally in severe cases.

Increased antinuclear antibody titers are found in 20% of patients. Rheumatoid factor test results are positive in 50% of patients.

Serum γ-globulin levels may be increased.

Associated carcinoma is present in ≤20% of patients and in ≤5% of patients older than 40 years (especially those with cancer of lung or breast). The polymyositis may antedate the neoplasm by up to 2 years.
Inclusion-body myositis shows characteristic biopsy findings of basophilic rimmed vacuoles with intranuclear filaments on electron microscopy. Serum CK level is normal or only slightly increased.

Disorders of Neuromuscular Transmission

Guillain-Barré Syndrome (Acute Inflammatory Demyelinating Polyradiculopathy)

Guillain-Barré syndrome is diagnosed by clinical and laboratory data.
It is characterized by paralysis that usually follows a nonspecific viral infection by approximately 10 days. Organisms that have been implicated include *Campylobacter jejuni*, *Mycoplasma pneumoniae*, enteroviruses, and Epstein-Barr virus. Weakness commonly begins in the lower extremities and progressively involves the trunk and upper extremities, usually in a symmetric pattern, and finally the bulbar muscles. In 50% of cases, tendon reflexes are lost early. Spontaneous recovery usually occurs in 2–3 weeks.
A congenital form with generalized hypotonia, weakness, and areflexia occurs in the neonate. There is gradual improvement over the first few months of life without evidence of residual disease at 1 year of age.

Laboratory Findings

Cerebrospinal fluid studies are essential in the diagnosis.
Cerebrospinal fluid:
Protein is increased to twice the normal level.
Glucose level is normal.
No pleocytosis is found.
Fewer than 10 WBCs/mm^3 are found.
Bacterial cultures give negative results.
Viral cultures rarely isolate specific viruses.
The dissociation of cerebrospinal fluid protein and lack of cellular response in a patient with acute or subacute polyneuropathy is diagnostic of Guillain-Barré syndrome.
Motor nerve conduction velocities are greatly reduced. Sensory nerve conduction time is usually slow. Electromyogram shows acute demarcation of muscle. Serum CK level is normal or mildly elevated.
Muscle and sural nerve biopsies are not usually required.

Myasthenia Gravis

Myasthenia gravis is one of the more common muscle diseases, affecting 1 in 40,000 persons in the United States. The most common age at onset is 20–40 years. There is a female preponderance when the disease occurs at <40 years of age.

Cause

Myasthenia gravis results from failure of neuromuscular transmission due to blockage of acetylcholine receptors by autoantibody.

- Acetylcholine receptor antibody is present in the serum of almost all patients. It is an immunoglobulin G antibody and may cross the placenta in pregnancy, causing neonatal myasthenia.
- Thymectomy often improves the condition, and it is believed that the thymus plays a role in the etiology of myasthenia gravis.
- The thymus is not the source of antibody, which is produced by the peripheral lymphoid tissue.

Neuropathy, Hereditary

Hereditary Neuropathy	Pattern of Inheritance
Hereditary motor and sensory neuropathy (HMSN)	
Type III, hypertrophic neuropathy of infancy (Dejerine-Sottas disease)	AR
Charcot-Marie-Tooth (HSMN type I)	AD
Hereditary sensory and autonomic neuropathy (HSAN)	
Type II, congenital sensory autonomic neuropathy	AR
Type III, familial dysautonomia (Riley-Day syndrome)	AR
Type IV, congenital insensitivity to pain	AR
Giant axonal neuropathy	AR
Infantile hypertrophic neuropathy	
Congenital hypomyelination neuropathy	
Metabolic storage disease	
Krabbe disease (globoid cell leukodystrophy)	AR
Metachromatic leukodystrophy, infantile	AR
Fabry disease	XL
Neuronal ceroid lipofuscinoses	AR
Adrenoleukodystrophy	AR
Refsum disease, infantile	AR

AD, autosomal dominant; AR, autosomal recessive; XL, X linked.

Diagnostic Tests

Diagnosed by sural nerve biopsy.

Specimen of sufficient length (25–30 mm) should be obtained for paraffin sections (light microscopy), electron microscopic examination, and nerve teasing.

Neuropathy, Peripheral

Abnormalities of peripheral nerves are rare in infants and young children and are often associated with systemic disease processes or diffuse central nervous system diseases that clinically overshadow the associated peripheral neuropathy. Examples include the mitochondrial encephalomyopathies and Leigh subacute necrotizing encephalomyelopathy. Clinical findings alone may be diagnostic, as in cases of Bell palsy, Möbius syndrome (bilateral congenital facial paralysis), and Erb palsy (branchial plexus injury); clinical history is often diagnostic, as in cases of the toxic neuropathies of diphtheria and botulism, or neuropathies induced by chemotherapy or antibiotics.

Diagnostic Tests

Sural nerve biopsy is helpful in evaluation of multiple mononeuropathies, such as may be associated with various types of vasculitis, but these conditions are not usually a significant consideration in infants. Guillain-Barré syndrome (acute inflammatory demyelinating polyradiculopathy) also is rare in infancy and may usually be diagnosed by clinical and laboratory data without the need for a nerve biopsy.

Instances in which a nerve biopsy is required are rare. Both skin biopsy samples (containing cutaneous twiglets) and muscle biopsy specimens (containing intramuscular motor nerve twiglets) may be used to study nerves by light and electron microscopy, without the need for sural nerve biopsy, and are especially useful when clinical features suggest a systemic metabolic storage disease associated with peripheral neuropathy. In a skin biopsy specimen, cutaneous nerve twiglets, fibrocytes, endothelial inflammatory cells, and sweat gland epithelium can all be evaluated for storage material at the ultrastructural level. In such instances, a skin biopsy is often the best source of diagnostic histologic material for electron microscopy. Conjunctival biopsy may serve a similar purpose. A muscle biopsy specimen often contains intramuscular motor nerve twiglets that can be readily studied for abnormalities.

Because an optimally processed muscle biopsy specimen has been snap-frozen and Epon embedded, both histochemical and ultrastructural studies can be done and can suggest appropriate biochemical studies for diagnostic confirmation. Epon sections of intramuscular nerves are excellent for evaluation of distribution and quantity of myelinated axons and for identification of "onion bulb" schwannian hypertrophy, as seen in hypertrophic neuropathy. Sural nerve biopsy may be considered in young children presenting with clinical findings of peripheral neuropathy that suggest one of the hereditary neuropathies and in whom nerve conduction abnormalities have already been documented. Sural nerve biopsy specimens should, if possible, be processed for Epon sections, nerve-teasing preparations, and paraffin sections. In infants and small children, obtaining sufficient specimen length (25–30 mm) for all three preparations may be difficult. In such cases, Epon embedding is a first priority, a nerve-teasing preparation second, followed by paraffin sections. Sural nerve biopsy specimens are excellent for evaluation of hereditary neuropathies or storage diseases. A major advantage of sural nerve specimens over skin or muscle samples is the possibility of performing nerve-teasing studies that can distinguish segmental demyelination from primary axonal degeneration and thereby help classify the pathologic process.

Biopsy Sites and Techniques

Biopsy Site	**Technique**	**Evaluation for**
Conjunctiva	Electron microscopy	Storage disease
Skin (cutaneous nerves)	Electron microscopy	Storage disease
Muscle (intramuscular nerves)	Histochemistry	Storage disease
	Epon sections and electron microscopy	
Sural nerve	Epon sections, electron microscopy	Storage disease
	Nerve teasing	Axonal and myelin abnormalities

Spinal Muscular Atrophy

The spinal muscular atrophies are second only to DMD as the most common severe neuromuscular diseases of childhood.

The infantile form (Werdnig-Hoffmann disease) has an incidence of 1 in 10,000 to 1 in 20,000.

Degeneration of anterior horn cells results in denervation, with weakness and atrophy of skeletal muscles and hypotonia. Trunk weakness and poor head control, fasciculations of the tongue, and absence of deep tendon reflexes are common symptoms. Death due to respiratory failure usually occurs by 2 years of age.

Clinical Types of Childhood Spinal Muscular Atrophy

	Onset	**Age at Death**
Type I (Werdnig-Hoffmann disease): acute	Birth to 2 mo	<2 yr
Type II: intermediate	3–15 mo	>2 yr
Type III (Kugelberg-Welander disease): mild	>24 months	Adult

Laboratory Findings

CK levels are normal or mildly elevated.

Electromyographic studies show neurogenic changes, and motor conduction may be minimally slowed. In the majority of cases, the disorder is due to an autosomal-recessive trait, and the defect has been mapped to chromosome band 5q11.2-13.3. All the various types are due to different mutations at the same locus on chromosome 5.

Prenatal diagnosis by DNA marker probes is possible.

Muscle biopsy findings include a diffuse population of rounded atrophic myofibers of <5 μm interspersed with extremely large hypertrophic myofibers of 50–80 μm, often in groups. It is unlike neurogenic atrophy in older children, in whom myofibrils are angulated with target fibrils.

Bone Disorders

Malignancy

Primary bone tumors (Ewing sarcoma, osteogenic sarcoma), leukemia, and neuroblastoma may all present with bone pain. The severity may range from mild pain and limping to severe, debilitating pain.

Osteomyelitis

The distal metaphysis of the long bones is a common site for osteomyelitis. The most common pathogens are those that cause septic arthritis. *Salmonella* infection is an additional consideration in those with sickle cell disease, and *Pseudomonas* infection should be suspected with osteomyelitis of the foot after puncture wounds through rubber shoes.

Bibliography

Barness L, Gilbert-Barness E. *Metabolic diseases: foundations of clinical management, genetics, and pathology.* Natick, MA: Eaton Pub, 2000.

Romansky SG. Diseases of muscle. In: Gilbert-Barness E, ed. *Potter's atlas of fetal and infant pathology.* St. Louis, MO: Mosby, 1998.

Romansky SG. Neuromuscular diseases. In: Gilbert-Barness E, ed. *Potter's pathology of the fetus and infant.* St. Louis, MO: Mosby, 1997.

Roscelki SB. Serum enzymes in diseases of skeletal muscle. *Clin Lab Med* 1989;9:767–781.

Wallach J. *Interpretation of diagnostic tests*, 7th ed. Philadelphia: Lippincott Williams & Wilkins, 2000.

14 Laboratory Studies in the Diagnosis of Pediatric Tumors

Biologic Markers with Increased Levels in Various Pediatric Malignancies

Acute lymphoblastic leukemia (ALL)	Lactate dehydrogenase (LDH) Interleukin-2 (IL-2) receptor Terminal deoxynucleotidyl transferase Ganglioside D_3
Non-Hodgkin lymphoma	LDH IL-2 receptor β_2-Microglobulin C-reactive protein
Hodgkin lymphoma	Ferritin β_2-Microglobulin C-reactive protein
Neuroblastoma	Catecholamines Cystathionine Aminoisobutyric acid Ferritin Neuron-specific enolase (NSE)
Wilms tumor	Hyaluronic acid Erythropoietin
Hepatoblastoma	α-Fetoprotein (AFP) Human chorionic gonadotropin (HCG)
Germ cell tumors	AFP HCG
Osteosarcoma	Alkaline phosphatase
Ewing sarcoma	LDH
Central nervous system tumors	NSE Polyamines

These studies may have prognostic significance.
Tissue diagnosis is definitive.

Biologic Markers Used in Diagnosis of Pediatric Tumors

α-Fetoprotein

AFP is produced during fetal life by the liver, yolk sac, and gastrointestinal tract and can be detected in high concentrations in fetal serum.

Increased serum concentrations of AFP have been documented in patients with hepatoblastoma, hepatocellular carcinoma, and gonadal and extragonadal germ cell tumors. Other nonmalignant conditions, such as hepatitis, cirrhosis, inflammatory bowel disease, ataxia telangiectasis, and tyrosinosis, are associated with increased serum concentrations of AFP.

Serum AFP concentrations peak during the thirteenth week of gestation, then decrease to approximately 30 μg/mL by term. By 6 months of age, serum concentrations generally are <50 ng/mL, and in normal children and adults rarely exceed 25 ng/mL.

In yolk sac tumors, hepatic tumors, and germ cell tumors, serum AFP concentrations typically range from 1,000 to 100,000 ng/mL.

Tumors with elevated AFP levels are classified into three groups: yolk sac type, hepatoblastoma type, and benign hepatic type.

Serial measurements of serum AFP level provides a reliable, noninvasive means of assessing the response to therapy and screening patients for early evidence of disease recurrence. AFP has been found to be a more reliable indicator than HCG of the extent of active disease.

Alkaline Phosphatase

Alkaline phosphatase activity is measured spectrophotometrically using a chromogenic substrate. In normal children, maximum serum concentrations range from 100 to 500 U/L, depending on the child's age and the specific methodology used. Maximum adult concentrations range from 50 to 100 U/L. Isoenzymes can be separated by electrophoresis, heat inactivation analysis, urea, or chemical inhibition by the use of specific antisera.

Alkaline phosphatase level is increased in patients with intrahepatic and extrahepatic biliary obstruction, hepatocellular damage, or increased osteoblastic activity. Increased concentrations of alkaline phosphatase can be demonstrated in both the serum and tumor tissue of patients with osteogenic sarcoma.

The risk of disease recurrence is higher with increased serum or tumor tissue concentrations of alkaline phosphatase.

C-Reactive Protein

C-reactive protein is an acute-phase reactant named for its ability to react with the C-polysaccharide on the cell wall of *Streptococcus pneumoniae*. It can be measured by RIA, radioimmunodiffusion, and rate nephelometry. The reference range is 80–800 μg/dL.

Creatine Kinase

Three dimeric isoenzymes of creatine kinase (CK) exist, each composed of a combination of M (muscle) and B (brain) subunits. CK-1 (BB) is found mainly in the brain, and CK-2 (MB) and CK-3 (MM) in heart and skeletal muscle. CK-3 is the predominant isoenzyme. Level is measured spectrophotometrically, and the normal range in the pediatric population is 40–380 U/L.

Increased concentrations of CK are seen in patients with inflammatory or degenerative muscle disorders, myocardial infarction, or damage to brain parenchyma (traumatic, ischemic, or inflammatory). Immunohistochemical studies have demonstrated M and B CK subunits in neuroblastoma and rhabdomyosarcoma cells and B subunits in Ewing sarcoma. Increased serum concentrations of CK-2 have been demonstrated in patients with rhabdomyosarcoma; however, its usefulness as a biologic marker has not been widely explored.

Cystathionine and Aminoisobutyric Acid

Cystathionine and aminoisobutyric acid are amino acids that are found in the urine of patients with neuroblastoma. Both can be measured by bidirectional paper chromatography, ion exchange, or high-pressure liquid chromatography (HPLC). Increased concentrations of cystathionine and aminoisobutyric acid have been demonstrated in approximately 60% of all patients with neuroblastoma (stages I–IV) and in up to 75% of patients with stage III and IV neuroblastoma.

Enolase

Neuron-specific enolase (NSE), composed of two δ subunits, is found primarily in neuronal, endocrine, and neuroendocrine cells. Nonneuronal enolase, consisting of two α subunits, is found in glial cells. A third hybrid form (α, δ) has also been identified.

Increase of NSE occurs in patients with neuroblastoma, medulloblastoma, and retinoblastoma. Concentrations found in association with the latter two tumors are generally <100 ng/mL.

Serum NSE level >100 ng/mL is predictive of a poor outcome in patients <2 years of age with stage III disease and in those <1 year of age with stage IV disease, but not in older patients or those with lower-stage disease. As is also true of serum ferritin, serum NSE concentrations are not increased in patients with stage IVS disease.

Erythropoietin

Erythropoietin is a hematopoietic growth factor that is produced by the kidney and regulates erythropoiesis. A glycoprotein, it is measured by RIA and enzyme-linked immunosorbent assay and is normally detectable in minute amounts in the serum and urine.

Erythropoietin has been detected in large amounts in both the serum and urine of patients with Wilms tumor. It is not associated with erythrocytosis. Erythropoietin level falls dramatically after resection of the primary mass but remains persistently present in patients with metastatic disease.

Ferritin

Ferritin is present in erythroid progenitors in the bone marrow, hepatic parenchymal cells, and reticuloendothelial cells of the liver, spleen, and bone marrow.

A sensitive indicator of total body iron stores, ferritin is decreased in the very early stages of iron deficiency. It is increased in states of iron overload (hemosiderosis and hemochromatosis) and in chronic inflammatory conditions (chronic infection, rheumatoid arthritis, chronic renal disease).

In some malignant conditions such as neuroblastoma, leukemia, Hodgkin lymphoma, and hepatocellular carcinoma, ferritin is produced by tumor cells, which results in an increase in total body ferritin and serum ferritin levels.

In patients with localized tumors and those with stage IVS neuroblastoma, serum ferritin concentrations are generally within the normal range. Approximately 50% of patients with advanced-stage disease (III and IV) have increased serum ferritin levels. In disseminated neuroblastoma, serum ferritin level is a reliable indicator of tumor burden and is therefore used in following response to therapy. Increased serum ferritin levels may correlate with poor prognosis.

Both acidic and basic isoferritins can be identified in patients with neuroblastoma, and recent evidence suggests that they may exert inhibitory effects on both T lymphocytes and granulocytes. In patients with Hodgkin disease, increased serum ferritin level at diagnosis appears to be associated with an increased risk of relapse.

Hormones

Increased hormone concentrations can be detected in a number of malignancies. Primary endocrine malignancies represent only 4–5% of all pediatric tumors. The tumors most commonly found are gonadal (45%), thyroid (30%), and pituitary (20%). The majority of these primary endocrine malignancies in children do not secrete hormones.

Neuroblastomas, germ cell tumors, and hepatic tumors are the nonendocrine tumors that may produce hormones. These hormones are HCG and the catecholamines.

Catecholamines

The catecholamines epinephrine, norepinephrine, and dopamine are produced by cells of neural crest origin in the adrenal medulla.

Pheochromocytoma is characterized by high circulating concentrations of epinephrine and norepinephrine and results in classical clinical symptoms including tachycardia, hypertension, weight loss, and flushing. Increased concentrations of epinephrine and norepinephrine can be detected in the serum, and their metabolites, vanillylmandelic acid (VMA) and the metanephrines, can be detected in the urine. It is necessary to assay for all intermediates in the catecholamine pathway, because pheochromocytomas may secrete a single intermediate.

Serum concentrations of epinephrine and norepinephrine are normal or minimally increased in children with neuroblastoma. VMA and 3-methoxy-4-hydroxyphenoglycol (MHPG), the major metabolites of norepinephrine, as well as homovanillic acid (HVA), the major metabolite of dopamine, are excreted in the urine in large amounts.

MHPG is measured by gas-liquid chromatography or HPLC. Normal urinary excretion is 1–2 mg per day. VMA can be measured spectrophotometrically, and both VMA and HVA can be measured by HPLC. Both metabolites can be measured simultaneously using bidirectional paper chromatography. Results generally are reported in terms of urine collection time or urine creatinine. Most commonly, HVA and VMA are measured in 24-hour urine collections. Normal urinary excretion is <10 mg/day each for HVA and VMA. The normal range for HVA is 1–40 μg/mg creatinine and for VMA is <7 μg/mg creatinine.

In neuroblastoma, the absolute value of the urinary VMA concentration and the ratio of VMA to HVA correlates directly with prognosis. Higher ratios of VMA to HVA tend to indicate better prognosis. Other catecholamine metabolites include vanillacetic acid, normetanephrine, and vanilglycol. Level of the dopamine metabolite vanillacetic acid correlates with a poorer prognosis. Levels of the epinephrine and norepinephrine metabolites normetanephrine and vanilglycol do not.

Human Chorionic Gonadotropin

HCG is composed of one α and one β subunit. The antigenic properties are dependent on distinct β subunits.

HCG is detected by RIA, using an antibody directed against the β subunit. Less than 5 IU/mL is detected in the serum of normal males and nonpregnant females. Increased concentrations are detected in pregnancies. In pathologic states, increased concentrations are observed most consistently in association with choriocarcinoma and nonseminomatous germ cell tumors and less, frequently, in association with seminomatous germ cell tumors and hepatomas.

The half-life of HCG in the serum is 12–20 hours. It is a useful indicator of response to therapy, with a dramatic decrease in serum concentrations often demonstrable within several hours of complete resection of an HCG-secreting tumor. Persistently increased HCG concentrations are present with residual or recurrent disease, except in children with virilizing hepatic tumors. AFP may be a more reliable indicator of disease status.

Hyaluronic Acid

Hyaluronic acid can be detected qualitatively by acetic acid precipitation and quantitatively by hyaluronidase degradation using colorimetric assay of disaccharide degradation products. It has been found in the serum of several patients with Wilms tumor.

Interleukin-2 Receptor

A soluble form of the IL-2 receptor, a membrane-associated cellular growth factor receptor, has been demonstrated in the serum by enzyme immunoassay. The range in normal children is 400–950 U/mL. Increased concentrations occur in ALL and non-Hodgkin lymphoma and correlate with increased LDH concentrations. Serum IL-2 receptor levels correlate inversely with prognosis.

Lactate Dehydrogenase

The highest concentrations of LDH are found in cardiac red blood cells. A tetrameric enzyme, LDH is composed of four polypeptide subunits.

Five isoenzymes have been identified, LDH_1 through LDH_5: LDH_1 and LDH_2 are found predominantly in kidney, cardiac muscle, and red blood cells; LDH_3 in a variety of tissues, including endocrine glands, spleen, lung, lymph nodes, and platelets; and LDH_4 and LDH_5 in liver and skeletal muscle.

LDH activity is measured spectrophotometrically. Increased serum LDH concentrations have been observed in leukemia, lymphoma rhabdomyosarcoma, Ewing sarcoma, neuroblastoma, hepatoma, and germ cell tumors. Among leukemia patients, those with lymphoblastic leukemias demonstrate higher serum concentrations of LDH than those with myeloid leukemias. Serum LDH concentrations appear to have prognostic value in ALL, nonlymphoblastic non-Hodgkin lymphoma, and Ewing sarcoma, with higher serum concentrations of LDH at diagnosis associated with a poorer prognosis.

In general, the lack of specificity of LDH limits its usefulness as a diagnostic tool, but the level of LDH can be used as a prognostic indicator.

Polyamines

The polyamines spermine, spermidine, and putrescine are produced in increased quantities by rapidly dividing tumors with high DNA turnover and have been demonstrated in the urine, serum, and cerebrospinal fluid of patients with central nervous system malignancies, especially medulloblastoma/primitive neuroepithelial tumor. Normal

Table 1. Immunophenotypic Analysis of Tissue from Metastatic Tumors in Marrow in Children

Tumor	Reactivity Expected with Immunohistochemical Preparations
Lymphoblastic lymphoma[a]	CD3, CD43
B-cell lymphoma	CD20
Anaplastic large-cell lymphoma	CD3, UCHL1, CD30
Hodgkin disease	CD15, CD30
Neuroblastoma	Synaptophysin, neuron-specific enolase
Rhabdomyosarcoma	Myo D1, myogenin, desmin, muscle-specific actin
Ewing sarcoma, peripheral neuroectodermal tumor[b]	013 (CD99), variable staining with neuron-specific enolase, synaptophysin
Synovial sarcoma	Vimentin, keratin

[a]More than 90% of cases show positive results for terminal deoxynucleotidyl transferase.
[b]Periodic acid–Schiff cytoplasmic positivity is usually manifested as small globules.

values in cerebrospinal fluid are spermidine, 77–293 pmol/mL, and putrescine, 58–278 pmol/mL. The polyamine N1,N12-diacetylspermine has been shown to be a diagnostic marker of leukemia, and its level correlates with tumor burden.

Terminal Deoxynucleotidyl Transferase

Terminal deoxynucleotidyl transferase functions in the normal state in immunoglobulin and T-cell leukemic lymphoblasts. It is not present in mature lymphocytes. Serum concentrations are measurable using quantitative enzyme assays or RIA. Increased concentrations are observed primarily in patients with T-cell and pre-B-cell ALL and chronic myelogenous leukemia.

Tumor-Associated Antigens

With the use of monoclonal antibodies, a number of tumor-associated antigens have been identified in pediatric patients. Tumor-associated antigens have been detected in the urine of several children with sarcomas of soft tissues and bone. Tumor-associated antigens may be useful in posttherapy follow-up; however, their utility as biologic markers has not been firmly established.

β_2-Microglobulin

Considered an acute-phase reactant, the peptide β_2-microglobulin constitutes the light chain of the HLA antigens. It is found freely circulating in the serum. It is measured by radioimmunoassay (RIA), with a normal reference range of 0.10–0.26 mg/dL. Increased concentrations occur in advanced-stage (III and IV) Hodgkin and non-Hodgkin lymphoma and correlate with disease remission and response to therapy.

Carcinoembryonic Antigen

Carcinoembryonic antigen (CEA) is measured by RIA or enzyme immunoassay. Normal concentrations range from 0 to 10 ng/mL.

Increased CEA levels in pediatric patients occurs with a variety of malignancies, including Wilms tumor, neuroblastoma, lymphoma, germ cell tumors, mesenchymal tumors, and retinoblastoma. The lack of specificity of CEA limits its utility as a diagnostic tool. If the level is initially increased, however, CEA concentration may be useful in monitoring response to therapy or as a noninvasive means of posttherapy follow-up.

Gangliosides

Two distinct gangliosides, D_2 and D_3, have been identified on the surfaces of neuroblastoma cells and T-cell ALL lymphoblasts, respectively. Ganglioside D_2 can be detected in the serum by HPLC in neuroblastoma. The usefulness of ganglioside D_2 and ganglioside D_3 levels as diagnostic and prognostic tools is not established.

Immunophenotypic Analysis of Metastatic Tumors in Marrow in Children

See Table 1.

Bibliography

Collins RD, Swerdlow SH, eds. *Pediatric hematopathology.* New York: Churchill Livingstone, 2001.

Hann HL, Lange BJ, Stalhut MW, et al. Serum ferritin and prognosis of childhood Hodgkin's disease. *Proc Am Soc Clin Oncol* 1987;66:190(abst).

Herlyn M, Menrad A, Kprowski H. Structure, function, and clinical significance of human tumor antigens. *J Natl Cancer Inst* 1990;82:1883–1889.

Hutton JJ, Coleman MS, Moffitt S, et al. Prognostic significance of terminal transferase activity in childhood acute lymphoblastic leukemia: a prospective analysis of 164 patients. *Blood* 1982;60:1267–1276.

Ishiguro Y, Kato K, Ito T, et al. Nervous system-specific enolase in serum as a marker for neuroblastoma. *Pediatrics* 1983;72:696–700.

Jaffe ES, Harris NL, Stein S, et al. *Tumors of hematopoietic and lymphoid tissue.* Lyon, France: International Agency for Research on Cancer Press, 2001. World Health Organization Classification of Tumors series.

Kaushansky K. Thrombopoietin: the primary regulator of platelet production. *Blood* 1995;86:419–431.

Kelly KM, Lange B. Oncologic emergencies. *Pediatr Clin North Am* 1997;44:809–830.

Kerbl R, Urban CE, Ambros PF, et al. Screening for neuroblastoma in late infancy by use of EIA (enzyme-linked immunoassay) method: 115,000 screened infants in Austria. *Eur J Cancer* 1996;32A:2298–2305.

Koren G, Ferrazini G, Sulh H, et al. Systemic exposure to mercaptopurine as a prognostic factor in acute lymphocytic leukemia in children. *N Engl J Med* 1990; 323:17–21.

Laug WE, Siegel SE, Shaw KNF, et al. Initial urinary catecholamine metabolite concentrations and prognosis in neuroblastoma. *Pediatrics* 1978;62:77–83.

Lee SH, Suh JW, Chung BC, et al. Polyamine profiles in the urine of patients with leukemia. *Cancer Lett* 1998;122:1–8.

Lin Ry, Argenta PA, Sullivan KM, et al. Urinary hyaluronic acid is a Wilms' tumor marker. *J Pediatr Surg* 1995;30:304–308.

Marsch JCW, Gibson FM, Prue RL, et al. Serum thrombopoietin levels in patients with aplastic anemia. *Br J Haematol* 1996;95:605–610.

Ortega JA, Siegel SE. Biological markers in pediatric cancer. In: Pizzo PA, Poplack DG, eds. *Principles and practice of pediatric oncology.* Philadelphia: JB Lippincott Co, 1989:149–162.

Pui CH, Dodge RK, Dahl GV, et al. Serum lactic dehydrogenase level has prognostic value in childhood acute lymphoblastic leukemia. *Blood* 1985;66:778–782.

Pui CH, Ip SH, Behm FG, et al. Serum interleukin 2 receptor levels in childhood acute lymphoblastic leukemia. *Blood* 1988;71:1135–1137.

Schulz G, Cheresh DA, Varki NM, et al. Detection of ganglioside G in tumor tissue and sera of neuroblastoma patients. *Cancer Res* 1984;44:5914–5920.

Tsuchida Y, Terada M, Honna T, et al. The role of subfractionation of alpha-fetoprotein in the treatment of pediatric malignancies. *J Pediatr Surg* 1997;32:514–517.

Van Turnout JM, Buckley JD, Quinn JJ, et al. Timing and magnitude of decline in alpha-fetoprotein levels in treated children with unresectable or metastatic hepatoblastoma are predictors of outcome: a report from the Children's Cancer Group. *J Clin Oncol* 1997;15:1190–1197.

Zeltzer PM, Marangos PJ, Evans AE, et al. Serum neuron-specific enolase in children with neuroblastoma: relationship to stage and disease course. *Cancer* 1986;57: 1230–1234.

15 Diseases of the Central and Peripheral Nervous System[1]

Laboratory Tests for Disorders of the Nervous System

Cerebrospinal Fluid Abnormalities

(See Chapter 1 for normal values.)
See Tables 1–3.

Gross Appearance

Turbidity of the cerebrospinal fluid (CSF) may be due to increased white blood cells (WBCs) (>200/mm^3) or red blood cells (RBCs) (>400/mm^3), or to the presence of bacteria (>10^5/mL) or other microorganisms (fungi, amebas), contrast media, or epidural fat aspirated during lumbar puncture.
Clots or pellicles indicate protein >150 mg/dL.
CSF with RBC >6,000/mm^3 appears grossly bloody; with RBC = 500–6,000/mm^3, it appears cloudy, xanthochromic, or pink-tinged (in bright light in clear glass tubes containing >1 mL of CSF).
Xanthochromia caused by bilirubin may be due to bleeding within 2–36 hours.
Serum bilirubin >6 mg/dL causes yellow fluid.

White Blood Cells

CSF WBCs may be corrected crudely for presence of blood (e.g., traumatic tap, subarachnoid hemorrhage) by subtracting 1 WBC for each 700 RBCs/mm^3 counted in CSF if the complete blood count is normal.
If significant anemia or leukocytosis is present:

$$\text{Corrected WBC} = \frac{\text{WBC in bloody CSF} - [\text{WBC (blood)} \times \text{RBC (CSF)}]}{[\text{RBC (blood)}]}$$

(RBC and WBC are cells/mm^3.)
This formula is used but usually is inaccurate.
CSF WBC count (>2,000–3,000/mm^3) with predominantly polymorphonuclear cells (PMNs) strongly suggests bacterial cause. When WBC <1,000/mm^3 in bacterial meningitis, one-third of cases have >50% lymphocytes or mononuclear cells. However, WBCs are usually PMNs in early stages of all types of meningitis; mononuclear cells only appear in a second specimen 18–24 hours later. Low WBC counts do not rule out acute bacterial meningitis.
Neutrophilic leukocytes are found in bacterial and some fungal infections (e.g., *Nocardia*, *Actinomyces*, *Arachnia*, *Brucella*).

[1]Portions of this chapter have been reproduced with permission from Wallach J. *Interpretation of diagnostic tests*, 7th ed. Philadelphia: Lippincott Williams & Wilkins, 2000.

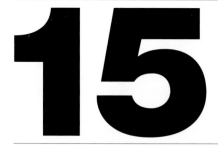

Table 1. Cerebrospinal Fluid Abnormalities[a]

	Normal	Abnormalities
Color	Clear, colorless	Yellow (xanthochromic): old hemorrhage, high protein level, complete subarachnoid obstruction Red: subarachnoid hemorrhage (if traumatic puncture is excluded) Turbid (purulent): bacterial meningitis Clear with clot on standing: high protein level, common in tuberculosis meningitis
Protein	20–50 mg/dL	Marked increase: infection, hemorrhage, tumor causing subarachnoid block Moderate increase: many causes
Oligoclonal protein bands[b]		Multiple sclerosis, syphilis
Serology		Results of VDRL test positive in neurosyphilis
Glucose	50–80 mg/dL (75% of blood glucose level)	Marked decrease in bacterial meningitis; increased in hyperglycemic states
Cells	0–5 (mostly lymphocytes); no neutrophils present	Increased neutrophils: bacterial infection Increased lymphocytes: viral, fungal, tuberculous meningitis, syphilis, cysticercosis, degenerative diseases Malignant cells: cancer (various types)
Gram stain of sediment	Negative	Useful test in meningitis; positive finding may provide immediate diagnosis
Culture	Negative	Positive with bacterial, mycobacterial, fungal, and viral infections

[a]Always check for evidence of raised intracranial pressure before lumbar puncture. If pressure is normal in a recumbent child ≥ 6 yr of age, remove 3-mL samples in three separate sterile containers for (a) chemical and serologic analysis, (b) culture, (c) cell count and cytologic analysis.
[b]Two to four immunoglobulin bands seen on electrophoresis of cerebrospinal fluid.
Reproduced with permission from Wallach J. *Interpretation of diagnostic tests*, 7th ed. Philadelphia: Lippincott Williams & Wilkins, 2000.

Cerebrospinal Fluid Chemistries

Glucose

Glucose level is decreased by use by bacteria (pyogens or tubercle bacilli), WBCs, or occasionally cancer cells in CSF.

Lags behind blood glucose by approximately 1 hour.

May rapidly become normal after onset of antibiotic therapy.

Is decreased in only approximately 50% of cases of bacterial meningitis.

Level <45 mg/dL is almost always abnormal.

Normal is 50–65% of blood glucose, which should always be measured on a blood sample drawn simultaneously. In acute bacterial meningitis, CSF/serum ratio of glucose is usually <0.5; a ratio <0.4 has 80% sensitivity and 96% specificity for distinguishing acute bacterial meningitis from acute viral meningitis; a ratio of <0.8 is significant in infants for bacterial meningitis.

May also be decreased in acute infection due to syphilis, Lyme disease, 10–20% of cases of lymphocytic choriomeningitis, and encephalitis due to mumps or herpes simplex virus (HSV). Generally not decreased in viral infections or parameningeal processes. May also be decreased in rheumatoid meningitis, lupus myelopathy, and other causes of chronic meningitis, fungal infection (*Cryptococcus*, *Coccidioides*), parasitic infection (e.g., *Taenia*), granulomatous meningitis (e.g., sarcoid), chemical meningitis, carcinomatous meningitis, hypoglycemia, and subarachnoid hemorrhage.

Table 2. Differential Diagnosis of Infectious Diseases of the Central Nervous System

CSF Finding	Encephalitis	Bacterial Meningitis[a]	Viral Meningitis	Tuberculous (Chronic) Meningitis	Brain Abscess
Pressure	Raised	Raised	Raised	Raised	May be very high
Gross appearance	Clear	Turbid	Clear	Clear; may clot	Clear
Protein	Slightly elevated	High	Slightly elevated	Very high	Elevated
Glucose	Normal	Very low	Normal	Low	Normal
Chloride	Normal	Low	Normal	Very low	Normal or low
Cells	Lymphocytes or normal	Neutrophils	Lymphocytes	Pleocytosis[b]	Pleocytosis
Gram stain	Negative	Positive in 90%	Negative	Negative	Occasionally positive
Acid-fast stain	Negative	Negative	Negative	Rarely positive	Negative
Bacterial culture	Negative	Positive in 90%	Negative	Negative	Occasionally positive
Mycobacterial culture	Negative	Negative	Negative	Positive	Negative
Viral culture	Positive in 30% or less	Negative	Positive in 70%	Negative	Negative

CSF, cerebrospinal fluid.
[a]Amebic and cryptococcal meningitis are diagnosed by the finding of these organisms in the smear.
[b]Pleocytosis is the presence of both neutrophils and lymphocytes in cerebrospinal fluid.
Reproduced with permission from Wallach J. *Interpretation of diagnostic tests*, 7th ed. Philadelphia: Lippincott Williams & Wilkins, 2000.

Protein

Total protein may be corrected for presence of blood (e.g., due to traumatic tap or intracerebral hemorrhage) by subtracting 1 mg/dL of protein for each 1,000 RBCs/mm^3 if serum protein and complete blood count are normal and CSF protein and cell count are determined on same tube of CSF. Serum protein levels must be normal to interpret any CSF protein values and should therefore always be measured concurrently.

May not be increased in early stages of many types of meningitis.

Normal in 10% of patients with bacterial meningitis (20% of cases of meningococcal meningitis).

Usually >150 mg/dL in bacterial meningitis. Increase occurs especially with *Streptococcus pneumoniae* infection.

Level >100 mg/dL distinguishes bacterial from aseptic meningitis (82% sensitivity and 98% specificity).

Level >500 mg/dL is infrequent and occurs chiefly in bacterial meningitis, bloody CSF, or cord tumor with spinal block and occasionally in polyneuritis and brain tumor.

Level >1,000 mg/dL suggests subarachnoid block; with complete spinal block, the lower the level of the cord tumor, the higher the protein concentration.

Rarely >200 mg/dL in viral meningitis.

When antibiotic treatment of bacterial meningitis is started before CSF is obtained, protein level may be only slightly elevated.

Table 3. Cerebrospinal Fluid Findings in Various Conditions

	Appearance	Protein (mg/dL)	Glucose (mg/dL)	WBC/mm^3	Microbiology/Serology/Other
Normal					
Ventricular		5–15			
Cisternal	C, colorless	10–25	45–80	0–10	
Lumbar	No clot	10–45			
TB meningitis	O, sl yellow, delicate clot	45–500	10–45	10–1,000, chiefly L	Acid-fast stain 25% sensitive Culture 60–80% sensitive PCR 100% specific
Tuberculoma		I		Small number of cells	
Acute pyogenic meningitis	O to Pu, sl yellow, delicate clot	50–1,500	0–45	25–10,000, chiefly P	Gram stain 60–90% sensitive Culture 80% sensitive, 100% specific Direct antigen/PCR 50–90% sensitive, 100% specific
Aseptic meningitis	C, T, or X	20 to >200	N	≤500, occ 2,000; first Ps, later mononuclear cells	All cultures negative
Viral meningitis		I	N	10–1,000, mostly L	Seroconversion Specific IgM Antigens PCR Culture 40–70% sensitive
AIDS		50–100	N	≥300	Culture 40–70% sensitive HIV antibodies, antigens
Acute anterior polio	C or sl O, may be sl yellow, may be delicate clot	20–350	N	10 to >500, L > P	Serologic tests Stool culture AST in CSF is always I
Mumps	N or O	20–125	N	0 to >2,000	IgM and IgG in blood and CSF Culture of CSF
Measles	N or O	sl I	N	≤500	Blood serology
Herpes zoster	N	20–110	N	≤300 in 40% of patients	PCR

Equine, St. Louis encephalitis, choriomeningitis	N or sl T	20 to >200	N	10–200; occ to 3,000	Blood serologic tests
Herpes simplex		I	N	10–1,000, chiefly L	CSF culture in congenital infection CSF serologic tests; brain biopsy
Rabies		N or sl I		N or ≤100 mononuclear cells	Serologic tests Cultures of brain or saliva Animal brain Tissue examination
Postinfectious	N	15–75	N	5–200, rarely ≤1,000	Serologic tests for specific viruses
Fungal					
Coccidioidomycoses		I	N early, then D	≤200 early; may be higher later	Antigen assay Culture 50% sensitive CF in CSF 75–90% sensitive Wet preparation in 20% KOH
Cryptococcal meningitis	N	≤500 in 90%	Moderate D in 55%	≤800 (L >P)	India ink stain 50% sensitive Cryptococcal antigen assay 90% sensitive Culture 90% sensitive
Toxoplasmosis	X	≤2,000	N	50–500; chiefly monocytes	Serologic tests in serum PCR Organism identified in sediment smear
Syphilis					Positive serologic test in blood and positive CSF VDRL PCR can detect treponemal DNA in CSF
Tabes dorsalis	N	25–100; I γ-globulin less marked than in general paresis	N	10–80	Early: VDRL titer may be low Late: 25% of patients may have normal CSF and negative VDRL in blood and CSF
Leptospirosis		I ≤80	N	≤500 M	
Lyme disease		I IgG and oligoclonal bands	N	≤450 L	*Borrelia burgdorferi* antibodies higher in CSF than in serum

(continued)

Table 3. (continued)

	Appearance	Protein (mg/dL)	Glucose (mg/dL)	WBC/mm³	Microbiology/Serology/Other
Primary amebic (*Naegleria*) meningitis	Sanguinopurulent, may be T or Pu	I	Usually D	400–21,000 mostly P; also RBC	Amebas seen on Wright stain of CSF
Chronic meningitis[a]					
Symptoms for 1–4 wk		Moderate to marked I	D	100–400, mostly L	
Cavernous sinus thrombophlebitis	Usually N; may be B		Usually N		
Brain abscess[b]		May be ≤75–300	N	25–300; P, L, RBCs	CSF cultures sterile Positive blood cultures in 10% Can be caused by almost any organism including fungi, *Nocardia*
Extradural abscess		100–400	N	Relatively few Ps and L	
Subdural empyema		I	N	Few hundred or less, mostly Ps	Negative smears and peripheral WBC I (≤25,000/mm³)
Cord tumor	C, occ X	≤3,500 in 85%; N in 15%	N	≤100, chiefly L; N in 60%	
Brain tumor[c]	C, occ X; B if hemorrhage into tumor	≤500	May be D if cells are present	≤150; N in 75%	Tumor cells in 20–40% of solid tumors; absence does not exclude meningeal tumor
Leukemia		I	D to 50% of blood level		Tumor cells identified by special methods
Pseudotumor cerebri	N	N	N	N	
Cerebral thrombosis	N	≤100, N in 60%	N	≤50, N in 75%, rarely ≤2,000	
Cerebral embolism[d]					
Bland	sl X in one-third of cases in a few days; may be B			May be 10,000 RBC	

Septic	sl X	I	N	≤200 with varying L and Ps; ≤1,000 RBCs	
Cerebral hemorrhage	N in 15%, X in 10%, B in 75%	Usually ≤2,000	N	Same as in blood; N in 10%	
Subarachnoid hemorrhage	B; X in 24 hr; no clot	Usually ≤1,000	N	Same as in blood	
Hypertensive encephalopathy		≤100			
Postoperative neurosurgery (especially posterior fossa)		I	<40	1,000–2,000, mostly Ps	CSF sterile unless postoperative infection
Traumatic tap	B	I by blood	N	Same as in blood	
Head trauma	N, B, or X	I if bloody	N	Same as in blood	
Acute epidural hemorrhage	C unless associated injuries				
Subdural hematoma	C, B, or X depending on associated injuries	N or sl I			Infants are often anemic
Chronic subdural hematoma	Usually X	300–2,000			
Polyneuritis					
Polyarteritis; porphyria; beriberi; alcohol effect; arsenic poisoning	N, X if protein very I	Usually N	N	N but albumino-cytologic dissociation in Guillain-Barré syndrome that may occur in heavy metal poisoning, infection, etc.	
Diabetes mellitus	Same as polyarteritis, etc.	Often ≤300	N	Same as polyarteritis, etc.	

(continued)

Table 3. (continued)

	Appearance	Protein (mg/dL)	Glucose (mg/dL)	WBC/mm^3	Microbiology/Serology/Other
Acute infection	Same as polyarteritis, etc.	≤1,500	N	Same as polyarteritis, etc.	
Lead encephalopathy	N or sl yellow	≤100	N	0–100	
Sarcoidosis (findings in ≤50%)		sl I; oligoclonal bands may be present	D in 10%	I in 40%	I ACE in serum or CSF in 50–70%
				Typically 10–100 but ≤6,000	
Behçet disease (25% have meningoencephalitis)		I	N	I	
Diabetic coma	N	N	I	Usually N	
Uremia	N	N or I	N or I	Usually N	
Epilepsy	N	N	N	N	
Eclampsia	May be B	Usually ≤200	N	May be RBCs	Uric acid I ≤3× N reflecting marked I in serum
Guillain-Barré syndrome		50–100 average; albuminocytologic dissociation	N		

ACE, angiotensin-converting enzyme; AIDS, acquired immunodeficiency syndrome; AST, aspartate aminotransferase; B, bloody; C, clear; CF, complement fixation; CSF, cerebrospinal fluid; D, decreased; HIV, human immunodeficiency virus; I, increased; IgG, immunoglobulin G; IgM, immunoglobulin M; L, lymphocytes; N, normal; O, opalescent; occ, occasionally; P, polymorphonuclear leukocyte; PCR, polymerase chain reaction; Pu, purulent; sl, slightly; RBC, red blood cell; T, turbid; WBC, white blood cell; X, xanthochromic.

[a]Possible underlying disorders:

Various infections: tuberculosis (most common cause), bacteria, spirochetes, fungi, protozoa, amebas, *Mycoplasma*, rickettsiae, helminths.

Systemic disorders (e.g., vasculitis, collagen vascular disease, sarcoid, neoplasm).

[b]Findings depend on stage and duration of abscess.

[c]Protein level is particularly increased with meningioma of the olfactory groove and with acoustic neuroma. Usually normal in brainstem gliomas and diencephalic syndrome of infants due to glioma of hypothalamus.

[d]Usually same as in cerebral thrombosis.

Modified with permission from Wallach J. *Interpretation of diagnostic tests*, 7th ed. Philadelphia: Lippincott Williams & Wilkins, 2000.

May show mild to moderate elevation in myxedema, uremia, connective tissue disorders, or Cushing syndrome.

Decreased CSF protein (3–20 mg/dL) may occur in hyperthyroidism, one-third of patients with benign intracranial hypertension, or after removal of large volumes of CSF in children 6–24 months of age.

Other Substances

CSF and serum angiotensin-converting enzyme levels are increased in 50–70% of cases of neurosarcoidosis.

CSF lactate level is useful to differentiate bacterial from viral meningitis; is independent of serum concentration. Due to sequelae of increased WBC.

- If <4 mmol/L (normal range), viral meningitis is likely.
- If >4.2 mmol/L, bacterial [including tuberculosis (TB)-associated] or fungal meningitis is likely.
- If 3–6 mmol/L with negative Gram stain finding and prior antibiotic therapy, partially treated bacterial meningitis is likely. In bacterial meningitis, level is still high after 1–2 days of antibiotic therapy.
- In cases with mild symptoms and negative Gram stain results with few PMNs, CSF lactate level may differentiate bacterial from early viral meningitis.
- May also be increased in non-Hodgkin lymphoma with meningeal involvement, cerebral malaria, head injury, and anoxia.

CSF chloride level reflects only blood chloride level, but in tuberculous meningitis a CSF decrease of 25% may exceed the serum chloride decrease because of dehydration and electrolyte loss.

CSF glutamine level of >35 mg/dL is associated with hepatic encephalopathy (due to conversion from ammonia).

Cerebrospinal Fluid Enzymes

Aspartate Aminotransferase

Present in 40% of central nervous system (CNS) tumors (various benign, malignant, and metastatic), depending on location, growth rate, and so on; chiefly useful as indicator of organic neurologic disease.

Lactate Dehydrogenase

Increased in cerebrovascular accidents—increase occurs frequently, reaches maximum level in 1–3 days, and is apparently not related to xanthochromia, RBC, WBC, protein, sugar, or chloride levels. Subarachnoid and subdural hemorrhage cause increase of all lactate dehydrogenase (LDH) isoenzymes, especially LDH_3, LDH_4, and LDH_5 (not due to hemolysis).

CNS tumors—LDH_5 >9% and LDH_1/LDH_5 ratio <2.5 in absence of infection or hemorrhage suggests tumor in meninges. LDH_5 >10% suggests higher grade malignancy. Increase in LDH_3, LDH_4, and occasionally LDH_5 may occur in leukemic and lymphomatous infiltration.

Meningitis—a sensitive indicator of meningitis (in specimen with no blood); normal or mild increase in viral meningitis; more marked increase in bacterial meningitis shows increase of LDH_1 and LDH_2; TB meningitis shows increase of LDH_1, LDH_2, LDH_3 (especially LDH_3); infection with human immunodeficiency virus (HIV) alone does not alter LDH isoenzyme pattern; isoenzyme changes may appear only in later stages and are of low sensitivity.

Tumor Markers

β-Glucuronidase has been reported to be increased in 60% of patients with acute myeloblastic leukemia involving CNS. Normal = <49 mU/L, indeterminate = 49–70 mU/L, suspicious = >70 mU/L.

Lysozyme (muramidase) is increased in various CNS tumors, especially myeloid and monocytic leukemias, but is also increased when neutrophils are increased (e.g., in bacterial meningitis).

γ-Aminobutyric acid is decreased in CSF in Huntington disease.

Immunoglobulin (Ig) G in CSF is increased 14–35% in two-thirds of patients with neurosyphilis. IgG oligoclonal bands are seen in neurosyphilis and multiple sclerosis.

In eclampsia, CSF shows gross or microscopic blood and increased protein (up to 200 mg/dL). Glucose is normal. Uric acid is increased (to three times normal level), which reflects the marked increase in serum level. (In normal pregnancy, CSF values have same reference range as in nonpregnant women.)

Microbiology and Serology

Gram stain of CSF sediment gives negative result in 20% of cases of bacterial meningitis because at least 10^5 bacteria/mL of CSF must be present to demonstrate 1–2 bacteria/100× microscopic field. Gram stain gives positive result in 90% of cases due to pneumococci, 85% of cases due to *Haemophilus influenzae*, 75% of cases due to meningococci, 50% of cases due to *Listeria monocytogenes*, and 30–50% of cases due to Gram-negative enteric bacilli. If antibiotics have been given before CSF was obtained, Gram stain results may be negative. Stain results are positive in <60% of cases of treated bacterial meningitis, <5% of cases of TB meningitis, 20–70% of cases of fungal meningitis, and <2% of cases of brain abscess. Sensitivity of Gram stain is increased by using fluorescent techniques with acridine orange.

Limulus amebocyte lysate is a rapid specific indicator of endotoxin produced by Gram-negative bacteria (*Neisseria meningitidis, H. influenzae* type b, *Escherichia coli, Pseudomonas*); is not affected by prior antibiotic therapy; is more rapid and sensitive than countercurrent immunoelectrophoresis (CIE).

Serologic methods are often preferred (e.g., positive results in 85% of coccidioidal cases compared with culture, which shows positive results in 37% of cases) especially in syphilis, brucellosis, Lyme disease.

Polymerase chain reaction is used to detect HSV and human enteroviruses in meningitis and encephalitis.

Antigen detection (latex agglutination) for *H. influenzae* type b, *Cryptococcus neoformans, N. meningitidis, S. pneumoniae, Streptococcus agalactiae* has replaced CIE.

False-positive results for group B streptococci may occur due to colonization of perineum.

Misleading positive results for *H. influenzae* type b may occur in both urine and CSF due to recent immunization with *H. influenzae* type b vaccine.

Lymphocytic cells are found due to bacteria, viruses, parasitic diseases, fungal infections, leukemia, parameningeal disorders, noninfectious disorders (e.g., neoplasms, sarcoidosis, multiple sclerosis, granulomatous arteritis)

Eosinophils are found in lymphoma, helminth infection (e.g., angiostrongyliasis, cysticercosis), rarely in other infections (e.g., TB, syphilis, Rocky Mountain spotted fever, coccidioidomycosis).

Special Tests

Prenatal Diagnosis

Amniocentesis: Increased α-fetoprotein in amniotic fluid (by 14 weeks) suggests open neural tube defects.

Ultrasonography: Hydrocephalus usually diagnosed readily. Other signs associated with Chiari II anomaly may be discernible (banana sign, callosal anomalies, mega choroid plexus).

Neonatal Diagnosis

Neurologic examination including pinprick examination of trunk, legs, and perineum. Functional integrity present if stimulus causes purposeful limb movements, arousal, crying, anal wink, and so on.

Myelomeningocele is usually apparent on physical examination.

Direct laryngoscopy is indicated for infants with stridor, an ominous sign suggesting the need for urgent CSF diversion or posterior fossa decompression or both.

Cranial ultrasonography is most efficient way to assess ventricular size promptly; may demonstrate associated anomalies (callosal agenesis, etc.).

Disorders of the Nervous System

See Tables 2 and 3.

Abscess, Brain

CSF shows WBC count of 25–300/mm^3 and increased neutrophils, lymphocytes, and RBCs.
- Protein level may be increased (75–300 mg/dL).
- Glucose level is normal.
- Bacterial cultures are negative in approximately 90% of cases.

Causes

Usually mixed anaerobic (e.g., streptococci or *Bacteroides*) and aerobic (e.g., streptococci, staphylococci, or *S. pneumoniae*) organisms and Gram-negative species (e.g., *Proteus, Klebsiella, Pseudomonas*)
- *Staphylococcus* infection predominates when due to penetrating trauma.
- *Toxoplasma* and *Nocardia* infections may be due to underlying acquired immunodeficiency syndrome (AIDS).
- Twenty percent of cultures are sterile.
- May be caused by almost any organism, including fungi and *Nocardia*.
- Findings depend on stage and duration of abscess.
- With rupture, acute purulent meningitis with many organisms.

Laboratory Findings

Laboratory findings due to associated primary disease.
- Ten percent of cases are due to penetrating skull trauma.
- Fifty percent of cases are due to contiguous spread from sinuses, mastoid, middle ear.
- Twenty percent of cases are cryptogenic.
- Twenty percent of cases are due to hematogenous spread, for example, from dental infections, primary septic lung disease (e.g., lung abscess, bronchiectasis, empyema), cyanotic congenital heart disease (e.g., septal defects), or other causes.

Abscess, Epidural of Spinal Cord/Extradural, Intracranial

CSF protein level is increased (usually 100–400 mg/dL), and relatively few WBCs are present (lymphocytes and neutrophils).

Most common causative organism is *S. aureus*, followed by *Streptococcus* and Gram-negative bacilli.

Laboratory findings due to preceding condition (e.g., adjacent osteomyelitis; bacteremia due to dental, respiratory, or skin infection).

Acquired Immunodeficiency Syndrome, Neurologic Manifestations

Dementia (also called subacute encephalitis) is most common neurologic syndrome in AIDS; occurs in >50% of cases; may be initial or later manifestation.

CSF abnormalities in 85% of cases
- Increased protein level (50–100 mg/dL) in 60% in patients
- Mild mononuclear pleocytosis (5–50 cells/mm^3) in 20% of patients

HIV antibodies

Aseptic meningitis—may occur early or late, or be chronic recurrent.

CSF may show
- Twenty to 300 cells/mm^3
- Increased protein (may be 50–100 mg/dL)
- HIV culture is usually positive.
- Increased CSF/serum antibody ratio, indicating local antibody production

Myelopathy—gradual onset; usually associated with dementia.
- Polymyositis is most common type.

Peripheral neuropathies, some of which may resemble Guillain-Barré syndrome
- CSF may show
  - Increased protein level (50–100 mg/dL)
  - Pleocytosis of 10–50 cells/mm^3

Opportunistic infections of CNS
- Viral [e.g., cytomegalovirus (CMV), HSV-1 and HSV-2, papovavirus]
- Nonviral (e.g., *Cryptococcus*, *Toxoplasma*, *Aspergillus fumigatus*, *Candida albicans*, *Coccidioides immitis*, *Mycobacterium avium-intracellulare*, and *Mycobacterium tuberculosis*, *Nocardia asteroides*, *Listeria*)

Neoplasms (e.g., Kaposi sarcoma, non-Hodgkin lymphoma)
Vascular (e.g., infarction, hemorrhage, vasculitis)
Associated diseases (e.g., neurosyphilis)

Ataxia, Cerebellar, Progressive, with Skin Telangiectasis (Louis-Bar Syndrome)

(Autosomal-recessive multisystem disease with cerebellar ataxia and oculocutaneous telangiectasia)
Some patients have
- Glucose intolerance
- Abnormal liver function test findings
- Decreased or absent serum IgA and IgE, which causes recurrent pulmonary infections; IgM is present.
- Increased serum α-fetoprotein levels

Bassen-Kornzweig Syndrome

Abnormal RBCs (acanthocytes) are present in the peripheral blood smear.
There may be
- Marked deficiency of serum β-lipoprotein and cholesterol
- Marked impairment of gastrointestinal fat absorption
- Low serum carotene levels
- Abnormal pattern of RBC phospholipids

Berry Aneurysm

In early subarachnoid hemorrhage (<8 hours after onset of symptoms), the test for occult blood may give positive results before xanthochromia develops. After bloody spinal fluid occurs, WBC/RBC ratio may be higher in CSF than in peripheral blood.

Bloody CSF clears by tenth day in 40% of patients. CSF is persistently abnormal after 21 days in 15% of patients. Five percent of cerebrovascular episodes due to hemorrhage are wholly within the parenchyma and CSF findings are normal.

Cerebrovascular Accident (Nontraumatic)

Causes

Hemorrhage
- Ruptured berry aneurysm (45% of patients)
- Hypertension (15% of patients)
- Angiomatous malformations (8% of patients)
- Miscellaneous causes (e.g., brain tumor, blood dyscrasia; infrequent)
- Undetermined cause (remainder of patients)

Occlusion (e.g., thrombosis, embolism, etc.) in 80% of patients
Especially if blood pressure is normal, ruptured berry aneurysm, hemorrhage into tumor, and angioma should be ruled out.

Coma and Stupor

Causes

Cerebral disorders
- Infection (e.g., meningitis, encephalitis)
- Brain contusions, hemorrhage, infarction, seizure, or aneurysm
- Brain mass (e.g., tumor, hematoma, abscess)
- Subdural or epidural hematoma
- Venous sinus occlusion
- Hydrocephalus
- Hypoxia

Decreased blood oxygen content and tension (e.g., lung disease, high altitude)
Decreased blood oxygen content with normal tension (e.g., anemia, carbon monoxide poisoning, methemoglobinemia)
Vascular abnormalities (e.g., subarachnoid hemorrhage, hypertensive encephalopathy, shock, acute myocardial infarction, aortic stenosis, Adams-Stokes syndrome, tachycardias)
Metabolic abnormalities
- Acid-base imbalance (acidosis, alkalosis)
- Electrolyte imbalance (increased or decreased sodium, potassium, calcium, magnesium)
- Porphyrias
- Aminoacidurias
- Uremia
- Hepatic encephalopathy
- Other disorders (e.g., leukodystrophies, lipid storage disease, niacin and pyridoxine deficiencies)

Endocrine abnormalities
- Pancreas (diabetic coma, hypoglycemia)
- Thyroid (myxedema, thyrotoxicosis)
- Adrenal gland (Addison disease, Cushing syndrome, pheochromocytoma)
- Pituitary (panhypopituitarism)
- Parathyroid (hypofunction or hyperfunction)

Poisons, drugs, or toxins
- Sedatives (especially alcohol, barbiturates)
- Enzyme inhibitors (especially salicylates, heavy metals, organic phosphates, cyanide)
- Other (e.g., paraldehyde, methyl alcohol, ethylene glycol)

Demyelinating Diseases

Disease	Comment
Multiple sclerosis	Possible viral or immune mediation.
Neuromyelitis optica (Devic disease)	Variant of multiple sclerosis with lesions focused in optic nerves, brainstem, and spinal cord.
Experimental allergic encephalomyelitis (EAE)	Demyelination induced in animal by immunization against brain tissue.
Acute disseminated encephalomyelitis	Apparent human analog of EAE; occurs postinfection with or postimmunization for smallpox, rabies, or pertussis.
Guillain-Barré syndrome	Resembles EAE but demyelination involves nerve roots and peripheral nerves; typically follows virus infection.
Progressive multifocal leukoencephalopathy	Papillomavirus infection.
Subacute sclerosing panencephalitis	Delayed injury caused by measles virus.
Diffuse sclerosis (Schilder disease)	Several variants, familial and sporadic; present early in life; may encompass several different entities.

Dysmyelinative disorders	Disorders of myelin metabolism; metachromatic leukodystrophy, lipidoses, phenylketonuria.
Demyelination secondary to systemic disease	Anoxia, toxic agents, nutritional disorders (e.g., vitamin B_{12} deficiency)

Embolism, Cerebral

Laboratory findings due to underlying causative disease
- Infective endocarditis
- Nonbacterial thrombotic vegetations on heart valves
- Chronic rheumatic mitral stenosis with atrial thrombi
- Mural thrombus due to underlying myocardial infarction
- Myxoma of left atrium
- Fat embolism in fracture of long bones
- Air embolism in neck, chest, or cardiac surgery

Empyema, Subdural, Acute

CSF
- Cell count is increased to a few hundred, with predominance of PMNs.
- Protein level is increased.
- Glucose level is normal.
- Bacterial smears and cultures give negative results.

WBC count is usually increased ($\leq$25,000/mm^3)
Laboratory findings due to preceding diseases
- Ear, nose, and throat infections, especially acute sinusitis or otitis media
- Intracranial surgery

Streptococci are the most common causative organisms when preceding condition is sinusitis. *Staphylococcus aureus* or Gram-negative organisms are the most common organisms after trauma or surgery.

Encephalopathy, Hypertensive

Laboratory findings due to changes in other organ systems and to other conditions.
- Cardiac
- Renal
- Endocrine
- Toxemia of pregnancy

Laboratory findings due to progressive changes that may occur (e.g., focal intracerebral hemorrhage).
CSF frequently shows increased pressure and protein level of $\geq$ 100 mg/dL.

Guillain-Barré Syndrome

CSF shows albumino-cytologic dissociation with normal cell count and increased protein (average 50–100 mg/dL). Protein increase parallels increasing clinical severity; increase may be prolonged. CSF may be normal at first.
Laboratory findings due to preceding disease may be present (e.g., acute infections of respiratory or gastrointestinal tract [such as Epstein-Barr virus (EBV), *Campylobacter*, varicella-zoster virus (VZV), *M. pneumoniae*, CMV, hepatitis virus, other viral, and rickettsial infections], Refsum disease, immune disorders, endocrine disturbances, exposure to toxins, neoplasms).

Headache

Many of the causes of headache are the same as in adults, but the relative frequencies may be very different. For example, brain tumors are the most commonly diagnosed solid tumor of childhood and many, especially posterior fossa tumors, present with characteristic headache.

Causes

Acute isolated headache	Infection Meningitis Encephalitis Sinusitis or mastoiditis Brain abscess Subarachnoid hemorrhage Systemic infection with fever
Acute recurrent headache	Brain tumor Vascular malformation Migraine, cluster headache Hypertension Metabolic abnormalities: hypoglycemia, etc. Sinusitis (rare in younger children) Drugs: alcohol, nitrates, calcium channel blockers, nonsteroidal antiinflammatory drugs
Posttraumatic headache	Concussion Subdural and epidural hemorrhage Cerebral contusion
Chronic progressive headache	Brain tumor Hydrocephalus Brain abscess Subdural hemorrhage Pseudotumor cerebri Acute angle-closure glaucoma
Chronic nonprogressive headache	Depression Stress, tension headache, anxiety Previous trauma School avoidance or attention seeking Temporomandibular joint syndrome

Hematoma, Subdural

CSF findings are variable—clear, bloody, or xanthochromic, depending on recent or old associated injuries (e.g., contusion, laceration).

Chronic subdural hematoma fluid is usually xanthochromic; protein content is 300–2,000 mg/dL.

Anemia is often present in infants.

Hemianopsia, Bitemporal

Laboratory findings due to causative disease

- Usually pituitary adenoma
- Metastatic tumor, sarcoidosis, Hand-Schüller-Christian disease, meningioma of sella, and aneurysm of circle of Willis

Hemorrhage, Cerebral

Bleeding may occur intracerebrally or in the subarachnoid or subdural areas. If papilledema or retinal hemorrhage is present, lumbar puncture should be withheld and cerebral imaging obtained.

WBC ($15,000–20,000/mm^3$) is higher than in cerebral infarct (e.g., embolism, thrombosis).

Erythrocyte sedimentation rate is usually increased.

CSF pressure usually is increased. If lumbar puncture is performed, pressure, presence of RBCs (ongoing bleed), and xanthochromia (previous bleed) should be noted. Protein level is usually increased.

Urine

- Transient glycosuria
- Laboratory findings of concomitant renal disease

Laboratory findings due to other causes of intracerebral hemorrhage [e.g., leukemia, aplastic anemia, purpuras, hemophilias, anticoagulant therapy, systemic lupus erythematosus (SLE), polyarteritis nodosa]

Laboratory findings due to other diseases that occur with increased frequency in association with berry aneurysm (e.g., coarctation of the aorta, polycystic kidneys, hypertension)

Differentiation between Bloody Cerebrospinal Fluid Due to Subarachnoid Hemorrhage and Traumatic Lumbar Puncture

CSF Finding	Subarachnoid Hemorrhage	Traumatic Lumbar Puncture
CSF pressure	Often increased	Low
Blood in tubes for collecting CSF	Mixture with blood is uniform in all tubes	Earlier tubes more bloody than later tubes; RBC count decreases in later tubes
CSF clotting	No clots	Often clots
Xanthochromia	Present if >8–12 hr since subarachnoid hemorrhage	Absent unless patient is icteric; may appear if CSF examination delayed ≥2 hr
Immediate repeat lumbar puncture at higher levels	CSF same as initial puncture	CSF clear

Hemorrhage, Epidural, Acute

CSF is usually under increased pressure; it is clear unless associated cerebral contusion, laceration, or subarachnoid hemorrhage is present.

Hydrocephalus

Causes

Noncommunicating hydrocephalus
- Congenital
- Aqueductal stenosis and atresia
- Dandy-Walker syndrome

Acquired
- Neoplasms and cysts obstructing cerebral aqueduct and the third ventricle
- Gliosis and chronic inflammation involving aqueduct
- Obstruction of fourth ventricle openings
- Organized subarachnoid hemorrhage, obstructing flow at base of brain
- Organized meningitis involving base of brain

Communicating hydrocephalus
- Choroid plexus papilloma (increased secretion)

Arnold-Chiari malformation

Deficient absorption of cerebrospinal fluid
- Dural sinus thrombosis
- Organized subarachnoid hemorrhage
- Organized meningitis
- ?Deficiency of arachnoid villi

Hypertension, Intracranial

Increased intracranial pressure is defined as elevation of the mean CSF pressure above 200 mm H_2O (15 mm Hg) when measured with the patient in the lateral decubitus position.

Causes

Obstructive hydrocephalus	
Infection	Abscess (mass effect and local edema). Meningitis, encephalitis.
Anoxia of any cause	
Hypoglycemia	
Hypertensive encephalopathy	Associated with altered capillaries of tumor, abscesses, toxins, (e.g., lead poisoning).
Uremia	
Infarction	With local edema or hemorrhage.
Neoplasm	Primary or secondary (mass effect and local edema)
Space-occupying lesions	Extradural, subdural, subarachnoid, or intracranial; rapidly expanding lesions produce greater rise in intracranial pressure than slowly expanding masses.
Hemorrhage or hematoma	
Cerebral edema	
Intracellular cytotoxic	Early manifestation of cell injury most commonly seen in ischemic states.
Extracellular vasogenic	Responsible for most cases of cerebral edema occurring in infections, trauma, neoplasms, and metabolic disorders.
Trauma	
Poisons	Vitamin A, lead, others.

Pseudotumor Cerebri

Benign intracranial hypertension with neurologic complex of headache and papilledema without mass lesion or ventricular obstruction.

CSF normal except for increased pressure.

Laboratory findings due to associated conditions (only obesity has been reported consistently) [e.g., Addison disease, infection, metabolic conditions (acute hypocalcemia and other electrolyte disturbances, empty sella syndrome, pregnancy), drugs (psychotherapeutic drugs, sex hormones and oral contraceptives, corticosteroid administration, usually after reduction of dosage or change to different preparation), immune diseases (SLE, polyarteritis nodosa, serum sickness), other conditions (sarcoidosis, Guillain-Barré syndrome, head trauma, various anemias), poisons (e.g., vitamin A toxicity)].

Leukemic Involvement of Central Nervous System

Intracranial hemorrhage is principal cause of death in leukemia (may be intracerebral, subarachnoid, subdural).

More frequent when WBC count is $>100,000/mm^3$ and with rapid increase in WBC count, especially in blastic crises.

Platelets frequently decreased.

Evidence of bleeding elsewhere.

CSF findings of intracranial hemorrhage

- Meningeal infiltration of leukemic cells

CNS is involved in 5% of patients with acute lymphoblastic leukemia at diagnosis and is the major site of relapse.

Meninges are involved in >30% of patients with malignant lymphoma; most prevalent in diffuse large-cell (histiocytic), lymphoblastic, and immunoblastic leukemia; occurs in one-third to one-half of patients with Burkitt lymphoma and 15–20% of patients with non-Hodgkin lymphoma. Hodgkin disease seldom involves CNS.

Involvement by chronic lymphoblastic leukemia, well-differentiated lymphocytic lymphoma, and plasmacytoid lymphomas is rare.

CSF may show

- Increased pressure and protein level.
- Glucose level decreased to <50% of blood level.

- Increased cells that are often not recognized as blast cells because of poor preservation and that may be identified by cytochemical, immunoenzymatic, immunofluorescent, and flow cytometry techniques.
- Malignant cells are found in 60–80% of patients with meningeal involvement.

Complicating meningeal infection (e.g., various bacteria, opportunistic fungi).

Meningitis, Aseptic (Viral Meningitis, Encephalomyelitis)

CSF

- Protein level is normal or slightly increased.
- Increased cell count shows predominantly PMNs at first, mononuclear cells seen later.
- Glucose level is normal.
- Bacterial culture results are negative.

If glucose levels are decreased, TB, cryptococcosis, leukemia, lymphoma, metastatic carcinoma, sarcoidosis, drug induction should be ruled out.

Causes

Infections

- Viral (especially poliomyelitis, infection with coxsackievirus, echovirus, HIV, EBV; lymphocytic choriomeningitis; and many others). Culture positive in 40% of cases, especially with enteroviruses.
- Bacterial (e.g., incompletely treated or very early bacterial meningitis, bacterial endocarditis, parameningeal infections such as brain abscess, epidural abscess, paranasal sinusitis).
- Spirochetal (e.g., leptospirosis, syphilis, Lyme disease).
- Tuberculous (CSF glucose levels may not be decreased until later stages).
- Fungal (e.g., infection with *Candida*, *Coccidioides*, *Cryptococcus*).
- Protozoan (e.g., toxoplasmosis).
- Amebic (e.g., *Naegleria* infection).
- Rickettsial (e.g., Rocky Mountain spotted fever)
- Helminthic

Chemical meningitis

Drug-induced meningitis (e.g., ibuprofen, trimethoprim, immune globulin, sulfadiazine, azathioprine, antineoplastic drugs); onset usually within 24 hours of drug ingestion.

Systemic disorders

- Vasculitis, collagen vascular disease
- Sarcoid
- Behçet syndrome
- Vogt-Koyanagi syndrome
- Harada syndrome
- Mollaret meningitis
- Neoplasm (e.g., leukemia, metastatic carcinoma)
- SLE

Vaccination has reduced the incidence of acute and postinfectious encephalitis due to measles, mumps, rubella, yellow fever, varicella, and poliomyelitis, but a few cases of vaccine-associated infections occur.

Coxsackievirus and echovirus usually cause benign aseptic meningitis.

Laboratory Findings

Laboratory findings due to preceding condition (e.g., measles) are noted.

- Polymerase chain reaction testing of CSF or fresh brain tissue for panel detection of HSV, VZV, enteroviruses, eastern equine encephalitis virus, St. Louis encephalitis virus, CMV, EBV, California serogroup viruses, and rabies (in saliva) makes 72-hour diagnosis possible on one sample and should replace culture, mouse inoculation, immunoassay, serology, and brain biopsy.
- Examination of paired serum samples during acute and convalescent periods may show seroconversion or fourfold increase in specific antibody titers.

- Enzyme-linked immunosorbent assay to detect IgM in CSF is sensitive and specific for Japanese B encephalitis; IgM is usually present at hospitalization and almost always present by third day of illness.
- HSV can be cultured from CSF in 50–75% of patients with meningitis and <5% with encephalitis.
- Detection of HSV antigen in CSF is reported to be 80% sensitive and 90% specific if testing is performed within 3 days of onset of illness. Brain biopsy is most sensitive and specific for HSV and its mimics.
- Brain biopsy is currently reserved for patients who do not respond to acyclovir therapy and have abnormality on computed tomographic (CT) scan or magnetic resonance imaging (MRI).

Meningitis, Bacterial

Blood culture results are usually positive if patient has not received antibiotics.

- Bacteria can be identified in CSF in 90% of patients.
- Culture is more reliable than Gram stain, although results of the stain offer a more immediate guide to therapy.
- Gram stain is positive in 70% of patients; sensitivity is increased by cytocentrifugation of specimen. When Gram stain yields positive results, CSF is more likely to show decreased glucose, increased protein, and increased RBCs. Seventy-five percent of cases are due to *N. meningitidis, S. pneumoniae, H. influenzae*.
- In *Listeria* meningitis, the Gram stain result is usually negative and the cellular response is usually monocytic, which may cause this meningitis to be mistakenly diagnosed as due to virus, syphilis, TB, Lyme disease, and so on.
- Gram stain of scrapings from petechial skin lesions demonstrate pathogen in 70% of patients with meningococcemia; Gram stain of buffy coat of peripheral blood and, less often, peripheral blood smear may reveal this organism.
- Detection of bacterial antigen in CSF (rapid latex agglutination assay has largely replaced CIE) for *S. pneumoniae*, group B *Streptococcus* (*S. agalactiae*), *H. influenzae*, some strains of *N. meningitidis*. Not affected by previous antimicrobial therapy that might inhibit growth in culture. *H. influenzae* infection is now rare due to routine immunization of children.
- False-positive result for *H. influenza* may occur due to recent immunization; test should not be performed if patient recently vaccinated.
- False-positive result for group B *Streptococcus* antigen in urine is common due to its colonization of perineum.

Table 4 shows the causes of bacterial meningitis by age.

The most useful test results that favor the diagnosis of acute bacterial meningitis rather than acute viral meningitis are

- CSF gives positive results with bacterial stain, culture, or antigen detection methods.
- Decreased CSF glucose level.
- Decreased CSF/serum ratio of glucose (<0.25 in <1% of acute viral meningitis cases and 44% of acute bacterial meningitis cases), even if CSF glucose is normal.
- Increased CSF protein level of >1.7 g/L (1% of acute viral meningitis and 50% of acute bacterial meningitis cases).
- CSF WBC >2,000/mm^3 in 38% of acute bacterial meningitis cases and PMN >1,180/mm^3, but low counts do not rule out acute bacterial meningitis.
- Peripheral WBC is useful only if WBC (>27,200/mm^3) and total PMN (>21,000/mm^3) counts are very high, which occurs in relatively few patients; leukopenia is common in infants and elderly patients.
- Combination of findings can exclude acute viral meningitis and rule in acute bacterial meningitis, but none of them can establish the diagnosis of acute viral meningitis, and absence of these findings cannot exclude acute bacterial meningitis.

Meningitis, Chronic

(Symptoms for >4 weeks)

CSF

- WBC of 100–400 WBC/mm^3, preponderance of lymphocytes.

Table 4. Causes of Bacterial Meningitis by Age

	Newborns	<1 Yr	1–5 Yr	5–14 Yr	>15 Yr
Most frequent	*Escherichia coli*	*Haemophilus influenzae*		*Neisseria meningitidis*	*Streptococcus pneumoniae*
Common	*Klebsiella-Aerobacter* β-Hemolytic streptococci *Listeria monocytogenes* *Staphylococcus aureus*	*Neisseria meningitidis* *Streptococcus pneumoniae*		*Haemophilus influenzae* *Streptococcus pneumoniae*	*Neisseria meningitidis* *Staphylococcus aureus*
Uncommon	Paracolon bacilli *Pseudomonas* species *Haemophilus influenzae*	*Pseudomonas* species *Staphylococcus aureus* β-Hemolytic streptococci *Escherichia coli*		β-Hemolytic streptococci	*Escherichia coli* *Pseudomonas* species
Rare	*Neisseria meningitidis*	*Klebsiella-Aerobacter*, paracolons, various other Gram-negative organisms			*Haemophilus influenzae*

The frequency of cases due to different organisms may vary from year to year, in the presence of epidemics, or by geographic location.
Occasionally more than one organism is recovered.
Haemophilus influenzae (almost always type b) formerly caused most cases between 6 mo and 3 yr of age but was unusual before 2 mo; now rare due to immunization.
Enteric bacteria are so rarely found in older children that, in their presence, immunologic defect or congenital dermal sinus should be ruled out. If surgery has not been performed and *Staphylococcus aureus* is present, congenital dermal sinus should be ruled out.
Gram stain of CSF should always be done in addition to culture because it provides a more immediate clue to the causative agent and the proper therapy and because the culture may be negative if the patient received antibiotics soon before the lumbar puncture.
Cultures should also be obtained from blood and from petechial skin lesions if present. Gram stain of buffy coat of blood is often useful.
CSF glucose level is very useful in differentiating bacterial from viral meningitis and is a good index to the severity of the infection, with a lower level in more severe infections.
Newborns with overwhelming pneumococcal infections may have no decrease in glucose level or increase of cells.
Repeat CSF examination in 24 hours if response to treatment is unsatisfactory or if *S. pneumoniae* partially resistant to penicillin was identified. Repeat CSF examination after treatment conclusion if original organism was a Gram-negative rod.
Reproduced with permission from Wallach J. *Interpretation of diagnostic tests*, 7th ed. Philadelphia: Lippincott Williams & Wilkins, 2000.

- Glucose level often decreased.
- Protein level is usually moderately or markedly increased.

Causes

Various infections
- TB is most common cause.
- Bacteria (e.g., *Brucella*).
- Spirochetes (e.g., *Leptospira interrogans*, *Treponema pallidum*, *Borrelia burgdorferi*).
- Fungi (e.g., *Candida*, *Coccidioides*, *Cryptococcus*).
- Protozoa (e.g., *T. gondii*).
- Amebas (e.g., *Naegleria*).
- Mycoplasma.
- Rickettsiae.
- Helminths.

Systemic disorders
- Vasculitis, collagen vascular disease
- Sarcoid
- Neoplasm (e.g., leukemia, lymphoma, metastatic carcinoma)
- Mollaret meningitis

Meningoencephalitis, Primary Amebic

Increased WBC, predominantly neutrophils

CSF
- Fluid may be cloudy, purulent, or sanguinopurulent.
- Protein level is increased.
- Glucose level is usually decreased, may be normal.
- Increased WBCs are chiefly PMNs. RBCs are frequently present. Motile amebas are seen in hemocytometer chamber or on wet mount using phase or diminished light.
- Amebas are seen on Wright, Giemsa, and hematoxylin-eosin stains. Results of Gram stain and cultures are negative for bacteria and fungi.
- Culture of tissue or CSF on agar or cell culture demonstrates organisms.

Electron microscopy allows precise classification of amebas.

Indirect immunofluorescent antibody and immunoperoxidase assays are reliable methods to identify amebas in tissue sections.

Meningomyelocele

Incomplete closure of the vertebral column during the first 4 weeks of embryogenesis, resulting in exposure of meninges and spinal cord.

Always associated with the constellation of findings known as the Chiari II malformation, which includes small posterior fossa, hindbrain herniation into the upper cervical spinal canal, dysgenesis or agenesis of the corpus callosum, neuronal migration disorders of varying degree, and hydrocephalus.

(Postneurulation defects develop after 25 days of intrauterine life, when neurulation is complete.)

Lesions include simple meningocele, lipomyelomeningocele, diastematomyelia, myelocystocele, neurenteric cyst, and intraspinal and pelvic meningoceles.

Genetics

Myelomeningocele, as well as the neural tube defects (anencephaly and encephalocele), represents examples of multifactorial inheritance.

Folic acid deficiency is an environmental factor strongly associated with neural tube defects.

Signs and Symptoms

The myelomeningocele is usually single and involves the lumbosacral spine.
Hydrocephalus requiring CSF diversion occurs in >80% of infants with Chiari II abnormality and myelomeningocele.
The Chiari II malformation (hindbrain herniation into the upper cervical spinal canal) requires surgical decompression in <20% of affected children.
If symptomatic, can impair cranial nerve control of swallowing and respiration, and, less frequently, cause pyramidal signs.
Syringomyelia, cystic expansion of the central spinal canal, is often present.
Surgical hindbrain decompression, if done promptly after onset of symptoms of hindbrain compression, may reverse or arrest these symptoms (stridor, respiratory difficulties, laryngomalacia), but the condition is often confused with respiratory infections, which thus delays treatment.

Risk Factors

First-trimester use of valproic acid and derivatives (valproate sodium)
High-risk pregnancy—previous children with spina bifida
Insufficient maternal levels of folic acid

Laboratory Tests

Prenatal: maternal serum α-fetoprotein level—elevated levels at 16–18 weeks suggest fetal open neural tube defects and indicate need for further prenatal evaluation and genetic counseling.
Causes rupture of perforating vessels passing from the basilar artery to the brainstem, which results in brainstem hemorrhages (Duret hemorrhage).
Herniation of the uncinate gyrus of the temporal lobe through the tentorial opening (tentorial herniation).
- Stretches and paralyzes the third nerve
- Compresses the pyramidal tract in the crus cerebri

Posterior fossa lesions cause herniation of the cerebellar tonsils through the foramen magnum, which leads to compression of the medulla, with cardiorespiratory failure and death.

Myelitis

CSF may be normal or may show increased protein and cells (20–1,000/mm^3 lymphocytes and mononuclear cells).
Laboratory findings due to causative condition (e.g., poliomyelitis, herpes zoster, TB, syphilis, parasitosis, abscess, multiple sclerosis, postvaccinal myelitis).
Nerve conduction velocity determines level of abnormality.
Electromyography distinguishes muscle from nerve disorder.

Neuralgia, Trigeminal (Tic Douloureux)

Laboratory findings due to causative disease
- Usually idiopathic.
- May also stem from multiple sclerosis or herpes zoster.

Neuritis of One Nerve or Plexus

Laboratory findings due to causative disease
- Infections (e.g., diphtheria, herpes zoster, leprosy)
- Sarcoidosis
- Tumor (leukemia, lymphoma, carcinomas); may find tumor cells in CSF
- Serum sickness
- Bell palsy
- Idiopathic

Neuritis/Neuropathy, Cranial Nerve, Multiple

Laboratory findings due to causative conditions

- Trauma
- Aneurysms
- Tumors (e.g., meningioma, neurofibroma, carcinoma, cholesteatoma, chordoma)
- Infections (e.g., herpes zoster)
- Benign polyneuritis associated with cervical lymph node tuberculosis or sarcoidosis

Neuritis/Neuropathy, Multiple

Nerve conduction velocity abnormal.
Laboratory findings due to causative disease.
Infections, for example,

- EBV (mononucleosis associated: CSF shows increased protein level and up to several hundred mononuclear cells).
- Diphtheria: CSF protein level is 50–200 mg/dL.
- Lyme disease.
- HIV-1.
- Hepatitis.

Postvaccinal effect.
Metabolic conditions (e.g., pellagra, beriberi, combined systemic disease, pregnancy, porphyria)—CSF usually normal. In 70% of patients with diabetic neuropathy, CSF protein level is increased to >200 mg/dL.
Uremia—CSF protein level is 50–200 mg/dL; occurs in a few cases of chronic uremia.
Collagen disease.

- Polyarteritis nodosa—CSF usually normal; nerve involvement in 10% of patients.
- SLE.

Neoplasm (leukemia)—CSF protein level often increased; may be associated with an occult primary neoplastic lesion outside CNS.
Sarcoidosis.
Toxic conditions due to drugs and chemicals (especially lead, arsenic, etc.).
Alcoholism—CSF usually normal.
Bassen-Kornzweig syndrome.
Refsum disease.
Chédiak-Higashi syndrome.
Guillain-Barré syndrome.

Neuropathy, Peripheral

Causes

Infections and postinfection syndromes
    Guillain-Barré syndrome
Metabolic neuropathies
    Deficiency of vitamins B_1, B_6, B_{12}, E
    Diabetic neuropathy*
    Porphyria
Hereditary neuropathies
    Refsum hypertrophic polyneuritis
    Peroneal muscular atrophy (Charcot-Marie-Tooth disease)
    X-linked dominant inheritance; distal leg muscles involved
    Neuropathies associated with heredofamilial amyloidosis
Ischemic neuropathies
    Diabetic neuropathy*
    Giant cell arteritis (high incidence of optic nerve involvement)

*Diabetic polyneuropathy may result from either axonal degeneration caused by the osmotic effect of sorbitol accumulating in the nerve or diabetic microangiopathy involving the vasa nervorum.

Neuropathy, Retrobulbar

CSF is normal or may show increased protein and ≤200/mm³ lymphocytes.
Multiple sclerosis ultimately develops in 75% of these patients.

Ophthalmoplegia

Laboratory findings due to causative disease
- Diabetes mellitus
- Myasthenia gravis
- Hyperthyroid exophthalmos

Palsy, Cerebral

The term *cerebral palsy* is used to describe a nonprogressive disorder of movement or posture that is the result of a CNS abnormality that occurred prenatally, perinatally, or during the first 3 years of life.

Causes

In 70% of cases, neither causes nor risk factors can be identified.
In utero infections, malformations, chromosomal abnormalities, and strokes are among suggested causes.
Risk factors are prematurity, hypoxic ischemia, encephalopathy in the perinatal period, seizures in the perinatal period, interventricular hemorrhage in the perinatal period, *in utero* infections, meningitis or encephalitis postnatally, child abuse.

Signs and Symptoms

Spastic
Associated and significant spasticity, and contractures, with or without aphonia, seizures, or mental retardation
Athetotic
Usually normal intelligence with choreiform movements, muscular hypertrophy
Ataxic
Normal intelligence, clumsy
Some patients are highly talkative (cocktail party syndrome).
Spastic Diplegic
Spares upper extremities, spastic lower extremities (scissor gait), and usually normal intelligence

Laboratory Tests

Laboratory data are not required to make the diagnosis.
Tests may help exclude metabolic diseases such as Tay-Sachs metachromatic leukodystrophy, mucopolysaccharidosis; radiography and brain imaging may help document brain injury; chromosome studies may document abnormalities.

Pathologic Findings

CT and MRI might show abnormalities of the brain, including cysts, cerebral atrophy, calcification, tumors, malformation, strokes, and so on.

Palsy, Facial, Peripheral Acute

Laboratory findings due to causative disease
- Infection
  Viral (e.g., VZV, HSV, HIV, EBV, poliomyelitis, mumps, rubella)
  Bacterial (e.g., Lyme disease, syphilis, leprosy, diphtheria, cat-scratch disease, *Mycoplasma pneumoniae*)
  Parasitic (e.g., malaria)
  Meningitis

Encephalitis
Local inflammation (otitis media, mastoiditis, osteomyelitis, petrositis)
- Trauma
- Tumor (acoustic neuromas, tumors invading the temporal bone)
- Granulomatous (e.g., sarcoidosis) and connective tissue diseases
- Diabetes mellitus
- Hypothyroidism
- Uremia
- Drug reaction
- Postvaccinal effect

Lyme disease and Guillain-Barré syndrome may produce bilateral palsy.

Refsum Disease

Rare hereditary recessive lipidosis of the nervous system with retinitis pigmentosa, peripheral neuropathy, cerebellar ataxia, nerve deafness, and ichthyosis.
CSF shows albuminocytologic dissociation (normal cell count with protein level usually increased to 100–700 mg/dL.

Retardation, Mental

Laboratory findings due to underlying causative condition

Prenatal Causes

Infections (e.g., syphilis, rubella, toxoplasmosis, CMV infections)
Metabolic abnormalities (e.g., diabetes mellitus, eclampsia, placental dysfunction)
Chromosomal disorders (e.g., Down syndrome, trisomy 18, cri du chat syndrome, Klinefelter syndrome)
Metabolic abnormalities
- Amino acid metabolism (e.g., phenylketonuria, maple syrup urine disease, hemocystinuria, cystathioninuria, hyperglycemia, argininosuccinic aciduria, citrullinemia, histidinemia, hyperprolinemia, oasthouse urine disease, Hartnup's disease, Joseph's syndrome, familial iminoglycinuria)
- Lipid metabolism (e.g., Batten disease, Tay-Sachs disease, Niemann-Pick disease, abetalipoproteinemia, Refsum disease, metachromatic leukodystrophy)
- Carbohydrate metabolism (e.g., galactosemia, mucopolysaccharidoses)
- Purine metabolism (e.g., Lesch-Nyhan syndrome, hereditary orotic aciduria)
- Mineral metabolism (e.g., idiopathic hypercalcemia, pseudohypoparathyroidism and pseudopseudohypoparathyroidism)

Perinatal Causes

Kernicterus
Prematurity
Anoxia
Trauma

Postnatal Causes

Poisoning (e.g., lead, arsenic, carbon monoxide)
Infections (e.g., meningitis, encephalitis)
Metabolic abnormalities (e.g., hypoglycemia)
Postvaccinal encephalitis
Cerebrovascular accidents
Trauma

Reye Syndrome

Acute noninflammatory encephalopathy with fatty changes in liver and kidney and rarely in heart and pancreas. Occurs typically in child recovering from influenza, varicella, or nonspecific viral illness and is associated with use of aspirin.

Diagnostic criteria

- CSF shows <8 WBC/mm^3.
- Low serum glucose level.
- Serum levels of aspartate aminotransferase, alanine aminotransferase, or ammonia three times or more the upper limit of normal.
- Fatty liver seen histologically.

Seizure[2]

Causes

Perinatal conditions
- Cerebral malformation
- Intrauterine infection
- Hypoxia-ischemia*
- Trauma
- Hemorrhage*

Infections
- Encephalitis*
- Meningitis*
- Brain abscess

Metabolic conditions
- Hypoglycemia*
- Hypocalcemia
- Hypomagnesemia
- Hyponatremia
- Storage diseases
- Reye's syndrome
- Degenerative disorders
- Porphyria
- Pyridoxine dependency (deficiency)

Poisoning
- Lead
- Drugs
- Drug withdrawal

Neurocutaneous syndromes
- Tuberous sclerosis
- Neurofibromatosis
- Sturge-Weber syndrome
- Klippel-Trenaunay-Weber syndrome
- Linear sebaceous nevus
- Incontinentia pigmenti

Systemic disorders
- Vasculitis (CNS or systemic)
- SLE
- Hypertensive encephalopathy
- Renal failure
- Hepatic encephalopathy

Other
- Trauma*
- Tumor
- Fever*
- Idiopathic*
- Familial

*Common.

Causes of Seizure That May Be Accompanied by Laboratory Abnormalities

Neoplasms

Circulatory disorders (e.g., thrombosis, hemorrhage, embolism, hypertensive, encephalopathy, vascular malformations)

Hematologic disorders (e.g., sickle cell anemia, leukemia)

Metabolic abnormalities

- Carbohydrate metabolism (e.g., hypoglycemia, glycogen storage disease)
- Amino acid metabolism (e.g., phenylketonuria, maple syrup urine disease)
- Lipid metabolism (e.g., leukodystrophies, lipidoses)
- Electrolyte balance (e.g., decreased sodium, calcium, and magnesium, increased sodium)
- Other disorders (e.g., porphyria)

Allergic disorders (e.g., drug reaction, postvaccinal reaction)

Infections

- Meningitis, encephalitis
- Postinfectious encephalitis (e.g., after measles, mumps)
- Fetal exposure (e.g., to rubella, measles, mumps)

Degenerative brain diseases

[2]Behrman RE, Kliegman R, eds. *Nelson essentials of pediatrics*, 2nd ed. Philadelphia: WB Saunders, 1994:681.

Spinal Cord Tumor

CSF protein level is increased. It may be very high and associated with xanthochromia when a block of the subarachnoid space is present.
With complete block, for cord tumors located at lower levels, protein concentration is higher.

Thrombosis, Cavernous Sinus

CSF is usually normal unless associated subdural empyema or meningitis is present, or it may show increased protein and WBC with normal glucose, or it may be hemorrhagic. Mucormycosis may cause this clinical appearance in diabetic patients.
Laboratory findings due to preceding infections, complications (e.g., meningitis, brain abscess), or other causes of venous thromboses (e.g., sickle cell disease, polycythemia, dehydration).

Thrombosis, Cerebral

Laboratory findings due to some diseases that may be causative.

- Hematologic disorders (e.g., polycythemia, sickle cell disease, thrombotic thrombopenia, macroglobulinemia)
- Arterial disorders (e.g., polyarteritis nodosa, Takayasu syndrome, dissecting aneurysm of aorta, syphilis, meningitis)
- Hypotension (e.g., myocardial infarction, shock)

CSF

- Protein may be normal or increased to ≤100 mg/dL.
- Cell count may be normal or ≥10 WBC/mm^3 during first 48 hours and rarely ≥2,000 WBC/mm^3 transiently on third day.

Trauma, Head

Laboratory findings due to single or various combinations of brain injuries

- Contusion, laceration, subdural hemorrhage, extradural hemorrhage, subarachnoid hemorrhage

Laboratory findings due to complications (e.g., pneumonia, meningitis)
In possible skull fractures

- CSF transferrin shows a double band but only a single transferrin band is seen in other fluids (serum, nasal secretions, saliva, tears, lymph).
- If enough (100 μL) fluid can be obtained to perform immunofixation, IgM is five times higher, prealbumin is 12 times higher, and transferrin is two times higher in CSF than in serum.
- The suggestion has been made that nasal secretions may be differentiated from CSF by absence of glucose (measured using test tapes or tablets) in nasal secretions, but this is not reliable because nasal secretions may normally contain glucose.

Tuberculoma of Brain

CSF shows increased protein with small number of cells. The tuberculoma may be transformed into TB meningitis with increased protein and cells (50–300/mm^3), and decreased glucose.

- MRI, CT, electroencephalogram abnormal.
- Laboratory findings due to TB elsewhere.

Tumor of Brain

Laboratory Findings

CSF

- CSF is clear but is occasionally xanthochromic or bloody if there is hemorrhage into the tumor.

- WBC may be increased ≤150 cells/mm^3 in 75% of patients; normal in others.
- Protein level is usually increased. Protein level is particularly increased with meningioma of the olfactory groove and with acoustic neuroma.
- Tumor cells may be demonstrable in 20–40% of patients with all types of solid tumors, but failure to find malignant cells does not exclude meningeal neoplasm.
- Glucose level may be decreased if cells are present.
- Brainstem gliomas, which are characteristically found in childhood, are usually associated with normal CSF.
- Usually normal in diencephalic syndrome of infants due to glioma of hypothalamus.

Laboratory findings due to underlying causative disease [e.g., primary brain tumors, metastatic tumors, leukemias and lymphomas, infections (tuberculoma, schistosomiasis, cryptococcosis, hydatid cyst), pituitary adenomas (CSF protein and pressure usually normal)].

Laboratory findings due to associated genetic conditions (e.g., tuberous sclerosis, neurofibromatosis, Turcot syndrome).

Electroencephalogram may have focal abnormalities.

Diagnostic Tests

MRI or CT of brain or both

Common Intracranial Neoplasms in Children Classified According to Location

Location	Children
Supratentorial	20%
Cerebral hemisphere	Rare
Suprasellar	Craniopharyngioma Juvenile astrocytoma
Pineal	Pineoblastoma Germ cell tumor (teratoma)
Infratentorial (posterior fossa) midline	70% Medulloblastoma Ependymoma
Cerebellar hemisphere	Juvenile astrocytoma
Cerebellopontine angle	Epidermoid cyst
Spinal cord	
Epidural	Rare
Intradural but extramedullary	Rare Neurofibroma Schwannoma Meningioma
Intramedullary	Ependymoma Astrocytoma

von Recklinghausen Disease (Multiple Neurofibroma)

CSF, MRI findings of brain tumor if acoustic neuroma occurs

Bibliography

Cacciola I, Pollicino T, Squadrito G, et al. Occult hepatitis B virus infection in patients with chronic hepatitis C liver disease. *N Engl J Med* 1999;341:22–26.

Czaja AJ. The variant forms of autoimmune hepatitis. *Ann Intern Med* 1996;125:588–598.

Cogswell ME, McDonnell SM, Khoury MJ, et al. Iron overload, public health, and genetics: evaluating the evidence for hemochromatosis screening. *Ann Intern Med* 1998;129:971–979.

De Lamballerie X, Charrel RN, Dussol B. Hepatitis GB virus C in patients on hemodialysis. *N Engl J Med* 1996;334:1549.

Edwards CQ, Kushner JP. Screen for hemochromatosis. *N Engl J Med* 1993;328:1616.

Fairfax MR, Merline JR, Podzorski RP. Check Sample Microbiology No. 97-1. American Society for Clinical Pathology, 1997.

Lemon SM. Type A viral hepatitis: epidemiology, diagnosis, and prevention. *Clin Chem* 1997;43:1494–1499.

Press RD, Flora K, Gross C, et al. Hepatic iron overload: direct HFE (HLA-H) mutation analysis vs quantitative iron assays for the diagnosis of hereditary hemochromatosis. *Am J Clin Pathol* 1998;109:577–584.

Sheth SG, Gordon FD, Chopra S. Nonalcoholic steatohepatitis. *Ann Intern Med* 1997;126:137–145.

U.S. Department of Health and Human Services. Recommendations for prevention and control of hepatitis C virus (HCV) infection and HCV-related chronic disease. Centers for Disease Control and Prevention. *MMWR Recomm Rep* 1998;47(RR-19):1–39.

16 Disorders of Lipid Metabolism

Tests of Lipid Metabolism

Diagnosis of Lipoprotein Disorders

The determination of lipid and lipoprotein concentrations is essential in the diagnosis and management of hyperlipoproteinemia. These tests are used in the assessment of risk of coronary heart disease (CHD). Increased concentration of total cholesterol, low-density lipoprotein cholesterol (LDL-C), and apolipoprotein (apo) B-100 and decreased concentrations of high-density lipoprotein cholesterol (HDL-C) and apo A-I are associated with increased risk of developing premature CHD. Lipoprotein (a) level is higher in children from families with premature CHD and is not affected by dietary therapy.

The National Cholesterol Education Program Laboratory Standardization Panel has issued specific recommendations to minimize the effect of preanalytical factors on lipid and lipoprotein test results. The panel recommends the following:

1. An individual's lipid and lipoprotein profile should be measured only when the individual is in a metabolic steady state.
2. Subjects should maintain their usual diet and weight for at least 2 weeks before the determination of lipid or lipoprotein levels.
3. Multiple measurements taken within 2 months, at least 1 week apart, should be performed before making a medical decision about further action.
4. Patients should not perform vigorous physical activity within the 24-hour period before testing.
5. Specimens drawn after fasting or nonfasting can be used for total cholesterol testing. However, a specimen drawn after 12 hours of fasting is required for measurement of triglycerides and lipoproteins.
6. The patient should be seated for at least 5 minutes before specimen collection.
7. The tourniquet should not be kept on more than 1 minute during venipuncture.
8. Total cholesterol, triglyceride, and HDL-C concentrations can be determined in either serum or plasma. When EDTA is used as the anticoagulant, plasma should be immediately cooled to 2–4°C to prevent changes in composition and values should be multiplied by 1.03.
9. For total cholesterol testing, serum can be transported either at 4°C or frozen. Storage of specimens at –20°C is adequate for total cholesterol measurement. However, specimens must be stored frozen at –70°C or lower for triglyceride and lipoprotein and apolipoprotein testing.
10. Blood specimens should always be considered potentially infectious and, therefore, must be handled accordingly.

Lipoprotein Electrophoresis

Used to identify rare familial disorders (e.g., types I, III, V hyperlipidemias) to anticipate problems in children. Shows a specific abnormal pattern in <2% of Americans (usually types II, IV).

Table 1. Serum Lipid Concentrations of Males and Females in the First Two Decades of Life

	LDL-C	VLDL-C	HDL-C	Triglycerides
Age/Sex	Range	Range	Range	Range
5–9 yr				
Female	1.76–3.63	0.03–0.62	0.93–1.89	0.36–1.19
Male	1.63–3.34	0–0.47	0.98–1.94	0.33–1.14
10–14 yr				
Female	1.76–3.52	0.05–0.60	0.96–1.81	0.48–1.48
Male	1.66–3.44	0.03–0.57	0.96–1.92	0.36–1.41
15–19 yr				
Female	1.53–3.55	0.05–0.62	0.91–1.92	0.44–1.49
Male	1.61–3.37	0.05–0.67	0.78–1.63	0.42–1.67

HDL-C, high-density lipoprotein cholesterol; LDL-C, low-density lipoprotein cholesterol; VLDL-C, very-low-density lipoprotein cholesterol.
Values are in millimols per liter (milligrams per deciliter).
Data compiled from Lipid Metabolism Branch of the National Heart, Lung, and Blood Institute. *The prevalence study.* Bethesda, MD: National Institutes of Health, 1980. *The Lipid Research Clinics population studies data book*, vol 1. NIH Publication No. 80-1527.

Indications
- Serum triglyceride levels are >300 mg/dL.
- Serum drawn after fasting is lipemic.
- Significant hyperglycemia, impaired glucose tolerance, or glycosuria exists.
- Serum uric acid is increased.
- Strong family history of premature coronary artery disease (CAD) is present.
- Clinical evidence of CAD or atherosclerosis is found in patient aged <40 years.

If lipoprotein electrophoresis is abnormal, tests should be performed to rule out secondary hyperlipidemias.

Lipid and Lipoprotein Cholesterol Concentrations in Children

See Table 1.

Mean serum cholesterol concentration increases from approximately 1.71 mmol/L (66 mg/dL) at birth to approximately 4.02 mmol/L (155 mg/dL) at age 3. Approximately half of serum cholesterol at birth is carried in HDL. The LDL-C concentration increases rapidly in the first weeks of life as LDL becomes the major carrier of serum cholesterol. At age 5, LDL-C concentration is approximately 2.5 mmol/L (97 mg/dL) and HDL-C is approximately 1.4 mmol/L (54 mg/dL). Later in life, males have higher LDL-C but lower HDL-C than females, a lipoprotein profile that places males at greater risk of CHD. Breast milk contains approximately two-thirds more cholesterol than infant formulas. Breast-fed human babies have higher serum cholesterol levels than bottle-fed babies.

Screening and Diagnosis

Traditionally, hypercholesterolemia in children and adolescents has been defined as a total cholesterol or LDL-C concentration higher than the 95th percentile [5.18 mmol/L (200 mg/dL) and 3.37 mmol/L (130 mg/dL), respectively]. The National Cholesterol Education Program Expert Panel on Blood Cholesterol Levels in Children and Adolescents of the National Institutes of Health and the American Academy of Pediatrics used a similar definition of high cholesterol [≥5.18 mmol/L (200 mg/dL)] and high LDL-C [≥3.37 mmol/L (130 mg/dL)] for children and adolescents from families with hypercholesterolemia or premature CHD. A borderline cholesterol concentration was defined as 4.40–5.15 mmol/L (170–199 mg/dL) and a borderline LDL-C concentration as 2.85–3.34 mmol/L (110–129 mg/dL). Borderline values are above the 75th percentile for both analytes.

Children tend to have higher HDL-C concentrations than adults. Therefore, it is important to determine LDL-C and HDL-C concentrations before classifying the child as hypercholesterolemic.

Measurement of Total Cholesterol Concentration

Almost all clinical laboratories in the United States measure cholesterol enzymatically. This reaction first involves the hydrolysis of cholesterol ester by cholesterol esterase. Free cholesterol is then oxidized in the presence of cholesterol oxidase and hydrogen peroxide is generated. The hydrogen peroxide is coupled with an enzymatic reaction to form a colored oxidation product or a reduced pyridine nucleotide. Incomplete hydrolysis of cholesterol ester leads to underestimation of the cholesterol concentration.

Cholesterol testing in the physician's office should be well regulated. Recommendations regarding cholesterol testing outside the clinical laboratories include

1. The use of accurate and precise analyzers (capable of determining cholesterol concentration within a 3% bias of reference values and 3% imprecision).
2. The use of a properly trained operator (ideally, a trained medical technician or technologist).
3. The institution of a quality control system and the participation in proficiency surveys.
4. The use of a system of split-sample analyses to routinely compare cholesterol testing done in the physician's office to that done in a qualified laboratory.
5. The use of a proper preparation procedure to minimize preanalytical variations.

*Cholesterol Decision Levels**

	Cholesterol (mg/dL)			
	LDL	HDL	Total	LDL/HDL Ratio
Desirable level/low risk	<130	>60	<200	0.5–3.0
Borderline level/moderate risk	130–159	35–60	200–239	3.0–6.0
Elevated level/high risk	≥160	<35	≥240	>6.0

*Measure serum total cholesterol, HDL-C, and triglycerides after 12- to 14-hour fast. Average results of two or three tests; if difference is ≥30 mg/dL, repeat test at interval of 1–8 weeks and average results of three tests. Use total cholesterol for initial case finding and classification and monitoring of diet therapy. Do not use age- or sex-specific cholesterol values as decision levels.

Apolipoproteins, Serum

Protein component of lipoproteins that regulates their metabolism; each of four major groups consists of a family of two or more immunologically distinct proteins.

Used to classify hyperlipidemias.

Apo A is the major protein of HDL; apo A-I and A-II constitute 90% of total HDL protein in ratio of 3:1.

Apo B is the major protein in LDL, important in regulating cholesterol synthesis and metabolism. Decreased by severe illness and abetalipoproteinemia.

Apo C-I, C-II, and C-III are associated with all lipoproteins except LDL; apo C-II is important in triglyceride metabolism.

Serum apo A-I and B levels are more highly correlated with severity and extent of CAD than total cholesterol and triglyceride levels.

Ratio of apo A-1 to apo B shows greater sensitivity and specificity for CAD than LDL/HDL ratio or HDL/triglyceride ratio or any of the individual components.

Because apo B is the only protein in LDL and apo A-I is the major protein constituent of HDL and very-low-density lipoprotein (VLDL), the ratio of apo B to apo A-I reflects the ratio of LDL to HDL and may be a better discriminator of CAD risk than the individual components; however, data on apolipoproteins are still limited.

Table 2. Serum Concentrations of Apolipoproteins A-I and B-100 Derived from the National Health and Nutrition Examination Survey III

	Apolipoprotein A-I (Percentile)					Apolipoprotein B-100 (Percentile)				
Age (yr)	10th	25th	50th	75th	90th	10th	25th	50th	75th	90th
Males										
4–5	112	122	132	149	159	62	69	79	89	98
6–11	117	126	141	155	168	61	69	76	89	99
12–19	106	116	128	141	153	58	67	75	85	98
Females										
4–5	111	118	130	140	155	64	72	82	91	99
6–11	117	125	135	145	157	61	70	81	90	101
12–19	111	120	132	146	165	58	67	79	92	104

Values are in milligrams per deciliter.
From Bachorik PS, Lovejoy KL, Carroll MD, et al. Apolipoprotein B and AI distributions in the United States, 1988–1991: results of the National Health and Nutrition Examination Survey III (NHANES III). *Clin Chem* 1997;43:2364–2368.

Table 2 shows the serum concentrations of apolipoproteins A-I and B-100 derived from the National Health and Nutrition Examination Survey III.

Measurement of Apolipoprotein Concentration

Apo A-I and B-100 are mainly measured in clinical laboratories by immunoturbidimetric or immunonephelometric assays. Other methods such as radioimmunoassay, radial immunodiffusion, and enzyme-linked immunosorbent assay are used in research settings and specialized lipid laboratories.

Cholesterol, High-Density Lipoprotein, Serum

Assessment of risk for CAD
Diagnosis of various lipoproteinemias

Increased In

(>60 mg/dL is negative risk factor for CAD)

- Vigorous exercise
- Increased clearance of triglyceride (VLDL)
- Moderate consumption of alcohol
- Insulin treatment
- Oral estrogen use
- Familial lipid disorders with protection against atherosclerosis (illustrate importance of measuring HDL to evaluate hypercholesterolemia)
- Hyperalphalipoproteinemia (HDL excess)
  - 1 in 20 adults with mild increased total cholesterol levels (240–300 mg/dL) secondary to increased HDL (>70 mg/dL).
  - LDL not increased.
  - Triglycerides are normal.
  - Inherited as simple autosomal dominant trait in families with longevity or may be caused by alcoholism, extensive exposure to chlorinated hydrocarbon pesticides, exogenous estrogen supplementation.
- Hypobetalipoproteinemia

Decreased In

Is inversely related to risk of CAD. For every 1 mg/dL decrease in HDL, risk for CAD increases by 2–3%.

Secondary causes

- Stress and recent illness [e.g., acute myocardial infarction (AMI), stroke, surgery, trauma].
- Starvation; nonfasting sample is 5–10% lower.
- Obesity.
- Lack of exercise.
- Cigarette smoking.
- Diabetes mellitus.
- Hypo- and hyperthyroidism.
- Acute and chronic liver disease.
- Nephrosis.
- Uremia.
- Various chronic anemias and myeloproliferative disorders.
- Use of certain drugs (e.g., anabolic steroids, progestins, antihypertensive β-blockers, thiazides, neomycin, phenothiazines).

Genetic disorders

- Familial hypertriglyceridemia.
- Familial hypoalphalipoproteinemia—common autosomal-dominant condition with premature CAD and stroke. One-third of patients with premature CAD may have this disorder. HDL <10th percentile (<30 mg/dL in men and <38 mg/dL in women of middle age).
- Homozygous Tangier disease.
- Familial lecithin-cholesterol acetyltransferase deficiency and fish eye disease.
- Nonneuropathic Niemann-Pick disease.
- HDL deficiency with planar xanthomas.
- Apo A-I and apo C-III deficiency variant I and variant II—rare genetic conditions associated with premature CAD and marked HDL deficiency.

Separation of High-Density Lipoprotein Fractions

The HDL fractions are separated from the other lipoproteins using precipitation techniques. Several precipitation reagents such as heparin–Mn^{2+}, phosphotungstate, and dextran sulfate–Mg^{2+} are commonly used to precipitate LDL and VLDL. The cholesterol concentration in the supernatant, which represents HDL-C, is then quantitated enzymatically.

The specificity of the assay can be determined by the demonstration of complete precipitation of LDL and VLDL or no coprecipitation of HDL, or both. This can be established by

Lipoprotein electrophoresis of the supernatant and resolubilized precipitate; the supernatant should have an HDL or α band only and no β or pre-β band, and the precipitate should have no HDL band.

Measurement of apo A-I and apo B-100 in the supernatant; the supernatant should only have apo A-I and not apo B-100.

Evaluation of the performance of the assay in the presence of high triglyceride concentration.

Direct assays for the determination of HDL-C are less affected by increased triglycerides and require <10 μL of sample. These assays have been shown to correlate highly with both the ultracentrifugation–dextran sulfate–Mg^{2+} method and the Centers for Disease Control and Prevention–designated comparison method and meet all performance criteria of regulatory goals for HDL-C measurement and the acceptable criteria established by the Clinical Laboratories Improvement Act of 1988.

Cholesterol, Low-Density Lipoprotein, Serum

Increased In

- Familial hypercholesterolemia
- Familial combined hyperlipidemia
- Diabetes mellitus
- Hypothyroidism
- Nephrotic syndrome

- Chronic renal failure
- Diet high in cholesterol and total and saturated fat
- Pregnancy
- Multiple myeloma, dysgammaglobulinemia
- Porphyria
- Pregnancy
- Wolman disease
- Cholesteryl ester storage disease
- Anorexia nervosa

Decreased In

- Severe illness
- Abetalipoproteinemia
- Oral estrogen use

Estimation of Low-Density Lipoprotein Cholesterol

The National Cholesterol Education Program guidelines require the use of LDL-C concentration in the diagnosis and management of hypercholesterolemia. LDL-C is not measured in most clinical laboratories but is estimated using the Friedewald equation:

LDL-C = total cholesterol – (HDL-C + VLDL-C)

VLDL-C = triglyceride/5 (for mg/dL or mg/L LDL-C values), or

VLDL-C = triglyceride/2.22 (for mmol/L LDL-C values)

Specimens drawn after fasting are required for the estimation of LDL-C by this formula. High triglyceride concentration can falsely overestimate VLDL-C and, therefore, underestimate LDL-C. Patients with type III hyperlipoproteinemia have VLDLs that are enriched with cholesterol relative to triglyceride. The presence of these abnormal particles can result in an underestimation of VLDL-C and an overestimation of LDL-C. This can be especially problematic because a patient with type III hyperlipoproteinemia can be misdiagnosed as having type IIb hyperlipoproteinemia and the treatments for the two disorders are different.

Immunologic assay for the direct determination of LDL-C uses monoclonal antibodies directed against apo A-I and apo E, HDL, and VLDL particles are removed, which leaves LDL in the supernatant. This assay presumably can be performed in samples drawn from nonfasting patients. A direct method for the determination of LDL-C has been introduced.

Cholesterol, Total, Serum

Monitoring for increased risk factor for CAD
Screening for primary and secondary hyperlipidemias
Monitoring of treatment for hyperlipidemias

Increased In

Hyperlipoproteinemias
- Hyperalphalipoproteinemia

Cholesteryl ester storage disease

Biliary obstruction
- Stone, carcinomas, etc., of duct
- Cholangiolitic cirrhosis
- Biliary cirrhosis
- Cholestasis

von Gierke disease

Hypothyroidism

Nephrosis (due to chronic nephritis, renal vein thrombosis, amyloidosis, systemic lupus erythematosus, periarteritis, diabetic glomerulosclerosis)

Pancreatic disease
- Diabetes mellitus
- Total pancreatectomy
- Chronic pancreatitis (some patients)

Pregnancy
Drug use (e.g., progestins, anabolic steroids, corticosteroids, some diuretics)
- Methodologic interference (Zlatkis-Zak reaction) (e.g., bromides, iodides, chlorpromazine, corticosteroids, viomycin, vitamin C, vitamin A)
- Ten percent of patients on long-term levodopa therapy
- Hepatotoxic effect (e.g., phenytoin sodium)
- Hormonal effect (e.g., corticosteroids, birth control pills, amiodarone hydrochloride)

Total fasting that induces ketosis leads to rapid increase.
Secondary causes should always be ruled out.

Decreased In

- Severe liver cell damage (due to chemicals, drugs, hepatitis)
- Hyperthyroidism
- Malnutrition (e.g., starvation, neoplasms, uremia, malabsorption in steatorrhea)
- Myeloproliferative disease
- Chronic anemia
- Pernicious anemia in relapse
- Hemolytic anemias
- Marked hypochromic anemia
- Cortisone and adrenocorticotropic hormone therapy
- Hypobeta- and abetalipoproteinemia
- Tangier disease
- Infection
- Inflammation
- Drug use
- Hepatotoxic effects (e.g., allopurinol, tetracyclines, erythromycin, isoniazid, monoamine oxidase inhibitors)
- Synthesis inhibition (e.g., androgens, chlorpropamide, clomiphene citrate, phenformin)
- Diminished synthesis (probable mechanism) (e.g., clofibrate)
- Other mechanisms (e.g., azathioprine, kanamycin sulfate, neomycin, oral estrogens, cholestyramine, cortisone and adrenocorticotropic hormone therapy)
- Methodologic interference (Zlatkis-Zak reaction) (e.g., thiouracil, nitrates)

Chylomicrons, Serum

Increased In

Lipoprotein lipase deficiency (autosomal-recessive disorder or due to deficient cofactor for lipoprotein lipase) presenting in children with pancreatitis, xanthomas, or hepatosplenomegaly.
Apo C-II deficiency (rare autosomal-recessive disorder due to absent or defective apo C-II). Accumulation of VLDL and chylomicrons increases risk of pancreatitis.
Type V hyperlipoproteinemia.

Triglycerides, Serum

Classification[1]

Normal	<200 mg/dL
Borderline high	200–400 mg/dL
High	400–1,000 mg/dL
Very high	>1,000 mg/dL

[1]Summary of the second report of the National Cholesterol Education Program Expert Panel on Detection, Evaluation, and Treatment of High Blood Cholesterol in Adults. *JAMA* 1993;269:3015–3023.

Increased In

- Genetic hyperlipidemias (e.g., lipoprotein lipase deficiency, apo C-II deficiency, familial hypertriglyceridemia, dysbetalipoproteinemia, cholesteryl ester storage disease, Wolman disease, von Gierke disease)
- Secondary hyperlipidemias
  Gout
  Pancreatitis
  Acute illness [e.g., AMI (rises to peak in 3 weeks and increase may persist for 1 year); cold, flu]
- Drug use (e.g., thiazide diuretics, anabolic steroids, cholestyramine, corticosteroids, amiodarone, interferon, alcohol)
- Pregnancy
- Concentrations associated with certain disorders
  250–500 mg/dL: associated with peripheral vascular disease; may be a marker for patients with genetic forms of hyperlipoproteinemias who need specific therapy.
  500 mg/dL: associated with high risk of pancreatitis.
  1,000 mg/dL: associated with hyperlipidemia, especially type I or type V; substantial risk of pancreatitis.
  5,000 mg/dL: associated with eruptive xanthoma, corneal arcus, lipemia retinalis, enlarged liver and spleen.

Decreased In

- Abetalipoproteinemia
- Malnutrition
- Dietary change (within 3 weeks)
- Recent weight loss
- Vigorous exercise (transient)
- Use of certain drugs (e.g., ascorbic acid, clofibrate, phenformin, asparaginase, metformin hydrochloride, progestins, aminosalicylic acid)

Total cholesterol and HDL-C levels are similar when the patient is fasting or nonfasting, but triglycerides should be measured after 12–14 hours of fasting. Serum levels are 3–5% higher than plasma levels.

Triglyceride levels are not a strong predictor of atherosclerosis or CAD and may not be an independent risk factor.

Measurement of Triglyceride Concentration

Most laboratories determine triglyceride concentration enzymatically. Triglycerides are hydrolyzed to glycerol in the presence of lipase. Complete triglyceride hydrolysis is essential for the accurate determination of levels of this analyte. Glycerol is then coupled by one or more enzymatic reactions to generate either a colored dye or an ultraviolet light–absorbing chemical. The intensity of the produced color or the increase in absorbance is proportional to the triglyceride concentration.

Disorders of Lipid Metabolism

See Tables 3–7.

Cholesteryl Ester Storage Disease

Rare inherited deficiency of lysosomal acid lipase; milder than Wolman disease.

Clinical and Laboratory Findings

Pattern similar to that of type II hyperlipidemia.

Increased LDL-C level and decreased HDL-C level.

Accelerated cardiovascular disease; absent xanthoma; enlarged liver and spleen.

Table 3. Hyperlipidemic Disorders

Type	Elevated Lipoprotein	Serum Cholesterol	Serum Triglyceride	Plasma on Standing[a]	Familial Disease (Inherited)	Secondary to
I	Chylomicrons	N	I	Creamy	Lipoprotein lipase deficiency (autosomal recessive)	—
II-a	LDL	I	N	Clear	Familial hypercholesterolemia (autosomal dominant, varies)	Hypothyroidism, nephrotic syndrome, diet, diabetes mellitus
II-b	LDL plus VLDL	I	I	Usually clear	Familial mixed lipoproteinemia (autosomal recessive)	—
III	β-VLDL	I	I	Turbid	Familial dysbetalipoproteinemia (autosomal recessive)	Obstructive jaundice
IV	VLDL	N	I	Clear or turbid	Familial triglyceridemia (variable)	Diabetes mellitus, alcoholism, diet
V	Chylomicrons plus VLDL	N	I	Creamy	Very rare	—

I, increased serum level; LDL, low-density lipoproteins (high content of triglyceride); N, normal serum level—normal levels are defined statistically for men and women, separately for different age groups; VLDL, very-low-density lipoproteins (high content of triglyceride).

[a]On standing, the plasma normally clears. Chylomicrons are large particles and tend to stay on the surface without precipitating, producing a creamy supernatant. This is a simple test to detect lipoprotein abnormalities.

Table 4. Lipoprotein Phenotyping by Electrophoresis (Fredrickson Classification)

Electrophoretic Lipoprotein Phenotype (Prevalence)	Elevated Lipoproteins	Plasma Cholesterol	Plasma Triglycerides	Appearance of Chilled Plasma	Primary Disorders	Secondary Disorders
Type I (rare)	Chylomicrons	Normal or slightly elevated	Markedly elevated	Creamy layer above clear or slightly turbid infranatant	Familial lipoprotein lipase deficiency	Systemic lupus erythematosus; not associated with atherosclerosis
Type II-a (moderately common)	LDLs	Moderately elevated	Normal	Clear	Familial hypercholesterolemia; familial combined hyperlipidemia; polygenic hypercholesterolemia	Nephrotic syndrome; hypothyroidism
Type II-b (common)	LDLs, VLDLs	Moderately elevated	Slightly elevated	Slight to moderate turbidity	Familial combined hyperlipidemia; polygenic hypercholesterolemia (dietary excess)	Nephrotic syndrome; stress induced
Type III (rare)	Broad β-lipoprotein	Moderately elevated	Moderately to markedly elevated	Turbid or opaque layer above turbid infranatant	Familial dysbetalipoproteinemia (broad β disease)	Hypothyroidism; monoclonal gammopathies
Type IV (common)	VLDLs	Normal or slightly elevated	Moderately to markedly elevated	Turbid to frankly opaque	Familial (mild); Tangier disease	Diabetes mellitus; alcoholism; uremia; stress; oral contraceptive use
Type V (fairly common)	Chylomicrons, VLDLs	Moderately elevated	Markedly elevated	Creamy layer over turbid to opaque infranatant	Familial combined hyperlipidemia	Alcoholism; oral contraceptive use; diabetes mellitus

LDL, low-density lipoprotein; VLDL, very-low-density lipoprotein.
Lipoprotein phenotyping results are based on the classifications of Fredrickson et al. using the lipid values in conjunction with the electrophoretic pattern.
Adapted from Havel RJ, et al. Lipoproteins and lipid transport. In: Bondy PK, Rosenberg LD, eds. *Metabolic control and disease*, 8th ed. Philadelphia: WB Saunders, 1980:393–494.

Table 5. Characteristics of Human Plasma Lipoproteins

Variable	Type I Chylomicron	Type II-a VLDL	Type II-b IDL	Type III LDL	Type IV HDL	Lipoprotein(a)
Density (g/mL)	<0.95	0.950–1.006	1.006–1.019	1.019–1.063	1.063–1.210	1.040–1.130
Electrophoretic mobility	Origin	Pre-β	Between data and pre-β	β	α	Pre-β
Molecular weight	$0.4–30.0 \times 10^9$	$5–10 \times 10^6$	$3.9–4.8 \times 10^6$	2.75×10^6	$1.8–3.6 \times 10^5$	$2.9–3.7 \times 10^6$
Diameter (nm)	>70	25–70	22–24	19–23	4–10	25–30
Lipid/protein ratio	99:1	90:10	85:15	80:20	50:50	75:25–64:36
Major lipids	Exogenous triglycerides	Endogenous triglycerides	Endogenous triglycerides, cholesteryl esters	Cholesteryl esters	Phospholipids	Cholesteryl esters, phospholipids
Composition	C 5%, TG 85%, PL 5%, P 2%	C 65%, TG 60%, PL 15%, P 10%		C 45%, TG 10%, PL 20%, P 25%	C 15%, TG 5%, PL 30%, P 5%	
Major proteins	A-I B-48 C-I C-II C-III	B-100 C-I C-II C-III E	B-100 E	B-100	A-I A-II	(a) B-100

C, cholesterol; HDL, high-density lipoprotein; IDL, intermediate-density lipoprotein; LDL, low-density lipoprotein; P, protein; PL, phospholipid; TG, triglyceride; VLDL, very-low-density lipoprotein.

Modified with permission from Rifai N. Lipoproteins and apolipoproteins: composition, metabolism, and association with coronary heart disease. *Arch Pathol Lab Med* 1986; 110:694–702.

Table 6. Disorders of Lipoproteins and Neutral Lipids

McKusick No.	Disorder	Inheritance	Enzyme or Protein Defect	Lipid Changes	Diagnostic Tissue	Prenatal Diagnosis
238600	Lipoprotein lipase deficiency, hyperlipoproteinemia type I	AR	Lipoprotein lipase	Plasma triglycerides increase	Posthepatin, plasma, adipose tissue	Not possible
144400	Familial hyperlipoproteinemia type II	AD	LDL receptor	Plasma LDL increases	Plasma	Possible
107741	Hyperlipoproteinemia type III (dysbetalipoproteinemia)	AR	Apo E	Plasma cholesterol and triglycerides increase	Plasma	Possible
144600	Hyperlipoproteinemia type IV	AD	Increased triglyceride synthesis	Plasma triglycerides increase	Plasma	Possible
144650	Hyperlipoproteinemia type V	AR	Increased triglyceride synthesis and decreased clearance	Plasma, triglycerides, chylomicrons increase	Plasma	Not possible
200100	Familial lipoprotein deficiency (abetalipoproteinemia)	AR	Apo B	Low plasma cholesterol	Plasma, erythrocytes	Not possible
205400	Tangier disease		High-density lipoprotein	Tissue cholesterol esters increase	Plasma	Not possible
207750	Apo C-II deficiency	AR	Apo C-II	Plasma triglycerides increase	Plasma	Not possible
144250	Familial combined hyperlipoproteinemia	AD	Increased Apo B synthesis	Plasma cholesterol and triglycerides increase	Plasma	Possible
245900	Lecithin-cholesterol acyltransferase deficiency	AR	Lecithin-cholesterol acyltransferase	Free cholesterol and phosphatidylcholine increase	Plasma	Not possible

143470	Hyperalphalipoproteinemia, cholesterol ester transfer protein deficiency	AR	Cholesterol ester transport protein	Plasma cholesterol increases, LDL decreases, HDL greatly increases, Apos A-I, E increase	Plasma	Possible
278000	Wolman disease	AR	Acid lipase	Lysosomal cholesterol esters, triglycerides increase	Fibroblasts, leukocytes	Possible
215000	Cholesterol ester storage disease	AR	Acid lipase	Lysosomal cholesterol esters increase	Fibroblasts, leukocytes	Possible
213700	Cerebrotendinous xanthomatosis	AR	C-sterol-27 hydroxylase	Tissue cholesterol and cholesterol increase	Fibroblasts, liver (plasma)	Possible
270400	Smith-Lemli-Opitz syndrome	AR	7-dehydrocholesterol reductase	Plasma 7-dehydrocholesterol increases	Enzyme, cholesterol levels	Possible

Apo, apolipoprotein; AD, autosomal dominant; AR, autosomal recessive; HDL, high-density lipoprotein; LDL, low-density lipoprotein.

Table 7. Comparison of Clinical, Genetic, and Biochemical Characteristics in Selected Lipid Disorders

Characteristic	Tangier Disease	Apo A-I Deficiency	Familial LCAT Deficiency	Fish Eye Disease
Affected gene	ABC1	Apo A-1	LCAT	LCAT
Corneal opacities	+	+/++/+++	+++	+++
Coronary risk	Normal	Normal or high	Normal	Normal
Other clinical findings	Abnormal tonsils Neuropathy Splenomegaly	Xanthomatosis	Uremia Proteinuria Anemia	None
Serum cholesterol	Low	Normal	Normal	Normal
Serum triglycerides	Increased	Low or increased	Increased	Increased
Cholesterol esters	Normal	Normal	Low	Low normal
LDL cholesterol	Low	Normal	Normal	Normal
HDL cholesterol	None	None	10%	10%
Apo A-I	2%	0–2%	15–30%	15–30%
β-LCAT activity	100%	50–80%	0%	50–100%
α-LCAT activity	50%	50%	0–10%	0%
LCAT mass	50%	50%	0–50%	10–50%
Specific LCAT activity	Normal	Normal	Decreased	Decreased

+, present; ++, severe; +++ very severe; Apo, apolipoprotein; HDL, high-density lipoprotein; LCAT, lecithin-cholesterol acyltransferase; LDL, low-density lipoprotein.

Hyperlipidemias, Primary

See Tables 3 and 8.

Familial Hypercholesterolemia (Type II)

Autosomal-dominant disorder

Diagnostic Studies

LDL receptors in fibroblasts or mononuclear blood cells are absent in homozygous patients and are at 50% of normal levels in heterozygous patients (test performed at specialized laboratories).

Homozygosity—Very rare condition (1 in 1 million) in which serum cholesterol level is very high (e.g., 600–1,000 mg/dL) with corresponding increase in LDL (six to eight times normal level). Both parents are heterozygous. Clinical manifestations of increased total cholesterol (xanthomata, corneal arcus, CAD that causes death, usually at <30 years).

Neonatal diagnosis requires finding increased LDL-C in cord blood; serum total cholesterol level is unreliable. Because of marked variation in serum total cholesterol levels during first year of life, diagnosis should be deferred until 1 year of age.

Heterozygosity—Increased serum total cholesterol (300–500 mg/dL) and LDL (two to three times normal level) with similar change in a parent or first-degree relative; levels of serum triglycerides and VLDL are normal in 90% and slightly increased in 10% of these cases. Gene frequency is 1 in 500 in general population. Premature CAD, tendinous xanthomas, and corneal arcus are often present. Plasma triglycerides are normal in type II-A but increased in type II-B.

Polygenic Hypercholesterolemia (Type II-A)

Clinical Findings

Persistent total cholesterol elevation (>240 mg/dL) and increased LDL without familial hypercholesterolemia or familial combined hypercholesterolemia.

Table 8. Comparison of Lipoproteinemias

Point of Comparison	Type I (Rarest)	Type II-a (Relatively Common)	Type II-b (Relatively Common)	Type III (Relatively Uncommon)	Type IV (Most Common)	Type V (Uncommon)
Origin	Exogenous hyperlipidemia due to deficient lipoprotein lipase	—	Overindulgence lipidemia	—	Endogenous hyperlipidemia	Mixed endogenous and exogenous hyperlipidemia (combined types I and IV)
Definition	Familial fat-induced hyperglyceridemia	Hyperbetalipoproteinemia (hypercholesterolemia)	Combined hyperlipidemia (mixed hyperlipidemia)	Carbohydrate-induced hyperglyceridemia with hypercholesterolemia	Carbohydrate-induced hyperglyceridemia without hypercholesterolemia	Combined fat- and carbohydrate-induced hypertriglyceridemia
Age	Usually <10 yr	—	—	Not known, <25 yr	Only occasionally seen in children	—
Gross appearance of plasma	On standing: supernatant	Clear (no cream layer on top)	No cream layer on top; clear to turbid infranatant	Clear, cloudy, or milky	Slightly turbid to cloudy; on standing: unchanged	Markedly turbid; on standing: supernatant, creamy, milky infranatant
Serum cholesterol	N or slightly I	Markedly I (300–600 mg/dL)	Markedly I (300–600 mg/dL)	Markedly I (300–600 mg/dL)	N or slightly I	I (250–500 mg/dL)
LDL cholesterol	N	I	I	I	N	N
HDL cholesterol	N to D	N to D	N to D	N to D	N to D	N to D
Apolipoprotein	I (B-48), I (A-IV), V (C-II)	I (B-100)	I (B-100)	I (E-II), D (E-III), D (E-IV)	V (C-II), I (B-100)	V (C-II), I (B-48), I (B-100)
Increased lipoprotein	Chylomicrons	LDL	LDL, VLDL	IDL	VLDL	VLDL, chylomicrons
Serum triglycerides	Markedly I (usually >2,000 mg/dL)	N	I ≤400 mg/dL	Markedly I (200–1,000 mg/dL)	Markedly I (500–1,500 mg/dL)	Markedly I (500–1,500 mg/dL)

(continued)

Table 8. (continued)

Point of Comparison	Type I (Rarest)	Type II-a (Relatively Common)	Type II-b (Relatively Common)	Type III (Relatively Uncommon)	Type IV (Most Common)	Type V (Uncommon)
Appearance of lipoprotein components visualized by electrophoresis						
Chylomicron	Marked I	0	0	0	0	I
β-Lipoprotein	N or D	I	I	I, floating β	N or I	N or I
Pre-β-lipoprotein	N or D	N	I	I	I	I
α-Lipoprotein	—	—	—	—	—	—
Other laboratory abnormalities	Glucose tolerance usually N			Hyperglycemia; glucose tolerance often abnormal; serum uric acid I	Glucose tolerance often abnormal; serum uric acid often I	Glucose tolerance usually abnormal; serum uric acid usually I
Triglyceride/cholesterol ratio	8	1	Variable	<2	1–5	>5
Lipid changes resembling primary hyperlipidemias						
Diet	—	—	Very high cholesterol diet	Same as for type II-a	Caffeine or alcohol before testing	—

Drugs	—	Triglyceride-lowering drugs in types III and IV	Same as for type II-a	Triglyceride-lowering drugs	Cholesterol-lowering drugs, chlorothiazide, birth control pills, or estrogens	—
Primary disease	—	Myxedema, nephrosis, obstructive liver disease, stress, porphyria, anorexia nervosa, idiopathic hypercalcemia	Same as for type II-a	Myxedema, dysgammaglobulinemia, liver disease	Nephrotic syndrome, hypothyroidism, pregnancy, glycogen storage disease	Myeloma macroglobulinemia, nephrosis

0, absent; D, decreased; HDL, high-density protein; I, increased; IDL, intermediate-density lipoprotein; LDL, low-density lipoprotein; N, normal; VLDL, very-low-density lipoprotein.

Because apoprotein (apo) B is the only protein in LDL and apo A-I is the major protein constituent of HDL and VLDL, the ratio of apo-B to apo A-I reflects the ratio of LDL to HDL and may be a better discriminator of coronary artery disease than the individual components; however, data on apolipoproteins are still limited. Obtain blood only after at least 12–14 hr of fasting and when patient has been on usual diet for at least 2 wk.

Rule out diabetes, pancreatitis, and hypothyroidism in all groups.

Increased susceptibility to coronary artery disease occurs in types II, III, and IV; accelerated peripheral vascular disease occurs in type III.

Xanthomas appear in types I, II, and III

Abdominal pain occurs in types I and V.

If dietary or drug treatment has begun, it may not be possible to classify the lipoproteinemia or the classification may be erroneous.

Type II-b is overindulgence hyperlipidemia; shows increased cholesterol and triglyceride levels, with increased β and pre-β; can be distinguished from type III only by detection of abnormal β-migrating lipoprotein in serum fraction with density >1.006.

From Office of Medical Application of Research, National Institutes of Health. Treatment of hypertriglyceridemia. *JAMA* 1984;251:1196.

Premature CAD occurs later in life than with familial combined hyperlipidemia.
Xanthomas are rare.

Diagnostic Studies

Polygenic hypercholesterolemia can be distinguished from familial hypercholesterolemia and hyperlipidemias in three ways: family studies (hyperlipidemia is present in no more than 10% of first-degree relatives in polygenic hypercholesterolemia, in contrast to 50% in the other two disorders); examination for tendon xanthomas (absent in polygenic hypercholesterolemia); and response to dietary restrictions of saturated fat and cholesterol that is more marked in the polygenic form.

Familial Combined Hyperlipidemia (Types II-B, IV, V)

Occurs in 0.5% of general population and 15% of survivors of AMI <60 years old.
Any combination of increased LDL and VLDL and chylomicrons may be found; HDL is often low; different family members may have increased levels of serum total cholesterol or triglycerides, or both.
Premature CAD occurs later in life (>30 years of age) than with familial hypercholesterolemia.
Xanthomas are rare.
Patients are often overweight.

Familial Dysbetalipoproteinemia (Type III)

Occurs in 1 in 5,000 in the population.

Diagnostic Studies

Abnormality of apo E with excess of abnormal lipoprotein (β-mobility-VLDL); total cholesterol level of >300 mg/dL plus triglyceride level of >400 mg/dL should suggest this diagnosis. VLDL-C/triglyceride ratio = 0.3.
Diagnosis by combination of ultracentrifugation and isoelectric focusing that shows abnormal apo E pattern.
Tuberous and tendinous xanthomas and palmar and plantar xanthomatous streaks are present.
Atherosclerosis is more common in peripheral than in coronary arteries.

Familial Hypertriglyceridemia (Type IV)

Autosomal-dominant condition present in 1% of general population and 5% of survivors of AMI aged <60 years.

Diagnostic Studies

Elevated levels of triglycerides (usually 200–500 mg/dL) and VLDL, with normal LDL and decreased HDL.
Distinction from familial combined hyperlipidemia is made only by extensive family screening.

Abetalipoproteinemia (Bassen-Kornzweig Syndrome)

Extremely rare autosomal-recessive disorder; fat malabsorption, steatorrhea, failure to thrive, neurologic symptoms, pigmented retinopathy, acanthocytosis.

Diagnostic Studies

Marked decreased in serum triglyceride level (<30 mg/dL) with little increase after ingestion of fat, and in total cholesterol (20–50 mg/dL).
Chylomicrons, LDL, VLDL, and apo B are absent; HDL level may be lower than in normal persons.
Plasma lipid levels are normal in heterozygotes.
Acanthocytes may be 50–90% of red blood cells (RBCs) and are characteristic.
Decreased RBC life span causes anemia, which may vary from severe hemolytic anemia to mild compensated anemia.
Low serum levels of carotene and other fat-soluble vitamins.
Results of biopsy of small intestine show characteristic lipid vacuolization; not pathognomonic (occasionally seen in celiac disease, tropical sprue, juvenile nutritional megaloblastic anemia).
Negative sweat test result distinguishes this disorder from cystic fibrosis.

Arteriosclerosis is absent.

A variant is normotriglyceridemic abetalipoproteinemia, in which patient can secrete apo B-48 but not apo B-100; this results in normal postprandial triglyceride values but marked hypocholesterolemia; associated with mental retardation and vitamin E deficiency.

Hypobetalipoproteinemia

Autosomal-codominant disorder with increased longevity and lower incidence of atherosclerosis; at least one parent shows decreased β-lipoprotein.

Diagnostic Studies

Marked decrease in LDL level and LDL/HDL ratio.

Homozygous patients have decreased levels of serum cholesterol (<60 mg/dL) and triglycerides and undetectable or trace amounts of chylomicrons, VLDL, and LDL.

Heterozygotes are asymptomatic and have serum total cholesterol, LDL, and apo B values of 50% of normal (consistent with codominant disorder). May also be caused by malabsorption of fats, infection, anemia, hepatic necrosis, hyperthyroidism, AMI, or acute trauma.

Hyperlipidemias, Secondary

Many secondary hyperlipidemias are combined hyperlipidemias.

- Diabetes mellitus*
  Increased VLDL with increased serum triglycerides, low HDL-C; LDL-C may be normal or mildly increased. (Higher triglyceride values correlate with hyperglycemia and poorer control of diabetes; reduced by insulin therapy.)
- Hypothyroidism†
  Increased LDL-C and total cholesterol. Patient should be tested for hypothyroidism whenever LDL-C is >190 mg/dL. Level rapidly becomes normal with treatment.
  Serum cholesterol is not always increased.
- Nephrotic syndrome*
  Increased serum total cholesterol and LDL-C are usual.
  Increased VLDL and, therefore, increased serum triglycerides may also occur.
- Other renal disorders (chronic uremia, hemodialysis, after transplantation)†
  Increased triglycerides and total cholesterol and low HDL-C may occur.
- Hepatic glycogenoses
  Increased serum lipoprotein is common in any of the forms, but the pattern cannot be used to differentiate the type of glycogen storage disease.
  Predominant increase in VLDL in glucose-6-phosphatase deficiency.
  Predominant increase in LDL in debrancher and phosphorylase deficiencies.
- Obstructive liver disease*
  Increased serum total cholesterol is common until liver failure develops.
  Resistant to conventional drug therapy. The type of lipoproteinemia is variable.
  In intrahepatic biliary atresia, there is often increase in lipoprotein X with marked increase in serum total cholesterol and even more marked increase in serum phospholipids.
- Chronic alcoholism†
  Marked increase in VLDL producing type IV or V patterns.
- Hyperlipoproteinemia of affluence (dietary)*
- Pregnancy*
- Drug effects
  Estrogens, steroids, β-blockers*
  Diuretics, cyclosporine†

*Predominantly hypertriglyceridemia.
†Predominantly hypercholesterolemia.

Hyperlipoproteinemias, Primary

- Familial combined hyperlipidemia (type V)
- Familial hyperbetalipoproteinemia (type II)

- Familial hypercholesterolemia
- Hyperprebetalipoproteinemia (type IV)

Clinical Findings

Neurologic symptoms, cardiac symptoms, dermatologic abnormalities after detection of hyperlipidemia by screening

Diagnostic Studies

Identification and quantitation of plasma lipids and lipoproteins

Definitive Diagnosis

Enzyme assay or DNA analysis, or both

Hypolipoproteinemias, Primary

- α-Lipoprotein deficiency (analphalipoproteinemia; Tangier disease)
- Hypobetalipoproteinemia/abetalipoproteinemia
- Lecithin-cholesterol acyltransferase deficiency

Clinical Findings

Neurologic symptoms, gastrointestinal disease, hematologic abnormalities, ophthalmologic disorders, renal dysfunction, and abnormal blood lipids detected by routine screening

Diagnostic Studies

Identification and quantitation of plasma lipids and lipoproteins

Definitive Diagnosis

Enzyme assay or DNA analysis, or both

Lecithin-Cholesterol Acyltransferase Deficiency (Familial)

Rare autosomal-recessive disorder. Corneal opacities lead to blindness.

Clinical Findings

Anemia with large RBCs that are frequently target cells.
Proteinuria.

Diagnostic Studies

Serum total cholesterol level is normal but cholesteryl esters are virtually absent. Plasma-free cholesterol level is extremely increased. HDL level is low.

L-Carnitine Deficiency

Rare metabolic disorder of fatty acid metabolism (β oxidation)

Clinical Findings

Low renal reabsorption (e.g., Fanconi syndrome); deficiency of medium-chain acyl–coenzyme A dehydrogenase; valproic acid therapy (inducing excretion of valproycarnitine in urine); excessive loss of free carnitine in urine due to failure of carnitine transport across cells of renal tubule, muscle, and fibroblasts; organic acidurias (e.g., methylmalonic aciduria, propionic acidemia); other conditions (e.g., maternal deficiency, prematurity).

Laboratory Findings

Two types:

Limited to muscle: normal levels in plasma and other tissues.

Myoglobinuria in older children or young adults. Biopsy specimen shows lipid deposits. Tissue homogenates do not support normal rates of β oxidation of long-chain fatty acids unless L-carnitine is added. Serum carnitine level is normal or slightly decreased.

Systemic: More acute clinical picture, presents earlier in life; may mimic Reye syndrome.

L-Carnitine depleted in blood and all tissues.

Tissue contains marked decreased activity of medium-chain acyl–coenzyme A dehydrogenase.

Hepatic encephalopathy.

Hypoglycemia without ketosis.

Hyperammonemia may be present.

Serum uric acid may be increased.

Lipodystrophy (Total), Congenital

Rare autosomal-recessive disorder characterized by absence of fat in skin and viscera, possibly due to deficiency in number or quality of insulin receptors.

Clinical Findings

No neonatal abnormalities. Later in life: marked insulin resistance, glucose intolerance, development of diabetes mellitus (although ketosis is unusual), increased serum triglyceride levels develop. Similar syndromes of leprechaunism and acquired and partial lipodystrophies.

Laboratory Findings

Laboratory findings due to fatty liver, cirrhosis, and acanthosis nigricans.

Smith-Lemli-Opitz Syndrome

Autosomal-recessive disorder of multiple congenital anomalies due to defective cholesterol biosynthesis; true metabolic malformation syndrome. The incidence of this disease has been estimated at 1 in 20,000 to 1 in 40,000. It is the second most frequent recessive disorder, after cystic fibrosis. The concentration of the cholesterol precursor 7-dehydrocholesterol is elevated >2,000-fold above normal in serum and tissues from patients with Smith-Lemli-Opitz syndrome (SLOS), whereas plasma cholesterol levels are markedly lower, which suggests that 7-dehydrocholesterol (7-DHC) reductase activity is defective. Patients with SLOS have an impaired ability to synthesize cholesterol. The LDL receptor expression is increased to compensate for this impairment. The clinical problems of these patients appear to arise from both a deficiency in available cholesterol and an excess of 7-dehydrocholesterol.

Diagnostic Studies

SLOS can be diagnosed pre- and postnatally by deficiency of 7-DHC reductase activity in cultured skin fibroblasts and chorionic villus samples.

It has been found that increased nuchal translucency at 11 weeks' gestation indicates accumulation of fluid in the neck area in a fetus subsequently shown to have SLOS. Prenatal ultrasonographic findings include growth retardation, oligohydramnios, mesomelic limb shortness, and cardiac, renal, and hand defects.

Serum levels of unconjugated estriol (MsuE3) are decreased in women carrying an affected fetus. There is an inverse relationship between clinical severity and levels of amniotic fluid and chorionic villus samples of 7-DHC and MsuE3, that is, the lower the MsuE3 level, the higher the 7-DHC level (as percentage of total sterols).

Maternal serum screening methods have defined a characteristic pattern of low MsuE3, low human chorionic gonadotropin, and low α-fetoprotein levels; this is also seen in trisomy 18. In such cases, the measurement of 7-DHC levels in amniotic fluid may confirm a diagnosis of SLOS.

Tangier Disease

Rare autosomal-recessive disorder causing defect in metabolism of apo A in which a marked decrease (heterozygous) or absence (homozygous) of HDL is seen.

Clinical Findings

Deposits of cholesteryl esters in reticuloendothelial cells cause enlarged liver, spleen, and lymph nodes, enlarged orange tonsils, small orange-brown spots in rectal mucosa; premature CAD, mild corneal opacification, and neuropathy may be present in homozygous type.

Diagnostic Studies

Plasma levels of apo A-I and A-II are extremely low. In homozygotes, HDL level is usually <10 mg/dL and apo A-I level is usually <5 mg/dL. In heterozygotes, HDL and apo A-I levels are approximately 50% of normal.

Pre-β-lipoprotein is absent.

Serum total cholesterol (<100 mg/dL), LDL-C, and phospholipid levels are decreased; triglyceride levels are normal or increased (100–250 mg/dL).

Wolman Disease

(See also Chapter 17, Metabolic and Hereditary Diseases.)

Rare autosomal-recessive deficiency of lysosomal acid lipase activity causing accumulation of cholesterol and triglycerides throughout body tissues and death within first 6 months.

Diagnostic Studies

Prominent anemia develops by 6 weeks of age.

Peripheral blood smear shows prominent vacuolation (in nucleus and cytoplasm) of leukocytes.

Characteristic foam cells in bone marrow resemble those in Niemann-Pick disease.

Abnormal accumulation of cholesteryl esters and triglycerides in tissue biopsy specimen (e.g., from liver) establishes the diagnosis; cirrhosis may also be present.

Assay shows absent acid lipase activity in many tissues, including leukocytes and cultured fibroblasts. Heterozygotes have enzyme activity of <50% of normal in leukocytes or cultured fibroblasts.

Prenatal diagnosis by demonstrating enzyme deficiency in cultured amniocytes.

Histologic findings due to organ involvement:

- Abnormal liver function test results (due to lipid accumulation)
- Malabsorption
- Decreased adrenal cortical function (diffuse calcification on computed tomography scan)

Bibliography

Aitman TJ, Godsland IF, Farren B, et al. Defects in insulin action in fatty acid and carbohydrate metabolism in familial combined hyperlipidemia. *Arterioscler Thromb Vasc Biol* 1997;17:748–754.

Assmann G, von Eckardstein A, Cullen P. Dyslipidemias. In: Fernandez J, Saudubray J-M, Van den Berghe G, eds. *Inborn metabolic diseases, diagnosis and treatment*, 2nd ed. New York: Springer, 1996.

Barness LA, Gilbert-Barness E. Metabolic diseases. In: Gilbert-Barness E, ed. *Potter's pathology of the fetus and infant*. St. Louis: Mosby–Year Book, 1997.

Bredie SJH, van Drongelar J, Kiemercy LA, et al. Segregation of analysis of plasma apolipoprotein B levels in familial combined hyperlipidemia. *Arterioscler Thromb Vasc Biol* 1997;17:834–840.

Dreon DM, Fernstrom HA, Miller B, et al. Low-density lipoprotein subclass patterns and lipoprotein response to a reduced-fat diet in man. *FASEB J* 1994;8:121–126.

Gilbert-Barness E, Barness L. Lipid disorders. In: Gilbert-Barness E, Barness L, eds. *Metabolic diseases: foundations of clinical management, genetics, and pathology.* Natick, MA: Eaton Publishing, 2000.

Kane JP, Havel RJ. Disorders of the biogenesis and secretion of lipoproteins containing the B apolipoproteins. In: Scriver CR, Beaudet AL, Sly WS, et al., eds. *The metabolic and molecular bases of inherited disease*, 7th ed. New York: McGraw-Hill, 1995:1853.

Olson RE. Discovery of the lipoproteins, their role in fat transport and their significance as risk factors. *J Nutr* 1998;128:439S–443S.

Wallach J. *Interpretation of diagnostic tests*, 7th ed. Philadelphia: Lippincott Williams & Wilkins, 2000.

17 Metabolic and Hereditary Diseases

Presentation and Categorization

The clinical features of inborn errors of metabolism are usually nonspecific and overlap those of a child with sepsis, severe viral infection (pre- or postnatal), central nervous system (CNS) disorders, and acute or chronic ingestion of a toxic substance.

Most Frequent Clinical Presentation of Metabolic Disease in the Neonate

Apparent sepsis
Hematologic abnormalities, including thrombocytopenia, neutropenia, and anemia in the presence of normal bone marrow findings
Poor feeding, projectile vomiting
Neurologic abnormalities, including seizures, coma, and myopathy
Dysmorphism (Menkes syndrome, pyruvate dehydrogenase deficiency, Zellweger syndrome, glutaric acidemia type II)
Metabolic acidosis with an increased anion gap

Most Frequent Presentation of Metabolic Disease in the Older Child

Unexplained mental retardation or developmental delay
Seizures of unknown cause
Failure to thrive, poor growth
Inappropriately severe response to a usually minor pediatric illness, such as upper respiratory tract or ear infection, that results in coma or significant metabolic acidosis
Abnormal laboratory findings, including excessive or deficient ketosis, acidosis or lactic acidosis, hypoglycemia, or hyperammonemia
Hypopigmentation or abnormal hair
Cataracts, corneal clouding, or other ophthalmologic abnormalities
Hepatic dysfunction, especially Reye syndrome–like disorders, including enlargement of the liver or spleen, fatty deposition in the liver or other tissues, or evidence of skeletal abnormalities on radiography (dysostosis multiplex)
Loss of previously attained motor skills, severe behavioral changes, difficulty with walking (ataxia)

Categories of Inborn Errors of Metabolism

Aminoacidopathies
Urea cycle defects
Organic acidemias
Fatty acid oxidation defects
Abnormalities of carbohydrate metabolism

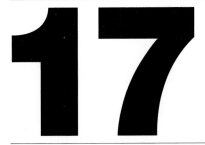

Mucopolysaccharidoses
Lysosomal storage disease
Mitochondrial disorders
Purine and pyridine disorders
Peroxisomal disorders
Nutritional disorders; vitamin and mineral metabolic disorder
Porphyrias

Amino Aciduria, Secondary

Inherited (generalized)
- Cystinosis
- Fanconi syndrome (idiopathic)
- Fructose intolerance
- Galactosemia
- Glycogen storage disease type 1 (rare)
- Lactose intolerance
- Lowe syndrome
- Tyrosinosis
- Wilson disease

Metabolic Errors That Cause Acidosis

Amino acid disorders
- Maple syrup urine disease
- Hypervalinemia
- Hyperleucine-isoleucinemia

Organic acid defects
- Isovaleric acidemia
- Propionic acidemia
- Methylmalonic acidemia
- Glutaric acidemia
- Combined carboxylase deficiency
- 3-Hydroxy-3-methylglutaric acidemia
- 2-Methyl-3-hydroxybutyric acidemia
- Acyl–coenzyme A (CoA) dehydrogenase deficiencies

Glycogen storage disease
- Type 1A
- Type 3

Ammonemia

Classes of Ammonemia

Urea Cycle Enzyme Defects

Carbamoyl phosphate synthetase (CPT) deficiency
Ornithine transcarbamylase (OTC) deficiency
Argininosuccinate synthetase deficiency (citrullinemia)
Arginase deficiency
N-acetylglutamate synthase deficiency

Transport Defects (Hyperornithinemia)

Lysinuric protein intolerance
Hyperammonemia-hyperornithinemia-homocitrullinemia

Fatty Acid Oxidation Defects

Medium-chain acyl-CoA dehydrogenase deficiency
Long-chain acyl-CoA dehydrogenase deficiency
Very-long-chain acyl-CoA dehydrogenase deficiency
Long-chain hydroxyacyl dehydrogenase deficiency
Systemic carnitine deficiency

Organic Acidemias

Propionic acidemia
Methylmalonic acidemia

Isovaleric acidemia
Glutaric acidemia type II
Acquired
Transient hyperammonemia of newborn
Reye syndrome
Liver failure
Herpes simplex in newborn
Toxin effects
Rett syndrome
Hyperinsulinism, hyperammonemia

Metabolic Errors Associated with Hyperammonemia in Children

Defects in urea cycle—severe hyperammonemia with respiratory alkalosis
- Arginosuccinate synthetase deficiency
- Arginosuccinate lyase deficiency
- Arginase deficiency
- Citrullinemia
- Ornithine transcarbamylase deficiency
- *N*-acetylglutamate synthetase deficiency
- Carbamoyl phosphate synthetase deficiency

Organic acid defects—mild to moderate hyperammonemia (≤500 mg/dL)
- Methylmalonic acidemia*
- Isovaleric acidemia*
- Multiple carboxylase deficiency*
- Propionic acidemia*
- Glutaric aciduria type II
- Ketothiolase deficiency

Hyperornithinemia
Transient hyperammonemia of newborn
Fatty acid oxidation defect

*Also characterized by lactic acidosis.

Laboratory Tests for Metabolic and Hereditary Diseases

Initial Laboratory Investigation of Suspected Inherited Metabolic Disease Presenting in the Newborn Period

See Tables 1 and 2 and Fig. 1.

Blood

Hemoglobin level, white blood cell (WBC) count, platelet count
Blood gases and plasma electrolyte levels (anion gap should be calculated)
Glucose level
Ammonium level
Lactate level
Calcium and magnesium levels
Liver function tests, including albumin and prothrombin and partial thromboplastin times
Amino acid analysis, *quantitative*
Carnitine level, total and free
Galactosemia screening test
Plasma sample for storage at –20°C; 10–20 mL

Urine

Dinitrophenylhydrazine test
Gas chromatography and mass spectrometry

Table 1. Investigations for Metabolic Disease in the Neonate

Presentation	Possible Metabolic Disorders	Suggested Investigations
Unexplained hypoglycemia	Organic acid disorders Amino acid disorders Glycogen storage disorder (type 1) Disorders of glyconeogenesis Congenital adrenal hyperplasia Congenital lactic acidosis Galactosemia	Organic acids (U) Amino acids (U, P) 3-Hydroxybutyrate (P) Free fatty acids (P) Lactate (P) Insulin (P) Cortisol (P) 17-Hydroxyprogesterone (P) Galactose-1-phosphate uridyltransferase (B)
Acid base imbalance		
Metabolic acidosis (exclude primary cardiac and respiratory disorders)	Organic acid disorders Congenital lactic acidosis	Organic acids (U) Lactate (P) Amino acids (U, P)
Respiratory alkalosis	Urea cycle disorders	Ammonia (P) Orotic acid (U) Amino acids (U, P)
Liver dysfunction (often associated with hypoglycemia and galactosuria)	Galactosemia Fructose 1,6-diphosphatase deficiency Hereditary fructose intolerance Tyrosinemia (type I) Glycogen storage disorder (type I) Disorders of gluconeogenesis α_1-Antitrypsin deficiency	Galactose-1-phosphate-uridyltransferase (B) Sugars (U) Amino acids (U, P) Succinyl acetone (U) α-Fetoprotein (P) Lactate (P) Oligosaccharides (U) Organic acids (U) α_1-Antitrypsin (P)
Neurologic dysfunction Seizures Depressed consciousness Hypotonia with Zellweger syndrome Organic acid disorders	Nonketotic hyperglycinemia Urea cycle disorders Xanthine/sulfine oxidase deficiency Homocystinuria (remethylation defect) Congenital lactic acidosis	Amino acids (U, P, C) Orotic acid (U) Ammonia (P) Urate (P, U) Sulfite (U) Lactate (P) Organic acids (U) Very-long-chain fatty acids (P)
Cardiomyopathy	Glycogen storage type 2 (Pompe disease) Fatty acid oxidation disorders Tyrosinemia (type I)	Lactate (P) 3-Hydroxybutyrate (P) Free fatty acids (P) Oligosaccharides (U) Organic acids (U) Carnitine (P) Amino acids (U, P)

B, whole blood; C, cerebrospinal fluid; P, plasma; U, urine.

Table 2. Newborn Screening

Disease	Level	Diagnostic Tests	Immediate Clinical Response
Phenylketonuria	Phe 4–6 mg/dL Phe 6–12 mg/dL Phe >12 mg/dL	Plasma amino acids (Phe, Tyr); phenyl acids; genotyping	For mild elevation: Evaluate nutritional, developmental, neurologic status, hepatic and renal function. Repeat screening test.
Maple syrup urine disease	Leu 4 mg/dL Leu 4–8 mg/dL Leu >8 mg/dL	Plasma amino acids (Val, Leu, Ileu)	For moderate elevation: Consult referral center and send frozen urine and plasma.
Homocystinuria	Meth 2–6 mg/dL Meth >6 mg/dL	Plasma amino acids (Tyr, Phe); blood spot for succinylacetone	For high levels: Arrange for hospitalization and diagnostic evaluation.
Tyrosinemia	Tyr 6–12 mg/dL Tyr 12–20 mg/dL Tyr >20 mg/dL		Repeat testings and treat.
Galactosemia	Beutler test, positive; *Escherichia coli* phage test, negative Beutler test, positive; *E. coli* phage test, positive	Galactose-1-phosphate uridyltransferase; galactokinase; uridine diphosphate galactose 4-epimerase; galactose-1-phosphate	Evaluate for jaundice, sepsis, cataracts, urine-reducing substances. Send blood for enzyme analysis. Remove lactose from diet.
Hypothyroidism	RIA: T_4 = 5.0–7.6 μg/dL; TSH <25 μIU/mL RIA: T_4 <5 μg/dL; TSH >25 μIU/mL	T_2, T_3, TSH, TBG, thyroid antibodies, bone age	Evaluate for hypothermia, hypoactivity, poor feeding, jaundice, constipation.

Ileu, isoleucine; Leu, leucine; Meth, methionine; Phe, phenylalanine; RIA, radioimmunoassay; T_2, diiodothyronine; T_3, triiodothyronine; T_4, thyroxine; TBG, thyroid-binding globulin; TSH, thyroid-stimulating hormone; Tyr, tyrosine; Val, valine.

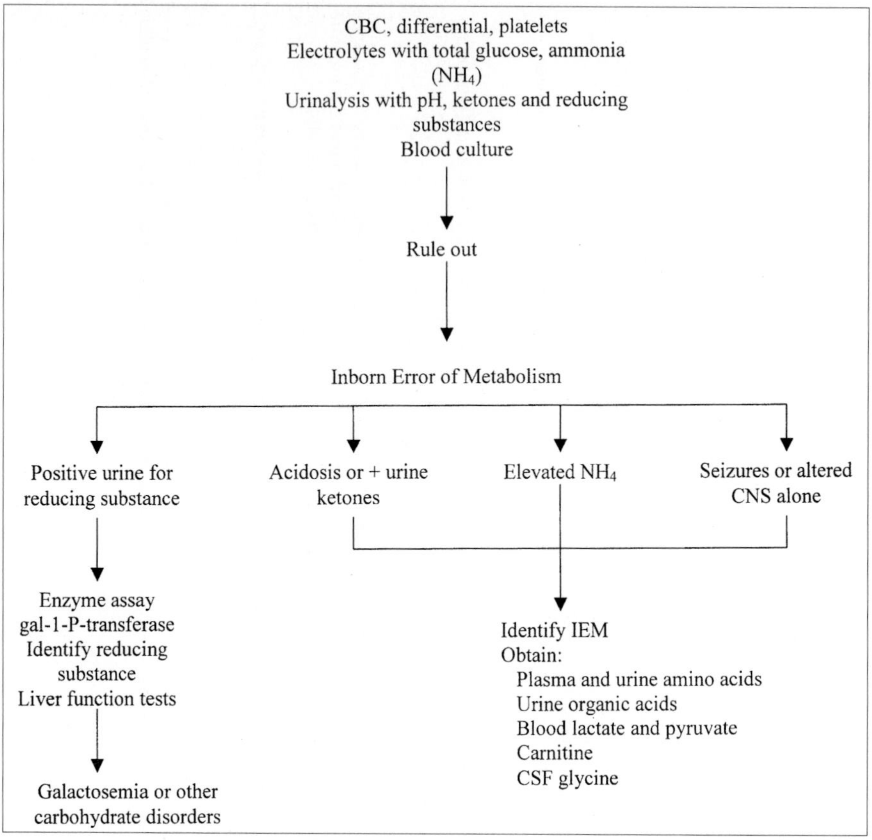

Fig. 1. Algorithm for diagnostic approach in suspected inborn error of metabolism (IEM) in a newborn. CBC, complete blood cell count; CNS, central nervous system; CSF, cerebrospinal fluid; gal-1-P-transferase, galactose-1-phosphate transferase.

Laboratory Tests in Metabolic Diseases

Initial Laboratory Tests

1. Blood
   a. Complete blood cell count (neutropenia, thrombocytopenia seen in organic acidemias)
   b. Serum electrolyte, glucose levels; anion gap
   c. Arterial blood gas concentrations
   d. Plasma ammonium level
2. Urine: Check odor; measure pH, ketone levels, levels of reducing substances

Acute Disease	**Urine Odors**
Maple syrup urine disease	Maple syrup, burned sugar
Isovaleric acidemia	Cheese or sweaty feet
Multiple carboxylase deficiency	Cat's urine
3-hydroxy-3-methylglutaryl-CoA lyase deficiency	Cat's urine
Nonacute Disease	
Phenylketonuria (PKU)	Musty
Hypermethioninemia	Rancid butter, rotten cabbage
Trimethylaminuria	Stale fish

Specific Studies

If any of the initial studies are abnormal:

1. Blood: Plasma amino acid levels, plasma carnitine levels (free and total)
2. Urine
   a. Metabolic screen: Includes pH; specific gravity; levels of protein, glucose, ketones, reducing substances (Clinitest); ferric chloride test; dinitrophenylhydrazine test (for α-ketoacids); nitrosonaphthol test (for tyrosine metabolites); nitroprusside test (for sulfhydryl groups); and mucopolysaccharide spot test.
   b. Tests for organic acids, amino acids.

Sample Collection

1. Tests for plasma amino acids and plasma carnitine each require 3 mL of blood collected in a green-top (sodium heparin) tube. Samples should be drawn after an overnight fast (or at least a 4-hour fast in an infant). Deliver on ice or separate and freeze plasma for later analysis.
2. Urine amino and organic acid assays each requires 5–10 mL of urine. If fresh urine cannot be delivered immediately to the laboratory, freeze samples.
3. Plasma ammonium values increase rapidly on standing. Collect sample on ice and deliver immediately to laboratory.
4. With skin biopsy for fibroblast studies, specimen should be stored in tissue culture medium at 4°C. When this medium is unavailable, store specimen in the patient's serum. Refrigerate, but do not freeze, specimen. Keep the tissue immersed in the culture medium.

Ferric Chloride Test

Ferric Chloride Reaction

1. Ferric iron forms colored derivatives when combined with many organic compounds. Results depend on methodology.
2. Place 2 drops of 10% ferric chloride in 1 mL of fresh urine; mix and observe color immediately and on standing.
3. The test is relatively insensitive and usually requires high concentration of the reacting metabolite. Phosphate ions yield cloudy precipitates, which may mask positive results.

Ferric Chloride Test Results[1]

Disorder	Compound	Color Reaction
PKU	Phenylpyruvic acid	Green
Tyrosinemia	4-Hydroxyphenylpyruvate	Fading green
Maple syrup urine disease	Branch chain ketoacids	Green/gray
Histidinemia	Imidazolepyruvate	Gray
Alkaptonuria	Homogentisic acid	Blue/green
Ketosis	Acetoacetate	Red/brown
Salicylates	Salicylic acid	Purple
Phenothiazines	Phenothiazines	Gray/green
Acetaminophen	Acetaminophen	Green

Genetic Testing

Karyotyping

Indications

1. Two or more major malformations (small size for gestational age and mental retardation are considered major malformations for this purpose).

[1]Soldin SJ, Rifai N, Hicks JM. *Biochemical basis of pediatric disease*, 3rd ed. Washington: American Association for Clinical Chemistry Press, 1998.

2. Features of specific chromosomal syndrome.
3. At risk for a familial chromosomal aberration.

Draw 3 mL of blood in a green-top tube that contains sodium heparin. Keep tube at room temperature.

DNA Testing

DNA-based diagnosis allows determination of a person's genotype without the need for a biochemical or enzymatic assay.

DNA-based diagnosis has a number of advantages. The specimen volume requirements are extremely small, and sufficient DNA can be obtained from a drop of blood or epithelial cells from cheek brushing or mouth washing. The relative stability of DNA also overcomes many of the problems of unstable or fastidious enzymes.

Two types of DNA-based diagnosis are direct gene evaluation and linkage analysis. In the former, an alteration is detected in a particular gene, either from study of a previously affected family member or from population screening. The exact mutation that produces the disease phenotype may not be identified without complete gene sequencing, which is technically impractical on a routine basis. In these cases, linkage analysis provides an alternative means for genetic diagnosis.

Direct DNA Analysis

Sickle cell disease (HbSS, HbSC)
Thalassemias
Hemophilia A and B
Gaucher disease
Fragile X syndrome
Retinoblastoma
α_1-Antitrypsin deficiency
Huntington disease
Charcot-Marie-Tooth disease type 1A
Spinal muscular atrophy
Cystic fibrosis
Fragile X syndrome
Medium-chain acyl-CoA dehydrogenase deficiency
Myotonic dystrophy
Muscular dystrophy (Duchenne or Becker)

Linkage Analysis

(Requires family members)

Linkage analysis reflects the physical distance on the chromosome between a genetic marker and disease locus. Linked genes are located close to each other on the same chromosome. Linkage analysis is used in diseases for which the abnormal gene has not yet been cloned but its chromosomal location is known. As information about the defective gene becomes available, diagnosis by direct gene analysis becomes preferable. The following are examples of diseases diagnosed by linkage analysis:

- Hemophilia A, B
- Muscular dystrophy (Duchenne or Becker)
- Neurofibromatosis, types 1, 2
- von Hippel-Lindau syndrome
- PKU
- Polycystic kidney disease
- Spinal muscular atrophy (Werdnig-Hoffmann disease)
- Hypertrophic cardiomyopathy

Polymerase Chain Reaction Testing

Polymerase chain reaction (PCR) analyses can be carried out with buccal washes, single hair bulbs, sperm, urinary sediment, and dried blood spots. In PCR the DNA sample used in the initial amplification steps may be unpurified, substantially degraded, fixed in formalin or mercury-based fixatives, or embedded in paraffin. DNA for PCR analysis has been obtained from stored screening cards that contain small circles of dried blood from newborns. This latter method is a convenient way to transport patient samples for future analysis or to bank DNA for patients with unknown or uncharacterized genetic disorders.

In many genetic diseases, the defective gene product is expressed in only one or a limited number of tissues; for example, urea cycle defect ornithine transcarbamylase deficiency and phenylalanine hydroxylase deficiency, in which the enzyme activity is expressed only in liver. PCR analysis of fetal DNA obtained by amniocentesis or chorionic villus biopsy provides a means for rapid, accurate diagnosis without the need to perform invasive tissue sampling or complex biochemical assays. PCR is a method for determining carrier status for inborn errors of metabolism. DNA analysis allows direct determination of alleles at a given genetic locus and genotype assignment by DNA sequence, which is generally more accurate than carrier status determination by enzymatic activity.

Electron Spray Tandem Mass Spectrometry

Electron spray tandem mass spectrometry plays a significant role in screening for inherited disorders because of its speed, sensitivity, accuracy, and multitasking capabilities. This technique has been expanded to include the diagnosis of very-long-chain fatty acid disorders, including peroxisomal disorders, defects of bile acids, and long-chain acyl dehydrogenase deficiency.

Expanded Supplemental Newborn Screening

The following disorders are detected by the expanded Supplemental Newborn Screening program (Neo Gen Screening Inc., Pittsburgh, PA):

- Cystic fibrosis (not valid after 3 months of age)
- Galactosemia
    - Galactokinase deficiency
    - Galactose-1-phosphate uridyltransferase deficiency
    - Galactose-4-epimerase deficiency
- Glucose-6-phosphate dehydrogenase deficiency
- Amino acid disorders
    - Maple syrup urine diseases
    - *Arginase deficiency
    - Acute neonatal citrullinemia
    - PKU
    - *Pyroglutamic aciduria
- Congenital adrenal hyperplasia:
    - Salt-wasting 21-hydroxylase deficiency
    - Simple virilizing 21-hydroxylase deficiency
- Biotinidase deficiency
- Adenosine deaminase deficiency (severe combine immunodeficiency)
- Acylcarnitine disorders
- Methylmalonic acidemias
    - Methylmalonyl-CoA mutase deficiencies (mut– and mut+)
- *Adenosylcobalamin synthesis defects
- *Combined adenosylcobalamin and methylcobalamin defects
    - Propionic acidemia
    - Isovaleric acidemia
    - Glutaric acidemia type I
    - *Multiple CoA carboxylase deficiency
    - 3-Methylcrotonyl-CoA lyase deficiency
    - *3-Ketothiolase deficiency
    - 3-Hydroxy-3-methylglutaryl-CoA lyase deficiency
    - *3-Methylglutaconyl-CoA hydratase deficiency
    - *3-Hydroxyisobutyryl-CoA hydrolase deficiency
    - *2,4-Dienoyl-CoA reductase deficiency
- Fatty acid oxidation
    - Medium-chain acyl-CoA dehydrogenase deficiency
    - Short-chain acyl-CoA dehydrogenase deficiency
    - *Long-chain acyl-CoA dehydrogenase deficiency
    - Long-chain hydroxy acyl-CoA dehydrogenase deficiency

*Carnitine palmitoyl transferase deficiency type II
Multiple acyl-CoA dehydrogenase deficiency (glutaric acidemia type II)

*Theoretically detectable in newborn period, but not yet identified in the SNS program.

Amino Acids, Pathologic Levels in Amino Acid Disorders

Disorder	Amino Acid	Abnormal Levels Plasma	Abnormal Levels Urine
Disorders of aromatic amino acid metabolism			
Hyperphenylalaninemia			
PKU: phenylalanine hydroxylase deficiency	Phenylalanine	I	I
Biopterin disorders	Phenylalanine	I	I
Tyrosinemia			
Transient neonatal	Tyrosine	I	I
Hepatorenal (type I)	Tyrosine	I	I
	Methionine	I	
	Other amino acids		I
Oculocutaneous (type II)	Tyrosine	I	I
Nonspecific liver damage	Tyrosine	I	I
	Methionine	I	
	Hawkinsin		I
Disorders of neutral amino acid metabolism			
Maple syrup urine disease			
Classic	Valine	I	I
	Alloisoleucine	Present	Present
	Isoleucine	I	I
	Leucine	I	I
	Alanine	D during severe episodes	
Intermittent, variable, intermediate thiamine-responsive	Above branched chain amino acids I during episodes but may be N to slightly I between episodes.		
3-Hydroxyisobutyryl-CoA deacylase deficiency	S-(2-carboxypropyl)-cysteine		I
	S-(2-carboxypropyl)-cysteamine		I
Nonketotic hyperglycinemia	Glycine	I	I
		[also I in cerebrospinal fluid (CSF)]	
Sarcosinemia	Sarcosine	I	I
Hartnup disease	Neutral amino acids	N to D	I
Disorders of basic amino acid metabolism			
Hyperlysinemia	Lysine	I	I
Pipecolic acid disorders	Pipecolic acid	I	
Saccharopinuria	Lysine	I	I
	Saccharopine	I	I
Lysinuric protein intolerance	Lysine	N to D	I
	Arginine	N to D	I
	Ornithine	N to D	
	A number of amino acids	I	
α-Aminoadipic aciduria	α-Aminoadipic acid	I	I
Hyperornithinemia-gyrate atrophy	Ornithine	I	I
Hyperornithinemia-hyperammonemia-homocitrullinuria syndrome	Ornithine	I	N
	Homocitrulline	N	I
Histidinemia	Histidine	I	I
Disorders of imino acid metabolism			
Hyperprolinemia			
Type I	Proline	I	I

	Hydroxyproline	N	I
	Glycine	N	I
Type II	Proline	I	I
	Hydroxyproline	N	I
	Glycine	N	I
	Δ'-pyrroline-5-carboxylic acid	I	I
	Δ'-pyrroline-3-hydroxy-5-carboxylic acid		I
Hyperhydroxyprolinemia	Hydroxyproline	I	I
Prolidase deficiency	Iminodipeptides of proline hydroxyproline		I
Neonatal iminoglycinuria	Proline, hydroxyproline, and glycine	N	I to age 6 mo
Familial renal iminoglycinuria	Proline		I
	Hydroxyproline		I
	Glycine		I
Disorders of sulfur amino acid metabolism			
Homocystinuria			
Cystathionine β-synthase deficiency	Homocystine	I	I
	Cysteine-homocysteine mixed disulfide	I	I
	Methionine	I	I
	Cystine	N to D	
	Cystathionine	N to D	
Cobalamin (cb) disorders: cb1C, cb1D, cb1E, cb1G, and B_{12} deficiency	Homocystine	I	I
	Cysteine-homocysteine mixed disulfide	I	I
	Methionine	N to D	
	Cystathionine	N to D	
5,10-Methylenetetrahydrofolate reductase deficiency	Homocystine	I	I
	Methionine	N to D	
	Cystathionine		N to I
Cystathioninuria	Cystathionine	N to I	I
Hypermethioninemia	Methionine	I	
	Methionine sulfoxides	I	
3-Mercaptolactic-cysteine disulfiduria mixed disulfide	3-Mercaptolactic-cysteine		I
Sulfite oxidase deficiency	S-Sulfocysteine		I
	Cystine	N to D	
Cystinuria	Cystine	N	I
	Dibasic amino acids (lysine, ornithine, arginine)	N	I
Cystinosis	Cystine	N (I in lysosomes of tissues)	N
Disorders of β- and γ-amino acid metabolism			
Hyper-β-alaninemia	β-Alanine	I	I
β-Aminoisobutyric aciduria	β-Aminoisobutyric acid	N to slightly I	I
γ-Aminobutyric acid aminotransferase deficiency	γ-Aminobutyric	I	
	β-Alanine		
	γ-Aminobutyric, β-alanine, and homocystine also I in CSF		
Carnosinase deficiency	Carnosine	I	I
	Anserine		I
Homocarnosinosis	Homocarnosine	N (I in CSF)	N

I, increased; D decreased; N, normal.

Organic Acids Excreted in Various Disorders

Disorder	Acid/Compound	Typical Abnormal Excretions (mmol/mol Creatinine)
Disorders of aromatic amino acid metabolism		
PKU	Phenylpyruvic	300–1,000
	Phenyllactic	200–1,000
	2-Hydroxyphenylacetic	50–2,000
Tyrosinemia		
Transient neonatal, oculocutaneous, and hepatorenal	4-Hydroxyphenylpyruvic	140–2,000
	4-Hydroxyphenyllactic	100–5,000
	4-Hydroxyphenylacetic	140–500
Hepatorenal only	*N*-acetyltyrosine	30–200
Hawkinsinuria	Succinylacetone	20–700
	4-Hydroxycyclohexylacetic	10–70
	5-Oxoproline	1,300–9,000
	4-Hydroxyphenylpyruvic	170–1,600
	4-Hydroxyphenyllactic	1,000–5,000
Alcaptonuria	Homogentisic	1,000–5,000
Disorders of branched chain amino acid metabolism		
Maple syrup urine disease	2-Oxoisocaproic	400–4,400
	2-Oxo-3-methylvaleric	500–2,500
	2-Oxoisovaleric	300–800
	2-Hydroxyisovaleric	850–3,600
	2-Hydroxyisocaproic	3–80
	2-Hydroxy-3-methylvaleric	60–400
Dihydrolipoyl dehydrogenase (E3) deficiency	Lactic	1,000–30,000
	2-Oxoglutaric	150–1,100
	2-Oxoisocaproic	0–200
	2-Oxo-3-methylvaleric	0–15
	2-Oxoisovaleric	0–3
	2-Hydroxyisovaleric	0–400
	2-Hydroxyisocaproic	0–70
	2-Hydroxy-3-methylvaleric	0–70
Isovaleric acidemia	Isovalerylglycine	2,000–9,000
	3-Hydroxyisovaleric	1,000–2,000
	4-Hydroxyisovaleric	20–300
3-Methylcrotonyl-CoA carboxylase	3-Hydroxyisovaleric	1,700–59,000
	3-Methylcrotonylglycine	400–1,000
Biotin-responsive multiple carboxylase deficiency		
Holocarboxylase synthetase deficiency	3-Hydroxyisovaleric acid	250–3,600
	3-Methylcrotonylglycine	30–260
	Methylcitric	15–200
	3-Hydroxypropionic	45–1,300
	Lactic	100–75,000
Biotinidase deficiency	Same as the above, but generally smaller elevations	
3-Methylglutaconic acidemia		
3-Methylglutaconyl-CoA hydratase	3-Methylglutaconic	500–100
	3-Hydroxyisovaleric	150–250
	3-Methylglutaric	5–10
Normal hydratase	3-Methylglutaconic	25–600
	3-Methylglutaric	10–85
3-Hydroxy-3-methylglutaric aciduria	3-Hydroxy-3-methylglutaric	200–11,000
	3-Methylglutaconic	140–10,000
	3-Methylglutaric	14–1,000
	3-Hydroxyisovaleric	60–4,000
	3-Methylcrotonylglycine	0–400

3-Oxothiolase deficiency		
Mitochondrial branched chain 3-oxothiolase deficiency	2-Methyl-3-hydroxybutyric	200–4,400
	2-Methylacetoacetic	0–650
	Tiglylglycine	0–1,000
Cytosolic 3-oxothiolase deficiency or succinyl-CoA/3-oxoacid-CoA transferase deficiency	3-Hydroxybutyric	Large amount
	Acetoacetic	Large amount
Propionic acidemia	Methylcitric	150–2,800
	3-Hydroxybutyric	20–2,000
	Propionylglycine	0–450
	3-Hydroxyvaleric	0–1,200
Methylmalonic acidemia	Methylmalonic	150–15,500
Mutase deficiency and cobalamin disorders	(Plus same metabolites as propionic acidemia)	
Malonyl-CoA decarboxylase deficiency	Malonic	50–4,000
	Methylmalonic	0–80
3-Hydroxyisobutyric aciduria	3-Hydroxyisobutyric	130–400
Disorders of dibasic amino acid metabolism		
2-Oxoadipic aciduria	2-Oxoadipic	20–220
	2-Hydroxyadipic	50–220
Glutaric aciduria type I	Glutaric	500–12,000
	3-Hydroxyglutaric	60–3,000
	Glutaconic	0–360
Hyperornithinemia-hyperammonemia-homocitrullinuria syndrome	Orotic	30–500
Lysinuric protein intolerance	Orotic	1–640
Disorders of pyrimidine metabolism		
Orotic aciduria	Orotic	1,400–5,600
Dihydropyrimidine dehydrogenase deficiency	Uracil	100–1,100
	Thymine	35–850
Disorders of fatty acid oxidation		
Long-chain hydroxyacyl-CoA dehydrogenase deficiency	3-Hydroxydecanedioic	Increased
	3-Hydroxydodecanedioic	Increased
	3-Hydroxytetradecanedioic	Increased
	3-Hydroxy-unsaturated dicarboxylic, saturated and unsaturated dicarboxylic	Increased
Very-long-chain acyl-CoA dehydrogenase deficiency	Suberic	0–20
	Sebacic	0–20
	Dodecamedioic and tetradecanedioic may be elevated.	
Medium-chain acyl-CoA dehydrogenase deficiency	Octanoic	2–20
	5-Hydroxyhexanoic	15–700
	7-Hydroxyoctanoic	4–300
	Adipic	5–5,200
	Suberic	6–5,000
	Octenedioic	0–250
	Sebacic	0–5,000
	Decenedioic	0–750
	Hexanoylglycine	2–730
	Phenylproionylglycine	1–90
	Suberylglycine	6–2,200
Short-chain acyl-CoA dehydrogenase deficiency	Ethylmalonic	180–1,150
	Methylsuccinic	20–60
	(Dicarboxylic acids variably elevated.)	
Multiple acyl-CoA dehydrogenase deficiency (glutaric aciduria type II)	Glutaric	0–22,000
	Ethylmalonic	10–1,400
	Adipic	0–1,600
	Suberic	0–200
	2-Hydroxyglutaric	180–8,250
	Isovalerylglycine	0–1,000

	Isobutyrylglycine	0–200
	2-Methylbutyrylgycine	0–200
	(Short-chain fatty acids may be elevated.)	
Normal dietary medium-chain triglycerides	Adipic	200–230
	Suberic	10–620
	Sebacic	0–750
	5-Hydroxyhexanoic	0–220
	7-Hydroxyoctanoic	25–150
Miscellaneous disorders		
4-Hydroxybutyric aciduria	4-Dihydroxybutyric	130–7,600
	3,4-Hydroxybutyric	5–225
Fumarase deficiency	Fumaric	3,000–4,000
2-Oxoglutaric dehydrogenase deficiency	2-Oxoglutaric	150–1,250
Mevalonic aciduria	Mevalonolactone, mevalonic acid	1,000–56,000
5-Oxoprolinuria	5-Oxoproline	4,000–30,000
Canavan disease	*N*-Acetylaspartic	1,000–7,000
D-Glyceric aciduria	D-Glyceric	10,000–20,000
Hyperoxaluria type I	Oxalic	90–350
	Glycolic	>100
	Glyoxylic	>10
Hyperoxaluria type II	Oxalic	90–350
	L-Glyceric	150–450
Glyceroluria	Glycerol	90,000–190,000
Lactic acidemia	Lactic	100–30,000
	Pyruvic	50–10,000
	2-Hydroxybutyric	10–1,000
	4-Hydroxyphenyllactic	50–500
Intestinal bacterial overgrowth	Lactic (D)	45–6,000
	3-Hydroxypropionic	100–6,400
	4-Hydroxyphenylacetic	100–2,000
Ketosis	3-Hydroxybutyric	100–50,000
	Acetoacetic	50–20,000
	3-Hydroxyisobutyric	50–3,000
	3-Hydroxyisovaleric	50–1,000
	3-Hydroxy-2-methylbutyric	10–200
	Adipic	15–450
	Suberic	0–100

Disorders of Amino Acid Metabolism

Branched-Chain Amino Acid Disorders

The three branched-chain amino acids, leucine, isoleucine, and valine, are essential amino acids and have similar metabolic pathways. In one group, deficiency of the branched-chain α-keto acid dehydrogenase complex results in the metabolic block of the three amino acids. This results in maple syrup urine disease. A group involving leucine transamination and decarboxylation results in the formation of a number of organic acids.

Tissue Required for Prenatal Diagnosis of Branched-Chain Aminoacidopathies[2]

Disorder	Tissue	Trimester of Pregnancy
Maple syrup urine disease	CV sampling, cultured AFC	I, II
Isovaleric acidemia	AF, cultured AFC	II

[2]Gibson KM, Elpeleg ON, Wappner RS. Disorders of leucine metabolism. In: Blau N, Duran M, Blaskovics ME, eds. *Physician's guide to the laboratory diagnosis of metabolic diseases.* London: Chapman and Hall, 1996.

Isolated 3-methylcrotonyl-CoA carboxylase deficiency	AF, cultured AFC, CV tissues	I, II
3-Methylglutaconic aciduria type I (3-methylglutaconyl-CoA hydratase deficiency)	AF, cultured AFC	II
3-Methylglutaconic aciduria, other types (3-methylglutaconyl-CoA hydratase, normal activity)	AF[a]	II
3-Hydroxy-3-methylglutaric aciduria (3-hydroxy-3-methyglutaryl-CoA lyase deficiency)	AF, cultured AF, CV tissue	I, II
Mevalonic aciduria (mevalonate kinase deficiency)	AF, cultured AFC, CV tissue	I, II

AF, amniotic fluid; AFC, amniotic fluid cells; CV, chorionic villus.
[a]Thus far, studies have been limited to patients categorized as having 3-methylglutaconic aciduria, unclassified form.

Hyperglycinemia, Nonketotic (Glycine Cleavage System Deficiency)

Clinical Symptoms
Acute neonatal crisis, neurologic symptoms, neurodegenerative symptoms, developmental delay, failure to thrive

Diagnostic Studies
Simultaneous quantitative amino acid studies in blood and spinal fluid. Urine amino acid analysis

Definitive Diagnosis
Enzymatic assay or DNA analysis or both

Isovaleric Acidemia

Clinical Symptoms
Episodic vomiting
Natural aversion to protein foods
Lethargy
Coma
Odor of sweaty feet
Psychomotor retardation
Seizures

Laboratory Findings
Acidosis
Ketosis
Anion gap increased
Ammonia (blood) increased
Neutropenia
Thrombocytopenia
Pancytopenia
Organic acids: isovalerylglycine and its metabolites in urine
Volatile short-chain organic acids: isovaleric acid in plasma
Abnormal levels of total and free carnitine (plasma)
Increased level of esterified carnitine (plasma)

Maple Syrup Urine Disease[3]

(Branched-chain α-ketodehydrogenase deficiency)

Maple syrup urine disease is an autosomal-recessive disorder of the mitochondrial multienzyme complex branched-chain α-keto acid dehydrogenase that results in increased concentrations of branched-chain amino acids and α-keto acids. Estimated incidence is 1 per 120,000 to 1 per 400,000 live births, and the disease is most common among the Mennonites of North America, in whom the incidence is 1 in 176. Untreated, the patient with classic maple syrup urine disease usually dies with apnea or coma.

[3]Gilson KM, Elpeleg ON, Wappner RS. Disorders of leucine metabolism. In: Blau N, Duran N, Blaskovics ME, eds. *Physician's guide to the laboratory diagnosis of metabolic diseases*. London: Chapman and Hall, 1996:125.

The odor of maple syrup, due to 2-oxo-3-methylvaleric acid, is detected in the urine, sweat, and saliva. A urine spot test with 2,4-dinitrophenylhydrazine and ferric chloride indicates the presence of ketoacids.

Abnormalities include neurodegenerative and acute neonatal neurologic symptoms, developmental delay, hepatocellular disease, gastrointestinal disease, failure to thrive, hypoglycemia, metabolic acidosis, hyperammonemia, and abnormal results on newborn screening tests.

Metabolic acidosis and ketoacidosis occur. Ferric chloride test of urine produces green-gray color. Hypoglycemia is usual. The disease may be severe or intermittent.

Patient should be monitored by daily urine testing with dinitrophenylhydrazine. Urine levels correlate with plasma levels; plasma levels can be measured once a month if urine test is negative or shows only traces (control plasma ranges: leucine = 180–700 μmol/L, isoleucine = 70–280 μmol/L, valine = 200–800 μmol/L).

Clinical Symptoms

Episodic vomiting
Lethargy
Irritability
Apnea
Poor feeding
Failure to thrive
Coma
Odor of maple syrup
Central nervous system symptoms
- Psychomotor retardation
- Central nervous system deterioration
- Cerebral edema
- Areflexia
- Hypotonia
- Hypertonia
- Ataxia
- Seizures

Laboratory Studies

Test for acidosis
Test for ketosis
Anion gap measurement
Glucose level (blood)
Ammonia level (blood)
2,4-Dinitrophenylhydrazine test (urine)
Ferric chloride test (urine)
Test for branched-chain amino acids (plasma or serum)
Test for organic acids, branched chain ketoacids (urine)

Diagnostic Studies

Chromatography of urine and plasma shows greatly increased urinary excretion of ketoacids of leucine, isoleucine, and valine. Presence of alloisoleucine (stereoisomeric metabolite of isoleucine) is characteristic.

Measurement of amount of defective enzyme in leukocytes and fibroblasts shows enzyme level 0–2% of normal; intermittent form (enzyme level, 2–8% of normal) and intermediate form (enzyme level, 8–16% of normal). Blood levels are normal in intermittent form except during acute episodes caused by infection, surgery, vaccination, or sudden increased intake of protein. Intermediate form shows persistent elevated levels of blood amino acids, which can be kept in normal range by maintaining dietary protein at <2 g/kg/day.

Prenatal diagnosis by measurement of enzyme concentration in cells cultured from amniotic fluid.

Definitive Diagnosis

Enzyme assay or DNA analysis or both

Molybdenum Metabolism Disorders

- Molybdenum cofactor deficiency
- Sulfite oxidase deficiency

Clinical Symptoms

Neurologic symptoms, developmental delay, gastrointestinal disease, ophthalmologic disorders, failure to thrive

Diagnostic Studies

Metabolite identification (amino and organic acids) and quantitation in blood and urine. Uric acid level.

Definitive Diagnosis

Enzymatic assay or DNA analysis or both

Other Branched-Chain and Organic Acid Disorders

Cytosolic acetoacetyl-CoA thiolase deficiency
3-Hydroxyisobutryl-CoA deacylase deficiency
3-Hydroxyisobutyric aciduria
3-Hydroxy-3-methylglutaryl CoA lyase deficiency
3-Methylcrotonyl-CoA carboxylase deficiency
3-Methylglutaconic acidurias
Barth syndrome (X-linked cardiomyopathy, neutropenia, and growth retardation)
3-methylglutaconyl-CoA hydratase deficiency
Unspecified 3-methylglutaconic aciduria
2-Methyl branched-chain acyl-CoA hydratase deficiency
Methylmalonic semialdehyde dehydrogenase deficiency
Mevalonate kinase deficiency (mevalonic aciduria)
Mitochondrial acetoacetyl-CoA thiolase deficiency
Succinyl-CoA/3-ketoacid CoA-transferase deficiency
Fatty acid oxidation disorders, for example, medium-chain, short-chain, long-chain, and very-long-chain acyl-CoA dehydrogenase deficiencies, long-chain hydroxyacyl dehydrogenase deficiency

Clinical Symptoms

Acute neonatal crisis, neurologic symptoms, visceromegaly, developmental delay, hepatocellular disease, renal dysfunction, gastrointestinal disease, skeletal myopathy and hypotonia, cardiomyopathy, failure to thrive, hypoglycemia, metabolic acidosis, hyperammonemia, immunologic abnormalities, dysmorphic features. Organic acids are usually excreted as carnitine esters.

Diagnostic Studies

Analysis of amino and organic acids in the blood and urine. Carnitine species identification and quantitation in blood and urine. Provocative tests in certain disorders.

Definitive Diagnosis

Enzymatic assay or DNA analysis or both

Glutamate Formiminotransferase Deficiency

Clinical Symptoms

Neurologic symptoms, developmental delay, failure to thrive, hematologic abnormalities

Diagnostic Studies

Amino and organic acid analysis of blood or urine, identification and quantitation. Decreased folic acid and glutamic acid levels in blood.

Definitive Diagnosis

Enzymatic assay or DNA analysis or both

Glutamic Acid Disorders

Disorders of the γ-glutamyl cycle

γ-Glutamylcysteine Synthase Deficiency

Clinical Symptoms

Chronic hemolytic anemia, peripheral and central neuropathy, metabolic acidosis

Diagnostic Studies

Generalized amino aciduria, decreased red cell glutathione, decreased red cell and glutamyl synthase

γ-Glutamyltranspeptidase Deficiency

Clinical Symptoms

Developmental delay and severe behavioral problems

Diagnostic Studies

Blood and urine glutathione levels high
Enzyme assay

Glutathione Synthase Deficiency (5-Oxoprolinuria, Pyroglutamic Acidemia)

5-Oxoprolinase deficiency. (No clear disease described.)

Clinical Symptoms

Acute neonatal crisis, neurologic symptoms, neurodegenerative symptoms, developmental delay, gastrointestinal disease, failure to thrive, hemolytic anemia, hypoglycemia, metabolic acidosis, or hyperammonemia

Diagnostic Studies

Blood and urine pyroglutamic acid level high; red cell glutathione level low. Amino acid studies in blood and urine. Organic acid analysis in urine.

Hartnup Disease

Hartnup disease is due to transport deficiency of neutral amino acids.

Clinical Symptoms

Dermatologic abnormalities similar to pellagra are usually present. Neurologic symptoms, developmental delay, psychiatric disorders occur rarely. Screening abnormality of urine amino acids.

Definitive Diagnosis

Neutral amino acids are found in excess in urine but not in blood. Urinary levels of proline, hydroxyproline, and arginine are normal, which distinguishes Hartnup disease from generalized amino acidurias of kidney disease, etc.

Hyperammonemia-Hyperornithinemia-Homocitrullinemia Syndrome

Clinical Symptoms

Signs of hyperammonemia, coma, weakness, hyperreflexia, developmental delay

Diagnostic Studies

Plasma levels of specific amino acids

Hypertyrosinemic Disorders

- Tyrosinemia type I
- Oculocutaneous tyrosinemia (tyrosinemia type II)
- Primary deficiency of 4-hydroxyphenylpyruvate dioxygenase (tyrosinemia type III)
- Transient tyrosinemia

- Hawkinsinuria
- Alkaptonuria

General Features

Clinical Symptoms
Developmental delay, ophthalmologic disorders, and dermatologic abnormalities in type II; neurologic symptoms, developmental delay, hepatocellular disease, hypoglycemia, metabolic acidosis and/or hyperammonemia in type III and Hawkinsinuria.

Diagnostic Studies
Amino acid quantitation in blood and urine. Blood or urine organic acid analysis with metabolite identification.

Definitive Diagnosis
Enzymatic assay or DNA analysis or both

Alkaptonuria (Homogentisic Acid Oxidase Deficiency)

Autosomal-recessive disorder in which absence of liver homogentisic acid oxidase causes excretion of homogentisic acid in urine.

Clinical Symptoms
Discolored urine, arthritis, skeletal abnormalities

Diagnostic Studies
Metabolite identification and quantitation in blood and urine.

Presumptive diagnosis by urine that becomes brown-black on standing and reduces Benedict solution (urine turns brown) and Fehling solution, but results of glucose-oxidase methods are negative. Ferric chloride test gives positive results (urine turns purple-black). Thin-layer chromatography and spectrophotometric assay identify urinary homogentisic acid but are not generally necessary for diagnosis.

Definitive Diagnosis
Enzymatic assay or DNA analysis or both

Hawkinsinuria

Infants <1 year develop lethargy, acidosis, failure to thrive; resolves after 1 year.

Diagnostic Studies
Urine levels of tyrosine and tyrosine metabolites are elevated. Urine contains 4-hydroxy cyclohexylacetic acid and hawkinsin, and smells like a swimming pool.

Tyrosinemia Type I (Fumarylacetoacetate Hydrolase Deficiency; Hepatorenal Tyrosinemia)

Clinical Symptoms
Acute neonatal crisis, neurologic symptoms, hepatocellular disease, visceromegaly, renal dysfunction, renal Fanconi syndrome, gastrointestinal disease, failure to thrive, hematologic abnormalities, hypoglycemia, metabolic acidosis or hyperammonemia, coagulation disorders, psychiatric disorders.

Diagnostic Studies
Amino acid quantitation in blood and urine. Increased blood and urine tyrosine and methionine levels. Increased blood phenylalanine level may cause positive test when screening for PKU. Urinary excretion of tyrosine metabolites *p*-hydroxyphenylpyruvic and *p*-hydroxyphenylacetic acids is increased; may be due to deficiency of enzyme fumarylacetoacetate hydrolase. May also be increased in myasthenia gravis, liver disease, ascorbic acid deficiency, malignancies. Carnitine metabolite identification. Specific identification of succinylacetone in blood or urine is diagnostic. Acetic and lactic acids may be increased in urine. Anemia, thrombocytopenia, and leukopenia are common. Urine δ-aminolevulinic acid level may be increased. Laboratory findings due to Fanconi syndrome, hepatic cirrhosis, and liver carcinoma are noted. Dietary restriction of tyrosine, phenylalanine, and methionine can correct biochemical and renal abnormalities but does not reverse or prevent progression of liver disease. Liver transplant can correct biochemical abnormalities. Prenatal diagnosis by measurement of succinylacetone in amniotic fluid has been used.

Definitive Diagnosis

Enzymatic assay or DNA analysis or both in liver biopsy or fibroblasts

Tyrosinemia Type II (Oculocutaneous)

Clinical Symptoms

Developmental delay, palmar and plantar hyperkeratosis, corneal ulcers, and photophobia may occur within the first months.

Diagnostic Studies

Tyrosinemia and tyrosyluria are suggestive; absent hepatic tyrosine transaminase is definitive.

Tyrosinemia Type III (4-Hydroxyphenylpyruvate Dioxygenase Deficiency)

Very rare, may be accompanied by developmental delay, seizures, ataxia, or self-mutilation

Diagnostic Studies

Tyrosinemia and tyrosyluria are moderate. Urine contains 4-hydroxyphenyl pyruvic, 4-hydroxyphenyl lactic, and 4-hydroxyphenylacetic acids. Enzyme activity decreased in liver biopsy specimen.

Transient Tyrosinemia

Due to incomplete development of tyrosine-oxidizing system, especially in premature or low-birth-weight infants. Usually asymptomatic but suggested by positive newborn phenylalanine screening test results.

Diagnostic Studies

Serum phenylalanine level is >4 mg/dL (5–20 mg/dL).

Serum tyrosine level is between 10 and 75 mg/dL.

Tyrosine metabolites in urine are ≤1 mg/mL (parahydroxyphenyl lactic and parahydroxyphenyl acetic acids); reversed within 24 hours by administration of ascorbic acid.

Lysine Oxidation Defects

Glutaryl-CoA dehydrogenase deficiency (glutaric acidemia I); 2-ketoadipic acid dehydrogenase deficiency (2-ketoadipic acidemia)

Clinical Symptoms

Acute neonatal crisis, neurologic symptoms, visceromegaly, developmental delay, hepatocellular disease, renal dysfunction, gastrointestinal disease, skeletal myopathy, dystonia, dyskinesia and hypotonia, failure to thrive, hypoglycemia, metabolic acidosis, hyperammonemia

Diagnostic Studies

Amino acids in blood and urine, and organic acids in urine are suggestive. Carnitine quantitation in blood and urine and ester identification are diagnostic.

Lysinuric Protein Intolerance

Clinical Symptoms

Gastrointestinal disease, hypoglycemia, metabolic acidosis, refusal to eat, hyperammonemia, and failure to thrive are prominent. Neurologic symptoms, developmental delay, hematologic abnormalities, coagulation disorders, pulmonary disease, renal dysfunction, and psychiatric disorders may occur.

Diagnostic Studies

Lysine, ornithine, arginine levels elevated in urine but decreased in blood.

Definitive Diagnosis

Demonstration of tissue transport defect and biochemical or DNA studies.

Organic Acidurias, Symptoms and Signs

General Symptoms Common to All Disorders

Decreased resistance to infections
Intermittent coma, Reye-like syndrome
Vomiting and failure to thrive
Hypotonia and lethargy
Hypoglycemia
Athetosis or ataxia
Peculiar odor
Myopathy
Neutropenia and thrombocytopenia
Isovaleric acidemia
Propionic acidemia
Methylmalonic acidemia
2-Methylacetoacetyl-CoA thiolase deficiency

Hypoglycemia

Maple syrup urine disease
3-Hydroxy-3-methylglutaconyl-CoA lyase deficiency
Methylmalonic acidemia
Glutaric acidemia types I and II
Ethylmalonic-adipic aciduria
Carnitine deficiency
Pyruvate carboxylase deficiency
Pyruvate dehydrogenase deficiency

Myopathy

Glycerol kinase deficiency
Carnitine deficiency
Glutaric acidemia type II

Phenylketonuria, Due to Phenylalanine Hydroxylase Deficiency (Mild, Moderate, or Severe)

Clinical Symptoms

Neurologic symptoms, neurodegenerative symptoms, developmental delay, failure to thrive, dermatologic abnormalities, newborn screening test abnormalities

Diagnostic Studies

Amino acid and pterin studies in blood and urine.

Normal blood phenylalanine = 2 mg/dL.

Classic PKU: High blood phenylalanine levels (usually >30 mg/dL and always >20 mg/dL in infancy) with phenylalanine and its metabolites in urine (incidence is 1 in 14,000); normal or decreased tyrosine concentration.

Less severe variant form of PKU: Blood phenylalanine levels are 15–30 mg/dL, and metabolites may appear in urine (incidence is 1 in 15,000).

Mild persistent hyperphenylalaninemia: Blood phenylalanine may be 2–12 mg/dL, and metabolites are not found in urine (incidence is 1 in 30,000); diet restriction is not required for this form.

For screening of newborns, urine phenylpyruvic acid level is no longer used. May not appear in urine until 2–3 weeks of age.

Preliminary blood screening tests (inhibition assay, fluorometry, paper chromatography) detect levels >4 mg/dL. Screening should be performed after protein-containing feedings have begun.

When repeat screening test results are positive, quantitative blood phenylalanine and tyrosine measurements confirm phenylalaninemia and exclude transient tyrosinemia of newborn. Diagnosis requires serum phenylalanine level ≥20 mg/dL. Urine ferric chloride test results are positive, and chromatography confirms presence of orthohydroxyphenylacetic acid.

Serial determinations should be performed in untreated borderline cases because blood levels may change markedly with time or due to stress and infection.

Definitive Diagnosis

DNA tests, liver phenylalanine hydroxylase levels

Phenylketonuria, Due to Disorders of Tetrahydrobiopterin Metabolism and Other Neurotransmitters

- Defects in biopterin synthesis
- Dihydropteridine reductase deficiency
- Guanosine triphosphate cyclohydrolase deficiency
- Segawa disease

Clinical Symptoms

Neurologic symptoms, neurodegenerative symptoms, developmental delay, failure to thrive, newborn screening test abnormality

Diagnostic Studies

Amino acid and pterin studies in blood and urine. Serum prolactin level. Metabolite identification and quantitation in blood, urine, and CSF.

Definitive Diagnosis

Enzymatic assay, DNA analysis if available (or both).

Pterins (Urine), Reference Ranges

	Xanthopterin (μmol/mol)	Neopterin (μmol/mol)	Total Biopterin (μmol/mol)	Tetrahydrobiopterin (% Total Biopterin)
Adult	100–350	250–400	450–1,000	20–65
Child	100–500	250–1,100	500–1,900	40–65

Sulfur Amino Acid (Cystine, Methionine) Disorders

Cobalamin Transport and Metabolism Disorders

Enterocyte cb1 malabsorption transcobalamin II deficiency
Intrinsic factor deficiency
R-binder deficiency

Clinical Symptoms

Neurologic symptoms, neurodegenerative symptoms, developmental delay, hepatocellular disease, gastrointestinal disease, skeletal myopathy, failure to thrive, hematologic abnormalities, hypoglycemia, metabolic acidosis or hyperammonemia, psychiatric disorders

Diagnostic Studies

Metabolite identification and quantitation in blood and urine. Amino acids in blood and organic acid analysis in blood or urine or both. Provocative tests or absorption studies or both.

Cystinuria

Clinical Symptoms

Renal calculi, urine amino acid abnormality

Diagnostic Studies

Amino acid quantitation in urine

Definitive Diagnosis

DNA analysis

Sulfite oxidase deficiency; see Molybdenum Metabolism Disorders.

Homocystinuria (Cystathionine Synthase Deficiency)

Clinical Symptoms

Failure to thrive, developmental delay, subluxed lenses and other eye defects, marfanoid stature, malar flush, osteoporosis, thromboembolism

Diagnostic Studies

Increased methionine and homocystine levels in blood and urine. Homocystine should be measured in fresh urine. Enzyme assay in liver biopsy specimen.

Response to vitamin B_6, folic acid, vitamin B_{12}, cysteine supplements, betaine; dietary methionine should be limited.

Other forms have specific defects in (a) methylcobalamin formation with megaloblastic anemia and hypomethioninemia (type II, complementation studies in fibroblasts) and (b) defect in methylene tetrahydrofolate reductase (type III, enzyme assay in fibroblast cultures or leukocytes).

Methionine Synthase Deficiency (cb1E and cb1G)

Clinical Symptoms

Neurologic symptoms, developmental delay, hematologic abnormalities

Diagnostic Studies

Metabolite identification and quantitation in blood and urine. Amino acid and organic acid analysis in blood or urine. Carnitine quantitation in blood or urine.

Definitive Diagnosis

Enzymatic assay or DNA analysis or both

Urea Cycle Defects

See Fig. 2 and Table 3.

The urea cycle consists of five enzymes responsible for the elimination of ammonia as urea: carbamoyl phosphate synthetase I (CPSI), OTC, argininosuccinate synthetase, argininosuccinate lyase (argininosuccinase), and arginase. CPSI and OTC are localized in the mitochondrial matrix; the other three enzymes are in the cytosol. The complete urea cycle is found only in the liver, where all five enzymes are induced in the perinatal period in a coordinated manner. Induction of the urea cycle enzymes is stimulated by dietary protein and hormones such as glucagon and glucocorticoids. In extrahepatic tissues, CPSI and OTC are expressed moderately in the small intestine, and argininosuccinate synthetase and argininosuccinate lyase are expressed strongly in the kidney and weakly in many other tissues.

Urea cycle disorders are characterized by the triad of encephalopathy, respiratory alkalosis, and hyperammonemia. A urea cycle disorder should be considered a diagnostic possibility in any patient of any age with occult encephalopathy. It is distinguished by absence of acidosis and ketosis and a very low serum urea level. At a few days of age, an affected infant develops lethargy, coma, convulsions after vomiting, and refusal to eat—signs frequently mistaken for infection or sepsis.

Hyperammonemia in the preterm infant may be due to transient hyperammonemia of the newborn, which is benign and responds to limitation of protein intake. In the newborn and older person, hyperammonemia occurs with many inborn errors of metabolism, including organic acidemias and fatty acid disorders.

Deficiencies of CPSI and OTC result in the more severe forms of urea cycle disorders. Argininosuccinate synthetase– and argininosuccinate lyase–deficient patients maintain the ability to excrete nitrogen in the form of citrulline, arginine, or argininosuccinic acid; presentation in these patients may be later in infancy. Although OTC deficiency presents in the neonatal period, both male patients with late onset and females may manifest a less severe form of the disease.

N-*Acetylglutamate Synthetase Deficiency*

Clinical Symptoms

Symptoms such as carbamoyl phosphate synthetase deficiency. Vomiting, lethargy, seizure.

Diagnostic Studies

Hyperammonemia, increased plasma levels of glutamate and alanine. Enzyme should be measured in liver biopsy specimen.

Ornithine Aminotransferase Deficiency

Gyrate atrophy of retina

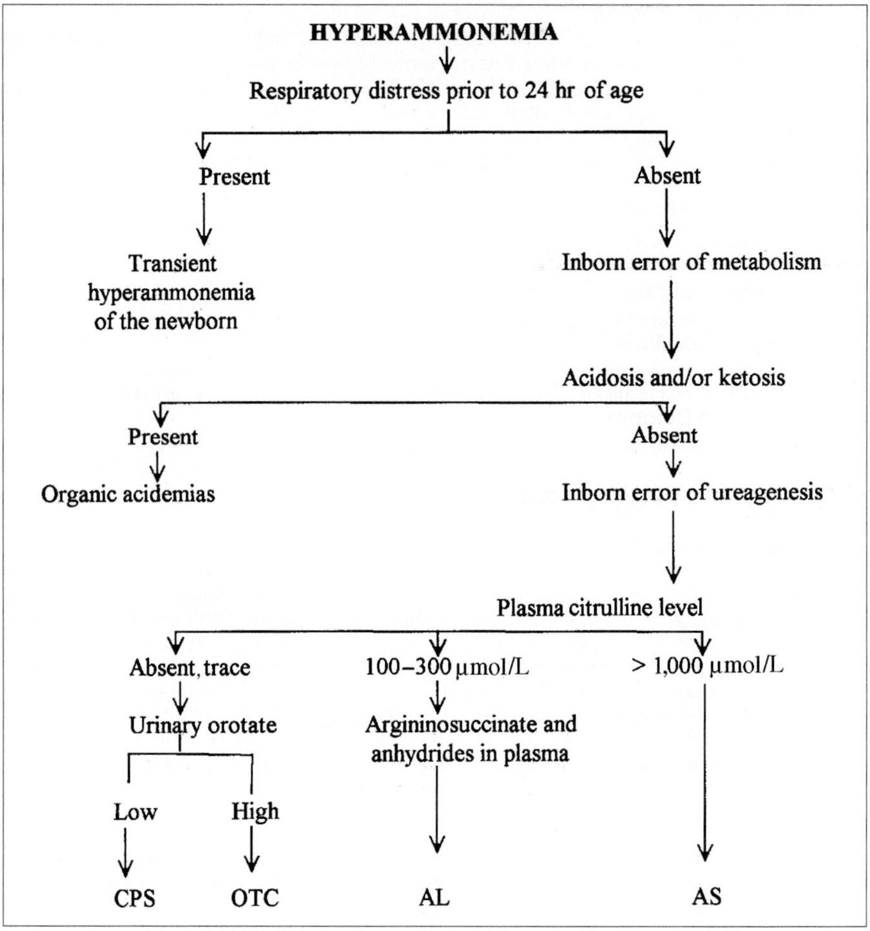

Fig. 2. Algorithm for determining the cause of hyperammonemia in a newborn. AL, argininosuccinase deficiency; AS, argininosuccinic acid synthetase deficiency; CPS, carbamoyl phosphate synthetase deficiency; OTC, ornithine transcarbamylase deficiency.

Clinical Symptoms

Ophthalmologic disorders, myopathy

Diagnostic Studies

Amino acids in blood and urine, enzymatic assay or DNA analysis or both

Fatty Acid Oxidation Disorders

See Table 4.

Common Laboratory Findings

Hypoglycemia
Hypoketosis (negative or 1+ urine ketones)
Elevated plasma levels of free fatty acids
Plasma free fatty acid level > β-hydroxybutyrate level

Table 3. Plasma Amino Acids, Urinary Orotic Acid, and Tissue for Enzyme Analysis in the Urea Cycle Disorders

Deficient Enzyme	Plasma Amino Acids	Urine Orotic Acid	Tissue for Enzyme Analysis
Urea cycle disorders			
Carbamoyl phosphate synthetase	↑Glutamic ↑Alanine ↓Citrulline ↓Arginine	Normal	Liver
Ornithine transcarbamylase	↑Glutamic ↑Alanine ↓Citrulline ↓Arginine	Increased	Liver
Argininosuccinate synthetase (argininosuccinate citrullinemia)	↑Citrulline ↓Arginine	Increased	Liver
Argininosuccinate lyase (argininosuccinic aciduria)	↑Citrulline ↑Argininosuccinate ↓Arginine	Increased	Red blood cells Liver
Arginase (argininemia)	↑Arginine	Increased	Red blood cells Liver
Related disorders			
N-acetylglutamine synthase	↑Glutamine ↑Arginine	Normal	Liver
Gyrate atrophy	↑Ornithine ↑Homocitrulline	Increased	Liver
Hyperornithinemia, hyperammonemia, homocitrullinuria	↑Ornithine ↑Homocitrulline	Increased	Liver
Lysinuric protein intolerance	↓Lysine ↓Arginine ↓Ornithine	Increased	Liver Intestine Cultured fibroblasts

↑, increased; ↓, decreased.

Acidosis
Mild to moderate increase in lactate level (especially in long-chain hydroxyacyl dehydrogenase deficiency)
Mild to moderate increase in aspartate aminotransferase (AST) and alanine aminotransferase (ALT) levels, usually without hyperbilirubinemia
Prothrombin time, partial thromboplastin time normal or mildly elevated
Elevated creatine phosphokinase level
Cardiac and skeletal muscle enzymes increased with episodic muscle weakness, rhabdomyolysis, myoglobinuria
Mild elevation of ammonia
Marked hyperuricemia
Low plasma carnitine level (except in carnitine palmitoyl transferase deficiency type I)
Elevated acylcarnitine level (except in carnitine palmitoyl transferase deficiency type I)
Specific accumulating acylcarnitines

Carnitine Metabolism Disorders

- Carnitine/acylcarnitine translocase deficiency
- Carnitine palmitoyltransferase deficiency (CPT I and II)
- Carnitine transport defect

Table 4. Characteristic Features of Fatty Acid Oxidation Defects

MIM No.	Disorder	Tissue Distribution	Chromosome Location	Symptoms and Signs	Laboratory Findings
212140	Carnitine deficiency	Kidney, heart, muscle, FB, liver		Cardiomyopathy, coma muscle weakness, Reye-like syndrome, sudden infant death	Glucose (P) ↓, ammonia (B) ↑, acidosis +, carnitine (P) ↑, long-chain acylcarnitine (P) N, cellular carnitine uptake ↓
255120	Carnitine palmitoyl	Liver, FB	11q22-q23	Coma, liver insufficiency, hepatomegaly	Glucose (P) ↓, ammonia (B) N or ↑, acidosis +, carnitine (P) N or ↑, long-chain acylcarnitine (P) N
212138	Acylcarnitine translocase	FB, liver, heart, muscle		Coma, cardiac abnormalities, liver insufficiency, vomiting	Glucose (P) ↓, ammonia (B) ↑, acidosis ±, free carnitine (P) ↓, acylcarnitine (P) ↑, long-chain acylcarnitine (P) ↑, seizures ±
255110	Carnitine palmitoyl	Muscle, heart, liver, FB	1p32	Coma, Reye-like syndrome, hepatomegaly, exercise intolerance, myalgia, cardiomyopathy, developmental delay ±, sudden death	Glucose (B) ↓, ketosis ↑,liver enzymes (P) ↑, CK (P) ↑, myoglobin (P, U) ↑, dicarboxylic acids (U) ±, carnitine (P) ↓, long-chain acylcarnitine (P) ↑
	Very-long-chain acyl-CoA dehydrogenase			Cardiomyopathy, coma, respiratory arrest, Reye-like syndrome, muscle weakness, muscle pain	Glucose (B) ↓, acidosis +, CK (P) ↑, dicarboxylic acids (U) ↑, $C_{14:1}$ acylcarnitine (P) ↑, carnitine (P) ↓, long-chain acylcarnitine (P) ↑
201450	Medium-chain acyl-CoA dehydrogenase	Muscle, liver, FB, WBC	1p31	Coma/lethargy, hepatopathy, hypotonia, apnea/respiratory arrest, sudden death, seizures ±, mental retardation, attention deficit disorder	Glucose (B) ↓, ketosis ±, acidosis +, transamines (P) ↑, ammonia (B) ↑, uric acid (P) ↑, dicarboxylic acids (U) N or ↑, glycine conjugates (U, P) ↑, decanoate (P) ↑, acylcarnitines (U) ↑, carnitine (P) N or ↓, long-chain acylcarnitine (P) N

201470	Short-chain acyl-CoA dehydrogenase	Muscle, liver, FB, WBC	12q22-qtr	Muscle weakness, lethargy, failure to thrive, mental retardation	Ketosis +, acidosis +, ethylmalonic acid (U) N or ↑, carnitine (P) ↓ or N
143450	Long-chain 3-hydroxyacyl-CoA	Liver, muscle, heart, FB, WBC	7	Coma/lethargy, hepatopathy, cardiomyopathy, neuropathy, retinopathy, muscle weakness, sudden death	Glucose (B) ↓, acidosis +, lactate (P) ↑, myoglobin (P, U) ↑, CK (P) ↑, dicarboxylic acids (U) ↑, hydroxy-dicarboxylic acids (U) ↑, long-chain 3-hydroxy fatty acids (P) ↑, carnitine (P) ↓, long-chain acylcarnitine (P) ↑
600890	Short-chain 3-hydroxyacyl-CoA dehydrogenase deficiency	Muscle, FB		Cardiomyopathy, muscle weakness, lethargy	Glucose (B) ↓, myoglobinuria +, CK (P) ↑, AST/ALT (P) ↑, ketosis +, ketones (U) ↑, dicarboxylic acids (U) N or ↑

↑, increased; ↓, decreased; +, present; ±, sometimes present; AST, aspartate transferase; ALT, alanine transferase; B, blood; CK, creatine kinase; CoA, coenzyme A; FB, fibroblasts; MIM, *Mendelian Inheritance in Man* system; N, normal; P, plasma; U, urine; WBC, white blood cells.

Children with organic acidemias excrete excess carnitine as esters and may present with signs of carnitine deficiency.

Clinical Symptoms

Acute neonatal crisis, neurologic symptoms, developmental delay, hepatocellular disease, visceromegaly, gastrointestinal disease, skeletal myopathy, cardiomyopathy, failure to thrive, hypoglycemia, metabolic acidosis, Reye syndrome, hyperammonemia.

Diagnostic Studies

Carnitine species identification and quantitation in blood, urine, or tissue. Amino and organic acid quantitation in blood or urine. Exercise physiology testing.

Definitive Diagnosis

Enzymatic assay or DNA analysis or both

Glutaric Acidemia Type I

Electron transfer flavoprotein deficiency
Electron transfer flavoprotein–ubiquinone oxidoreductase deficiency

Clinical Symptoms

Acute neonatal crisis, neurologic symptoms, visceromegaly, developmental delay, hepatocellular disease, renal dysfunction, gastrointestinal disease, skeletal myopathy and hypotonia, cardiomyopathy, failure to thrive, hypoglycemia, metabolic acidosis, hyperammonemia, immunologic abnormalities, dysmorphic features.

Diagnostic Studies

Amino and organic acid identification and quantitation in blood and urine. Carnitine species identification and quantitation in blood or urine.

Definitive Diagnosis

Enzymatic assay or DNA analysis or both

Disorders of Carbohydrate Metabolism

Urine-Reducing Substance

Galactose: galactosemia, galactokinase deficiency, severe liver disease
Fructose: hereditary fructose intolerance, essential fructosuria
Glucose: diabetes mellitus, renal glycosuria, Fanconi-type renal tubular acidosis
p-Hydroxyphenyl pyruvic acid: tyrosinemia
Xylose: pentosuria

Carbohydrate-Deficient Glycoprotein Syndrome

Carbohydrate-deficient glycoprotein syndrome encompasses a group of autosomal-recessive disorders resulting from defect in synthesis of the carbohydrate fraction of glycoproteins.

Developmental delay and growth failure are associated with dysmorphic features, including inverted nipples, prominent jaw and ears, skin dimples, and prominent fat pads. Infants may have hypotonia, hyperreflexia, strokelike episodes, and, later, ataxia and muscle atrophy of the lower extremities. Strabismus and retinitis pigmentosa are common.

Diagnostic Studies

Magnetic resonance imaging examination of brain reveals cerebellar hypoplasia; blood mannose level is decreased. Carbohydrate-deficient transferrin in serum and CSF determined by isoelectric focusing is diagnostic.

Fructose Metabolism Disorders

- Fructose-1,6-biphosphatase deficiency
- Fructose-1-phosphate aldolase deficiency (hereditary fructose intolerance)

Clinical Symptoms

Acute neonatal crises, hypoglycemia, metabolic acidosis, hepatocellular disease, renal Fanconi syndrome, failure to thrive, and recurrent vomiting

Diagnostic Studies

Reducing substances in urine; amino acids in blood and urine. Fructose tolerance tests contraindicated and dangerous. Metabolite identification in blood or urine, history of avoidance of sugar-containing foods.

Definitive Diagnosis

Enzyme assay or DNA analysis or both

Galactose Metabolism Disorders

Defects in liver and RBCs of galactose 1-phosphate uridyltransferase, which converts galactose to glucose, resulting in accumulation of galactose-1-phosphate

Normal blood levels for metabolic diseases

Galactose in urine	Not detectable
In blood	0–450
In urine	0–1,500
Galactose-1-phosphate in erythrocytes	
Nongalactosemic	5–49 µg/g Hb
Galactosemic (galactose-restricted diet)	80–125 µg/g Hb
Galactosemic (unrestricted diet)	>125 µg/g Hb
Galactose-1-phosphate uridyltransferase (galactosemia) in whole blood	18.5–28.5 U/g Hb
Galactokinase in whole blood	
<2 yr old	20–80 mU/g Hb
≥2 yr old	12–40 mU/g Hb

General Features

Clinical Symptoms

Acute neonatal crisis, neurologic symptoms, developmental delay, hepatocellular disease, visceromegaly, renal dysfunction, renal Fanconi syndrome, gastrointestinal disease, failure to thrive, ophthalmologic disorders, hypoglycemia, metabolic acidosis, coagulation disorders, cataracts, gonadal dysfunction.

Diagnostic Studies

Increased blood galactose of ≥300 mg/dL (normal is <5 mg/dL).

Increased urine galactose of 500–2,000 mg/dL (normal is <5 mg/dL). Positive urine reaction with Clinitest but negative with Clinistix and Tes-Tape; may be useful for pediatric screening up to 1 year of age.

Reduced RBC galactose-1-phosphate uridyltransferase establishes diagnosis.

Serum glucose may appear to be elevated in fasting state but falls as galactose increases; hypoglycemia is usual.

Galactose tolerance test is positive but not necessary for diagnosis and may be hazardous because of induced hypoglycemia and hypokalemia.

- Use an oral dose of 35 g of galactose/m^2 of body area.
- Normal: Serum galactose increases to 30–50 mg/dL; returns to normal within 3 hours.
- Galactosemia: Serum increase is greater, and return to baseline level is delayed.
- Heterozygous carrier: Response is intermediate.
- The test is not specific or sensitive enough for genetic studies.

Albuminuria.

General ammoaciduria is identified by chromatography.

Laboratory findings due to complications

- Jaundice (onset at age 4–10 days)
- Liver biopsy—dilated canaliculus filled with bile pigment with surrounding rosette of liver cells
- Severe hemolysis
- Coagulation abnormalities
- Vomiting, diarrhea, failure to thrive
- Hyperchloremic metabolic acidosis
- Cataracts
- Mental and physical retardation
- Decreased immunity (~25% of infants develop *Escherichia coli* sepsis that may cause death)

Findings disappear (but are not reversed) when galactose (e.g., milk) is eliminated from diet. Efficacy of diet is monitored by measuring RBC level of galactose-1-phosphate (desired range <4 mg/dL or <180 μg/g hemoglobin).

Screening incidence is 1 in 62,000 live births. Cord blood is preferred, but this prevents also screening for PKU, because latter test is normal in neonatal cord blood. Filter paper blood may show false-positive results for PKU, tyrosinemia, and homocystinuria. Test is invalidated by exchange transfusion.

Prenatal diagnosis is made by measurement of galactose-1-phosphate uridyltransferase in cell culture from amniotic fluid. Parents show <50% enzyme activity in RBCs.

Definitive Diagnosis

Enzymatic assay or DNA analysis or both

Galactokinase Deficiency

Clinical Symptoms

Cataracts, newborn screening test result abnormalities

Diagnostic Studies

Metabolite identification and quantitation in blood and urine

Definitive Diagnosis

Enzymatic assay or DNA analysis or both

Galactosemia

Diagnostic Studies

1. Elevated blood level of galactose and red blood cell (RBC) and tissue levels of galactose-1-phosphate.
2. Elevated urine levels of galactose, galactitol, and galactonic acid.
3. Aminoaciduria, typically gross and generalized.
4. Albuminuria.
5. Hyperchloremic acidosis.
6. Hyperbilirubinemia is predominantly due to liver damage but sometimes to hemolysis associated with Gram-negative bacterial sepsis in the neonate. The coincidence of the relatively frequent Gilbert gene and differences in degree of neonatal maturation of bilirubin glucuronyl transferase activity influence level of bilirubin.
7. Hypoglycemia is relatively infrequent.

Uridine 5'-Diphosphate Galactose-4-Epimerase Deficiency

Clinical Symptoms

Hepatocellular disease, developmental delay, newborn screening test abnormalities

Diagnostic Studies

Metabolite identification and quantitation in blood and urine

Definitive Diagnosis

Enzymatic assay or DNA analysis or both

Glycolytic Disorders

[Disorders of glycolysis (Embden-Meyerhof pathway) and the pentose monophosphate shunt in erythrocytes or muscles]

- Aldolase deficiency (RBC, muscle)
- Diphosphoglycerate mutase deficiency (RBC)
- Diphosphoglycerate phosphatase deficiency (RBC)
- Enolase deficiency (RBC)
- Glucose-6-phosphate dehydrogenase deficiency (RBC)
- Glucosephosphate isomerase deficiency (RBC, muscle)
- Lactate dehydrogenase deficiency (RBC, muscle)
- Lactate transporter deficiency (muscle)
- Phosphofructokinase deficiency (muscle) (glycogen storage disease type 7)
- Phosphoglycerate kinase deficiency (RBC, muscle)
- Phosphoglycerate mutase deficiency (RBC, muscle)
- Pyruvate kinase deficiency (RBC)
- Triose phosphate isomerase deficiency (RBC, muscle)

Clinical Symptoms

Hematologic abnormalities (RBC), myopathy (muscle), failure to thrive, hypoglycemia, metabolic acidosis

Diagnostic Studies

Myopathic: plasma creatine phosphokinase, carnitine levels, amino acid studies in blood and urine. Organic acid analysis in blood or urine or both. Exercise physiology testing. For RBC glycolytic disorders: RBC physiologic studies.

Definitive Diagnosis

Enzymatic assay or DNA analysis or both

Glycogen Storage Diseases

See Tables 5–7.

Glycogen Synthetase Deficiency (Glycogen Storage Disease Type 0)

Clinical Symptoms

Developmental delay, failure to thrive, hypoglycemia, labile hypoglycemia or hyperglycemia

Diagnostic Studies

Amino acid studies in blood and urine, organic acid analysis in blood or urine. Tolerance tests (including glucagon tolerance test). Confirmation by glycogen content in liver.

Definitive Diagnosis

Enzymatic assay or DNA analysis or both

Table 5. Glycogen Storage Diseases

MIM No.	Type	Inheritance	Enzyme Defect	Clinical/Pathologic Features	Pathology	Tissue for Diagnosis[a]
240600	0	AR	Glycogen synthetase	Hypoglycemia, failure to thrive, liver fibrosis	Glycogen is present (0.5% after meal)	Liver, muscle, RBC
232200	1a (von Gierke disease)	AR	Glucose-6-phosphatase	Hepatosplenomegaly, hypoglycemia, hyperlipidemia, acidosis, eruptive xanthomas, hepatic adenomas, hepatocellular carcinoma, no response to glucagon or epinephrine, kidney and GI mucosa involved	Uniform distribution of glycogen with distention of liver cells, mosaic pattern, small and large fat vacuoles, nuclear glycogenation; electron microscopy—uniform increase in normal-appearing glycogen, lipid droplets with glycogen particles within them, normal muscle	Liver
232210	1s (1asp)	AR	Stabilizing protein for glucose-6-phosphatase	Very early clinical onset		Liver
232220	1b	AR	Glucose-6-phosphate transporter protein	Like 1a plus neutropenia, recurrent infections, Crohn disease	Similar to type 1a	Liver
232240	1c		Microsomal phosphate transporter	Hepatomegaly	Uniform distribution of glycogen, mosaic pattern	Liver
232500	1d		Microsomal glucose transporter	Hepatomegaly	Uniform distribution of glycogen, mosaic pattern	Liver
232300	2 (Pompe disease)	AR	α-1,4-glycosidase (acid maltase)	Cardiomegaly, hepatomegaly, hypotonia, no hypoglycemia, macroglossia, generalized glycogenosis, CNS involvement, death usually by 1–2 yr	Uniform slight distention of liver cells, microvacuolation due to accumulation, nonmosaic pattern, fat absent; electron microscopy—glycogen vesicles surrounded by membranes (so-called lysosomes), muscle-marked glycogen deposition; muscle electron microscopy—excessive glycogen (free and in vesicles), loss of myofibrils	Liver, muscle, WBC, amniocytes, fibroblasts

232330	2b	?AR vs. XLR	Not established	Cardiac glycogenesis with survival to 2nd decade	Similar to type 2	Liver, muscle, WBC, amniocytes, fibroblasts
	2 (Antopol disease)	AD	Not established	Survival to 2nd to 4th decade	Similar to but milder changes than in type 2	Liver, muscle, WBC, amniocytes, fibroblasts
	2 (skeletal muscle type)	AR	Acid maltase	Childhood/adult onset, muscle weakness, cerebral aneurysms in adults	Changes in muscle similar to those in type 2	Muscle, WBC, amniocytes, fibroblasts
232400	3 (Forbes disease/Cori disease/limit dextrinosis)	AR	Amylo-1,6-glucosidase	Liver, skeletal muscle, heart involvement, hypoglycemia Response to glucagon	Uniform distension of liver cells due to glycogen, mosaic pattern, nuclear glycogenation, fibrous septa formation, small droplets of fat; electron microscopy—same as type 1 (lipid vacuoles less frequent); muscle electron microscopy—glycogen subsarcolemmal and between myofibrils	Liver, muscle, WBC
232500	4 (Andersen disease/amylopectinosis)	AR	Amylo-1,4-1,6-transglucosidase (brancher enzyme)	Cirrhosis, jaundice hepatosplenomegaly, CNS involvement, portal hypertension, sudden death in infancy; adult females with cardiomyopathy are heterozygotes; allelic form with clinical picture like muscular dystrophy in adults	Liver—pale, amphophilic, hyaline or vacuolated, PAS-positive, diastase-resistant material (amylopectin), particularly in periportal hepatocytes; variable, large lipid vacuoles, prominent septa formation progressing to cirrhosis; electron microscopy—fibrillar appearance of amylopectin; muscle—amylopectin deposits	Muscle, WBC, amniocytes, fibroblasts
232600	5 (McArdle disease)	AR	Myophosphorylase (1,4α-D-glucan, orthophosphate α-glucosyl transferase, D-glycanorthophosphatase-α-D-glucosyl transferase)	Muscle pain, weakness after exercise, myoglobinuria, good prognosis	Muscle—subsarcolemmal glycogen; electron microscopy—same as in light microscopy; liver—normal	Muscle enzyme histochemistry

(continued)

Table 5. (continued)

MIM No.	Type	Inheritance	Enzyme Defect	Clinical/Pathologic Features	Pathology	Tissue for Diagnosis[a]
232700	6 (Hers disease)	AR	Hepatophosphorylase	Hepatomegaly, mild to moderate hypoglycemia, good prognosis	Liver—nonuniform distention of hepatocytes due to glycogen, mosaic pattern, septa formation, small fat droplets; electron microscopy—burst appearance of glycogen, rosettes, lipid vacuoles with glycogen; muscle—normal	Liver, WBC, RBC
232800	7 (Tarui disease)	AR	Muscle phosphofructokinase	Muscle cramps, myoglobinuria, good prognosis	Muscle—subsarcolemmal glycogen; electron microscopy—same as in light microscopy	Muscle enzyme histochemistry
261750	8	AR	Hepatic phosphorylase	Hepatomegaly, growth retardation, lipidemia, progressive neurologic deterioration	Nonuniform distention of hepatocytes due to glycogen, mosaic pattern; electron microscopy—same as in type 6, less frequent lipid vacuoles with glycogen in them; muscle—subsarcolemmal glycogen; electron microscopy—same as in light microscopy	Liver, CNS (glucogen in axons)
306000		XLR	b Kinase			
306000	9	AR	Hepatic phosphorylase kinase	Marked hepatomegaly, mild hypoglycemia, good prognosis	Nonuniform distention of hepatocytes due to glycogen, mosaic pattern, septa formation, small lipid droplets; electron microscopy—same as in type 6, frequent lipid vacuoles with glycogen in them; muscle—normal	Liver
	10	AR	Cyclic 3',5' AMP-dependent kinase	Hepatomegaly, liver and muscle involvement, good prognosis	Nonuniform distention of hepatocytes due to glycogen, mosaic pattern, septa formation, small lipid droplets; electron microscopy—same as in type 6; muscle—subsarcolemmal glycogen	Liver, muscle

(continued)

Other forms of glycogen disease						
261740	Cardiac glycogenesis	AR	Cardiac, phosphorylase kinase	Causes early death	Cardiac glycogenosis	Cardiac muscle
	Glycogenesis of liver/skeletal muscle			Hepatomegaly, muscle weakness	Glycogenosis of liver and skeletal muscle	Liver, skeletal muscle
	(a)	AR	Phosphorylase kinase			
	(b)	AR	Phosphoglucomutase			
	Glycogen myopathy with hemolytic anemia	AR	Hexokinase	Muscle weakness	Glycogenosis of muscle	Muscle
	Hepatic glycogenesis, hemolytic anemia, mental retardation	AR	Aldolase 1 (aldolase A)	Hepatomegaly hemolytic anemia	Hepatic glycogenosis	Liver
138550	Cerebral glycogenosis	AR	Brain glycogen phosphorylase	CNS symptoms	Involvement of cerebral cortex deep nuclei, cerebellar cortex, glycogen in neurons and astrocytic processes PAS-positive, diastase sensitive	Brain
138550	Glycogen storage disease with renal tubular dysfunction	AR	Unknown (defective galactose oxidation)	Failure to thrive, hepatomegaly, hypophosphatemic rickets	Glycogen accumulation in liver and proximal renal tubular cells	Liver, kidney

AD, autosomal dominant; AMP, adenosine monophosphate; AR, autosomal recessive; CNS, central nervous system; MIM, *Mendelian Inheritance in Man* system; PAS, periodic acid–Schiff; RBC, red blood cells; WBC, white blood cells; XLR, X-linked recessive.

[a]Tissues should be fixed in alcohol for preservation of glycogen. Lipid stains should be done on frozen sections. Tests for absence of myophosphorylase in type 5 and phosphofructokinase in type 7 done on snap-frozen (–70°C) muscle biopsy specimen by enzyme histochemistry. Biochemical studies done on tissue wrapped in aluminum foil and fresh-frozen (–70°C) (liver or muscle). Transport on dry ice by overnight mail to reference laboratory. WBC skin fibroblasts and amniocytes should be shipped at room temperature; avoid freezing or overheating.

Table 6. Morphologic Differentiation of Glycogenoses

Types	Lobular Pattern	Liver Nuclear Hyperglycogenation	Septa Formation	Cytoplasmic Lipid	Muscle
1	Uniform, mosaic	+	–	Prominent large vacuoles plus small droplets	Normal
2	Uniform, nonmosaic; cytoplasmic, microvesiculation	–	–	Absent	Massive glycogen deposits with loss of myofibrils
3	Uniform, mosaic	+	+	Small droplets	Subsarcolemmal glycogen or normal
4	Peripheral amylopectin deposits	–	+ (cirrhosis)	Variable, large vacuoles	Focal basophilic deposits
5	Normal	–	–	Absent	Subsarcolemmal glycogen
6	Nonuniform, mosaic	–	+	Small droplets	Normal
7	Normal	–	–	–	Subsarcolemmal glycogen
8	Nonuniform, mosaic	–	–	Absent	Normal
9	Nonuniform, mosaic	–	+	Small droplets	Normal
10	Nonuniform, mosaic	–	+	Small droplets	Subsarcolemmal glycogen

+, present; –, absent.
From McAdams AJ, Hug G, Bove KE. Glycogen storage disease, types I to X. *Hum Pathol* 1974;5:463.

Glycogen Storage Disease Type 1A (von Gierke Disease)

In glycogen storage disease type 1A, patients present with enlarged liver and kidneys and a tendency to episodes of hypoglycemia. Patients have a "doll" face and stunted growth, hypoglycemia, ketosis, lactic acidosis, hyperlipidemia, hyperuricemia, gout, and, occasionally, bleeding episodes. Xanthomas are common. A variant of type 1A is due to a deficiency of stabilizing protein.

Diagnostic Studies

Note: Glucose oxidase filter strip detects only glucose; Benedict solution detects all sugars.

Blood glucose level is markedly decreased.

After overnight fast, marked hypoglycemia and increased blood lactate and occasionally pyruvate with severe metabolic acidosis, ketonemia, and ketonuria. (Recurrent acidosis is most common cause for hospital admission.)

Blood triglyceride levels are high; cholesterol level is moderately increased, and serum free fatty acid levels are increased with xanthomas and lipid-laden cells in bone marrow.

Mild anemia is present. Impaired platelet function may cause bleeding tendency. Serum uric acid level increased with nephrocalcinosis, proteinuria. Serum phosphorus and

Table 7. Tissues Useful in Diagnosis of Storage Diseases

Organ or Tissue	Manifestation	Disease to Be Considered	Presumptive Test	Diagnostic Test
Liver	Increased size; disordered liver function test results in some, but not all, patients with the disease	α_1-Antitrypsin deficiency	Plasma α_1-antitrypsin	Electrophoresis and inorganic phosphate typing; immunopathology, electron microscopy on liver biopsy specimen
		Cholesteryl ester storage disease	Liver biopsy	Fibroblast acid lipase
		Mucopolysaccharidoses	Urine mucopolysaccharide quantitation; electron microscopy of conjunctival biopsy	Specific enzyme analysis
		Glycoproteinoses	Urine oligosaccharides; electron microscopy of conjunctival biopsy	Specific enzyme analysis
		Mucolipidoses types II, III	Urine oligosaccharides; electron microscopy of conjunctival biopsy	Fibroblasts, lysosomal enzymes
		Glycogen storage disease	Conjunctival biopsy (type 2), liver biopsy, electron microscopy	Electron microscopy (type 2)
		Niemann-Pick disease	Conjunctival biopsy, liver biopsy, electron microscopy	Leukocyte or fibroblast sphingomyelinase
		Gaucher disease	Gaucher cells in liver, bone marrow; increased serum total hexosaminidase or acid phosphatase	Leukocyte or fibro-β-glucosidase; electron microscopy
		Wolman disease	Liver biopsy	Fibroblast acid lipase
Spleen	Increased size	Mucopolysaccharidoses	Urine mucopolysaccharide quantitation; electron microscopy of conjunctival biopsy specimen	Specific enzyme analysis
		Gaucher disease	Gaucher cells in bone marrow	Leukocyte or fibroblast β-glucosidase; electron microscopy
		Niemann-Pick disease	Conjunctiva, bone marrow, or liver biopsy; electron microscopy	Leukocyte or fibroblast sphingomyelinase

(continued)

Table 7. (continued)

Organ or Tissue	Manifestation	Disease to Be Considered	Presumptive Test	Diagnostic Test
Bone and joint	Dysostosis multiplex, other radiographic changes	Mucopolysaccharidoses	Urine mucopolysaccharide quantitation; electron analysis microscopy of conjunctival biopsy specimen	Specific enzyme
		Glycoproteinoses	Urine oligosaccharide determination; electron microscopy of conjunctival biopsy specimen	Specific enzyme analysis
	Swollen joints, soft tissue nodules	Farber disease	Tissue biopsy for electron microscopy	Fibroblast culture; lysosomal acid ceramidase
Eye	Macular cherry-red spot	Tay-Sachs disease	Serum hexosaminidase A	Leukocyte or fibroblast hexosaminidase A
		Sandhoff disease	Serum total hexosaminidase	Leukocyte or fibroblast total hexosaminidase
		Niemann-Pick disease	Conjunctival, bone marrow, or liver biopsy; electron microscopy	Leukocyte or fibroblast sphingomyelinase
		Generalized gangliosidosis	White cell β-galactosidase, occasionally urine oligosaccharide increases can be seen by thin layer chromatography; conjunctival, bone marrow biopsies; electron microscopy	Leukocyte or fibroblast β-galactosidase
		Sialidoses	Urinary oligosaccharide excretion, conjunctival biopsy for electron microscopy	Fibroblast sialidase
	Corneal clouding	Mucopolysaccharidoses (Hunter, Scheie, Morquio, Maroteaux-Lamy syndromes, β-glucuronidase deficiency)	Urine mucopolysaccharides; conjunctival biopsy for electron microscopy	Specific enzyme analysis
		Mucolipidoses types II, III	Urinary oligosaccharide excretion; conjunctival biopsy for electron microscopy	Fibroblast lysosomal enzymes
	Crystal in lens	Cystinosis	Cystine crystals in tissues	Cystine in leukocytes, fibroblasts
Adrenal gland	Bilateral adrenal calcification	Wolman disease	Liver biopsy	Fibroblast acid lipase

Muscle—cardiac, skeletal	Cardiomegaly; heart failure	Pompe disease	Electron microscopy of conjunctiva, lymphocytes, or skin	Lymphocyte or fibroblast α-glucosidase; electron microscopy
	Myopathy involving skeletal muscle	Glycogen storage disease types 3, 4	Liver biopsy for electron microscopy	Specific enzyme analysis
Brain	Progressive mental and motor dysfunction; retardation	Krabbe disease	Conjunctival biopsy for microscopy CSF protein (increased)	Galactocerebroside β-galactosidase, leukocytes, or fibroblast culture
		Metachromatic leukodystrophy	Conjunctival biopsy for electron microscopy; CSF protein (increased); sural nerve biopsy; nerve conduction studies	Arylsulfatase A, fibroblast culture
		Neuronal ceroid lipofuscinoses		Peripheral blood lymphocyte, skin, conjunctival biopsy for electron microscopy
		Niemann-Pick disease	Conjunctival, bone marrow, or liver biopsy	Leukocyte or fibroblast sphingomyelinase
		Gaucher disease	Gaucher cells in bone marrow, liver	Leukocyte or fibroblast; β-glucosidase; electron microscopy
		Mucopolysaccharidoses	Urine mucopolysaccharide quantitations; electron microscopy of several tissues from biopsy including conjunctiva	Specific enzyme analysis
		Glycoproteinoses	Urine oligosaccharide determination; electron microscopy of conjunctival biopsy specimen	Specific enzyme analysis
		Tay-Sachs disease	Serum hexosaminidase A	Leukocyte or fibroblast hexosaminidase A
		Sandhoff disease	Serum total hexosaminidase	Leukocyte or fibroblast total hexosaminidase
		Generalized gangliosidosis	White cell β-galactosidase; urine oligosaccharide thin layer chromatography; conjunctival, bone marrow biopsy for electron microscopy	Leukocyte or fibroblast β-galactosidase

CSF, cerebrospinal fluid.

alkaline phosphatase levels are decreased. Urinary levels of nonspecific amino acids are increased, without increase in blood amino acid levels. Fanconi syndrome is rare.

Liver function test results (other than those related to carbohydrate metabolism) are relatively normal, but serum γ-glutamyltransferase, AST, and ALT levels may be increased.

Glucose tolerance may be normal or diabetic type; diabetic type is more frequent in older children and adults.

Functional Tests

Administer 1 mg of glucagon intravenously or intramuscularly after 8-hour fast. Blood glucose level increases 50–60% in 10–20 minutes in the normal person. Little or no increase occurs in infants or young children with von Gierke disease; delayed response may occur in older children and adults.

Intravenous administration of glucose precursors (e.g., galactose or fructose) causes no rise in blood glucose level, which demonstrates block in gluconeogenesis, but normal rise occurs in limit dextrinosis (type 3 glycogen storage disease).

Biopsy of liver: biochemical studies.

Absent or markedly decreased glucose-6-phosphatase level on assay of frozen liver provides definitive diagnosis.

- Increased glycogen content (>4% by weight) but normal biochemically and structurally.
- Other enzymes (other glycogen storage diseases) are present in normal amounts.

Histologic findings are not diagnostic; vacuolization of hepatic cells and abundant glycogen granules are seen.

Biopsy of jejunum

- Intestinal glucose-6-phosphatase is decreased or absent.

Biopsy of muscle shows no abnormality of enzyme activity or glycogen content.

Definitive Diagnosis

Enzyme assay, deficient hepatic glucose-6-phosphatase, or DNA analysis.

Glycogen Storage Disease Type 1B

Glycogen storage disease type 1B shows all the clinical and biochemical features of von Gierke disease except that liver biopsy specimen does not show deficiency of glucose-6-phosphatase.

Clinical Symptoms

Patient may have maturation-arrest neutropenia; varies from mild to agranulocytosis; usually constant but may be cyclic. Associated increased frequency of staphylococcal and *Candida* infection.

Diagnostic Studies

Established by finding of impaired function of glucose-6-phosphatase activity in granulocytes.

Glycogen Storage Disease Type 2 (Pompe Disease)

Clinical Symptoms

Classic infantile form (type 2A) characterized by neurologic, cardiac, and muscle involvement, frequently by liver enlargement, death within first year; juvenile form (type 2B) shows muscle disease resembling pseudohypertrophic dystrophy; adult form (type 2C) characterized by progressive myopathy.

Diagnostic Studies

Aerobic and anaerobic exercise physiology testing. Muscle biopsy. Fasting blood glucose level, glucose tolerance test, glucagon response test, and rises in blood glucose after fructose infusion are normal. Acetonuria is not present. General hematologic findings are normal. Staining of circulating leukocytes for glycogen shows massive deposition of glycogen.

Diagnosis confirmed by finding of an absence of α-1,4-glucosidase in muscle and liver biopsy specimens of cultured fibroblasts. Assay in amniotic cell culture.

Definitive Diagnosis

Enzyme assay (acid maltase), deficient lysosomal and glucosidase, or DNA analysis.

Glycogen Storage Disease Type 3

Autosomal-recessive disease with enlarged liver, retarded growth, chemical changes, and benign course.

Diagnostic Studies

Serum creatine kinase level may be increased. Mild increase in cholesterol and triglycerides. Marked fasting acetonuria (as in starvation). Fasting hypoglycemia is less severe than in type 1 disease. Normal blood lactate level; uric acid level is usually normal. Serum AST and ALT levels are increased in children but normal in adults. Diabetic type of glucose tolerance curve with associated glucosuria.

Infusion of gluconeogenic precursors (e.g., galactose, fructose) causes a normal hyperglycemic response unlike in type 1 disease. Low fasting blood sugar does not show expected rise after administration of subcutaneous glucagon or epinephrine but does increase 2 hours after high-carbohydrate meal.

Diagnosis confirmed by liver and muscle biopsy specimens that show biochemical findings of increased glycogen, abnormal glycogen structure, absence of specific enzyme activity. Normal phosphorylase and glucose-6-phosphatase activity. Deficient amylo-1-6-glucosidase (debrancher enzyme).

Glycogen Storage Disease Type 4 (Andersen Disease; Brancher Deficiency; Amylopectinosis)

Due to absence of amylo(1,4→1,6)-transglucosidase. Hypoglycemia is not present.

Diagnostic Studies

Liver function test results may be altered as in other types of cirrhosis (e.g., slight increase in serum bilirubin level, reversed albumin/globulin ratio, increased AST level, decreased cholesterol level). Blood glucose response to epinephrine and glucagon may be flat.

Biopsy specimen from liver may show a cirrhotic reaction to glycogen of abnormal structure, which stains with Best carmine and periodic acid–Schiff stains.

WBC may be increased and hemoglobin may be decreased.

Definitive Diagnosis

Enzyme assay

Glycogen Storage Disease Type 5 (McArdle Disease; Myophosphorylase Deficiency)

Autosomal-recessive disease due to absent myophosphorylase in skeletal muscle; patient shows very limited ischemic muscle exercise tolerance despite normal appearance of muscle.

Diagnostic Studies

Administration of epinephrine or glucagon causes a normal hyperglycemic response.

Muscle biopsy specimen is microscopically normal in young; vacuolation and necrosis are seen in later years. Increased glycogen is present.

Exercise quickly causes muscle cramping and weakness. Regional blood lactate and pyruvate levels do not increase. Similar abnormal response occurs in type 3 disease involving muscle and in types 7, 8, 10.

Myoglobulinuria may occur after strenuous exercise. Increased serum levels of muscle enzymes (e.g., lactate dehydrogenase, creatine kinase, aldolase) for several hours after strenuous exercise.

Definitive Diagnosis

Enzyme assay or DNA analysis or both

Glycogen Storage Disease Type 6 (Hepatic Phosphorylase Deficiency)

Clinical Symptoms

Enlarged liver present from birth. Hypoglycemia uncommon.

Diagnostic Studies

Serum levels of cholesterol and triglycerides are mildly increased. Serum uric acid and lactic acid levels are normal. Liver function test results are normal. Fructose tolerance is normal. Response to glucagon and epinephrine is variable but tends to be poor.

Diagnosis is based on decreased phosphorylase activity in liver, leukocytes, and RBC hemolysate, but muscle phosphorylase is normal.

Glycogen Storage Disease Type 7

Autosomal-recessive disease with deficiency of muscle phosphofructokinase.

Diagnostic Studies

Fasting hypoglycemia is marked. RBCs show 50% decrease in phosphofructokinase activity.

Other members of family may have reduced tolerance to glucose.

Clinically identical to type 5 disease.

Definitive Diagnosis

Muscle biopsy specimen shows marked decrease in phosphofructokinase activity (1–3% of normal).

Glycogenosis Type 8

Hepatomegaly from very early childhood with progressive degeneration of the CNS. Initial truncal ataxia, nystagmus, hypotonia, and catecholaminuria are typically followed by spasticity and progress to decerebration. The disease is fatal in childhood. There is no hypoglycemia, and the blood glucose response to epinephrine or glycogen is normal.

Definitive Diagnosis

The diagnosis is confirmed by the demonstration of low liver phosphorylase activity despite normal levels of total liver phosphorylase (i.e., active and inactive) and an intact phosphorylase activating system.

Glycogenosis Type 9 (Liver Phosphorylase Kinase Deficiency)

Hepatomegaly with mild hypoglycemia is found. Skeletal muscle is normal biochemically and morphologically. Glycogen-distended hepatocytes tend to be in periportal locations. The cell membranes appear coarse and may be undulated. Septa formation is prominent, and there may be low-grade inflammatory changes. There is no nuclear hyperglycogenation. Cytoplasmic vacuoles are prominent. There is no hypoglycemia.

By electron microscopy, the appearance of the liver cells is very similar to that in types 6 and 10 except that lipid bodies with glycogen inclusions may be more frequent.

Definitive Diagnosis

The low phosphorylase activity in type 9 glycogenosis is due not to phosphorylase deficiency but to deficient activity of phosphorylase kinase.

Glycogenosis Type 10

Asymptomatic hepatomegaly with no hypoglycemia and no blood glucose rise after glucagon administration.

Unlike in glycogenosis types 6, 8, and 9, there is also increased glycogen in the muscle.

Definitive Diagnosis

Demonstration in liver and muscle of normal total phosphorylase level. Complete inactivation of muscle phosphorylase is the result of deficient activity of cyclic adenosine monophosphate–dependent kinase.

Lysosomal Storage Disorders

See Table 7.

Glycoprotein Metabolism Disorders

See Table 8.

- Mucolipidosis II (I-cell disease)
- Mucolipidosis III (pseudo-Hurler polydystrophy)
- α-*N*-acetylgalactosaminidase deficiency (Schindler disease)
- α-Mannosidosis
- β-Mannosidase deficiency (β-mannosidosis)
- α-Fucosidase deficiency (fucosidosis)
- Aspartylglycosaminuria
- Neuraminidase deficiency (sialidosis)

Aspartylglycosaminuria

Aspartylglycosaminuria is due to deficient activity of aspartylglucosaminidase. It manifests as a dysmorphic syndrome resembling Hurler disease at approximately 1 year of age. This disorder occurs primarily in Finland.

Infants with this disorder are healthy for the first few months of life. Recurrent infections, diarrhea, and hernias are noted during the first year. Head circumference and stature are decreased later in childhood and sometimes hepatomegaly is observed. Coarsening of the facies and sagging skin folds are subtle in the first decade. Acne and sun sensitivity occur. Crystal-like lens opacities, joint laxity, macroglossia, hoarse voice, short stature, skeletal dysplasia, and brachycephaly occur. Mental development is relatively normal until 5 years of age, except for delayed speech. Mental deterioration occurs with intelligence quotient values usually <40 in adults. Clumsiness, hypotonia, and spasticity, and cardiac valvular involvement and angiokeratomas have been reported. Death occurs in the fourth or fifth decade.

Radiographic changes show very mild dysostosis multiplex, with wedge-shaped vertebral bodies later in life and thickening of the cortex of the skull. Cerebral atrophy may occur.

Diagnostic Studies

Diagnosis of aspartylglycosaminuria is based on the measurement of aspartylglucosaminidase activity in an easily obtained tissue source, such as sonicates of WBCs, fibroblasts, or amniotic fluid cells.

Prenatal Diagnosis

Cultured amniotic fluid cells as well as chorionic villus samples show aspartylglucosaminidase activity, and a DNA-based test suitable for the detection of the mutation is available.

Table 8. Clinical Features of Mannosidosis, Fucosidosis, Sialidosis, and Aspartylglycosaminuria

Disorder	Age of Onset	Facies	Dysostosis Multiplex	Neurologic Findings	Hepatosplenomegaly	Eye Findings	Hematologic Findings	Other Findings
Mannosidosis/α-mannosidosis/glycoproteins with α-linked mannose residues								
Type I	3–12 mo	Coarse	+++	Severe mental retardation	+++	Cataracts, corneal opacities	Vacuolated lymphocytes	Hearing loss
Type II	1–4 yr	Coarse	++	Mental retardation	++	Cataracts, corneal opacities	Vacuolated lymphocytes	Hearing loss prominent
β-Mannosidosis	<1–6 yr	Some dysmorphism	±	Mental retardation	–	–	–	Angiokeratomas, recurrent infection
Fucosidosis/α-fucosidase/ fucose-containing sphingolipids, glycoproteins, oligosaccharides								
Type I	3–18 mo	Mild coarsening	++	Mental retardation, seizures	++	Infrequent	Vacuolated lymphocytes	Sweat, NaCl increased
Type II	1–2 yr	Mild coarsening	++	Mental retardation	++	Tortuous conjunctival vessels	Vacuolated lymphocytes	Angiokeratoma, anhidrosis

Sialidosis/neuraminidase/glycoproteins, oligosaccharides								
Type I	8–25 yr	Normal	–	Severe myoclonus, generalized seizures, neuropathy, deep tendon reflexes	–	Blindness, cherry-red spots	Vacuolated lymphocytes rarely	
Type II juvenile	2–20 yr	Mild coarsening	++	Myoclonus, mental retardation	–	Reduced acuity, cherry-red spots	Vacuolated lymphocytes	Angiokeratoma
Sialic acid storage disease								
Infantile	0–12 mo	Coarse	+++	Mental retardation	±	Cherry-red spots	Vacuolated lymphocytes	Renal involvement
Congenital	In utero	Coarse	+++	Mental retardation	++	?	Vacuolated lymphocytes	Hydrops fetalis, stillbirth
Aspartylglucosaminuria/aspartylglucosaminidase/glycoproteins with aspartyglucosamine moieties	1–5 yr	Coarse, sagging skin	+	Mental retardation	–	Lens opacities	Vacuolated lymphocytes	Acne, sun sensitivity

++, pronounced; +++, severe; –, not present; ±, sometimes present.

Fucosidosis

Fucosidosis is caused by deficiency of α-L-fucosidase that leads to the accumulation of fucose-containing sphingolipids, glycoproteins, and oligosaccharides. Clinical onset ranges from infancy to adolescence. It is panethnic, but the majority of reported patients have been from Italy or the southwestern part of the United States. The more severely affected patients (type I, fatal infantile) develop symptoms within the first year of life, with the onset of psychomotor retardation, coarse facies, growth retardation, cardiomegaly, dysostosis multiplex, neurologic retardation, and increase in sweat sodium chloride level. The milder phenotypes (type II) are characterized by signs occurring at 1–2 years of age, presence of angiokeratoma, longer survival, and a more normal level of sweat sodium chloride.

Diagnostic Studies

A modified thin-layer chromatography method is based on the simultaneous detection of both urinary oligosaccharides and glycopeptides or analysis by high-pressure liquid chromatography. Lymphocytes are vacuolated.

Diagnosis is based on the enzymatic assay of α-L-fucosidase in any available cell type, particularly WBCs and cultured fibroblasts.

Fucosidase activity and protein concentration measured by an enzyme-linked immunosorbent assay may yield more definitive clinical results.

Mannosidosis

Mannosidosis is a lysosomal storage disease characterized by a deficiency in the lysosomal enzyme α-mannosidase, which results in an excessive accumulation of mannose-containing oligosaccharides in the cells of the nervous system, liver, spleen, and bone marrow. Patients with the disease have a Hurler-like facies, show mental retardation, and lack motor coordination. The clinical course is relatively benign compared to that of many of the other storage diseases that involve the CNS.

Diagnostic Studies

Patients affected with α-mannosidosis excrete increased amounts of oligosaccharides, particularly Man (α1→3) Man (β1→4)GlcNAc. Urinary screening for oligosaccharides by high-pressure liquid chromatography quantitates oligosaccharides in urine and fibroblasts.

Acid α-mannosidase activity, determined in WBCs, fibroblasts, or cultured amniotic fluid cells or trophoblasts, is severely reduced. Direct measurement of α-mannosidase in plasma has been less reliable because of the presence of forms of mannosidase enzymes in plasma that are not decreased in patients with mannosidosis.

Laboratory findings include vacuolated lymphocytes with globular inclusions in vacuoles testing positive for acid phosphatase. Most patients do not have mucopolysacchariduria. Decreased serum levels of immunoglobulin G can occur, and a decreased PR interval on electrocardiogram is reported.

Mucolipidoses

I-cell disease is differentiated from Hurler syndrome by the absence of mucopolysacchariduria. I-cell (inclusion-cell) disease is so named because of numerous phase-dense inclusions in the cytoplasm of cultured fibroblasts from affected individuals. Similar inclusions have since been seen in cells from patients with mucolipidosis I and pseudo-Hurler polydystrophy (mucolipidosis III).

Mucolipidosis II is characterized by a deficiency of multiple lysosomal enzymes in cultured fibroblasts and an increased concentration in culture medium, serum, and other body fluids.

Diagnostic Studies

The diagnosis of both mucolipidosis II and mucolipidosis III can be confirmed by measuring the activities of lysosomal enzymes in serum or in cultured fibroblasts. Tenfold to 20-fold increases in β-hexosaminidase, iduronate sulfatase, and arylsulfatase A are characteristic of both mucolipidosis II and mucolipidosis III. Lysosomal enzyme activities in WBCs are not reliable for diagnosis. The level of *N*-acetylglucosamine phosphotransferase activity in WBCs or cultured fibroblasts can be measured directly with commercially available substrates.

Activity of plasma hyaluronidase, an endoglycosidase of presumably lysosomal origin, is not increased in the plasma from individuals with mucolipidosis II and III, unlike most lysosomal enzymes.

Sialic Acid Storage Disease

- Infantile sialic acid storage disease
- Salla disease
- Sialuria
- Mucolipidosis IV
- Galactosialidosis

Clinical Symptoms

Children present with hepatosplenomegaly, coarse facies, and massive urinary excretion of sialic acid, dysostosis multiplex, and early death. The chronic form with a prolonged life span is known as *Salla disease*. The more severe infantile sialic acid storage disease is less common and does not show ethnic prevalence.

Infantile sialic acid storage disease is a lysosomal storage disorder characterized by accumulation of free sialic acid within lysosomes, which results in progressive neurologic degeneration, multiorgan failure, and death in early childhood. Disease onset is between 3 and 6 months of age, with lag of developmental milestones, delay or absence of walking, impaired speech development, and severe mental retardation.

Diagnostic Studies

The diagnostic test for both Salla disease and infantile sialic acid storage disease is demonstration of elevated levels of free sialic acid in the urine by thin-layer chromatography and the direct measurement of sialidase activity in fresh tissue samples, fibroblasts, cultured amniotic fluid cells, or WBCs. Tissue samples should not be frozen or exposed to prolonged sonication. The substrate is 4-methylumbelliferyl-β-*N*-acetylneuraminic acid. Measurement of carboxypeptidase activity distinguishes galactosialidosis patients from sialidosis patients.

Prenatal Diagnosis

Prenatal diagnosis of Salla disease and infantile sialic acid storage disease can be made by chorionic villus biopsy or amniocentesis as early as 9–10 weeks by demonstration of increased free sialic acid or sialated oligosaccharides either in the amniotic fluid, cultured amniotic fluid cells, or chorionic villus sample, or by biochemical or ultrastructural analysis of the placenta. Neuraminidase activity is detectable in fresh normal cultured amniotic fluid cells as well as in chorionic villus samples. The cells must be handled with special care because enzyme activity is quickly destroyed by freezing, sonication, or exposure to temperatures of above 37°C.

Mucopolysaccharidoses

Disorders of glycosaminoglycan (GAG) metabolism

- α-L-Iduronidase deficiency [mucopolysaccharidosis (MPS) type I]
- Hurler disease (MPS IH)
- Scheie disease (MPS IS)
- Hurler-Scheie disease (MPS I H/S)
- Iduronate sulfate deficiency (Hunter syndrome; MPS II)
- Sanfilippo syndrome (MPS III)
- Heparan *N*-sulfatase deficiency (Sanfilippo syndrome type A; MPS IIIA)
- α-*N*-acetylglucosaminidase deficiency (Sanfilippo syndrome type B; MPS IIIB)
- Acetyl CoA–α-glucosaminide acetyltransferase deficiency (Sanfilippo syndrome type C; MPS IIIC)
- *N*-acetylglucosamine-6-sulfatase deficiency (Sanfilippo syndrome type D; MPS IIID)
- Galactose-6-sulfatase deficiency (Morquio syndrome type A; MPS IVA) [for Morquio syndrome type B (MPS IVB), see G_{M1} Gangliosidoses]
- Acetylgalactosamine-4-sulfatase deficiency (aryl-sulfatase B) (Maroteaux-Lamy syndrome; MPS VI)
- β-Glucuronidase deficiency (Sly syndrome; MPS VII)

Clinical Symptoms

The MPSs are a group of lysosomal storage diseases resulting from a genetic defect of hydrolases that hydrolyze carbohydrates. They are distinguished by storage of GAGs or mucopolysaccharides and glycolipids in the lysosomes of different cell types, including fibroblasts, macrophages, WBCs, and parenchymal cells of liver, kidneys, brain, and other organs and neurons, and by excretion of mucopolysaccharides in the urine.

Diagnostic Studies

Urinary GAG excretion is age dependent and may be present in normal infants up to 1 year of age. In the MPSs, an increased GAG concentration may be present in amniotic fluid and in urine at birth.

Good screening results have been obtained with a diagnostic test based on dimethylmethylene blue. The test allows direct measurement of GAGs. Keratin sulfate exhibits the same reactivity as dermatan and chondroitin by addition of Tris base (dimethylmethylene blue–Tris). False-negative screening test results occur.

GAG concentrations should be given as GAG/creatinine ratios.

Prenatal Diagnosis

Prenatal diagnosis is possible for all the MPSs. Enzyme assays for cultured fibroblasts may be used on cells grown from amniotic fluid.

Chorionic villus biopsy samples are used for the rapid diagnosis of MPS II, IIIA, IIIB, IIIC, and IVA. Diagnosis of MPS I presents some difficulty because even normal villi have low activity.

Carrier testing using DNA analysis is practical.

Chromosomal Location	MIM No.	MPS Type	Enzyme Defect[a]
4p16.3	252800	I (Hurler-Scheie, Hamrick-Barness diseases)	α-L-Iduronidase
X.q28	309900	II (Hunter syndrome)	Iduronate-2-sulfatase
	252900	IIIA (Sanfilippo syndrome A)	*N*-Sulfoglucosamine sulfase
	252920	IIIB (Sanfilippo syndrome B)	α-*N*-Acetylglucosaminidase
	252930	IIIC (Sanfilippo syndrome C)	α-Glucosamine *N*-acetyltransferase
12q14	252940	IIID (Sanfilippo syndrome D)	*N*-Acetylglucosamine-6-sulfatase
16q24	253000	IVA (Morquio syndrome A)	*N*-Acetylgalactosamine-6-sulfatase
3p21-cen	253010	IVB (Morquio B)	β-Galactosidase
5q11-q13	253200	VI (Maroteaux-Lamy syndrome)	*N*-Acetylgalactosamine-4-sulfatase (arylsulfatase B)
7q21.11	253229	VII (Sly syndrome)	β-Glucuronidase
Not assigned	253230	VIII (DiFerrante's disease)	Glucosamine-6-sulfate sulfatase

MIM, *Mendelian Inheritance in Man* system.
Note: MPS V not assigned.
[a]Enzyme detectable in WBCs, lymphocytes, fibroblasts, chorionic villi, and cultured amniotic fluid cells.

Lipid Storage Disorders

- Acid lipase deficiency (cholesteryl ester storage disease; Wolman disease)
- Ceramidase deficiency (Farber lipogranulomatosis)
- α-Galactosidase A deficiency (Fabry disease)
- Galactosylceramidase deficiency (Krabbe disease)
- β-Glucosidase deficiency (Gaucher disease)
- G_{M1} gangliosidosis (β-galactosidase deficiency)
- Infantile (type I) G_{M1} gangliosidosis
- Late infantile/juvenile (type III) G_{M1} gangliosidosis

- Morquio syndrome type B (MPS IVB)
- G_{M2} gangliosidosis
- G_{M2} activator deficiency
- Hexosaminidase A deficiency (Tay-Sachs disease)
- Hexosaminidase B deficiency (Sandhoff disease)
- Niemann-Pick disease types A and B (acid sphingomyelinase types A and B)
- Niemann-Pick disease type C (defect of lysosomal trafficking of cholesterol)
- Niemann-Pick disease type D
- Arylsulfatase A deficiency (multiple sulfatase deficiency, metachromatic leukodystrophy)

General Diagnostic Studies

See Table 7.

Initial studies appropriate for neurologic symptoms, neurodegenerative symptoms, developmental delay, hepatocellular disease, visceromegaly, gastrointestinal disease, cardiomyopathy, skeletal abnormalities, failure to thrive, ophthalmologic disorders, deafness, dermatologic abnormalities, psychiatric disorders.

Diagnostic studies: metabolite identification and quantitation in blood and urine or tissue biopsy specimen for electron microscopy.

Cholesteryl Ester Storage Disease

See Chapter 16, Disorders of Lipid Metabolism.

Fabry Disease

Fabry disease is an X-linked inborn error of glycosphingolipid catabolism resulting from deficient activity of the lysosomal hydrolase α-galactosidase A in tissues and fluids of affected hemizygous males. Most heterozygous female carriers have an intermediate level of enzymatic activity.

The enzyme defect leads to the systemic deposition of glycosphingolipids with terminal α-galactosyl moieties, predominantly globotriaosylceramide and, to a lesser extent, galactosylceramide and blood group B substances. Symptoms are worse in patients with blood group B or AB. Deposition occurs in ganglion cells and in cell types in the heart, kidneys, eyes, and most other tissues. Severe joint pain beginning in early adolescence is the common presentation.

Definitive Diagnosis

Determination of enzyme in fibroblasts or DNA analysis.

Farber Disease

Farber disease is an autosomal-recessive disorder caused by lysosomal acid ceramidase deficiency that results in ceramide accumulation. It is manifested clinically by the diagnostic triad of hoarseness, painful and swollen joints, and periarticular and subcutaneous nodules, particularly near the joints and over pressure points. Most cases lack significant visceral involvement. This illness often leads to death within the first few years of life.

During infancy, hoarseness, respiratory difficulty, vomiting, swollen painful joints, failure to thrive, and death due to respiratory infections occur.

Definitive Diagnosis

Definitive diagnosis is made by determining lysosomal ceramidase activity and ceramide content in cultured fibroblasts. Examination of biopsy specimens from periarticular tissues may be diagnostic.

Gangliosidoses

The gangliosidoses are autosomal-recessive conditions and are divided into two major groups, G_{M1} gangliosidoses and G_{M2} gangliosidoses; cases of later onset have been described as late infantile-juvenile form (type 2) or adult-chronic form (type 3). The diverse clinical phenotypes stem from mutations in the genes coding for β-hexosaminidases. β-hexosaminidase has an α subunit and a β subunit, each encoded by separate genes or a small acidic protein. Combinations of these subunits lead to isoenzyme diversity. To stabilize the enzyme-substrate complex, a G_{M2} activator protein is essential. The accumulation of lysosomal G_{M2} ganglioside and glycosphingolipids leads to progressive cerebral degeneration.

All the gangliosidoses and their variants can be diagnosed prenatally from amniotic fluid cells or chorionic villus biopsy samples.

G_{M1} Gangliosidoses

G_{M1} Gangliosidosis Type 1 (Generalized Gangliosidosis)

G_{M1} gangliosidosis is a neurosomatic disease manifesting in early infancy (infantile form, type 1). Developmental arrest is observed a few months after birth, followed by progressive neurologic deterioration and generalized spasticity with sensorimotor and psychointellectual dysfunctions. Macular cherry-red spots occur in 50% of patients; facial dysmorphism, hepatosplenomegaly, and generalized skeletal dysplasia are present in infantile cases. Extrapyramidal signs of protracted course, presenting as dystonia, are the major neurologic manifestations in adults with G_{M1} gangliosidosis.

The human β-galactosidase gene has been mapped to chromosome 3. Heterogeneous gene mutations in patients with infantile G_{M1} gangliosidosis were found in Japanese and white patients with late infantile-juvenile G_{M1}, with adult-chronic G_{M1} gangliosidosis, and with Morquio syndrome type B.

Glycoconjugates with terminal B-galactose are increased in tissues and urine from patients with G_{M1} gangliosidosis and Morquio syndrome type B. Ganglioside G_{M1} and its asialo derivative G_{A1} accumulate in the brains of patients with G_{M1} gangliosidosis. Levels of oligosaccharides derived from keratan sulfate or glycoproteins are elevated in visceral organs and urine in patients with G_{M1} gangliosidosis or Morquio syndrome type B, which appears to be a variant of G_{M1} gangliosidoses.

G_{M1} Gangliosidosis Type 2 (Juvenile)

G_{M1} gangliosidosis type 2 (juvenile) usually becomes apparent at approximately 1 year of age and is clinically and pathologically similar to type 1 gangliosidosis.

The facial features are characteristic with prominent philtrum and hypertrophic gingivae. Mental and motor deterioration begins after the first year of life; death occurs during the first decade. Viscera are usually not significantly enlarged, and only subtle bone changes may be present with radiologic features of dysostosis multiplex. Deficiency of β-galactosidase results in excessive accumulation of G_{M1} ganglioside and its asialo derivative in the CNS and of a keratan sulfate–like galactose-containing proteoglycan in viscera. Both forms of the disease are due to the homozygous state of autosomal-recessive genes without apparent ethnic predilection.

Prenatal Diagnosis

G_{M1} gangliosidosis type 2 has been diagnosed *in utero* by enzyme assay of amniotic cells, and the pathologic features of the disease have been confirmed by examination of the therapeutically aborted fetus.

G_{M2} Gangliosidoses

The G_{M2} gangliosidoses are a group of inherited disorders caused by excessive intralysosomal accumulation of ganglioside G_{M2} and related glycolipids, particularly in neuronal cells.

G_{M2} Gangliosidosis Type 1 (Tay-Sachs Disease)

At least three forms of G_{M2} gangliosidosis type 1 are known. Two feature mutations of the α subunit of β-hexosaminidase (types B and B1), and another stems from mutation of the gene for saposin, the hexosaminidase activator protein (AB form). The prototype, type B, manifests a striking incidence in children of Eastern European Jewish origin. Because the α subunit but not the β-hexosaminidase is mutated, the total amount of β-hexosaminidase is normal.

Although affected infants are normal at birth, in the first year of life they develop rapidly progressive psychomotor deterioration, seizures, hypotonia, blindness with cherry-red spot in the macula, dementia, and death by 3–5 years. The red macula represents a normal segment of the retina rendered vivid by contiguous white areas, which contain the stored material. Ganglioside accumulation results in the characteristic neuropathologic finding of ballooning of neurons with massive intralysosomal accumulation of lipophilic membranous bodies and membranous concentric bodies by electron microscopy. The brain is first enlarged due to the accumulation of storage material in the neurons but later becomes atrophic. Carrier screening and prenatal diagnosis are available. Carrier rate in the Ashkenazi Jewish population is 1 in 30 to 40, with an incidence of disease of 1 in 4,000. Screening programs for Tay-Sachs disease have been instituted in Jewish population centers.

G_{M2} Gangliosidosis Type 2 (Sandhoff Disease)

Five phenotypes occur within the type 2 group of G_{M2} gangliosidoses, which feature a total deficiency of β-hexosaminidase leading to the extensive neuronal and visceral storage of G_{M2} gangliosides, glycolipids, glycoproteins, and oligosaccharides. Both α and β subunit mutations have been described. The pattern of inheritance is autosomal recessive. The reported heterozygote frequency indicates a birth incidence for this disorder of approximately 1 in 1,000,000 among Jewish infants in North America and approximately 1 in 700,000 among non-Jewish infants.

The clinical course is similar to that of Tay-Sachs disease. In addition to the CNS involvement as in type 1 G_{M2} gangliosidosis, there is extraneural visceral storage in histiocytes of the spleen, lymph nodes, bone marrow, lung, and pancreatic acinar cells.

Diagnostic Studies

The diagnosis of homozygosity is made by the hexosaminidase assay of serum or cultured fibroblasts. Detection of heterozygosity can be made on serum. Low level of total hexosaminidases with a low percentage of hexosaminidase B is used as the criterion for the diagnosis of an affected individual or a carrier.

Gaucher Disease

Gaucher Disease Type I

Type I (nonneuronopathic) is the chronic form of Gaucher disease. Clinical manifestations are highly variable. The disease has been diagnosed from infancy to adulthood. The incidence in the Ashkenazi Jewish population is between 1 in 600 and 1 in 2,500. The disease is inherited as an autosomal-recessive trait.

Painless splenomegaly, thrombocytopenia, anemia, and leukopenia are the usual initial presenting symptoms. Platelet counts may be $<50 \times 10^9$/L without an accompanying bleeding diathesis. The liver frequently does not become significantly enlarged until later in the course of the disease. Erlenmeyer flask deformity of the distal ends of the femur is considered diagnostic of Gaucher disease. Diffuse yellow-brown skin pigmentation may involve the face and legs. Renal involvement, pulmonary hypertension, and cardiac abnormalities are less frequent.

Gaucher Disease Type II

Type II Gaucher disease (acute neuronopathic, infantile), an autosomal-recessive disorder, has no ethnic predilection. It is rapidly progressive, with severe neurologic complications and signs of cranial nerve nuclei and extrapyramidal tract involvement beginning by 3–6 months after birth. The brain is the site of extensive neuronal cell death, reactive gliosis, and the perivascular accumulation of Gaucher cells. The CNS deterioration is manifest by strabismus, trismus, and retroflexion of the head. The condition is due to the deficiency of the lysosomal enzyme glucocerebrosidase.

Patients with type II Gaucher disease initially have symptoms during infancy, and all die before 3 years of age.

Hematologic Findings

Bleeding is a common presenting symptom.

Thrombocytopenia
- Most common peripheral blood abnormality
- Usually due to splenic sequestration and responds to splenectomy

Anemia—normocytic, normochromic
- Usually mild, with hemoglobin level >8 mg/dL
- Splenic sequestration
- Marrow replacement with Gaucher cells

Leukopenia

Clotting Factors
- Prolonged bleeding time
- Acquired von Willebrand factor deficiency
- Factor IX deficiency
- Factor XI deficiency

Bone Marrow

Gaucher cells in marrow is the hallmark of the disease.
- Iron storage is increased.
- Bone marrow can be entirely replaced by Gaucher cells.
- Definitive diagnosis requires demonstration of glucocerebrosidase deficiency.

Gaucher cells can be seen in other conditions and lymphoproliferative disorders
- Chronic myelogenous leukemia
- Hodgkin lymphoma
- Multiple myeloma
- Thalassemia
- Acquired immunodeficiency syndrome

Microscopic Pathologic Findings
- Necrosis
- Marrow replacement by Gaucher cells

Biochemical Abnormalities
- Elevated serum β-hexosaminidase level
- Elevated plasma tartrate-resistant acid phosphatase level
- Increased plasma angiotensin-converting enzyme level
- Increased plasma cholesterol level
- Increased plasma glucocerebroside level
- Marked deficiency of lysosomal glucocerebrosidase in leukocytes, fibroblasts, or tissues

Gaucher Disease Type III (Juvenile)

Gaucher disease type III is a subacute form of neuronopathic disease intermediate in severity between types I and II. Presentation is in childhood.

Diagnosis of Gaucher Disease

Enzymatic Assay
- β-Glucocerebrosidase activity is measured in peripheral blood leukocytes.
- Leukocytes are disrupted, incubated with a commercially available fluorescent substrate, and the resulting fluorescence is measured with a fluorometer.
- A reduction to ≤30% in measured activity is diagnostic of the disease.
- A lesser degree of reduction is characteristic of carriers, who average approximately 50% of normal β-glucocerebrosidase activity.
- This assay has a substantial rate of false-negative readings among carriers.
- Some 20% of carriers demonstrate enzyme activity in the normal range.
- Cultures of skin fibroblasts, amniotic fluid cells, and chorionic villi can also be used for diagnosis.
- DNA analysis provides greater accuracy in detecting heterozygotes.

DNA Analysis
- Has some advantages over enzymatic diagnosis.
- Results are qualitative rather than quantitative.
- Provides greater accuracy in detection of heterozygotes.
- PCR is used to detect Gaucher mutations.

- Allele-specific oligonucleotide (ASO) hybridization: Regions containing mutations are amplified via PCR. ASO probes are added and hybridize to a mutated allele. Mutant ASO hybridizes only to a mutated allele. Normal ASOs hybridize only to normal alleles.

Ancillary Studies

- Serum levels of some enzymes may be elevated.
- Acid phosphatase: Lysosomal enzyme that may reflect overall macrophage activity. Elevation is suggestive of Gaucher disease when possibility of metastatic prostate carcinoma has been eliminated
- Angiotensin-converting enzyme level may be increased.
- Elevated plasma ferritin levels are commonly seen.
- Decreased plasma cholesterol levels may be seen in unsplenectomized patients.

Krabbe Disease (Globoid Cell Leukodystrophy)

Krabbe disease is an autosomal-recessive disorder caused by deficiency of galactocerebrosidase, the lysosomal enzyme responsible for the degradation of galactocerebroside. Galactocerebroside (galactosylceramide) is a sphingoglycolipid consisting of sphingosine, fatty acid, and galactose, and is normally present almost exclusively in the myelin sheath.

This disorder usually presents between 3 and 6 months of life after a normal neonatal period and has a rapidly progressive course with irritability, hypersensitivity to external stimuli, and severe mental and motor deterioration. Patients rarely survive beyond 2 years. Hypertonicity with hyperactive reflexes presents in the early stages, but patients later become flaccid and hypotonic. Blindness, deafness, and seizures are common. Peripheral neuropathy is almost always detectable. Galactosylceramide accumulates in the peripheral system and CNS.

Diagnostic Studies

Enzyme assay to document enzyme deficiency.

- Cultured peripheral leukocytes or fibroblasts.
- Cultured amniotic fluid cells or biopsied chorionic villi (preferred).
- Can be used to identify heterozygous carriers.

Examination of brain and peripheral nerve biopsy specimens has been superseded by the enzyme assay.

Metachromatic Leukodystrophy

Metachromatic leukodystrophy is an autosomal-recessive lysosomal storage disease caused by deficiency of the enzyme arylsulfatase A. Frequency is estimated to be 1 in 40,000. Arylsulfatase A is involved in the degradation of sulfated glycolipids, and one of its major substrates is cerebroside 3-sulfatase. This lipid is found mainly in the myelin membranes, where it accounts for 3–4% of total membrane lipids. Arylsulfatase A initiates the degradation of this lipid by desulfation of a sulfated galactose residue. In this reaction, arylsulfatase A requires a small acidic protein or saposin B.

Clinical Manifestations

General

- Progressive clinical course

Early stages

- Gait disturbance
- Mental regression
- Urinary incontinence
- Speech disturbances

Late stages

- Bedridden condition, quadriplegia

- Severe mental deficits
- Lack of awareness of surroundings

Diagnostic Studies

Diagnosis is made by enzyme assay in peripheral WBCs or cultured fibroblasts, although some patients may have normal activity attributed to deficiency of the enzyme activator protein or a Km mutant. Enzyme may be measured in sural nerve biopsy. Some normal individuals may have low enzyme activity (pseudo–arylsulfatase A deficiency). Cerebroside sulfate loading test, examination of nerve biopsy specimen, or detection of urinary sulfatide excretion by the presence of brown metachromasia on a filter paper urine spot with cresyl violet may be used for diagnosis.

Prenatal Diagnosis

Prenatal diagnosis is based on assay of arylsulfatase A activity in cultured amniotic fluid or chorionic villus. Cerebroside sulfate loading of such cells is used if the pseudodeficiency gene is present in the family.

Sphingomyelin Storage Diseases (Sphingomyelinase Deficiency; Niemann-Pick Diseases)

Sphingomyelinase deficiency results in storage of sphingomyelin.

Niemann-Pick Disease Types A and B

The most common and severe variant of Niemann-Pick disease is type A, the acute neuropathic form. These patients, often of Eastern European Jewish ancestry, present early in life. Often the skin has a yellow-brown pigmentation, lymph nodes are enlarged, and ocular manifestations (cherry-red macula and corneal opacifications) are evident. Few survive beyond 4 years of age.

The type B variant (an allele variant of type A) features a pattern of visceral involvement similar to that in type A yet spares the CNS. These children present at a later age with isolated splenomegaly. In time, a more generalized visceral pattern of involvement is manifest, yet many patients survive several decades. Neonates may present with ascites and meconium ileus, and some have developed biliary atresia or, more commonly, neonatal hepatitis. Hepatic storage of glycogen has been described in type B. Storage cells are more prominent in type A. Storage material is found in reticuloendothelial cells, hepatocytes, and pulmonary macrophages, sometimes with calcification, and in syncytiotrophoblast and villus stromal cells.

Diagnostic Studies

The diagnosis of types A and B Niemann-Pick disease can be made by enzymatic determination of sphingomyelinase activity in cell or tissue extracts. Detection of heterozygosity by enzyme assay is unreliable, however, and molecular studies are required. Prenatal diagnosis by enzymatic or molecular analyses of cultured amniocytes and chorionic villus sampling has been accomplished.

Niemann-Pick Disease Types C and D

Patients with Niemann-Pick disease types C and D may present with neonatal jaundice, appear to recover, then suffer progressive neurodegeneration. Hepatosplenomegaly is not as severe as in types A and B. Patients may survive to adulthood. In addition to sphingomyelinase deficiency, these patients have a defect in cholesterol transport.

Neurologic signs appear later in type D and are less severe than in type C. Many of these patients can trace lineage to Nova Scotia. The defect is similar to that of type C.

Diagnostic Studies

Sphingomyelinase activity is measured in peripheral WBCs, cultured fibroblasts, or lymphoblasts.

Wolman Disease

Deficiency of acid lipase results in storage of cholesterol esters and triglycerides in lysosomes. Clinically, infants fail to thrive and show pernicious vomiting, hepatosplenomegaly, and steatorrhea. Adrenal glands are calcified. Death occurs early in the severe form of the disease.

Definitive Diagnosis

Enzyme measurement in WBCs, fibroblasts, chorionic villus sample, or amniocytes

Mitochondrial Disorders

Mitochondria are present in all eukaryotic cells dependent on aerobic metabolism and generate most of the cellular adenosine triphosphate. They also regulate cytoplasmic calcium levels. By electron microscopy, mitochondria show a smooth spherical outer membrane and an inner membrane with numerous infoldings, known as cristae. The membranes divide the content of mitochondria into separate compartments, each harboring specific biochemical structures for transport and processing of chemical compounds.

Mitochondria not related to adenosine triphosphate are required for most of the major metabolic pathways used by a cell to build, break down, and recycle its molecular building blocks. Mitochondria contain the rate-limiting enzymes for pyrimidine biosynthesis (dihydroorotate dehydrogenase) and heme synthesis (δ-aminolevulinic acid synthetase) required to make hemoglobin. In the liver, mitochondria are specialized to detoxify ammonia in the urea cycle. Mitochondria are also required for cholesterol metabolism, estrogen and testosterone synthesis, neurotransmitter metabolism, and free radical production and detoxification. They oxidize fat, protein, and carbohydrates.

Mitochondrial Disorders of Oxidative Phosphorylation

Disorders of the Nuclear OXPHOS Genes

The term *mitochondrial disease* can apply to disorders of energy metabolism, including mitochondrial transport, substrate use, Krebs cycle, and the respiratory chain. Mitochondrial disorders involving other pathways appear under discussions of organic acidemia and the urea cycle. The most important function of the mitochondrion is oxidative phosphorylation in which oxidative metabolism is coupled through the electron transport chain to the production of adenosine triphosphate.

Mitochondrial DNA Point Mutations

- Antibiotic-induced sensorineural deafness
- Hypertrophic cardiomyopathy and myopathy
- Leber hereditary optic neuropathy
- Leber hereditary optic neuropathy and infantile bilateral striatal necrosis
- Leber hereditary optic neuropathy and multiple systems degeneration
- Leigh disease
- Maternally inherited sensorineural deafness
- Mitochondrial myopathy, encephalopathy, lactic acidosis, and strokelike episodes
- Myoclonic epilepsy and ragged-red-fiber disease
- Neurogenic ataxia, retinitis pigmentosa

Mitochondrial DNA Deletions and Duplications

- Chronic progressive external ophthalmoplegia syndrome
- Diabetes mellitus and deafness
- Kearns-Sayre syndrome

- Mitochondrial encephalopathy, lactic acidosis, and stroke
- Pearson syndrome
- Idiopathic dystonia
- Lethal infantile cardiomyopathy
- Luft disease
- Mitochondrial myopathy
- Myoneurogastrointestinal disorder and encephalopathy
- Progressive infantile poliodystrophy (Alpers disease)

Examples of Mitochondrial Disorders[4]

Disorder	Systemic Lesions	CNS Lesions
Leigh disease	None reported	Deep and periventricular gray matter spongy change; vascular proliferation; cystic lesions
Pyruvate dehydrogenase complex		
Pyruvate decarboxylase deficiency	None reported	Cerebrum; deep and periventricular gray matter cystic lesions in white more than in gray matter
Pyruvate carboxylase deficiency	Hepatic steatosis	Cerebral white matter; neocortex; paucity of myelin; neuronal loss
Glioneuronal dystrophy (some cases of Alpers disease)	Hepatic fibrosis	Neocortex spongy change and neuronal loss
Respiratory chain enzymes deficiency	Cardiomyopathy	
Biotin-dependent enzymes; biotinidase deficiency	Skin rash; alopecia	Insufficient data
Carnitine deficiency	Lipid myopathy	None reported
Carnitine palmitoyl transferase deficiency	Rhabdomyolysis	None reported
Ragged-red-fiber–related diseases		
Kearns-Sayre disease	Ragged red fibers	Brainstem, cerebellar white matter; spongy change
Luft disease	Ragged red fibers	None reported
MERRF	Ragged red fibers	Dentate nucleus; brainstem neuronal loss; tract degeneration
MELAS	Ragged red fibers	Neocortex microinfarcts

MELAS, mitochondrial encephalopathy, lactic acidosis, and stroke; MERRF, myoclonic epilepsy with ragged red fibers.

General Features of Mitochondrial Disorders

Clinical Symptoms

Acute neonatal crisis, neurologic symptoms, neurodegenerative symptoms, developmental delay, hepatocellular disease, visceromegaly, renal Fanconi syndrome, gastrointestinal disease, skeletal myopathy, cardiomyopathy, cardiac symptoms, failure to thrive, ophthalmologic disorders, deafness, hypoglycemia, metabolic acidosis or hyperammonemia (or both), diabetes, psychiatric disorders at any age. Healthy relatives who are silent carriers may have no symptoms.

[4]Powers JM, Haroupian DS. Central nervous system. In: Damijanov I, Linder J, eds. *Anderson's pathology.* St. Louis: Mosby, 1996.

Laboratory Findings

Lactic acidemia
Nonketotic hypoglycemia
Dicarboxylic aciduria
Organic aciduria
Amino aciduria
Myoglobinuria
Decreased levels of free and total carnitine

Diagnostic Studies

An electroencephalogram, brain magnetic resonance imaging, and specialized muscle biopsy are frequently required for the diagnosis. Fresh—not frozen or fixed—muscle tissue for isolation of mitochondria is essential for a reliable diagnosis.

Most mitochondrial DNA point mutations can be identified in blood cells, so that muscle biopsy is unnecessary. However, secure diagnosis of disorders due to mitochondrial DNA deletions, such as Kearns-Sayre syndrome and sporadic progressive external ophthalmoplegia with ragged red fibers, requires muscle biopsy.

Electrospray tandem mass spectrometry is an important method for rapid pinpointing of diagnoses in symptomatic patients with mitochondrial disorders as well as for routine detection of the presence of these disorders in presymptomatic newborns and children at a time when early intervention or treatment can significantly improve their prognosis.

Exercise physiology testing, nuclear magnetic resonance phosphorus-31 spectroscopy, and muscle biopsy for histochemistry, electron microscopy, and biochemical, nuclear, and mitochondrial DNA analysis are helpful.

Specific Tests for the Diagnosis of Mitochondriopathies

DNA chip technology offers the promise of automation of detection for DNA mutations. In this technique, large groups, or arrays, of different short wild-type genetic sequences are placed on a solid support, or chip. These arrays are then chemically joined, or hybridized, with samples of DNA from patients and their family members after PCR amplification. The presence of mutations causes incomplete hybridization that is demonstrated by variations in fluorescence, which can then be rapidly analyzed by a scanner.

These miniature chips allow comparison of mutant and wild-type genetic sequences. Arrays can be tagged by fluorescence for multicolor detection. Enzymes are used to facilitate identification of mutations, acting as tagged targets for comparison. Hybridization patterns of long PCR products of the entire mitochondrial genome have been imaged in <10 minutes, identifying 99% of the mitochondrial sequence correctly.

Magnetic resonance imaging with specific substrate detection (lactate and pyruvate) is a technique that has not been widely used as yet but offers potential.

The measurement of oxygen consumption using tissue oximetry.

Definitive Diagnosis

Enzymatic assay or DNA analysis or both

Pyruvate Metabolism Disorders

Lipoamide dehydrogenase deficiency
Phosphoenolpyruvate carboxykinase deficiency
Pyruvate dehydrogenase deficiency, including E1, E2, E3, and X components
Pyruvate carboxylase deficiency
Pyruvate dehydrogenase phosphatase deficiency

Clinical Symptoms

Acute neonatal crisis, neurologic symptoms, neurodegenerative symptoms, developmental delay, hepatocellular disease, visceromegaly, skeletal myopathy, gastrointestinal disease, cardiomyopathy, failure to thrive, ophthalmologic disorders, hypoglycemia, metabolic acidosis or hyperammonemia or both, psychiatric disorders

Diagnostic Studies

Lactate, pyruvate and amino acid studies in blood, urine, or CSF. Metabolite identification and quantitation in blood and urine or carnitine quantitation and species identification in blood or urine or both.

Definitive Diagnosis

Enzyme assay or DNA and analysis or both

Disorders of Pyrimidine and Purine Metabolism

General Features

Clinical Symptoms

Renal or bladder calculi, gout, uric acid calculi, gouty arthritis

Clinical Signs and Laboratory Data

Clinical Sign	Diagnostic Possibilities
Psychomotor delay	PRPP synthetase superactivity Adenylosuccinase deficiency Combined xanthine and sulfite oxidase deficiency HGPRT deficiency (complete) UMP synthase deficiency Dihydropyrimidine dehydrogenase deficiency
Ataxia	HGPRT deficiency (complete)
Autism	PRPP synthetase superactivity Adenylosuccinase deficiency Dihydropyrimidine dehydrogenase deficiency
Self-mutilation	HGPRT deficiency
Deafness	PRPP synthetase superactivity
Growth retardation	Adenylosuccinase deficiency ADA deficiency UMP synthase deficiency
Recurrent infections	ADA deficiency PNP deficiency
Renal insufficiency	PRPP synthetase superactivity HGPRT deficiency APRT deficiency
Arthritis	PRP synthetase superactivity HGPRT deficiency (partial)
Renal stones	PRPP synthetase superactivity (uric acid) Xanthine oxidase deficiency (xanthine)
Muscle wasting	Adenylosuccinase deficiency
Muscle cramps	Myoadenylate deaminase deficiency
Laboratory Data	
Anemia	UMP synthase deficiency
Lymphopenia	
Deficient B and T cells	ADA deficiency
Deficient T cells	PNP deficiency
Hyperuricemia	PRPP synthetase superactivity HGPRT deficiency (complete or partial)
Hypouricemia	PNP deficiency Xanthine oxidase deficiency (isolated or combined with sulfite oxidase deficiency)
Orotic aciduria	UMP synthase deficiency

ADA, adenosine deaminase; APRT, adenine phosphoribosyltransferase; HGPRT, hypoxanthine-guanine phosphoribosyltransferase; PNP, purine nucleotide phosphorylase; PRPP, phosphoribosyl pyrophosphate; UMP, uridine monophosphate.

Diagnostic Studies

Metabolite identification and quantitation in blood and urine. Blood uric acid level. Radiography of joints.

Definitive Diagnosis

Enzymatic assay or DNA analysis or both

Adenosine Deaminase Deficiency and Purine Nucleoside Phosphorylase Deficiency

Clinical Symptoms

Severe combined immunodeficiency. Immunologic or autoimmune abnormalities, skeletal or neurologic abnormalities or both, failure to thrive. Absent T- and B-cell function.

Diagnostic Studies

Metabolite identification and quantitation in blood and urine. Studies of B-cell and T-cell function. Adenosine deaminase deficiency—urinary uric acid level normal or increased; purine nucleoside phosphorylase deficiency—urinary uric acid level very low.

Definitive Diagnosis

Enzymatic assay or DNA analysis or both. Measurement of T- and B-cell activity.

Hypouricemia

The following diseases and conditions associated with hypouricemia in children:

1. Decreased uric acid production
   a. Xanthine oxidase deficiency
   b. Liver disease
   c. Purine nucleoside phosphorylase deficiency
   d. Molybdenum cofactor deficiency
   e. Lymphoma
   f. Diabetes mellitus
   g. Volume expansion
2. Increased renal excretion of uric acid
   a. Fanconi syndrome
   b. Fanconi-like renal tubular defect
      i. Cystinosis
      ii. Cytochrome *c* oxidase deficiency
      iii. Galactosemia
      iv. Glycogen storage disease type 1
      v. Heavy metal intoxication
      vi. Hereditary fructose intolerance
      vii. Lowe syndrome
      viii. Tyrosinemia
      ix. Wilson disease
   c. Drugs
      i. Glyceryl guaiacolate
      ii. Phenylbutazone
      iii. Probenecid
      iv. Radiographic contrast materials
      v. Salicylates
      vi. Sulfinpyrazone
      vii. Total parenteral nutrition

Lesch-Nyhan Syndrome (Hypoxanthine-Guanine Phosphoribosyl-Transferase Deficiency)

Lesch-Nyhan syndrome, and X-linked recessive disorder, is characterized by hyperuricemia, choreoathetosis, spasticity, mental retardation, and compulsive self-mutilation.

Individuals with a partial deficiency of hypoxanthine-guanine phosphoribosyltransferase (HGPRT) have hyperuricemia and gouty arthritis but are generally spared the neurologic consequences of Lesch-Nyhan syndrome. Gouty arthritis symptoms in individuals with partial HGPRT deficiency usually appear in adult life.

Affected children generally appear normal during the first few months of life. At 3–4 months of age, a neurologic syndrome evolves, including delayed motor development, choreoathetoid movements, and spasticity with hyperreflexia and scissoring of gait. Patients develop a striking, compulsive self-destructive behavior, including biting of their fingers and lips, which leads to mutilating loss of tissue. Speech is hampered by athetoid dysarthria.

Diagnostic Studies

Lack of enzyme HGPRT in RBCs, fibroblasts, other tissues

Definitive Diagnosis

Enzymatic assay or DNA analysis or both

Myoadenylate Deaminase Deficiency

Clinical Symptoms

Muscle weakness, fatigue, myalgia

Diagnostic Studies

Muscle biopsy for histochemistry. Anaerobic exercise testing. Myoglobinuria with increased uric acid.

Definitive Diagnosis

Enzyme assay or DNA analysis in muscle biopsy specimen. Creatine phosphokinase level is increased.

Orotic Aciduria (Orotate Phosphoribosyltransferase and Orotidine-5'-Monophosphate Decarboxylase Deficiency; Uridine Monophosphate Synthase Deficiency)

Clinical Symptoms

Renal dysfunction, macrocytic hypochromic anemia, failure to thrive, developmental delay, gastrointestinal disease, cardiac symptoms, strabismus, crystalluria, immunologic abnormalities

Diagnostic Studies

Metabolite identification in liver, fibroblasts, WBCs. Organic acid analysis in blood or urine or both.

Definitive Diagnosis

Enzymatic assay or DNA analysis or both

Pyrimidine-5'-Nucleotidase Deficiency, Dihydropyrimidine Dehydrogenase Deficiency, and Dihydropyrimidinuria (Dihydropyrimidase Deficiency)

Clinical Symptoms

Seizures, hypertonia, hyperreflexia, autism
Hematologic abnormalities, developmental delay

Diagnostic Studies

Metabolite identification and quantitation, uracil and thymine levels in blood and urine

Definitive Diagnosis

Enzymatic assay in cultured fibroblasts and leukoblasts, DNA analysis, or both

Xanthine and Sulfite Oxidases Deficiency

Clinical Symptoms

Seizures, feeding difficulty

Definitive Diagnosis

Enzymatic assay

Xanthinuria (Xanthine Oxidase Deficiency)

Clinical Symptoms

Renal or bladder calculi, skeletal myopathy, arthropathy, duodenal ulcers

Diagnostic Studies

Metabolite quantitation in urine

Definitive Diagnosis

Enzymatic assay or DNA analysis or both

Peroxisomal Disorders

Peroxisomes are organelles bound by single membranes that contain finely granular or flocculent, electron-dense matrices. The peroxisome derives its name from its content of catalase and at least one hydrogen peroxide–producing oxidase enzyme. Peroxisomes are present predominately in liver and kidney but also in heart, adrenal cortex, muscle, brown adipose tissue, lung, intestine, and spleen, and are probably ubiquitous in animal cells except for mature erythrocytes.

Classification[5]

Peroxisomal disorders can be subdivided into three groups. In the first group, the organelle fails to be formed or maintained, which results in the defective function of multiple peroxisomal enzymes. These diseases form a spectrum of severity; infants with Zellweger syndrome are the most profoundly affected and those with infantile Refsum disease are the least affected. Increased plasma and tissue very-long-chain fatty acids, defective bile acid oxidation, abnormal metabolism of phytanic and pipecolic acid, and impaired plasmalogen synthesis characterize this group. In the second group there is a genetically determined deficiency of a single peroxisomal enzyme and peroxisome structure is intact. The third group includes RCDP, in which peroxisomes are present but there are multiple defects. The incidence of peroxisomal disorders has been estimated as 1 in 25,000 to 1 in 50,000.

Defect	Some Distinguishing Clinical Features
Absence of peroxisomes	
Zellweger syndrome	Severe peroxisomal phenotype with characteristic facial dysmorphism, disturbances of neuronal migration (polymicrogyria, neuronal heterotopias), corneal clouding, nystagmus, cataracts, congenital heart disease, poor feeding, failure to thrive, death within a few months.

[5]Clark JTR. *Clinical guide to inherited metabolic disease*. New York: Cambridge University Press, 1996.

Neonatal adrenoleukodystrophy	Severe peroxisomal phenotype with more subtle facial dysmorphism, disturbances of neuronal migration (polymicrogyria, neuronal heterotopias), chemical evidence of adrenal insufficiency, poor feeding, failure to thrive, survival for up to a few years.
Infantile Refsum disease (IRD)	Severe peroxisomal phenotype with facial dysmorphism, subtle disturbances or neuronal migration (polymicrogyria, neuronal heterotopias), decreased plasma cholesterol, prominent retinal degeneration and sensorineural hearing impairment, survival for up to many years.
Hyperpipecolic acidemia	Severe peroxisomal phenotype with prominent retinal degeneration, cirrhosis, survival for up to many years.
Single enzyme defects	
Dihydroxyacetone phosphate acyltransferase deficiency	Identical to classic rhizomelic chondrodysplasia punctata.
Acyl-CoA oxidase deficiency Bifunctional enzyme deficiency 3-Ketoacyl-CoA thiolase deficiency Dihydroxy- and trihydroxycholestanoic acidemia	Phenotype to Zellweger syndrome with neuronal heterotopias, polymicrogyria with or without facial dysmorphism, renal cysts, neuronal heterotopias, early death with subtle facial dysmorphism and liver disease, survival variable.
Multiple defects with peroxisomes present	
Rhizomelic chondrodysplasia punctata	Severe peroxisomal phenotype with facial dysmorphism, severe shortening of proximal limbs, chondrodysplasia punctata (stippled epiphyses), skin lesions, cataracts, survival highly variable.

General Features

Clinical Symptoms

Dysmorphic features, acute neonatal presentation, neurologic symptoms, neurodegenerative symptoms, hypotonia, developmental delay, hepatocellular disease, visceromegaly, renal dysfunction, gastrointestinal disease, skeletal myopathy, skeletal abnormalities, failure to thrive, ophthalmologic disorders, deafness, coagulation disorders, endocrine disorders.

Diagnostic Studies

Serum assays of very-long-chain fatty acids and phytanic acid identify most patients. All peroxisomal diseases, except rhizomelic chondrodysplasia punctata (RCDP), are accompanied by increased serum values of very-long-chain fatty acids. Patients with RCDP have elevated phytanic acid levels when their diets include enough dairy products to expose them to chlorophyll-derived phytosis. Patients with infantile Refsum disease have increased serum concentrations of pristanic acid as well as phytanic acid.

Diagnostic tests for peroxisomal disorders include the following:

1. Increased levels of long-chain fatty acids in plasma, RBCs, or cultured skin fibroblasts, except in RCDP.
2. Diminished levels of plasmalogen in RBCs and defective plasmalogen synthesis. These are features of peroxisome biogenesis and represent the most striking single abnormality in RCDP.
3. Elevated pipecolic acid levels in plasma, present in nearly all patients with disorders of peroxisomes.
4. Elevated levels of plasma phytanic acid, which are the prime and characteristic abnormality in Refsum disease.
5. Absent or abnormal peroxisomes in liver biopsy specimens by electron microscopy.

Peroxisomal enzyme activities and immunoblot studies of peroxisomal fatty acid oxidation enzymes are performed in a rectal mucosal biopsy specimen.

Diagnostic Assays for Specific Peroxisomal Disorders[6]

Disease	Maternal	Type of Assay
All peroxisomal disorders	Plasma	VLCFAs, bile acids, phytanic acid, pristanic acid, polyunsaturated fatty acids
Classic Zellweger syndrome	RBC	Plasmalogens
Neonatal adrenoleukodystrophy Infantile Refsum disease Zellweger-like disorder Pseudo–infantile Refsum disease	Fibroblasts	Plasmalogens biosynthesis, DHAPAT, alkyl DHAP synthase, particle-bound catalase, VLCFA β-oxidation, immunoblotting β-oxidation proteins, phytanic acid oxidation
Rhizomelic chondrodysplasia punctata (classic/atypical phenotypes	Plasma, RBC, fibroblasts	Phytanic acid, plasmalogens, DHAPAT, alkyl DHAP synthase, phytanic acid oxidation
Isolated defect of bile acid synthesis	Plasma, liver	Bile acids, THCA-CoA oxidase
Isolated pipecolic acidemia	Plasma, liver	Pipecolic acid, pipecolic acid oxidase
Classic Refsum disease	Plasma, fibroblasts	Phytanic acid, phytanic acid oxidation
Hyperoxaluria type I	Urine, liver	Organic acids, AGT
Acatalasemia	RBC	Catalase

AGT, alanine-glyoxylate aminotransferase; DHAP, dihydroxyacetone phosphate; DHAPAT, dihydroxyacetone phosphate acyltransferase; RBC, red blood cells; THCA, trihydroxycholestanoic acid; VLCFA, very-long-chain fatty acid.

Prenatal Diagnosis

Except for type I hyperoxaluria, all peroxisomal disorders can be identified prenatally in the first or second trimester of pregnancy by measurement of very-long-chain fatty acids and bile acid intermediates, and by assays of plasmalogen synthesis in cultured amniocytes or cultured chorionic villus cells.

The prenatal diagnosis of the group I disorders (absent peroxisomes) uses cultured cells from amniotic fluid or biopsied chorionic villus tissue to measure very-long-chain fatty acid levels, sedimentable (i.e., peroxisome-localized) catalase level, plasmalogen synthesis, and phytanic acid oxidation and to directly visualize peroxisomes using immunofluorescence microscopy. Plasmalogen synthesis and phytanic acid oxidation are measured in the prenatal diagnosis of RCDP. X-ALD is diagnosed by analysis of very-long-chain fatty acids in cell cultures. DNA linkage studies can be used for prenatal diagnosis in families in which the DNA haplotypes are informative. The prenatal diagnosis of type I hyperoxaluria requires measurement of alanine-glyoxylate aminotransferase activity in biopsy specimens of fetal liver due to absent or minimal activity of the enzyme in fibroblasts and in cell cultures from chorionic villus biopsy specimens or amniotic fluid.

Adrenoleukodystrophy and Adrenomyeloneuropathy, X-Linked

Clinical Symptoms

Neurologic symptoms, neurodegenerative symptoms, developmental delay, hypoglycemia, metabolic acidosis, adrenal failure, psychiatric disorders

Diagnostic Studies

Plasma very-long-chain fatty acid levels

[6]Poll-The BT, Saudubray JM. Peroxisomal disorders. In: Fernandez J, Saudubray J-M, Van den Berghe G, eds. *Inborn metabolic diseases*, 3rd ed. Berlin: Springer-Verlag, 2000.

Definitive Diagnosis

Enzymatic (dihydroxyacetone phosphate acyltransferase) assay or DNA analysis or both

Disorders of Bile Acid Biosynthesis and Storage of Sterols Other Than Cholesterol

- 27-Hydroxylase deficiency (cerebrotendinous xanthomatosis)
- 3-β-Hydroxy-C27 steroid dehydrogenase deficiency
- 3-β-Hydroxysteroid-Δ^5-oxidoreductase-isomerase deficiency
- 3-Oxo-Δ^4-steroid 5-β-reductase deficiency
- Phytosterolemia (sitosterolemia)

Clinical Symptoms

Hepatocellular disease, xanthomas, visceromegaly, renal dysfunction, failure to thrive, coagulation disorders, and, in cerebrotendinous xanthomatosis, neurologic symptoms and failure to thrive

Diagnostic Studies

Identification of bile acid intermediates in blood, tissues, or urine. Exclusion of other hepatic pathology.

Definitive Diagnosis

Enzymatic assay or DNA analysis or both

Hyperoxaluria, Primary, Types I and II

Clinical Symptoms

Hepatocellular disease, visceromegaly, renal dysfunction, gastrointestinal disease, skeletal myopathy, failure to thrive, ophthalmologic disorders, skeletal abnormalities

Diagnostic Studies

Amino acid studies in blood and urine. Metabolite identification and quantitation in blood, urine, or tissues. Organic acid analysis in blood or urine or both.

Definitive Diagnosis

Enzymatic (alanine-glyoxylate aminotransferase) assay or DNA analysis or both

Refsum Disease

Clinical Symptoms

Neurologic symptoms, neurodegenerative symptoms, cardiomyopathy, cardiac symptoms, ophthalmologic disorders, deafness

Diagnostic Studies

Plasma phytanic acid level

Definitive Diagnosis

Enzymatic (dihydroxyacetone phosphate acyltransferase) assay or DNA analysis or both

Porphyrias

See Table 9.

Porphyria results from partial deficiency of one of the enzymes of heme biosynthesis. The human genes for these enzymes have been cloned, and molecular genetic methods are used to identify and characterize mutations and define the extent of heterogeneity at the DNA level in these conditions.

In normal cells, the concentrations of the intermediates of heme biosynthesis appear to be lower than the Michaelis constants of the enzymes that metabolize them. A partial enzyme deficiency can therefore be compensated and the rate of formation of heme maintained by increasing the concentration of the substrate of the defective enzyme.

At least 80% of individuals who inherit one of the autosomal-dominant enzyme deficiencies remain asymptomatic throughout life and are considered to have latent porphyria. Many of these persons may show no evidence of heme precursor overproduction. Symptoms tend to start at a young age and persist in those who are affected.

Acute neurovisceral attacks are associated with increased excretion of the porphyrin precursor aminolevulinic acid (ALA), accompanied by porphobilinogen (PBG) except in the very rare condition PBG synthase deficiency porphyria. Acute attacks do not occur in porphyrias in which neither PBG nor ALA excretion is increased. Skin lesions in porphyria are the consequence of overproduction of porphyrins, which, except in erythropoietic protoporphyria, are derived from oxidation of accumulated porphyrinogens. They are not seen in the two conditions acute intermittent porphyria and PBG synthase deficiency porphyria due to porphyrin overproduction.

General Features

Enzyme Deficiencies and Inheritance in the Porphyrias

Disorder	Enzyme Deficiency	Inheritance	Location	cDNA Cloned
PBG synthase deficiency	PBG synthase	AR	9q34	Yes
Acute intermittent porphyria	PBG deaminase[a]	AD	11q24.1-24.2	Yes
Congenital erythropoietic porphyria	Uroporphyrinogen III	AR	10q25.2-26.3	Yes
Porphyria cutanea tarda				
Type I (sporadic)	Uroporphyrinogen decarboxylase	Polygenic		
Type II (familial)	Uroporphyrinogen decarboxylase	AD	1p34	Yes
Toxic	Uroporphyrinogen decarboxylase	Not inherited		
Hereditary coproporphyria	Coproporphyrinogen oxidase	AD	3q12	Yes
Variegate porphyria	Protoporphyrinogen oxidase	AD	1q21-23	Yes
Protoporphyria	Ferrochelatase	AD	18q21.3	Yes

AD, autosomal dominant; AR, autosomal recessive.
[a]Synonyms: hydroxymethylbilane, uroporphyrinogen-I-synthase.

Main Types of Porphyria

Disorder	Acute Attacks	Skin Lesions	Estimated Prevalence of Overt Cases (All Ages)
PBG synthase deficiency porphyria	+	–	—
Acute intermittent porphyria	+	–	1–2 in 100,000
Congenital erythropoietic porphyria	–	+	<1 in 1,000,000
Porphyria cutanea tarda	–	+	1 in 25,000
Hereditary coproporphyria	+	+	<1 in 250,000
Variegate porphyria	+	+	1 in 250,000
Erythropoietic protoporphyria	–	+	1 in 200,000

+, occurs; –, does not occur.
In hereditary coproporphyria and variegate porphyria, skin lesions and acute attacks may occur together or separately.

Table 9. Disorders of Porphyrin Metabolism

McKusick No.	Pathway Intermediate	Inheritance	Enzyme	Porphyrias	Metabolites (ALA, PBG)
	Glycine + succinyl-CoA				
	↓		ALA synthase		
125270	ALA	AR		Doss porphyria	+++
	↓		ALA dehydrase		
176000	PBG	AD		Acute intermittent porphyria	+++
	↓		PBG deaminase		(++)
263700	Uroporphyrinogen I (Uroporphyrin I)	AR		Congenital erythropoietic porphyria	
	↓		Urocosynthase		
176100	Uroporphyrinogen III (Uroporphyrin III)	AD		Porphyria cutanea tarda	+++
	↓		Urodecarboxylase		
				Hepatoerythropoietic porphyria	+++
121300	Coproporphyrinogen III (Coproporphyrin)	AR		Hereditary coproporphyria	+++
	↓		Coprooxidase		(+)
176200	Protoporphyrinogen IX (Protoporphyrinogen)	AR		Variable porphyria	+++
	↓		Protooxidase		(+)
177000	Protoporphyrin IX (Protoporphyrin)	AD		Erythropoietic protoporphyria	
	↓		Ferrochelatase		
	Heme				

+, present; ++, moderately increased; +++, markedly increased; $\pm$, sometimes increased; AD, autosomal dominant; ALA, Δ aminolevulinic acid; AR, autosomal recessive; CoA, coenzyme A; Copro, coproporphyrin; PBG, porphobilinogen; Proto, protoporphyrin; Uro, uroporphyrin.

Urine (Uro)	Feces (Copro)	Erythrocytes						Gene Locus
		Uro	Copro	Proto	Uro	Copro	Proto	
++	+++					+	++	? 11q23qter
++	++	++	+					
	(+)							
+++	+++	++	+++	+	+++	++	++	
+++	++	++	+					1pter-p34
		(+)						
+	++	++						++
++	+++	++	+++	+				9
	(+)							
++	+++		+++	+++				?
	(+)							
	±		±	+++		+	+++	18q21.3

Diagnostic Studies

The most reliable method of diagnosis is to measure total erythrocyte porphyrin level by a quantitative fluorometric method.

Diagnostic tests for the porphyrias are the following:

Disorder	Urine PBG/ALA	Porphyrins	Porphyrins in Feces	Porphyrins in Erythrocytes
PBG synthase deficiency[a]	ALA	Copro II	Not increased	Zn-proto
Acute intermittent porphyria	PBG > ALA	(Porphyrin mainly from PBG)	Normal, occasionally slight increase (copro, proto)	Not increased
Congenital erythropoietic porphyria	Not increased	Uro I > copro I	Copro I	Zn-proto, copro, uro
Porphyria cutanea tarda	Not increased	Uro > Hepta[b]	Isocopro, Hepta[b]	Not increased
Hereditary coproporphyria	PBG > ALA[c]	Copro III (porphyrin from PBG)	Copro III	Not increased
Variegate porphyria	PBG > ALA	Copro III (porphyrin from PBG)	Proto IX > copro III, X porphyrin	Not increased
Protoporphyria	Not increased	Not increased	± Proto	Proto

±, sometimes present; copro, coproporphyrin; isocopro, isocoproporphyrin; proto, protoporphyrin; uro, uroporphyrin; Zn-proto, zinc protoporphyrin.
[a]Lead poisoning produces an identical overproduction pattern.
[b]Hexa- and pentacarboxylic porphyrins and coproporphyrin are increased to a smaller extent.
[c]PBG and ALA excretion may be normal when only skin lesions are present.

Cutaneous Porphyrias in Children

Congenital Erythropoietic Porphyria

Congenital erythropoietic porphyria, Günther disease, is an uncommon cutaneous porphyria in which massive overproduction of porphyrins, mainly within the erythropoietic system, produces a severe photodermatosis, hemolytic anemia, and marked porphyrinuria. It is most striking and severe in its cutaneous manifestations.

Clinical Symptoms

Congenital erythropoietic porphyria occurs worldwide and with equal frequency in both sexes. It usually presents in infancy, and the first symptom is often red discoloration of the diapers that is noticed at or soon after birth. Such infants may be photosensitive and develop erythema and bullae in areas of skin exposed to sunlight either directly or through window glass. Severe cutaneous reactions to phototherapy for hyperbilirubinemia have been reported in cases of congenital erythropoietic porphyria. By the second year of life, most affected children have characteristic porphyric lesions on light-exposed skin: subepidermal bullae, hypertrichosis, and superficial erosions resulting from increased mechanical fragility.

In older children and adults, there is often extensive scarring due to repeated infection of blisters and erosions, with atrophy and extensive areas of sclerodermatous change that may progress to severe photomutilation with atrophy of ears, nose, and digits; damage around the eyes may lead to corneal ulcerations and blindness.

Almost all patients have erythrodontia, with both the deciduous and permanent teeth being colored reddish brown. The teeth show bright red fluorescence on exposure to long-wave ultraviolet light. Porphyrin also accumulates in erythrocytes, and accelerated destruction of photo-damaged erythrocytes in the spleen explains the hemolysis and splenomegaly that is present in many patients. The hemolytic anemia is characteristically intermittent and is usually mild or moderate in severity, only rarely becoming life threatening.

Diagnostic Studies

Uroporphyrinogen III synthase activity is decreased by 70–90% in patients with congenital erythropoietic porphyria and is intermediate between this range and normal values in obligatory carriers. Over 20 point mutations have been identified in the uroporphyrinogen III synthase gene, for which patients are either homozygous or compound heterozygous.

Prenatal Diagnosis

Assays to measure porphyrins in amniotic fluid and uroporphyrinogen III synthase in amnion cells are available. Such testing is likely to be superseded by recombinant DNA methods for direct detection of mutations.

Porphyria Cutanea Tarda

Less than 1% of patients with porphyria cutanea tarda (PCT) develop skin lesions during childhood. These may appear as early as the second year of life. The lesions are much less severe than in congenital erythropoietic porphyria and similar to those seen in adults with PCT: skin fragility, subepidermal bullae, and hypertrichosis on the backs of the hands, face, and other sun-exposed areas. Unlike in adults with PCT, evidence of coexistent liver disease is uncommon in children.

Affected children probably have the type II or familial form of PCT in which uroporphyrinogen decarboxylase deficiency is present in all tissues and is inherited in an autosomal-dominant fashion. Most individuals who inherit the gene are asymptomatic, and therefore it is not unusual for patients to be the only clinically affected members of their families. The diagnosis of type II PCT can be established by demonstrating a 50% decrease in level of erythrocyte uroporphyrinogen decarboxylase. Children, like adults with PCT, may be homozygous for the hemochromatosis C282Y mutation and should be screened for its presence, particularly if they are of northern European descent.

Erythropoietic Protoporphyria

Erythropoietic protoporphyria (EPP) is the third most common porphyria and the most common form of porphyria in children. Onset of EPP after childhood is uncommon. The condition is produced by accumulation of protoporphyrin IX secondary to decreased ferrochelatase activity. Acute photosensitivity is prominent, and the condition is clinically distinguishable from all other cutaneous porphyrias.

Clinical Symptoms

Patients present with acute photosensitivity that usually starts in early childhood, often before age 2 years. An intense pricking, itching, burning sensation usually occurs within 5–30 minutes of exposure to sunlight, and blends into burning pain. Erythema, edema, and petechiae follow. Small vesicles may appear and acute photo-oncolysis may occur. After repeat attacks, the skin may become thickened, waxy, and pitted with small circular or linear scars, especially over the bridge of the nose, around the mouth, and over the knuckles. Some patients may develop pigmented protoporphyrin gallstones.

Carriers of the EPP gene are often asymptomatic as in other autosomal-dominant porphyrias. Affected individuals may have no relatives with overt EPP.

Progressive hepatic failure is an uncommon but well-recognized complication that results from liver damage caused by accumulation of protoporphyrin in hepatocytes. Liver disease does not occur in asymptomatic gene carriers.

Diagnostic Studies

Free protoporphyrin concentration is increased in erythrocytes. Protoporphyrin concentration may be increased in plasma and in feces. Urinary porphyrin concentrations are normal, except when liver disease leads to secondary coproporphyrinuria. Ferrochelatase activities are decreased in lymphocytes and other nucleated cells. Detection of asymptomatic gene carriers may require enzyme measurement by DNA analysis. Over 30 mutations of the ferrochelatase gene have been identified in EPP. Most are inherited in an autosomal-dominant pattern. Patients with overt disease may be homoallelic for several mutations. Inheritance of two disabling ferrochelatase mutations may predispose to liver disease in EPP.

Liver function should be assessed and persistent abnormalities investigated by biopsy. Very high and increasing erythrocyte porphyrin concentrations (>20–30 µmol/L), high plasma porphyrin concentrations, and relatively low fecal protoporphyrin excretion reflect impaired biliary secretion and suggest liver disease.

Hepatoerythropoietic Porphyria

Hepatoerythropoietic porphyria (HEP) is a rare form of cutaneous porphyria that results from severe uroporphyrinogen decarboxylase deficiency. Skin fragility and blisters, often accompanied by hypertrichosis and clinically indistinguishable from the lesions of PCT and chronic erythropoietic porphyria, are usually first noticed between the ages of 2 and 5. The skin lesions are usually more severe than in PCT and, with progression, may resemble those of chronic erythropoietic porphyria with photomutilation. Porphyrinuria is less marked and may not be sufficient to color the urine; erythrodontia is infrequent, and hemolytic anemia with splenomegaly has been reported in only two patients.

Urinary and fecal porphyrin excretion patterns resemble those of PCT. Unlike in PCT, the erythrocyte porphyrin concentration is invariably raised, due to increased zinc-protoporphyrin concentrations.

Differentiation between PCT and HEP depends on measurement of uroporphyrinogen decarboxylase. In erythrocytes, enzyme activity is decreased by at least 70%. These low activities, together with the finding that both parents of affected individuals have enzyme activities around 50% of normal, suggest that patients with HEP may be homozygous for the enzyme defect that causes type II PCT.

Hereditary Coproporphyria

Hereditary coproporphyria (HCP) is a disease caused by a deficiency of coproporphyrinogen oxidase (coprooxidase) activity, which is inherited as an autosomal-dominant trait. Although similar to AIP, HCP may be associated with photosensitivity in addition to neurologic symptoms. Clinical expression of HCP depends on the same metabolic and chemical factors that influence expression of the genetic defect in AIP. Coprooxidase is a mitochondrial enzyme that catalyzes the removal of the carboxyl group and two hydrogens from the propionic groups of pyrrole rings A and B of coproporphyrinogen to form vinyl groups at these positions. The reaction thus yields a divinyl compound—protoporphyrinogen. The gene encoding human coprooxidase has been assigned to chromosome 9.

Clinical Signs and Symptoms

Symptoms similar to AIP are abdominal pain, vomiting, constipation, neuropathies, and psychiatric manifestations. Cutaneous photosensitivity occurs in approximately 30% of cases. Attacks have been precipitated by pregnancy, the onset of menstruation, and contraceptive steroids, but the most common precipitating factor has been drug administration, most notably barbiturates. Neuropathies may be associated with abnormalities detected by electromyographic nerve conduction studies and tests of autonomic nervous system function.

The biochemical hallmark of HCP is hyperexcretion of coproporphyrin (predominantly type III) into the urine and feces. However, minimal elevation in urinary coproporphyrin is the most common biochemical abnormality of the heme biosynthetic pathway.

Diagnosis

Urine ALA and PBG are increased, as are coproporphyrins; this situation is similar to that found in VP, but fecal predominance of coproporphyrin is more suggestive of HCP, in contrast to VP, in which fecal coproporphyrin and protoporphyrin concentrations are usually approximately equal. In the absence of the availability of the enzyme determination, the best index for screening family members is the demonstration of substantially elevated coproporphyrin in the urine and the stool.

Coprooxidase is decreased to approximately 50% of normal in liver, fibroblasts, lymphocytes, and leucocytes. Considerable excess of coprooxidase activity in liver cells probably explains why patients with acute attacks are rare, whereas several asymptomatic carriers are found in their kindred when the enzyme is assayed.

There is a sensitive radiochemical method for determination of coprooxidase activity[7] and a fluorometric assay for coprooxidase.[8]

Homozygous Forms of the Acute Autosomal-Dominant Porphyrias

Homozygous forms of acute intermittent porphyria, variegate porphyria, and hereditary coproporphyria have been described in children with enzyme deficiencies of ≥80% and patterns of overproduction of heme precursors resembling those of the corresponding autosomal-dominant disorders. Typical acute attacks of porphyria are unusual. None have an anemia attributable to defective heme biosynthesis, although erythrocyte zinc-protoporphyrin concentrations are increased.

Overt Acute Porphyria in Children

Acute attacks of acute intermittent porphyria, hereditary coproporphyria, or variegate porphyria may occur near the age of puberty but are uncommon earlier in childhood. Attacks are precipitated by anticonvulsant therapy. The clinical features and treatment are the same as for adults. Diagnosis depends on demonstration of excess PBG in urine, followed by analysis of fecal porphyrins to distinguish between acute intermittent porphyria, hereditary coproporphyria, and variegate porphyria.

Homozygous Acute Intermittent Porphyria

Homozygous acute intermittent porphyria is the most severe of the homozygous variants of the autosomal-dominant porphyrias. Four children with homozygous acute intermittent porphyria have been described. All had excessive excretion of PBG from birth with PBG deaminase activities of <20% of normal. Clinically, the condition is characterized by progressive neurologic deterioration with leukodystrophy and, in most patients, convulsions and bilateral cataracts.

Homozygous Variegate Porphyria

Homozygous variegate porphyria is characterized by skin lesions of varying severity early in childhood, usually before the age of 1 year. Blisters, skin fragility, hypertrichosis, and skeletal abnormalities of the hands are prominent features.

Homozygous Hereditary Coproporphyria

Two types of homozygous hereditary coproporphyria have been described. Type I is associated with excessive excretion of coproporphyrin III. Type II is characterized by excretion of a tricarboxylic intermediate of the coproporphyrinogen oxidase reaction. Affected children have severe hyperbilirubinemia. Mild photosensitivity and compensated hemolytic anemia may persist after the neonatal period.

Laboratory Investigation of Porphyria

None of the porphyrias has clinical features that are sufficiently distinctive to enable the diagnosis to be made without laboratory investigations.

The essential investigation is examination of the urine for excess PBG. Screening tests such as the Watson-Schwartz test, which depend on the reaction of PBG with *p*-dimethyl-aminobenzaldehyde in acid to form a red color that is insoluble in organic solvents, have been criticized because of poor sensitivity, but if carefully carried out can detect as little as 35–50 μmol PBG/L. If results of this test are negative while symptoms are present, the child is very unlikely to have an acute porphyria. If doubt remains or if the child is seen between recurrent attacks and the screening test results are negative, PBG level should be measured by a quantitative method.

[7]Elder GH, Evans JO. A radiochemical method for the measurement of coproporphyrinogen oxidase and utilization of substrates other than coproporphyinogen III by the enzyme from rat liver. *Biochem J* 1978;169:205.

[8]Labbe P, Camadro JM, Chambon H. Fluorometric assays for coproporphyrinogen oxidase and protoporphyrinogen oxidase. *Anal Biochem* 1985;149:248.

A normal PBG concentration excludes acute intermittent porphyria. In variegate porphyria and hereditary coproporphyria, PBG level may return to normal after an acute attack, but fecal porphyrin excretion remains high; these conditions can be excluded by measuring fecal and plasma porphyrin levels. An increase in fecal porphyrin concentration without any evidence of heme precursor overproduction is almost always explained by an increased concentration of heme in the gut, either from the diet or from occult gastrointestinal bleeding, the heme being metabolized to porphyrins by bacteria.

Measurement of urinary porphyrins is usually unhelpful. Increase in PBG excretion does not differentiate between acute intermittent porphyria, variegate porphyria, and hereditary coproporphyria; fecal and plasma porphyrin measurements are required for this purpose. If PBG concentration is normal, the most frequent cause of increased urinary porphyrin excretion is coproporphyrinuria. The usual reason is cholestasis, but occasionally lead poisoning or hepatic enzyme induction due, for example, to long-term treatment with anticonvulsants may be responsible.

Detection of Gene Carriers

Enzymatic detection of carriers of the variegate porphyria and hereditary coproporphyria genes during childhood depends on measurement of protoporphyrinogen and coporphyrinogen oxidases, respectively. Both measurements require nucleated cells, such as lymphocyte, lymphoblastoid, or fibroblast cell lines. Tests are technically difficult and results do not always distinguish between affected and unaffected individuals. DNA methods are available for both conditions. In South Africa, where the high prevalence of variegate porphyria among persons of African descent is caused by a founder effect, most patients have the same mutation (R59W) in the protoporphyrinogen oxidase gene. Elsewhere, variegate porphyria shows the extensive allelic heterogeneity that is characteristic of acute intermittent porphyria, hereditary coproporphyria, and other porphyrias.

Children who are known or suspected carriers of the genes for acute intermittent porphyria, variegate porphyria, or hereditary coproporphyria should be managed in a similar fashion to adult carriers. They or their parents should ensure that drugs known to precipitate acute porphyria are avoided. In addition, they should wear a bracelet or necklace indicating that they have porphyria to prevent, for example, administration of an inappropriate anesthetic after an accident.

Other Metabolic and Hereditary Disorders

Canavan Disease (Aspartoacylase Deficiency)

Aspartoacylase hydrolyzes *N*-acetylaspartate to acetic and aspartic acids. The enzyme is reported to be cytosolic or membrane associated and is solubilized by detergent of *N*-acetylaspartate, which accumulates in tissues and fluids. Patients are asymptomatic for the first month of life although enzymatic and metabolite abnormalities are present prenatally. Poor head control, seizures, and abnormal muscle tone begin in the second to fourth month, and the infant becomes neurologically abnormal before 6 months of age in association with delayed closure of the anterior fontanelle.

Clinical Symptoms

Normal in first month of life, poor head control and hypotonia at 2–4 months, generalized seizures, opisthotonus, loss of very early milestone skills, increased head circumference, leukodystrophy on magnetic resonance imaging or CT, hypotonia progressing to spasticity, decerebrate or decorticate posturing late.

Diagnostic Studies

Identification and quantitation of metabolite (*N*-acetyl-L-aspartic acid) in urine

Definitive Diagnosis

Enzyme assay or DNA analysis or both

Copper Metabolism Disorders

Wilson Disease (Hepatolenticular Degeneration)

See Chapter 10, Liver Disease.

Kinky Hair Syndrome (Menkes Syndrome) and Occipital Horn Syndromes

X-linked recessive error of copper metabolism causing accumulation of excess copper in a low-molecular-weight protein; syndrome of neonatal hyperthermia, feeding difficulties, and sometimes prolonged jaundice; at 2–3 months, seizures and progressive change of hair from normal to steel wool–like texture with light color; striking facial appearance, increasing mental deterioration, infections, failure to thrive; changes in elastica interna of arteries; death in early infancy.

Diagnostic Studies

Decreased copper level in serum and liver; normal in RBCs.

Glycerol Metabolism Disorders

- Glycerol kinase deficiency
- Glycerol intolerance syndrome

Clinical Symptoms

Acute neonatal crisis, skeletal myopathy, developmental delay, and Addison disease caused by a contiguous gene deletion.

Diagnostic Studies

Metabolite identification and quantitation in blood and urine. Carnitine quantitation in blood or urine or both.

Definitive Diagnosis

Enzymatic assay or DNA analysis or both

Neuronal Ceroid Lipofuscinoses (Batten Disease)

See Table 10.

- Haltia-Santavuori disease [infantile neuronal ceroid lipofuscinosis (NCL)]
- Jansky-Bielschowsky disease (late infantile NCL)
- Kufs disease (adult type I; the juvenile form of NCL is the most common)
- Spielmeyer-Vogt disease (juvenile NCL)

Clinical Symptoms

Neurologic symptoms, neurodegenerative symptoms, developmental delay, hepatocellular disease, visceromegaly, gastrointestinal disease, cardiomyopathy, skeletal abnormalities, failure to thrive, ophthalmologic disorders, deafness, dermatologic abnormalities, and psychiatric disorders.

NCL is probably the most common hereditary progressive neurodegenerative disorder in children.

Diagnostic Studies

Metabolic identification and quantitation in blood and urine, tissue biopsy to obtain sample for electron microscopy, DNA analysis, or DNA linkage studies.

A diagnosis of NCL should not be made on the finding of a cytosome in a single cell. Demonstration of vacuolated lymphocytes found in juvenile NCL is a highly suggestive finding, although vacuolated lymphocytes are found in several storage disorders other than NCL. Lymphocytes may also be examined by electron microscopy. Biopsy sites are skin and conjunctiva. The biopsy specimen should include secretory coils of the sweat glands located at the border of the dermis and the subcutaneous adipose tissue. Lipofuscin accumulates in the lysosomes. It gives positive autofluorescence and stains positively with periodic acid–Schiff, Sudan

Table 10. Clinical, Neurophysiologic, and Morphologic Features of Neuronal Ceroid Lipofuscinosis

	INCL	LINCL	JNCL	Adult NCL
Eponym	Haltia-Santavuori disease	Jansky-Bielschowsky disease	Spielmeyer-Vogt disease	Kufs disease
Age of onset	8–18 mo	2–4 yr	4–8 yr	30 yr
Mental retardation	Early	Early	Late	Late
Visual failure	Relatively early	Late	Early, leading symptom	Not present
Ataxia	Moderate to marked	Marked	Marked	Variable
Myoclonus	Constant	Constant	Mild to moderate	Severe symptoms in some patients
Nonambulatory	8–30 mo	3–5 yr	13–28 yr	>35 yr
Retinal pigment aggregations	Negative	Rare	Positive	Not present
EEG	Isoelectric by 3 yr	Spikes inducible by low photic stimulation	Nonspecific	Sensitivity to low photic stimulation
VEP	Abolished by 2–4 yr	Early high	Early abnormal	High
SEP	Low	High	Variable	Variable, high
Vacuolated lymphocytes	Negative	Negative	Positive	Negative
Ultrastructure of particles	Amorphic granular	CCP	CFP	Curvilinear profiles

CCP, cytosolic curvilinear profiles; CFP, cytosolic fingerprint profiles; EEG, electroencephalogram; INCL infantile neuronal ceroid lipofuscinosis; JNCL, juvenile neuronal ceroid lipofuscinosis; LINCL, late infantile neuronal ceroid lipofuscinosis; NCL, neuronal ceroid lipofuscinosis; SEP, somatosensory evoked potential (cases from the past have been diagnosed by this method); VEP, visual evoked potential.
From Gilbert-Barness E, Barness LA. Neuronal ceroid lipofuscinosis. In: *Metabolic diseases: foundations of clinical management, genetics and pathology.* Natick, MA: Eaton Publishing, 2000.

black B, oil red O, and fuchsin. The lipopigment granules show intense acid phosphatase activity. Suction biopsy of rectal mucosa to obtain neural cells of the submucosal autonomic ganglions usually requires anesthesia. Culture of glomeruli from a kidney biopsy specimen or autopsy tissue when examined by electron microscopy is usually diagnostic for NCL and is the cornerstone for the diagnosis.

Selected Signs and Symptoms

Disorders Associated with Dysmorphic Features

Disorder	Dysmorphic Features	Other Features	Specific Investigations
Maternal PKU	Microcephaly	Congenital heart disease	Plasma phenylalanine in mother
Congenital lactic acidosis (pyruvate dehydrogenase deficiency)	Abnormal facies Microcephaly	Acidosis Hypotonia Seizures Abnormal brain (absence of corpus callosum)	Blood (and CSF) lactate Fibroblast studies Pyruvate oxidation DNA analysis

Zellweger syndrome and related disorders	High forehead Shallow supraorbital ridges Epicanthic folds Abnormal ear helices High arched palate Micrognathia Large fontanelle	Hypotonia Hepatomegaly Seizures Calcific stippling of epiphyses	RBC membrane plasmalogens Platelet and fibroblast dihydroxyacetone phosphate acyl transferase Plasma C26/C24 fatty acid ratios
Glutaric aciduria type II (multiple acyl-CoA dehydrogenase deficiency)	Macrocephaly Abnormal facies	Hypotonia Hypoglycemia Polycystic kidneys	Urinary organic acids Lymphocyte/fibroblast fatty acid oxidation
Sulfite/xanthine oxidase deficiency (molybdenum cofactor deficiency)	Abnormal facies	Seizures Hypotonia	Urine sulfite Plasma urate Urine urate/creatinine
Congenital adrenal hyperplasia	Ambiguous genitalia in females	Salt loss Recurrent vomiting Dehydration Hyponatremia	Plasma 17-hydroxyprogesterone
Congenital hypothyroidism	Coarse facies	Jaundice Constipation	Serum thyroid-stimulating hormone and free thyroxine
G_{M1} gangliosidosis	Frontal bossing Depressed nasal bridge Low-set ears	Feeding difficulties Hypoactivity Hypotonia Edema	Urinary GAGs White cell/fibroblast β-Galactosidase
Mucolipidosis type II (I-cell disease)	Course facies Depressed nasal bridge Large tongue	Restricted joint movement Radiologic changes	Plasma arylsulfatase A (I-cell screen)
Mucolipidosis type I (sialidosis)	Course facies Depressed nasal bridge Large tongue	Radiologic changes Cherry-red spot Myoclonus	White cell/fibroblast neuraminidase Urinary oligosaccharides
Mucopolysaccharidosis type VII (Sly syndrome)	Course facies Depressed nasal bridge Large tongue	Hydrops fetalis Hepatomegaly	White cell/fibroblast β-glucuronidase Note: GAGs are not always normal
Multiple sulfatase deficiency (Austin's variant)	Coarse facies Depressed nasal bridge Large tongue	Ichthyosis Hepatomegaly Radiologic changes Corneal clouding	White cell/fibroblast sulfatase (e.g., arylsulfatase A) Urinary GAGs
Mevalonate kinase deficiency	Abnormal facies	Hypotonia Hepatosplenomegaly Anemia	Urinary organic acids
Menkes disease	Abnormal facies	Hypothermia Fine hair Trichorrhexis nodosa Seizures	Serum copper and ceruloplasmin

GAG, glycosaminoglycan.

Disorders Presenting as Nonimmune Fetal Hydrops

Hematologic disorders
- Glucose-6-phosphate dehydrogenase deficiency
- Pyruvate kinase deficiency
- Glucose phosphate isomerase deficiency
- Perinatal iron storage disease

Lysosomal storage diseases
- G_{M1} gangliosidosis
- Gaucher disease
- Niemann-Pick disease
- Sialidosis
- Galactosialidosis
- I-cell disease
- Sialic acid storage disorder
- Morquio disease (mucopolysaccharidosis type IV)
- Sly syndrome (mucopolysaccharidosis type VII)

Carnitine deficiency
Wolman disease
β-Glucuronidase deficiency
Neuraminidase deficiency
Myotonic dystrophy
Perinatal iron storage syndrome

Disorders with Recognized Pathology of Peripheral Blood, Bone Marrow, and Conjunctiva and Skin

See Table 11.

Special Testing

Laboratories Performing Specialized Studies

A list of a number of laboratories performing metabolic studies can be accessed at biochemgen.ucsd.edu/.

A list of biochemical genetics laboratory services can be found at http://www.simd.org/ucsdw3bg/.

A directory of medical genetics laboratories can be obtained at http://www3.ncbi.nlm.nih.gov/Omim/searchomim.html, the National Center for Biotechnology Information.

Filter paper screening for over 25 metabolic diseases may be obtained from
Neo Gen Screening
90 Emerson Lane, Suite 1403
Abele Business Park
Bridgeville, PA 15017
Phone: 412-220-2300

A list of disorders detectable by the Newborn Screening Program is available at http://www.neogenscreening.com/disscreened.cfm.

One source of laboratories that offer molecular testing for specific genetic disorders is GeneTests/Gene Clinics, a medical genetics knowledge database providing information on genetic tests for diagnosis, management, and counseling of patients with inherited disorders.

Services are free to health care providers but require registration.

	GeneTests	**GeneClinics**
Internet:	http://www.genetests.org	http://www.geneclinics.org
Phone:	206-527-5742	206-221-4674
Fax:	206-527-5743	206-221-4679
E-mail:	genetests@genetests.org	genetests@genetests.org

Table 11. Inherited Metabolic Disorders with Recognized Pathology of Peripheral Blood, Bone Marrow, and Conjunctiva and Skin

	Bone Marrow		Conjunctival/Skin Biopsy	
Disease	Peripheral WBC	Foamy Histiocytes	Electron Microscopy Inclusion Type	Site
Niemann-Pick disease	VL	+	Pleomorphic, dense-lucent lamellar	EP, EN, M, N
Gaucher disease		+		
Krabbe disease			Crystal-like	N
Metachromatic leukodystrophy			Herringbone	N
Farber disease		+	Tubular, "banana bodies" granular membranous	M, EN, N
G_M gangliosidosis	VL	+	Fibrillogranular, membranous	EP, EN, M, N
Tay-Sachs disease			Membranous, granular	N, EN, M
Sandhoff disease			Membranous, granular	N, EN, M
Fabry disease	–	+	Lamellar	EN, M
Wolman disease	VL	+		
Mucopolysaccharidoses types I, II, III	NG, VL	+	Fibrillogranular, membranous	EP, M, N, EN
Sialic acid storage disease	VL	+	Granular, sparse	EN, M
Mucolipidosis type II	VL		Fibrillogranular, lamellar	M, EN, N
Mucolipidosis type III	VL		Fibrillogranular, lamellar	M, EN, N
Mucolipidosis type IV	VL		Fibrillogranular, lamellar	EP, EN, M, N
Fucosidosis	VL	+	Fine granular, sparse	EP, EN, M, N
Mannosidosis	VL	+	Fibrillogranular	M, EN, N
Aspartylglucosaminuria	VL		Fibrillogranular	EN, M, N
Galactosialidosis	VL		Fibrillogranular, sparse	EP, M
Cystinosis		+	Crystals	M

+, present; –, not present; EN, endocardial; EP, epithelial; M, mesenchymal (histiocytes); N, neural; NG, neutrophil granules; VL, vacuolated lymphocytes; WBC, white blood cells.

A catalog of genetics syndromes with updated references is available at Online Mendelian Inheritance in Man (OMIM), http://www3.ncbi.nlm.nih.gov/omim/. In general, OMIM does not provide specific testing sites, but it often discusses the potential for molecular testing and gives references that can be used to contact experts in the field.

Enzyme Tests

The following enzyme tests are available from the Laboratory of Medical Genetics, University of Alabama at Birmingham. Office telephone number: 205-934-4983.

Enzyme	Disease	Sample Source
Acetyl-CoA–α-glucosaminide *N*-acetyltransferase	Sanfilippo syndrome type C	FIB

Arylsulfatase A	Metachromic leukodystrophy	FIB, WBC
Arylsulfatase A (serum screen)	Mucolipidosis type II or III	SER
Arylsulfatase B	Maroteaux-Lamy syndrome	FIB, WBC
Aspartylglucosaminidase	Aspartylglucosaminuria	FIB, WBC
α-Fucosidase	Fucosidosis	FIB, WBC, SER
α-Galactosidase A	Fabry disease	FIB, WBC
β-Galactosidase	G_{M1} gangliosidosis/Morquio syndrome type B	FIB, WBC
α-Glucosidase	Pompe disease	FIB
β-Glucosidase	Gaucher disease	FIB, WBC
β-Glucuronidase	Sly syndrome	FIB, WBC
Heparin sulfamidase	Sanfilippo syndrome type A	FIB, WBC
β-Hexosaminidase (total activity)	Sandhoff disease	FIB, WBC, SER
β-Hexosaminidase A	Tay-Sachs disease	FIB, WBC, SER
Iduronate 2-sulfatase	Hunter syndrome	FIB, SER
α-Iduronidase	Hurler syndrome	FIB, WBC
α-Mannosidase	α-Mannosidosis	FIB, WBC
β-Mannosidosis	β-Mannosidosis	FIB, WBC, SER
N-acetylgalactosamine-6-sulfatase	Morquio syndrome type A	FIB
N-acetylglucosamine-6-sulfatase	Sanfilippo syndrome type D	FIB
N-acetyl-α-D-glucosaminidase	Sanfilippo syndrome type B	FIB, WBC, SER
Sialidase (neuraminidase)	Sialidosis	FIB
N-acetyl-α-D-galactosaminidase	Schindler disease	FIB, WBC, SER
Urinary sialic acid analysis	Salla disease	Urine

FIB, fibroblasts; SER, serum; WBC, white blood cells.

Bibliography

Barness LA, Gilbert-Barness E. Metabolic diseases. In: Gilbert-Barness E, ed. *Potter's pathology of the fetus and infant*. Philadelphia: Mosby–Year Book, 1997.

Beulter E, Grabowski GA. Gaucher disease. In: Scriver CR, Beaudet AL, Sly WS, et al., eds. *The metabolic and molecular bases of inherited disease*, 8th ed. New York: McGraw-Hill, 2000.

Bhala A, Willi SM, Rinaldo P, et al. Clinical and biochemical characterization of short-chain acyl-coenzyme A dehydrogenase deficiency. *J Pediatr* 1995;126:910.

Black J, Stapleton FB, Roy S III, et al. Varied types of urinary calculi in a patient with cystinosis without renal tubular acidosis. *Pediatrics* 1986;78:295.

Blom HJ, Anderson HC, Krasnewich DM, et al. Pulsed amperometric detection of carbohydrates in lysosomal storage disease fibroblasts: a new screening technique for carbohydrate storage diseases. *J Chromatogr* 1990;533:11.

Bootsma AH, Overmars H, van Rooij A, et al. Rapid analysis of conjugated bile acids in plasma using electrospray tandem mass spectrometry: application for selective screening of peroxisomal disorders. *J Inherit Metab Dis* 1999;22:307.

Bory C, Boulieu R, Chantin C, et al. Diagnosis of alcaptonuria: rapid analysis of homogentisic acid by HPLC. *Clin Chim Acta* 1990;189:7.

Boustany R-MN, Alroy J, Kolodny EH. Clinical classification of neuronal ceroid-lipofuscinosis subtypes. *Am J Med Genet Suppl* 1988;5:47.

Brady RO. Gaucher's disease: past, present and future. *Baillieres Clin Haematol* 1997;10:612.

Brenner DA, Bloomer JR. A fluorometric assay for measurement of protoporphyrinogen oxidase activity in mammalian tissue. *Clin Chim Acta* 1980;100:259.

Brusilow SW, Horwich AL. Urea cycle enzymes. In: Scriver C, Beaudet A, Sly W, et al., eds. *Metabolic and molecular bases of inherited disease*, 7th ed. New York: McGraw-Hill, 1995:1187.

Brusilow SW. Urea cycle disorders: clinical paradigm of hyperammonemic encephalopathy. In: Boyer JL, Ockner RK, eds. *Progress in liver disease*, vol 5. Philadelphia: WB Saunders, 1995.

Brusilow SW, Maestri NE. Urea cycle disorders: diagnosis, pathophysiology, and therapy. In: Barness LA, ed. *Advances in pediatrics*, vol 43. St. Louis: Mosby–Year Book, 1996:127.

Cederbaum SD. SIDS and disorders of fatty acid oxidation: where do we go from here? *J Pediatr* 1998;132:913.

Chen YT, Burchell A. Glycogen storage disease. In: Scriver CR, Beaudet AL, Sly WS, et al., eds. *The metabolic and molecular basis of inherited diseases*, 8th ed. New York: McGraw-Hill, 2000.

Chuang DT. Maple syrup urine disease: it has come a long way. *J Pediatr* 1998;132:517.

Chuang DT, Shih VE. Disorders of branched chain amino acid and keto acid metabolism. In: Scriver CR, Beaudet AL, Sly WS, et al., eds. Scriver CR, Beaudet AL, Sly WS, et al., eds. *The metabolic and molecular basis of inherited diseases*, 8th ed. New York: McGraw-Hill, 2000.

Clarke JTR. *A clinical guide to inherited metabolic diseases*. Cambridge: Cambridge University Press, 1996.

Clarke LA, Dimmick JE, Applegarth DA. Pathology of inherited metabolic disease. In: Dimmick JE, Kalousek DK, eds. *Developmental pathology of the embryo and fetus*. Philadelphia: JB Lippincott Co, 1993.

Davidson BL, Tarlé SA, van Antwerp M, et al. Identification of 17 independent mutations responsible for human hypoxanthine-guanine phosphoribosyltransferase (HPRT) deficiency. *Am J Hum Genet* 1991;48:951.

Demaugre F, Bonnefont J-P, Colonna M, et al. Infantile form of carnitine palmitoyltransferase II deficiency with hepatomuscular symptoms and sudden death. Physiopathological approach to carnitine palmitoyltransferase II deficiencies. *J Clin Invest* 1991;87:859.

DeVivo DC. The expanding clinical spectrum of mitochondrial diseases. *Brain Dev* 1993;15:1.

DeVivo DC, Tein I. Primary and secondary disorder of carnitine metabolism. *Int Pediatr* 1990;5:2.

DiMauro S. Promising avenues of investigation in the diagnosis and treatment of mitochondrial defects. In: Shaw Weeber K, ed. *A primary care physician's guide*. Psy-Ed Corporation Publishers, 1997.

DiMauro S, Bonilla E. Mitochondrial encephalomyopathies. In: DiMauro S, Barchi RL, eds. *The molecular and genetic basis of neurological disease* Boston: Butterworth–Heinemann, 1997:201.

Dimmick JE, Applegarth DA. Inherited metabolic diseases. In: Stocker JT, Dehner LP, eds. *Pediatric pathology*, 2nd ed. Philadelphia: JB Lippincott Co, 2001.

Dimmick JE, Applegarth DA. Pathology of inherited metabolic disease. In: Stocker J, Dehner L, eds. *Pediatric pathology*. Philadelphia: JB Lippincott Co, 1992.

Khan KM, Brooks SS, Pullarkat RK. Abnormal acid phosphatases in neuronal ceroidlipofuscinoses. *Am J Med Genet* 1995;57:285.

Fernandes J, Saudubray JM, Van den Berghe G. *Inborn metabolic diseases: diagnosis and treatment*. New York: Springer-Verlag, 2000.

Finegold D. Diagnosis: the promise of DNA analysis in understanding mitochondrial disease. In: Shaw Weeber K, ed. *A primary care physician's guide*. Psy-Ed Corporation Publishers, 1997.

Finocchiaro G, Taroni F, Rocchi M, et al. cDNA cloning, sequence analysis, and chromosomal localization of the gene from human carnitine palmitoyltransferase. *Proc Natl Acad Sci U S A* 1991;88:661.

Folkerth RD, Alroy J, Lomakina I, et al. Mucolipidosis IV: morphology and histochemistry of an autopsy case. *J Neuropathol Exp Neurol* 1995;54:154.

Gahl WA. Cystinosis coming of age. *Adv Pediatr* 1986;33:95.

Gibson KM, Bennett MJ, Naylor EW, et al. 3-Methyl-crotonylcoenzyme A carboxylase deficiency in Amish/Mennonite adults identified by detection of increased acylcarnitines in blood spots of their children. *J Pediatr* 1998;132:519.

Gibson KM, ten Brink HJ, Schor DS, et al. Stable-isotope dilution analysis of D- and L-2-hydroxy-glutaric acid: application to the detection and prenatal diagnosis of D- and L-2-hydroxyglutaric acidemias. *Pediatr Res* 1993;34:277.

Gieselmann V, von Figura K. Advances in the molecular genetics of metachromatic leukodystrophy. *J Inherit Metab Dis* 1990;13:560.

Gilbert-Barness E, Barness LA. Isovaleric acidemia. *Pediatr Dev Pathol* 1999;2:286.

Gilbert-Barness E, Barness L. *Metabolic diseases: foundations of clinical management, genetics and pathology*. Natick, MA: Eaton Publishing, 2000.

Gilbert-Barness E, Barness LA. The mucolipidoses. In: Landing B, Haust M, Bernstein J, et al., eds. *Genetic metabolic diseases*. Basel: Karger, 1993.

Goebel HH. The neuronal ceroid-lipofuscinoses. *J Child Neurol* 1995;10:424.

Goldin E, Blanchette-Mackie EJ, Dwyer NK, et al. Cultured skin fibroblasts derived from patients with mucolipidosis 4 are auto-fluorescent. *Pediatr Res* 1995;37:687.

Goodman SI, Markey SP. *Diagnosis of organic acidemias by gas chromatography-mass spectrometry,* 6th ed. New York: Alan R. Liss, 1981.

Griffiths GM, Isaaz S. Granzymes A and B are targeted to the lytic granules of lymphocytes by the mannose-6-phosphate receptor. *J Cell Biol* 1993;120:885.

Hammans SR, Morgan-Hughes JA. Mitochondrial myopathies: clinical features, investigation, treatment and genetic counseling. In: Schapira AHV, DiMauro S, eds. *Mitochondrial disorders in neurology.* Oxford: Butterworth–Heineman, 1994:49.

Hirano M, DiMauro S. Clinical features of mitochondrial myopathies and encephalomyopathies. In: Lane RJM, ed. *Handbook of muscle disease*. New York: Marcel Dekker, 1996:479.

Hoffmann GF, Aramaki S, Blum-Hoffmann E, et al. Quantitative analysis for organic acids in biological samples: batch isolation followed by gas chromatographic-mass spectrometric analysis. *Clin Chem* 1989;38:32.

Holtzapple PG, Genel M, Yakovac WC, et al. Diagnosis of cystinosis by rectal biopsy. *N Engl J Med* 1969;281:143.

Hommes FA, Varghese M. High-performance liquid chromatography of urinary oligosaccharides in the diagnosis of glycoprotein degradation disorders. *Clin Chim Acta* 1991;203:21.

Hopwood JJ, Brooks DA. An introduction to the basic science and biology of the lysosome and storage disorders. In: Applegarth DA, Dimmick JE, Hall JG, eds. *Organelle disorders*. New York: Chapman and Hall, 1997:7.

Ijlst L, Wanders RJ, Ushikubo S, et al. Molecular basis of long-chain 3-hydroxyacyl-CoA dehydrogenase deficiency: identification of the major disease-causing mutation in the alpha-subunit of the mitochondrial trifunctional protein. *Biochim Biophys Acta* 1994;1215:347.

Ikonen E, Syvänen A-C, Peltonen L. Dissection of the molecular pathology of aspartylglucosaminuria provides the basis for DNA diagnostics and future therapeutic interventions. *Scand J Clin Lab Invest* 1993;53:19.

Jakobs C, Stellaard F, Kvittingen EA, et al. First trimester prenatal diagnosis of tyrosinemia type I by amniotic fluid succinylacetone determination. *Prenat Diagn* 1990;10:133.

Jenkinson CP, Grody WW, Cederbaum SD. Comparative properties of arginases. *Comp Biochem Physiol B Biochem Mol Biol* 1996;114:107.

Johnson DW. A rapid screening procedure for the diagnosis of peroxisomal disorders: quantification of very long-chain fatty acids, as dimethylaminoethyl esters, in plasma and blood spots, by electrospray tandem mass spectrometry. *J Inherit Metab Dis* 2000;23:475.

Johnson DW. Dimethylaminoethyl esters for trace, rapid analysis of fatty acids by electrospray tandem mass spectrometry. *Rapid Commun Mass Spectrom* 1999;13:2388.

Johnson DW. Alkyldimethylaminoethyl ester iodides for improved analysis of fatty acids by electrospray ionization tandem mass spectrometry. *Rapid Commun Mass Spectrom* 2000;14(21):2019.

Kamoun P, Poggi F, Saudubray JM, et al. Paradoxical hyperammonemia with hypocitrullinemia, hypoornithinemia and hypoprolinemia (PHHH syndrome). Paper presented at: *Advances in inherited urea cycle disorders; May 20–21, 1997; Vienna, Austria.*

Kappas A, Sassa S, Galbraith RA, et al. The porphyrias. In: Scriver CR, Beaudet AL, Sly WS, et al., eds. *The metabolic and molecular bases of inherited diseases*, 8th ed. New York: McGraw-Hill, 2000:2103.

Kvittingen EA. Hereditary tyrosinemia type I: an overview. *Scand J Clin Lab Invest* 1986;184:27.

Laberge C, Griener A, Valet JP, et al. Fumarylacetoacetase measurement as a mass-screening procedure for hereditary tyrosinemia type I. *Am J Hum Genet* 1990;47:325.

La Du BN. Alkaptonuria. In: Scriver CR, Beaudet AL, Sly WS, et al., eds. *The metabolic and molecular bases of inherited diseases*, 7th ed. New York: McGraw-Hill, 1995:1371.

Lake BD. Lysosomal enzyme deficiencies. In: Graham DI, Lantos PL, eds. *Greenfield's neuropathology*. London: Arnold Publishing, 1997.

Landing BH, Ang SM, Villarreal-Engelhardt G, et al. Galactosemia: clinical and pathologic features, tissue staining patterns with labeled galactose- and galactosamine-binding lectins, and possible loci of nonenzymatic galactosylation. *Perspect Pediatr Pathol* 1993;17:99.

Long WW, Pawel B, Morrow G. Hereditary fructose intolerance. Pathological case of the month. *Arch Pediatr Adolesc Med* 1997;151:1166.

Masataka M. Regulation of the urea cycle genes in urea and nitric oxide synthesis. Paper presented at: *Advances in inherited urea cycle disorders*; *May 20–21, 1997; Vienna, Austria.* (abstr)

Meikle PJ, Hopwood JJ, Clague AE, et al. Prevalence of lysosomal storage disorders. *JAMA* 1999;281:249.

Millington DS, Ming-Lui H, Stevens RD, et al. In vitro text for diagnosis of long-chain fatty acid oxidation. Paper presented at: *Society for Inherited Metabolic Disorders annual meeting; March 12–15, 1999; Lake Lanier Islands, GA*.

Mitchell GA, Lambert M, Tanguay RM. Hypertyrosinemia. In: Scriver CR, Beaudet AL, Sly WS, et al., eds. *The metabolic and molecular bases of inherited diseases*, 7th ed. New York: McGraw-Hill, 1995:1077.

Mole SE. Recent advances in the molecular genetics of neuronal ceroid lipofuscinosis. *J Inherit Metab Dis* 1996;19:269.

Morales LE. Gaucher's disease: a review. *Ann Pharmacother* 1996;30:381.

Morrow G, Barness LA, Efron ML. Citrullinemia with defective urea production. *Pediatrics* 1967;40:565.

Moser HW. Peroxisomal diseases. *Adv Pediatr* 1989;36:1.

Mudd SH, Levy HL, Skorby F. Disorders of transsulfuration. In: Scriver CR, Beaudet AL, Sly WS, et al., eds. *The metabolic and molecular bases of inherited diseases*, 7th ed. New York: McGraw-Hill, 1995:1279.

Natowicz MR. Clinical and biochemical manifestations of hyaluronidase deficiency. *N Engl J Med* 1996;335:1029.

Naviaux MD. The spectrum of mitochondrial disease. In: Shaw Weeber K, ed. *A primary care physician's guide*. Psy-Ed Corporation Publishers, 1997.

Naylor EW. Electrospray tandem mass spectrometry screening for mitochondrial and metabolic diseases. In: Shaw Weeber K, ed. *A primary care physician's guide*. Psy-Ed Corporation Publishers, 1997.

Neufeld EF, Meunzer J. The mucopolysaccharidoses. In: Scriver CR, Beaudet AL, Sly WS, et al., eds. *The metabolic and molecular bases of inherited diseases*, 7th ed. New York: McGraw-Hill, 1995:2465.

Nordmann Y, Deybach J-C. Human hereditary porphyrias. In: Daley H, ed. *Biosynthesis of heme and chlorophylls*. New York: McGraw-Hill, 1990:491–542.

O'Brien JS, Willems PJ, Fukushima H, et al. Molecular biology of the α-L-fucosidase gene and fucosidosis. *Enzyme* 1987;38:45.

Passarge E. *Color atlas of genetics*, 2nd ed. New York: Thieme Medical Publishing, 2001.

Petushkova NA, Ivleva TS, Voxniy YAM. Human chorionic β-mannosidase: comparison with β-mannosidase from human cultured fibroblasts. *Prenat Diagn* 1992;12:835.

Poh-Fitzpatrick MB. A plasma porphyrin fluorescence marker for variegate porphyria. *J Am Acad Dermatol* 1983;8:115.

Poll-The BT, Saudubray J-M. Peroxisomal disorders. In: Fernades J, Saudubray J-M, Van den Berghe G, eds. *Inborn metabolic diseases*, 2nd ed. Berlin: Springer-Verlag, 1996.

Prence EM, Natowicz MR. Diagnosis of α-mannosidase in plasma. *Clin Chem* 1992;38:501.

Proceedings of the Fifth International Conference on Neuronal Ceroid Lipofuscinosis. Special Issue: Ceroid Lipofuscinoses, Batten Disease and Allied Disorders. *Am J Med Genet* 1995;57:121.

Rapola J. Neuronal ceroid-lipofuscinoses in childhood. In: Landing BH, Haust MD, Bernstein J, et al., eds. *Genetic metabolic diseases*. Basel: Karger, 1993:7. Perspectives in Pediatric Pathology, vol 17.

Rapola J, Salonen R, Ammälä P, et al. Prenatal diagnosis of the infantile type of neuronal ceroid lipofuscinosis by electron microscopic investigation of human chorionic villi. *Prenat Diagn* 1990;10:553.

Recio L, Cochrane J, Simpson D, et al. DNA sequence analysis of in vivo HPRT mutation in human T lymphocytes. *Mutagenesis* 1990;5:505.

Roe CR, Coates PM. Mitochondrial fatty acid oxidation disorders. In: Scriver CR, Beaudet AL, Sly WS, et al., eds. *The metabolic and molecular bases of inherited disease*, 7th ed. New York: McGraw-Hill, 1995:1051.

Rossiter BJF, Caskey C. Hypoxanthine-guanine phosphoribosyltransferase deficiency: Lesch-Nyhan syndrome and gout. In: Scriver CR, Beaudet AL, Sly WS, et al., eds. *The metabolic and molecular bases of inherited disease,* 8th ed. New York: McGraw-Hill, 2000.

Santos M, Clevers HC, Marx JJM. Mutations of the hereditary hemochromatosis candidate gene HLA-H in porphyria cutanea tarda. *N Engl J Med* 1997;36:1329.

Saudubray J, Charpentier C. Clinical phenotypes: diagnosis/algorithms. In: Scriver CR, Beaudet AL, Sly WS, et al., eds. *The metabolic and molecular bases of inherited disease*, 7th ed. New York: McGraw-Hill, 1995.

Schindler D, Kanzaki T, Desnick RJ. A method for the rapid detection of urinary glycopeptides in α-*N*-acetylgalactosaminidase deficiency and other lysosomal storage disease. *Clin Chim Acta* 1990;190:81.

Schuchman EH, Desnick RJ. Niemann-Pick disease types A and B: acid sphingomyelinase deficiencies: In: Scriver CR, Beaudet AL, Sly WS, et al., eds. *The metabolic and molecular bases of inherited disease,* 8th ed. New York: McGraw-Hill, 2000.

Scriver CR, Beaudet AL, Sly WS, et al., eds. *The metabolic and molecular bases of inherited disease*, 7th ed. New York: McGraw-Hill, 1995.

Scriver CR, Beaudet AL, Sly WS, et al. *The metabolic and molecular bases of inherited disease,* 8th ed. New York: McGraw-Hill, 2000.

Scriver CR, Krugman S, Eisensmith RC. The hyperphenylalaninemias. In: Segal S, Berry GT. Disorders of galactose metabolism. In: Scriver CR, Beaudet AL, Sly WS, et al., eds. *The metabolic and molecular bases of inherited disease,* 8th ed. New York: McGraw-Hill, 2000.

Sidransky E, Fartasch M, Lee RE, et al. Epidermal abnormalities may distinguish type 2 from type 1 and type 3 of Gaucher disease. *Pediatr Res* 1996;39:134.

Stanley CA, KeLeeuw S, Coates PM, et al. Chronic cardiomyopathy and weakness or acute coma in children with a defect in carnitine uptake. *Ann Neurol* 1991;30:709.

Stanley CA, Sunaryo F, Hale DE, et al. Elevated plasma carnitine in the hepatic form of carnitine palmitoyltransferase-1 deficiency. *J Inherit Metab Dis* 1992;15:785.

Stibler H, Skovby F. Failure to diagnose carbohydrate-deficient glycoprotein syndrome prenatally. *Pediatr Neurol* 1994;11:71.

Sweetman L. Organic acid analysis. In: Hommes FA, ed. Techniques in diagnostic human biochemical genetics: a laboratory manual. New York: Wiley-Liss, 1991:143.

Tanaka K, Rosenberg LE. Disorders of branched chain amino acid and organic acid metabolism. In: Stanbury JB, Wyngaarden JB, Frederickson DS, et al., eds. *The metabolic basis of inherited disease*, 5th ed. New York: McGraw-Hill, 1983:440.

Taschner PEM, de Vos N, Post JG, et al. Carrier detection of Batten disease (juvenile neuronal ceroid-lipofuscinosis). *Am J Med Genet* 1995;57:333.

Treacy EP, Delente JJ, Elkas G, et al. Analysis of phenylalanine hydroxylase genotypes and hyperphenylalaninemia phenotypes using L-(1-13C) phenylalanine oxidation rates in vivo: a pilot study. *Pediatr Res* 1997;42:430(abst).

Vallance H, Applegarth D. An improved method for quantification of very long chain fatty acids in plasma. *Clin Biochem* 1994;27:183.

Van den Berghe G, Vincent MF. Disorders of purine and pyrimidine metabolism. In: Fernades J, Saudebray J-M, Van den Berghe G, eds. *Inborn metabolic disease*, 2nd ed. Basel: Springer-Verlag, 1996.

Van Gennip H, Driedijk PC, Elzinga A, et al. Screening for defects of dihydropyrimidine degradation by analysis of amino acids in urine before and after acid hydrolysis. *Int J Pur Pyr Res* 1991;2[Suppl 1]:41.

Vladutiu GD, Smail D. Mutant haplotypes and biochemical correlations in CPT II deficiency. Paper presented at: *Society for Inherited Metabolic Disorders Annual Meeting; March 12–15, 1999; Lake Lanier Islands, GA*.

Vockley JG, Jenkinson CP, Shukla H, et al. Cloning and characterization of the human type II arginase gene. *Genomics* 1996;38:118.

Wallace DC. Diseases of the mitochondrial DNA. *Annu Rev Biochem* 1992;61:1175.

Wallace DC. Maternal genes: mitochondrial diseases. *Birth Defects* 1987;23:137.
Wang Y, Ye J, Ganapathy V, et al. Mutations in the organic cation/carnitine transporter OCTN2 in primary carnitine deficiency. *Proc Natl Acad Sci U S A* 1999;96:2346.
Wisniewski KE, Rapin I, Heaney-Kieras J. Clinico-pathological variability in the childhood neuronal ceroid-lipofuscinoses and new observations on glycoprotein abnormalities. *Am J Med Genet* 1988;29:27.
Wohlers TM, Christacos NC, Harreman MT, et al. Identification and characterization of a mutation, in the human UDP-galactose-4-epimerase gene, associated with generalized epimerase-deficiency galactosemia. *Am J Hum Genet* 1999;64:462.
Young EP. Prenatal diagnosis of Hurler disease by analysis of α-L-iduronidase in chorionic villi. *J Inherit Metab Dis* 1992;15:224.
Zeigler M, Bargel R, Suri V, et al. Mucolipidosis type IV: accumulation of phospholipids and gangliosides in cultured amniotic cells. A tool for prenatal diagnosis. *Prenat Diagn* 1992;12:1037.
Zimran A, Elstein D, Abrahamov A, et al. Prenatal molecular diagnosis of Gaucher disease. *Prenat Diagn* 1995;15:1185.

18 Endocrine Disorders

Pediatric Endocrine Testing

Pediatric Reference Intervals for Selected Hormones

Test	Age	Reference Interval
Aldosterone, serum (ng/dL) (M, F)	<1 yr	5–132
	1–3 yr	5–60
	4–7 yr	4–76
	8–11 yr	3–28
	12–16 yr	1–18
Aldosterone, urine (μg/d) (M, F)	Newborn	0.7–11.0
	Infant	0.62–22.00
	Child	2.3–16.0
Androstenedione (ng/dL)	0–5 mo	5–45 (M) 5–35 (F)
	6–12 mo	5–30 (M) 5–25 (F)
	1–5 yr	5–45 (M) 5–40 (F)
	6–9 yr	5–55 (M) 5–45 (F)
	10–11 yr	10–30 (M) 25–80 (F)
	12–14 yr	20–85 (M) 15–175 (F)
	15–17 yr	35–100 (M) 55–200 (F)
Cortisol (μg/dL) (M, F)	5 d	0.6–19.8
	2 mo to 13 yr	2.5–22.9
Dehydroepiandrosterone (DHEA) (ng/dL)	<6 yr	26–72 (M) 19–42 (F)
	6–7 yr	29–66 (M) 73–165 (F)
	8–9 yr	53–135 (M) 74–180 (F)
	10–11 yr	183–383 (M) 234–529 (F)
	12–14 yr	240–520 (M) 224–611 (F)
Dehydroepiandrosterone sulfate (DHEAS) μg/dL)	0–5 mo	0–148 (M) 0–147 (F)
	6 mo to 7 yr	0–18 (M) 0–37 (F)
	8–9 yr	0–110 (M, F)
	10–12 yr	5–137 (M) 3–111 (F)
	13–15 yr	3–188 (M) 4–171 (F)

	16–18 yr	26–189 (M)
		10–237 (F)
Erythropoietin (mIU/mL)	1–3 yr	1.7–17.9 (M)
		2.1–15.9 (F)
	4–6 yr	3.5–21.9 (M)
		2.9–8.5 (F)
	7–9 yr	1.0–13.5 (M)
		2.1–8.2 (F)
	10–12 yr	1–14 (M)
		1.1–9.1 (F)
	13–15 yr	2.2–14.4 (M)
		3.8–20.5 (F)
Estradiol (pg/mL)	1–6 yr	<15 (M, F)
	7–10 yr	<15 (M)
		<70 (F)
	11–12 yr	<40 (M)
		10–300 (F)
	13–15 yr	<45 (M)
		10–300 (F)
Estrone (pg/mL)	<6 yr	18–53 (M)
		19–46 (F)
	6–7 yr	17–48 (M)
		17–44 (F)
	8–9 yr	20–54 (M)
		31–70 (F)
	10–11 yr	21–49 (M)
		28–68 (F)
	12–14 yr	17–44 (M)
		57–140 (F)
Follicle-stimulating hormone (FSH) (mIU/mL)	5 d	<0.2–4.6 (M, F)
	2 mo to 9 yr	0.2–2.7 (M)
	2 mo to 3 yr	1.4–9.2 (F)
	4–6 yr	0.4–6.6 (F)
	7–9 yr	0.4–5.0 (F)
	10–11 yr	0.4–5.0 (M)
	12–13 yr	0.4–6.6 (M)
	14–15 yr	0.7–13.2 (M)
Gastrin (pg/mL) (M, F)	1–12 d	69–190
	1.5–22 mo	55–100
17α-Hydroxyprogesterone (ng/dL)	0–1 d	170–2,500
	1–7 d	30–350
	7–28 d	0–250
	1–12 mo	0–170
	1–9 yr	0–100
	10–11 yr	0–130
	12–14 yr	30–200
	15–17 yr	30–230
17-Hydroxyprogesterone (ng/dL)	0–1 mo	53–86 (M)
		17–204 (F)
	1–5 mo	35–157 (M)
		25–110 (F)
	6–12 mo	6–40 (M)
		5–47 (F)
	1–3 yr	2–19 (M)
		3–51 (F)
	4–6 yr	1–34 (M)
		4–34 (F)
	7–9 yr	1–45 (M)
		4–44 (F)
	10–12 yr	1–34 (M)
		3–33 (F)

	13–15 yr	23–82 (M) 2–72 (F)
	16–18 yr	8–100 (M) 3–91 (F)
Insulin-like growth factor (IGF) (ng/mL)	<2 mo	Not established (M, F)
	2 mo to 5.9 yr	17–248 (M, F)
	6–8.9 yr	88–474 (M, F)
	9–11.9 yr	110–565 (M)
	9–11.9 yr	117–771 (F)
	12–15.9 yr	202–957 (M)
	12–15.9 yr	261–1,096 (F)
	16–24.9 yr	182–780 (M, F)
	25–39.9 yr	114–492 (M, F)
	40–54.9 yr	90–360 (M, F)
	≥55 yr	71–290 (M, F)
Luteinizing hormone (LH) (mIU/mL)	0–2 yr	0.5–1.9 (M) 0–0.5 (F)
	2–10 yr	0–0.5 (M, F)
	11–20 yr	0.5–5.3 (M) 0.5–9.0 (F)
Prolactin (ng/mL)	<1 mo	3.7–81.2 (M) 0.3–95.0 (F)
	1–12 mo	0.3–28.9 (M) 0.2–29.9 (F)
	1–3 yr	2.3–13.2 (M) 1–17 (F)
	4–6 yr	0.8–16.9 (M) 1.6–13.1 (F)
	7–9 yr	1.9–11.6 (M) 0.3–12.9 (F)
	10–12 yr	0.9–12.9 (M) 1.9–9.6 (F)
	13–15 yr	1.6–16.6 (M) 3.0–14.4 (F)
Testosterone (ng/dL)	1–5 mo	1–177 (M) 1–5 (F)
	6–11 mo	2–7 (M) 2–5 (F)
	1–6 yr	0–10 (M, F)
	6–8 yr	0–20 (M) 0–10 (F)
	8–11 yr	0–25 (M) 0–30 (F)
	11–13 yr	0–350 (M) 0–50 (F)
	13–15 yr	15–500 (M) 0–50 (F)
Thyroglobulin (ng/mL) (M, F)		
	Term infants	
	Cord blood	5–65
	1 d	6–93
	3 d	9–148
	Premature infants (27–31 weeks' gestation)	
	1 d	107–395
	10 d	49–163
	30 d	17–63
	Premature infants (31–34 weeks' gestation)	
	1 d	147–277
	10 d	32–112

	30 d	19–51
	7–12 yr	20–50
	13–18 yr	9–27
Thyroid-stimulating hormone (TSH) (μIU/mL)	1–30 d	0.52–16.00 (M) 0.72–13.10 (F)
	1 mo to 5 yr	0.55–7.10 (M) 0.46–810 (F)
Thyroxine (T_4) (μg/dL)	1–30 d	5.9–21.5 (M) 6.3–21.5 (F)
	1–11 mo	6.4–13.9 (M) 4.9–13.7 (F)
	1–3 yr	7.0–13.1 (M) 7.1–14.1 (F)
	4–6 yr	6.1–12.6 (M) 7.2–14.0 (F)
	7–12 yr	6.7–13.4 (M) 6.1–12.1 (F)
	13–15 yr	4.8–11.5 (M) 5.8–11.2 (F)
T_4, free by equilibrium dialysis, serum (ng/dL)	Birth to 4 d	2.2–5.3
	2–20 wk	0.9–2.2
	21 wk to 24 mo	0.7–1.9
	25 mo to 7 yr	0.8–2.3
	8–20 yr	0.6–2.0
	21–87 yr	0.8–2.7
	Pregnancy	
	First trimester	0.7–2.0
	Second trimester	0.5–1.6
	Third trimester	0.5–1.6
T_4, free (direct) (ng/dL) (M, F)	<6 yr	0.94–1.59
	7–12 yr	0.94–1.50
Vanillylmandelic acid, random urine (mg/g creatinine)	0–1 yr	0–18.8 (M, F)
	2–4 yr	0–11 (M, F)
	5–19 yr	0–8.3 (M, F)

Pituitary Diseases and Growth Disorders

Defects in pituitary function may be responsible for defects in growth rate and defects in the function of any or all other endocrine glands.

Assays for Pituitary and Related Hormones

Growth Hormone Assays

Growth hormone (GH) in plasma consists of various molecular forms that may not be equally recognized in different assays. Technical improvements have led to new assays such as immunoradiometric assay with monoclonal or polyclonal antibodies, immunoenzymometric assay or enzyme-linked immunosorbent assay, immunofluorometric assay, and oligoclonal assay.

The commonly used stimuli for GH secretion include clonidine, L-Dopa, ornithine, glucagon-propranolol, and insulin induction of hypoglycemia. The last two may induce severe hypoglycemia and their use requires close follow-up. The arginine stimulation test is less potent and gives more false-negative results. By convention, failure to achieve a maximum stimulated GH concentration of 7 or 10 mg/mL using conventional radioimmunoassays (RIAs) defines classical GH deficiency. Cutoff value is lower when some of the monoclonal assays are used.

Assessment of maximum spontaneous GH secretion is by sampling at frequent intervals or by continuous withdrawal during 12- to 24-hour periods, with results expressed as spontaneous peak values or integrated concentrations of GH (IC-GH). Some children with low GH concentrations after GH stimulation have spontaneous GH profiles and IC-GH in the normal range.

To interpret the individual data, one must be aware of the large range of IC-GH values obtained in normal children.

In boys with delayed puberty, transient low GH secretion may be corrected by administration of testosterone as a depot preparation 50 mg intramuscularly (i.m.) or 100 mg/m^2 every 2 weeks for 2 months. Alternatively, in both sexes, and especially in patients with pubertal delay, sex steroid priming at first stimulation test may be performed by giving ethinyl-estradiol 40 μg/m^2 divided in three doses for 2 days preceding the GH stimulation test. The peak GH values are then increased to the pubertal range, which improves the diagnostic value of the stimulation test. A negative correlation exists between GH concentration and adiposity expressed as body mass index or percentage of body fat.

Insulin-Like Growth Factor Assays

Immunoradiometric assays using simple extraction techniques allow an accurate determination of plasma IGF-I levels in most clinical conditions. High-affinity antisera are needed for the RIA. Use of recombinant IGF-I as a reference standard now allows expression of concentrations in nanograms per milliliter and comparison among laboratories. The possibility of significant interferences of IGF-I–binding proteins occurs in patients with chronic renal failure.

For IGF-II measurement, variable antibodies have been used: polyclonal antibody with minimal cross reactivity with IGF-I, specific antibody prepared against a synthetic peptide derived from the C domain of IGF-II, or a competitive protein-binding assay. IGF-II does not play a significant role in postnatal growth.

IGF-I serum levels show differences in absolute values with a progressive increase in concentration during childhood and a marked increase at puberty.

Diabetes Insipidus

Diabetes insipidus is due to defective regulation of water balance secondary to decreased secretion of or failure of response to vasopressin.

Signs and Symptoms

Signs and symptoms include thirst/polydipsia, polyuria, nocturia, dehydration, headache, and visual disturbance. Skin should be examined for café-au-lait spots indicating neurofibromatosis petechial lesions suggestive of histiocytosis. Inadequate secretion of vasopressin may be due to loss or malfunction of the neurosecretory neurons that make up the neurohypophysis (posterior pituitary). Insensitivity to vasopressin—a disorder of renal tubular function—results in inability to respond to vasopressin in absorption of water. Lithium carbonate, demeclocycline hydrochloride, and methoxyflurane may produce vasopressin insensitivity. Also, hypokalemia and hypercalcemia alter ability to concentrate urine.

Familial cases of vasopressin deficiency may occur (commonly with autosomal-dominant inheritance). The disease is usually isolated and often secondary to other disorders.

Nephrogenic diabetes insipidus is usually inherited as a sex-linked recessive trait, expressed in males and rarely in females, and is usually manifest in infancy.

Excessive water intake (primary polydipsia) usually is of functional origin.

Diagnostic Studies

Test for hypernatremia (particularly in infants and children)

Test for inability to concentrate urine (measured by osmolality rather than specific gravity)

Urinary glucose level (to rule out diabetes mellitus)

Plasma vasopressin or urinary vasopressin level after osmotic stimulus such as fluid restriction or administration of hypertonic saline

Special Tests

Testing of the ability to concentrate urine in the face of water deprivation is done by measuring urine and plasma osmolality before and after a 6-hour period of thirst. It is not wise to perform overnight thirst tests, particularly in children, as severe dehydration may occur, leading to central nervous system damage.

The most valuable measurements are the urine/plasma osmolality ratio and plasma vasopressin concentrations. The results are sometimes difficult to interpret because low ratios may be found in patients with primary polydipsia. If results support the diagnosis, desmopressin should be administered to test renal concentrating ability.

Imaging Studies

Computed tomography (CT) or magnetic resonance imaging (MRI) of brain may detect tumor.

Growth Hormone, Urinary

GH is excreted in the urine as natural 22-kilodalton GH. A small fraction of injected GH is recovered in the urine. GH excretion is significantly diminished in children with hypopituitarism.

Growth Hormone–Binding Protein

The high-affinity GH-binding protein can be measured in plasma as the plasma GH-binding activity. RIA techniques allow a more thorough evaluation of its physiologic and clinical significance. Its concentration is very low at birth, rises during childhood, and reaches adult values by age 25 years. Its measurement provides useful clinical information for rare genetic conditions of GH insensitivity; it is undetectable in most patients with Laron-type dwarfism because of mutations in extracellular binding domains of the GH receptor. In certain short populations, such as the African pygmies and New Guinea people, a decreased concentration of GH-binding protein has been found, which possibly indicates a partial end-organ resistance.

Growth Hormone Deficiency

Children with GH deficiency have retarded bone age and decreased growth rate (below 4.5 cm/year before puberty), documented during at least a year's follow-up.

The diagnostic procedure usually begins with a GH stimulation test eventually conducted after sex steroid priming. If the GH responses are discrepant, it is necessary to further investigate the patient's condition by measuring plasma IGF-I levels.

If GH deficiency is documented, MRI should be performed to detect a craniopharyngioma or a less frequent tumor, or to document pituitary anatomy. Pituitary stalk interruption with an ectopic posterior hypophyseal bright spot and anterior pituitary hypoplasia indicates that GH deficiency, generally part of idiopathic multiple pituitary deficiencies, will be permanent and requires long-term GH therapy. Transient GH deficiency is seen mostly in boys with pubertal delay. GH treatment is rarely required in these children.

Growth Retardation

See Table 1.

Table 1. Evaluation of Growth Retardation

Cause	Clinical Signs	Plasma Biochemical/ Hormonal Signs	Possible Diagnosis
Familial and neonatal history	Parental short stature and/or pubertal delay	Normal	Genetic/constitutional growth retardation
	Poor economic status	Normal GH, low IGF-I	Calorie/protein deficiency
	Disturbed family, child abuse	Normal GH, low IGF-I	Psychosocial dwarfism
	Small for date and/or dysmorphic features	Normal	Intrauterine growth retardation
		Normal	Chromosomal, skeletal disorders
Endocrine causes	GH deficiency features, hypoglycemia or growth retardation associated with midline defects or perinatal asphyxia secondary to cranial irradiation or brain tumor, isolated (sporadic or familial)	Low GH, low IFG-I	Isolated GH deficiency or multiple pituitary deficiencies
		Low GH, low IGF I	Isolated GH deficiency (GRF deficiency); GH gene deletion
		High GH, low IFG-I	GH receptor mutation: GH insensitivity
	Hypothyroidism	Low T_4/T_3, high TSH	Primary hypothyroidism
	Obesity, osteoporosis	High plasma/urinary cortisol	Cushing syndrome
	Corticoid therapy	Low DHEAS	Iatrogenic
	Delayed puberty	Lack of sex steroid secretion	Delayed puberty (transient or organic)
Polyuria, polydipsia	Failure to concentrate urines	Diabetes insipidus with vasopressin deficiency	
Diabetes mellitus	Normal GH low IGF-I	Poor control	
Nonendocrine causes	Anemia, rickets	Low 25OHD3, anemia, low iron	Vitamin D deficiency and iron deficiency
	Turner features (girl)	46,XO karyotype	Turner syndrome
	Low weight for height	Normal GH, low IGF-I	Malnutrition, anorexia nervosa
	Chronic diarrhea	Antigliadin antibodies, low folate	Celiac disease
	Abdominal pain, fever	Accelerated sedimentation rate	Crohn ileitis
	Anemia, edema	Increased creatinine, urea	Chronic renal failure
	Polyuria, polydipsia	Failure to respond to vasopressin	Diabetes insipidus with vasopressin resistance

DHEAS, dehydroepiandrosterone sulfate; GH, growth hormone; GRF, growth hormone–releasing factor; IGF-I, insulin-like growth factor I; 25OHD3, 25-hydroxyvitamin D_3; T_3, triiodothyronine; T_4, thyroxine.

Causes by Age

Infancy	Intrauterine growth retardation
	Calorie deficiency (malnutrition, malabsorption)
	Essential nutrient deficiency or excess (unbalanced diet)
	Metabolic diseases, renal failure
	Hypothyroidism
	Hypopituitarism
Childhood	Genetic short stature
	Calorie deficiency (psychosocial dwarfism, malabsorption)
	Chronic diseases
	GH deficiency
	Inflammatory bowel diseases
	Hypothyroidism
	Essential nutrient deficiency or excess
	Genetic bone disease
	Syndromes: (girls)
	Turner syndrome
	Hypercorticism, hyperandrogenism
	Cushing syndrome
Puberty	Constitutional delay
	Turner syndrome
	Essential nutrient deficiency or excess
	Hypopituitarism
	Anorexia nervosa
	Chronic diseases

Growth Retardation Due to Abnormalities of Growth Hormone and Insulin-Like Growth Factor I

Low Growth Hormone, Low Insulin-Like Growth Factor I

Primary GH deficiency	
Genetic	Autosomal dominant or recessive, X-linked recessive
	GH gene mutation, gonadotropin-releasing factor receptor gene mutation
Idiopathic	Isolated GH deficiency (probably GH-releasing hormone deficiency)
Primary multiple pituitary hormone deficiency	
Genetic	Autosomal or X-linked, recessive
Developmental	Midline defects (cleft lip and palate)
	Pituitary aplasia
	Optic-septum dysplasia
Organic	Cranial irradiation
	Hypothalamic-pituitary tumors
	Trauma
Idiopathic	Perinatal trauma and asphyxia
	Pituitary stalk interruption (on MRI)
Secondary GH deficiency	
Chronic malnutrition	
Hemochromatosis, psychosocial dwarfism, thalassemia	

High Growth Hormone, Low Insulin-Like Growth Factor I

Primary GH insensitivity
- Laron-type dwarfism (GH receptor gene mutation and absent plasma GH-binding protein)
- Genetic dwarfism with low GH receptor activity (pygmy)

Secondary GH insensitivity
- Acute fasting
- Chronic malnutrition, protein-calorie deficiency
- Bioinactive but immunoreactive GH

High Growth Hormone, Normal to High Insulin-Like Growth Factor I

Chronic renal failure with excess in IGF-binding protein 3 (IGFBP-3) (supposed resistance to GH and IGF-I)

Primary IGF-I receptor defect (not demonstrated)

Hypercortisolism, Pituitary-Dependent

Diffuse, symmetric hyperplasia due to an oversecretion of adrenocorticotropic hormone (ACTH) by the pituitary is the most common cause of hypercortisolism.

Adrenal glands are usually no more than twice the normal weight.

The cortex is diffusely, but usually mildly, thickened, with a yellow outer zone and a brownish inner zone. Scattered small nodules may be present.

Whereas Cushing syndrome in adults, which usually occurs in the third and fourth decades, is most often due to a pituitary adenoma, children <8 years of age are more likely to have an adrenocortical adenoma.

Most patients with pituitary-dependent hypercortisolism have a pituitary adenoma that secretes ACTH; the female/male ratio is 3:1. In a small number of patients, no pituitary tumor can be identified; pituitary hyperplasia or hypothalamic dysfunction is believed to be responsible for the disorder in the small group without a demonstrable adenoma.

Insulin-Like Hormone–Binding Protein 3 and Other Insulin-Like Hormone–Binding Proteins

IGFBP-3 secretion is GH dependent, with low levels in patients with GH deficiency or genetic insensitivity. Its plasma concentrations measured by RIA increase soon after birth and remain constant thereafter until puberty; there is no circadian variation. Most of the IGFBP-3 is bound to the large 150-kilodalton complex and does not cross the capillary barrier. Large variability in IGFBP-3 levels is found in patients with hypopituitarism. A characteristic feature of chronic renal failure is an increase in IGFBP-3. It is decreased in chronic malnutrition and during prolonged fasting. IGFBP-1 circulating levels decline from birth to puberty, with considerable diurnal variations and a nocturnal peak. It is found in amniotic fluid and maternal serum during gestation. It is increased during fasting, chronic malnutrition, and noncontrolled diabetes. In GH-deficient children, there is an increased correlation between IGFBP-1 levels and GH levels. IGFBP-1 concentrations are inversely correlated with plasma insulin levels, and low IGFBP-1 values are reported in states of insulin resistance.

Table 2 shows serum levels of IGFBP-3 in healthy children at various ages.

Short Stature

Failure to grow or short stature, or both, may be the presenting symptoms of endocrine disorders or chronic diseases. The key sign is a growth rate that is low for the child's age.

One should focus on treatable causes of short stature. It may be advisable to perform a laboratory screening for diseases such as renal failure and celiac disease and to consider the possibility of thyroid or GH deficiency.

Diagnostic Studies

Elements of routine evaluation of a child with short stature or decreased growth rate and failure to thrive are the following:

- History, including calorie intake calculation and physical examination
- Skull radiography, bone age on left hand
- Complete blood count, folate level, carotene level, endomysial antibody level, erythrocyte sedimentation rate, vitamin E level
- Serum electrolyte levels, creatinine level, blood urea nitrogen level, urinalysis
- Karyotype in girls
- Thyroid function: T_4, TSH

Table 2. Serum Levels of Insulin-Like Growth Factor–Binding Protein 3 in Healthy Children at Various Ages

	Percentile		
Age Group (Male/Female Combined)	5th	50th	95th
0–1 wk	0.42	0.77	1.39
1–4 wk	0.77	1.29	2.09
1–3 mo	0.87	1.48	2.54
3–6 mo	0.98	1.61	2.64
6–12 mo	1.07	1.72	2.76
1–3 yr	1.41	2.05	2.97
3–5 yr	1.52	2.25	3.32
5–7 yr	1.66	2.44	3.59
7–9 yr	1.82	2.63	3.80
9–11 yr	2.12	3.01	4.26
11–13 yr	2.22	3.30	4.89
13–15 yr	2.31	3.48	5.24
15–17 yr	2.33	3.39	4.95
20–30 yr	2.20	3.29	4.93

Values are in milligrams per liter.
Adapted from Blum WF, Ranke MB, Kietzmann K, et al. A specific radioimmunoassay for the growth hormone (GH)–dependent somatomedin-binding protein: its use for diagnosis of GH deficiency. *J Clin Endocrinol Metab* 1990;70:1292–1298.

GH response to pharmacologic stimulation or spontaneous profiles on nighttime or 24-hour testing
IGF-I and IGFBP-3 levels
Tuberculin skin test
Sweat test or gene tests for the common growth factor mutations (e.g., ΔF 508, etc.)

See also Table 3.

Tall Stature

As is the case with short stature, the diagnosis of tall stature is largely based on the clinical assessment. In most cases, children presenting with tall stature have no

Table 3. Growth Disturbance in Relation to Abnormal Puberty

Clinical Presentation	Estradiol,[a] Testosterone	LH, FSH	Diagnosis
Delayed puberty (retarded growth and bone maturation)	Low	Low	Delayed puberty hypogonadotropism
	Low	High	Primary gonadal failure
Precocious puberty (accelerated growth and bone maturation)	High	Pubertal level	Central precocious puberty
	High	Low	Primary gonadal hyperfunction
	DHEAS high	Normal	Premature pubarche
	17-OHP high	Normal	Congenital virilizing adrenal hyperplasia

DHEAS, dehydroepiandrosterone sulfate; FSH, follicle-stimulating hormone; LH, luteinizing hormone; 17-OHP, 17-hydroxyprogesterone.
[a]Concentration compared with normal level for chronologic age.

disease but represent extremes of normal variation. However, accelerated growth with advanced bone maturation in a child who was initially of normal stature suggests primary endocrine disorders, and hormonal evaluation is required using various approaches that depend on the age, sex, and pubertal status of the child. The main causes are true precocious puberty (more frequent in girls than boys), virilization due to late-onset congenital adrenal hypoplasia, and hyperthyroidism related to Graves disease. GH hypersecretion is rare during childhood and results in gigantism and acromegaly.

See also Table 3.

Thyroid Disorders

Thyroid hormone homeostasis is controlled by the hypothalamus and anterior pituitary gland. Thyrotropin-releasing hormone (TRH) is produced by several hypothalamic nuclei and is secreted into the hypophyseal portal system and carried to the anterior pituitary to bind to cell membrane receptors on thyrotrophic cells. It stimulates the thyroid cells to increase the synthesis and release of L-3,5,3'-triiodothyronine (T_3) and T_4. These hormones, in turn, feed back on the pituitary thyrotroph to suppress synthesis of TSH.

Pituitary TSH is detectable at 8–10 weeks of gestation in the human fetus. TSH concentrations are low until 16 weeks of gestation and are increased significantly at 28 weeks. Serum TSH is detectable at 10 weeks of gestation.

In infants, children, and adolescents, serum TSH concentrations exhibit a circadian rhythm, with declining values throughout the morning, nadir values in the afternoon, and an approximate doubling, or surge, at night.

The thyroid has two main endocrine functions: secretion of the thyroid hormones T_4 and T_3 by the follicular cells, and secretion of calcitonin by the C cells. Thyroid hormones are first synthesized as a prohormone, thyroglobulin, which is released by the thyroid and constitutes a normal plasma component measured by RIA.

After iodide is absorbed from the gastrointestinal tract, it enters the iodine pool and is removed by trapping in the follicular cells of the thyroid gland or excreted in the urine.

T_4 and T_3 are secreted by the thyroid gland in a T_4/T_3 ratio of 10:1. Twenty percent of T_3 is directly secreted by the thyroid, whereas 80% is converted from T_4 by peripheral deiodination, catalyzed by T_4-5'-deiodinase. T_3 comes from direct thyroid secretion. T_3 is three to four times more potent than T_4.

Extrathyroidal T_3 production is decreased by starvation and virtually all illnesses, increased by overfeeding, decreased in hypothyroidism, and increased in hyperthyroidism.

Diagnosis of Thyroid Disorders

Measurement of TSH level and estimation of free T_4 (FT_4) level are recommended for diagnosis of both hypothyroidism and hyperthyroidism. A TRH suppression test, T_3 level , or free T_3 level may be needed to confirm hyperthyroidism if FT_4 is within normal limits. To establish the cause of hypothyroidism, radioactive iodine uptake or scan may be performed. Antithyroid antibodies, preferably antithyroid peroxidase (anti-TPO), may establish an autoimmune mechanism.

Central Hypothyroidism

Levels of both TSH and FT_4 and other hormones related to pituitary function (e.g., cortisol, LH, FSH, prolactin) should be measured.

Treatment of Primary Hypothyroidism

TSH should be monitored until normalized and at change of drug dosage or change of symptoms. TSH level should be obtained annually.

Table 4. Normal Values for Serum Thyroxine and Triiodothyronine by Age

Age	T_4 nmol/L (μg/dL)	T_3 nmol/L (ng/dL)
Cord blood		
25 wk	78.7–216.7 (6.1–16.8)	
30 wk	73.5–201.2 (5.7–15.6)	0.08–2.17 (5–141)
40 wk	85.1–233.5 (6.6–18.1)	
45 wk	91.6–250.3 (7.1–19.4)	
1–5 d	180.2–365.5 (14.0–28.4)	1.54–11.40 (100–740)
1–11 mo	92.7–2,020.1 (7.2–15.7)	1.62–3.77 (105–245)
1–4 yr		1.62–4.14 (105–269)
5–9 yr		1.45–3.71 (94–241)
1–9 yr	77.2–182.8 (6.0–14.2)	
10–14 yr		1.26–3.28 (82–213)
15–19 yr		1.23–3.23 (80–210)
10–20 yr	60.5–159.6 (4.7–12.4)	

From: Fisher DA. The thyroid gland. In: Brook CGD, ed. *Clinical pediatric endocrinology,* 2nd ed. Oxford: Blackwell Scientific Publications and San Juan Capistrano, CA: Nichols Institute Reference Laboratories, 1989:313.

Treatment of Hypopituitarism

Hormone replacement should be monitored by measuring FT_4 level.

Treatment of Hyperthyroidism with Antithyroid Drugs

Level of FT_4 (and T_3 if needed) should be measured initially.

Iatrogenic Hypothyroidism (After Thyroid Ablation)

Thyroid hormone replacement should be monitored by measuring TSH level.

Reference Intervals for Thyroid Function Indicators*

See Table 4.

Thyroglobulin, Quantitative

Specimen: serum
Unit: ng/mL

Term Infants	**Male/Female**
Cord blood	5–65
1 d	6–93
10 d	9–148
Premature Infants (27–31 wk)	**Male/Female**
1 d	107–395
3 d	49–163
30 d	17–63
Premature Infants (31–34 wk)	**Male/Female**
1 d	147–277
10 d	32–112
30 d	19–51

*Physicians are urged to base their treatment decisions on the reference intervals furnished by the clinical laboratory.

7–12 yr	20–50
13–18 yr	9–27

Thyroid-Stimulating Hormone

Specimen: serum
Unit: μIU/mL

Age	Male	Female
1–30 d	0.52–16.00	0.72–13.10
1 mo to 5 yr	0.55–7.10	0.46–8.10
6–18 yr	0.37–6.00	0.36–5.80

Thyroxine

Specimen: serum
Unit: μg/dL

Age	Male	Female
<1 mo	5.9–21.5	6.3–21.5
1–11 mo	6.4–13.9	4.9–13.7
1–3 yr	7.0–13.1	7.1–14.1
4–6 yr	6.1–12.6	7.2–14.0
7–12 yr	6.7–13.4	6.1–12.1
13–15 yr	4.8–11.5	5.8–11.2

Thyroxine, Free, Direct

Specimen: serum
Unit: ng/dL

Age	Male	Female
1–3 d	0.80–2.78	0.88–1.93
4–30 d	0.48–2.32	0.61–1.93
1–11 mo	0.76–2.00	0.88–1.84
1–5 yr	0.90–1.59	1.02–1.72
6–10 yr	0.81–1.68	0.82–1.58
11–15 yr	0.92–1.57	0.79–1.49
16–18 yr	0.92–1.53	0.83–1.44

Thyroxine-Binding Globulin

Specimen: serum
Unit: μg/mL

Age	Male	Female
1–11 mo	16–33	18–32
1–3 yr	16–32	19–34
4–6 yr	17–30	18–31
7–12 yr	17–29	15–29
13–18 yr	13–26	14–29

Triiodothyronine

Specimen: serum
Unit: ng/mL

Age	Male	Female
0–1 mo	15–210	15–200
2–11 mo	95–275	50–264
1–5 yr	80–253	126–258
6–10 yr	96–232	104–227
11–15 yr	73–199	96–211
16–18 yr	69–201	91–164

Triiodothyronine, Free

Specimen: serum
Unit: pg/mL

Age	Male	Female
1–3 d	1.4–4.8	1.4–5.4
4–30 d	1.4–5.5	1.5–5.0
1–11 mo	2.0–2.9	2.5–6.5
1–5 yr	2.4–6.7	3–6
6–10 yr	2.9–6.0	2.7–6.2
11–15 yr	3.1–5.9	2.6–5.7
16–18 yr	3.5–5.7	2.8–5.2

Serum Thyroid-Stimulating Hormone Values Determined by Immunoradiometric Assay[1]

Age	Serum TSH (μU/L)
Premature infants (gestational age)	
25–27 wk	0.2–30.3
28–30 wk	0.2–30.6
31–33 wk	0.7–27.9
34–36 wk	1.1–21.6
Infants, children, and adults	
1–4 d	1–39
2–20 wk	1.7–9.1
5–24 mo	0.8–8.1
2–7 yr	0.7–5.7
8–20 yr	0.7–5.7
21–45 yr	0.4–4.2

Thyroid Hormone–Binding Ratio

Age	Thyroid Hormone–Binding Ratio
Cord	0.70–1.11
1–3 d	0.83–1.17
1 wk	0.70–1.05
1–12 mo	0.70–1.05
1–3 yr	0.78–1.14
3–10 yr	0.75–1.18
Pubertal children and adults	0.85–1.15

Thyroid Function Tests

See Table 5.

Radioactive Thyroid Uptake, Scintiscanning, and Ultrasonography

Thyroid scintiscanning may be useful in determining the cause of congenital hypothyroidism (i.e., ectopia or aplasia of the thyroid gland) and in evaluating nodules of the thyroid gland and goiters.

Ultrasonography is useful for determining thyroid size and the cause of diffuse goiters.

Thyrotropin-Releasing Hormone Stimulation Test

Serum TSH values increase in normal children and adolescents within 10 minutes after intravenous (i.v.) administration of TRH, peak at 20–45 minutes, and then decline to baseline values by 2 hours. The TRH test distinguishes hypothalamic TRH deficiency

[1]Serum obtained during first week of life. Adams LM, Emery JR, Clark SJ, et al. Reference ranges for newer thyroid function tests in premature infants. *J Pediatr* 1994;126:122–127. Nelson JC, Clark SJ, Borut DL, et al. Age-related changes in serum free thyroxine during childhood and adolescence. *J Pediatr* 1993;123:899–905.

Table 5. Recommendations for Thyroid Function Testing in Pediatric Patients

Clinical Findings	Test
Hyperthyroid, symptomatic	FT_4, TSH
After therapy	FT_4 (T_3)
Hypothyroid, symptomatic	TSH, FT_4 (anti-TPO)
Subclinical	TSH first (T_4, anti-TPO)
Monitoring of replacement therapy	TSH
Hypopituitary	TSH and FT_4
Acutely ill	None unless suspicion
Pregnant, diagnosis of hypothyroidism	TSH, FT_4
Treated	TSH
Elderly, healthy	None
Ill	None
Women >60 yr	TSH
High risk[a]	TSH
Healthy adults	None unless suspicion or risk

Anti-TPO, anti-thyroid peroxidase; FT_4, free thyroxine; T_3, triiodothyronine; TSH, thyroid-stimulating hormone.
[a]Ambiguous symptoms, concurrent illness associated with thyroid disease, use of drugs associated with thyroid dysfunction.
Based on the consensus recommendations for thyroid testing from the American Thyroid Association, the National Academy of Clinical Biochemistry, and the Royal College of Physicians of London.

from pituitary TSH deficiency, as in the case of hypothyroidism, evaluates pituitary TSH reserve, and offers a confirmatory test for hyperthyroidism.

Thyroid Antibody Testing

Autoimmune Disorders

Patients with thyroid autoimmune disease develop antibodies to three major classes of antigen: thyroglobulin; thyroid microsomal antigen, specifically thyroid peroxidase; and the thyroid cell TSH receptor protein.

TSH receptor–stimulating immunoglobulins (TSIs) produce the hyperthyroid state in Graves disease.

Very high serum concentrations of TSI before the start of therapy in patients with Graves disease indicate probability of failure of therapy or relapse at the end of the drug treatment.

Autoimmunity substantially contributes to the pathogenesis of a number of thyroid disorders, such as Hashimoto thyroiditis, primary myxedema, and Graves thyrotoxicosis. One frequently finds autoantibodies directed against thyroglobulin, microsomal antigens (TPO), and TSH receptors.

Anti-TPO antibodies are an indicator of autoimmune thyroid disease, one of the most common causes of hypothyroidism.

Antibodies to Thyroxine and Triiodothyronine

On very rare occasions, certain patients, particularly those with Graves disease, chronic lymphocytic thyroiditis, and nonthyroidal illnesses, may have serum antibodies to T_4 or T_3. Radiobinding assays for detection of anti-T_4 and anti-T_3 autoantibodies are available from commercial laboratories.

Thyroid-Stimulating Hormone

A normal serum TSH value in ambulatory patients virtually excludes the diagnosis of thyroid disease. Transiently elevated TSH values may be found in patients recovering from major physiologic stress.

Serum TSH can be measured by RIA. The assay can identify patients with primary hypothyroidism and allows differentiation of patients with nonthyroidal illnesses and low serum TSH values from those with hyperthyroidism. Increased TSH level is highly predictive of a suppressed response to TRH stimulation.

Serum TSH concentration is increased at birth. An acute increase in values occurs within the first few minutes of life, and peak values are observed approximately 30 minutes after delivery. Values decrease rapidly thereafter, falling to 50% of the peak values by 2 hours of life. Serum TSH concentrations decrease further, so that by 48 hours of age levels are only slightly higher than cord blood values.

TSH level in serum is used for evaluating suspected thyroid disease. Values <0.1 μIU/mL are suggestive of hyperthyroidism. For these patients, FT_4 and third- or fourth-generation TSH tests may be useful. As T_3 toxicosis is an occasional cause of hyperthyroidism, free T_3 measurement is suggested for patients with suppressed TSH and normal FT_4 levels.

Thyroxine

Peak serum concentration of T_4 is reached 24 hours after birth and the level then slowly decreases over the first weeks of life. Serum T_4 values are significantly lower in infants who are small for gestational age (SGA) than in full-term infants, and even lower values are present in premature infants. After approximately 50 days of age, comparable serum T_4 concentrations are present in the three groups of infants. Between 1 and 15 years of age, concentration of T_4 decreases gradually with increasing age.

Thyroxine, Free

In vitro methods of measuring FT_4 include the following:

1. FT_4 index methods that correct total T_4 values using an assessment of T_4-binding proteins.
2. Equilibrium dialysis or ultrafiltration methods that separate FT_4 from bound hormone using a semipermeable membrane.

Serum FT_4 concentrations peak at 24 hours of life and then decrease slowly over the first weeks of life. Similar to T_4 levels, serum FT_4 concentrations correlate positively with increasing gestational age and birth weight. FT_4 concentrations decrease progressively with age during childhood.

Thyroxine-Binding Globulin

The T_4-binding globulin (TBG) concentration is high in cord blood and decreases to adult values by 20 years of age. Serum TBG values are higher in healthy, full-term newborns than in SGA newborns. A positive correlation is present between serum TBG and thyroid hormone concentrations.

Serum concentrations of T_4-binding proteins (T_4-binding prealbumin, or TBPA) are higher in full-term newborns than in SGA newborns; however, the serum concentration of TBPA is lower in SGA newborns than in premature newborns.

Table 6 lists causes of abnormal serum concentrations of TBG and T_4-binding proteins.

Reverse Triiodothyronine

T_4 is the major secretory product of the thyroid gland and is metabolized in peripheral tissues to either T_3 or 3,3',5'-triiodothyronine reverse T_3. Reverse T_3 is metabolically inactive. A variety of disorders and drugs can inhibit the conversion of T_4 to T_3, which results in low serum T_3 levels. These include uncontrolled diabetes mellitus, chronic liver disease, renal failure, malnutrition, trauma, burns, propanolol, and glucocorticoids. Collectively, these conditions are referred to as nonthyroidal illness.

Table 6. Causes of Abnormal Serum Concentration of Thyroxine-Binding Globulin or Thyroxine-Binding Proteins

	TBG	TBPA
Hypothyroidism	↑	—
Genetic disorder	↑ or ↓	N
Estrogens	↑	↓
Pregnancy	↑	↓
Hepatic disease	↑ or ↓ or N	↓
Androgens	↓	—
Anabolic steroids	↓	—
Nephrosis	↓	—
Severe hypoproteinemia	↓	—
Phenytoin (Dilantin)	↓	—
Glucocorticoids (high dosage)	↓	↓
Salicylate (aspirin)	N	↓
Heroin	↑	—
Methadone	↑	—
Acute stress	—	↓
Chronic illness	—	↓
Thyrotoxicosis	—	↓

↑, increased; ↓, decreased; N, normal; TBG, thyroxine-binding globulin; TBPA, thyroxine-binding proteins.

Reference level for reverse T_3 is as follows[2]:

Age	Reverse T_3 [nmol/L (ng/dL)]
1 mo to 20 yr	0.15–0.54 (10–35)

Hypothyroidism

Neonatal Screening

The incidence of congenital hypothyroidism in nonendemic areas of the world is approximately 1 in 4,000 live births. Congenital hypothyroidism is the most common endocrine cause of infant mental retardation that is preventable with early therapy. Blood spots are collected on filter paper in the neonatal period and the eluates used for measurement of TSH and T_4. In most screening programs in the United States, the primary screening test is T_4 measurement, and in those samples with T_4 values in the lower 10%, a follow-up measurement of TSH in the same sample is performed. For all neonates for whom screening test results suggest the possibility of hypothyroidism, follow-up measurement of serum TSH and T_4 levels is required before a definitive diagnosis of hypothyroidism is made.

Signs and Symptoms

The infant may be lethargic, constipated, and bradycardic, with a persistent large umbilical hernia and neonatal jaundice. The older child may be lethargic, short, anorexic, cold intolerant, bradycardic, and have nonpitting edema and constipation. Umbilical hernia may be persistent.

[2]Nichols Institute Reference Laboratories, San Juan Capistrano, CA.

Causes of Decreased Serum Thyroid Binding or Hypothyroxinemia in Pediatric Patients

I. Hypothyroidism
II. Decreased T_4-binding proteins
  A. T_4-binding globulin
    1. Androgens
    2. Anabolic steroid hormones
    3. Inherited complete or partial TBG deficiency
    4. Nonthyroidal illnesses
    5. Glucocorticoids
  B. TBPA
    1. Nonthyroidal illnesses
    2. Glucocorticoids
  C. T_4-binding albumin
    1. Nonthyroidal illnesses
III. Drug-related inhibition of binding
  A. Salicylates in high doses
  B. Furosemide in high doses
IV. Illness-related inhibition of binding
  A. Protein inhibitors
  B. Fatty acid inhibitors

Hyperthyroidism

In >90% of pediatric patients, hyperthyroidism is due to Graves disease. Graves disease is an autoimmune disease in which TSI antibodies bind to TSH receptors on follicular cells of the thyroid and stimulate thyroid hormone synthesis, which results in the clinical manifestations of thyrotoxicosis.

Clinical signs and symptoms of thyrotoxicosis include nervousness, fatigue, weakness, heat intolerance, increased perspiration, hyperactivity, tachycardia, arrhythmias, palpitation, systolic hypertension, increased appetite, loss of weight, diarrhea, warm and moist skin, hyperreflexia, tremor, muscle weakness, and menstrual disturbances.

Types of hyperthyroidism include the following:

- Graves disease, the most common form, is an autosomal disease. TSIs of the immunoglobulin G class are produced and bind to TSH receptors on the thyroid gland. The TSIs mimic the action of TSH and cause excess secretion of T_4 and T_3. Goiter and ophthalmopathy (Graves ophthalmopathy) are common characteristics.
- Toxic multinodular goiter occurs late in life. Nodules are insidious and almost never malignant; no ophthalmopathy or localized myxedema is present.
- Toxic uninodular goiter, solitary nodule with autonomous function, is almost always benign.
- Other causes include TSH-secreting and pituitary tumors; surreptitious ingestion of T_4 or T_3; functioning trophoblastic tumors; iodine-induced hyperthyroidism, especially from the cardiac drug amiodarone hydrochloride; subacute thyroiditis; thyroid cancer; and ectopic thyroid tissue.
- Secondary hyperthyroidism with excess TSI production is seen in patients with some pituitary tumors.

Causes of Hyperthyroxinemia in Children

I. Hyperthyroidism
II. Increased serum binding of thyroid hormones
  A. TBG
  B. T_4-binding albumin
    1. Familial dysalbuminemic hyperthyroxinemia
  C. TBPA
    1. Inherited abnormal TBPA
  D. Anti-T_4 antibodies

III. Nonthyroidal illnesses
  A. Medical illnesses
  B. Psychiatric illnesses
IV. Drug-induced hyperthyroxinemia
V. Generalized thyroid hormone resistance

Laboratory Findings

Biochemical confirmation of thyrotoxicosis can be determined by the presence of elevated levels of serum total and free T_4 and T_3 and decreased serum TSH levels; biochemical confirmation of thyrotoxicosis does not include confirmation of the cause of disease.
Most patients with thyrotoxicosis have overt clinical biochemical disease, but thyrotoxicosis may also be subclinical (normal serum T_4 and T_3 levels and decreased TSH concentration).
Elderly patients with thyrotoxicosis may present with predominant involvement of one organ system and with the classic signs and symptoms of thyrotoxicosis; this is referred to as apathetic thyrotoxicosis.
T_3: total T_3 by immunometric assay >200 ng/mL
T_4: by immunometric assay >12.5 μg/dL (161 nmol/L)
Free T_4 index: >12
TSH: below normal
Radioiodine uptake: high in Graves disease, high or normal in toxic nodules

Drugs That May Alter Laboratory Results

Drugs that may alter laboratory results include the following:
- Anabolic steroids
- Androgens
- Estrogens
- Heparin
- Iodine-containing compounds
- Phenytoin
- Rifampin
- Salicylates
- T_4
- Triiodothyronine
- Thyroid scans using radioiodine: diffuse in Graves disease, focal in toxic nodule

The diagnosis of thyroid function disorder can be difficult when patients are taking medications that can alter results of thyroid function tests. Phenytoin treatment of euthyroid patients results in a 30–40% decrease in serum T_4 and free T_4 levels and either normal or slightly decreased concentrations of T_3 and free T_3. Treatment with carbamazepine or rifampin also results in subnormal serum free T_4 concentrations. Several pharmacologic agents appear to act predominantly by decreasing the rate of production of T_3 from T_4 in peripheral tissues. These agents include glucocorticoids or propranolol hydrochloride in high doses, oral cholecystographic radiopaque agents, and amiodarone.

Disorders of Calcium and Phosphorus Metabolism

See Tables 7 and 8.

Bone Turnover Markers

Markers for Bone Formation

In the evaluation of bone formation, measurements of total alkaline phosphatase (may also come from the liver, intestine, and placenta), bone-specific alkaline phosphatase, osteocalcin, type I procollagen carboxy-terminal propeptide, and type I procollagen amino terminal propeptide are useful.

Table 7. Some Biochemical Changes in Disorders of Calcium and Phosphorus Metabolism in Infancy and Childhood

Disorder	Serum Phosphorus Concentration	Parathyroid Hormone Concentration	Serum 1,25 $(OH)_2D$ Concentration	Serum 25-OHD Concentration	Urinary Calcium Excretion	Urinary Phosphorus Excretion
Hypocalcemia						
Parathyroid disorders						
Hypoparathyroidism						
Congenital	↑	↓	↓	N	↓	↓
Transient or functional	↑	↓	↓	N	↓	↓
Pseudohypoparathyroidism	↑	↑	↓	N	↓	↓
Vitamin D disorders						
Vitamin D deficiency	↓	↑	N, ↑	↓	↓, Var	↓
Hepatic disease	↓	↑	N, ↓	↓	↓, Var	↓
Renal disease	↑	↑	↓	N	↓, Var	↓
Vitamin D–dependent rickets, type I	↓	↑	↓	N, ↑	↑, Var	↓
Vitamin D–dependent rickets, type II	↓	↑	Very ↑	N, ↑	↓, Var	↓
Mineral disorders						
Hypomagnesemia	N	N, ↓	N, ↓	N	↓	N
High phosphate load	↑	↑	↓	N	↓	↑
Hypercalcemia						
Iatrogenic	N	↓	↓	N	↑	N
Low phosphorus intake	↓	↓	↑	N	↑	↓
Hyperparathyroidism	↓	↑	↑	N	↑	↑

Vitamin D intoxication	N, ↑	↓	N, ↑	↑	↑	↑
Subcutaneous fat necrosis	N	↓	N, ↓	N	↑	N
Idiopathic hypercalcemia of infancy	N	↓	N, ↓	N	↑	N
Benign familial hypocalciuric hypercalcemia	N	N, ↑	N	N	↑	N
Immobilization	N	↓	N, ↓	N	↑	N
Hypophosphatemia						
Inadequate phosphorus intake	N, ↑	↓	↑	N	↑	↓
Hyperparathyroidism	↑	↓	↑	N	↑	↑
Hypophosphatemic rickets	N	N	N, ↓	N	N	↑
Hyperphosphatemia						
Parathyroid disorders						
Hypoparathyroidism	↓	↓	↓	N	↓	↓
Pseudohypoparathyroidism	↓	↑	↓	N	↓	↓
Thyrotoxicosis	N, ↑	N, ↑	N, ↓	N	N, ↑	N, ↑
High phosphate intake (cow's milk formula)	↓	↑	↓	N	↓	↑
Renal failure	↓	↑	↓	N	↓	↓

↑, increased; ↓, decreased; N, normal; Var, variable.
From Soldin SJ, Rifai N, Hicks JM. *Biochemical basis of pediatric disease*, 3rd ed. Washington: American Association for Clinical Chemistry Press, 1998:259.

Table 8. Normal Values of Calcium, Phosphorus, Parathyroid Hormone, Calcitonin, and Vitamin D

	Ca mmol/L (mg/dL)	iCa mmol/L (mg/dL)	P mmol/L (mg/dL)	PTH ng/L (pg/mL)	CT ng/L (pg/mL)	$1,25(OH)_2D$ pmol/L (pg/mL)	25-OHD nmol/L (ng/mL)	UCa excretion (mg/kg/d	TRP mmol/L (mg/dL)
Cord blood	255.00 ± 0.15 (10.2 ± 0.6)[a]	1.45 ± 0.07 (5.83 ± 0.30)[a]	1.56 ± 0.20 (4.8 ± 0.6)[b]	3.40 ± 0.91[b]	58 ± 19[c]	81.4 ± 23.0 (33.9 ± 9.8)[b]	33 ± 8 (13 ± 3)[d]		
0–18 mo[e]									
Black	2.43 ± 0.15 (9.73 ± 0.60)	1.31 ± 0.04 (5.24 ± 0.18)	2.08 ± 0.22 (6.47 ± 0.69)	11.5 ± 0.4	65 ± 35	168 ± 62 (70 ± 26)	133 ± 45 (53 ± 18)		
White	2.41 ± 0.15 (9.67 ± 0.59)	1.30 ± 0.06 (5.22 ± 0.25)	2.19 ± 0.29 (6.78 ± 0.92)	12.3 ± 0.5	61 ± 34	137 ± 15 (57 ± 25)	128 ± 43 (51 ± 17)		
Summer	2.36 ± 0.14 (9.46 ± 0.56)	1.30 ± 0.04 (5.21 ± 0.17)	2.20 ± 0.26 (6.83 ± 0.81)	12.5 ± 0.3	75 ± 35	146 ± 41 (61 ± 17)	133 ± 40 (53 ± 16)		
Winter	2.47 ± 0.11 (9.91 ± 0.44)	1.30 ± 0.04 (5.23 ± 0.18)	2.08 ± 0.26 (6.44 ± 0.80)	11.0 ± 0.5	46 ± 30	173 ± 62 (72 ± 26)	113 ± 45 (45 ± 18)		
Children	2.35 ± 0.17 (9.4 ± 0.7)[f]	1.14 ± 0.13 (4.59 ± 0.52)[g]	1.13 ± 0.22 (3.5 ± 0.7)[f]	11 – 35[h]	32 ± 22[i]	120 ± 13 (50.0 ± 5.5)	88 ± 23 (35.2 ± 9.2)[j]	2.4[k]	1.15–2.44
Summer						73 ± 5 (30.4 ± 2.3)	66 ± 6 (26.5 ± 2.4)		
Winter						56 ± 5 (23.4 ± 2.3)	49 ± 5 (19.4 ± 2.1)		

iCa, ionized calcium; PTH, parathyroid hormone; CT, calcitonin; 1,25(OH_2)D, 1,25-dihydroxyvitamin D; 25-OHD, 25-hydroxyvitamin D; TRP, tubular reabsorption of phosphate per liter of glomerular filtrate; UCa, urinary calcium.

Values are Mean ± 1 standard deviation unless otherwise indicated.

Sources:

[a]Loughead JL, Mimouni F, Tsang RC. Serum ionized calcium concentrations in normal neonates. *Am J Dis Child* 1988;142:516–518.

[b]Namgung R, Tsang RC, Specker BL, et al. Low bone mineral content and high serum osteocalcin and 1,25-dihydroxyvitamin D in summer- versus winter-born newborn infants: an early fetal effect? *J Pediatr Gastroenterol Nutr* 1994;19:220–227.

[c]Loughead JL, Mimouni F, Ross R, et al. Postnatal changes in serum osteocalcin and parathyroid hormone concentrations. *J Am Coll Nutr* 1990;9:358–362.

[d]Delmas PD, Glorieux FH, Delvin EE, et al. Perinatal serum bone Gla-protein and vitamin D metabolites in preterm and full-term neonates. *J Clin Endocrinol Metab* 1987;65:588–591.

[e]Specker BL, Lichtenstein P, Mimani F, et al. Calcium-regulating hormones and minerals from birth to 18 months of age: a cross-sectional study. II. Effects of sex, race, age, season, and diet on serum minerals, parathyroid hormone, and calcitonin. *Pediatrics* 1986;77:891–896.

[f]Cherian AG, Hill JG. Percentile estimates of reference values for fourteen chemical constituents in sera of children and adolescents. *Am J Clin Pathol* 1978;69:24–31.

[g]Arnaud SB, Goldsmith RS, Stickler GB, et al. Serum parathyroid hormone and blood minerals: interrelationships in normal children. *Pediatr Res* 1973;7:485–493.

[h]Shaw NJ, Wheeldon J, Brocklebank JT. Indices of intact serum parathyroid hormone and renal excretion of calcium, phosphate, and magnesium. *Arch Dis Child* 1991;65:1208–1211.

[i]Shainkin-Kerstenbaum R; Funkenstein B, Conforti A, et al. Serum calcitonin and blood mineral interrelationships in normal children aged six to twelve years. *Pediatr Res* 1977;11:112–116.

[j]Weisman Y, Reiter E, Rott A. Measurement of 24,25 dihydroxyvitamin D in sera of neonates and children. *J Pediatr* 1977;91(6):904–908.

[k]Ghazali S, Barratt TM. Urinary excretion of calcium and magnesium in children. *Arch Dis Child* 1974;49:97–101.

Markers for Bone Resorption

Markers of bone resorption include the urine calcium/creatinine ratio, urine hydroxyproline/creatinine ratio, and acid phosphatase level. Assays that measure urinary pyridinium cross links of type I collagen have largely replaced the older assays. These fragments of collagen are more accurate indicators of bone resorption, as they are almost exclusively derived from bone type I collagen. High-pressure liquid chromatography of total pyridinoline and deoxypyridinoline are the most accurate tests. Several commercial assays, including free deoxypyridinoline, and N-telopeptide and C-telopeptide (peptide-bound) cross links are available.

Calcium and Phosphorus Levels in the Newborn

The third trimester is the time of maximal intrauterine calcium and phosphorus accretion. Daily accretion rates of 117–150 mg calcium/kg and 74 mg P/kg have been estimated for near-term fetuses. Interruption of the placental supply of these minerals at the time of delivery therefore predisposes the neonate to hypocalcemia at a time when oral feeding is limited. Parathyroid hormone (PTH) level increases markedly after birth.

Serum 1,25-dihydroxyvitamin D (1,25$(OH)_2$D) concentrations rise steadily during the first day of life.

Calcium-Regulating Hormones

See Table 9.

Measurements of hormones involved in the regulation of calcium metabolism are very helpful in the diagnosis of metabolic bone disease.

Parathyroid Hormone

Assays available for PTH include RIAs and two-site immunoradiometric assays or immunochemiluminometric assays. The three regions specific to PTH RIAs include

Table 9. Clinically Useful Assays of Calcium Regulatory Hormones

Hormone	Indicator for Assay	Interpretation/Comment
Parathyroid hormone (PTH)	↑ Serum calcium	Normal or elevated PTH in the presence of normal renal function is diagnostic of primary hyperparathyroidism.
	Chronic renal failure	Used for investigation of renal bone disease.
	↓ Serum calcium	Decreased in hypoparathyroidism.
		Elevated in pseudohypoparathyroidism (PTH resistance).
PTH–related peptide	↑ Serum calcium	Elevated level highly suggestive of humoral hypercalcemia of malignancy.
Calcitonin	Thyroid nodule	Diagnosis of medullary thyroid carcinoma.
		Useful as tumor marker.
25-Hydroxyvitamin D	Fracture, osteoporosis ↓ Serum calcium or phosphate	Best indicator of vitamin D deficiency and osteomalacia.
1,25-Dihydroxyvitamin D	Disorders of vitamin D metabolism	Diagnosis of osteomalacia and rickets.

↑, increased; ↓, decreased.

carboxy-terminal, amino-terminal, and midmolecule regions. Midmolecule assays measure all important circulating PTH fragments.

Parathyroid Hormone–Related Peptide

Elevated levels of PTH-related peptide are highly suggestive of an underlying tumor.

Vitamin D

Measurement of vitamin D metabolites should be confined to 25-hydroxyvitamin D, the storage form of this vitamin. This metabolite formed from calciferol in the liver has a long half-life (15–60 days).

Hypercalcemia

Hypercalcemia is defined as total serum calcium concentration of >2.7 mmol/L (10.8 mg/dL) or serum ionized calcium concentration of >1.4 mmol/L (5.6 mg/dL). In pathologic hypercalcemia, elevation of serum Ca^{2+} usually occurs simultaneously with elevation of total calcium; however, elevated total calcium may occur without elevation of Ca^{2+}. Hypercalcemia in the neonate is usually iatrogenic and due to administration of calcium salts for treatment of hypocalcemia or for prophylaxis during exchange transfusions; the use of thiazide diuretics, which depress urinary calcium excretion; and hyperalimentation errors, either excess calcium or insufficient phosphorus. Human milk feeding of preterm infants may lead to hypophosphatemia because of the low phosphorus content of human milk relative to the needs of preterm infants, and this, in turn, may cause secondary hypercalcemia.

Hypercalcemia, Familial Hypocalciuric

Familial hypocalciuric (or benign) hypercalcemia is characterized by lifelong hypercalcemia with normal urinary calcium excretion. It is inherited as an autosomal-dominant trait. It is caused by insensitivity of the parathyroid cells to inhibition by serum calcium.

The hypercalcemia persists after subtotal parathyroidectomy; such surgery is contraindicated. Parathyroid cell hyperfunction is polyclonal and nonneoplastic. The presence of normal urinary calcium excretion despite hypercalcemia is an effect of the mutated calcium-sensing receptors in the kidneys.

Hyperphosphatemia

Hyperphosphatemia in infants up to 18 months of age is defined as serum phosphorus concentrations of >2.7 mmol/L (8.4 mg/dL). In older children and adolescents, serum phosphorus concentrations >2 mmol/L (6 mg/dL) are considered to be in the hyperphosphatemic range. Hyperphosphatemia may be caused by a decrease in urinary phosphorus excretion or by sudden release of intracellular phosphorus into the extracellular space.

Hypocalcemia

Neonatal hypocalcemia is defined as a total serum calcium level of <2 mmol/L (8 mg/dL) for term infants or <1.75 mmol/L (7.0 mg/dL) for preterm infants, and serum ionized calcium level of <1.1 mmol/L (4.4 mg/dL) measured using the ion-selective electrode method.

Neonatal hypocalcemia is classified as either early or late. Early neonatal hypocalcemia occurs during the first 48 hours of life, whereas late neonatal hypocalcemia occurs toward the end of the first week of life.

Early neonatal hypocalcemia occurs as a result of the inability of the neonate to adequately compensate for the sudden cessation of placental calcium supply after birth. Preterm infants may not exhibit the surge in PTH secretion observed in term infants at birth. Birth asphyxia may result in an increase in serum calcium concentration and may delay enteral feeding, both of which may theoretically aggravate neonatal hypocalcemia. Early neonatal hypocalcemia in infants of diabetic mothers may be related to Mg insufficiency and, consequently, to impaired PTH secretory activity.

Hypomagnesemia, whether transient or due to hereditary intestinal Mg malabsorption or renal Mg losses, is associated with resistant hypocalcemia.

Hypophosphatemia

Hypophosphatemia is usually defined as serum phosphorus concentrations of <1.55 mmol/L (4.8 mg/dL) in infants <18 months of age. Transient causes include respiratory alkalosis (with mechanical ventilation) and low dietary phosphorus intake. The latter may occur in a preterm infant fed human milk. Vitamin D deficiency results in hypophosphatemia. Dietary phosphorus deficiency is unusual in children. In the clinically or chronically ill child, inadequate phosphorus in total parenteral nutrition, frequent dosing with P-binding antacids (aluminum binds phosphorus in the gut), or excessive stool losses can cause hypophosphatemia.

Nutritional Causes of Calcium and Phosphorus Disorders

In preterm infants, calcium and phosphorus requirements are high because of mineral deprivation associated with early delivery, poor intestinal absorption of cow's milk–based formula, and use of calciuretic medication, especially in sick preterm infants. Inadequate provision of these minerals can increase the risk of hypocalcemia, hypophosphatemia, hypercalciuria, and rickets in these infants.

In term infants, the relatively high phosphorus content of standard commercial formulas (due to the naturally high phosphorus content of the cow's milk from which these formulas are derived) may result in hyperphosphatemia and secondary hypocalcemia. Evaporated milks have high phosphorus content and readily cause hypocalcemia. Some of these hypocalcemic infants will develop neonatal tetany and seizures.

The high phosphorus and fiber load of many cereals given to infants as first foods increases calcium-phosphorus complexing and may cause competition with calcium absorption. The resultant inadequate calcium absorption may lead to hypocalcemia. Higher serum PTH concentrations have been found in infants fed cereal at age 4 months than in those who were started on cereal at age 6 months, but there is no apparent effect on bone mineral content.

Parathyroid Disorders

Hyperparathyroidism, Neonatal

Primary neonatal hyperparathyroidism is usually caused by an autosomal-recessive gene, although it may also be familial or occur as part of multiple endocrine adenomatosis. The condition is associated with failure to thrive (poor weight gain and growth), increased serum PTH concentrations, hypercalcemia, hyperphosphaturia leading to hypophosphatemia, and hypercalciuria sometimes leading to nephrocalcinosis. Skeletal demineralization may occur in untreated cases as calcium is continually leached out from bone by excessive amounts of circulating PTH. Surgical removal of the parathyroid glands is crucial. Both neonatal severe hyperparathyroidism and familial hypocalciuric hypercalcemia appear to occur secondary to mutations in the human Ca^{2+}-sensing receptor gene on chromosome 3. Patients with neonatal severe hyperparathyroidism are homozygous and those with familial hypocalciuric hypercalcemia are heterozygous for the defective genes.

Secondary hyperparathyroidism may occur in infants of mothers with untreated hypoparathyroidism and in the presence of maternal and neonatal renal tubular acidosis. Hypocalcemia in the mother leads to compensatory fetal parathyroid gland hyperplasia, with subsequent increased PTH secretion.

Hyperparathyroidism in Older Children

Diagnosis Studies

Hyperchloremic acidosis due to excess PTH and increased alkaline phosphatase due to increased bone turnover are present. Aminoaciduria and level of urinary cyclic adenosine monophosphate excretion may be increased. Increased PTH concentration is best determined by intact PTH molecule assay.

Hyperparathyroidism, Primary

See Table 10.

The parathyroids are small endocrine glands, and increases in their size or enhancements of their function have no effect on neighboring tissues. Effects of excessive secretion of PTH are manifested chemically as abnormal fluxes of calcium and phosphorus in bone, in the kidneys, and in the gastrointestinal tract. This results in hypercalcemia, hypercalciuria, and increased rates of bone turnover.

Primary hyperparathyroidism is usually first suspected when a patient is found on biochemical screening to have hypercalcemia; less often it is suspected because nephrolithiasis or osteopenia is present. The anticalciuric effect of thiazide drugs can raise serum calcium concentrations slightly and thereby uncover occult hyperparathyroidism.

Most patients with primary hyperparathyroidism have high serum PTH concentrations and high serum ionized calcium concentrations. Diagnostic tests for this disorder are measurements of serum PTH and ionized calcium.

Causes of Sporadic Primary Hyperparathyroidism

Solitary parathyroid adenomas account for 85% of cases of primary hyperparathyroidism; hyperfunction in multiple parathyroid glands (a category that includes hyperplasia, multiple adenomas, and polyclonal hyperfunction) occurs in most of the remainder; a few patients (<1%) have parathyroid carcinoma. Approximately 75% of patients with sporadic primary hyperparathyroidism are women. Sporadic primary hyperparathyroidism may result from external irradiation of the neck. Mild hyperparathyroidism occurs in approximately 5% of patients receiving long-term lithium therapy, and it often persists after the therapy is discontinued.

Syndromes of Hereditary Primary Hyperparathyroidism

Among the patients with primary hyperparathyroidism caused by hyperfunction of multiple parathyroid glands, the disorder is inherited in approximately 20%. Any of these hereditary syndromes, such as multiple endocrine neoplasia type 1, may present as isolated hyperparathyroidism in some families.

Neonatal Severe Primary Hyperparathyroidism

Neonatal severe primary hyperparathyroidism is a rare and potentially lethal disorder. Affected neonates have a marked enlargement of all parathyroid glands, very high serum PTH concentrations, and marked hypercalcemia [calcium concentration of >16 mg/dL (4 mmol/L)].

Diagnostic Studies

Measurements of serum calcium, PTH, 25-hydroxyvitamin D, and $1,25(OH)_2D$ are used in the diagnosis and treatment of hyperparathyroidism and hypoparathyroidism. Serum calcium level should usually be measured at the same time as serum PTH level; because the ionized fraction of serum calcium is the biologically active form, it is the preferred index of hyper- and hypoparathyroidism.

Current assays for serum PTH are two-site assays designed to detect both amino-terminal and carboxy-terminal epitopes of the peptide. Approximately half of the PTH detected in the serum of patients with chronic renal disease is biologically inactive.

PTH can be measured in fluid obtained from a lesion by fine-needle aspiration (usually guided ultrasonographically) or in serum from the veins of the neck and mediastinum, catheterized selectively. Serum test results that can be obtained in 10–15 minutes allow physicians to assess the completeness of the removal of hyperfunctioning parathyroid tissue during the operation for parathyroid tumors.

Table 10. Categories of Primary Hyperparathyroidism

Characteristic Inheritance	Sporadic Adenoma Not Inherited	Multiple Endocrine Neoplasia Type I Autosomal Dominant	Familial Hypocalciuric Hypercalcemia Autosomal Dominant	Neonatal Severe Primary Hyperparathyroidism Autosomal Dominant
Age at onset of hypercalcemia	55 yr	25 yr	Birth	Birth
Urinary calcium excretion	Normal to high	Normal to high	Low to normal	Low to normal
Serum parathyroid hormone concentration	High	High	Normal	Very high
Parathyroid glands				
No. abnormal	One	Multiple	Multiple	Multiple
Enlargement	20 times normal size	5 times normal size	Minimally enlarged	Very enlarged
Clonality	Monoclonal or oligoclonal	Monoclonal or oligoclonal	Polyclonal	Polyclonal
Effectiveness of parathyroidectomy	95% cured	90% cured, but many recur	Surgery not indicated	Total parathyroidectomy required
Pathophysiology	Stepwise acquired mutations of certain genes, such as MEN1, promote the emergence of a neoplastic clone in parathyroid glands.	Sequential inactivation of both copies (first copy by inheritance) of the MEN1 gene leads to the growth of one or more neoplastic clones in parathyroid glands.	Monoallelic inherited inactivation of the calcium-sensing receptor gene decreases the sensing of serum calcium by parathyroid cells and by renal tubules.	Biallelic inactivation of calcium-sensing receptor gene impairs calcium sensing in parathyroid cells more than does monallelic inactivation.

MEN, multiple endocrine neoplasia.
All entries are typical for the given disorder. Ranges are broad, with overlap (not shown) among categories.
From Marx SJ. Hyperparathyroid and hypoparathyroid disorders. *N Engl J Med* 2000;343(25):1863–1875.

Hyperparathyroidism, Secondary and Tertiary

Hypocalcemia from any cause stimulates PTH secretion, and chronic hypocalcemia also stimulates the growth of the parathyroid glands. Secondary hyperparathyroidism often lasts longer and is more severe in patients with chronic renal failure than in patients with other hypocalcemic disorders, such as a deficiency or malabsorption of vitamin D. Eventually, either before or after renal transplantation, secondary hyperparathyroidism can develop into a disorder of oversecretion of PTH with hypercalcemia (tertiary hyperparathyroidism).

Hypoparathyroidism

Deficiency of PTH from disease, injury, or congenital malfunction of the parathyroid glands manifests as hypocalcemia producing neuromuscular symptoms ranging from paresthesia to tetany.

Classification

Hypoparathyroidism (follows accidental removal of or damage to parathyroid glands during surgery; may be transient or permanent)
Idiopathic (parathyroid glands absent or atrophied)
Pseudohypoparathyroidism (no PTH deficiency, but target organs do not respond to its action)

Signs and Symptoms

Chronic hypocalcemia, possibly asymptomatic
Neuromuscular excitability, such as carpopedal spasm
Increased deep tendon reflexes
Chvostek sign: hyperirritability of the facial nerve when tapped
Trousseau sign: carpopedal spasm within 2 minutes of inflating a blood pressure cuff over systolic pressure
Dysphagia
Organic brain syndrome
Psychosis
Mental deficiency (children)
Tetany (paresthesias, pain, difficulty walking, laryngospasm, stridor, cyanosis, seizures)
Dry hair
Brittle fingernails
Cataracts
Dry, scaly skin
Cardiac arrhythmias

Causes of Hypoparathyroidism

Idiopathic
- Di George syndrome
- Congenital absence of parathyroid glands
- Late onset, autoimmune

Surgery (may be transient)
Infiltrative effects—metastatic carcinoma and others
Irradiation
Hypomagnesemia
Alcohol

Risk Factors

Neck surgery
Neck trauma
Head and neck malignancies

Laboratory Findings

Serum total and ionized calcium levels are decreased.
Serum phosphorus level is increased [>5.4 mg/dL (>1.74 mmol/L)].
RIA for PTH shows decreased levels.

Pathologic Findings

Complete or almost complete replacement of parathyroid gland parenchymal tissue by fat
Brain blood vessels calcified
Possible early posterior lenticular cataract formation on slit-lamp examination

Imaging Studies

Radiography
- Increased bone density
- Tooth roots absent
- Calcification of cerebellum, choroid plexus, cerebral basal ganglia

Hypoparathyroidism, Neonatal

Neonatal hypoparathyroidism may be transient or permanent. Transient neonatal hypoparathyroidism may occur in preterm infants and in infants of insulin-dependent diabetic mothers in whom there may be a blunted PTH response to low serum calcium concentrations. This phenomenon has been termed *functional hypoparathyroidism*. Approximately 30% of preterm infants and 50% of infants born to insulin-dependent diabetic mothers present with hypocalcemia in the first few days of life and may manifest jitteriness, tetany, seizures, or cardiac arrhythmias.

Transient neonatal hypoparathyroidism may occur in infants of untreated hyperparathyroid mothers. Maternal hypercalcemia secondary to excess PTH activity leads to fetal hypocalcemia, which inhibits fetal parathyroid gland hormone production. The management is similar to the management of the hypocalcemic preterm infant or infant of a diabetic mother. The disorder may last for several weeks.

Transient neonatal hypoparathyroidism has been linked to a deletion within chromosome band 22q11, identified in patients with DiGeorge syndrome and the velocardiofacial (Shprintzen) syndrome.

Signs and Symptoms

Congenital hypoparathyroidism is a permanent condition accompanied by hypocalcemia. It is associated with agenesis, dysgenesis, or hypoplasia of the parathyroid glands. The disorder may be transmitted as an X-linked or autosomal-dominant trait but may also occur as a sporadic mutation (known as idiopathic hypoparathyroidism). These infants present with unremitting hypocalcemia and very low or undetectable serum PTH concentrations (hormone deficiency hypoparathyroidism) and increased serum phosphorus concentrations.

Hypocalcemia may be associated with cardiac arrhythmias, tetany, seizures, and mental retardation. *Candida* infection of the nails and mouth occur in one-sixth of patients. A feature of untreated early hypoparathyroidism in later infancy and childhood is dental hypoplasia.

Pseudohypoparathyroidism is a variant of parathyroid gland dysfunction. Unlike in idiopathic hypoparathyroidism, parathyroid glands are hyperplastic and actively secrete increased amounts of PTH. End-organ responsiveness to PTH is deficient (hormone-resistant hypoparathyroidism). In contrast to individuals with idiopathic hypoparathyroidism, who have no dysmorphic features, individuals with pseudohypoparathyroidism are characteristically short and thickset, with round facies, short necks, and short fingers and toes at birth. Hypocalcemia, subcutaneous soft tissue calcific nodules, dental hypoplasia, and developmental delay and mental retardation may develop later in infancy and childhood.

Diagnostic Studies

Diagnosis is based on the presence of persistent hypocalcemia and markedly increased (rather than low) serum PTH concentrations, in association with hyperphosphatemia and the characteristic physical stigmata. Confirmation of the diagnosis requires an i.v. PTH infusion test in which skeletal or renal cell response, or both, to PTH is assessed: in normal individuals, urinary excretion of cyclic adenosine monophosphate (an index of PTH effect on plasma membrane adenyl cyclase activity) or phosphate, or both, are increased in response to the PTH challenge. This response is diminished or nearly absent in individuals with pseudohypoparathyroidism.

Other Genetic Disorders of Parathyroid Hormone Action

Blomstrand Chondrodystrophy

Blomstrand chondrodystrophy is characterized by growth impairment, primarily in the form of short limbs. It has been lethal prenatally, and, therefore, the regulation of serum calcium has not been evaluated *in vivo*. It is caused by inactivating mutations of the type I PTH receptor and is inherited as an autosomal-recessive trait.

The growth plates show accelerated calcification and a near absence of proliferating chondrocytes.

Jansen Chondrodystrophy

Jansen chondrodystrophy is characterized by short limbs, mild hypercalcemia, and low serum PTH concentrations. It is caused by activating mutations of the type I PTH receptor and is inherited as an autosomal-dominant trait. It is associated with increased proliferation and delayed maturation of chondrocytes, which may weaken the growth plates and thereby cause the short limbs.

Hyperparathyroidism–Jaw Tumor Syndrome

The hyperparathyroidism–jaw tumor syndrome is rare and is characterized by hyperparathyroidism, cemento-ossifying fibromas of the jaw, renal cysts, Wilms tumor, and renal hamartomas. By age 40, approximately 80% of patients with this syndrome have hyperparathyroidism and approximately 10% of those have a parathyroid carcinoma. It is inherited as an autosomal-dominant trait.

Pseudohypoparathyroidism

See Table 11. This is a heterogeneous group of inherited disorders with renal resistance to PTH.

Pseudohypoparathyroidism Type Ia

Pseudohypoparathyroidism type Ia is characterized by mental retardation, short stature, round facies, short metacarpals and metatarsals, and other skeletal abnormalities, which are known collectively as Albright hereditary osteodystrophy, and by hypocalcemia and high serum concentrations of PTH. It is caused by inactivating mutations in the α subunit of *GNAS1* and is inherited as an autosomal-dominant trait.

Pseudohypoparathyroidism Type Ib

Pseudohypoparathyroidism type Ib is characterized by isolated resistance to PTH without the accompanying Albright osteodystrophy. It is associated with defective methylation within *GNAS1*, which is caused by a mutation in or near *GNAS1*.

Pseudopseudohypoparathyroidism

Pseudopseudohypoparathyroidism occurs in families with pseudohypoparathyroidism type Ia. It consists of a combination of inactivating mutations of *GNAS1* and Albright osteodystrophy without the resistance to multiple hormones that characterizes pseudohypoparathyroidism. The hormone resistance is suppressed when the mutated *GNAS1* gene is inherited from the father (i.e., paternal imprinting, or suppression, of the mutant copy occurs in selected tissues). Serum potassium and urine calcium, phosphorus, and ALP are normal.

Rickets

Rickets is a disease of growing bone and is a mineralization defect of bone and cartilage. Disturbances in vitamin D, PTH, calcium, phosphorus, and alkaline phosphatase homeostasis can contribute to poor bone mineralization.

Vitamin D deficiency may occur in the presence of severely restricted sunlight exposure or increased skin pigmentation in temperate climates, the skin being the major organ of vitamin D production. Deficiency may occur with decreased dietary vitamin D intake and vitamin D malabsorption. In children of strict vegetarians, diets already deficient in vitamin D may be made worse by the binding of vitamin D with dietary fiber, which inhibits its absorption.

Deficiency or absence of the hepatic microsomal enzyme 25-hydroxylase may occur with hepatocellular failure (hepatic rickets), whereas renal 25-hydroxyvitamin D 1α-hydroxylase deficiency may occur as an autosomal-recessive disorder (vitamin D–dependent rickets type I) or in the presence of renal failure (renal rickets). In vitamin D–dependent rickets type II, $1,25(OH)_2D$ is normally produced but is inactive due to an absence or defective functioning of the vitamin D receptor. This disorder is inherited in an autosomal-recessive manner and is secondary to a point mutation in the vitamin D receptor gene. Rickets may occur in infants and children on long-term anticonvulsant therapy, especially with phenytoin (Dilantin) and phenobarbitone.

Hypophosphatemic rickets is an X-linked dominant disorder characterized by decreased proximal renal tubular phosphorus reabsorption. Rickets occurs at a few months of age and is usually associated with normal or elevated PTH level, normal or low $1,25(OH)_2D$ level, and normal or low serum calcium level. Rickets associated

Table 11. Pseudohypoparathyroidism

MIM No.	Disorder	Incidence	Inheritance	Biochemical Defect	Chromosome Locus	Defects	Effects
103580	Pseudohypoparathyroidism type Ia	Unknown; over 100 cases	Autosomal dominant	α Subunit of stimulatory guanine nucleotide-binding protein associated with adenyl cyclase	20q13	Reduced synthesis of protein	Deficiency of protein leads to generalized hormone resistance with hypoparathyroidism and hypogonadism most prominent clinically. Other abnormalities include obesity, short stature, mental retardation, and bony anomalies collectively termed Albright osteodystrophy.
603233	Pseudohypoparathyroidism type Ib	Unknown	Unknown	Unknown	Unknown	Unknown	Isolated resistance to parathyroid hormone due to defect in receptor adenylate cyclase complex leads to hypoparathyroidism.

MIM, Mendelian Inheritance in Man system.

with hypophosphatemia is commonly encountered in preterm infants who are fed human milk exclusively and in those on parenteral nutrition.

Rickets is observed in alkaline phosphatase deficiency, which may present in the infantile (autosomal-recessive) or childhood (unknown inheritance) form with decreased bone and serum alkaline phosphatase activity with normal serum calcium and phosphorus levels.

Diagnostic Studies

The typical metaphyseal widening and fraying with disruption of the growth plate are most prominent in weight-bearing joints with proximal muscle hypotonia and weakness. Amino aciduria is commonly found in those cases related to vitamin D deficiency with associated elevations of PTH.

Adrenocortical Disorders

The adrenal cortex is divided into three zones: the subcapsular glomerulosa; the zona reticularis, next to the adrenal medulla; and, separating these two, the zona fasciculata.

Functionally, the glomerulosa acts as a separate gland. The absence of P450c17 results in the production solely of mineralocorticoids and, in particular, aldosterone. Cells of the glomerulosa are the only site of P450c18 activity; aldosterone is not produced elsewhere in the adrenal gland. In the human, the function of the fasciculata and reticularis is to produce glucocorticoids and adrenal androgens, respectively, although the separation of this function is not absolute.

Tests of Adrenal Function

Adrenocorticotropic Hormone Stimulation Test, Rapid (Cosyntropin Test)

Draw blood for measurement of baseline cortisol or steroidogenesis precursors (17-hydroxypregnenolone (17-PREG), 17-hydroxyprogesterone (17-OHP), 11-deoxycortisol). Inject cosyntropin 0.25 mg i.m. or i.v. (if i.v., dilute cosyntropin in 2–5 mL of sterile saline and inject over 2 minutes). Draw blood for measurement of serum cortisol or steroidogenesis precursors 30 and 60 minutes after injection if indicated.

A normal cortisol response is considered to be one or more of the following:

- a doubling of the baseline value at 60 minutes unless the baseline value is already above the normal range;
- a rise of 10 μg/dL; an absolute 1-hour cortisol level >18 μg/dL.

A normal cortisol response usually rules out primary adrenal insufficiency but not secondary adrenal insufficiency. Estrogen, spironolactone, and cortisol derivatives can elevate baseline levels, causing test interference. Stimulated plasma concentrations of 17-PREG, 17-OHP, and 11-deoxycortisol of >2,000 ng/dL, 1,500 ng/dL, and 1,500 ng/dL, respectively, indicate 3β-hydroxysteroid dehydrogenase, 21-hydroxylase, and 11-hydroxylase deficiency.

Adrenocorticotropic Hormone Stimulation Test, Prolonged

Used to differentiate primary and secondary adrenocortical insufficiency.

Procedure:

Day 1: Starting at 8 a.m., obtain 24-hour urine sample for measurement of 17-hydroxycorticosteroids and creatinine.

Day 2: Repeat urine measurements as performed on day 1.

Day 3: Starting at 8 a.m., insert i.v. line and give 250 μg synthetic ACTH (cosyntropin) in 250 mL normal saline over 8–12 hours. Repeat 24-hour urine testing as on days 1 and 2. (An alternative to i.v. cosyntropin is ACTH gel, 20 U/m^2 IM every 12 hours; or cosyntropin, 800 μg/24 hours, can be infused i.v. for 2–3 consecutive days.)

Days 4 and 5: Repeat 24-hour urine testing as on previous days.

In normal individuals urinary 17-hydroxycorticosteroid excretion increases to two to five times baseline (days 1 and 2) after synthetic cosyntropin infusion. Patients with primary adrenal insufficiency do not respond, whereas individuals with secondary insufficiency have low baseline 17-hydroxycorticosteroids levels that progressively increase after ACTH is given. Patients may eat a regular diet and remain ambulatory during the test. In those individuals strongly suspected of having primary adrenal insufficiency, dexamethasone 20 μg/kg/day can be given to prevent adrenal crisis. This will not interfere with the test.

Dexamethasone Suppression Test, Low-Dose and High-Dose

Used to differentiate Cushing disease (pituitary hypersecretion of ACTH) from other types of endogenous hypercortisolism (Cushing syndrome)

- Day 1: Beginning at 8 a.m., obtain 24-hour urine levels for 17-hydroxycorticosteroids, urinary free cortisol level, and creatinine excretion. Repeat measurements daily until end of test.
- Day 2: Repeat urine measurements as performed on day 1.
- Day 3: Draw blood for measurement of ACTH and cortisol levels at 8 a.m. Begin oral administration of dexamethasone 0.5 mg every 6 hours for 2 days (2 mg/day in adults; 5 μg/kg up to 0.5 mg per dose in children).
- Day 4: Draw blood for measurement of ACTH and cortisol levels at 8 a.m. Continue dexamethasone as on day 3.
- Day 5: Draw blood for measurement of ACTH and cortisol levels at 8 a.m. Begin oral administration of dexamethasone 2 mg every 6 hours for 2 more days (8 mg/day in adults; 40 μg/kg up to 2.0 mg per dose in children).
- Day 6: Repeat blood and urine tests as on day 5. Continue high-dose dexamethasone administration.
- Day 7: Draw blood for measurement of ACTH and cortisol levels at 8 a.m.

This test is used to discriminate between different causes of hypercortisolism. Patients with normal pituitary corticotrophs (normal subjects or those with pseudo–Cushing syndrome) show suppression after low-dose dexamethasone administration. Patients with abnormal corticotrophs (Cushing disease) show suppression only after high doses of dexamethasone; patients with ectopic ACTH syndrome or Cushing syndrome secondary to cortisol-secreting adrenal tumors usually fail to respond even to the high-dose dexamethasone administration. On low-dose dexamethasone (2 mg/day), suppression of urinary 17-hydroxycorticosteroid level to <4 mg/day or to <2.5 mg/g creatinine during the second day of dexamethasone, suppression of urinary free cortisol level to <50% of baseline, or a blood cortisol level of <5 μg/dL indicates normal regulation of ACTH. High-dose dexamethasone suppression is suggestive of Cushing disease if urinary 17-hydroxycorticosteroid levels are suppressed to <50% of baseline, urinary free cortisol levels decrease at least 90% from baseline concentrations, and blood cortisol level falls to <5 μg/dL. ACTH levels are suppressed to <5 pg/mL on either dose. Patients with Cushing syndrome due to adenoma, carcinoma, or ectopic ACTH production rarely show suppression. No dietary or activity restrictions are necessary during this test. Severely depressed patients or those taking phenytoin may not show suppression on low-dose dexamethasone but usually do so to high-dose dexamethasone.

General Features of Adrenal Gland Disorders

Adrenal Defects

Each inherited disorder has been associated with several gene defects. This decreases the usefulness of genetic analysis in establishing the primary diagnosis. When the genetic defect has been identified in a known patient, the information is of use in family studies, genetic counseling, and prenatal diagnosis.

Classification of Pediatric Adrenocortical Disorders

Primary Adrenocortical Disorders

Adrenocortical Hyperfunction

Glucocorticoid excess
- Adrenal adenoma
- Adrenal carcinoma

Adrenocortical Hypofunction

Glucocorticoid deficiency
- Steroid biosynthetic defects:
  - 21-Hydroxylase deficiency

Mineralocorticoid excess
- Adrenal glomerulosa adenoma (Conn syndrome)
- Adrenocortical nodular hyperplasia
- Steroid biosynthetic defects:
  - 17α-Hydroxylase deficiency
  - 11β-Hydroxylase deficiency

Adrenal tumors secreting deoxycorticosterone or corticosterone
Dexamethasone suppressible hyperaldosteronism
Adrenal androgen excess
- Adrenal adenoma
- Adrenal carcinoma
- Steroid biosynthetic defects
- 21-hydroxylase deficiency
- 11β-Hydroxylase deficiency

Mixed adrenal hormone excess
- Adrenal tumors
  - 17α-Hydroxylase deficiency
  - 11β-Hydroxylase deficiency

Congenital unresponsiveness to ACTH
Mineralocorticoid deficiency
- Steroid biosynthetic defects
  - Corticosterone methyl oxidase deficiency types I and II
  - Adrenal androgen deficiency
  - Steroid biosynthetic defect
  - 17,20-Desmolase deficiency

Delayed adrenarche
Mixed adrenal steroid deficiency
- Steroid biosynthetic defects
- 20,22-Desmolase deficiency
- 3β-Hydroxysteroid dehydrogenase deficiency
- 21-Hydroxylase deficiency
- Combined 17α-hydroxylase and 17,20-desmolase deficiency

Congenital adrenal hypoplasia
Adrenoleukodystrophy
Wolman disease
Adrenal crisis of acute infection (Waterhouse-Friderichsen syndrome)
Autoimmune adrenal disease

Secondary Adrenocortical Disorders

Adrenocortical Hypofunction
Hypopituitarism
Isolated ACTH deficiency
Hypothalamic defect
Intracranial tumor, craniopharyngioma
Adrenal suppression as a consequence of glucocorticoid therapy
Hypofunction after removal of unilateral adrenal tumor
Steroid therapy in mother during pregnancy

Adrenocortical Hyperfunction
Pituitary tumor
Ectopic ACTH-secreting tumor
Hyperaldosteronism secondary to renal disease
Pseudohyperaldosteronism

Adrenal Hyperplasia, Congenital

Congenital adrenal hyperplasia (CAH) is a complex of disorders transmitted as autosomal-recessive traits involving multiple steps in the adrenocortical synthesis of cortisol (hydrocortisone). As a consequence of impaired cortisol production, there is a compensatory increase in the secretion of ACTH that leads to an increase in adrenocortical cell number (hyperplasia) and size (hypertrophy) and an increase in steroidogenesis up to the point of blockage in the pathway. Clinical manifestations depend on the site of block and the products produced by the adrenal cortex *in utero*. Blocks early in the steroid pathway lead to abnormalities of genital formation, often in both male and female fetuses, whereas those later in the pathway (21-hydroxylase) result in virilization of female genitalia but not male genitalia.

Steroidogenic Acute Regulatory Protein Deficiency (Congenital Lipoid Adrenal Hyperplasia; Congenital Adrenal Hyperplasia Type I)

Because the steroidogenic acute regulatory protein is essential for the initial step of cholesterol transport into adrenal and gonadal mitochondria before its hydroxylation and cleavage by cytochrome P450scc (encoded by CYP 11A located on chromosome 15q23–q24) and its redox partners (adrenodoxin, adrenodoxin reductase) to pregnenolone, failure of this step impairs synthesis of glucocorticoids, mineralocorticoids, androgens, and estrogens, and the enlarged adrenals are filled with cholesterol [Online Mendelian Inheritance in Man (OMIM) 201710, 600617]. Thus, 46,XY individuals fail to masculinize (external genitalia are often completely feminine), whereas müllerian duct differentiation is inhibited. The 46,XX fetus has normal female external and internal genitalia. Frequently these patients have signs of severe adrenal insufficiency manifested by poor feeding and vomiting, hypotension due to hypovolemia, hyponatremia, and hyperkalemia.

Clinical and Laboratory Findings

Signs of glucocorticoid deficiency (lethargy, vomiting) and mineralocorticoid deficiency (hyponatremia, hyperkalemia, hypovolemia); very low levels of all intermediates of the glucocorticoid, mineralocorticoid, androgen/estrogen biosynthetic pathways in basal and stimulated [ACTH, human chorionic gonadotropin (hCG)] pathways.

3β-Hydroxysteroid Dehydrogenase Deficiency (Congenital Adrenal Hyperplasia Type II), Δ^{5-4} Oxosteroid Isomerase Deficiency

The steroid 3β-hydroxysteroid dehydrogenase mediates the conversion of pregnenolone to progesterone, of 17α-hydroxypregnenolone (17-PREG) to 17α-hydroxyprogesterone (17-OHP), and of DHEA to androstenedione. Its gene (HSD3B2) is encoded on chromosome band 1p13.1 and is pivotal for synthesis of glucocorticoids, mineralocorticoids, androgens, and estrogens. The enzyme is found in adrenal gland, ovary, testes, and brain. In affected 46,XY individuals the external genitalia are incompletely masculinized, whereas in 46,XX patients the genitalia are often partially virilized due to the action of the weak androgen DHEA or low levels of its metabolite androstenedione (OMIM 201810). Signs of glucocorticoid and mineralocorticoid deficiency are frequently present in the postnatal period and require immediate intervention. In milder forms of 3β-hydroxysteroid dehydrogenase deficiency, children may present with premature pubarche and adult females with hirsutism and infertility as a variant of the polycystic ovary syndrome.

Diagnostic Studies

Diagnosis is made by measuring the Δ^5 steroids 17-PREG and pregnenolone in plasma or the Δ^5/Δ^4 ratio of steroid metabolites in urine: levels of pregnenolone, 17-PREG, and DHEA are high and levels of all other intermediates in the glucocorticoid, mineralocorticoid, and androgen/estrogen biosynthetic pathways in basal and stimulated (ACTH/hCG) pathways are low. In older subjects with less severe forms of this disorder, there should be elevated levels of pregnenolone, 17-PREG, and DHEA in pre- and post-ACTH stimulation specimens.

Cytochrome P450c21 (21-Hydroxylase) Deficiency (Congenital Adrenal Hyperplasia Type III)

Deficiency of microsomal P450c21 is the most common form of CAH (accounting for 95% of cases of this disorder); it occurs with a frequency of 1 in 10,000 to 1 in 18,000 live births. The gene encoding cytochrome P450c21 (CYP21) is located on the short arm of chromosome 6 in the midst of the HLA complex. It is paired with a pseudogene (CYP21P) with 98% homology with CYP21 in the zona fasciculata (site of glucocorticoid and androgen synthesis) of the adrenal cortex. Because 17-OHP cannot be converted to desoxycortisol and cortisol, ACTH is increased, the adrenal cortex enlarges, cortisol precursors accumulate, and the metabolism of 17-OHP is directed into the androgen pathway. Progesterone cannot be converted to deoxycorticosterone and then to aldosterone in (OMIM 201910).

Classic 21-hydroxylase deficiency is characterized by excessive secretion of adrenal androgens (primarily testosterone), which leads to virilization of female external genitalia *in utero* and pseudoisosexual precocious puberty in male children. The internal genitalia of both sexes are normal for genotype. If the deficiency of P450c21 activity is severe, aldosterone production is also impaired, which results in the salt-wasting form of CAH (occurring in approximately 75% of patients with classical P450c21 CAH).

Nonclassical P450c21 deficiency manifests as late-onset hyperandrogenism—as premature pubarche or excessive acne in children and adolescents or as a cause of the polycystic ovary syndrome in adult women. The cryptic form of P450c21 deficiency is identified only by family survey, in which a family member is found to have an identical functional defect but no clinical manifestation of hyperandrogenism.

Diagnostic Studies

Measurement of plasma 17-OHP concentrations by immunoassay has replaced urinary pregnenolone estimation in diagnosis of CAH due to 21-hydroxylase deficiency. Concentration of 17-OHP is normally greatly increased in infantile forms. Patients with nonclassical CAH may have basal plasma 17-OHP levels within the normal range. Differentiation of these groups can be aided by using a short ACTH stimulation test, with measurement of 17-OHP, cortisol, and 11-deoxycortisol. Nonclassical CAH patients have an increase of 17-OHP of >40 nmol/L (normal levels are <15 nmol/L) at 30 minutes. Differentiation of heterozygotes is accomplished by the measurement of 17-OHP/deoxycortisol ratios, which are increased above the normal value of <12 at 30 minutes.

Increased 17-OHP concentrations are found in sick full-term or healthy premature infants who may be hyponatremic and gives rise to diagnostic confusion. It may be necessary to do several 17-OHP estimations and perform a short ACTH test. Patients with 21-hydroxylase deficiency may have basal plasma cortisol levels within the normal range and some increase on ACTH stimulation. Increased 17-OHP levels have been reported in other steroid biosynthetic defects, for example, 11β-hydroxylase and 3β-hydroxysteroid dehydrogenase defects, and have led to reports of combined 11β- and 21-hydroxylase deficiencies.

Prenatal Screening

Many states now screen for cytochrome P450c21 deficiency CAH by measuring 17-OHP in filter paper dried blood samples. Abnormal neonatal screening study results must be confirmed by measurement of serum 17-OHP concentrations.

Sex of fetuses is identified by chromosome analysis and by a combination of amniotic fluid 17-OHP concentration and HLA typing of amniotic cells or by DNA analysis.

Cytochrome P450c11 (11β-Hydroxylase) Deficiency (Congenital Adrenal Hyperplasia Type IV)

Deficiency of 11β-hydroxylase is the second most common inborn error of steroid biosynthesis but accounts for only 5–15% of cases. Mutations in CYP 1161 (chromosome 8q21 and its product P450c11 lead to defective conversion of deoxycortisol to cortisol and of deoxycortisol to corticosterone, and to excessive secretion of deoxycortisol, a potent mineralocorticoid (OMIM 202010). Presentation is similar to that of 21-hydroxylase deficiency, but hypertension is present in most cases. Patients may have hypoglycemia and alkalosis. Elevated levels of androgens lead to virilization of girls and pseudoisosexual precocity in boys. Biochemical diagnosis is established by finding an increased plasma deoxycortisol concentration or a raised urinary excretion of tetrahydrodeoxycortisol.

In the severe form, it appears that 11β-hydroxylation of both 17-hydroxy and 17-deoxysteroids is affected, whereas in milder forms only 11β-hydroxylation of 17-hydroxysteroids is reduced.

Cytochrome P450c17 (17α-Hydroxylase/17,20-Lyase) (Congenital Adrenal Hyperplasia Type V)

One microsomal enzyme protein with two functional domains catalyzes the actions of 17α-hydroxylation and cleavage of 21-carbon to 19-carbon structures (17,20-lyase). The gene for P450c17 (CYP17) is located on chromosome band 10q24.3. P450c17 catalyzes the conversion of pregnenolone to 17-PREG. Although the secretion of cortisol, androgens, and estrogens is restricted, the mineralocortical pathway is intact. In 46,XY patients there is incomplete masculinization of the external genitalia and absence of müllerian duct structures (OMIM 202110). The internal and external genitalia of the 46,XX patient are normal. Both have hypokalemic hypertension, excessive kaliuria, and sodium and fluid retention, the consequence of increased secretion of the mineralocorticoid desoxycorticosterone, and no evidence of glucocorticoid insufficiency because of the secretion of glucocorticoid. Affected girls fail to feminize at puberty and present with sexual immaturity, whereas affected boys may have normal feminine or ambiguous external genitalia and fail to virilize at adolescence. Some affected boys may even develop gynecomastia when the deficiency of P450c17 is partial.

Diagnostic Studies

In patients with combined enzyme deficiencies, findings are hypertension and absence of sexual maturation in 46,XX individuals; feminine or ambiguous genitalia in 46,XY patients; high levels of pregnenolone, progesterone, desoxycorticosterone, and corticosterone; and low levels of all other intermediates in the glucocorticoid and androgen/estrogen biosynthetic pathways in basal and stimulated (ACTH, hCG) pathways. In patients with isolated 17,20-lyase deficiency, glucocorticoid and mineralocorticoid pathways are intact; pregnenolone and progesterone levels are high with low 17-OHP, 17-PREG, DHEA, androstenedione, and testosterone values.

Adrenal Tumors, Steroid-Producing

Adrenal tumors producing steroids are rare. Approximately 5% of all pediatric adrenal tumors arise in the cortex, and the incidence is between 0.1 and 0.4 in 1 million each year. Increased incidence in early childhood and female/male ratios between 2:1 and 5:1 are reported. Adrenocortical carcinoma may be more common than adenoma.

Signs and Symptoms

The clinical presentation of adrenal tumors in children is predominantly one of precocious puberty or virilization or both. This may be associated with signs of hypercortisolism (Cushing syndrome) or even occasionally feminization. Aldosterone-secreting tumors and asymptomatic (non–hormone producing) tumors comprise a higher proportion of adrenal tumors in adults.

Measurement of plasma and urinary steroid levels, measurement of responses to trophic hormones, and suppression tests have been used.

Two major patterns of steroid secretion have been observed in pediatric virilizing adrenal tumors. In the first, urinary ketosteroid excretion is high (>50 μmol/24 hours), serum testosterone level is markedly raised for age, and the principal steroid produced is DHEA. In the second major pattern, urinary ketosteroid excretion is lower (<20 μmol/24 hours), serum testosterone level is moderately raised, and the major steroid produced is 11β-hydroxyandrosterone. Both patterns can be associated with either adenoma or carcinoma.

Tumors detected in early infancy are sometimes associated with increased excretion of 16-oxygenated-3β-hydroxyl-5-ene steroids, which are produced normally in the neonatal period. These tumors lack 3β-hydroxysteroid dehydrogenase activity.

Adrenocortical Hypofunction

Decreased production of one or more of the adrenal steroid hormones may be caused by primary diseases of the adrenal glands or may be secondary, resulting from decreased stimulation by either ACTH or renin as a consequence of hypothalamic-pituitary disease or renal disease, respectively.

The biochemical diagnosis of adrenocortical hypofunction is established by use of tests of basal steroid hormone excretion, of the intactness of the hypothalamic-pituitary-adrenal axis, and by the response of the adrenal gland to the stimulus of exogenous ACTH. The measurement of plasma ACTH level is extremely helpful in distinguishing primary from secondary adrenal failure. Diurnal rhythm of ACTH and cortisol secretion is often maintained in primary and secondary disease and its measurement is not a useful test. The insulin stress test should be used with caution in the diagnosis of adrenal failure because of the danger of severe hypoglycemia, and in most cases of severe hypoadrenalism the short ACTH test is an adequate substitute.

Results of adrenal hypofunction from primary disease (partial or complete destruction) of the adrenal gland are inadequate secretion of glucocorticoids and mineralocorticoids. An autoimmune process is the most common cause (80% of the cases) followed by tuberculosis. AIDS is becoming a more frequent cause. The hypofunction is characterized by weakness, fatigue, tiredness, weight loss, dizziness, low blood pressure, orthostatic hypotension, increased pigmentation (on extensor surfaces, hand creases, dental-gingival margins, buccal and vaginal mucosa, lips, areola, pressure points, scars; "tanning"; freckles; vitiligo), anorexia, nausea, vomiting, chronic diarrhea, abdominal pain, decreased cold tolerance, salt craving, hair loss in females, and depression.

Addisonian crisis is an acute complication of adrenal insufficiency with circulatory collapse, dehydration, hypotension, nausea, vomiting, and hypoglycemia, usually precipitated by acute physiologic stress such as surgery, systemic illness, or acute withdrawal of long-term corticosteroid therapy.

Autoimmune adrenal insufficiency shows some hereditary disposition. Familial glucocorticoid insufficiency may have a recessive pattern; adrenomyeloneuropathy is X-linked.

Causes

Adrenal insufficiency may be caused by bacterial infection, fungal disease, bilateral adrenal hemorrhage, and infarction; antiphospholipid syndrome; surgical adrenalectomy; sarcoidosis; adrenoleukodystrophy; adrenomyelodystrophy; polyglandular endocrine syndromes and congenital disorders (enzyme defects, hypoplasia, familial glucocorticoid insufficiency).

Laboratory Findings

Laboratory findings include low serum sodium level, elevated serum potassium level, elevated blood urea nitrogen level, increased creatinine, elevated serum calcium level, hypoglycemia, and metabolic acidosis. Low cortisol level (between 8 and 9 a.m.), elevated ACTH level, moderate neutropenia, eosinophilia, relative lymphocytosis, anemia, and adrenal cortex autoantibody (ACA/21) are found.

Special Tests

Rapid ACTH stimulation test: administer cosyntropin 0.25 mg i.v. and measure cortisol levels preinjection and 60 minutes postinjection. Patients with Addison disease have low to normal values that do not rise.

Plasma cortisol level.

Metapyrone test.

Basal ACTH level; elevation suggests primary adrenal failure.

Insulin-induced hypoglycemia test.

Measurement of corticotropin-releasing hormone level may help distinguish secondary from tertiary adrenal insufficiency.

Autoantibody tests.

- 21-Hydroxylase (most specific)
- 17-Hydroxylase
- 17-α-Hydroxylase (may not be associated)

Synacthen Stimulation Test

The Synacthen stimulation test is the gold standard for investigation of suspected primary or secondary adrenocortical hypofunction.

Specimen: 5 mL of blood in EDTA for cortisol and ACTH assays before a dose of 250 µg aqueous Synacthen (ACTH 1-24), given by i.m. injection.

Plasma cortisol level:

- Baseline (before Synacthen): 200–650 nmol/L.
- After Synacthen: an increase of ≥270 nmol/L over the baseline level to a level of ≥500 nmol/L indicates a normal response.

Failure to respond indicates adrenal insufficiency. If basal ACTH level is elevated, this suggests primary adrenal failure. The test may be done after 3 days of priming the adrenal cortex with 1 mg of depot Synacthen daily.

Imaging Studies

Abdominal CT scan reveals small adrenal glands in autoimmune adrenalitis, enlarged adrenal glands in infiltrative and hemorrhagic disorders.

Abdominal radiograph may show adrenal calcifications.

Chest radiograph may show adrenal calcifications, small heart size, calcification of cartilage.
The low-dose ACTH test is useful in assessing responsiveness in patients currently taking steroids.

Aldosterone Synthetase Deficiency

Aldosterone synthetase is the product of CYP O11B2 (chromosome 8q21); it is also called corticosterone methyl oxidase (CMO), an enzyme with two functions: CMO I (or 18-hydroxylase) converts corticosterone to 18-hydroxycorticosterone; CMO II (or 18-hydroxysteroid dehydrogenase) converts the latter to aldosterone. Inability to secrete aldosterone leads to poor growth due to a salt-wasting state with hyponatremia and hyperkalemia but without glucocorticoid deficiency.

Diagnosis

Elevated levels of 18-hydroxycorticosterone and increased ratio of 18-hydroxycorticosterone to aldosterone are the biochemical hallmarks of this disorder.
In pseudohypoaldosteronism, aldosterone is increased in plasma and urine. Renin is increased, and hyponatremia and hyperchloremia are markedly decreased.
Aldosteronism is characterized by hypertension, hypokalemia, and decreased renin. It may be due to aldosterone-secreting adrenal adenoma or adrenal hyperplasia. Some forms may be suppressed by glucocorticoid treatment.
Levels of electrolytes, renin, cortisol, deoxycorticosterone acetate, and urine and plasma aldosterone should be measured.

Cushing Syndrome in Children

Clinical abnormalities are associated with chronic exposure to excessive amounts of cortisol. The most frequent cause is prolonged use of exogenous glucocorticoids. The syndrome occurs with MEN (multiple endocrine neoplasia) 1, Carney complex, exogenous ACTH exposure, ACTH-secreting pituitary tumor, adrenal adenoma, adrenal carcinoma, macro- and micronodular hyperplasia, and other neuroendocrine tumors, such as carcinoid. Cushing syndrome may result from overproduction of ACTH as a consequence of hypothalamic-pituitary disease (Cushing disease) or ectopic ACTH secretion from nonadrenal tumors. Due to increased circulating levels of ACTH, the patients have bilateral adrenal hyperplasia. Approximately 50% of all pediatric cases of Cushing syndrome are ACTH dependent, with the majority of these being in the older age group. Other cases are ACTH independent and are caused by adrenal adenomas or carcinomas. Rare syndromes causing ACTH-independent disease are primary adrenal micronodular dysplasia and McCune-Albright syndrome.
The disorder affects girls more frequently than boys.

Signs and Symptoms

Moon face (facial adiposity), increased adipose tissue in neck and trunk, central weight gain, emotional lability, hypertension, osteoporosis, purple striae on the skin, and diabetes or glucose intolerance with fasting hyperglycemia or glycosuria or both. Muscle weakness due to loss of muscle mass from increased catabolism, skeletal growth retardation in children, easy bruising, and hirsutism occur.

Laboratory Tests

The most useful initial screening tests are the 24-hour urine free cortisol excretion test and the overnight dexamethasone test.
Other laboratory tests are
  Plasma cortisol level (a.m. and p.m.)
  Plasma ACTH concentration
  Tests for

Glycosuria (possible)
Neutrophilia
Lymphopenia
Hyperglycemia
Hyperlipidemia
Hypokalemia

Pathologic Findings

Hyalinization of basophilic cells (anterior pituitary)—Crooke hyaline changes
Muscular atrophy
Nephrosclerosis

Diagnostic Procedures

Not all tests are indicated for every case. Choice of diagnostic procedure is dependent on circumstances and judgment.

To differentiate causes of Cushing syndrome, the following procedures are recommended:

- Plasma ACTH concentration
- High-dose dexamethasone suppression test
- Imaging of the pituitary and adrenal areas

Unmeasurable plasma ACTH is diagnostic of primary adrenal disease, usually a tumor.

Imaging Studies

Radiography of the lumbar spine—osteoporosis is common.
If pituitary tumor suspected, pituitary MRI scan.
If adrenal disease suspected, abdominal CT scan.
If ectopic ACTH secretion suspected, chest CT scan.

Hypercortisolism

See Table 12.

Table 12. Etiology of Hypercortisolism: Laboratory Differential Diagnosis

	Pituitary Based	Adrenal Cortical Neoplasm	Ectopic ACTH	Primary Adrenal Hyperplasia
Plasma cortisol	High, no diurnal variation	High, no diurnal variation	High, no diurnal variation	High, no diurnal variation
Plasma ACTH	High	Low	High	Low
Response to ACTH with glucocorticoid production	Rise	None	Usually none	Variable, may rise
Dexamethasone suppression	Suppresses with high dose only	No suppression	No suppression	No suppression
Response to metyrapone	Rise in 12-deoxycortisol	No response	No response, usually	Variable, often rises in 12-deoxycortisol

ACTH, adrenocorticotropic hormone.

Adrenomedullary Disorders

Adrenal Medulla

Disorders of the adrenal medulla include neuroblastoma and pheochromocytoma. The diagnosis of these conditions depends principally on the measurement of their metabolites.

Catecholamine Synthesis

The adrenal medulla produces two principal catecholamines, norepinephrine (noradrenaline) and its methylated derivative, epinephrine, in the ratio of 1:9. These are produced from the amino acid tyrosine. Tyrosine hydroxylase converts tyrosine to dihydroxyphenylalanine, which is then metabolized to the physiologically active metabolite dopamine through the activity of dihydroxyphenylalanine decarboxylase. Norepinephrine and epinephrine are produced from dopamine.

Catecholamine Metabolism

Metabolites of catecholamines include normetanephrine and metanephrine, produced from norepinephrine and epinephrine, respectively, and usually measured as total metanephrines; homovanillic acid (HVA, 4-hydroxy-3-methoxy-phenylacetic acid), and 4-hydroxy-3-methoxy-mandelic acid (HMMA), also known as vanillylmandelic acid. These metabolites are produced by the action of two enzymes, catechol-O-methyl transferase and monoamine oxidase. Catecholamines and their O-methylated derivatives are excreted in the urine, partly as sulphate and glucuronide conjugates.

Evaluation of Adrenal Medullary Function

Total catecholamines, free catecholamines (norepinephrine, epinephrine, and dopamine), metadrenalines, and HVA and HMMA excretion in urine are used to diagnose neuroblastoma and pheochromocytoma. Total metadrenaline excretion remains useful as a preliminary screening test for pheochromocytoma. High-pressure liquid chromatography allows specific differentiation of the individual catecholamines and overcomes the problems of interferences from drugs and dietary substances.

Because of problems in collecting 24-hour urine specimens from very young children, random urine collections are used and the results are expressed as creatinine ratios.

Urine samples must be acidified to pH 1 immediately after voiding. HVA and vanillylmandelic acid appear to be stable in unacidified urine collected onto filter paper for population screening.

The measurement of total HVA (free plus conjugated HVA) has been proposed as a useful alternative investigation when the free urinary HVA level is borderline.

Plasma determination of catecholamine levels is unsatisfactory due to their lack of stability.

Reference Ranges for Catecholamines and Their Metabolites

See Table 13.

Neuroblastoma

Neuroblastoma accounts for 7–10% of all pediatric malignancies and is predominantly a disease of infancy. It is the most common nonhematopoietic tumor in the first 2 years of life.

Neuroblastomas are tumors derived from cells of neuroectodermal origin. They are classified clinically into types I to IV, depending on the primary site and degree of spread. This classification has prognostic significance.

Table 13. Reference Ranges for Catecholamines and Their Metabolites

	Upper Limit[a] of Normal Excretion [mmol/mol creatinine (µg/mg creatinine)]			
Age	Norepinephrine	Dopamine	HMMA (VMA)	HVA
<1 yr	0.25 (0.37)	1.8 (2.4)	15.0 (26.3)	22.0 (35.5)
1–2 yr	0.2 (0.3)	1.5 (2.0)	12.0 (21.1)	17.0 (27.4)
3–4 yr	0.15 (0.22)	0.90 (1.22)	8 (14)	15.0 (24.2)
5–9 yr	0.14 (0.21)	0.80 (1.08)	7.0 (12.3)	10.0 (16.1)
10–15 yr	0.11 (0.16)	0.70 (0.95)	7.0 (12.3)	7.0 (11.3)

Note: These reference ranges were derived from urine collected over 18–24 hr into sufficient acid to reduce pH to <3.0. The reference population consisted of patients in whom an adrenal medullary tumor was suspected but whose final diagnosis excluded neuroblastoma or pheochromocytoma. Analysis was by high-pressure liquid chromatography with electrochemical detection.
HMMA, 4-hydroxy-3-methoxymandelic acid; HVA, homovanillic acid; VMA, vanillylmandelic acid.
[a]The upper limit of normal is defined as the 0.95 fractile, determined using nonparametric methods.

Diagnostic Studies

Diagnosis of neuroblastomas relies on the measurement of HVA and HMMA in 24-hour urine collections by high-pressure liquid chromatography. Five percent to 10% of patients are referred to as "nonsecretors."

Screening for Neuroblastoma

Because neuroblastoma may spontaneously regress, especially in early infancy, newborn screening has not been accepted as a screening test.

Pheochromocytoma

Pheochromocytomas are catecholamine-secreting tumors. Patients present with headache, hypertension, profuse sweating, and diarrhea.

Tumors are found more frequently in boys (male/female ratio 1.8:1.0), and 35–40% are single tumors of the adrenal medulla. Ten percent of children have bilateral adrenal tumors; 10% of the tumors are malignant.

Familial pheochromocytomas are recognized either as a separate entity or in association with disorders such as MEN, neurofibromatosis, and von Hippel–Lindau syndrome.

Elevated levels of total metadrenalines and free catecholamine in 24-hour urine tests are diagnostic.

Gonadal Disorders

Hormone Assays

In the normal male infant the concentrations of testosterone are approximately half of the values in adult males; levels then tend to decrease somewhat until age 6–7 days, when they rise to 5.2–10.4 nmol/L (150–300 ng/dL) for the next 8–12 weeks of life. This is followed by very low concentrations during infancy and childhood until puberty.

By measuring the ratio of androstenedione to testosterone (in a normal male at 1–2 weeks of age, usually <1) and of testosterone to dihydrotestosterone (range, 2.5–7.5), it is possible to determine whether there is a deficiency of 17-ketoreductase and 5α-reductase, respectively. Direct assay of samples in the first 6 months of life may result in spurious levels. Androgens can arise from the fetus (CAH) or from the mother.

The placenta secretes large amounts of progesterone and 17-OHP; these steroids cross to the fetus, and their concentrations at birth in cord blood and in the infant are high. Their half-life is short, and by the third day of life measured values are representative of the infant's secretion of these steroids.

The concentrations of plasma 17-OHP are important to the diagnosis of CAH due to 21-hydroxylase deficiency. Normal newborns have huge concentrations of Δ^5-steroids conjugated as sulfates, which have a markedly prolonged half-life, and this interferes with the assay of 17-OHP. The concentrations of Δ^5-steroid sulfates decrease slowly with age, so that their interferences become minimal by 2–4 months of age. Most laboratories use a purification procedure for the determination of this steroid in infants up to 4–6 months of age.

Abnormal Sexual Differentiation

Diagnosis of Disorders of Gonadal Differentiation

See Fig. 1.

The genetic control of gonadal differentiation is dependent on testis determination in the presence of the sex-determining region of the Y chromosome (SRY) or a muta-

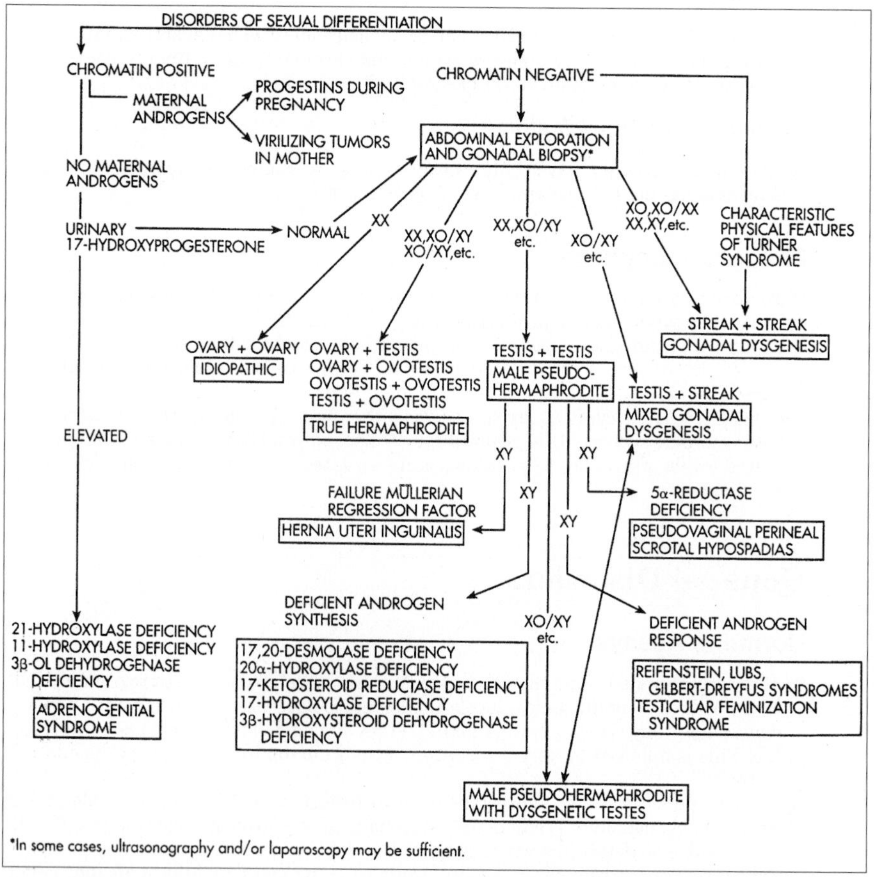

Fig. 1. Schematic diagram of disorders of sexual differentiation. 3β-OL, 3β-hydroxysteroid. [From Allen TD. Disorders of sexual differentiation. *Urology* 1976;7(Suppl 1):1–32.]

Table 14. Conditions with Absent SRY Gene Product

	Normal Female, 46,XX	"Superfemale," 47,XXX	Turner Syndrome 45,X, 45,X/46,XX (Variants)	46,XY Female, 46,XY[–]
External genitalia	F	F	F	F
Internal ducts	F	F	F	F
Gonads				
In utero	Ovaries	Ovaries	Ovaries	Ovaries
Adult	Ovaries	Ovaries	Streaks (ovaries rarely)	Streaks
Fertility	Yes	Yes (limited)	No (yes rarely)	No

F, female; SRY, sex-determining region of the Y chromosome.

tion that permits testis determination even in the absence of SRY. If SRY is absent or SRY action fails to occur, ovarian determination proceeds.

The SRY gene can be identified using polymerase chain reaction amplification and sequencing of this gene. This permits the detection of the presence of this gene, as in 46,XX males, or of its deletion or mutation, as in 46,XY females.

Another application of this technique is being investigated for the study of the androgen receptor gene. Polymerase chain reaction amplification of each of the eight exons of this gene, along with techniques that permit detection of point mutations, can be used to rule out androgen insensitivity.

Disorders Related to Abnormal Gonadal Differentiation

At the level of present knowledge, classification is based on the presence or absence of normal testis-determining genes. Conditions in which testis determination is lacking include normal 46,XX female karyotype; 47,XXX "superfemale" karyotype; 45,X Turner syndrome and its variants; and the 46,XY female karyotype (complete or pure gonadal dysgenesis or Swyer syndrome). The conditions with normal or partial testis determination include normal 46,XY male karyotype; 47,XXY Klinefelter syndrome; 45,X male karyotype; 46,XX male karyotype; 46,XX true hermaphrodite karyotype; mosaic 45,X/46,XY,46XY true hermaphrodite karyotype; and 46,XY partial gonadal dysgenesis.

Table 14 lists conditions with absent SRY gene product.

Table 15 shows conditions with normal or partial testis-determining function.

Ambiguous Genitalia

Evaluation of the Neonate with Ambiguous Genitalia

The evaluation of an infant with ambiguous genitalia must be carried out as an emergency procedure: first, because life-threatening symptoms such as salt loss can develop; and second, because a decision must be made as rapidly as possible about whether the infant will be reared as male or female.

History: family history; maternal exposure to toxic agents; endogenous androgen production.

Physical examination: associated congenital anomalies, perineal orifice(s), phallic size, gonads palpable or not palpable.

Normal-appearing male may have an abnormal karyotype such as 47,XXY (Klinefelter syndrome) or, rarely, 46,XX (46,XX male). Deficiency or partial deficiency of one of the enzymes needed for cortisol biosynthesis can result in masculinization of the genitalia of a female fetus, except that no gonads are palpated in the scrotum.

Table 15. Conditions with Normal or Partial Testis-Determining Function

	46,XY Normal	47,XXY Klinefelter Syndrome	45,X Male	46,XX Male	46,XX True H	45,X/46,XY	46,XY True H	46,XY Partial Gonadal Dysgenesis
External genitalia	M	M	M	M	Amb	M/Amb/F	Amb	Amb
Internal ducts	M	M	M	M	Variable	Variable	Variable	Variable
Gonads								
In utero	Testes	Testes	Testes	Testes	Ovotestes	Variable	Ovotestes	Ovotestes?
Adults	Testes	Testes[a] (no sperm)	Testes (no sperm)	Testes[a] (no sperm)	Ovotestes	Variable	Ovotestes	Dysgenetic gonads
Fertility	Yes	No	No	No	Variable	Variable	Variable	No

Amb, ambiguous; F, female; H, hermaphrodite; M, male.
[a]Hyalinized tubules.

Gonads not palpable, müllerian structures present, 46,XX: increased 17-OHP, 21-hydroxylase deficiency CAH; measure sodium level, potassium level, plasma renin activity.

17-Hydroxyprogesterone normal: measure pregnenolone, 17-OHP (low—deficiency of steroidogenic acute regulatory protein; elevated—deficiency of 3β-hydroxysteroid dehydrogenase), 11-deoxycortisol (elevated—deficiency of 11-hydroxylase).

Gonads palpable, müllerian duct structures present, 46,XY or variant: measure müllerian inhibitory hormone level.

Gonads palpable, müllerian duct structures absent, 46,XY or variant: measure intermediates of testosterone and dihydrotestosterone synthesis in basal specimens and after hCG administration; assess androgen receptor.

No diagnosis: gonadal biopsy for true hermaphroditism.

Measure testosterone, dihydrotestosterone, and the precursors of androgens; obtain a karyotype; and evaluate the genital structures by sonograms and genitogram. Following is a recommended schedule for tests.

- Day 1 or 2: Karyotype, including study of fluorescent Y chromosome and of possible mosaicism. Measurement of concentrations of testosterone and dihydrotestosterone in single blood sample to compare the values of these two steroids.
- Day 3 or 4: Measurement of concentration of 17-OHP, 17-PREG, and androstenedione, also in a single blood sample.
- Day 5 or 6: Sonogram of the gonads and internal ducts followed by genitogram (retrograde injection of contrast substance through the urogenital sinus).
- Day 10 to 12: Repeat concentrations of 17-OHP, 17-PREG, androstenedione, testosterone, and dihydrotestosterone.

Throughout the period of evaluation, concentrations of serum electrolytes and blood glucose should be checked at least once a day to detect the possible development of an adrenal crisis with salt loss and hypoglycemia.

In infants with a 46,XY karyotype, male pseudohermaphroditism, true hermaphroditism, and partial gonadal dysgenesis should be considered. In 46,XY patients with low testosterone concentrations, increased androgen precursor values permit determination of the enzyme deficiency involved; low precursor values suggest partial gonadal dysgenesis or true hermaphroditism. In 46,XY individuals with normal male concentrations of testosterone, a high testosterone/dihydrotestosterone ratio (>12 in newborns) indicates the diagnosis of 5α-reductase deficiency; a normal testosterone/dihydrotestosterone ratio suggests either androgen insensitivity (i.e., androgen receptor abnormality) or a timing defect.

Ultrasonography of the pelvis and abdomen will determine whether a uterus is present, whether anomalies of the kidneys are present, and (with experienced examiners) whether the adrenal glands are unusually enlarged (in the term newborn, the adrenal glands are one-third as large as the kidneys themselves). The presence of müllerian duct structures implies abnormal secretion or action of müllerian inhibitory hormone and, hence, testicular Sertoli cell function in early fetal life. The karyotype is then determined and the serum concentration of 17-OHP measured, because virilizing 21-hydroxylase deficient CAH is among the most common causes of genital ambiguity. It is essential that the 17-OHP level be measured in a laboratory that uses serum purification methods (extraction and chromatography) before assay of this metabolite.

Analysis of the genome of the androgen receptor is required for specific identification of androgen insensitivity disorders. Serum concentrations of LH and FSH are often elevated in patients with anorchia or other forms of gonadal dysgenesis and androgen insensitivity syndromes. Surgical exploration and gonadal biopsy are usually necessary to establish the diagnosis of true hermaphroditism.

XX Sex Reversal

Phenotypically normal male with 46,XX karyotype characterized often by short stature, small testes, primary hypogonadism, and the presence of translocated Y-specific DNA (including SRY) found on the distal portion of Xp.

XY Sex Reversal

Phenotypically normal female with 46,XY karyotype; the condition may be associated with pure gonadal dysgenesis characterized by delayed puberty, tall stature, ovarian stroma without oogonia, increased risk for development of gonadoblastoma, and in some patients a mutation in SRY. Other examples of XY sex reversal with normal female phenotype include complete androgen insensitivity syndrome and complete deficiency of 17α-hydroxylase.

XY Gonadal Dysgenesis

XY gonadal dysgenesis, also termed "mixed" gonadal dysgenesis, is associated with the 45,X/46,XY karyotype and a phenotype that may vary from that of Turner syndrome to that of a male with short stature and hypoplastic testes. One dysgenetic testis and a streak gonad are most commonly present in these patients.

True Hermaphroditism

Ambiguity of internal and external genitalia as well as microscopic evidence of both ovarian and testicular tissue (either as separate structures or an ovotestis) are present in the patient with true hermaphroditism. The karyotype of these patients is most frequently 46,XX, often with Y DNA translocated to one of the X chromosomes.

Male Pseudohermaphroditism

In the male pseudohermaphrodite, the external and internal genitalia are ambiguous (incompletely masculinized), but the gonads are recognizable as testes, albeit often primitive; karyotype is 46,XY.

Causes

Dysgenetic testes
Variant of 46,XY, 45,X/46,XY, 46,XYp– gonadal dysgenesis (associated with degenerative renal disease)
Disorders of androgen synthesis
Leydig cell hypoplasia—inactivating mutation of the LH receptor

Specific Disorders Associated with Male Pseudohermaphroditism

- Abnormal cholesterol transport
  - Steroidogenic acute regulatory protein (chromosome band 8q11.2): congenital lipoid adrenal hyperplasia
- Deficiencies of steroidogenic enzyme activity
  - 7-Dehydrocholesterol reductase deficiency—Smith-Lemli-Opitz syndrome (chromosome band 7q32.1)
  - 3β-Hydroxysteroid dehydrogenase type 2 deficiency (chromosome band 1p13.1)
  - 17α-Hydroxylase/17,20-lyase deficiency (chromosome band 10q24.3)
  - 17β-Hydroxysteroid dehydrogenase type 3 deficiency (chromosome band 9q22)
  - 5α-Reductase type 2 deficiency (chromosome band 2p23)
- Abnormal androgen receptor synthesis or function
  - Complete androgen insensitivity
  - Partial androgen insensitivity
- Maternal estrogens or progestins
- Eponymic syndromes
  - Denys-Drash syndrome (WT1)
  - Campomelic dysplasia (SOX9)
- Persistent müllerian duct syndrome
- Vanishing testes syndrome

Female Pseudohermaphroditism

In the female pseudohermaphrodite, the external genitalia are masculinized; the internal genitalia are feminine in the majority of subjects and absent in a few patients.

Specific Disorders Associated with Female Pseudohermaphroditism

- Deficiencies of enzyme activity
  - 3β-Hydroxysteroid dehydrogenase type 2 deficiency (chromosome band 1p13.1)

21-Hydroxylase deficiency (chromosome band 6p21.3)
11β-Hydroxylase type I deficiency (chromosome band 8q21)
Deficiency of placental aromatase
Maternal androgen
Virilizing luteoma
CAH
Ingestion of androgens, synthesis of estrogens
Eponymic syndromes
Fraser syndrome (cryptophthalmos, ambiguous internal and external genitalia)
VACTERL syndromes (vertebral, anal, cardiac, tracheoesophageal fistula, radial, renal, limb anomalies)

Classification of Female Pseudohermaphroditism in Subjects with 46,XX Karyotype

Excess fetal androgen
21-Hydroxylase deficiency
Partial pseudohermaphroditism (simple virilizing form)
More complete pseudohermaphroditism (salt-losing form)
11-Hydroxylase deficiency (hypertensive form)
3β-Hydroxysteroid dehydrogenase deficiency
Excess maternal androgen
Iatrogenic causes
Virilizing tumor of ovary or adrenal gland
Congenital abnormalities
Structural or teratogenic factors

Androgen Synthesis Abnormalities

Androgen Insensitivity

Mutations in the transcription factor androgen receptor (AR gene, chromosome band Xq11-q12) lead to complete or incomplete forms of androgen insensitivity with varying degrees of feminization of the external genitalia of a 46,XY fetus, but absence of müllerian duct structures (OMIM 300068, 313700). This is an X-linked recessive disorder. Partial androgen insensitivity has also been recorded in undervirilized males and in infertile males with normal secondary sexual characteristics.

5α-Reductase Type 2 Deficiency

Conversion of testosterone to dihydrotestosterone in genital epithelium is essential for masculinization of the external genitalia catalyzed by 5α-reductase type 2 (SRD5A2 gene, chromosome band 2p23). Deficiency of this enzyme during embryogenesis leads to autosomal-recessive pseudovaginal perineoscrotal hypospadias (OMIM 264600). Ambiguous genitalia or normal female genitalia are present in the affected male infant, with a shallow blind "vaginal" pouch and a perineal urethral orifice. At puberty these patients masculinize as testosterone production is normal. Deletions and point mutations in SRD5A2 have been found in these patients.

17β-Hydroxysteroid Dehydrogenase Type 3 Deficiency

Deficiency of 17β-hydroxysteroid dehydrogenase (17β-HSD) type 3 (HSD17B3 gene, chromosome band 9q22) impairs conversion of androstenedione to testosterone and leads to incomplete masculinization of fetal male external genitalia. (Synonyms for this enzyme include: 17β-hydroxysteroid oxidoreductase and 17-ketosteroid reductase.) There are three isoenzymes of 17β-HSD; type 3 is expressed in the gonads. If unrecognized, these patients develop gynecomastia but also virilize at puberty due to restoration of testosterone synthesis by peripheral 17β-HSD isoenzymes (types 1 and 2) during childhood and puberty (OMIM 264300). In females with deficiency of 17β-HSD type 3, hyperandrogenism occurs at puberty as androstenedione production increases, but splice junction mutations have been found in HSD17B3 in patients with deficiency of 17β-HSD type 3.

7-Dehydrocholesterol Reductase Deficiency

Smith-Lemli-Opitz syndrome (chromosome band 7q32.1) is an autosomal-recessive disorder characterized by microcephaly, developmental delay, hypotonia, distinctive facies (square forehead, blepharoptosis, short nose with anteverted nostrils, cleft palate, micrognathia), polydactyly, syndactyly, incomplete masculinization of male external genitalia, and occasionally retention of müllerian duct derivative structures (OMIM 270400) with striking hypocholesterolemia. The important functions of this lipid in signal transduction, cell membrane formation, myelinization of the nervous system, and hormone synthesis are impaired.

Leydig Cell Hypoplasia

Inactivating mutations in the 7-transmembrane LH–choriogonadotrophin receptor (LHGR gene, chromosome band 2p21) lead to Leydig cell hypoplasia and aplasia, and hence defective androgen synthesis (OMIM 152790). Affected neonatal males have micropenis and ambiguous or female external genitalia but no müllerian duct derivatives. In affected females, growth and sexual maturation, including menarche, are normal, but secondary amenorrhea ensues. Deletions and nonsense mutations lead to inactive LH–choriogonadotrophin receptors in this autosomal-recessive disorder.

Persistent Müllerian Duct Syndrome

In persistent müllerian duct syndrome, due to an abnormality of müllerian inhibitory hormone synthesis or to a defect in its receptor, müllerian duct regression fails to occur and a genotypic-phenotypic male shows rudimentary uterus and fallopian tubes, usually in a hernia sac.

Vanishing Testes Syndrome

The vanishing testes syndrome occurs in phenotypic males with 46,XY karyotype and normal wolffian duct structures but absent or rudimentary testes; it is likely that the testes were normally formed and fully functional in the first trimester but then deteriorated, either because of a transplacentally transmitted environmental toxic agent or because of a genetic error (as yet unidentified) in factors necessary to maintain testicular integrity.

Aromatase Deficiency

Aromatase deficiency may occur only during gestation or may be lifelong. Aromatase (P450arom) is essential for conversion of androgens to estrogens during gestation. Placental aromatase deficiency during pregnancy leads to virilization of the affected mother and masculinization of the external genitalia of the female fetus (phallic enlargement, fusion of the labioscrotal folds). In females with somatic mutations in the gene encoding P450arom (CYP19) there is female pseudohermaphroditism, excessive growth, failure of feminine pubertal maturation, and progressive virilization at puberty with polycystic ovaries by ultrasonographic examination.

Clinical and Laboratory Findings

Serum concentrations of LH, FSH, testosterone, and androstenedione are elevated and estradiol levels are low. In affected males, genital development is normal; there is a tall, eunuchoid stature and normal virilization, but osteopenia and incomplete skeletal maturation (OMIM 107910).

Hirsutism

Excessive male-pattern hair growth due to increased androgenic hormones.
Often accompanied by menstrual irregularities.

Extreme androgenic effects (deep voice, clitorimegaly, balding) are known as *virilization*.
Incidence in United States is 8% of adult women.
Predominant age group affected is postpubertal females.

Signs and Symptoms

Hair thickens and darkens in male pattern—beard, moustache, chest hair.
Usually accompanied by irregular menses and anovulation.
Usually accompanied by acne.
May be accompanied by infertility.
Onset is usually gradual.

Causes

Excessive androgenic effects
- Excessive hormone production from the ovary or adrenal gland
- Increased peripheral sensitivity to androgens
- Decreased sex hormone–binding globulin

Causes with persistent anovulation
- Polycystic ovary disease
- Hypothyroidism
- Hyperprolactinemia

Ovarian causes
- Polycystic ovaries
- Ovarian tumors
- Premature ovarian failure

Adrenal causes
- Tumor (rare)
- Cushing disease (rare)
- Late-onset CAH

Other Risk Factors

Family history.
Anovulation.
A specific cause often is not found.

Diagnostic Studies

Basic workup—total testosterone, DHEAS, 17-OHP, TSH prolactin levels.
If testosterone level is >200 ng/dL, ovarian tumor workup is needed.
If DHEAS level is >700 μg/dL, adrenal tumor workup is needed.
LH/FSH ratio is elevated in 75% of cases of polycystic ovary syndrome.

Special Tests

Measurement of fasting glucose/insulin ratio is used to rule out insulin resistance in polycystic ovary syndrome.

If there is a strong suspicion of Cushing disease, 1 mg dexamethasone should be given by mouth in evening and a blood sample drawn for plasma cortisol measurement at 8:00 a.m. Cortisol level of >5 mg/dL is borderline; level of >10 mg/dL is abnormal (dexamethasone suppression test).

If 17-OHP level is 300–800 ng/dL, ACTH (cosyntropin) test should be performed (ACTH 0.25 mg is given i.v. and 17-OHP level is checked at 0 and 1 hour).

If DHEAS level is high but not in tumor range, low dose dexamethasone test is performed (0.5 mg dexamethasone is given four times daily for 5 days, then DHEAS and testosterone levels are rechecked; levels decrease if androgens are adrenal and do not if they are ovarian).

Imaging Studies

If testosterone level is >200 ng/dL or DHEAS level is >700 μg/dL, CT of ovaries or adrenal glands is needed.

Ultrasonography can image polycystic ovaries as a supplement to clinical diagnosis.

Table 16. Causes of Delayed Puberty

	Site of Defect	Gonadotropin	LH/FSH Response to GnRH	Gonadal Steroids
Constitutional delay, reversible hypogonadotropism	Delayed maturation or hypothalamus	Low	Prepubertal	Low
Permanent hypogonadotropism	Hypothalamus or pituitary	Low	Prepubertal or absent	Low
Hypogonadotropism related to increased androgens	Adrenal or gonadal androgens	Low	Prepubertal	Elevated
Hypergonadotropic hypogonadism	Gonads	Elevated	Accentuated	Low

FSH, follicle-stimulating hormone; GnRH, gonadotropin-releasing hormone; LH, luteinizing hormone.

Puberty, Delayed

See Table 3.

Puberty is usually considered to be delayed in boys if there is no noticeable testicular enlargement by the age of 14 years and in girls if there is no breast development by the age of 13 years; in girls, puberty is considered delayed if menstruation does not commence within approximately 3 years of the onset of breast development.

In many cases the delayed puberty will eventually resolve and result in normal maturation. In other cases the delayed puberty is associated with hypogonadism.

Causes

See Table 16.

Diagnostic Testing

Gonadotropin function should be determined by measuring LH and FSH concentration in serum and the response to the administration of gonadotropin-releasing hormone (GnRH). The methods used are similar to those described for sexual precocity.

With hypogonadotropism, whether the cause is a hypersecretion of androgens, including adrenal androgens (DHEA, DHEAS, and androstenedione) and testosterone, should be determined. If 21-hydroxylase deficiency is considered, then plasma 17-OHP concentration should be measured. If 11-hydroxylase deficiency is possible, plasma 11-deoxycortisol concentration should be determined. Complete androgen suppression will be obtained in a dexamethasone suppression test in CAH, but no suppression will be observed in cases of virilizing adrenal or ovarian tumors.

Constitutional Delay and Reversible Hypogonadotropism

The term *constitutional delay* applies to subjects whose pubertal maturation occurs after the normal average age but is eventually established. This is the most common cause of pubertal delay, particularly in boys.

Certain conditions result in delayed secretion of gonadotropins that is reversible after the correction of the original condition, such as malnutrition as in starvation or anorexia nervosa, and involvement in competitive sports like gymnastics, swimming, and running. A number of systemic diseases (severe cardiovascular or respiratory disorders, inflammatory bowel disease, renal tubular acidosis, poorly controlled diabetes mellitus), as well as psychopathology, can result in delay of gonadotropin secretion.

Table 17. Normal Serum Levels of Testosterone and Related Androgens

	Male		Female	
	Prepubertal	Adult (Age Related)	Prepubertal	Adult (Age Related)
Free testosterone (pmol/L)	—	170–510	—	<4
Total testosterone (nmol/L)	<0.5	8–35	<0.5	<4
Sex hormone–binding globulin (nmol/L)	55–100	10–50	55–100	30–90; (250–500 in the third trimester of pregnancy)
Dihydrotestosterone (nmol/L)	—	1.0–2.5	—	—

Permanent Hypogonadotrophic Hypogonadism

Tumors as well as other destructive disorders of the pituitary-hypothalamic area can result in an inability to secrete GnRH or LH and FSH. Various congenital anomalies of the central nervous system can result in hypogonadotropism. Some are associated with various syndromes such as septo-optic dysplasia, Kallmann syndrome, and some cases of Prader-Willi syndrome. In some patients, the anatomical anomaly cannot be determined and the cause is termed *idiopathic hypopituitarism*.

Causes of Permanent Hypogonadotrophic Hypogonadism Leading to Delayed Puberty

Tumors of pituitary gland, hypothalamus, optic chiasma, third ventricle, adenoma, craniopharyngioma
- Glioma
- Dysgerminoma

Destructive disorders
- Histiocytosis
- Sarcoidosis
- Lupus erythematosus

Head trauma: hemorrhage

Congenital anomalies
- Pituitary aplasia
- Deficient LH and FSH or GnRH secretion related to various syndromes
- Idiopathic hypopituitarism

Hypogonadotropism Related to Increased Androgen Secretion

See Table 17.

In some cases of hypogonadotropism related to increased androgen secretion, the androgens arise from the adrenal glands (virilizing adrenal tumor of CAH due to 21-hydroxylase deficiency or to 1-hydroxylase deficiency). In other cases the androgens are gonadal in origin. The disorder can be related to polycystic ovaries or ovarian tumors (adrenal rest tumor, hilar cell tumor, arrhenoblastoma) in girls and to Leydig cell tumors in boys.

Presentation is that of androgen effects, including virilism without estrogenic effect in girls and without testicular development in boys. Treatment is to remove or suppress the origin of androgen hypersecretion.

Hypergonadotropic Hypogonadism with Normal-Appearing Female External Genitalia

In 46,XX gonadal dysgenesis, the abdominal sonogram shows the presence of streak gonads. The steroid enzyme deficiencies are characterized by an inability to synthesize androgens and estrogens. Patients with ovarian disorders have a history of autoimmune abnormality, chemotherapy, radiation therapy, or surgical operation for bilateral ovarian torsion or tumor. The syndrome of resistant ovaries is usually diagnosed by exclusion.

In 46,XY pure gonadal dysgenesis, the gonadal tissue disappears early in fetal life, which results in completely normal female phenotype and streak gonads detected by sonography. With 46,XY karyotype, steroid enzyme deficiencies must be complete to result in a female phenotype. Androgen insensitivity is X-linked and is characterized by the presence of testes in the abdomen or the labial folds with normal male testosterone secretion but lack of androgen receptor function. Although there is a short vagina, there are no müllerian structures and few or no wolffian structures. The LH concentrations are always elevated, but much less than in other conditions of hypergonadotrophic hypogonadism. At puberty, breast development occurs but usually there is no pubic or axillary hair and no menstruation.

The karyotype 45,X is characterized by streak gonads and short stature with increased incidence of cardiovascular malformations, particularly coarctation of the aorta, and increased incidence of thyroid antibodies, hypothyroidism, and congenital kidney malformations, especially horseshoe kidney. The karyotype 47,XXX is sometimes termed "superfemale." Some of these patients have a delayed puberty, and many of them have premature menopause.

Hypergonadotropic Hypogonadism with Normal Male External Genitalia

With karyotype 46,XY, vanishing testes are diagnosed if gonads cannot be localized, due to destruction of the testes after gonadal differentiation. Noonan syndrome is associated with "male Turner syndrome" and a number of the congenital malformations found in 45,X karyotype, including short stature. The testicular function may be normal with normal Leydig cell function. Most patients are azoospermic. Partial testicular dysgenesis is a poorly understood syndrome characterized by partial but variable malformation of the testes, usually with variably decreased Leydig cell function.

Karyotype 46,XY

Anorchia (vanishing testes)
Noonan syndrome (male Turner syndrome)
Partial testicular dysgenesis
Other testicular disorders
Inflammation (autoimmune)
Bilateral trauma or tumor
Radiation or chemotherapy

Karyotype 46,XX

46,XX males
Some 47,XYY individuals
Some 45,X/46,XY individuals

Puberty, Precocious

See Table 3.

Precocious puberty is the onset of puberty in girls before age 8 years or in boys before age 9 years. These children present with tall stature for their age and secondary sex characteristics. Central precocious puberty is a premature activation of the hypothalamic GnRH pulse generator, whereas peripheral precocious puberty is independent of GnRH function. In contrasexual precocity, there is excessive production of estrogens in males or excessive production of androgens in females.

In central precocious puberty, the early activation of the hypothalamic GnRH pulse generator results in a pubertal LH-FSH pulse pattern. Idiopathic forms are more frequent in girls than in boys. The incidence of precocious puberty due to an identifiable central nervous system lesion is approximately the same in both sexes.

Fig. 2 shows the workup procedure for children with signs of precocious puberty.

Central Precocious Puberty

Causes

Idiopathic
Central nervous system involvement

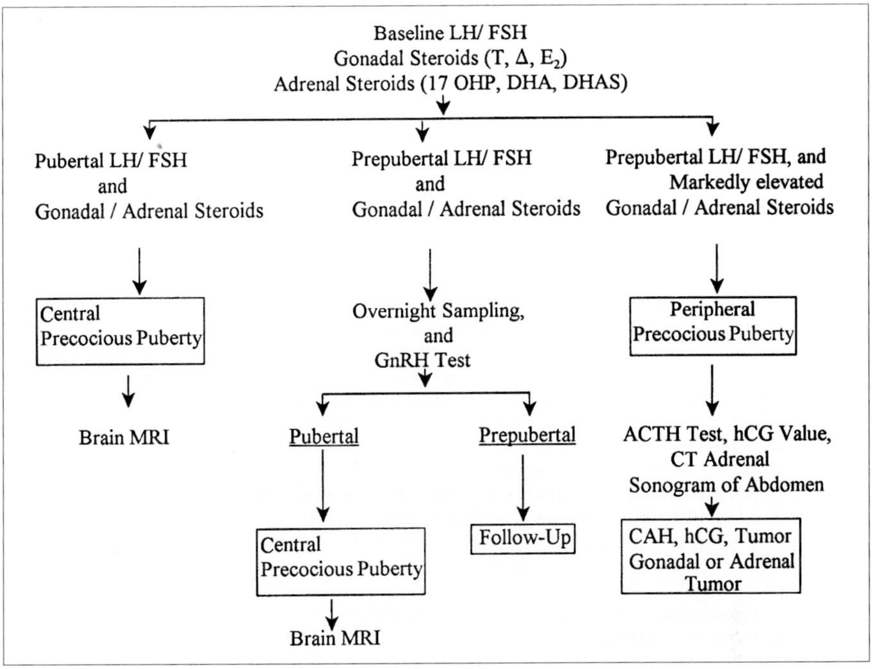

Fig. 2. Workup for signs of precocious puberty in children. ACTH, adrenocorticotropic hormone; CAH, congenital adrenal hyperplasia; CT, computed tomography; Δ, androstenedione; DHA, dehydroepiandrosterone; DHAS, dehydroepiandrosterone sulfate; E_2, estradiol; FSH, follicle-stimulating hormone; GnRH, gonadotropin-releasing hormone; hCG, human chorionic gonadotropin; LH, luteinizing hormone; MRI, magnetic resonance imaging; 17-OHP, 17α-hydroxyprogesterone; T, testosterone. (From Seldin SJ, Rifain, Hicks JM, ed. *Biochemical basis of pediatric disease*, 3rd ed. Washington: American Association for Clinical Chemistry Press, 1998:197.)

Tumor: hamartoma, astrocytoma, glioma
Neurofibromatosis
Injuries: hydrocephalus, meningitis, encephalitis, head trauma
Severe primary hypothyroidism

Peripheral Precocious Puberty

Children with peripheral precocious puberty do not have a mature hypothalamic-pituitary-gonadal axis. Rather, the stimulus for sex steroid production is independent of the GnRH pulse generator. In girls the sexual precocity is due to estrogen exposure, whereas in boys the sexual precocity is due to androgen exposure.

Both gonadal and adrenal tumors are rare in both sexes. McCune-Albright syndrome is thought to be due to an abnormality of a G-protein subunit associated with the LH receptor that results in the secretion of gonadal steroids despite the absence of LH stimulation. Some cases of premature Leydig cell maturation or familial male precocious puberty have been due to mutations in the LH receptor.

Causes

Girls

McCune-Albright syndrome (café-au-lait spots, precocious puberty and fibrous dysplasia)

Boys

McCune-Albright syndrome
Testicular tumors
Masculinizing tumors

Ovarian tumors (cysts)
Feminizing adrenal tumors
Ectopic hCG tumors

CAH
Ectopic hCG tumors
Premature Leydig cell maturation

Contrasexual Precocious Puberty

Gynecomastia appearing before the onset of puberty in a male is rare and may be caused by an estrogen-secreting adrenal tumor. Virilization and hirsutism in prepubertal girls are also rare and may be due to CAH or an androgen-secreting adrenal or ovarian tumor.

Incomplete Precocious Puberty

Premature thelarche is the isolated development of breasts in girls before age 8 years. It usually occurs in the first 4 years of life and often it regresses completely. A transient increase in LH, FSH, and estradiol concentrations may be observed. Gonadotropin and steroid concentrations are usually low, and there is no activation of the GnRH pulse generator, no estrogenization of the vaginal mucosa, and no significant advancement in bone age. One small ovarian cyst can be found by pelvic sonogram in some cases. The cyst is the source of estrogens. Rupture and disappearance of the cyst result in breast regression.

Premature adrenarche occurs between ages 4 and 8 years, with predominantly pubic hair development, often only on the labia in girls. In addition, there may be apocrine odor and axillary hair and mild to moderate acceleration of growth velocity with a slight advancement of bone age. Estrogen, testosterone, and gonadotropin concentrations are prepubertal. Concentration of adrenal androgens, particularly DHEA and DHEAS, is increased and may rise to pubertal values. Puberty occurs at a normal time.

Diagnostic Studies

Initial laboratory evaluation determines whether precocious puberty involves gonadotropins (LH, FSH), gonadal steroids (testosterone, estradiol), and adrenal steroids (17-OHP, androstenedione, DHEA, and DHEAS). Test for bone age and thyroid function tests (T_4, RIA, T_3 resin uptake, T_{index}, and TSH) should be obtained.

If prepubertal values of LH, FSH, and steroids are reported, an overnight blood sampling (every 20 minutes from 2 a.m. to 6 a.m. for LH and FSH, every hour for gonadal steroids) and a GnRH test (at 8 a.m., an i.v. slow push of 100 μg of GnRH is given, followed by blood sampling every 20 minutes for 2 hours) should be performed. Because LH and FSH are secreted only at night in the early stages of puberty, a daytime sampling may give misleading information. The GnRH test will result in LH-FSH concentrations in the adult range if the subject is in early puberty (stage II). When the results of the overnight sampling and GnRH tests are indicative of a prepubertal status, the patient should be followed closely.

Markedly increased levels of gonadal or adrenal steroids with prepubertal LH and FSH levels suggest a peripheral cause for the sexual precocity. An ACTH test (0.25 mg of ACTH 1-24, i.v. slow push, followed by blood sampling at 0, 30, and 60 minutes for 17-OHP and progesterone) helps determine whether CAH is the cause of precocity. An increased hCG concentration suggests an hCG-producing tumor. CT of the adrenal glands and sonography of abdomen and pelvis may be indicated.

Other Endocrine Disorders

Endocrine Abnormalities Associated with Human Immunodeficiency Virus Infection and Acquired Immunodeficiency Syndrome

Human immunodeficiency virus–associated endocrine dysfunctions may present early in the disease course with subtle clinical manifestations, or they may be part of the severe systemic disease occurring in the latter stages of acquired immunodeficiency syndrome (AIDS) and may be marked.

Clinical manifestations vary and may include manifestations related to

- Adrenal gland: adrenal insufficiency.
- Hypothalamic-pituitary axis: hyponatremia, growth failure (in pediatric AIDS).

Thyroid gland: primary hypothyroidism; euthyroid sick syndrome, in which the thyroid gland is normal but, due to severe systemic nonthyroidal illness, alternations in thyroid physiology occur, including decreased circulating T_3 levels as a consequence of impaired conversion of T_4 to T_3 and T_4 levels that vary and may be increased.

Pancreas: acute pancreatitis, chronic pancreatitis, pancreatic abscess, hyperamylasemia due to nephropathy, glucose intolerance, diabetes mellitus, steatorrhea, and obstructive jaundice.

Parathyroid glands: hypercalcemia.

Gonads: decreased levels of circulating sex steroids, including testosterone, estradiol, or progesterone; very high levels of pituitary gonadotropins, including LH and FSH. Chronic disease results in gonadal atrophy with disturbances in menstrual function and ovulation and reduced spermatogenesis.

Hypoglycemic Disorders of Infants and Children

Causes

Abnormal hormone secretion
- Transient neonatal hyperinsulinism
- Infant of diabetic mother
- Erythroblastosis fetalis
- Beckwith-Wiedemann syndrome

Persistent/sustained hyperinsulinism
- Mutation in SUR/Kir6.2 gene
- Hyperinsulinism/hyperammonemia syndrome
- Insulinoma

Drug-induced hyperinsulinism
- Insulin, oral hypoglycemic agents
- GH deficiency
- ACTH or cortisol deficiency
- ? Glucagon deficiency
- ? Somatostatin deficiency
- ? Thyroid hormone deficiency

Small Size for Gestational Age

Many SGA infants develop transient neonatal hypoglycemia.

Other Causes

Salicylate compounds may produce hypoglycemia and increased ketones. A history of salicylate ingestion should be sought in all acutely hypoglycemic infants. Ethyl alcohol inhibits hepatic gluconeogenesis and may also produce hypoglycemia. Hypoglycemia in cyanotic congenital heart disease may be due to poor hepatic perfusion, which results in a decreased rate of hepatic glucose production.

Reye syndrome often follows a viral illness (influenza A or B, varicella) and may be compounded by the administration of aspirin. Hypoglycemia is prominent in younger children.

Diagnostic Studies

See Table 18.

The diagnosis of hypoglycemia depends on the accurate laboratory measurement of plasma glucose concentration. Demonstration of a plasma glucose concentration <2.2–2.5 mmol/L (40–45 mg/dL) should trigger further evaluation.

The presence of hypoglycemia in the absence of ketonuria or ketonemia is strongly suggestive of hyperinsulinism. In these infants, a glucagon stimulation test (0.03 mg/kg i.v.) performed at the time of hypoglycemia will result in a significant glycemic response (up to 1.1–1.7 mmol/L or 20–30 mg/dL increment in the first 10 minutes). The hyperresponsiveness to glucagon is due to the presence of excess hepatic glucose deposition resulting from the hyperinsulinism.

Table 18. Investigation of Hypoglycemia in Childhood

	Hyper-insulinism	Inborn Error	Ketotic Hypoglycemia	Hormone (GH/ Cortisol Deficiency)
Glucose	↓	↓	↓	↓
Lactate	N	↑	N	N
B-hydroxy-butyrate	↓	N	↑	↑
Free fatty acids	↓	N	↑	↑
GH	N, ↑	↑	↑	N, ↓
Cortisol	N, ↑	↑	↑	N, ↓
Insulin	↑[a]	↓	↓	↓
Associated features	LGA	Hepatomegaly Developmental/ growth delay Metabolic acidosis Hyperlipidemia Hyperuricemia		Newborn: Micropenis Hyperbilirubinemia Hypothyroidism Older: Short stature

↑, increased; ↓, decreased; GH, growth hormone; LGA, large for gestational age.
[a]May be within the "usual" physiologic range.

Hypoglycemia and hypoketonemia may also be seen in disorders of ketogenesis, that is, fatty acid oxidation defects. In these children, measurement of plasma carnitine concentrations and a search for urinary organic acids may prove helpful.

Multiple Endocrine Neoplasia Syndromes

MEN is a genetic predisposition to hyperplasia and tumors, or both, in two or more endocrine organs. The disease may appear simultaneously or sequentially in different organs. Some distinct forms of MEN are MEN type 1, MEN type 2A, and MEN type 2B.

Multiple Endocrine Neoplasia Type 1 (Wermer Syndrome)

See Table 19.

Patients with MEN 1 have various combinations of parathyroid, pancreatic, anterior pituitary, and other tumors. MEN 1 is caused by an inactivating germline mutation of tumor-suppressor gene (the MEN1 gene) inherited as an autosomal-dominant trait.

Endocrine tumors (carcinoids) of the stomach, ileum, lung, and thymus and adrenocortical hyperplasia or tumors, thyroid disease, lipomas, and pinealomas may occur.

Components	Frequency of Involvement
Parathyroid hyperplasia or adenoma	90–100%
Pancreatic or gastrointestinal neuroendocrine hyperplasia or neoplasm	75%
Pituitary edema	66%

Multiple Endocrine Neoplasia Type 2

The MEN 2 syndromes include MEN 2A and MEN 2B. These are dominant disorders that are due to mutations in the RET (receptor tyrosine kinase) protooncogene. Calcitonin-producing C cells in the thyroid are hyperplastic and result from the proliferative stimulus of the mutant RET.

Table 19. Multiple Endocrine Neoplasia Type 1

Organ/Pathology	Approximate Incidence	Hormones	Symptoms
Parathyroid glands	>90%	Parathyroid hormone	Hyperparathyroidism
Diffuse or nodular hyperplasia with adenomatosis			
Endocrine pancreas/ duodenum	50–85%	Multihormonal	
Diffuse microadenomatosis of the pancreas with or without one of several macrotumors (>0.5 cm)			
PPoma	Most frequent	Pancreatic polypeptide	
Insulinoma	10–30%	Insulin	Hypoglycemia
VIPoma	2–10%	Vasoactive intestinal polypeptide	Verner-Morrison syndrome
Glucagonoma	Rare	Glucagon	Glucagonoma syndrome
Somatostatinoma	30–50%	Somatostatin	GH inhibition
Gastrinoma of the duodenum	30–65%	Gastrin	Hypergastrinemia, Zollinger-Ellison syndrome
Anterior pituitary gland			
Inactive or GH adenoma	70%	Often inactive, GH	Local symptoms, hypopituitarism, acromegaly
GH adenoma, prolactinoma	25%	Growth hormone, prolactin	Acromegaly, hyperprolactinemia, Cushing disease
ACTH adenoma	Rare	ACTH	
Gastrointestinal and thymic endocrine cells	5%		
Carcinoids			
Adrenal cortex			
Nodular hyperplasia, adenoma	40%	Hypercorticism	
Thyroid gland			
Follicular adenoma	20%	Hyperthyroidism, mild	

ACTH, adrenocorticotropic hormone; GH, growth hormone.

Multiple Endocrine Neoplasia Type 2A (Sipple Syndrome)

See Table 20.

Diffuse or nodular adrenal medullary hyperplasia occurs in the majority of patients with MEN 2A. Pheochromocytomas are mostly multicentric and bilateral and rarely show malignant behavior. Nodular hyperplasia of chief cells of the parathyroid glands occurs in up to 60% of patients with MEN 2A. Thyroid tumors occur in over 90%.

Components	**Frequency of Involvement**
C-cell hyperplasia or medullary thyroid carcinoma (MTC)	Approximately 100%
Pheochromocytoma	50%
Parathyroid hyperplasia or adenoma	25%

Table 20. Multiple Endocrine Neoplasia Type 2A

Organ/Pathology	Approximate Incidence	Hormones	Symptoms
Thyroid	>90%	Calcitonin, calcitonin gene	
Multifocal diffuse and nodular C-cell hyperplasia			
Thyroid medullary carcinoma (bilateral)			Diarrhea, tends to progress
Adrenal medulla	20–40%		
Medullary hyperplasia	85–90%		
Pheochromocytoma	85–90%		Hypertension
Bilateral	70–80%	Epinephrine, norepinephrine	
Extrarenal	10–15%		
Parathyroid glands			
Chief cell hyperplasia	60%	Parathyroid hormone	Hyperparathyroidism, often asymptomatic

Multiple Endocrine Neoplasia Type 2B (or Type 3; Gorlin Syndrome)

See Table 21.

MEN 2B is a familial form of MTC that becomes clinically apparent at a young age and is often multiple and bilateral. It is invariably accompanied by C-cell hyperplasia in the residual gland.

Components	Frequency of Involvement
C-cell hyperplasia or MTC; increased calcitonin	Approximately 100%
Pheochromocytoma	34%
Parathyroid hyperplasia or adenoma	4%

Once an MEN syndrome has been diagnosed in a family member, all other at-risk family members should be screened. A screening method for determination of increased serum calcitonin includes a 50-second infusion of calcium gluconate, followed by a 10-second bolus of pentagastrin, followed by measurement of calcitonin levels at 2, 3, 5, and 10 minutes; peak levels occur at the 2- and 3-minute points.

Calcitonin Stimulation Tests

Used to detect and manage MTC or C-cell hyperplasia (neoplastic precursor of MTC)

Pentagastrin Stimulation Test

Draw blood for measurement of baseline calcitonin level.

Inject pentagastrin 0.5 μg/kg i.v. push (5 seconds).

Draw blood for repeat measurement of calcitonin level at 1 or 2 and 5 minutes.

Combined or Pentagastrin-Calcium Infusion Test

Draw blood for measurement of baseline calcitonin level.

Inject pentagastrin 0.5 μg/kg i.v. push (5 seconds).

Inject calcium 2 mg/kg i.v. over 1 minute.

Draw blood for repeat measurement of calcitonin level at 1, 2, 5, 10, and 30 minutes.

Interpretation

Although most patients with MTC have elevated baseline calcitonin levels, a significant number (≥30%) have normal or borderline levels. In patients with MTC and a normal baseline calcitonin concentration, stimulated levels are often markedly increased, usually 3–20 times baseline. In the familial form of MTC (autosomal dominant with

Table 21. Multiple Endocrine Neoplasia Type 2B

Organ/Pathology	Approximate Incidence	Hormone	Symptoms
Thyroid	>90%		
Multifocal diffuse and nodular C-cell hyperplasia		Calcitonin, calcitonin gene-related peptide	
Thyroid medullary carcinoma (bilateral)			Diarrhea tends to develop early and progress rapidly
Adrenal medulla	20–40%		
Medullary hyperplasia	85–90%		
Pheochromocytoma	85–90%		Hypertension
Bilateral	70–80%	Epinephrine, norepinephrine	
Extraadrenal	10–15%		
Parathyroid glands	Rarely		No hyperparathyroidism
Chief-cell hyperplasia		Parathyroid hormone	
Peripheral neural system	100%		
Marfanoid habitus	100%		
Mucosal neuromas	100%		
Intestinal ganglioneuromatosis	40–50%		Diarrhea or constipation

variable penetrance), all family members should be tested semiannually or yearly from not later than age 5 until at least age 40. These tests are not specific for MTC, as increased levels of calcitonin can be seen in other conditions, including other tumors (oat cell tumor of lung, breast), pregnancy, renal failure, subacute thyroiditis, various bone diseases, and pernicious anemia. False-negative results have also been reported. Side effects are less common with the rapid infusions of these chemicals and are generally brief (lasting only a few minutes) if they occur. Those reported are often vague, poorly defined unpleasant sensations: nausea, vomiting, diarrhea, headache, weakness, flushing, lightheadedness, and burning.

Bibliography

Abraham GE, Swerdloff RS, Tulchinsky D, et al. Radioimmunoassay of plasma 17-hydroxyprogesterone. *J Clin Endocrinol Metab* 1971;33:42–46.

Ashcraft MW, Van Herle AJ, Vener SL, et al. Serum cortisol levels in Cushing's syndrome after low- and high-dose dexamethasone suppression. *Ann Intern Med* 1982;87:21–26.

Atkinson MA, MacLaren NK. The pathogenesis of insulin-dependent diabetes mellitus. *N Engl J Med* 1994;331:1428–1436.

Balbalola AA, Ellis G. Serum dehydroepiandrosterone sulfate in a normal pediatric population. *Clin Biochem* 1985;18:184–189.

Baumann G. Growth hormone binding proteins and various forms of growth hormone: implications for measurements. *Acta Paediatr Scand* 1990;370:72–80.

Berkovitz GD, Fechner PY, Marcantonio SM, et al. The role of the sex-determining region of the Y chromosome (SRY) in the etiology of 46,XX true hermaphroditism. *Hum Genet* 1992;88:411–416.

Bottazzo GF, Florin-Christensen A, Doniach D. Islet cell antibodies in diabetes mellitus with autoimmune polyendocrine deficiencies. *Lancet* 1974;2:1279–1283.

Buster JE, Chang RJ, Preston DL, et al. Interrelationships of circulating maternal steroid concentrations in third trimester pregnancies. I. C21 steroids: progesterone, 16 alpha-hydroxyprogesterone, 17 alpha-hydroxyprogesterone, 20 alpha-dihydroprogesterone, delta 5-pregnenolone, delta 5-pregnenolone sulfate, and 17-hydroxy delta 5-pregnenolone. *J Clin Endocrinol Metab* 1979;48(1):133–138.

Butler J, Moore P, Mieli-Vergani G, et al. Serum free thyroxine and free tri-iodothyronine in normal children. *Ann Clin Biochem* 1988;25:536–539.

Cook JF, Hicks JM, Godwin ID, et al. *Clin Chem* 1992;38:959.

Ducharme JR, Forest MG, DePeretti E, et al. Plasma adrenal and gonadal sex steroids in human pubertal development. *J Clin Endocrinol Metab* 1976;42:468–476.

Eisenbarth GS. Type I diabetes: a chronic autoimmune disease. *N Engl J Med* 1986;314:1360–1368.

Feldkamp CS. Thyroid testing algorithms: a rational design can improve patient care and reduce costs. *Clin Lab News* 1997;23:7.

Gharib H, Kao PC, Heath HH III. Determination of silica-purified plasma calcitonin for the detection and management of medullary thyroid carcinoma. Comparison of two provocative tests. *Mayo Clin Proc* 1987;62:373–378.

Grumbach MM, Conte FA. Disorders of sexual differentiation. In: Wilson JD, Foster DW, eds. *Williams textbook of endocrinology,* 8th ed. Philadelphia: WB Saunders, 1992:853–951.

Gwinup G, Johnson B. Clinical testing of the hypothalamic-pituitary-adrenocortical system in state of hypo- and hypercortisolism. *Metabolism* 1975;24:777–791.

Hennessy JF. A comparison of pentagastrin injection and calcium as provocative agents for the detection of medullary carcinoma of the thyroid. *J Clin Endocrinol Metab* 1974;39:487–495.

Johnson GF. Laboratory diagnosis and screening of thyroid disease. American Society of Clinical Pathologists teleconference series 1996;24:1–16.

Jonetz-Mentzel L, Wiedemann G. *Eur J Clin Chem Clin Biochem* 1993;31:525–529.

Liddle GW. Tests of pituitary-adrenal suppressibility in the diagnosis of Cushing's syndrome. *J Clin Endocrinol Metab* 1960;20:1539.

Lindholm J, Kehlet H. Re-evaluation of the clinical value of the 30-minute ACTH test in assessing the hypothalamic-pituitary-adrenocortical function. *Clin Endocrinol* 1987;26:53–59.

Liu N, Garon J. A new generation of thyroid testing. *Adv Admin Lab* 1999;11:29–30.

Marx SJ. Hyperparathyroid and hypoparathyroid disorders. *N Engl J Med* 2000;343(25):1863–75.

May ME, Carey RM. Rapid adrenocorticotropic hormone test in practice. *Am J Med* 1985;69:679.

Meites S, ed. *Pediatric clinical chemistry, reference (normal) values*, 3rd ed. Washington: American Association for Clinical Chemistry Press, 1989.

Melby JC. Assessment of adrenocortical function. *N Engl J Med* 1971;285:735–739.

Migeon CJ, Berkovitz GD, Brown TR. Sexual differentiation and ambiguity. In: Kappy MS, Blizzard RM, Migeon CJ, eds. *Wilkins' the diagnosis and treatment of endocrine disorders in childhood and adolescence*, 4th ed. Springfield, IL: Charles C Thomas, 1994:573–715.

Migeon CJ, Berkovitz GD. Congenital defects of the external genitalia in the newborn and prepubertal child. In: Carpenter SE, Rock J, eds. *Pediatric and adolescent gynecology.* New York: Raven Press, 1992:77–94.

Miller WL. Molecular biology of steroid hormone synthesis. *Endocr Rev* 1988;9:295–318.

Nelson JC, Tindall DJ. A comparison of the adrenal response to hypoglycemia, metyrapone, and ACTH. *Am J Med Sci* 1978;275:165–172.

Parthemore JG. A short calcium infusion in the diagnosis of medullary thyroid carcinoma. *J Clin Endocrinol Metab* 1974;39:108–111.

Rafferty B, Gaines Das R. Comparison of pituitary and recombinant human thyroid-stimulating hormone (rh TSH) in a multicenter collaborative study: establishment of the first World Health Organization reference reagent for rh TSH. *Clin Chem* 1999;45(12):2207–2208.

Report of the Expert Committee on the Diagnosis and the Classification of Diabetes Mellitus. *Diabetes Care* 1997;20:1183–1197.

Rifai N, Morales A, Albalos F, et al. *Clin Chem* 1993;39:1170–1171.

Rossini AA, Greiner DL, Friedman HP, et al. Immunopathogenesis of diabetes mellitus. *Diabetes Rev* 1993:1;43–75.

Sealfon MS. A review of thyroid testing. *Adv Lab* September 2000:89–93.

Shuman CR. Diabetes mellitus: definition, classification and diagnosis. In: Galloway J, Potvin J, Shuman C. *Diabetes mellitus*, 9th ed. Indianapolis, IN: Lilly, 1988:1–14.

Soldin SJ, Hicks JM, eds. *Pediatric reference ranges*. Washington: American Association for Clinical Chemistry Press, 1995:127.

Soldin SJ, Hill JG. Liquid-chromatographic analysis for urinary 4-hydroxy-3-methoxymandelic acid and 4-hydroxy-3-methoxyphenylacetic acid, and its use in investigation of neural crest tumors. *Clin Chem* 1981;27:502–503.

Speckart PF, Nicoloff JT, Bethune JE. Screening for adrenocortical insufficiency with cosyntropin. *Arch Intern Med* 1971;128:761.

Stark P, Beckerhoff R, Leumann EP, et al. *Helv Pediatr Acta*, 1976;30:349–356.

Surks MI, Chopra IJ, Mariash CN, et al. American Thyroid Association guidelines for use of laboratory tests in thyroid disorders. *JAMA* 1990;263:1529–1532.

Tannenbaum GS, Painson JC, Lapointe M, et al. Pituitary hypothalamic somatostatin. Interplay of somatostatin and growth hormone-releasing hormone in genesis of episodic growth hormone secretion. *Metabolism* 1990;39:35–39.

Tri-Delta Diagnostics. *TPO antibodies: quantitative enzyme immunoassay for the determination of thyroid peroxidase antibodies in serum or plasma samples*. Osceola, WI: Elias UAS; 1992.

Wallach J. *Interpretation of diagnostic tests*, 7th ed. Philadelphia: Lippincott Williams & Wilkins, 2000.

19 Urinary Diseases

Urinary System

The kidney maintains the fluid and electrolyte composition of the body within a narrow range of normal despite wide fluctuations in intake and excretion of fluid and solute by a process of filtration, reabsorption, and secretion of electrolytes, solutes, and water, mediated by various hormonal systems. Approximately 20% of the cardiac output is delivered to the filtering unit of the kidney, the glomeruli, of which there are 1.2 million in each kidney. Passage of water through the glomeruli occurs freely, whereas passage of electrolytes and solutes is determined by their size and charge. As water and solute travel along the tubular system of the nephron, varying amounts are reabsorbed and secreted to maintain homeostasis.

Tests of Urinary Function

Urine Specimen Collection and Preparation

Collection of urine (e.g., catheter, bag, midstream, and suprapubic methods) is discussed in the section Urinary Tract Infection.

Use a freshly voided urine specimen, first-morning urine specimen, or postprandial urine specimen. Collect the urine specimen in a clean container. Collection of a "clean-catch" urine specimen is recommended to prevent the possibility of a positive leukocyte test result caused by leukocytes external to the urinary system. Perform testing as soon as possible after collection. *Do not* centrifuge or add preservatives to the urine specimen. Bilirubin in urine is unstable at room temperature and when exposed to light. If testing cannot be performed within 1 hour after collection, refrigerate the specimen at 2–8°C immediately. Bring refrigerated specimens to room temperature before testing. Mix thoroughly before use.

Examination of Urine

See Table 1.

Clarity

Turbidity usually is normal due to crystal formation at room temperature. Uric acid crystals (Fig. 1) form in acidic urine, phosphate crystals in alkaline urine. Cellular material and bacteria can also cause turbidity.

Dipsticks and Test Tapes

IRIS Chemstrips (Roche; Basel, Switzerland) and Multistix (Bayer; Tarrytown, NY)

For the determination of specific gravity, pH, leukocytes, nitrite, protein, glucose, ketones, urobilinogen, bilirubin, and blood in urine.

Storage and Stability

Store IRIStrips at temperatures below 30°C. Do not freeze. Opened IRIStrips are stable until the expiration date when stored in the original capped vial. The vial must be closed immediately after removal of each strip.

Table 1. Visual Appearance of Urine

Color	Cause
Dark yellow	Concentrated urine, bile pigments, riboflavin
Red	Doxorubicin hydrochloride (Adriamycin), methyldopa, beets in anemic individuals, blackberries, deferoxamine mesylate (with elevated serum iron), phenytoin, red food coloring, hemoglobulin, phenazopyridine hydrochloride (acid urine), phenolphthalein (alkaline urine), phenothiazines, porphyrins, chloroquine, rifampin, phenazopyridine hydrochloride (Pyridium), pyrvinium pamoate (Povan), red blood cells, red diaper syndrome (nonpathogenic *Serratia marcescens*), urates
Yellow-brown	Antimalarials (pamaquine, primaquine, quinacrine), sulfasalazine (Azulfidine) (alkaline urine), B-complex vitamins, bilirubin, carotene, cascara, metronidazole, nitrofurantoin, sulfonamides
Brown-black	Hemosiderin, homogentisic acid (alkaptonuria), melanin (especially in alkaline urine), myoglobin, old blood, quinine sulfate
Purple-brown	Porphyrins (old urine)
Orange	Phenazopyridine, rifampin, urates, warfarin sodium
Blue-green	Doxorubicin hydrochloride, amitriptyline hydrochloride, blue diaper syndrome (familial metabolic disease, nephrocalcinosis), biliverdin (seen in chronic obstructive jaundice), indomethacin, methylene blue, *Pseudomonas* urinary tract infection (rare), riboflavin

Procedure

Dip test areas in urine completely but briefly to avoid dissolving out the reagents. If using strips visually, read test results carefully at the times specified, in a good light (such as fluorescent) and with the test area held near the appropriate color chart on the bottle label.

After dipping the strip, check the pH area. If the color on the pad is not uniform, read the reagent area immediately, comparing the darkest color to the appropriate color chart. All reagent areas except leukocyte areas may be read between 1 and 2 minutes after dipping to identify negative specimens and to determine the pH and specific gravity. A positive reaction (a reading of "small" or greater) at <2 minutes on the leukocyte test may be regarded as a positive indication of leukocytes in urine. Color changes that occur after 2 minutes are of no diagnostic value. If the strips are analyzed instrumentally, the instrument will automatically read each reagent area at the specified time.

The following table lists the generally detectable levels of analytes in urine; however, because of the inherent variability of clinical urines, lesser concentrations may be detected under certain conditions.

Reagent Area	**Sensitivity**
Glucose	75–125 mg/dL glucose
Bilirubin	0.4–0.8 mg/dL bilirubin
Ketone	5–10 mg/dL acetoacetic acid
Blood	0.015–0.062 mg/dL hemoglobin
Protein	15–30 mg/dL albumin
Nitrite	0.06–0.1 mg/dL nitrite ion
Leukocytes	5–15 cells/high-power field (hpf) in clinical urine

Urine Parameters

pH

In the presence of cations, protons are released by a complexing agent in the urine test strip and produce a color change. The indicator bromthymol blue changes from blue to blue-green to yellow. Normal pH is 4.5–8.0.

The test strip contains the indicators methyl red and bromthymol blue. These indicators give clearly distinguishable colors over the pH range of 5–9.

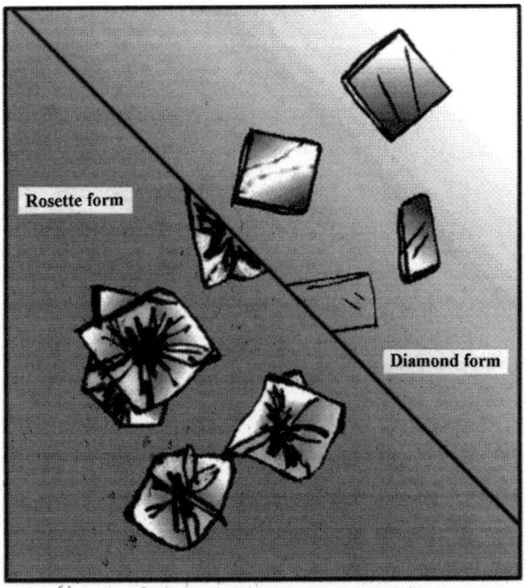

Fig. 1. Uric acid crystals.

Specific Gravity

Normal Values

Normal urine specific gravity is ≥1.001–1.030.

As renal impairment becomes more severe, specific gravity is fixed at approximately 1.010.

Specific Gravity Measurement

Hydrometer/urinometer: Requires at least 15 mL of urine at room temperature. Device must be free-floating in the sample.

Refractometer: Requires only one drop of urine. Based on the principle that the refractive index of a solution is related to the content of dissolved solids. Presence of glucose, protein, and iodine-containing contrast material can lead to falsely high readings.

IRIS Chemstrips: Results for randomly collected urine specimens vary from 1.001 to 1.035. Because of the chemical principle of the test, results may be slightly different than results obtained with other specific gravity measurement methods when elevated amounts of certain urine constituents are present. Glucose and urea concentrations >1% may cause a low specific gravity reading relative to that obtained with other methods. In the presence of moderate amounts of protein (100–500 mg/dL) or ketoacidosis, readings may be elevated.

Leukocytes

Leukocytes in urine are detected in test strips by the action of esterase, present in granulocytic leukocytes, which catalyzes the hydrolysis of an indoxyl carbonic acid ester to indoxyl. The indoxyl formed reacts with a diazonium salt to produce a purple color.

Test Limitations

This test is not affected by erythrocytes in concentrations up to 10,000/μL or by bacteria common in urine. Do not collect specimens in containers that have been cleaned with strong oxidizing agents. Do not use preservatives. The drugs cephalexin and gentamicin sulfate have been found to interfere with this test. High levels of albumin (>500 mg/dL) in the urine may interfere with the test results.

Table 2. Twenty-Four-Hour Protein Excretion in Children of Different Ages

Age	Protein Concentration (mg/L)	Protein Excretion (mg/24 hr) Mean (Range)	Protein Excretion (mg/24 hr/m² BSA) Mean (Range)
Premature (5–30 d)	88–845	29 (14–60)	182 (88–371)
Full term	94–455	32 (15–68)	145 (68–309)
2–12 mo	70–315	38 (17–85)	109 (48–244)
2–4 yr	45–217	49 (20–121)	91 (37–223)
4–10 yr	50–223	71 (26–194)	85 (31–234)
10–16 yr	45–391	83 (29–238)	63 (22–181)

BSA, body surface area.

Expected Values

Normal urine should produce no color reaction. A trace reaction indicates a possible borderline situation, and the test should be repeated on a fresh urine sample from the same patient. Positive and repeated trace findings indicate the need for further testing of the patient or urine sample in accordance with the medically accepted procedures for pyuria.

Nitrite

The nitrite test is useful for detection of urinary tract infection (UTI). A red-violet color on the test strip indicates infection.

The nitrite test used in the test strip is a refinement of previous methods and exhibits increased sensitivity. Nitrite, if present, reacts with an aromatic amine to give a diazonium salt, which by coupling with a further compound in the strip, yields a red-violet azo dye.

Protein

See Table 2.

The presence of an abnormal quantity of protein in the urine is a reliable marker of renal parenchymal disease. Healthy individuals excrete <100–150 mg (60 mg/m^2 of body surface area) of protein per day. The newborn may transiently have proteinuria of up to 1 g/day.

Tamm-Horsfall glycoprotein is the main protein constituent of normal urine. Changes in Tamm-Horsfall glycoprotein excretion unfortunately do not correlate with renal pathology. In the future, it may become possible to measure various urinary proteins and renal cell proteins using monoclonal antibodies to specific renal antigens.

Tests for Protein in Urine

Significant proteinuria, as determined by the first three tests, should be confirmed by testing a 24-hour collection specimen.

1. Dipstick test: Detects only albumin. Significant if ≥1+ (30 mg/dL) on two of three random samples taken 1 week apart when the urine specific gravity is <1.015 or if ≥2+ (100 mg/dL) on similarly collected urine when the specific gravity is >1.015. False-positive results can occur with highly concentrated alkaline urine (pH >8), gross hematuria, pyuria, or bacteriuria; in the presence of quaternary ammonium chloride (e.g., antiseptics, chlorhexidine, or benzalkonium); with very dilute or acidic urine (pH 4.5); and in cases of nonalbumin proteinuria, which can be detected by sulfosalicylic acid.
2. Sulfosalicylic acid test: Add 0.5–0.8 mL (5–8 drops) of 20% sulfosalicylic acid to 5 mL of urine (pH 4.5–6.5) and examine for turbidity. Barely evident turbidity is graded as trace; increasing amounts of turbidity are graded as 1–4+. False-positive results occur due to concentrated urine, gross hematuria, intravenous contrast material, periodic acid–Schiff stain, cephalosporins, penicillins, phosphates, sulfonamides, and tolbutamide.
3. Protein/creatinine ratio: Determine concentrations in a randomly collected spot urine sample during normal ambulation. The normal urinary protein/urinary

Table 3. Albuminuria

	Normal	Microalbuminuria[a]	Advanced Nephropathy
Albumin concentration (g/mL)	<0.01	0.02–0.2	>0.2
Albumin/creatinine ratio (μg/mL)			
Volume 1,000 mL/d	<15	30	>30
Volume 1,500 mL/d	<10	20	>20
Albumin excretion rate			
μg/min	<10	20–200	>200
mg/d	<15	30–300[b]	>300[c]

[a]Amounts defined in consensus statement of American Diabetes Association.
[b]Albuminuria of ≥300 mg/d.
[c]Creatinine clearance of <70 mL/min/1.73 m^2 of body surface area.

creatinine ratio is <0.2 in older children and <0.5 during the first few months of life. A urinary protein/urinary creatinine ratio >2.0 is suggestive of the nephrotic range of proteinuria. All aberrant ratios should be confirmed with testing of a 24-hour urine collection for proteinuria.

4. Twenty-four-hour urine collection: Normal, ≤4 mg of protein/m^2/hour; abnormal, 4–40 mg/m^2/hour; nephrotic range, ≥40 mg/m^2/hour.

Tests for Microalbuminuria

Routine urinalysis dipstick testing for protein (albumin) cannot detect microalbuminuria. Laboratory methods such as radioimmunoassay and nephelometry measure very low concentrations of urinary albumin. Normoalbuminuria is defined as a urine albumin excretion rate of <15 μg/minute, and microabluminuria as a raised urine albumin excretion of 15–200 μg/minute. To screen for microalbuminuria, a short timed (e.g., 1-hour) urine collection can be used. False-negative results are extremely rare; the predictive value of a negative test is 96% and its specificity is 81% in insulin-dependent diabetic children. Positive test results (urine albumin excretion >15 μg/minute) need to be confirmed with positive test results on at least two of three 24-hour urine collections. Exercise must be avoided during the collection period.

Microalbuminuria is the earliest sign of diabetic nephropathy (Table 3).

Urine shows many hyaline and granular casts and double refractile fat bodies.

Hematuria is rare. Azotemia develops gradually after several years of proteinuria.

- Biopsy of kidney is diagnostic.

Sugars

Normally, urine does not contain sugars. Glucosuria is suggestive but not diagnostic of diabetes mellitus or proximal renal tubular disease. The presence of other reducing sugars can be confirmed by chromatography.

Dipstick: Detects only glucose. False-positive results occur with high levels of ascorbic acids (used as preservative in antibiotics).

Clinitest tablet: Identifies all reducing substances in urine, including reducing sugars (glucose, fructose, galactose, pentoses, lactose), several amino acids, ascorbic acid, chloral hydrate, chloramphenicol, cysteine, glucuronates, hippurate, homogentisic acid, isoniazid, ketone bodies, nitrofurantoin, oxalate, penicillin, salicylates, streptomycin, sulfonamides, tetracycline, and uric acid. Sucrose is not a reducing sugar, and it is not detected by Clinitest.

Method: Use five drops of urine, 10 drops of water, one tablet. Compare with standard scale (Table 4).

Ketones

Except with trace amounts of ketones, ketonuria suggests ketoacidosis, usually from either diabetes mellitus or catabolism of fat induced by inadequate calorie intake. Neonatal ketoacidosis may occur with a metabolic defect such as propionic aci-

Table 4. Standard Scale for Interpretation of Clinitest Results

Color	% Reducing Substance
Blue	None
Greenish blue	Trace
Green	0.5
Greenish brown	1.0
Yellow	1.5
Brick red	2.0

demia, methylmalonic aciduria, or a glycogen storage disease. Decreased or absent ketones in children or infants with malnutrition and acidosis may suggest an inborn error of fat metabolism.

Dipstick: Detects acetoacetic acid best, acetone less well; does not detect β-hydroxybutyrate. False-positive results may occur after phthalein administration or with phenylketonuria.

Acetest tablet (Ames Co.): Detects only acetoacetic acid and acetone.

Hemoglobin, Myoglobin

Centrifuged urine usually contains <five red blood cells (RBCs)/hpf. Significant hematuria is 5–10 RBCs/hpf and corresponds to a Chemstrip reading of 50 RBCs/hpf or a Labstix (Roche Diagnostics, Indianapolis, Indiana) reading of "trace hemolyzed" or "small."

Dipstick testing: Positive result with intact RBCs, hemoglobin, and myoglobin; can detect as few as three to four RBCs/hpf. False-positive result can occur with the presence of bacterial peroxidases, high ascorbic acid concentrations, and povidone iodine (Betadine; e.g., from fingers of medical staff).

Microscopy: Used to differentiate hemoglobinuria or myoglobinuria from hematurias (intact RBCs). Examination of RBC morphology by phase-contrast microscopy may help to localize the source of bleeding. Distorted small RBCs suggest upper tract bleeding origin, whereas normal RBCs suggest lower tract bleeding. Red cell casts or doughnut-shaped RBC with bulbous projections suggests glomerular source. Blood clots or terminal hematuria suggests a lower urinary tract cause.

Differentiation of hemoglobinuria and myoglobinuria

1. History: Hemoglobinuria is seen with intravascular hemolysis or in hematuric urine that has been standing for an extended period. Myoglobinuria is seen after crush injuries, vigorous exercise, or major motor seizures and in fever, malignant hyperthermia, electrocution, snakebites, ischemia, muscle and metabolic disorders, and some infections.
2. Clinical laboratories may use many techniques to measure hemoglobin or myoglobin directly. In nephropathy from myoglobinuria, the blood urea nitrogen (BUN)/creatinine ratio is low (creatinine is released from damaged muscles), and creatine phosphokinase is high.

Microscopic hematuria occurs in 0.5–1.0% of children, macroscopic hematuria in 0.1%. Coexistence of hematuria and proteinuria, or a brown or smoky color to the urine, implies a glomerular source.

Bilirubin and Urobilinogen

Dipstick test: Both are normally present in the urine in only very small amounts.

Correlating the results of both bilirubin and urobilinogen tests can provide very helpful diagnostic information (Table 5).

Sediment

Using light microscopy, unstained, centrifuged urine can be examined for formed elements, including casts, cells, and crystals. Centrifuge 10 mL for 5 minutes, then decant 9 mL of supernatant. Resuspend sediment in remaining 1 mL of urine.

Table 5. Correlation of Bilirubin and Urobilinogen Test Results

	Normal	Hemolytic Disease	Hepatitic Disease	Biliary Obstruction
Urine urobilogen	Normal	Increased	Increased	Decreased
Urine bilirubin	Negative	Negative	Positive or negative	Positive

Place drop on glass slide; use coverslip. Best results are obtained with subdued light. Focus particularly on the edge of the coverslip, because formed elements collect there.

Urinary Findings in Various Diseases

See Table 6.

Renal Function Tests

Tests of Glomerular Function

Creatinine

Creatinine clearance

$$\text{Creatinine clearance (mL/minute)} = \frac{[\text{UCr (mg/mL)} \times \text{V (mL/minute)}]}{\text{PCr (mg/minute)}}$$

where UCr = urine concentration of creatinine, V = urine flow rate, and PCr = plasma concentration of creatinine.

$$\text{Corrected creatinine clearance} = \text{creatinine clearance (mL/minute)} \times \frac{1.73}{m^2}$$

Normal newborn	40–65 mL/minute/1.73 m^2
Child, adult	88–137 mL/minute/1.73 m^2

Timed urine specimen: Standard measure of glomerular filtration rate (GFR).

Method: Have patient empty bladder (discard specimen) before beginning the collection. Collect urine over any time period; record interval to the nearest minute. Draw the blood sample at the beginning and end of the period and use the average.

Estimation of GFR from plasma creatinine level: Useful when a timed specimen cannot be collected; correlates well with standard GFR for children with relatively normal body habitus.

Estimated GFR (mL/minute/1.73 m^2) = kL/PCr

where k = proportionality constant[1]; L = height (cm); PCr = plasma creatinine (mg/dL).

Low birth weight, 1 year	0.33 mL/minute/1.73^2
Appropriate weight for gestation age, first year	0.45 mL/minute/1.73^2
Children and adolescent girls	0.55 mL/minute/1.73^2
Adolescent boys	0.70 mL/minute/1.73^2

Creatinine clearance is normal until >50% of renal parenchyma is inactivated. With renal insufficiency, test results parallel the parenchymal destruction.

Urinary acidification is impaired in chronic renal disease with azotemia. It is decreased without parallel impairment of GFR in renal tubular acidosis (RTA), some cases of Fanconi syndrome, and some cases of acquired nephrocalcinosis.

Proximal tubular malfunction is indicated by urinary excretion of substances normally reabsorbed by tubules, for example, renal glycosuria (blood glucose <180

[1]Schwartz GJ, Brion LP, Spitzer A. The use of plasma creatinine concentration for estimating glomerular filtration rate in infants, children, and adolescents. *Pediatr Clin North Am* 1987; 34:571.

Table 6. Urinary Findings in Various Diseases

Disease	Volume	Specific Gravity	Protein[a]	RBCs[b]	WBCs and Epithelial Cells[b]	Casts[c,d]	Comments
Normal	600–2,500 mL	1.003–1.030	0 (0.05)	0 or occ. (0–0.130)	0–0.65	0 or occ. (2,000/24 hr)	—
Acute febrile condition	↓	↑	Trace to positive			Few	—
Orthostatic proteinuria	N	N	↑ (≤1 g)	N (0–0.130)	0–3	Var; H&G	Normal when recumbent; abnormalities after upright posture
Glomerulonephritis							
Acute	↓	↑	2–4+(0.5–5.0)	1–4+ (1–1,000)	1–400	2–4+; H&G; RBC, epithelial, mixed RBC and epithelial	Gross hematuria or "smoky" urine
Latent			(0.1–2.0)	(1–100)	1–20	RBC, H&G	
Nephrosis (nephrotic stage)	↓	↑	4+ (4–40)	0–few (0.5–50.0)	20–1,000	Epithelial, fatty, waxy; H&G	Fat-laden epithelial cells, anisotropic fat in epithelial cells and casts
Terminal	↑ or ↓	↓; fixed	1–2+ (2–7)	Trace–1+ (0.5–10.0)	1–50	1–3+ broad, waxy, H&G, epithelial	—
Pyelonephritis							
Acute	N	N	0–2+ (0.5–2.0)	Few (0–1)	20–2,000	WBC, H&G, bacteria	Bacteria, many WBCs in clumps
Chronic	N or ↓	N or ↓	2–4+ (0–5)	Few (0–1)	0.5–50.0	Same as acute; often few or none	Same as acute; findings may be intermittent
Renal tuberculosis			(0.1–3.0)	(1–20)	1–50	WBC, H&G	Tubercle bacilli
Disseminated lupus erythematosus	Var	N or ↓	1–4+ (0.5–20.0)	1–4+ (1–100)	1–100	1–4+ RBC, fatty, waxy, H&G	—
Toxemia of pregnancy	↓	↑	3–4+ (0.5–10.0)	0–1+ (0–1)	1–5	3–4+ H&G	—

↑, increased; ↓, decreased; H&G, hyaline and granular casts; occ., occasionally; N, normal; Var, variable.
[a]Protein quantitative values in parentheses are given as grams/24 hr.
[b]Quantitative values in parentheses are given as cells × 10^6/24 hr.
[c]Detection of casts requires examination of fresh or preserved urine and acid pH.
[d]Italics denote most important or diagnostic finding.

mg/dL as in Fanconi syndrome, heavy metal poisoning), aminoaciduria, phosphaturia.

Serum creatinine and BUN levels are not useful in discovering early renal insufficiency because they do not become abnormal until 50% of renal function has been lost.

Serum creatinine increase occurs in 10–20% of patients taking aminoglycosides and up to 20% of patients taking penicillins (especially methicillin).

Cystatin C: A New Marker for Glomerular Filtration Rate

Creatinine is not a good marker for measuring glomerular filtration rate in neonates and infants because its serum concentration is more highly dependent on muscle mass, which is rapidly changing in these age groups, than on the filtration rate. Cystatin C is a 13,600-d cysteine protease synthesized by all cells and handled by the kidney in much the same manner as creatinine. Cystatin C is measured by particle-enhanced nephelometric immunoassay.

Glomerular function is determined by nuclear scans

Normal values of GFR are measured by inulin clearance

Tests of Tubular Function

Proximal Tubule

Proximal tubule reabsorption: the proximal tubule is responsible for the reabsorption of electrolytes, glucose, and amino acids. Studies to determine proximal tubular function compare urine and blood levels of specific compounds to arrive at a percent tubular reabsorption (Tx):

$$Tx = 1 - \frac{Ux/Px}{UCr/PCr} \times 100$$

where Ux = concentration of compound in urine; Px = concentration of compound in plasma; UCr = concentration of creatinine in urine; and PCr = concentration of creatinine in plasma. This formula is also used for amino acids, electrolytes, calcium, and phosphorus.

Glucose reabsorption: The glucose threshold is the plasma glucose concentration at which significant amounts of glucose appear in the urine. The presence of glucosuria must be interpreted in relation to simultaneously determined plasma glucose concentration. If the plasma glucose concentration is <120 mg/dL and glucose is present in the urine, this implies incompetent tubular reabsorption of glucose and proximal renal tubular disease.

Urine calcium: Hypercalciuria is seen with RTA, vitamin D intoxication, hyperparathyroidism, steroid use, immobilization, excessive calcium intake, and loop diuretic use. It may be idiopathic (associated with hematuria and renal calculi).

Twenty-Four-Hour Urine

Calcium excretion of >4 mg/kg/24 hours or positive result on spot urine test: Determine Ca^{2+}/creatinine ratio. It is recommended that an abnormally elevated spot urine Ca^{2+}/creatinine ratio be followed with a 24-hour urine calcium determination.

Bicarbonate reabsorption (proximal RTA): The majority of bicarbonate reabsorption occurs in the proximal tubule. Abnormalities in reabsorption lead to type 2 RTA. These patients have high fractional excretion of bicarbonate in their urine at normal serum bicarbonate levels. They can acidify their urine, however, when faced with metabolic acidosis.

Distal Tubule

Urine acidification (distal RTA): A urine acidification defect should be suspected when random urine pH values are >6 in the presence of moderate systemic metabolic acidosis. Acidification defects should be confirmed by simultaneous measurement of venous or arterial pH, plasma bicarbonate concentration, and the pH of fresh urine (determined by pH meter, not dipstick).

Urine concentration: A urine specific gravity of ≥ 1.023 for a randomly obtained specimen indicates intact concentrating ability. Within limits, clinical overnight fast is adequate to test concentrating ability.

Spot urine: Determine Ca^{2+}/creatinine ratio. It is recommended that an abnormally elevated spot urine Ca^{2+}/creatinine ratio be followed with a 24-hour urine calcium determination.

Age-Related Calcium/Creatinine Ratios

Age	Ca^{2+}/Cr ratio (mg/mg), 95th percentile for age
<7 mo	0.86
7–18 mo	0.60
19 mo to 6 yr	0.42
Adults	0.22

Renal Biopsy

Should be preceded by

- Confirmation that two kidneys are present
- Confirmation that no renal infection is present
- Confirmation that no bleeding disorder is present (complete blood count, prothrombin time, activated partial thromboplastin time, possibly bleeding time)

Examination should include histologic analysis [staining with hematoxylin and eosin, trichrome, periodic acid–Schiff, silver, other stains (e.g., for amyloid) when indicated], immunofluorescence testing (with antisera specific for IgG, IgA, IgM, C1q, C3, C4, fibrinogen, albumin), and electron microscopy (e.g., necessary for diagnosis for Alport syndrome, thin basement membrane nephritis).

Contraindications for Percutaneous Renal Biopsy

Absolute contraindications for percutaneous biopsy occur in a few circumstances: single kidney, small kidney, large renal cyst. In cases of bleeding diathesis or anticoagulant therapy in children, biopsy should be either postponed (by 10 days if the patient is receiving heparin sodium) or performed after temporary correction of the bleeding disorder by appropriate factors, and washed red blood cells should be on hand for transfusion. Open biopsy techniques using cup biopsy forceps are reported to be safe in patients with clotting disorders. Other factors: renal artery aneurysm, renal neoplasm, acute pyelonephritis, uncontrolled hypertension, end-stage renal disease, asymptomatic hematuria without proteinuria.

Indications for Renal Biopsy

Hematuria

Primary acute nephritic syndrome (hematuria, proteinuria, edema, hypertension)
Suspicion of rapidly progressive glomerulonephritis (GN)
Persistence of impaired renal function, hypertension, and low complement (C3) levels beyond a few weeks
Systemic disorders associated with features of acute nephritis or vasculitis
Systemic lupus erythematosus (SLE) with abnormal urinalysis results or impaired function
Suspected Wegener granulomatosis, polyarteritis nodosa with evidence of renal involvement
Severe Henoch-Schönlein purpura
Immunoglobulin nephropathy (Berger disease)
  With impaired renal function
  With nephrotic syndrome
Isolated gross or microscopic hematuria
Suspected familial nephritis (Alport syndrome)
Parental anxiety

Proteinuria

Nephrotic Syndrome

Onset in first year or after 12 years
Resistance to a 6- to 8-week course of steroids
Candidate for cytotoxic drugs for treatment of steroid dependency or frequent relapse of nephrotic syndrome
Unusual clinical and laboratory features such as hypertension, hypocomplementemia, gross hematuria, or persistent abnormal renal function
Asymptomatic (nonorthostatic) persistent proteinuria >1,000 mg/24 hours
Normal renal function, if diagnosis is still uncertain after 6 months

Impaired renal function at presentation, if diagnosis is uncertain or in the presence of microscopic hematuria or hypertension
Acute renal allograft dysfunction
Primary nonfunction for 10–14 days, unexplained deterioration of function, unexplained proteinuria, or before beginning antilymphocyte therapy to confirm diagnosis of rejection

Acute Renal Failure

Unknown cause for renal failure
Rapidly progressive GN
Severe oliguria, anuria lasting >1–2 weeks
Suspected acute interstitial nephritis
Presence of extrarenal manifestations of a diffuse renal disease

Chronic Renal Failure

The kidney is only moderately decreased in size and the diagnosis is uncertain

Urinary Disorders

Acidosis, Renal Tubular

See Tables 7–9.

RTA is characterized by a normal anion gap and hyperchloremic metabolic acidosis. It may be due to an increased fractional excretion of bicarbonate [type 2 (proximal) RTA] or may be associated with hyperkalemia (type 4 RTA).

Other tests such as the ammonium chloride loading test or furosemide test may be useful in assessing a urinary acidification defect.

Diagnostic Studies

Studies	Interpretation
Fresh, spot urine pH	Type 1 RTA, urine pH consistently >5.5. Type 2 RTA, urine pH <5.5.
Serum electrolytes	Metabolic acidosis with serum total CO_2 <17.5 mEq/L.
24-hr urine collection for calcium, citrate, potassium, and oxalate	Hypercalciuria, hypocitraturia, and potassium wasting are associated with type 1 RTA. Rule out hyperoxaluria.
Ultrasonography of the kidneys	Nephrocalcinosis in undiagnosed, untreated, or inadequately treated RTA.
Urine minus blood Pco_2	Normal value, >20 mm Hg; Distal, type 1 RTA, <20 mm Hg.
Tubular reabsorption of bicarbonate (TRB)	Bicarbonate wasting or TRB >15% in type 2 RTA and <5% in type 1 RTA at normalized serum total CO_2.
Tubular reabsorption of phosphate (TRP)	TRP <60% filtered load of phosphate in Fanconi syndrome and other proximal tubular defects in reabsorption and other proximal tubular defects in reabsorption of phosphate. If Fanconi syndrome is suspected, 24-hr urine collection is needed to confirm the aminoaciduria and potassium wasting.
Renal acidification studies	If metabolic acidosis is clearly present, with total CO_2 <17.5 mEq/L (17.5 mmol/L), there is no need for further acidification. If the metabolic acidosis is unclear, renal ability to acidify can be tested maximally after ammonium chloride or arginine hydrochloride acid loading. The net 1.73 m^2 confirms a distal tubular acidification defect.

Type 1 (Distal 1)

(Collecting ducts do not secrete sufficient H^+ to form ammonium or secreted H^+ backleaks out of collecting tubule lumen.)

Table 7. Laboratory Findings in Renal Tubular Acidosis

Findings	RTA Type 1	RTA Type 2	RTA Type 4
Non–anion gap acidosis	Yes	Yes	Yes
Minimum urine pH	>5.5	<5.5	<5.5
Percentage filtered urine HCO_3 excreted	<10%	>15%	<10%
Serum potassium level	Low	Low	High
Fanconi syndrome of malabsorption	No	Yes	No
Stone or nephrocalcinosis	Yes	No	No
Daily acid excretion	Low	Normal	Low
Ammonium excretion	High for pH	Normal	Low for pH
Daily HCO_3 replacement needs	<4 mmol/kg	>4 mmol/kg	<4 mmol/kg

RTA, renal tubular acidosis.

Table 8. Urinary Findings in Renal Tubular Acidosis

Test	Proximal	Distal	Hyperkalemic
During acidosis			
Urine net charge	Negative	Positive	Positive
Urine pH	<5.5	>5.5	<5.5
Alkali loading			
$FeHCO_3$	>10–15%	<5%	>5–10%
Urine P_{CO_2} (mm Hg)	>70	<55	≥70
Associated defects of tubular infection	Present	Absent	Absent
Hypercalciuria, nephrocalcinosis	Absent	Present	Absent

$FeHCO_3$, fractional excretion of bicarbonate = [(urine HCO_3/plasma HCO_3)(urine creatinine/plasma creatinine)] × 100; P_{CO_2}, partial pressure of CO_2.

Clinical and Laboratory Findings

- Hyperchloremic acidosis, low plasma bicarbonate concentration; should be suspected in any patient with metabolic acidosis with normal anion gap and inappropriately high urine pH (>5.3 in adults, >5.6 in children). Incomplete type 1 RTA should be suspected with normal plasma bicarbonate concentration, urine pH persistently >5.3, and calcium stone disease or positive family history.
- Alkaline urine (pH 6.5–7.0) that persists at any level of plasma bicarbonate.
- Ammonium loading test (ammonium chloride, 0.1 g/kg) shows inability to acidify urine below pH 6.5 and depressed rates of excretion of titratable acid and ammonium.

Often presents with complications (e.g., nephrocalcinosis, interstitial nephritis, renal calculi, rickets, osteomalacia, as well as growth retardation).

Secondary distal RTA type 1 can be due to a number of disorders.

Clinical Spectrum of Secondary Type 1, Distal RTA[2]

- Tubular interstitial renal disorders
    - Obstructive uropathy
    - Medullary sponge kidney
    - Renal transplantation
    - Nephrocalcinosis induced by metabolic and endocrine disorders
        - Vitamin D intoxication

[2]Hanna JC, Santos F, Chan JCM. Renal tubular acidosis. In: *Clinical pediatric nephrology.* New York: McGraw-Hill, 1992:665–698.

Table 9. Biochemical and Clinical Characteristics of Various Types of Renal Tubular Acidosis

	Distal Type 1	Type 1 with HCO_3^- Wasting	Proximal Type 2	Hyperkalemic Type 4
At subnormal (HCO_3^-)[a]				
Minimal urine pH	>5.5	>5.5	<5.5	<5.5
TA and NH_4^+ excretion	↓	↓	N or ↓	↓
Urinary citrate excretion	↓	↓	↑	?
Plasma K^+ concentration	N or ↓	N or ↓	Usually ↓	↑
Renal K^+ clearance	>20%	>20%	>20%	<20%
Urine anion gap[b]	Positive	Positive	Positive or ? negative	Positive
At normal (HCO_3^-)				
TA and NH_4^+ excretion	↓	↓	↓	↓
Fractional HCO_3^- excretion	3–5%	5–10%	>15%	1–15%
Urinary citrate excretion	N	N	↑	?
Plasma K^+ concentration	N	N	N or ↓	N or ↑
U – B PCO_2 (mm Hg)	<20	<20	>20	<20
Therapeutic alkali requirement (mEq/kg/d)	1–3	5–10	5–20	1–5
Osteomalacia	Rare	Rare	Frequent	Absent
Nephrocalcinosis, nephrolithiasis	Common	Common	Rare	Absent

↑, increased; ↓, decreased; N, normal; TA, titratable acid; U – B PCO_2, urine partial pressure of CO_2 (PCO_2) minus blood PCO_2 during bicarbonate loading, when urine pH > blood pH.
[a]Plasma bicarbonate concentration.
[b]Urine anion gap = [Na] + [K^+] + [Cl] (based on urine electrolytes).
From Holliday MA, Barratt TM, Avner ED, eds. *Pediatric nephrology*, 3rd ed. Baltimore: Williams & Wilkins; 1994.

Hyperparathyroidism
Idiopathic hypercalciuria
Wilson disease
Hyperthyroidism

- Genetically transmitted systemic diseases
  - Ehlers-Danlos syndrome
  - Marfan syndrome
  - Osteopetrosis with associated nerve deafness
  - Sickle cell anemia
  - Elliptocytosis
    - Carbonic anhydrase deficiency
    - Hereditary fructose intolerance
    - Fabry disease
- Autoimmune disease
  - Sjögren syndrome
  - Hypergammaglobulinemic disorders
  - SLE
  - Chronic active hepatitis
  - Thyroiditis
- Toxin- or drug-induced disease
  - Amphotericin B
  - Lithium
  - Analgesics
  - Cyclamate
  - Toluene

- Hyponatruric states
  - Nephrotic syndrome
  - Hepatic cirrhosis

Type 2 (Proximal)

Clinical and Laboratory Findings

Hypokalemic or normokalemic type
Low plasma bicarbonate. Hyperchloremic acidosis, growth failure
Primary (inability of tubular cell to secrete enough H^+)
Secondary

- Increased serum globulins (especially γ-globulin) (e.g., Sjögren syndrome, Hodgkin disease, sarcoidosis, chronic active hepatitis, cryoglobulinemia)
- Pyelonephritis
- Medullary sponge kidney, medullary cystic disease
- Ureterosigmoidostomy
- Hypercalcemia, hypoparathyroidism, vitamin D, intoxication
- Starvation, malnutrition, rickets, heavy metal intoxication
- Fanconi syndrome, Lowe syndrome, tyrosinemia, Wilson disease, hereditary fructose intolerance, old tetracycline ingestion, cystinosis

Clinical Spectrum of Type 2, Proximal RTA[3]

- Isolated RTA
  - Primary (sporadic or familial)
  - Carbonic anhydrase inhibition
    - Acetazolamide
    - Mafenide acetate (Sulfamylon)
    - Carbonic anhydrase deficiency
    - Osteopetrosis with carbonic anhydrase II deficiency
- Generalized
  - Primary (sporadic or familial)
  - Inborn error of metabolism
    - Cystinosis
    - Lowe syndrome
    - Hereditary fructose intolerance
    - Tyrosinemia
    - Galactosemia
    - Wilson disease
    - Pyruvate carboxylase deficiency
    - Metachromatic leukodystrophy
    - Glycogen storage disease
- Dysproteinemic states
  - Multiple myeloma
  - Light-chain disease
  - Monoclonal gammopathy
  - Amyloidosis
- Vitamin D deficiency, dependence, or resistance
- Interstitial renal disease
  - Sjögren syndrome
  - Medullary cystic disease
  - Renal transplantation rejection (early)
  - Balkan nephropathy
  - Chronic renal vein thrombosis
- Toxins
  - Outdated tetracyclines
  - Lead
  - Mercury
  - Gentamicin

[3]Hanna JD, Santos F, Chan ICM. Renal tubular acidosis. In: *Clinical pediatric nephrology.* New York: McGraw-Hill, 1992:665–698.

Cadmium
Maleic acid
Warfarin sodium (Coumarin)
Streptozocin

- Miscellaneous
  Nephrotic syndrome
  Paroxysmal nocturnal hemoglobinuria
  Malignancy
  Congenital heart disease

Type 3 (Mild Form of Type 1, Distal)

Hyperkalemic type (due to impaired sodium reabsorption in cortical collecting tubules)

- Hypoaldosteronism
- Obstructive nephropathy
- SLE
- Sickle cell nephropathy
- Cyclosporine toxicity

Type 4 (Aldosteronism)

Consists of a variety of conditions characterized by

- Mild to moderate renal impairment
- Hyperchloremic acidosis
- Hyperkalemia
- Acid urine pH
- Reduced ammonium secretion
- Frequently, tendency to lose sodium in urine
- Decreased mineralocorticoid secretion in some patients due to isolated hypoaldosteronism; decreased tubular response to aldosterone in others

Follow-Up Studies for Renal Tubular Acidosis

Studies	Interpretation
Serum total CO_2	Adequate base therapy to maintain serum total CO_2 >22 mEq/L (22 mmol/L)
Spot urine calcium/creatinine ratio	Adequate base therapy to maintain urine calcium/creatinine ratio at <0.20 mg/mg
Ultrasonography of the kidneys	Monitoring of nephrocalcinosis

Alport Syndrome

Alport syndrome, or hereditary nephritis, is associated with high-frequency nerve deafness and ocular abnormalities and usually has an X-linked mode of inheritance. Diagnosis is based on multilaminar splitting of the glomerular capillary basement membrane and absence of the Goodpasture antigen on the basement membrane.

Antineutrophil Cytoplasmic Antibody–Associated Renal Disease

Antineutrophil cytoplasmic antibody (ANCA), described in 1982 in patients with pauci-immune necrotizing GN and systemic vasculitis, is specific for constituents of neutrophil azurophilic granule and monocyte lysosomes. The antibodies are useful in the classification of rapidly progressive GN and small-vessel vasculitis and can be used to monitor response to therapy. Two patterns have been identified: c-ANCA, which produces cytoplasmic staining of neutrophils and is specific for proteinase e, and p-ANCA, which artifactually redistributes around the cell nucleus when fixed in alcohol and is specific for myeloperoxidase. c-ANCA is a sensitive marker for Wegener granulomatosis. Patients with disease limited to the kidneys have a higher frequency of p-ANCA, whereas those with pulmonary and sinus involve-

Table 10. Clinical and Laboratory Features of Neonatal Bartter Syndrome, "Classic" Bartter Syndrome, and Gitelman Syndrome

	Neonatal Bartter Syndrome	"Classic" Bartter Syndrome	Gitelman Syndrome
Polyhydramnios, prematurity	+++	++	ϕ
Presentation in adolescence	ϕ	ϕ	+++
Impaired urinary concentration	+++	+++	+
Polyuria, polydipsia	+++	+++	+
Hyperrenin, hyperaldosteronism	+++	+++	++
Elevated prostaglandins levels	+++	+++	ϕ
Hypokalemia	+++	+++	+++
Metabolic alkalosis	+++	+++	++
Hypercalciuria	+++	++	ϕ
Hypocalciuria	ϕ	ϕ	+++
Nephrocalcinosis	+++	ϕ	ϕ
Hypomagnesemia	+	+	+++
Growth retardation	+++	+++	+

+++, severe or almost always present; ++, moderate or frequently present; +, mild or occasionally present; ϕ, absent.

ment have a higher incidence of c-ANCA. ANCA may also be found in patients with other diseases such as ulcerative colitis.

Bartter Syndrome

See Table 10.

Children with Bartter syndrome present with hypokalemia, normal blood pressure, and elevated plasma concentrations of renin and aldosterone. Urine potassium level is elevated.

Berger Disease (Immunoglobulin A Nephropathy)

(A focal proliferative GN; immunologic mediation; probably the most common form of GN.)

Persistent or intermittent microscopic hematuria with episodes of painless gross hematuria and minimal proteinuria, often associated with (rather than following by 4–10 days) infection of any type.

Plasma IgA increased in ≤50% of patients.

Progression to renal failure in 5–25 years in 20–40% of cases.

Diagnosis is based on examination of renal biopsy specimen, with immunofluorescence showing predominant mesangial IgA, IgG, and C3.

May be associated with celiac disease, dermatitis herpetiformis, some liver diseases.

May be related to Henoch-Schönlein purpura.

Calculi, Urinary Tract

Investigate for recurrent calculi.

Urine pH, microscopy, and culture. Identify crystals if present. Measure levels of serum electrolytes, calcium, phosphate, uric acid, oxalate, protein, amino acids, cystine (Fig. 2), creatinine; analyze calculus if available.

Causes

Hypercalciuria is most common noninfectious cause (especially idiopathic but also due to distal RTA and therapy with furosemide, prednisone, or adrenocorticotropic hormone).

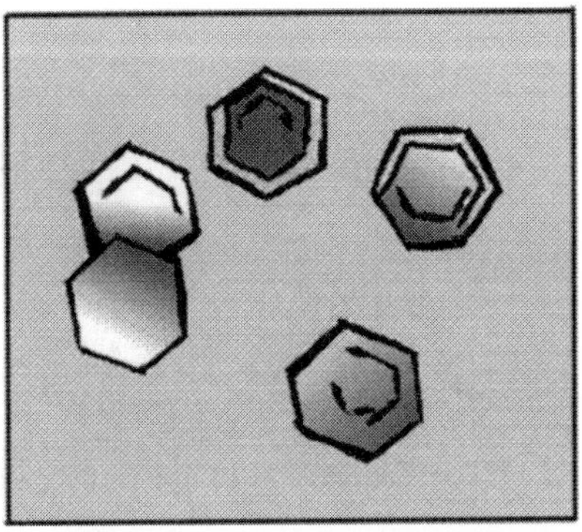

Fig. 2. Hexagonal cystine crystals.

May be familial; may accompany hyperparathyroidism, metastatic bone disease, Cushing syndrome, sarcoidosis.
Oxaluria accounts for 3–13% of stones.
Uric acid stones comprise 4% of stones.
Cystinuria is found in 5–7% of children with stones.
Hypocitraturia is found in 10% of children with stones.
Xanthine is found in 1–3% of children with stones.
Crystalluria can aid diagnosis when cystine crystals (occur only in homozygous or heterozygous cystinuria) or struvite crystals (magnesium, calcium, ammonium, phosphate) are found. Presence of calcium oxalate (Fig. 3), phosphate (Fig. 4), and

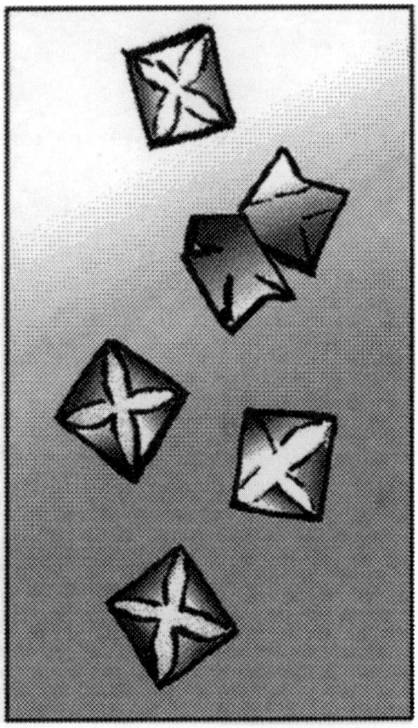

Fig. 3. Calcium oxalate crystals—maltese crosses.

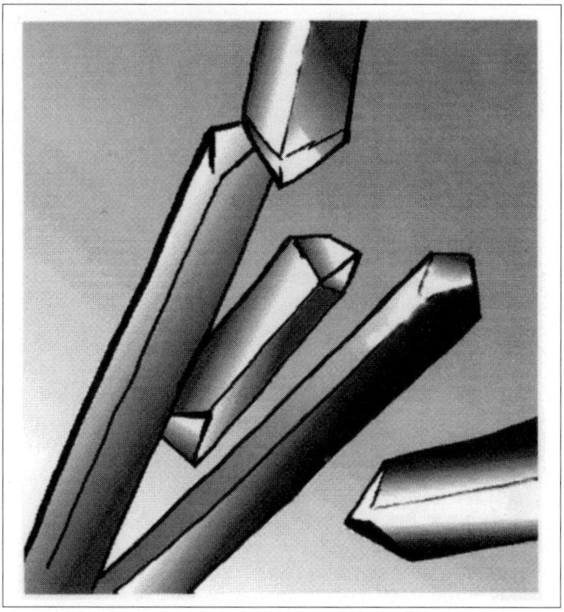

Fig. 4. Triple phosphate crystals.

uric acid should arouse suspicion about possible cause of stones, but they may occur in normal urines.

Glomerulonephritis

See Tables 11 and 12.

Causes

Poststreptococcal GN	1–2% of cases progress to chronic GN
Rapidly progressive GN	90% of cases progress to chronic GN
Membranous GN	50% of cases progress to chronic GN
Focal glomerulosclerosis	50–80% of cases progress to chronic GN
Membranoproliferative GN	50% of cases progress to chronic GN
IgA nephropathy	30–50% of cases progress to chronic GN

Laboratory Findings

The presence of red cell casts with or without proteinuria is usual. Measurement of the third component of the complement system, C3, used in conjunction with measurements of C4 and total hemolytic complement (C5H50), helps distinguish the type of GN. Activation of the classical pathway results in low concentrations of C3 and C4, whereas activation of the alternate pathway leads only to low C3 values. Deficiencies of other complement components result in normal C3 and C4 levels, but a low C5H50 level. The GNs commonly associated with low C3 concentrations include SLE, membranoproliferative GN, GN caused by chronic infections such as bacterial endocarditis or infected ventriculoperitoneal shunts, postinfectious nephritis, and inherited abnormalities of the complement system. Diseases usually associated with normal C3 concentrations include Henoch-Schönlein purpura, Berger disease [immunoglobulin (Ig) A nephropathy], epidemic hemolytic-uremic syndrome, Goodpasture syndrome, and hereditary nephritis.

Table 11. Differentiation of Types of Glomerulonephritis

Clinical Manifestations	Poststreptococcal Glomerulonephritis	IgA Nephropathy	Membranoproliferative Glomerulonephritis	Idiopathic Rapidly Progressive Glomerulonephritis (RPGN)
Age and sex	All ages, mean 7 yr, 2:1 male	15–35 yr, 2:1 male	15–30 yr, 6:1 male	Mean 58 yr, 2:1 male
Acute nephritic syndrome	90%	50%	90%	90%
Asymptomatic hematuria	Occasionally	50%	Rare	Rare
Nephrotic syndrome	10–20%	Rare	Rare	10–20%
Hypertension	70%	30–50%	Rare	25%
Acute renal failure	50% (transient)	Very rare	50%	60%
Other	Latent period of 1–3 wk	Follows viral syndromes	Pulmonary hemorrhage; iron deficiency anemia	None
Laboratory findings	↑ ASO titers (70%) Positive streptozyme (95%) ↑ C3–C9, normal C1, C4	↑ Serum IgA (50%) IgA in dermal capillaries	Positive anti-GBM antibody	Positive ANCA
Immunogenetics	HLA-B12, D "EN"	HLA-Bw 35, DR4	HLA-DR2	None established
Renal pathology				
Light microscopy	Diffuse proliferation	Focal proliferation	Focal → diffuse proliferation with crescents	Crescentic GN
Immunofluorescence	Granular IgG, C3	Diffuse mesangial IgA	Linear IgG, C3	No immune deposits
Electron microscopy	Subepithelial humps	Mesangial deposits	No deposits	No deposits
Prognosis	95% resolve spontaneously; 5% RPGN or slowly progressive	Slow progression in 25–50%	75% stabilize or improve if treated early	75% stabilize or improve if treated early
Treatment	Supportive	None established	Plasma exchange, steroids, cyclophosphamide	Steroid pulse therapy

↑, increased; ANCA, antineutrophil cytoplasm antibody; ASO, antistreptolysin-O; GBM, glomerular basement membrane; GN, glomerulonephritis; IgA, immunoglobulin A; IgG, immunoglobulin G.

[a]Relative risk.

Modified from Couser WG. Glomerular disorders. In: Wyngaarden JB, Smith LH, Bennett JC, eds. *Cecil textbook of medicine*, 19th ed. Vol 1. Philadelphia: WB Saunders, 1992.

Table 12. Glomerular Diseases

		Hematuria (% of Cases)		Proteinuria (% of Cases)			
Glomerular Disorder	May Be Found in	Micro Present	RBC Casts Present	1–3 g Present	>3 g Present	Renal Function Decreased	Comments
IgA nephropathy (Berger disease)	Focal proliferative GN	100	50	75	25	25% or NS; N in 75%	—
IgM mesangial nephropathy	—	50	Rare	50	50	>75% or NS	—
Acute GN secondary to infection (focal GN)	SBE, bacterial pneumonia, viral infections, infection of implanted devices	100	50	75	25	100%	—
Crescentic (rapidly progressive) GN, anti-GBM	Goodpasture syndrome in two-thirds of patients	100	50	50	50	100%	90% have HLA-DR2 antigen + anti-GBM
Immune complex	SLE, mixed cryoglobulinemia, Henoch-Schönlein purpura	100	50	50	50	100%	—
Nonimmune complex	Wegener granulomatosis, polyarteritis	—	—	—	—	—	$ANCA^+$
GN and vasculitis	Wegener granulomatosis, Henoch-Schönlein purpura, mixed cryoglobulinemia; Goodpasture syndrome may occur	100	50	50	100%	—	$ANCA^+$
SLE							
Mesangial	—	15	—	10	—	N	Most frequent type in SLE + ANA
Focal proliferative	—	50	—	25	—	N or ↓	—
Membranous	—	50	—	—	85	N or ↓	—
Diffuse proliferative (<25% of SLE patients)	—	75	—	—	75	Usually ↓; uremia develops in 50–75%	—

Minimal-change disease	Lipid nephrosis, nil disease	20	—	—	100	N	85% respond to steroid therapy Most common cause of NS in children
Focal sclerosis		75	—	25	75	Usually ↓	Frequent cause of NS
Membranous nephropathy	Usually idiopathic; occasionally due to heavy metal toxicity (e.g., gold, mercury), persistent hepatitis B infection, other viruses (e.g., measles, varicella, coxsackievirus), other infections (e.g., malaria, syphilis, leprosy, schistosomiasis), neoplasias (e.g., colon carcinoma, lymphoma, leukemia), sarcoidosis, SLE, others	50	—	25	75	N early; ↓ late	Frequent cause of NS Strong association with HLA-DR3 Spontaneous remission in 25–50% Persistent proteinuria without progression in 25% Progressive glomerular sclerosis causing renal failure in 50%
Membranoproliferative GN							Common in adults; uncommon in children
Type 1 (idiopathic)	SBE, essential cryoglobulinemia, Henoch-Schönlein purpura, SLE, sickle cell disease, hepatitis and cirrhosis, C2 deficiency, α_1-antitrypsin deficiency, infected shunts (*Staphylococcus*, *Corynebacterium*)	75	25	50	50	Usually ↓; NS at onset in 75%	Renal failure within 5 yr common in adults but may be delayed 0–20 yr Persistent, marked proteinuria is poor prognostic sign Renal vein thrombosis may occur
Type 2 (idiopathic)	Infection with streptococci, pneumococci, *Candida*; lipodystrophy	—	—	—	—	—	—

↓, decreased; ANCA, antineutrophil cytoplasmic antibody; ANA, antinuclear antibody; GBM, glomerular basement membrane; GN, glomerulonephritis; Ig, immunoglobulin; N, normal; NS nephrotic syndrome; RBC, red blood cell; SBE, subacute endocarditis; SLE, systemic lupus erythematosus.

Goodpasture syndrome occurs in <5% of cases of GN.

From Border WA, Glassock RJ. Progress in treating glomerulonephritis. *Drug Therapy* April 1981:97; Miller TR, Anderson RJ, Linas SL, et al. Urinary diagnostic indices in acute renal failure: a prospective study. *Ann Intern Med* 1978;89:47; and Oken DE. On the differential diagnosis of acute renal failure. *Am J Med* 1981;71:916.

Normal Serum Complement Values

C3	Age 0–5 d	0.39–1.56 g/L (39–156 mg/dL)
	Age >5 d	0.77–1.43 g/L (77–143 mg/dL)
C4	Age 0–5 d	0.05–0.33 g/L (5–33 mg/dL)
	Age >5 d	0.07–0.40 g/L (7–40 mg/dL)
C5H50		1:24 (serial dilution bioassay)

Serum Complement Values in Acute Nephritis

Disorder	Approximate Percentage of Cases
Depressed serum C3 or hemolytic complement levels	
Systemic disease	
SLE (focal)	75
SLE (diffuse)	90
Subacute bacterial endocarditis	90
"Shunt" nephritis	90
Cryoglobulinemia	85
Renal disease	
Acute poststreptococcal GN	90
Membranoproliferative GN	
Type 1	50–80
Type 2	80–90
Normal serum complement level	
Systemic disease	
Polyarteritis nodosa	
Wegener granulomatosis	
Hypersensitivity vasculitis	
Henoch-Schönlein purpura	
Goodpasture syndrome	
Visceral abscess	
Renal disease	
IgG-IgA nephropathy	
Idiopathic rapidly progressive GN	
Antiglomerular basement membrane disease	
Immune complex disease	
Negative immunofluorescence findings	

Glomerulonephritis, Focal Proliferative

Attacks of hematuria usually occurs at height of upper respiratory tract infection (bacterial or viral).

Prognosis is usually good, especially in children. Progressive nephritis causing renal failure is more common in adults.

Serum IgA level is often increased.

Azotemia is usually absent.

Proteinuria is slight or absent.

Glomerulonephritis, Membranoproliferative

Clinical course may be active, or periods of remission may occur; 50% of patients have chronic renal insufficiency in 10 years.

Marked proteinuria and nephrotic type of syndrome is found in 70% of patients.

Normal serum C4 level but prolonged or permanent depression of C3 is found in 60–80% of patients; clinical course is not related to serum complement levels.

Renal biopsy and immunofluorescent antibody findings are typical.

GFR is <80 mL/minute/1.73 m^2 in two-thirds of patients.

Glomerulonephritis, Poststreptococcal, Acute

Evidence of infection with group A β-hemolytic *Streptococcus* by

- Culture of throat swab specimen.

- Serologic findings indicative of recent streptococcal infection.
  - ASOT of >250 Todd units (increased in 80% of patients). Rise begins 10–14 days after infection, peaks in 4–6 weeks, declines in next 4–6 months. Usually develops 7–21 days after a β-hemolytic streptococcal infection. Titer results unreliable after streptococcal pyoderma. Increased in 20% of cases of membranoproliferative GN. Early use of penicillin prevents rise of ASOT in either condition.
  - Antihyaluronidase
  - Anti–desoxyribonuclease-β
  - Antistreptokinase
  - Anti–diphosphopyridine nucleotidase
  - Anti–nicotinamide adenine dinucleotidase, and so on
- Combined use of serologic tests establish recent streptococcal infection.

Urine
- Hematuria—gross or only microscopic. Microscopic hematuria may occur during the initial febrile upper respiratory tract infection and then reappear with nephritis in 1–2 weeks. It lasts 2–12 months; usual duration is 2 months.
- RBC casts are glomerular origin of hematuria.
- White blood cell (WBC) casts and WBCs are inflammatory.
- Granular and epithelial cell casts are present.
- Fatty casts and lipid droplets occur several weeks later, not related to hyperlipemia.
- Proteinuria is usually <2 g/day. May disappear although RBC casts and RBCs still occur.
- Decreased urinary aldosterone occurs in the presence of edema.
- Oliguria is frequent.

Blood
- Azotemia is found in approximately 50% of patients.
- Erythrocyte sedimentation rate is increased.
- Leukocytosis with increased polymorphonuclear cells.
- Mild anemia is seen, especially when edema is present (may be due to hemodilution, bone marrow depression, or increased destruction of RBCs).
- Serum protein levels are normal, or nonspecific decrease of albumin and increase of α_2- and sometimes of β- and γ-globulins are noted.
- Serum cholesterol level may be increased.
- Serum C3 and total hemolytic complement levels fall 24 hours before onset of hematuria and return to normal within approximately 8 weeks when hematuria subsides. If C3 is low for >8 weeks, consider lupus nephritis or membranoproliferative GN.
- Antihuman kidney antibodies are present in serum in 50% of patients.

Renal biopsy shows characteristic findings with electron microscopy and immunofluorescence.

Chronic renal insufficiency reported in <2% of patients.

Azotemia with high urine specific gravity and normal phenolsulfonphthalein excretion usually means chronic GN.

Glomerulonephritis, Rapidly Progressive

Type I idiopathic (5–20%): mediated by antibodies against the glomerular basement membrane (linear deposits of Ig).

Type II idiopathic (30–40%): immune complex mediated (granular deposits of Ig), tends to occur in older patients.

Type III: few or no immune deposits (“pauci-immune”).

ANCA induced.

Glomerulonephritis, Rapidly Progressive (Nonstreptococcal)

Preceded by systemic disease in many patients
- Poststreptococcal GN
- Infective endocarditis
- Sepsis
- Hepatitis B, C

- Drugs to treat human immunodeficiency virus infection, for example, penicillamine

Preceded by multisystem diseases

- SLE
- Goodpasture syndrome
- Necrotizing vasculitis
- Polyarteritis nodosa
- Wegener granulomatosis
- Henoch-Schönlein purpura
- Cryoglobulinemia

No cultural or serologic (e.g., ASOT) evidence of recent streptococcal infection.

Oliguria is present with urine volume often <400 mL/day.

Hematuria is often gross.

RBCs, WBCs, and casts are present in urine.

Proteinuria is usually >3 g/day.

Renal function declines rapidly. Azotemia is usually marked with BUN >80 mg/dL and serum creatinine >10 mg/dL (in poststreptococcal type, BUN is usually 30–100 mg/dL and serum creatinine 1.5–4.0 mg/dL).

Serum complement levels are normal.

Renal biopsy and immunofluorescent antibody findings; extracapillary proliferation. Progress is poor.

Goodpasture Syndrome

Goodpasture syndrome presents with pulmonary hemorrhage and renal disease. The diagnosis is confirmed by detection of a circulating anti–glomerular basement membrane antibody or by renal biopsy findings. Complement disorders may be associated with recurrent infections and various forms of renal disease.

Hematuria

Causes of Hematuria in Children

Anatomic abnormalities
Congenital abnormalities
Trauma
Polycystic kidneys
Vascular abnormalities
Tumors
Stones
Hematologic disorders
- Coagulopathies
- Thrombocytopenia
- Sickle cell disease
- Renal vein thrombosis

Birth asphyxia with tubular necrosis
Infection
- Bacterial infection
- Tuberculosis
- Viral infection

Cystitis
Glomerular diseases
- Recurrent gross hematuria syndrome
- IgA nephropathy
- Idiopathic (benign familial) hematuria
- Alport syndrome
- Acute poststreptococcal GN
- Membranous glomerulopathy
- Nephritis of chronic infection
- Rapidly progressive GN
- Goodpasture syndrome
- Anaphylactoid purpura

Table 13. Evaluation of the Child with Hematuria

Initial studies (studies performed on all patients)
Complete blood cell count
Urine culture
Serum creatinine level
24-hr urine collection for
Creatinine
Protein
Calcium
Serum C3 level
Ultrasonography or intravenous pyelography
Studies performed on selected patients
Deoxyribonuclease B titer or streptozyme test if hematuria is of <6 mo duration
Skin or throat specimen cultures when appropriate
Antinuclear antibody titer
Urine erythrocyte morphology
Coagulation studies, platelet count when suggested by history
Sickle cell screen
Voiding cystourethrography when infection is present or a lower tract lesion is suspected
Doppler ultrasonography or radionuclide studies for suspected renal vein thrombosis
Renal biopsy: indicated for
Persistent high-grade microscopic hematuria
Microscopic hematuria plus any of the following
Diminished renal function
Proteinuria exceeding 150 mg/24 hr (0.15 g/24 hr)
Hypertension
Second episode of gross hematuria
Cystoscopy: indicated for
Pink to red hematuria
Dysuria
Sterile urine culture

Modified from Behrman RE, Kliegman RM, Jenson HB, eds. *Nelson textbook of pediatrics*, 16th ed. Philadelphia: WB Saunders, 2000.

Hemolytic-uremic syndrome
Henoch-Schönlein purpura
Drugs
Excessive exercise

Diagnostic Studies

See Table 13.
Suggested evaluation of persistent hematuria

1. Examination of urine sediment, urine dipstick testing for protein, urine culture, sickle cell screen, urine calcium/creatinine ratio, family history, medication history, and audiology screen (if appropriate).
2. Measurement of serum electrolytes, BUN, serum creatinine, serum total protein and albumin; complete blood count with smear; and serologic tests for hepatitis, human immunodeficiency virus.
3. Antistreptolysin-O titers (ASOTs), C3 and C4 levels, antinuclear antibody test.
4. Renal ultrasonography and other indicated imaging studies.
5. Referral to a pediatric nephrologist.

Hypercalciuria, Familial

Increased excretion of urinary calcium of >350 mg/24 hours on diet containing 600–800 mg/day.

- >4 mg/kg/24 hours.
- >140 mg/g of urinary creatinine is most useful criterion in short or obese patients.

Normal blood calcium level.

Serum 1,25-dihydroxyvitamin D_3 levels are usually high.

Four types of hypercalciuria, as shown by findings from 2-hour urine collection after fasting:

- Renal: calcium/creatinine ratio >0.15. Hypercalciuria persists despite absent dietary calcium in intestine after fasting. One-tenth as common as absorptive type. Due to abnormality of renal tubular reabsorption.
- Absorptive: <20 mg calcium or calcium/creatinine ratio <0.15; 24-hour urine level falls to <200 mg/24 hours after ingestion of low-calcium diet (400 mg/day) for 3–4 days. Almost always due to primary increase in intestinal calcium absorption. Probably autosomal dominant is most common type.
- Resorptive (nonabsorptive): >30 mg calcium or calcium/creatinine ratio >0.15. Due to primary hyperparathyroidism.
- Indeterminate: calcium is 20–30 mg/2-hour urine sample.

Calcium/Creatinine Ratios with Random Urine Collection[4]

		Calcium/Creatinine Ratio [μmol/μmol (mg/mg)]	
Age	**n**	**Mean**	**95th Percentile**
<7 mo	103	0.67 (0.24)	2.42 (0.86)
7–18 mo	40	0.56 (0.20)	1.69 (0.60)
19 mo to 3 yr	41	0.30 (0.11)	1.18 (0.42)
Adult	31	0.27 (0.10)	0.61 (0.22)

Hypertension, Renovascular

Renin-Angiotensin System

Renin is a proteolytic enzyme (molecular weight 31,000–40,000 d) predominantly formed and stored in the juxtaglomerular apparatus of the kidney and released into the renal vein and lymph. When released into the circulation, renin acts on its substrate angiotensinogen, an α_2-globulin made mainly in the liver, to form a relatively inactive decapeptide, angiotensin I. Passage through the pulmonary circulation cleaves angiotensin I by a converting enzyme, which yields the octapeptide angiotensin II. A potent vasoconstrictor, angiotensin II also stimulates thirst and secretion of aldosterone, antidiuretic hormone, and catecholamines.

A number of factors control renin release, including renal tubular sodium concentration, renal perfusion pressure, and α-adrenergic vascular tone.

When renal nerves are stimulated, renin release increases. Sympathectomy decreases baseline renin activity and decreases renin secretion in response to sodium depletion. Central nervous system stimulation modulates renin release with renal nerves intact.

Hypertension

Normal blood pressure is defined as systolic and diastolic pressure less than the 90th percentile for age and sex. The causes of hypertension are distinctly different for children and for adults. Most infants and children with hypertension have a secondary cause. Hypertension in the neonatal period is not rare. It may be secondary to a renal artery thrombosis from an improperly placed umbilical artery catheter. Congenital coarctation of the aorta may be diagnosed at birth or shortly thereafter. In a number of hypertensive infants, the cause is unknown; however, they may outgrow the problem by age 1 year (transient neonatal hypertension). Hypertension in the older adolescent is more like that in the adult in that the

[4]Sargent JD, Stukel TA, Kresel J, et al. Normal values for random urinary calcium to creatinine ratios in infancy. *J Pediatr* 1993;123:393–397.

most common cause is essential or primary hypertension. Renal disorders are the most common cause. Abnormal physical signs include abdominal bruit in renal artery stenosis, café-au-lait skin lesions in neurofibromatosis, or a cushingoid appearance in cases of adrenal corticosteroid excess. Plasma electrolyte and acid-base measurements demonstrating a hypokalemic metabolic alkalosis suggest activation of the renin-angiotensin system, which is assessed by measuring renin level in a blood sample from a peripheral vein and sodium level in a 24-hour urine sample. Pheochromocytoma should be excluded in all patients by measuring vanillylmandelic acid and catecholamines in a 24-hour urine sample. If the screen result is positive, computed tomography or magnetic resonance imaging (MRI) of the abdomen should be requested. Metaiodobenzylguanidine scintigraphy can detect elusive or multiple tumors. When renal artery stenosis is suspected, a renal arteriogram should be obtained.

Factors Influencing Renin Release[5]

Increase in Renin Release

- Drugs
  - Vasodilators
  - Diuretics
  - β-Adrenergic stimulators
  - EDTA (via calcium efflux)
- Hormones
  - Glucagon
  - Prostaglandins
  - Norepinephrine and other catecholamines
- Diet
  - Sodium deprivation or loss

Decrease in Renin Release

- Drugs
  - β-Adrenergic blockers
  - Mineralocorticoids
  - α-Adrenergic stimulators
  - Lanthanum
- Hormones
  - Mineralocorticoids
  - Vasopressin
    - Angiotensin
    - Atrial natriuretic factor
- Diet
- Salt load

Causes of Hypertension in Children

See Table 14.

Renal

- Parenchymal causes
  - Chronic pyelonephritis
  - Acute or chronic GN
  - Congenital defects
    - Polycystic kidney disease
    - Segmental hypoplasia
    - Ask-Upmark kidney
  - Hemolytic-uremic syndrome
  - Renal transplant
- Renovascular
  - Intrinsic renal artery disease
    - Fibromuscular lesions: intimal, medial, perimedial
    - Neurofibromatosis
    - Arteritis
  - Extrinsic renal artery disease
    - Paraaortic tumors
    - Paraaortic lymph nodes
    - Paraaortic neurofibromata

Endocrine

- Pheochromocytoma
- Congenital adrenal hyperplasia
- Hyperthyroidism
- Primary aldosteronism

Vascular system

- Coarctation of the aorta
- Takayasu arteritis

Drug related

- Corticosteroid use
- Amphetamine overdose

[5]Ingelfinger JR. *Hypertension*. Philadelphia: WB Saunders, 1982:48.

	Licorice ingestion
	Oral contraceptive use
	Street drug use
Miscellaneous	Essential hypertension
	Wilms tumor
	Neuroblastoma
	Burns
	Increased intracranial pressure
	Hypercalcemia

Nephritis, Hereditary

Familial autosomal-dominant disease associated with nerve deafness and lens defects (Alport syndrome) is rare. Renal disease is progressive.

Hematuria, gross or microscopic, is common; more marked after occurrence of unrelated infection. Other laboratory findings are the same as in other types of nephritis.

Nephritis, Interstitial, Chronic

Due to infections
- Pyelonephritis

Not due to infections
- Analgesic abuse
- Diabetes mellitus
- Use of certain drugs
  - Allergic response (e.g., antibiotics, diuretics, phenytoin, cimetidine, NSAIDs)
  - Toxicity (e.g., cyclosporine, lithium, cisplatin, amphotericin B)

Table 14. Causes of Hypertension by Age Group

	Cause	
Age	Most common	Less Common
Neonates, infants	Renal artery thrombosis after umbilical artery catheterization Coarctation of the aorta Renal artery stenosis	Bronchopulmonary dysplasia Medications Patent ductus arteriosus
1–10 yr	Renal parenchymal disease Coarctation of aorta	Renal artery stenosis Hypercalcemia Neurofibromatosis Neurogenic tumors Pheochromocytoma Mineralocorticoid increase Hyperthyroidism Transient hypertension Hypertension induced by immobilization Sleep apnea Essential hypertension Medications
11 yr to adult	Renal parenchymal disease Essential hypertension	All causes listed above

Table 15. Comparison of Clinical and Morphologic Types of Systemic Lupus Erythematosus Nephritis

	Mesangial Changes (% of Patients)	Focal Proliferative GN (% of Patients)	Diffuse Proliferative GN (% of Patients)	Membranous GN (% of Patients)
Percentage of all patients	39	27	16	18
Hematuria, pyuria	13	53	78	50
Proteinuria	36	67	89	100
Nephrotic syndrome	0	27	56	90
Azotemia	13	20	22	10
Decreased complement	54	77	100	75
Increased anti-DNA	45	75	80	33
Decreased complement and increased anti-DNA	36	63	80	33
Hypertension	22	40	56	50
Prognosis	Better	Worse	Worse	Better

GN, glomerulonephritis.
From Appel GB. The course of management of lupus nephritis. *Intern Med* 1981;2:82.

- Toxic substances
  - Exogenous (e.g., lead, mercury, cadmium)
  - Endogenous, for example,
    - Uric acid
    - Hypercalcemic nephropathy, nephrocalcinosis
    - Oxalate
- Irradiation nephritis
- Sarcoidosis
- Others

Nephritis Associated with Systemic Lupus Erythematosus

See Table 15.

Renal involvement occurs in two-third of patients with SLE.

Nephritis of SLE may occur as acute, latent, or chronic GN, nephrosis, or asymptomatic albuminuria or hematuria. Histology may be mesangial, focal or diffuse proliferative, or membranous GN.

Urine findings are as in chronic active GN. Azotemia or marked proteinuria usually indicates death in 1–3 years.

Laboratory findings of SLE may disappear during active nephritis, nephrosis, or uremia.

Examination of needle biopsy specimen should always include immunofluorescence and electron microscopy as well as light microscopy. May show normal or minimal disease, mesangial lesions, focal proliferative GN, diffuse proliferative GN, or membranous GN.

Laboratory findings due to drug therapy

- Prednisone
- Cytotoxic drugs (e.g., azathioprine, cyclophosphamide)
  - Leukopenia—nadir WBC kept at 1,500–4,000/mm^3
  - Infection (e.g., herpes zoster, opportunistic organisms)
  - Gonadal toxicity

Hemorrhagic cystitis
Neoplasia

Nephronophthisis

Nephronophthisis is characterized by polyuria and polydipsia, anemia, and failure to thrive. The proteinuria may be a tubular pattern with a predominance of β_2-microglobulin. There is a tendency to renal salt wasting. The urine sediment is unremarkable.

Nephrotic Syndrome

Manifestations

Proteinuria is in excess of 3.5 g/1.73 m^2/day.
Hypoalbuminemia (loss, enhanced renal catabolism, decreased hepatic synthesis).
Hyperlipidemia (stimulated by decreased plasma oncotic pressure).
Insidious onset of edema (loss of intravascular volume).
Homeostatic adjustments to correct the resulting deficit in effective plasma volume lead to an increase in sodium or water retention.

- Activation of renin-angiotensin-aldosterone system
- Enhanced vasopressin secretion
- Sympathetic nervous system stimulation
- Alteration in secretion or in the renal response to atrial natriuretic peptide
- Loss of important proteins in addition to albumin

Thyroid-binding globulin abnormality (abnormal thyroid function test results or clinical hypothyroidism).
Cholecalciferol-binding protein abnormality (vitamin D deficiency and secondary hyperparathyroidism leading to hypocalcemia, hypocalciuria).
Transferrin abnormality (iron-resistant microcytic, hypochromic anemia).
Metal-binding protein abnormalities (deficiency of zinc and copper).
Multifactorial hypercoagulable state: loss of antithrombin III, protein C, protein S, fibrinogen; enhanced platelet aggregation; increased α- and β-globulins.

Minimal-Change Disease

Ninety percent of children respond to prednisone treatment.
Nonresponse suggests focal glomerulosclerosis.
Cyclophosphamide may produce remission in cases with frequent relapses.
Male preponderance is seen.
If diagnosis is in doubt, renal biopsy should be performed.

Causes of Nephrotic Syndrome

Primary glomerular diseases
- Minimal-change disease (70–80% of affected children, 15–20% of adults) caused by foot process defects (formerly called lipid nephrosis or nil disease)
- Mesangial proliferative GN
- Focal and segmental glomerulosclerosis
- Membranous GN
- Membranoproliferative GN
- Other proliferative GNs (e.g., focal, IgA nephropathy, mesangial)
- Rapidly progressive GN

Infection
- Poststreptococcal GN, malaria, hepatitis B, infectious mononucleosis, secondary syphilis, acquired immunodeficiency syndrome

Drugs
- Organic gold, penicillamine, NSAIDs, contrast media
- Probenecid, captopril
- Contrast media

Mercury (organic, inorganic, and elemental)
Street heroin (including impurities)
Antivenoms and antitoxins
Neoplasia
Hodgkin disease, non-Hodgkin disease, melanoma, lymphoma, and leukemias
Wilms tumor
Multisystem diseases
SLE, Henoch-Schönlein purpura, vasculitides, dermatomyositis, rheumatoid arthritis, Goodpasture syndrome, Alport syndrome
Diabetic glomerulosclerosis
Amyloidosis
Hereditofamilial or congenital diseases
Malignant obesity
Renovascular hypertension
Thyroiditis
Chronic allograft rejection
Myxedema
Bee sting allergies
Chronic interstitial nephritis with vesicoureteric reflux
Sickle cell disease
Preeclamptic toxemia
Berger disease
Polyarteritis (rare)
Takayasu disease
Sarcoidosis
Sjögren syndrome
Wegener granulomatosis (rare)
Cryoglobulinemia
Venous obstruction
Obstruction of inferior vena cava (thrombosis, tumor)
Constrictive pericarditis
Tricuspid stenosis
Congestive heart failure

Table 16 provides a summary of primary renal diseases that present as idiopathic nephrotic syndrome.

Obstructive Uropathy

Partial obstruction of both kidneys may cause

- Increasing azotemia with normal or increased urinary output (due to decreased renal concentrating ability).
- In unilateral obstruction, BUN usually remains normal unless underlying renal disease is present.
- Obstruction of bladder [e.g., urethral stricture, neurogenic bladder dysfunction (multiple sclerosis, diabetic neuropathy)]
- Obstruction of both ureters [e.g., infiltrating neoplasm (especially of uterine cervix), bilateral calculi, congenital anomalies, retroperitoneal fibrosis]

If ureter is obstructed for >4 months, functional recovery is unlikely.
Laboratory findings are due to the underlying disease.

Oxalosis

(Rare autosomal-recessive inherited disorders of metabolism of glyoxylate, a liver enzyme causing recurrent calcium oxalate renal lithiasis, nephrocalcinosis, and uremia)

Primary

Urinary oxalate is usually >100 mg/24 hours unless renal function is diminished.
Urinary glycolic and glyoxylic acid are elevated.

Table 16. Primary Renal Diseases Presenting as Idiopathic Nephrotic Syndrome

				Membranoproliferative Glomerulonephritis	
	Minimal-Change Nephrotic Syndrome	Focal Segmental Sclerosis	Membranous Nephropathy	Type 1	Type 2
Frequency[a]					
Children	75%	10%	<5%	10%	10%
Adults	15%	15%	50%	10%	10%
Clinical manifestations					
Age (yr)	2–6, some adults	2–10, some adults	40–50	5–15	5–15
Sex	2:1 male	1.2:1.0 male	2:1 male	Male-female	Male-female
Nephrotic syndrome	100%	90%	80%	60%	60%
Asymptomatic proteinuria	0	10%	20%	40%	40%
Hematuria	10–20%	60–80%	60%	80%	80%
Hypertension	10%	20% early	Infrequent	35%	35%
Rate of progression of renal failure	Does not progress	10 yr	50% in 10–20 yr	10–20 yr	5–15 yr
Associated conditions	Allergy? Hodgkin disease, usually none	None	Renal vein thrombosis, cancer, SLE, hepatitis B virus	None	Partial lipodystrophy
Laboratory findings	Manifestations of nephrotic syndrome ↑ BUN in 15–30%	Manifestations of nephrotic syndrome ↑ BUN in 20–40%	Manifestations of nephrotic syndrome	Low C1, C4, C3–C9	Normal C1, Low C4
Immunogenetics	HLA-B8, B12 (3.5)[b]	Not established	HLA-DRW3 (12–32)[b]	Not established	C3 nephritis factor

					Not established
Renal pathology					
Light microscopy	Normal	Focal sclerotic lesions	Thickened GBM, spikes	Thickened GBM, proliferation	Lobulation
Immunofluorescence	Negative	IgM, C3 in lesions	Fine granular IgG,	Granular IgG, C3	C3 only
Electron microscopy	Foot process fusion	Foot process fusion	Subepithelial deposits of C3	Mesangial and subendothelial deposits	Dense deposits
Response to steroids	90%	15–20%	May be slow progression	Not established	Not established

↑, elevated; BUN, blood urea nitrogen; GBM, glomerular basement membrane; Ig, immunoglobulin; SLE, systemic lupus erythematosus.

[a]Frequency as a cause of idiopathic nephrotic syndrome. Approximately 10% of adult nephrotic syndrome cases are due to various diseases that usually present with acute glomerulonephritis.

[b]Relative risk.

Modified from Couser WG. Glomerular disorders. In: Wyngaarden JB, Smith LH, Bennett JC, eds. *Cecil textbook of medicine*, 19th ed. Philadelphia: WB Saunders, 1992:560.

Secondary Oxalosis

May be due to ingestion of oxalate-containing foods, for example, green leafy vegetables, chocolate, tea, ascorbic acid; ethylene glycol poisoning; methoxyflurane anesthesia; Crohn disease, pancreatitis, bypass surgery.

Uric Acid Excretion

Usually associated with hyperuricemia.
Hyperuricemia in hereditary conditions (X-linked Lesch-Nyhan syndrome).
May accompany dehydration, leukemia, allopurinol therapy.

Cystine Excretion

Cystinuria >300 mg/day.

Polycystic Kidney Disease

Occurs in two forms:

Autosomal-dominant form is usually slowly progressive and asymptomatic until patient is >50 years old; accounts for approximately 10% of transplant or dialysis cases.

Usually does not manifest until adult life. Some cases have been diagnosed in the neonatal period and in childhood. It may present as polyuria.

- Polyuria is present.
- Hematuria may be gross and episodic or an incidental microscopical finding (50% of patients).
- Proteinuria occurs in approximately one-third of patients and is mild (<1 mg/24 hours).
- Renal calculi may be associated (≤30% of patients with autosomal-dominant polycystic kidney disease).
- Hypertension may be present (affects 30% of children, affects ≤60% of adults before onset of renal insufficiency and >80% with end-stage renal failure).
- Anemia of renal failure is less severe than that in other forms of kidney disease.
- Prenatal diagnosis is possible using DNA obtained by amniocentesis or chorionic villus sampling.

Autosomal-recessive form is usually more severe and becomes manifest earlier with fewer patients surviving as adults. It is characterized by very large cystic kidneys that can be diagnosed prenatally. It is associated with oligohydramnios. The Potter sequence and pulmonary hypoplasia are incompatible with life. Some patients have undergone successful kidney transplantation at birth.

Polyuria

(Increased urine excretion)
Diabetes insipidus (antidiuretic hormone insufficiency)
Diabetes mellitus (polydipsia and polyuria)
Acute, tubular necrosis
Psychogenic polydipsia
Diuretic therapy
Chronic renal failure

Central Diabetes Insipidus

Urine specific gravity is 1.001–1.010, urine osmolality 50–300 mOsm/kg.
Other renal functions are usually normal. Water deprivation results in severe dehydration.

Serum sodium level is markedly elevated when patient is dehydrated. Serum vasopressin level is decreased.
Administration of deamino-D-arginine-vasopressin results in increased urine specific gravity and osmolality.
MRI of head may reveal calcification or tumor in area of hypoplasia.

Nephrogenic Diabetes Insipidus

Signs and symptoms are similar to those of central diabetes insipidus except that there is little or no response to deamino-D-arginine-vasopressin, and other signs of chronic renal disease (elevated BUN and creatinine) are present.

Psychogenic Diabetes Insipidus

Urine specific gravity and osmolality are similar to those in central diabetes insipidus. Careful observation during water deprivation results in decreased urine volume and increased urine concentration.

Proteinuria, Persistent, Asymptomatic

Asymptomatic persistent proteinuria is defined as constant proteinuria of >250 mg/day in infants and >500 mg/day in children. The long-term prognosis in children is not known, so they should be carefully followed every 3–6 months, with measurement of blood pressure and plasma creatinine level. A renal biopsy is not necessary as long as the patient is stable. If hematuria is present, the prognosis is guarded.
Types of proteinuria include
- Glomerular proteinuria
- Tubular proteinuria
- Tissue proteinuria

Glomerular Proteinuria

Transient proteinuria (nonpathologic): Most common in children. Associated with exercise, stress, dehydration, postural changes, cold exposure, fever, seizures, congestive heart failure, and use of vasoactive drugs. Serial urine tests should give negative results for protein.
Orthostatic proteinuria: Common, not associated with renal pathology. Rarely exceeds 1 g/day. Obtain first morning specimen then have patient walk for 7–10 minutes. Only the second specimen contains protein.
Proteinuria secondary to glomerulopathies
- Primary glomerular disease: minimal-change disease, focal segmental GN, membranous nephropathy, membranoproliferative GN, IgM nephropathy, IgA nephropathy
- Secondary glomerular disease: medication induced [nonsteroidal antiinflammatory drugs (NSAIDs), captopril, lithium (citrate or carbonate), etc.], postinfectious (streptococcal infections, hepatitis B, chronic shunt infections, subacute bacterial endocarditis), infectious (bacterial, fungal, viral), neoplastic (solid tumors, leukemia), multisystem (SLE, Henoch-Schönlein purpura, sickle cell disease), reflux nephropathy, congenital nephrotic syndrome

Tubular Proteinuria

Overload proteinuria: Occurs when excessive amount of low-molecular-weight proteins overwhelms the tubular reabsorption capacity (e.g., light chains: multiple myeloma; lysozyme: monocytic and myelocytic leukemia; myoglobin: hemolysis).
Tubular dysfunction or disorders: Occurs when normal amounts of low-molecular-weight proteins are not adequately reabsorbed because of damaged or dysfunctional tubular cells [Fanconi syndrome, Lowe syndrome, reflux nephropathy, cystinosis, effects of drugs or heavy metals (mercury, lead, cadmium, outdated tetracyclines)], ischemic tubular injury, and renal hypoplasia or dysplasia.

The identifying characteristic of tubular proteinuria is the presence of 25–60% protein of low molecular weight. This proteinuria may result from failure of tubular reabsorption of plasma proteins.

The measurement of β_2-microglobulin (molecular weight of 11,815 d) is an index of tubular proteinuria. The ratio of urine albumin to β_2-microglobulin is <15 in tubular proteinuria, whereas in glomerular proteinuria the ratio is >1,000.

Retinol-binding protein (molecular weight of 21,200 d) provides a measurement of low molecular weight proteinuria, because, unlike β_2-microglobulin, it is stable in acid urine. The high-molecular-weight lysosomal enzyme *N*-acetyl-β-D-glucosaminidase is not specifically a renal protein but is highly active in proximal tubular cells. In states of proximal tubular injury from disease or nephrotoxins, urinary *N*-acetyl-β-D-glucosaminidase level is increased. *N*-acetyl-β-D-glucosaminidase is measured colorimetrically; dietary substances can interfere with the assay.

Tissue Proteinuria

Acute inflammation of urinary tract
Uroepithelial tumors

Purpura, Henoch-Schönlein

Henoch-Schönlein purpura is a clinical diagnosis based on the presence of a purpuric skin rash, usually of the lower extremities, arthralgias, abdominal pain, and renal involvement, which may range from microscopic hematuria to a mixed nephritic and nephrotic syndrome. Patients may demonstrate signs of IgA nephropathy.

Stenosis, Renal Artery

- Mild proteinuria occurs often.
- Hypertension.
- BUN and creatinine levels increased.
- Plasma renin activity in peripheral vein is increased, may cause hypokalemic metabolic alkalosis.
- Urine sodium concentration may be low.
- Asymmetrical renal function or size (e.g., scan, ultrasonography, pyelogram).
- Intravenous pyelogram, arteriography, MRI, Doppler ultrasonography of renal arteries support diagnosis.
- Late-onset (age >55 years) or early-onset (age <20 years) hypertension is often severe.

Thrombosis, Renal Vein

May occur in the newborn, particularly in infants of diabetic mothers.

- Hematuria, microscopic pyuria, and variable proteinuria and decreased creatinine clearance.
- Postprandial glycosuria, nephrotic syndrome, hyperchloremic acidosis (RTA), hyperosmolarity, anemia; platelet count may be decreased; oliguria and uremic death if infarction is extensive.
- Increased fibrin degradation products in blood may be more than three times the normal limits (disseminated intravascular coagulation).
- Laboratory findings due to thromboembolic disease elsewhere (e.g., pulmonary).
- Laboratory findings due to underlying causative conditions (e.g., nephrotic syndrome, hypernephroma, metastatic cancer, trauma, amyloidosis, diabetic glomerulosclerosis, hypertension, papillary necrosis, disseminated intravascular coagulation, sickle cell disease, polycythemia, heart failure, etc.).

Tubular Interstitial Diseases

Defects in Tubular Function

Defects in proximal tubule function: selective reabsorption defects leading to hypokalemia, amino aciduria, glycosuria, phosphaturia, uricosuria, bicarbonaturia (i.e., RTA type 2). Proteinuria is usually mild (<2 g/day). The combination of these is Fanconi syndrome.

Defects in urinary acidification and concentrating ability: hyperchloremic metabolic acidosis with urine of maximum acidity (i.e., pH of ≤5.3), usually from a reduced ability to generate and excrete ammonia due to the loss in renal mass.

Damage to collecting ducts: can lead to distal or type 1 RTA. This is characterized by high urine pH (>5.5) during either spontaneous or ammonium chloride–induced metabolic acidosis.

Causes

Extrinsic toxins or inherent metabolic toxins
- Chronic use or abuse of analgesics
- Lead poisoning
- Acute uric acid nephropathy
- Gouty nephropathy
- Hypokalemia
- Hypercalcemia
- Cystinosis
- Fabry disease
- Drug exposure (antibiotics, lithium, CSA, radiographic contrast media, heavy metals)

Neoplasia
- Lymphoma
- Leukemia
- Multiple myeloma

Immune disorders
- Hypersensitivity nephropathy
- Sjögren syndrome
- Amyloidosis
- Transplant rejection
- Immune disorders associated with GN
- Acquired immunodeficiency syndrome

Vascular disorders
- Arteriolar nephrosclerosis
- Atheroembolic disease
- Sickle cell nephropathy
- Acute tubular necrosis

Hereditary renal diseases
- Hereditary nephritis (Alport syndrome)
- Medullary cystic disease
- Medullary sponge kidney
- Polycystic kidney disease

Infectious injury
- Acute pyelonephritis
- Chronic pyelonephritis
- Chronic urinary tract obstruction
- Vesicoureteral reflux
- Radiation nephritis
- Parenchymal disease associated with extrarenal neoplasm: leukemia, lymphoma, multiple myeloma

Tubular Necrosis, Acute

Nonoliguric form is usually due to nephrotoxic agents. Mortality is approximately 25%.

Oliguric form is usually due to ischemic events (e.g., renovascular occlusion, bilateral cortical necrosis), rapidly progressive GN, obstructive uropathy. Mortality is approximately 50%.

Usually multiple causes (e.g., hypotension, sepsis, nephrotoxic drugs, radiographic contrast material, volume depletion).

Sudden progressive increase in BUN and serum creatinine levels with ratio of <20:1.

In patients with oliguric type who have not had recent diuretic therapy, urine osmolality is <350 mOsm/kg H_2O and spot sodium is >20 mEq/L.

Urine sodium concentration usually is >40 mEq/L but may be <20 mEq/L in nonoliguric patients.

Fractional excretion of sodium (FE_{Na}) is usually >1% in both oliguric and nonoliguric patients.

Uremia

Pathologic Findings

- Toxins are by-products of protein and amino acid metabolism.
- Increased levels of parathyroid hormone, insulin, glucagon, growth hormone, lactate dehydrogenase, prolactin, aldosterone.
- Decreased transcellular ion transport (sodium–potassium–adenosine triphosphatase) leads to increased intracellular sodium, decreased intracellular potassium, and decreased magnitude of transcellular voltage. Changes are secondary to osmotically induced overhydration of cells, increased total body water, and increased intracellular/extracellular water ratio.
- Metabolic acidosis leads to efflux of potassium from cells, which causes a normal or high serum potassium level despite decreased intracellular potassium.
- Hypothermia from decreased sodium–potassium–adenosine triphosphatase activity (greater part of energy production)
- Azotemic pseudodiabetes (i.e., with normal fasting blood sugar levels), which does not necessarily require therapy.
  - Decreased utilization of peripheral glucose
    - Decreased intracellular potassium level
    - Increased levels of catecholamines
    - Decreased insulin sensitivity
- Metabolic acidosis
    - Increased growth hormone
    - Increased prolactin level
    - Increased glucagon level
- Triglycerides increased (from the lipogenic effect of hyperinsulinism), with decreased high-density lipoprotein, and a normal cholesterol level.

Urinary Tract Infection

UTI is common, affecting 3% of girls and 1% of boys in the pediatric age group. The risk of recurrence is 30% after the first UTI and increases to 75% after subsequent infections. The majority of UTIs occur in the absence of an anatomical urinary tract abnormality. The occurrence of an infection in the presence of urinary obstruction (incidence, 10%) or vesicoureteric reflux may predispose to renal scarring.

UTIs may be classified on the basis of symptoms, the presence of an underlying anatomic or functional abnormality, or the site of infection. Symptoms of cystitis include dysuria, frequency, and urgency, and may be accompanied by foul-smelling or cloudy urine. Pyelonephritis may manifest as flank or abdominal pain, fever, and rigors. UTI is often accompanied by septicemia and potentially life-threatening metabolic abnormalities in infants.

Diagnostic Studies

The diagnosis of UTI is based on finding significant numbers of microorganisms on urine culture.

Urine Collection Methods

Significant bacteriuria separates true infection from bacterial contamination. Indicators of contamination include low bacterial colony counts, multiple types of organisms, different organisms on serial culture, or the detection of nonpathogenic organisms. False-negative culture results or low colony counts may occur in cases of dilute urine from a patient with a urinary concentrating defect, high rate of urinary flow, low urine specific gravity or pH, or prior administration of antibacterial drugs, or use of inappropriate culture medium, for example, media for tubercle bacilli, *Mycoplasma*, *Ureaplasma*, *Chlamydia*, anaerobes.

Various methods of obtaining urine for culture in children have evolved.

Catheter Specimen

Careful adherence to aseptic technique is essential in collection of a specimen via catheter. Introduction of bacteria into the bladder and trauma to the urethra may occur at the time of catheterization. Bacterial growth of $\geq 10^3$ colony-forming units (CFU)/mL ($\geq 1 \times 10^6$ CFU/L) is significant, especially when associated with pyuria or symptoms.

Bag Sample

After cleansing of the genitalia, urine is obtained by affixing a sterile bag. Contamination frequently occurs, and a bag sample is most useful when it gives negative results for significant bacterial growth.

Midstream Urine Specimen

A midstream urine sample is obtained by cleansing the genitalia and periurethral area and collecting the midportion of the urinary stream to reduce contamination from urethral or prostatic secretions.

- Count of >100,000 bacteria/mL indicates active infection (>85% sensitivity).
- Count of <10,000/mL in the absence of therapy largely rules out bacteriuria.
- Count of 10,000–100,000/mL indicates that sampling should be repeated and specimen should be cultured.
- Count of <100,000/mL with clinical findings of acute pyelonephritis with no obvious explanation, such as recent use of antibiotics, suggests urinary tract obstruction or perinephric abscess.

Suprapubic Specimen

Suprapubic sterile needle aspiration is the most accurate method of urine collection, and is simpler and less traumatic in infants than catheterization. The infant should not have voided for at least 1 hour and is restrained. Skin 1–2 cm above the symphysis pubis is cleaned with alcohol. A syringe with a 1-in No. 22G needle is inserted almost perpendicular to the skin, and gentle pressure is applied. The presence of any organism on culture of such a specimen is diagnostic of UTI. Compared to urethral catheterization in adults, the method is simpler, less traumatic, and more accurate.

Dipstick Testing

Urine is prepared for culture, and a dipstick is placed in a small amount of urine for tests as previously described.

Urine Culture

Method

Urine is cultured for organism identification and determination of antibiotic sensitivity. Once obtained, urine for bacterial culture should be plated immediately, using a calibrated loop, onto 5% sheep's blood agar and a medium selective for Gram-negative bacilli such as MacConkey agar. The culture is incubated for 24 hours to obtain a colony count; a further 12–24 hours of incubation is necessary for *in vitro* antibiotic sensitivity testing. If immediate plating is not possible, refrigeration at 4°C will maintain stable colony counts for 24 hours. When urine remains at room temperature, the number of bacteria doubles every 30–45 minutes.

Automated, rapid culture methods have been developed. They have low sensitivity, however, especially for low colony counts and slow-growing organisms, which makes them inappropriate for investigation of nosocomial infections and evaluation of patients with low-grade bacteriuria.

Interpretation of Results

Method of Collection	Quantitative Culture: Criterion for Presence of UTI
Suprapubic aspiration	Growth of Gram-negative urinary pathogens in any number (the exception is up to 2–3 $\times 10^3$ CFU/mL of coagulase-negative staphylococci).
Catheterization	Febrile infants or children usually have $\geq 50 \times 10^3$ CFU/mL of a single urinary pathogen, but infection may be present with counts of 10×10^3 to 50×10^3 CFU/mL.
Midstream clean catch	
Symptomatic patients	Symptomatic patients usually have $\geq 10^5$ CFU/mL of a single urinary tract pathogen.
Asymptomatic patients	At least two specimens collected on different days show $\geq 10^5$ CFU/mL of the same organism.

Pyuria

Pyuria is defined clinically as ≥10 WBC/mm³ (≥10 × 10^6 WBC/L) of uncentrifuged urine, counted with a hemocytometer, or >10 WBC/hpf of centrifuged urine. The presence of pyuria is suggestive of, but not diagnostic for, UTI.

Leukocyte esterase detected by the dipstick correlates with pyuria rather than UTI. *Trichomonas* may cause a positive reaction. Leukocyte esterase and nitrite assays should not substitute for direct microscopy or culture in the detection of UTI.

Dipstick test for pyuria (measures leukocyte esterase of neutrophil granules; does not detect lymphocytes) has negative predictive value of >90% and positive predictive value of 50% for bacterial infection. Sensitivity is 100% for >50 WBCs/hpf, 90% for 21–50 WBCs, 60% for 12–20 WBCs, and 44% for 6–12 WBCs.

Dipstick test of first-catch urine is a cost-effective way to detect asymptomatic urethritis (*Chlamydia, Neisseria*) in males.

Urinary Nitrite

Urinary nitrite is produced by the reduction of dietary nitrate by certain bacteria. It is measured using an amine-impregnated dipstick, which produces a pink color reaction when results are positive. False-negatives occur in the presence of dilute urine, inadequate dietary nitrates, high doses of vitamin C, and non–nitrate reducing bacteria such as *Staphylococcus* and *Enterococcus*. The test is insensitive at colony counts of <10^5 CFU/mL (<100 × 10^6 CFU/L). Dipstick testing of first-catch urine is a cost-effective way to detect asymptomatic urethritis (*Chlamydia, Neisseria*) in males.

Microscopy for Bacteria

Direct microscopic examination of uncentrifuged urine, either unstained or Gram-stained, that shows one polymorphonuclear cell/hpf or one organism/hpf has sensitivity of 85% and specificity of 60% for bacteriuria. It may yield >10% false-positive results. One organism/oil immersion field (threshold of detection for microscopy) in uncentrifuged urine correlates with a count of ≥10,000 colonies/mL. Gram staining of cytospin specimens has >90% sensitivity and >80% specificity for a count of ≥100,000/mL. With pyuria and bacteriuria, Gram staining to differentiate Gram-positive cocci (e.g., enterococci or staphylococci) from Gram-negative bacilli suggests appropriate immediate initial therapy. Patients with chronic UTI and asymptomatic bacteriuria may not show significant numbers of WBCs on urine microscopic examination; however, pyuria is associated with bacteriuria in 90% of cases. The presence of large numbers of squamous epithelial cells may indicate that the specimen contains greater numbers of bacteria from the vagina or the perineum rather than from the urinary tract. Bacteriuria and pyuria are often intermittent; in the chronic atrophic stage of pyelonephritis, they are often absent. In acute pyelonephritis, marked pyuria and bacteriuria are almost always present; hematuria and proteinuria may also be present during the first few days of infection. The presence of WBC casts is very suggestive of pyelonephritis. Glitter cells may be seen. Coliforms are more likely to be detected than enterococci. Bacteria and hematuria without proteinuria are suggestive of lower UTI.

- If culture shows a common Gram-positive saprophyte, culture should be repeated, because the second culture is often negative.
- Causative bacteria are usually enteric organisms; <10% are Gram-positive cocci.
- Positive significant results in a single culture or a finding of a predominant organism should be considered a positive test result in symptomatic patients (95% reliable), and repeat culture is unnecessary.
- A finding of three or more species with none being predominant (i.e., >80% of the growth) almost always represents specimen contamination and culture should be repeated; however, true mixed infection may occur after instrumentation or with chronic infection.
- Presence of *Pseudomonas* or *Proteus* may indicate that the patient has an anatomic abnormality. If an organism other than *Escherichia coli* is found, patient probably has chronic pyelonephritis, even if this is the first clinical episode of infection.
- In women, >80% of UTIs are due to *E. coli* and a smaller percentage are due to *Staphylococcus saprophyticus*; UTIs are less often due to other aerobic Gram-negative bacilli. In men, Gram-negative bacilli cause 75% of UTIs, but *E. coli* causes only 25% of infections in men and <50% of infections in boys.
- Other common Gram-negative bacilli are *Proteus* and *Providencia* species. Gram-positive organisms (especially enterococci and coagulase-negative staphylococci)

cause 20% of infections in men and boys but *S. saprophyticus* infection is rare. Infection due to *Gardnerella vaginalis* is found in <3% of men with bacteriuria.

- If *Candida* organisms are isolated, rule out contaminated specimen, diabetes mellitus, papillary necrosis, indwelling catheter, broad-spectrum antibiotic exposure, immunosuppressive chemotherapy, malignancy, malnutrition.
- Presence of "sterile" pyuria (≥10 WBCs/hpf in centrifuged urine) and absence of bacilli should cast doubt on diagnosis of untreated bacterial UTI and may occur in renal tuberculosis, chemical inflammation, mechanical inflammation (e.g., due to calculi, instrumentation), early acute GN before appearance of hematuria or proteinuria, polycystic kidney disease, papillary necrosis, interstitial cystitis, transplant rejection, sarcoidosis, genitourinary (GU) tract neoplasm, the presence of uric acid, and hypercalcemic nephropathy, lithium and heavy metal toxicity, extreme dehydration, hyperchloremic renal acidosis, genital herpes, nonbacterial gastroenteritis, and respiratory tract infections, as well as after administration of oral polio vaccine.
- When urine cultures are persistently negative in the presence of other evidence of pyelonephritis, specific search should be made for tubercle bacilli.

With pyuria and bacteriuria, persistent alkaline pH may indicate infection with urea-splitting organism (e.g., *Proteus*, or less often *Pseudomonas* or *Klebsiella*).

Bacteria should be cleared from urine within 48 hours of initiation of antibiotic therapy; persistence indicates need to change antibiotic treatment or to search for another explanation.

Asymptomatic bacteriuria occurs in ≤15% of pregnant women. Routine urinalysis is done on first prenatal visit because 20–40% of untreated patients with positive cultures develop acute pyelonephritis during pregnancy (occurs in only 1% of women with negative cultures). Persistent or recurrent infection may be due to stones or obstruction.

Acute pyelonephritis shows two consecutive colony counts of ≥100,000 organisms/mL with or without upper GU tract symptoms (flank pain, fever, costovertebral angle tenderness, fever, chills, nausea, vomiting, leukocytosis).

Acute urethral syndrome and acute cystitis show a colony count of ≥100 organisms/mL and lower GU tract symptoms (dysuria, frequency, urgency, suprapubic pain). Urine dipstick test for WBC (leukocyte esterase) detects 8–10 WBC/hpf. Pyuria is rarely present unless a bacterial count is >10,000/mL.

With catheterization for <30 days or intermittent catheterization, the criterion for bacteriuria is ≥100 organisms/mL; multiple organisms are common.

With catheterization for >30 days, mixed infections with >100,000 organisms/mL occur in >75% of cases. Organisms constantly change, with new ones appearing approximately every 2 weeks.

Decreased glucose (<2 mg/dL) in properly collected first-morning urine (no food or fluid intake after 10 p.m., no urination during night) correlates well with high colony count.

Positive test result for antibody-coated bacteria (using fluorescein-conjugated antihuman globulin) is said to indicate bacteria of renal origin and to be 81% predictive of upper GU tract infection. Result is negative in lower tract infection. False-positives may occur with heavy proteinuria, prostatitis, or contamination with vaginal or rectal bacteria. False-negatives may occur early in infection. Test is less reliable for children and adults with neurogenic bladder. Test is not recommended for routine use.

Albuminuria is usually <2 g/24 hours (≤2+ qualitative); this finding therefore helps to differentiate pyelonephritis from glomerular disease, in which albuminuria is usually >2 g/24 hours; may be undetectable in a very dilute urine associated with fixed specific gravity.

β_2-microglobulin is increased in 24-hour urine specimen in pyelonephritis (due to tubular damage) but not in cystitis.

Decreased concentrating ability occurs relatively early in chronic renal infection but not in bladder infections. Persistent dilute urine suggests renal rather than bladder infection. It is not a sensitive or specific test.

Renal blood flow and GFR show a parallel decrease proportional to progress of renal disease. Comparison of function in right and left kidneys shows more disparity in pyelonephritis than in diffuse renal disease (e.g., nephrosclerosis, GN). Fluctuation in renal function (e.g., due to recurrent infection, dehydration) with considerable recovery is more marked and frequent in pyelonephritis than in other renal diseases. Twenty-four-hour creatinine clearance decreases before BUN and blood creatinine levels rise. UTI in infants <1 year old is associated with an underlying GU tract anomaly in 55% of males and 35% of females.

Lactate dehydrogenase 4 and *lactate dehydrogenase 5* are increased in urine in renal medullary damage (pyelonephritis); less useful than β_2-microglobulin to distinguish upper from lower urinary tract damage.

Hyperchloremic acidosis (due to impaired renal acid excretion and bicarbonate reabsorption) occurs more often in chronic pyelonephritis than in GN.

Patients with UTIs should be followed with routine periodic urinalysis and colony counts for at least 2 years because asymptomatic recurrence of bacteriuria is common.

Imaging Studies

Imaging with first documented UTI should be pursued in all boys, in girls <5 years, and in older girls with pyelonephritis or recurrent infections. Referral to a pediatric urologist is also recommended if studies reveal obstructive lesion, high-grade (IV or V) vesicoureteral reflux (VUR), or progressive changes in dimercaptosuccinic acid (DMSA) imaging or voiding cystourethrography (VCUG) on follow-up studies.

1. Abdominal radiograph: for checking stool patterns or if suspicion of spinal dysraphism.
2. Renal sonography: a noninvasive nonionizing evaluation for gross structural defects, lesions that are obstructive, positional abnormalities, and renal size and growth.
3. VCUG: test for evaluation of VUR and bladder and urethral anatomy. Perform when patient is asymptomatic and cleared of bacteruria. Indicated in all boys, girls <5 years, and girls >5 years with recurrent or febrile UTIs. Repeat in 6–12 months if initial study is positive for reflux. Radionucleotide cystography: has 1/100th the radiation exposure of a VCUG and increased sensitivity for transient reflux; may substitute for VCUG. Radionucleotide cystography does not visualize urethral anatomy, is not sensitive for low-grade reflux, and cannot grade reflux.
4. DMSA imaging: technetium 99m DMSA normally taken up by renal tubules; defects on DMSA image indicate tubular defects. Best for radiographic documentation of acute or chronic pyelonephritis. Indicated in patients with febrile UTI, abnormal VCUG or renal sonography, prenatally diagnosed vesicoureteral reflux. Repeat in 6 months if initial study is positive for acute pyelonephritis to rule out scars.
5. Diethylenetriamine pentaacetic acid/mercaptotriglycine imaging: may also be used for indications given above for use of DMSA imaging. Provides quantitative assessment of renal function.

Renal Failure

Tests for Evaluation of Renal Failure

Renal Function Tests

Measurement of renal plasma flow and tubular function:

Para-aminohippurate	
Males	560–800 mL/min
Females	500–700 mL/min
Diodrast	600–800 mL/min
Filtration fraction—GFR/RPF	
Males	17–21%
Females	17–23%
Maximal Diodrast excretory capacity	
Males	43–59 mg/min
Females	33–51 mg/min

RPF, renal plasma flow.

Table 17. Laboratory Guide to Evaluation of Renal Impairment

Condition	Renal Clearance of Endogenous Creatinine[a] (Glomerular Filtration Rate)	Urinary Excretion of IV PSP in 15 Min (Renal Tubular Transport Mechanisms)
Normal	15–180 L/24 hr (80–125 mL/min)	≥25%
Slight impairment	75–90 L/24 hr (52.0–62.5 mL/min)	15–25%
Mild impairment	60–75 L/24 hr (42–52 mL/min)	10–15%
Moderate impairment	40–60 L/24 hr (28–42 mL/min)	5–10%
Marked impairment	<40 L/24 hr (<28 mL/min)	<5%

PSP, phenolsulfonphthalein.
[a]Creatinine clearance is normally less in females than in males, and it usually decreases with age, starting at 20 yr.

Laboratory Studies to Assess Renal Failure

See Table 17.
Urinary output—normal urine output is 0.5–3.0 mL/kg/hour.
Serum potassium level: hyperkalemia.
Cardiac monitoring mandatory: peaked T waves, prolonged PR interval, loss of P waves, widening of QRS, ventricular fibrillation arrhythmia.
Serum sodium level: hypernatremia primarily related to fluid overload more than total body Na loss.
- Symptomatic (mental status changes, loss of consciousness, seizures) or Na <120 mEq/dL:
  - Estimate Na deficit: 0.6 × body weight × (130 – Na).
  - Replace with 3% NaCl (0.5 mEq/mL) if symptomatic: 2.5 mEq/kg/hour.
- Asymptomatic
  - Estimate Na deficit as earlier, replace deficit at 0.5 mEq/kg/hour.

Serum calcium level: Monitor ionized Ca whenever possible.
If ionized Ca <3 mg/dL or patient is symptomatic (seizures, tetany, arrhythmias), give calcium gluconate (dilution 100 mg/mL): 200–500 mg/kg/day intravenously [start with 100 mg/kg (1 mL/kg) over 4–6 hours and reassess].
Constantly monitor heart rate.
Blood pressure: Estimate of 95th percentile for age:
- Systolic: 100 + (2.5 × age)
- Diastolic: 70 + (1.5 × age)

Acid-base status
- Renal failure is associated with a metabolic acidosis; if there is a respiratory component to acidosis, other causes must be considered. If pH <7.25 or HCO_3 <12 mmol/L, base deficit should be corrected.

Glomerular Filtration Rate

Estimate GFR from serum creatinine level and height: k × height (cm)/creatinine (mg/dL)
Proportionality constant for calculating GFR:

	***k* Value**
Low birth weight, during first year of life	0.33
Term, appropriate weight for gestational age, during first year of life	0.45
Children and adolescent girls	0.55
Adolescent boys	0.70

Creatinine Clearance

Age (yr)	**Mean Creatinine Clearance (mL/min/1.73 m² body surface area)**
0–1	72
1	45
2	55

3	60
4	71
5	73
6	64
7	67
8	72
9	83
10	89
11	92
12	109
13–14	86

Osmolality, Urine

Urine osmolality may be impaired when other tests are normal (Fishberg concentration test, BUN, phenolsulfonphthalein excretion, creatinine clearance, intravenous pyelogram); may be especially useful in diabetes mellitus, essential hypertension, silent pyelonephritis.

Blood Urea Nitrogen/Creatinine

Normal: 10–15 mg/dL
Prerenal azotemia or gastrointestinal (GI) bleeding: >20 mg/dL
Liver disease, starvation, inborn error of metabolism: <5 mg/dL

Laboratory Differentiation of Oliguria Due to Different Causes

(Numbers in parentheses are for neonates.)

Test	Prenatal Oliguria		Low-Output Failure		Antidiuretic Hormone Secretion
Urine sodium mmol/L	<20	(<40)	>40	(>40)	>40
Specific gravity	<1.020	(1.015)	<1.010	(<1.015)	>1.020
Osmolality (mOsm/L)	>500	(>400)	<350	(<400)	>500
Urine/plasma osmolality ratio	>1.3		<1.3		>2
Urea nitrogen mg/dL	>20		<10		>15
Creatinine mg/dL	>40	(>20)	<20	(<15)	>30
RFI	<1	(<3)	>1	(>3.0)	>1
FE_{Na}	<1	(<2.5)	>1	(>3.0)	Close to 1

FE_{Na}, fractional excretion of sodium = (UNa/PNa)/(UCr/PCr) × 100, where UNa is urine sodium level, PNa is plasma sodium level, UCr is urine creatinine level, and PCr is plasma creatinine level; RFI, renal failure index = UNa/(UCr/PCr).

Electrolytes

Sodium

Reference value for serum sodium level is 135–143 mmol/L (mEq/L) for children and 132–142 mmol/L (mEq/L) for infants. Limits are reduced in renal insufficiency.

Hyponatremia [Na <130 mmol/L (mEq/L)] implies a dilution of body solute, either as a result of sodium loss or water retention and extracellular fluid (ECF) volume expansion. Pseudohyponatremia may result from hyperlipidemia, hyperglycemia, or hyperproteinemia. Ion-specific electrodes are preferred to flame photometry for the measurement of sodium and potassium. For every 3.4 mmol/L (62 mg/dL) increment in the plasma glucose concentration, water will be drawn out of the cells to reduce the plasma Na concentration by 1 mmol/L (mEq/L).

Hypernatremia [Na >150 mmol/L (mEq/L)] is usually secondary to a water deficit and is seen in some infants with diarrhea and in infants with diabetes insipidus of pituitary or renal origin.

Potassium

Reference range for a plasma potassium level is 3.5–5.0 mmol/L (mEq/L) for children and 4.5–6.5 mmol/L (mEq/L) for premature and term infants. Maintenance of the ECF potassium concentration is related to hormone control, drugs, disease, and, to a lesser extent, dietary intake.

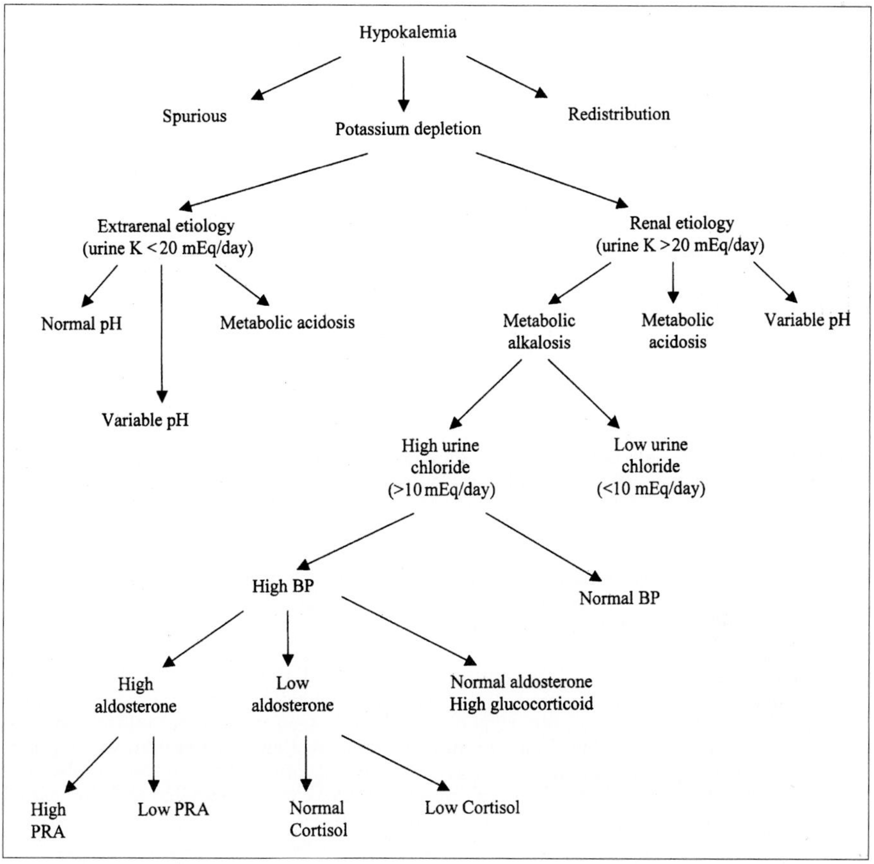

Fig. 5. Flow diagram for the differential diagnosis of hypokalemia. BP, blood pressure; PRA, plasma renin activity.

Hyperkalemia [K >5.0 mmol/L (mEq/L)] can be the result of excessive potassium intake in patients with renal failure or hypoaldosteronism. Spurious hyperkalemia can occur with thrombocytosis and hemolysis.

Hypokalemia [K <3.5 mmol/L (mEq/L)] is seen in renal tubular disorders such as RTA (Fanconi syndrome), in diuretic use, and in hyperaldosteronism. See Figs. 5–7.

Calcium

Reference range for total plasma calcium level is 2.25–2.62 mmol/L (9.0–10.5 mg/dL) for children, 1.8–2.5 mmol/L (7.2–10.0 mg/dL) for premature infants, and 2.0–2.75 mmol/L (8–11 mg/dL) for term infants. The range for ionized calcium level is 1.14–1.29 mmol/L (4.6–5.2 mg/dL) for children, and 1.10–1.5 mmol/L (4.4–6.0 mg/dL) for infants. Much of the plasma calcium is bound to protein (40%) and the remainder exists as free or ionized calcium (50%) or in complex with other ions (10%). Ionized calcium is physiologically active. In hypoalbuminemic states, the total calcium level is reduced. If measurement of ionized calcium is not available, one can adjust the result by adding 0.023 mmol/L (0.09 mg/dL) for every 1 g/L (0.1 g/dL) that the albumin is <46 g/L (4.6 g/dL). An alternate formula is

$$\text{Corrected calcium} = [\text{Ca} - (\text{albumin} \times 40)] + 1$$

where albumin is in g/L and Ca is in mmol/L

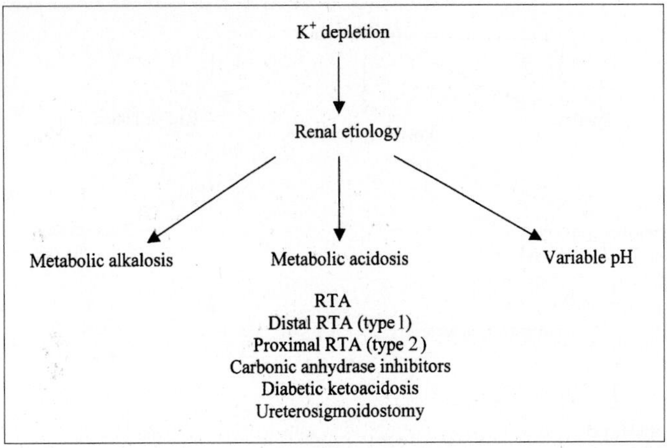

Fig. 6. Flow diagram for the differential diagnosis of potassium depletion of renal cause with metabolic acidosis. RTA, renal tubular acidosis.

Hypocalcemia may present with tetany and occurs with hypoparathyroidism and vitamin D deficiency rickets. Hypercalcemia occurs with vitamin D toxicity, hyperparathyroidism, and some malignancies.

Magnesium

Reference range for plasma magnesium level is 0.75–1.15 mmol/L (1.5–2.3 mEq/L) for newborns, 0.70–0.95 mmol/L (1.4–1.9 mEq/L) for children, and 0.65–1.00 mmol/L (1.3–2.0 mEq/L) for adults. Hypomagnesemia is seen in neonatal tetany, diseases with increased GI fluid loss, and diuretic therapy. Renal magnesium wasting can occur with Gitelman syndrome, a renal tubular disorder in which there is also urinary potassium wasting. Magnesium wasting also can be associated with the use of drugs such as aminoglycosides and *cis* platinum.

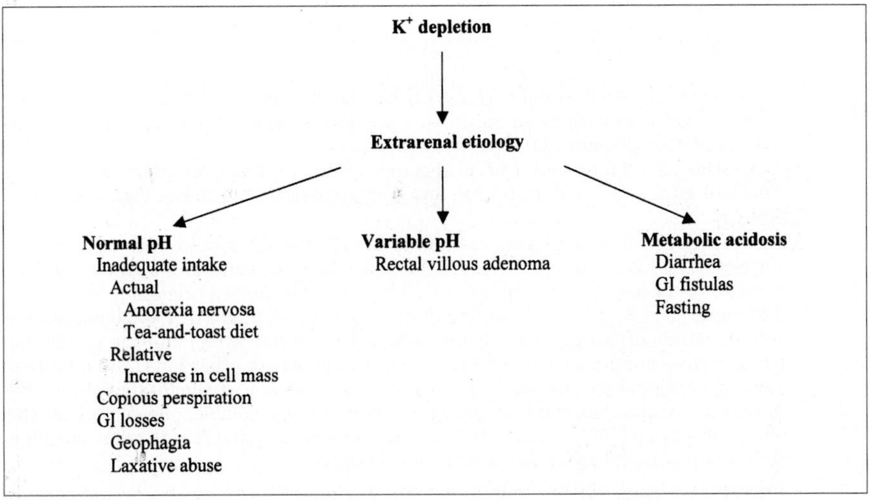

Fig. 7. Flow diagram for the differential diagnosis of potassium depletion of extrarenal cause. GI, gastrointestinal.

Urea

Reference range for plasma urea level is 2–10 mmol/L (5.6–28 mg/dL) for newborns, 1.8–5.4 mmol/L (5–15 mg/dL) for children 1–2 years of age, and 2.9–7.1 mmol/L (8–20 mg/dL) for children 2–16 years of age. Urea is the main nitrogen-containing metabolite of protein catabolism. It is synthesized in the liver from ammonia by hepatic enzymes of the urea cycle. Over 90% is excreted by the kidney. Because of tubular reabsorption of urea, especially in the presence of oliguria, urea clearance underestimates GFR. Although plasma urea level does not give a good reflection of GFR, it does give important metabolic data. It is increased in babies who are fed excessive protein or insufficient water, and in states of acute reversible renal failure from dehydration. It is decreased in infants with urea cycle defects and in infants fed low or no protein. Assessment of the diet of patients with chronic renal failure is aided by knowing the plasma urea value. Each gram of protein leads to the excretion of 0.3 g of urea.

Creatinine

Creatinine is an endogenous product of muscle metabolism. Its rate of production is proportional to muscle mass and it is excreted predominantly by glomerular filtration (90%), with a small and varying component excreted via renal tubular secretion (10%). Under normal circumstances, the rates of production and excretion are fairly constant. The repeated measurement of plasma creatinine concentration is a useful test of GFR. Serum creatinine level normally is 0.5–1.0 mg/dL.

Bicarbonate

Normally 80–90% of filtered bicarbonate is reabsorbed in the proximal tubule. A further 15–50% is reabsorbed distally so that very little bicarbonate escapes into the urine (fractional excretion <5%). In proximal RTA, bicarbonate reabsorption is impaired, which results in an increased fractional excretion of bicarbonate, <10–15%. Proximal RTA most often occurs in conjunction with a generalized proximal tubular disorder. The bicarbonate loading test measures bicarbonate excretion and reabsorption at different filtered loads of bicarbonate. During bicarbonate infusion, plasma and urine bicarbonate and creatinine concentrations are measured and plotted against the plasma bicarbonate to determine the bicarbonate threshold.

Glucose

The proximal tubular glucose concentration is the same as the plasma concentration, as glucose is freely filtered. Ninety percent of filtered glucose is reabsorbed against a concentration gradient in the proximal tubule via a sodium-coupled active transport mechanism. The glucose receptors are saturable. As blood glucose level rises, so does the glucose concentration in the tubular fluid. Proximal glucose reabsorption increases linearly until the receptors are saturated, at which point a maximum value of glucose transport is reached, that is, the tubular maximum. The tubular maximum for adults, children, and infants is 16 mmol/minute/1.73 m^2 (300 mg/minute/1.73m^2) and occurs at a plasma glucose level of 10 mmol/L (180 mg/dL). The normal 24-hour excretion of glucose should be <2.8 mmol/day (0.5 g/day).

Phosphate

Eighty-five percent to 95% of filtered phosphate is reabsorbed by the proximal tubule via an active transport system. The 24-hour excretion of phosphate is diet dependent but averages 10–15% of the filtered load. Thus, a normal tubular reabsorption of phosphate (TRP) is >85% and is calculated as follows:

$$\text{TRP}(\%) = 1 - \frac{\text{UPO}_4}{\text{PPO}_4} \times \frac{\text{PCr}}{\text{UCr}} \times 100$$

where UPO_4 and PPO_4 = urine and plasma phosphate level, respectively, and UCr and PCr = plasma and urine creatinine levels, respectively.

Amino acids

Normally, 85% of filtered amino acids are reabsorbed in the proximal tubule. Fractional clearances for most amino acids are <1%, with the exception of aspartate, serine, glycine, histidine, and taurine, for which clearances range from 2% to 9%. Thus, amounts in excess of 5% of the filtered load are abnormal. Amino aciduria may be generalized and associated with renal Fanconi syndrome. Alternately, it may be due to abnormalities in the transport of neutral amino acids (Hartnup disease), acidic amino acids (benign condition), or cystine (cystinuria) and the basic amino acids (ornithine, arginine, and lysine), which predisposes to urolithiasis. The presence of cystine causes a positive result on the urinary cyanide nitroprusside test.

Chloride

The urinary excretion of chloride is dependent on dietary intake and the state of hydration. With ECF volume contraction, the urinary chloride level will be low [<10 mmol/L (mEq/L)] unless the volume contraction is secondary to diarrhea. With acute diuretic use, chloride level will be high in the presence of ECF volume contraction, as is the case in Bartter syndrome.

Urine pH

The major value of urinary pH measurement is in the detection of bicarbonaturia (pH >7). It is not a reliable indicator of distal ammonium excretion. Once a low distal ammonium excretion is suggested by a positive urine net charge, however, the urine pH will help differentiate low ammonium generation (acid pH) from low distal hydrogen ion secretion (alkaline pH). Urine pH must be measured in a fresh, anaerobically collected sample. This may require urinary catheterization in infants.

Renal Failure, Acute

Acute renal failure is defined as a sudden decrease in renal function, accompanied by the accumulation of nitrogenous wastes within the body. It may be accompanied by anuria, oliguria, or polyuria. The serum creatinine level is increased by ≥0.5 mg/dL or >50% over baseline value, or creatinine clearance is decreased by 50%. Five major clinical syndromes are associated with an acute decline in glomerular filtration and need for dialysis.

Prerenal disorders (approximately 40% of hospital-acquired and approximately 70% of community-acquired cases)

- Hypotension (e.g., shock, sepsis)
- Hypoxia
- Volume contraction (e.g., hemorrhage, dehydration, burns)
- Severe heart failure (e.g., myocardial infarction, cardiac tamponade, pulmonary emboli)
- Respiratory distress syndrome
- Hepatorenal syndrome
- Drug effects (e.g., cyclosporine, amphotericin B)
- Combinations of insults (such as NSAID treatment in the presence of congestive heart failure, aminoglycoside exposure in patients with sepsis, use of radiocontrast agents in patients receiving angiotensin-converting enzyme inhibitors)
- Occlusion of renal artery or vein (due to thrombosis, embolism, severe stenosis, or dissecting aneurysm)

Renal disorders (intrinsic renal disorders)

Congenital renal abnormalities, for example, dysplastic, polycystic kidneys

Acute tubular necrosis

- Acute interstitial nephritis causes approximately 10% of cases.

Drug effects (e.g., methicillin)

Infection

Cancer (e.g., lymphoma, leukemia)

Other (e.g., sarcoidosis)

Toxic agents (approximately 35% of cases)

Heavy metals (e.g., lead mercury, *cis* platinum, arsenic, cadmium, bismuth)

Organic solvents (e.g., carbon tetrachloride, ethylene glycol)

Antibiotics (e.g., aminoglycosides, tetracyclines, penicillins, amphotericin B)

Radiographic contrast media (especially in diabetic persons or those with preexisting renal insufficiency).

Pesticides, fungicides

Other drugs (e.g., phenylbutazone, phenytoin, calcium)

Hemoglobin, myoglobin

Intratubular obstruction (e.g., myeloma light chains; crystals such as uric acid, calcium oxalate; acyclovir, sulfonamide, methotrexate sodium)—5% of cases

Vasculitis

Acute poststreptococcal
SLE
Subacute bacterial endocarditis
Henoch-Schönlein purpura
Goodpasture syndrome
Malignant hypertension
Hemolytic-uremic syndrome
Thrombotic thrombocytopenic purpura
Drug-related vasculitis

- Large-vessel disease
  - Bilateral renal vein occlusion (thrombosis, tumor infiltration)
  - Renal artery occlusion (embolism, thrombosis, stenosis, aortic dissection, trauma to renal arteries)
- Small-vessel disease (malignant hypertension, vasculitis, sickle cell anemia, hemolytic-uremic syndrome, toxemia of pregnancy, scleroderma, atheroembolism, hypercalcemia, transplant rejection)

Postrenal disorders

- Bladder obstruction (e.g., benign prostatic hypertrophy, carcinoma, urethral valves, stricture, trauma)
- Bilateral obstruction of ureters or renal pelves (e.g., carcinoma, calculi, papillary necrosis, blood clots)
- Neurogenic bladder

Early Stage

- Urine is scant in volume (often <50 mL/day) for ≤2 weeks; anuria for >24 hours is unusual. Usually bloody. Specific gravity may be high because RBCs and protein are present. Urine sodium concentration is usually >50 mEq/L.
- BUN rises 20 mg/dL/day in transfusion reaction. It rises 50 mg/dL/day in overwhelming infection or severe crushing injuries.
- Serum creatinine level is increased.

Serum uric acid level is often increased; may be >20 mg/dL in some types (e.g., rhabdomyolysis).
Hypocalcemia may occur.
Disproportionately increased serum phosphorus and creatinine levels indicate tissue necrosis.
Serum amylase and lipase levels may be increased without evidence of pancreatitis.
Metabolic acidosis is present.
WBCs are increased even without infection.

Second Week

- Urine becomes clear several days after onset of acute renal failure, and a small daily increase in volume occurs. Daily volume of 400 mL indicates onset of tubular recovery. Daily volume of 1,000 mL occurs in several days or ≤2 weeks. RBCs and large hematin casts are present. Protein is slight or absent.
- Azotemia increases. BUN level continues to rise for several days after onset of diuresis.

Metabolic acidosis increases.
Serum potassium is increased. Electrocardiographic changes are always found when serum potassium is >9 mEq/L but are rarely found when it is <7 mEq/L.
Anemia usually appears during second week.
Bleeding tendency is frequent, with decreased platelet counts, abnormal prothrombin consumption, and so on.

Diuretic Stage

High urinary potassium excretion may cause decreased serum potassium level.
Urine sodium concentration is 50–75 mEq/L.
Serum sodium and chloride levels may increase because of dehydration from diuresis if replacement of water is inadequate.

Hypercalcemia may occur in some patients with muscle damage.
Azotemia disappears 1–3 weeks after onset of diuresis.

Later Findings

Anemia may persist for weeks or months.
Pyelonephritis may first occur during this stage.
Renal blood flow and GFR do not usually become completely normal.
Recovery from renal necrosis complicating pregnancy may be followed by renal calcification, contraction of kidneys, and death from malignant hypertension in 1–2 years.

Urinary Diagnostic Indices in Acute Renal Failure

See Tables 18 and 19.
Urinary sodium levels between 20 and 40 mEq/L may be found in all forms of acute renal failure.

$$FE_{Na} = 100 \times \frac{\text{(urine sodium/plasma sodium)}}{\text{(urine creatinine/plasma creatinine)}}$$

Urine sodium level is an index of renal ability to conserve sodium and represents percentage of filtered sodium to reach the urine. It is considered the most reliable test to distinguish prerenal azotemia from acute tubular necrosis with oliguria.
Causes of FE_{Na} <1%

- Prerenal azotemia
- Acute GN
- Early acute urinary tract obstruction (first few hours)
- Early sepsis
- Some cases of acute tubular necrosis due to radiographic contrast material or myoglobinuria due to rhabdomyolysis
- Ten percent of cases of nonoliguric acute tubular necrosis

Some causes of FE_{Na} >1% (injured tubules)

- 90% of cases of acute tubular necrosis
- Later urinary tract obstruction (days to months)
- Diuretic administration
- Preexisting chronic renal failure
- Diuresis due to mannitol, glycosuria, or bicarbonaturia

Renal failure index = urine sodium/(urine creatinine/plasma creatinine); measures sodium conservation and concentrating ability.
Indices (especially renal failure index and FE_{Na}) are chiefly of value in oliguric patients for the early differentiation of prerenal azotemia from acute tubular necrosis.
Values ≤1 for renal failure index and FE_{Na} suggest prerenal azotemia and values ≥3 suggest acute tubular necrosis; values of 1–3 are less definitive; values for nonoli-

Table 18. Dehydration and Decreased Renal Perfusion versus Acute Renal Failure

	Dehydration/Reduced Perfusion		Acute Renal Failure	
	Child	Newborn	Child	Newborn
U_{Na} (mEq/L)	<10	≤20	>50	>50
FE_{Na} (%)	≤1	≤2.5	>2	>3
U_{Osm}	≥500	≥350	≤300	≤300
U/P_{Osm}	≥1.5	≥1.2	0.8–1.2	0.8–1.2
BUN/creatinine	>20	>10	Both ↑	Both ↑
Fluid push	Urine ↑	Urine ↑	No change	No change

↑, increased; BUN, blood urea nitrogen; FE_{Na}, fractional excretion of sodium = 100 × [(urine sodium concentration/plasma sodium concentration)/(urine creatinine level/plasma creatinine level)]; U_{Na}, urine sodium concentration; U_{Osm}, urine osmolality; U/P_{Osm}, urine/plasma osmolality.

Table 19. Urinary Diagnostic Indices in Acute Renal Failure

	Prerenal Azotemia	Postrenal (Acute Obstructive)	Acute GN and Vasculitis	Acute Interstitial Nephritis	Acute Tubular Necrosis		Renal Vascular Occlusion	
					Oliguric	Nonoliguric	Arterial	Venous
Urine volume (mL/24 hr)	~500[a]	Usually <500; fluctuates from day to day	<500	Var	<350	1,000–2,000	Var Anuria if bilateral/complete	Var
Urine specific gravity	H (>1.015)	—	—	—	L; <1.010	—	—	—
Urine osmolality (mOsm/kg H_2O)	>500	Var; usually <500	<500	Var	<350	350	Var	Var
Urine sodium (mEq/L)	L;<20	H;>40	L; usually <20	Var	>40	Var	Var	Var
U/P osmolality	>1.5	<1.2	—	—	<1.2	<1.2	—	—
U/P urea nitrogen	>8	Usually >8	>8	—	<3	<8	—	—
U/P creatinine	>40	<20	>40	—	<20	<20	—	—
Renal failure index	<1 (90% of cases)	>2 (95% of cases)	<1	—	>2 (95% of cases)	>3	—	—
FE_{Na}	<1 (≤94% of cases)	>1	<1	Var	>1	>1	Var	Var
BUN/creatinine ratio	>20:1	>20:1	>20:1	>20:1	>20:1	>20:1	>20:1	>20:1
Urine sediment	Hyaline casts	N; RBCs, WBCs, crystals may be present	RBCs, RBC casts	WBCs, WBC casts, eosinophils	Granular casts, renal tubular epithelial cells, cell debris, pigment, crystals		Var	Var
Comments	Decreased renal perfusion	Evidence of GU tract obstruction	Biopsy findings classify disease	Eosinophilia, thrombocytopenia	Renal hypoperfusion, nephrotoxin	Nephrotoxin	Aortic injury, atheromatous emboli	Renal vein occlusion with nephrotic syndrome

BUN, blood urea nitrogen; FE_{Na}, fractional excretion of sodium; GN, glomerulonephritis; GU, genitourinary; H, high; L, low; N, normal; RBC, red blood cell; U/P, urine/plasma ratio; Var, variable; WBC, white blood cell.

[a]Polyuria may be present.

From Andreoli TE et al., eds. *Cecil essentials of medicine*, 2nd ed. Philadelphia: WB Saunders, 1990:212; Okun DE. On the differential diagnosis of acute renal failure. *Am J Med* 1981;71:916; Schrier RW. Acute renal failure: pathogenesis, diagnosis, and management. *Hosp Pract* March 1981:93; and Miller TR, Anderson RJ, Linas SL, et al. Urinary diagnostic indices in acute renal failure: a prospective study. *Ann Intern Med* 1978;89:47.

guric acute renal failure frequently are intermediate between those for prerenal azotemia and oliguric renal failure.

Values are usually >1 in cases of urinary obstruction or acute interstitial nephritis; values are usually <1 in acute GN.

Diagnostic indices for patients with reversible acute obstructive uropathy often resemble indices for patients with acute tubular necrosis or prerenal azotemia; indices for patients with obstructive uropathy depend on duration of obstruction and severity of azotemia.

Interferences

Specimens used to compute urinary indices should be obtained before onset of treatment if possible; several therapies may make results uninterpretable, especially administration of dopamine, mannitol or other diuretics, glucose, or radiographic contrast material. A timed 12- to 24-hour urine specimen need not be obtained. In patients with acute renal failure, urine sodium level and osmolality cannot vary significantly from hour to hour; a randomly collected specimen is sufficient.

Urine Sediment in Acute Renal Failure

Examination of the urine sediment is crucial in evaluating the patient with acute renal failure. A sediment containing renal tubular epithelial cells (or cellular casts) and pigmented granular casts with hematuria and proteinuria supports a diagnosis of acute tubular necrosis. RBC casts are found in GN. Leukocyturia, especially with eosinophiluria, supports a diagnosis of interstitial nephritis. Detection of eosinophils in the urine sediment after Wright staining is considered a useful indicator of acute interstitial nephritis. The use of Hansel stain greatly enhances the recognition of urinary eosinophils. Dipstick-detected hematuria without cellular elements on microscopy is suggestive of hemoglobinuria or myoglobinuria. In acute renal failure, urinary sodium concentration differentiates between prerenal causes [Na <10 mmol/L (10 mEq/L)] and intrinsic renal disease (Na >20 mmol/L). Urine sodium concentration may also be used to assess the adequacy of fluid replacement in the volume-contracted patient. Once the ECF space is replete, urinary sodium level will begin to rise. With intrinsic renal disease, the urinary sodium level is a guide to the appropriate sodium concentrations of replacement fluid.

Present in approximately 80% of patients; urine sodium is >20 mEq/L.

Sediment may be normal in cases with prerenal or postrenal causes with minimal or absent proteinuria. Eosinophils, increased WBCs and WBC casts, minimal proteinuria may be found in acute interstitial nephritis. RBC casts indicate GN, vasculitis, or microembolic disease. Myoglobin casts indicate myoglobinuria. WBCs in hyaline casts indicate renal parenchymal infection rather than lower GU tract infection.

In a patient with two functioning kidneys, obstruction of only one ureter should cause serum creatinine to rise to 2 mg/dL; acute renal failure that is postrenal with creatinine level of >2 mg/dL suggests that obstruction is bilateral or that patient has only one functioning kidney.

Total anuria for >2 days is uncommon in acute tubular necrosis and should suggest other possibilities (e.g., ruptured bladder, urinary tract obstruction, micro- or large-vessel disease, renal cortical necrosis, GN, allergic interstitial nephritis).

Dehydration in Patients with Renal Failure

Assessment of fluid status

- Examine pulse and blood pressure, orthostatic pulse and blood pressure, body weight, skin turgor, capillary refill, cardiac status (congestive heart failure), pulmonary edema, peripheral edema, mental status.
- Patients with peripheral edema can still be intravascularly depleted.
- Check serum levels of electrolytes, BUN, and creatinine, and osmolality; check urine levels of electrolytes and creatinine, osmolality.

The normal response of a kidney to dehydration is to conserve water and sodium to maintain intravascular volume; in renal failure, the kidney loses its ability to conserve sodium and to concentrate the urine.

Urine Concentration

Specific gravity in a randomly obtained urine sample of ≥1.023 indicates intact concentrating ability within the limits of clinical testing; no further tests are indicated. Use of a first-voided specimen after overnight fast is adequate to test concentrating ability.

Urine Osmolality

Measurement of urine osmolality during water restriction is an accurate, sensitive test of decreased renal function.

Normal: concentration >800 mOsm/kg.

Hypervolemia: 400–600 mOsm/kg.

Syndrome of inappropriate secretion of antidiuretic hormone: 200–300 mOsm/kg.

Severe impairment: <400 mOsm/kg.

Causes of Acute Renal Failure[6]

Prerenal

- Hypovolemia
  - Hemorrhage
  - GI losses
  - Hypoproteinemia
  - Burns
- Adrenal disease with salt wasting
- Shock
  - Septicemia
  - Disseminated intravascular coagulation
  - Hypothermia
  - Hemorrhage
  - Heart failure
- Hypoxia
  - Pneumonia
  - Aortic clamping
  - Respiratory distress syndrome

Renal

- GN
  - Poststreptococcal
  - SLE related
  - Membranoproliferative
  - Idiopathic rapidly progressive
- Henoch-Schönlein purpura
  - Localized intravascular coagulation
  - Renal vein thrombosis
    - Cortical necrosis
  - Hemolytic-uremic syndrome
- Acute tubular necrosis
  - Heavy metals
  - Chemicals
  - Drugs
  - Hemoglobin, myoglobin
  - Hereditary nephritis
  - Acute interstitial nephritis
  - Infection
  - Drugs
- Tumors
  - Renal parenchymal infiltration
  - Uric acid nephropathy
- Developmental abnormalities
  - Cystic disease
  - Hypoplasia-dysplasia

Postrenal

- Obstructive uropathy
  - Ureteropelvic junction
  - Ureterocele
  - Urethral valves
  - Tumor
- Vesicoureteral reflux
- Acquired
  - Stones
  - Blood clot

Azotemia, Prerenal

Prerenal azotemia is caused by hypotension, hypovolemia, or inadequate renal perfusion such as may occur with hemorrhage or congestive heart failure. Physiologic responses result in a reduction in GFR and increased tubular reabsorption of salt and water. Restoration of adequate circulating volume reverses the acute renal failure.

Azotemia, Postrenal (Obstructive Uropathy)

Postrenal azotemia results from obstruction in the collecting system and may be due to intratubular obstruction (e.g., methotrexate sodium, uric acid) or to extrinsic compression (e.g., tumor). Relief of the obstruction restores GFR to normal.

Glomerulonephritis, Acute

Acute GN results in a diminished GFR due to vascular inflammation. The most common lesions in children are acute poststreptococcal nephritis and hemolytic-uremic syndrome. Recovery of renal failure depends on the underlying disease process.

Hemolytic-Uremic Syndrome

Hemolytic-uremic syndrome is based on a microangiopathic hemolytic anemia, thrombocytopenia, and acute renal failure with hematuria and proteinuria. Levels of liver

[6]From Behrman RE, Kliegman R, Jenson HB. *Nelson textbook of pediatrics*, 16th ed. Philadelphia: WB Saunders, 2000.

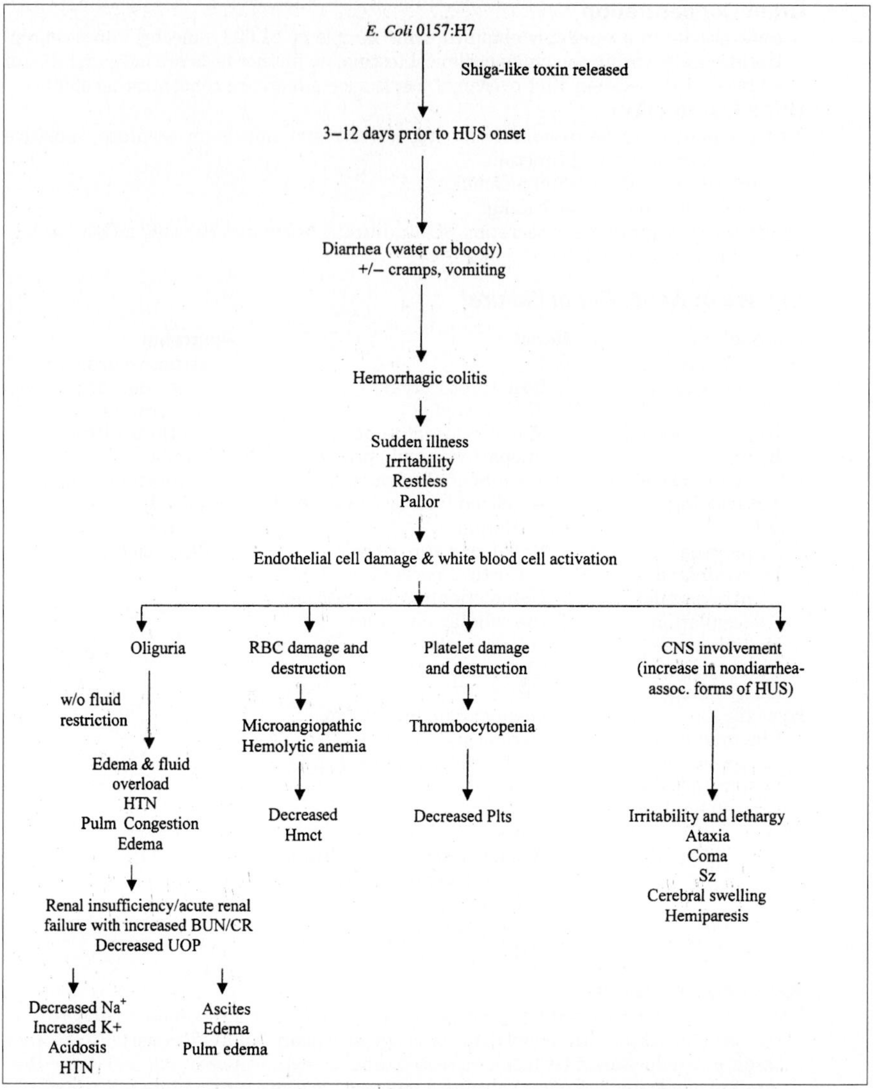

Fig. 8. Signs and symptoms of hemolytic-uremic syndrome (HUS). BUN, blood urea nitrogen; CNS, central nervous system; CR, creatinine; Hmct, hematocrit; HTN, hypertension; Plts, platelets; Pulm, pulmonary; RBC, red blood cell; Sz, seizure; UOP, urinary output.

transferases and serum amylase may be increased, with biochemical abnormalities of acute renal failure. Therapy is supportive with early institution of dialysis.

Signs and Symptoms

See Fig. 8.

Hepatorenal Syndrome

Usually appears in patients with laboratory findings of decompensated cirrhosis with moderate to marked ascites, especially after fluid loss (e.g., GI hemorrhage, diarrhea, forced diuresis).

Hyponatremia, hyperkalemia, hepatic encephalopathy, coma may be present.

Must be differentiated from renal failure due to toxins, drugs (e.g., NSAIDs, acetaminophen, carbon tetrachloride); infection; acute tubular necrosis; obstructive nephropathy.

Oliguria is marked.

Progressive azotemia (serum creatinine >2.5 mg/dL).

Urine sodium is decreased to almost absent (<10 mEq/L; often 1–2 mEq/L). Urine is acid, concentrated, with high specific gravity and urine/plasma osmolality ratio >1.0, and a small amount of protein. Few hyaline and granular casts, few RBCs (<50/hpf) may be found.

Urine indices resemble those of prerenal azotemia and contrast with acute tubular necrosis, in which urine has low fixed specific gravity and high sodium content and a characteristic sediment may be found.

Nephritis, Interstitial, Acute

Acute interstitial nephritis causes a decrease in GFR because of interstitial inflammation. It is seen frequently in nonoliguric renal failure, is often related to drugs or toxins, and is more common in adults.

Renovascular Disease, Acute

For renovascular disease to cause acute renal failure, it must be a bilateral process or occur in a solitary kidney. A common cause in infants is renal vein thrombosis.

Tubular Necrosis, Acute

Acute tubular necrosis occurs as a result of hypoperfusion, a nephrotoxic injury, or a combination of the two. Removal of the insult does not result in immediate improvement in renal function.

Renal Failure, Chronic

Chronic renal insufficiency is defined as a serum creatinine level of 1.5–3.0 mg/dL.

Chronic renal failure is defined as a serum creatinine level of >3.0 mg/dL.

BUN is increased, and renal function tests show impairment.

Creatinine clearance levels:

>30 mL/min/1.73 m^2	Usually asymptomatic
<30 mL/min/1.73 m^2	Usually symptomatic
<15 mL/min/1.73 m^2	Metabolic disturbances requiring intervention
<5 mL/min/1.73 m^2	End-stage renal disease requiring dialysis and transplantation

Loss of renal concentrating ability (nocturia, polyuria, polydipsia) is an early manifestation of progressive renal functional impairment. Abnormal urinalysis results are usually the first finding. Variable abnormalities include proteinuria, hematuria, pyuria, and presence of granular and cellular casts, and may be found in asymptomatic patients.

Serum sodium level is decreased with increased urine sodium levels (>5–10 mEq sodium/L).

Serum potassium level is increased with increased loss in urine (>15–20 mEq/L). Occurs in primary aldosteronism and may also occur in malignant hypertension, tubular acidosis, Fanconi syndrome, nephrocalcinosis, diuresis during recovery from tubular necrosis.

Acidosis is present due to renal failure to secrete acid as NH_4^+ and to reabsorb filtered bicarbonate, and to decreased production of tubular bicarbonate.

Serum calcium level is decreased. Secondary parathyroid hyperplasia may occur, but hypercalcemia is not found.

Serum phosphorus level increases when creatinine clearance falls to approximately 25 mL/minute.

Serum alkaline phosphatase may be normal or may be increased with renal osteodystrophy.

Serum uric acid level is increased but is usually <10 mg/dL.

Increased serum amylase occurs frequently.

Serum creatine kinase level may be increased; uremic patients may have a persistently increased creatine kinase MB fraction is present without evidence of cardiac disease.

Increased serum levels of triglycerides, cholesterol, and very-low-density lipoproteins (pre-β) are common as renal failure progresses.
Blood levels of organic acids, phenols, indoles, and homocysteine are increased.
Normochromic normocytic anemia is usually proportionate to the degree of azotemia.
Bleeding tendency is evident. GI hemorrhage from ulcers anywhere in GI tract may be severe.
Laboratory findings due to uremic pericarditis, pleuritis, and pancreatitis are noted. (BUN is usually >100 mg/dL).
Serum albumin and total protein are decreased.

Chronic Renal Failure with Normal Urine May Occur in

Nephrosclerosis (e.g., aging, hypertension)
Renal tubular acidosis
Interstitial nephritis
Hypercalcemia
Potassium deficiency
Uric acid nephropathy
Obstruction (including retroperitoneal fibrosis)

Dialysis

Indications

Uremia
Progressive metabolic encephalopathy
Uncontrolled hyperkalemia
Pericarditis
Intractable fluid overload
Poisoning with chemicals and drugs (of limited use because of large volume of distributions)

Techniques

Peritoneal dialysis: may be used short as well as long term, as in continuous ambulatory or continuous cycling peritoneal dialysis.
Hemodialysis: requires placement of special vascular access devices. May be the method of choice with exposure to certain toxins (e.g., ammonia, uric acid, or poisons) or when there are contraindications to peritoneal dialysis.
Continuous arteriovenous hemofiltration and hemodialysis and continuous venovenous hemofiltration and hemodialysis: these are therapies with the primary goal of continuous generation of a plasma ultrafiltrate. Indications include fluid management, renal failure with profound hemodynamic instability, electrolyte disturbance, and intoxication with substances that are freely filtered across the particular ultrafiltration membrane used. Continuous arteriovenous and continuous venovenous hemofiltration and hemodialysis can be helpful in the management of oliguric patients who are in need of better nutritional support, postoperative cardiac patients, and patients with septicemia. These therapies also require special vascular access devices.

Transplantation of Kidney

Before transplantation, the donor is selected.
Three successive urinalysis and culture results must be negative.
Donor and recipient must show
- ABO and Rh blood group compatibility
- Leukoagglutinin compatibility
- Platelet agglutinin compatibility

After transplantation, rejection is suspected if
- Total urine output decreases, proteinuria increases.
- Cellular or granular casts appear, urine osmolality is decreased.

- BUN and creatinine levels increase.
- Hyperchloremic RTA may be an early sign of rejection or indicate smoldering rejection activity.
- Renal clearance values decrease, renogram obtained with iodohippurate sodium tagged with iodine 131 shows alteration, and kidney biopsy specimen shows a characteristic microscopic appearance allowing definitive diagnosis.

Bibliography

Birch DE, et al. *A color atlas of urine microscopy.* London: Chapman & Hall Medical, 1994.

Cilento B, Stock J, Kaplan G. Hematuria in children: a practical approach. *Urol Clin North Am* 1995;22:43.

Cruz C, Spitzer A. When you find protein or blood in urine. *Contemp Pediatr* 1998;15(9):89.

Feigin RD, Cherry JD, eds. *Textbook of pediatric infectious diseases*, 3rd ed. Philadelphia: WB Saunders, 1992:483.

Fitzwater D, Wyatt R. Hematuria. *Pediatr Rev* 1994;15:102.

Greenhill A, Gruskin AB. Laboratory evaluation of renal function. *Pediatr Clin North Am* 1976;23:661.

Hellerstein S. Urinary tract infections: old and new concepts. *Pediatr Clin North Am* 1995;42:1143.

Henry JB. *Clinical diagnosis and management by laboratory methods*. Philadelphia: WB Saunders, 1984.

Holliday MA, Barratt TM, Avner ED. *Pediatric nephrology.* Baltimore: Williams & Wilkins, 1994.

Netter FH, Shapter RK, Yonkman FF. *The CIBA collection of medical illustrations*, vol 6. Summit, NJ: Ciba Pharmaceutical Products, 1973:80.

Norman ME. An office approach to hematuria and proteinuria. *Pediatr Clin North Am* 1987;34:545.

Rushton H. Urinary tract infections in children: epidemiology, evaluation and management. *Pediatr Clin North Am* 1997;44:5.

Sadowski R, Falkner B. Hypertension in pediatric patients. *Am J Kidney Dis* 1996;27:3.

Schwartz GJ, Brion LP, Spitzer A. The use of plasma creatinine concentration for estimating glomerular filtration rate in infants, children, and adolescents. *Pediatr Clin North Am* 1987;34:571.

Sinaiko A. Hypertension in children. *N Engl J Med* 1996;335:26.

Wallach J. *Interpretation of diagnostic tests*, 7th ed. Philadelphia: Lippincott Williams & Wilkins, 2000.

20 Nutritional Diseases

Biotin Metabolism Disorders

- Biotinidase deficiency
- Holocarboxylase synthase deficiency

Clinical Symptoms

Neurologic symptoms, developmental delay, skeletal myopathy, failure to thrive, ophthalmologic disorders, deafness, alopecia, dermatologic abnormalities, immunologic abnormalities, hypoglycemia, metabolic acidosis or hyperammonemia, ataxia

Diagnostic Studies

Amino acid studies in blood and urine. Organic acid analysis in blood or urine or both. Carnitine quantitation in blood or urine or both. Carnitine species identification.

Definitive Diagnosis

Enzymatic assay or DNA analysis or both.

These are metabolic errors. Nutritional biotin deficiency is extremely rare—seen after consuming raw egg white that contains avidin, a biotin antagonist.

Deficiency, Copper, Nutritional

Found in patients on total parenteral nutrition (TPN) and in neonates, premature infants, and children recovering from severe protein-calorie malnutrition fed iron-fortified milk formula with cane sugar and cottonseed oil.

Microcytic anemia not responsive to iron and vitamins.

Low serum albumin level.

Leukopenia with white blood cell (WBC) count $<5{,}000/mm^3$ and neutropenia ($<1{,}500/mm^3$).

Copper administration corrects neutropenia in 3 weeks and anemia responds with reticulocytosis.

Decreased copper and ceruloplasmin in plasma and decreased hepatic copper confirm diagnosis.

Serum Copper Increased In

Anemias
- Pernicious anemia
- Megaloblastic anemia of pregnancy
- Iron-deficiency anemia
- Aplastic anemia

Leukemia, acute and chronic

Infection, acute and chronic

Malignant lymphoma

Biliary cirrhosis

Hemochromatosis

Collagen diseases (including systemic lupus erythematosus, rheumatoid arthritis, acute rheumatic fever, glomerulonephritis)

Hypothyroidism
Hyperthyroidism
Frequently associated with increased levels of C-reactive protein
Ingestion of oral contraceptives and estrogens
Pregnancy

Deficiency, Folate

Macrocytic or megaloblastic anemia
Neural tube defects in offspring of folate-deficient (or metabolically deficient) mothers

Diagnostic Studies

Serum folate level

Deficiency, Niacin (Pellagra)

Whole blood niacin level <24 µmol/L
Decreased excretion of niacin metabolites (nicotinamide) in 6- or 24-hour urine sample
Plasma tryptophan level elevated or decreased

Deficiency, Riboflavin

Decreased riboflavin level in plasma, red blood cells (RBCs), WBCs.
RBC glutathione reductase activity coefficient is ≥1.20.

Deficiency, Thiamine (Beriberi)

Increased blood pyruvic acid level.
Laboratory findings due to complications (e.g., heart failure).
Laboratory findings due to underlying conditions (e.g., chronic diarrhea, inadequate intake, alcoholism).
Decreased thiamine level in blood and urine; becomes normal within 24 hours after therapy begins (thus baseline levels should be established first).
RBC transketolase <8 U (baseline), addition of thiamine pyrophosphate causes >20% increase.

Deficiency, Vitamin A

Nyctalopia, optic abnormalities, increased infection
Decreased plasma level of vitamin A

Deficiency, Vitamin B_6 (Pyridoxine)

Decreased pyridoxic acid level in urine
Decreased serum levels of vitamin B_6
Microcytic anemia
Urine xanthurenic acid

Deficiency, Vitamin B_{12} and Folic Acid

See Table 1.

Deficiency, Vitamin C (Scurvy)

Rumpel-Leede test gives positive result.
Microscopic hematuria is present in one-third of patients.
Stool may give positive results for occult blood.

Table 1. Laboratory Tests in Differential Diagnosis of Vitamin B_{12} and Folic Acid Deficiencies

	Vitamin B_{12} Deficiency	Folate Deficiency	Vitamin B_{12} and Folate Deficiency
Serum folate	N or I	D	D
Serum vitamin B_{12}	D	N or D	D
Red blood cell folate	N or D	D	D
Methylmalonic acid	I	N	I
Homocysteine	I	I	I

D, decreased; I, increased; N, normal.

Laboratory findings due to associated deficiencies (e.g., anemia due to folic acid deficiency).

Plasma level of ascorbic acid is decreased—usually 0 in frank scurvy. (Normal level is 0.5–1.5 mg/dL, but lower level does not prove diagnosis.) Ascorbic acid in buffy coat (WBC) is decreased—usually absent in clinical scurvy. (Normal level is 30 mg/dL.)

Tyrosyl compounds (phenols) are present in urine (detected by Millon reagent) in patients with scurvy but are absent in normal persons after protein consumption and administration of tyrosine.

Deficiency (or Excess), Vitamin D

1,25-Dihydroxyvitamin D

Formed from 25-hydroxyvitamin D by kidney, placenta, granulomas

Use

Differential diagnosis of hypocalcemic disorders
Monitoring of patients with renal osteodystrophy

Increased In

Hyperparathyroidism
Chronic granulomatous disorders
Hypercalcemia associated with lymphoma

Decreased In

Vitamin D deficiency
Hypercalcemia of malignancy (except lymphoma)
Tumor-induced osteomalacia
Hypoparathyroidism
Pseudohypoparathyroidism
Renal osteodystrophy
Type I vitamin D–resistant rickets

25-Hydroxyvitamin D

Use

Evaluation of vitamin D intoxication or deficiency

Increased In

Vitamin D intoxication (distinguishes this from other causes of hypercalcemia)

Decreased In

Rickets
Osteomalacia
Secondary hyperparathyroidism
Malabsorption of vitamin D (e.g., severe liver disease, cholestasis)
Diseases that increase vitamin D metabolism (e.g., tuberculosis, sarcoidosis, primary hyperparathyroidism)

Hydroxylase Deficiencies and Disorders of Vitamin D Resistance

- 1-α,25- and 25-hydroxylase deficiencies (autosomal recessive)
- Resistance to 1,25-dihydroxyvitamin D (groups of genetic disorders)

Clinical Symptoms

Skeletal abnormalities, rickets, failure to thrive, growth failure

Diagnostic Studies

Serum alkaline phosphatase (high), serum calcium (low or normal), phosphate (very low)

Identification and quantitation of vitamin D and its metabolites in blood, parathyroid hormone assay

Definitive Diagnosis

Enzyme assay or DNA analysis or both

Hypophosphatemic Rickets (Vitamin D–Resistant Rickets)

Clinical Symptoms

Skeletal abnormalities, growth failure (often familial), skeletal myopathy

Diagnostic Studies

Serum calcium (low normal), phosphate (low), alkaline phosphate (low-high)

Assessments of renal phosphate transport, calciferol metabolites in plasma

Imaging Studies

Radiography (wrist, knee, or ankle)

Definitive Diagnosis

DNA analysis

Deficiency, Vitamin E

Hemolytic anemia, ceroid deposition in muscle fat.

Plasma tocopherol <0.4 mg/dL, in adults; <0.15 mg/dL in infants aged 1 month.

Laboratory findings due to underlying conditions (e.g., malabsorption in adults; diet high in polyunsaturated fatty acids in premature infants).

Rose-Györgyi hemolysis test gives positive result.

Deficiency, Vitamin K

See Table 2.

Due to a variety of transient defects in clotting; more commonly seen in low-birth-weight premature infants and anoxic or septic neonates, liver disease.

Prothrombin time is markedly increased.

Partial thromboplastin time is increased.

Table 2. Comparison of Hemorrhagic Diseases of the Newborn

Test	Hemorrhagic Disease of the Newborn Due to Vitamin K Deficiency	Secondary Hemorrhagic Disease of the Newborn
Capillary fragility	Normal	Usually abnormal
Bleeding time	Normal	Often increased
Clotting time	Increased	Variable
One-stage prothrombin	Marked increase (≤5%)	Moderate increase (usually 5–25%)
Factor V	Normal	Often decreased (<50%)
Fibrinogen	Normal	Occasionally marked decrease
Platelet count	Normal	Occasionally decreased
Response to vitamin K	Improvement in clotting factors appears in 2–4 hr; almost complete correction in 24 hr	Little or no response

Coagulation time is increased.
Bleeding time is normal; may be slightly increased.
Capillary fragility, prothrombin consumption, and platelet count are normal.
Laboratory findings due to blood loss.

Deficiency, Zinc

Causes

- Acrodermatitis enteropathica (rare autosomal-recessive disease of infancy due to block in intestinal absorption of zinc)
- Inadequate nutrition (e.g., parenteral alimentation)
- Decreased absorption or availability
- Increased losses
- Iatrogenic causes
- Copper administration

Laboratory Findings

Plasma zinc levels do not always reflect nutritional status.
Findings of decreased or very excessive urinary zinc excretion may be helpful.
Plasma, RBC, or WBC zinc levels are insensitive markers for zinc status.
Plasma concentrations
- Normal range = 70–120 μg/dL
- Moderate depletion = 40–60 μg/dL
- Severe depletion = 20 μg/dL

Failure to Thrive

Causes

	% of Cases
Inadequate caloric intake	87.0
Maternal deprivation (e.g., caloric restriction, child abuse, emotional disorders)	
Congenital abnormalities (e.g., cleft lip or palate, tracheoesophageal fistula, esophageal webs, macroglossia, achalasia)	
Acquired abnormalities (e.g., esophageal stricture, subdural hematoma, hypoxia, diabetes insipidus)	
Increased use of calories	3.0
Infant of narcotic-addicted mother	
Prolonged fever (e.g., chronic infections)	
Excessive crying	
Congenital heart disease	
Decreased intestinal function	
Abnormal digestion, e.g.,	3.0
Cystic fibrosis	
Trypsin deficiency	
Mono- and disaccharidase deficiencies	
Abnormal absorption, e.g.,	0.5
Celiac syndrome	
Gastroenteritis	
Biliary atresia	
Megacolon	
Giardiasis	
Protein-losing enteropathy	
Renal loss of calories	
Chronic renal disease, e.g.,	0.5
Renal tubular acidosis	
Pyelonephritis	
Polycystic disease	
Congenital or acquired nephritis	

Congenital nephrosis
Nephrogenic diabetes insipidus

Other 6.0

Anemia
- Fetal-maternal transfusion
- Hemoglobinopathies
- Iron deficiency

Hypercalcemia

Hyperparathyroidism
- Vitamin A or D intoxication
- Idiopathic

Endocrine abnormalities
- Hypothyroidism
- Hypoadrenalism
- Hyposomatotropism
- Congenital hyperthyroidism

Metabolic abnormalities
- Glycogen storage disease
- Galactosemia, amino aciduria
- Hypophosphatasia
- Mucopolysaccharidosis
- Rickets

Central nervous system lesions
- Subdural hematoma
- Intracerebral hemorrhage
- Tumors

Congenital abnormalities
- Congenital heart disease
- Chromosomal abnormalities
- Ectodermal dysplasia

Unknown

Diagnostic Studies

Initial tests
- Pathologic examination of placenta for intrauterine growth retardation
- Complete blood count (anemia, hemoglobinopathy)
- Urine—test for urine-reducing substances, ferric chloride test, pH, specific gravity, microscopic examination, colony count, and bacterial culture
- Stool—occult blood, ova and parasites, pH
- Serum—levels of sodium, potassium, chloride, bicarbonate, creatinine, calcium, immunoglobulin G, immunoglobulin A

More detailed tests
- Sweat chloride level
- Serum thyroid-stimulating hormone and thyroxine (hypothyroidism)
- Serum and urine amino acid levels (amino acidurias)
- Tuberculin test
- Serologic tests for congenital infection (rubella, cytomegalovirus infection, toxoplasmosis, syphilis)
- Duodenal enzyme measurements
- Chromosomal studies

Premature infants (shortened gestational period) should be differentiated from infants whose weight is below that expected for gestational age.

Intrauterine Growth Retardation

Causes

Chronic hypertension, especially with renal involvement and proteinuria
Chronic renal disease
Severe diabetes mellitus
Preeclampsia and eclampsia with underlying chronic vascular disease

Hypoxia, for example,
- Cyanotic heart disease
- Pregnancy at high altitudes
- Hemoglobinopathies, especially sickle cell disease

Maternal protein-calorie malnutrition

Placental conditions
- Extensive infarction
- Parabiotic transfusion syndrome
- Hemangioma of placenta or cord
- Abnormal cord insertion

Fetal factors
- Chromosomal abnormalities
- Malformations of gastrointestinal tract that interfere with swallowing
- Chronic intrauterine infections (e.g., rubella, cytomegalovirus and herpesvirus infection, syphilis, toxoplasmosis)

Unexplained
- No specific diagnostic laboratory tests are available.

Initial Tests

- Pathologic examination of placenta, complete blood count

Malnutrition, Protein-Calorie (Kwashiorkor)

Occurs in patients with inadequate protein intake in presence of low caloric intake, or normal caloric intake and increased catabolism (e.g., trauma, severe burns, respiratory or renal failure, nonmalignant gastrointestinal tract disease); may develop quickly. Major loss of protein from visceral compartments may impair organ function.

Decreased serum albumin (2.1–3.0 g/dL in moderate deficiencies, <2.1 g/dL in severe deficiencies.

Decreased serum prealbumin (transthyretin) is a more sensitive measure than decreased albumin due to shorter half-life (normal range is 18–36 mg/dL; severe malnutrition is <10.7 mg/dL; moderate malnutrition is 10.7–16.0 mg/dL). With therapy, increases >1 mg/dL daily. Other proteins with short half-lives are retinol-binding protein and fibronectin. Effective in monitoring growth rate in preterm infants. Also decreased in impaired liver function (e.g., hepatitis, cirrhosis, obstructive jaundice) and some types of amyloidosis.

Decreased serum transferrin (150–200 mg/dL in mild, 100–150 mg/dL in moderate, <100 mg/dL in severe deficiencies) or transferrin iron-binding concentration. Increase in transferrin due to inflammation decreases diagnostic utility.

All serum complement components except C4 and sometimes C5 are decreased.

Decreased total lymphocyte count evidencing diminished immunologic resistance (2,000–3,500/mm^3 is normal; <1,500/mm^3 is indication for further assessment; 800–1,200/mm^3 is moderate; <800/mm^3 is severe; should always be interpreted with total WBC count).

Diminished delayed hypersensitivity reaction (measure by skin testing).

Essential amino acids (serum) decreased.

Vitamin and mineral serum levels decreased.

Normal anthropometric measurements (e.g., weight and height, triceps skinfold, arm circumference measurements).

Marasmus

Chronic deficiency in total energy and protein intake as in wasting illnesses (e.g., cancer).

Normal serum protein levels.

Impaired immune function.

Clinically, patient shows severe wasting of skeletal muscle and fat; edema rare. May progress to marasmic kwashiorkor.

Laboratory findings due to underlying diseases (e.g., cancer) or complications (e.g., infections).

Monitoring of Nutritional Therapy

Weekly 24-hour urine nitrogen excretion reflects degree of hypermetabolism and correction of deficits.

Increase of serum prealbumin and retinol-binding proteins by 1 mg/dL/day indicates good response. Measure two or three times per week. May precede improvement in albumin levels by 7–10 days.

Somatomedin C level may be used for monitoring.

Nutritional Factors in Young Children (Laboratory Indicators)

Folate—serum folate <6 μg/dL suggests low intake. RBC <20 μg/dL or increased excretion of formiminoglutamic acid in urine after histidine load suggests poor nutritional status.

Iodine—<50 μg/g of creatinine in urine suggests recent low intake of iodine.

Glutathione reductase–flavin adenine dinucleotide effect, expressed as ratio, of >1.2:1.0 suggests poor nutritional status.

Calcium, phosphorus, alkaline phosphatase—rickets.

Thiamine—<125 μg/g of creatinine in urine suggests low intake of thiamine. Transketolase-thiamine pyrophosphate effect, expressed as a ratio, of >1.5:1.0 suggests poor nutritional status.

Vitamin A—serum carotene <40 μg/dL suggests recent low intake. Serum vitamin A <20 μg/dL suggests low stores of vitamin A or may indicate failure of retinol transport out of liver into circulation.

Ascorbic acid—serum ascorbate <0.3 mg/dL suggests recent low intake. Whole blood ascorbate <0.3 mg/dL indicates low intake and reduction in body pool of ascorbic acid. Leukocyte ascorbic acid <20 mg/dL suggests poor nutritional status.

Riboflavin—<250 μg/g of creatinine in urine suggests low recent intake of riboflavin.

Serum albumin <3.2 g/dL suggests low protein intake, but this is a rather insensitive, nonspecific indicator of protein status.

Blood urea nitrogen <6 mg/dL or urine <8 mg/g of creatinine suggests recent low protein intake or metabolic error in urea cycle.

Obesity, Associated Diseases

See Table 3.

Total Parenteral Nutrition, Metabolic Complications

Laboratory Findings

Serum cholesterol level decreases rapidly during first 2 days, then remains at low level. Apolipoprotein A level decreases 30–50% after long-term TPN but apolipoprotein B level is usually unchanged.

Hyperglycemia (which may cause osmotic diuresis and hyperosmolarity) or hypoglycemia may be present.

Serum electrolyte levels are usually unchanged but sodium may decrease slightly and potassium may increase slightly after fifth day. Changes depend on solution composition and infusion rate. Frequent monitoring is indicated.

Ketosis develops if insufficient calories or low glucose concentration; may indicate onset of infection.

Hyperosmolarity may occur due to TPN infusion.

Lactic or hyperchloremic metabolic acidosis develops in some patients.

Serum creatinine level and creatinine clearance are not significantly changed.

Serum uric acid level decreases markedly after 2–17 days of TPN and returns to pretreatment level 3–7 days after cessation of TPN.

Plasma amino acid levels may be abnormal.

Deficiency of essential fatty acids (on fat-free TPN), zinc, or copper may develop.

Transient increase is seen in serum levels of aspartate aminotransferase (three to four times), alanine aminotransferase (three to seven times), alkaline phosphatase (two times), and γ-glutamyltransferase (markedly increased).

Table 3. Diseases Associated with Obesity

Disease	Mechanism	Clinical Effects
Type 2 diabetes mellitus	Obesity leads to increased resistance to insulin action, which leads to glucose intolerance. Diabetes mellitus occurs in genetically susceptible individuals.	B-cell (pancreatic islet) hyperplasia followed by atrophy. Complications of diabetes mellitus (e.g., retinopathy, neuropathy). Risk factor for atherosclerosis.
Hypertension	Statistical association with obesity but no clear mechanism elucidated. Increased secretion of adrenal glucocorticosteroids is a minor factor.	Risk factor for atherosclerosis, cerebral hemorrhage (stroke).
Hyperlipidemia	Increased fat mobilization from adipose stores results in increased lipoprotein synthesis in liver.	Risk factor for atherosclerosis. Hypertriglyceridemia, hypercholesterolemia, increased very-low-density lipoprotein level.
Atherosclerotic arterial disease	Statistical association with obesity along with other risk factors (diabetes, hypertension, hyperlipidemia).	Myocardial infarction (ischemic heart disease) (heart attack); cerebral thromboses and infarction (stroke).
Cholelithiasis (gallstones)	Increased cholesterol excretion in bile.	Acute and chronic and cholecystitis.
Osteoarthrosis	Increased body weight causes cartilage degeneration in weight-bearing joints.	Lumbar spine, hips, and knees most commonly affected.

Direct bilirubin level is normal or slightly increased. Improves 1 week after cessation of TPN and returns to normal in 1–4 months.
Serum folate level falls 50% if not supplemented.
Sixty-seven percent of children show eosinophilia (>140/mm^3) after 9 days of TPN.
Laboratory findings of sepsis due to infection of catheter.

Monitoring of Patients on Total Parenteral Nutrition

Twice weekly: chemistry profile, electrolyte levels, transthyretin level.
Weekly: complete blood count, urinalysis, chemistry and acid-base profiles, levels of iron, zinc, copper, magnesium, triglycerides, ammonia.
Every 2 weeks: folate, vitamin B_{12} levels.
Baseline: all of the above tests.
Unstable clinical condition may require testing daily or more often.

Vitamin Reference Ranges (Blood)*

Limited utility because blood levels may not reflect tissue stores.

Vitamin A	
Retinol	360–1,200 μg/L <20 μg/dL indicates low intake and tissue stores 20–36 μg/dL indeterminate
Retinyl esters	≤1.0 μg/dL
Carotene	48–200 μg/dL
Vitamin C (ascorbic acid)	0.2–2.0 mg/dL <0.2 mg/dL represents deficiency

*Values are for serum unless otherwise indicated.

Vitamin D	Indirect estimate by measuring serum alkaline phosphatase, calcium, and phosphorus
Total 25-hydroxyvitamin D	14–42 ng/mL (winter)
1,25-dihydroxyvitamin D	15–80 ng/mL (summer)
Vitamin E (α-tocopherol)	
Children	3.0–15.0 μg/dL
Adults	5.5–17.0 μg/dL
Deficiency	<3.0 μg/mL
Excess	>40 μg/mL
Vitamin B_1 (thiamine)	5.3–7.9 μg/dL
Vitamin B_2 (riboflavin)	3.7–13.7 μg/dL
Vitamin B_{12} (cobalamin)	
Low	<150 pg/mL
Normal	190–900 pg/mL
Urine methylmalonate	0.0–4.0 μmol/dL
Unsaturated vitamin B_{12}–binding capacity	870–1,800 pg/mL
Folate, serum	≥3.5 ng/mL
RBC	
<1 yr	74–995 ng/mL
1–11 yr	96–362 ng/mL
≥12 yr	180–600 ng/mL

Bibliography

Barness LA. Nutritional diseases. In: Gilbert-Barness E, ed. *Potter's atlas of fetal and infant pathology.* St. Louis: Mosby–Year Book, 1998.

Barness LA. Nutritional diseases. In: Gilbert-Barness E, ed. *Potter's pathology of the fetus and infant*. St. Louis: Mosby–Year Book, 1997.

Wallach J. *Interpretation of diagnostic tests*, 7th ed. Philadelphia: Lippincott Williams & Wilkins, 2000.

21 Disorders of the Skin

Tests for Evaluation of Skin Disorders

Laboratory tests such as Gram staining of smears, culture of skin specimen, potassium hydroxide (KOH) preparation, Tzanck testing of smears, hair mounts, scabies preparations, and direct fluorescent antibody (DFA) testing can identify pathogenic organisms that enable directed therapy for skin disorders. Skin biopsy specimens can provide invaluable information when histopathologic examination is appropriately combined with special stains, immunofluorescence, polymerase chain reaction (PCR) testing, immunohistochemistry, or electron microscopy.

Many genetic skin diseases can be diagnosed prenatally with the aid of specific genetic and metabolic tests such as PCR or fluorescent *in situ* hybridization (FISH). Chromosomal analysis may be helpful in the diagnosis of certain congenital dermatologic diseases.

Most skin disorders can be diagnosed by the clinical appearance but some require a diagnostic biopsy.

Bacterial Cultures

Scraping or cotton swab specimen should be plated on blood agar and inoculated into a thioglycollate (anaerobic) broth. If infection with Gram-negative rods is suspected, MacConkey or eosin-methylene blue agar plates should be inoculated. If meningococcal or gonococcal infection is suspected, the specimen should be plated on Thayer-Martin or chocolate agar plates in a carbon dioxide atmosphere. Culture specimens for suspected anaerobic *Streptococcus*, *Bacteroides*, and *Clostridium* should be plated on blood agar.

Early identification of infectious organisms is critical in certain rapidly progressive skin infections such as necrotizing fasciitis. Gram stain and culture of overlying skin have a low yield; the growth of organisms takes several days, even when cultures are positive. The use of a rapid *Streptococcus* test can be helpful in the early identification of streptococcal infection in necrotizing fasciitis.

Biopsy of the Skin

Punch biopsy is the common method of skin sampling used in dermatology. This approach is excellent for complete removal of small lesions (<6 mm) and for skin sampling for diagnostic purposes by routine histology, immunofluorescence, electron microscopy, or culture.

Punch biopsies are performed with reusable sterile Keyes skin punches or more commonly with inexpensive, extremely sharp disposable punches. Punches can be purchased in sizes ranging from 2 to 6 mm. Typically, a 3- or 4-mm punch biopsy is performed for diagnostic purposes.

Fibroblast Culture

Clean skin with iodine-containing solution. Wash with alcohol. Obtain biopsy specimen as indicated earlier. Place skin in sterile tube or in a tube with transport medium. Specimen can be maintain at 70°C or grown at 28°C.

Special Stains

Routine skin biopsy specimens are usually stained with hematoxylin and eosin stain. For the identification of bacteria, a Gram stain is used, and for fungi identification periodic acid–Schiff and methenamine silver stains are used.

Darkfield Examination

Darkfield examination is an infrequently performed examination used to detect *Treponema pallidum*, the pathologic organism in syphilis.

Sample Collection

The spirochete is most likely to be detected in nasal discharge or scrapings from moist mucocutaneous lesions. Specimens from the mouth should be avoided because of the presence of normal oral spirochetes, which can be mistaken for *T. pallidum.*

Preparation Technique

1. While wearing gloves, clean the surface of the lesion with dry gauze.
2. Touch a coverslip to serous fluid expressed from a lesion.
3. Place the coverslip on a drop of saline on a glass slide.
4. Examine immediately (if possible at the bedside); do not let the specimen dry out.
5. Spirochetes, if present, are seen as undulating and rotating corkscrew-shaped organisms.

Direct Fluorescent Antibody Test for Diagnosis of Herpesvirus Infection

The DFA test is a rapid, cost-effective, sensitive, and highly specific method for detecting and distinguishing cutaneous herpes simplex virus (types 1 and 2) and varicella-zoster virus infections. Direct immunofluorescence is most sensitive on vesicles, less sensitive on pustules, and even less on crusted lesions. DFA testing uses monoclonal antibodies directed against type-specific glycoprotein epitopes of the herpesvirus envelope.

The base of a blister, erosion, or ulcer is aggressively scraped. The material is then smeared on a glass slide and sent to the laboratory. Slides are prepared with a few drops of fluorescein-conjugated murine monoclonal antibodies against herpes simplex virus 1 and 2 (prepared as a 1:1 mixture) or varicella-zoster virus. After approximately 30 minutes the slides are rinsed and examined by epifluorescence microscopy. Emission of bright green cytoplasmic fluorescence indicates positive results.

Electron Microscopy

Electron microscopy may be very useful in establishing the diagnoses of several diseases, such as Langerhans cell histiocytosis and epidermolysis bullosa. Specimens for electron microscopy are placed in glutaraldehyde. Electron microscopy allows for precise localization of the ultrastructural level of cleavage, which allows differentiation of simplex, junctional, and dystrophic types of epidermolysis bullosa.

Fluorescent *In Situ* Hybridization

With FISH, specific regions of the genome can be detected by applying complementary labeled nucleic acid probes. After denaturation of the DNA, the probes can hybridize to target sequences on chromosomes and form a new DNA duplex.

DNA probes can be used to identify foreign genes, including bacteria, viruses, and fungi. Detection of infectious agents with FISH techniques has been reported for human immunodeficiency virus, cytomegalovirus, herpes simplex virus, hepatitis B virus, and Epstein-Barr virus.

Prenatal Diagnosis

DNA-based prenatal diagnosis has largely superseded older techniques such as fetoscopy and fetal skin biopsy. PCR-based prenatal diagnosis of dystrophic and junctional epidermolysis bullosa has been performed through analysis of type VII collagen and laminin 5 genes of dystrophic and junctional epidermolysis bullosa, respectively, and of keratin 10 for epidermolytic hyperkeratosis. Testing can be done using chorionic villus sampling at 10–15 weeks' gestation in families at risk for recurrence of epidermolysis bullosa. Percutaneous umbilical vein blood samples taken during the early weeks of pregnancy may provide an even earlier diagnosis.

Preimplantation genetic diagnosis is an alternative to conventional approaches to prenatal diagnosis. The genetic abnormality in question is diagnosed before implantation of the fetus, which allows for selection of nonaffected, healthy fetuses. DNA analysis and *in vitro* fertilization are used to select for a normal genotype before implantation. At the six- to ten-cell stage, one cell is removed for DNA extraction and PCR amplification. Removal of one or two cells at this stage does not affect viability or the rate of development of the embryo. After analysis of DNA, only the embryos with normal DNA are implanted. This technique has been used in families at risk for cystic fibrosis and epidermolysis bullosa.

The Online Mendelian Inheritance in Man Web site, http://www.ncbi.nlm.nih.gov/Omim, is a database of human genes and genetic disorders. The database contains textual information, pictures, and valuable information. It also contains extensive links to the Entrez database of the National Center for Biochemical Information. GeneTests/GeneClinics is a medical genetics information resource providing laboratory and clinic directories and educational materials at http://www.genetests.org or http://www.geneclinics.org.

Fungal Cultures and Potassium Hydroxide Preparation

KOH examination of skin, hair, and nails for suspected fungal infection is a commonly used diagnostic procedure.

Sample Collection

Scrapings of the skin for KOH preparation and fungal culture should be collected from the margins of the lesions because this is the area of active growth of the fungus. Do not cleanse with alcohol because it removes much of the scale, which makes collection of adequate material difficult. The use of antibiotics in the fungal culture media is a preferable method for preventing bacterial overgrowth of cultures.

If blisters are present, use curved iris scissors to remove the blister roof for examination. India ink–containing KOH preparations (Swartz-Lamkin) are available to enhance the hyphae and increase the yield of positive results.

Scalp scrapings can be obtained in a similar manner. If culture material is needed, a toothbrush, a gynecologic viral collection brush, or a wet cotton-tipped applicator can be rubbed against the scalp surface and placed in the collection container or directly on the culture medium.

For collection of fungal samples from the nails, a 2- or 3-mm skin curette may be used to scrape out subungual debris, which may be more accessible when the nail is trimmed.

Mycosel agar (BD Biosciences, Sparks, Maryland) is commonly used for fungal culture media composed of Sabouraud dextrose agar containing chloramphenicol and cycloheximide to reduce bacterial overgrowth.

Dermatophyte test medium is a simplified culture system for the detection of dermatophytes. When the culture results are positive, dye in the medium turns red. Certain nondermatophytes, such as *Aspergillus* species, can also turn the media red, so colony morphology should be evaluated. For most fungi, inoculated media can be kept at room temperature. The bottle caps should be kept locked to allow air into the culture bottle. Some diphasic fungi such as *Cryptococcus* species grow poorly at room temperature and should be incubated at 37°C. For deep fungi, a skin biopsy must be performed.

Preparation Technique

1. Select an area of the lesion. The margin of a lesion is recommended.
2. Using a No. 15 blade, edge of a microscopic slide, or Fomon blade, scrape gently across the edge of the scaling skin plaque, nail parings, subinguinal debris, or short hair stubs using the motion of a knife spreading butter on bread.
3. Gently drop the skin scrapings onto a glass slide by tapping the edge of the blade against the glass. Material may be swept into a pile using the blade or coverslip, and coverslip applied.
4. Apply a few drops of 10–20% KOH to the edge of the coverslip. Heat slide gently or set slid on microscopic stage with light turned on.
5. Apply gentle pressure to the surface to flatten the scales. Absorb excess KOH with a paper towel and apply pressure with a pencil eraser to flatten thick specimen.
6. Rack down the substage condenser and put the light on low.
7. Scan and focus the smear with 4–100× objectives, scanning the material at low power until suspicious areas are identified and then switching to higher power to confirm the presence of hyphae or yeast.

Hair Examination by Microscopy

Hair can be examined with the light microscope, both with and without the use of polarizing lenses.

Sample Collection

Hair obtained for microscopic examination should be snipped rather than pulled. Most hair abnormalities seen in the neonate involve scalp hair. The hair changes of Netherton syndrome, however, are variable and are often absent from scalp hair. The diagnosis of Netherton syndrome can be made in these patients by sampling eyebrow or eyelash hair.

Identification of Some Hair Abnormalities

Conditions	Microscopic Hair Findings
Trichothiodystrophy	Light microscopy: wavy, irregular outline with a flattened shaft with folded ribbon configuration. Polarized microscopy: light and dark bands or "tiger tail" pattern.
Chédiak-Higashi syndrome	Light microscopy: evenly distributed small, granular melanin aggregates.
Griscelli syndrome	Light microscopy: large, unevenly distributed melanin aggregates, primarily located in the medulla.
Netherton syndrome	Light microscopy: "ball and socket" configuration or trichorrhexis invaginata may include golf-tee or tulip-like configurations; may show circumferential strictures (earliest stage of invagination).
Menkes syndrome	Light microscopy: classically reveals pili torti or twisted hair, but monilethrix and trichorrhexis nodosa also reported.

Immunofluorescence Tests

Direct immunofluorescence testing detects immunoreactants localized in the tissues of the patient's skin or mucous membrane. Indirect immunofluorescence testing detects circulating antibodies in the patient's serum.

Direct Immunofluorescent Microscopy

Direct immunofluorescent microscopy is useful for the diagnosis of immune-mediated vesiculobullous diseases, lupus erythematosus, and leukocytoclastic vasculitis. Biopsy of a perilesional area (next to but not including a fresh blister) should be performed. Frozen sections are incubated with fluorescent-linked antibodies to human immunoglobulin (Ig) G, IgA, IgM, and C3, as well as other antibodies. Specimens may be frozen until testing or kept in transport medium (Michel medium:

ammonium sulfate, *N*-ethylmaleimide, and magnesium sulfate in a citrate buffer) for at least 2 weeks without loss of reactivity.

Biopsy Technique for Direct Immunofluorescence

1. Perilesional (normal) skin is most desirable. Never biopsy the base of an ulcer or center of a blister.
2. Biopsy the freshest, most recent lesion.
3. If the epidermis and dermis become detached during the procedure, submit both in separately labeled containers.
4. Place specimens in transport medium (Michel transport medium or Zeus fixative). Never place the specimen in formalin.
5. If transport medium is not available, cover skin biopsy with saline-soaked gauze and transport immediately to immunofluorescence laboratory for processing.

Indirect Immunofluorescent Microscopy

In indirect immunofluorescent microscopy various dilutions of the patient's serum are incubated on an epithelial substrate, usually primate esophagus. This diagnostic technique is useful for diagnosis of pemphigus vulgaris, pemphigus foliaceus, bullous pemphigoid, and other autoimmune blistering disorders.

For diagnosis of epidermolysis bullosa, a skin biopsy specimen is submitted for immunofluorescent antigenic mapping. Through this technique, the ultrastructural level of a blister can be determined based on the binding of antibodies having known ultrastructural binding sites. The three most commonly used antibodies are those directed against bullous pemphigoid antigen, laminin, and type IV collagen.

The specimen should be placed in an immunofluorescence transfer medium (Michel, Zeus) and forwarded to a reference laboratory experienced in antigenic mapping. Immunofluorescence antigenic mapping can be completed within 2 hours of receipt of a specimen. Immunofluorescence antigenic mapping is available at no cost for any patient enrolled in the National Epidermolysis Bullosa Registry: phone: 919-966-2007; fax: 919-966-7080; E-mail: Ijohnson@med.unc.edu; Web site: http://www.med.unc.edu/derm/nebr_site/index.htm.

Polymerase Chain Reaction Testing

PCR is used for the detection of foreign DNA in the diagnosis of infectious diseases.

PCR is also useful to detect genetic mutations for genetic disease diagnosis and for oncology and to detect chromosomal translocations in leukemias and lymphomas in children. PCR is 100,000 times more sensitive than cytogenetic studies and 10,000 times more sensitive than flow cytometry or Southern blotting techniques in detecting chromosomal translocations.

PCR is of immense value in the prenatal diagnosis of a number of genetic disorders, including dermatologic diseases.

A major advantage of PCR is that it can be performed on minimal amounts of tissue. Both the quantitative sample requirements and the transport medium requirements for PCR are liberal. For identification of herpes simplex virus DNA, for example, the amount of tissue used for a Tzanck smear is sufficient. Viral culture medium is effective for transport. Fresh, fresh-frozen, formalin-fixed, and even paraffin-embedded specimens are acceptable for PCR testing.

Scabies and Ectoparasite Preparations

In ectoparasitic infections, a linear burrow is a good place to scrape for specimens but may prove hard to identify. On young infants and children, where mites abound, the palms are a fruitful location because hands and fingers are used for rubbing and scratching. Finger webs, wrists, feet, axillae, vesicles, and untouched pink papules are good sites for scraping.

A fresh burrow can be identified as a 5- to 10-mm elongated papule with a vesicle or pustule at one end. A small dark spot resembling a fleck of pepper may be seen in the vesicle. This spot is the mite, and it can be lifted out of the burrow with a needle or the point of a scalpel. Usually it is best to scrape the burrow vigorously while the skin is held taut between the thumb and index finger. Although this may induce a small amount of bleeding, if performed with multiple short, rapid strokes, it is usually painless. A drop of mineral oil should be applied to the skin before scraping to ensure adherence of the scrapings to the blade. The scrapings are placed on a slide; another drop of mineral oil is added, and a coverslip is applied. Gentle pressure with a pencil eraser may be used to flatten thick specimens.

Mites are 0.2–0.4 mm in size with four pairs of legs and can be easily identified using the scanning power of a microscope. Eggs are oval and one-half of the size of the mite. Feces are also oval but are golden brown in color and usually occur in clumps. Ova and feces are usually oval and should be distinguished from air bubbles.

Lice are six-legged insects visible to the unaided eye. They are commonly found on the scalp, eyelashes, and pubic areas. Pubic lice are short and broad, with claws spaced far apart to grasp the sparse hairs on the trunk, pubic area, and eyelashes. Scalp lice are long and thin, with claws closer together to grasp the denser hairs found on the head. The lice are best identified close to the skin where eggs are more numerous and more obvious. Diagnosis can be made by identifying the louse or by plucking hairs and confirming the presence of nits (eggs) by microscopic examination.

Technique for Mineral Oil Scraping for Scabies Identification

1. Select a good site such as palms, web spaces, wrists, or obvious burrows that are not excoriated.
2. Apply mineral oil to a No. 15 blade. The lesion to be sampled may also be covered with mineral oil to reduce pain and friction.
3. Scrape the lesion vigorously five or six times to remove the stratum corneum. Punctate bleeding demonstrates that the depth is correct.
4. Apply mineral oil to a glass slide.
5. Immerse the No. 15 blade in the oil and transfer onto the glass slide.
6. Add a coverslip to the glass slide.
7. View under microscope on low power (4× or 10×). Mites, eggs, and feces are all recognizable.

Tzanck Preparation

Microscopic examination of cells obtained from the base of a vesicle or bulla (Tzanck smear) is used primarily for the diagnosis of viral processes, including herpes simplex and varicella-zoster viruses. The diagnosis of toxic epidermal necrolysis, staphylococcal scalded skin syndrome, pemphigus vulgaris, and Langerhans cell histiocytosis can be made by this procedure.

The smear is obtained by removing the roof of a blister with a curved scalpel blade and scraping the face of the blister to obtain the moist cloudy debris. The material is placed on a glass slide. The tissue on the slide can be air dried, heat fixed, or fixed in methanol before staining with stains such as Giemsa, crystal violet, toluidine blue, Papanicolaou, immunofluorescence. Multinucleated giant cells are seen on high power and can be diagnostic of varicella and herpes simplex infection. To indicate a positive result, epidermal nuclei should be "molded" together with nuclear membranes that appear to be indenting each other.

Preparation Technique

1. Select a lesion. The yield for obtaining positive results from a smear is highest from a fresh vesicle, followed by a pustule, and then a crusted lesion.
2. Wipe the lesion with alcohol and allow it to dry for 1 minute.
3. Using a No. 15 blade, either remove the crust or unroof the vesicle or pustule.
4. Using a No. 15 blade at an angle of <90 degrees, scrape the lesion base with the edge of the blade.
5. Gently transfer the material from the blade to a glass slide by repeatedly and gently touching the blade to the slide (forceful smearing will grind the cells, which results in crushed nuclei).

6. Allow the smear to air dry (alternately, tissue may be heat fixed or fixed in methanol).
7. Flood the slide with staining solution for 30–60 seconds. Use either Giemsa, Wright, methylene blue, or toluidine blue stain.
8. Rinse excess stain off the slide with tap water and allow the stain to air dry.
9. Apply one or two drops of immersion oil or tap water, then place coverslip over the slide.
10. Rack up the substage condenser toward the stage and adjust the field diaphragm for optimal illumination and resolution.

Findings

The following are findings of Tzanck smear of blister scrapings and Wright and Gram stains of blister fluid contents in some neonatal cutaneous conditions:

Condition	**Findings**
Transient neonatal pustular melanosis	Large numbers of polymorphonuclear leukocytes
Pustular psoriasis	Large numbers of polymorphonuclear leukocytes
Acropustulosis of infancy	Large numbers of polymorphonuclear leukocytes
Incontinentia pigmenti	Large numbers of eosinophils
Erythema toxicum neonatorum	Large numbers of eosinophils
Eosinophilic pustular folliculitis	Large numbers of eosinophils
Toxic epidermal necrolysis	Cuboidal cells with high nuclear to cytoplasmic ratio; inflammatory cells present
Staphylococcal scalded skin syndrome	Broad epidermal cells without inflammation
Histiocytosis	Histiocytes with oval nuclei with longitudinal grooves or kidney-bean shape
Varicella or herpes simplex	Multinucleated giant cells

Viral Cultures

Although Tzanck smears and the DFA technique can provide rapid results in cases of suspected viral infection, the gold standard remains viral culture. After the specimen is taken, the applicator should be placed in a sterile tube containing at least 3 mL of viral transport medium (buffered isotonic balanced salt solution containing penicillin and streptomycin or gentamicin to prevent bacterial contamination). (When vancomycin hydrochloride and amikacin sulfate are added, specimens should be refrigerated or transported on ice for best results.)

Herpes simplex virus produces identifiable changes in culture cells in 2 to 3 days. Varicella-zoster virus is more difficult to culture; culture can take 7–14 days, and false-negative results are frequent.

Studies using PCR in the identification of herpes infection in keratoconjunctivitis and in primary genital herpes have found the assay to be superior to viral culture in sensitivity and in ease of specimen collection.

Wood Light Examination

The Wood lamp is helpful in the clinical evaluation of cutaneous pigmentary disease, selected cutaneous infections, and porphyria.

Early subclinical hypopigmented macules of tuberous sclerosis and streaky hypopigmentation seen in hypomelanosis of Ito are often detected with the Wood lamp. Various dermatologic conditions have characteristic fluorescent patterns, including yellow-green fluorescence of hair in selected dermatophyte infections (e.g., *Microsporum canis*).

Erythrasma is a superficial bacterial infection of moist skin of the groin, axilla, and toe webs. It appears as a brown or red flat plaque and is caused by a *Corynebacterium* that excrete a pigment containing a porphyrin. This pigment fluoresces coral red or pink under Wood light. Tinea versicolor, a superficial fungal infection with hypopigmented macules and plaques on the trunk, fluoresces under Wood light with a green-yellow color. *Pseudomonas* infection of the toe web space and colonization of the skin in burn patients fluoresces yellow-green. Patients with porphyria cutanea tarda excrete uroporphyrins in their urine, and examination of a urine specimen shows an orange-yellow fluorescence. Adequate blood levels of tetracycline hydrochloride produce yellow fluorescence in the opening of hair follicles, whereas lack of fluorescence indicates poor intestinal absorption or poor patient compliance.

The Wood lamp also emits purple light in the visible spectrum. This wavelength can be used to accentuate subtle changes in pigmentation. The purple light is absorbed by melanin in the skin and is variably reflected by patches of hypopigmentation and depigmentation. This may be particularly useful in evaluating light-pigmented individuals with vitiligo or ash leaf macules.

Skin Disorders

Dermatitis, Atopic

Chronic pruritic eczematous condition affecting characteristic sites, associated with family history of atopy (asthma, allergic rhinitis, atopic dermatitis).

Predominant age: mainly a childhood disease. Affects 5% of all children, usually appearing in the first year of life and gradually subsiding over subsequent years.

Predominant sex: affects males and females equally (females tend to have somewhat worse prognosis).

Signs and Symptoms

Pruritus is the most common symptom.

Distribution of Lesions

Infants—trunk, face, and extensor surfaces

Children—antecubital and popliteal fossae

Adults—face, neck, upper chest, and genital areas

Morphology of Lesions

Infants—erythema and papules; may develop oozing, crusting vesicles.

Children and adults—lichenification and scaling are typical with chronic eczema.

Family history of atopic dermatitis may be more useful than morphology in making the diagnosis.

Associated Features

Facial erythema, mild to moderate

Perioral pallor

Infraorbital fold (Dennie sign, Morgan line)

Dry skin

Increased palmar linear markings

Pityriasis alba (hypopigmented asymptomatic areas on face and shoulders)

Keratosis pilaris

Laboratory Findings

Serum IgE levels are frequently elevated.

Differential Diagnosis

Photosensitivity rashes

Contact dermatitis (especially if only the face is involved)

Scabies

Seborrheic dermatitis (especially in infants)

Psoriasis or lichen simplex chronicus if only localized disease is present in adults

Rare conditions of infancy: histiocytosis X, Wiskott-Aldrich syndrome, ataxia telangiectasia syndrome

Ichthyosis vulgaris

Dermatitis, Contact

The cutaneous reaction to an external substance.

1. Primary irritant dermatitis is due to direct injury of the skin. It affects individuals exposed to specific irritants and generally produces discomfort immediately after exposure.
2. Allergic contact dermatitis affects only individuals previously sensitized to the contactant. It represents a delayed hypersensitivity reaction and several hours are required for the cascade of cellular immunity to be completed to manifest itself.

Signs and Symptoms

Acute

Papules, vesicles, bullae with surrounding erythema.
Crusting and oozing may be present.
Pruritus.

Chronic

Erythematous base
Thickening with lichenification
Scaling
Fissuring

Distribution

Areas where epidermis is thinner (eyelids, genitalia).
Areas of contact with offending agent (e.g., nail polish).
Palms and soles are more resistant.
Deeper skinfolds are spared.
Linear arrays of lesions are present.
Lesions with sharp borders and sharp angles are pathognomonic.

Differential Diagnosis

1. Based on clinical impression—appearance, periodicity, localization
2. Groups of vesicles—herpes simplex
3. Diffuse bullous or vesicular lesions—bullous pemphigoid
4. Photo distribution—phototoxic or allergic reaction to systemic allergen
5. Eyelids—seborrheic dermatitis
6. Scaly eczematous lesions—atopic dermatitis, nummular eczema, lichen simplex chronicus, stasis dermatitis, xerosis

Special Tests

Patch tests for allergic contact dermatitis (use of systemic corticosteroids or recent aggressive use of topical steroids may alter results).

Dermatitis, Diaper

Diaper dermatitis is a rash occurring on the area covered by a diaper. The rash may be an irritant contact dermatitis, candidiasis, atopic dermatitis, or seborrheic dermatitis.

Signs and Symptoms

- Diaper dermatitis
  Prominent rashes on buttocks and pubic skin.
  Creases of skin are relatively spared.
  Rash is dusky red and shiny.
  Skin seems chapped.
  Weeping, crusting, and excoriations are not prominent.
- Candidiasis diaper rash
  Initial involvement of creases with rapid extension.
  Bright red color.

Accompanying edema.
Isolated satellite papules and pustules at margins of inflammatory plaques.
Excoriations are prominent.
Positive results on KOH preparation.
Positive results on cultures.

- Atopic diaper dermatitis
  Distribution spares creases.
  Genitalia frequently involved.
  Itch-scratch cycle with excoriations is prominent.
  Child scratches vigorously at night.
  Weeping, crusting, excoriations sometimes present; secondary bacterial infection can occur.
- Seborrheic diaper dermatitis
  Dusky red patches and plaques deep within skin creases.
  Nonintertriginous skin is relatively spared.
  Weeping, crusting, excoriations are not prominent.
  Other sites of seborrheic dermatitis are frequently present: retroauricular, axillary folds, scalp.

Laboratory Findings

Culture will reveal *Candida*, if present.

Special Laboratory Tests

KOH preparation, culture of pustules if present

Bibliography

Bianchi DW. Prenatal diagnosis by analysis of fetal cells in maternal blood. *J Pediatr* 1995;127:847–856.

Chen CL, Chow KC, Wong CK, et al. A study on Epstein-Barr virus in erythema multiforme. *Arch Dermatol Res* 1998;290:446–449.

Christiano AM, LaForgia S, Paller AS, et al. Prenatal diagnosis for recessive dystrophic epidermolysis bullosa in 10 families by mutation and haplotype analysis in the type VII collagen gene (COC 7A1). *Mol Med* 1996;2:59–76.

Colon-Fontanez F, Eichenfield LE, Krous HF, et al. Congenital Langerhans cell histiocytosis: the utility of the Tzanck test as a diagnostic screening tool. *Arch Dermatol* 1998;134:1039–1040.

Detlefs RL, Friedsen IJ, Berger TG, et al. Eosinophil fluorescence: a cause of false positive slide tests for herpes simplex virus. *Pediatr Dermatol* 1987;4:129–133.

Eichenfield LF, Frieden IJ, Esterly NB. *The textbook of neonatal dermatology.* Philadelphia: WB Saunders, 2001.

Eisenstein BI. The polymerase chain reaction: a new method of using molecular genetics for medical diagnosis. *N Engl J Med* 1990;322:178–183.

Elenitsas R, Jaworsky C, Murphy GF. Diagnostic methodology: immunofluorescence. In: Murphy GF, ed. *Dermatopathology: a practical guide to common disorders*. Philadelphia: WB Saunders, 1995:29–45.

Erlich KS. Laboratory diagnosis of herpesvirus infections. *Clin Lab Med* 1987;7:759–776.

Fine JD, Gay S. LDA-1 monoclonal antibody: an excellent reagent for immunofluorescence mapping studies in patients with epidermolysis bullosa. *Arch Dermatol* 1986;122:48–51.

Friedlander SF, Pickering B, Cunningham BB, et al. Use of cotton swab method in diagnosing tinea capitis. *Pediatrics* 1999;104:276–279.

Gilchrest BA, Fitzpatrick TB, Anderson BB, et al. Localization of melanin pigment on the skin with a Wood's lamp. *Br J Dermatol* 1977;96:245–248.

Greer CE, Peterson SL, Kiviat NB, et al. PCR amplification from paraffin-embedded tissues. Effects of fixative and fixation time. *Am J Clin Pathol* 1991;95:117–124.

Hidalgo F, Melon S, de Ona M, et al. Diagnosis of herpetic keratoconjunctivitis by nested polymerase chain reaction in human tear film. *Eur J Clin Microbiol Infect Dis* 1998;17:120–123.

Hurwitz S. Hair disorders. In: Schachner LA, Hansen RC, eds. *Pediatric dermatology.* 2nd ed. New York: Churchill Livingstone, 1995:583–614.
Kurban RS, Mihm MC. Dermatopathology: cutaneous reaction patterns and the use of specialized laboratory techniques. In: Moshella SL, Hurley HJ, eds. *Dermatology,* 3rd ed. Philadelphia: WB Saunders 1992:125–148.
Lo AC, Feldman SR. Polymerase chain reaction: basic concepts and clinical applications in dermatology. *J Am Acad Dermatol* 1994;30:250–260.
McGarth JA, Handyside AH. Preimplantation genetic diagnosis of severe inherited skin diseases. *Exp Dermatol* 1998;7:65–72.
Nahass GT, Goldstein BA, Shu WY, et al. Comparison of Tzanck smear, viral culture, and DNA diagnostic methods in detection of herpes simplex and varicella-zoster infection. *JAMA* 1992;268:2541–2544.
Ou CY, Kwok S, Mitchell SW, et al. DNA amplification for direct detection of HIV-1 in DNA of peripheral blood mononuclear cells. *Science* 1988;239:295–297.
Rogers M. Hair shaft abnormalities. Part II. *Aust J Dermatol* 1996;37:1–11.
Rogers MF, Ou CY, Rayfield M, et al. Use of the polymerase chain reaction for the early detection of the proviral sequences of human immunodeficiency virus in infants born to seropositive mothers. New York City collaborative study of maternal HIV transmission and Montefiore Medical Center HIV perinatal transmission study group. *N Engl J Med* 1989;320:1649–1654.
Schlesinger Y, Tebas P, Gaudreault-Keener M, et al. Herpes simplex virus type 2 meningitis in the absence of genital lesions: improved recognition with use of the polymerase chain reaction. *Clin Infect Dis* 1995;20:842–848.
Shoji H, Koga M, Kusuhara T, et al. Differentiation of herpes simplex virus 1 and 2 in cerebrospinal fluid of patients with HSV encephalitis and meningitis by stringent hybridization of PCR-amplified DNAs. *J Neurol* 1994;241:526–530.
Solomon AR. New diagnostic tests for herpes simplex and varicella zoster infection. *J Am Acad Dermatol* 1988;18:218–221.
Tanphaichitr A, Brodell RT. How to spot scabies in infants. *Postgrad Med* 1999;105: 191–192.
Tremblay C, Coutlee F, Weiss J, et al. Evaluation of a nonisotopic polymerase chain reaction assay for detection in clinical specimens of herpes simplex virus type 2 DNA. Canadian Women's HIV Study Group. *Clin Diagn Virol* 1997;8:53–62.
Zirn JR, Tompkins SD, Huie C, et al. Rapid detection and distinction of cutaneous herpesvirus infections by direct immunofluorescence. *J Am Acad Dermatol* 1995;33:724–728.

22 Diseases of the Eye

Blepharitis

An inflammatory reaction of the eyelid margin. It usually occurs as seborrheic (nonulcerative) or as staphylococcal (ulcerative) blepharitis. Both types may coexist.

Signs and Symptoms

Staphylococcus aureus blepharitis
- Itching
- Lacrimation (tearing)
- Burning
- Photophobia (light sensitivity)
- Usually worse in morning
- Recurrent stye (external hordeolum or internal hordeolum)
- Recurrent chalazia (chronic inflammation of meibomian glands)
- Fine epithelial keratitis, lower half of cornea
- Ulcerations at base of eyelashes
- Broken, sparse, misdirected eyelashes (trichiasis)

Seborrheic blepharitis
- Lid margin erythema
- Dry flakes, oily secretions on lid margins or lashes, or both
- Associated dandruff of scalp, eyebrows
- Sometimes nasolabial erythema, scaling

Mixed blepharitis (seborrheic with associated *S. aureus* infection)
- Most common type of blepharitis
- Symptoms and signs of both staphylococcal and seborrheic blepharitis

Causes

Seborrheic
- Accelerated shedding of skin cells with associated sebaceous gland dysfunction.
- Pityrosporum ovale and Pityrosporum orbiculare yeasts often colonize.
- Oil and skin cells foster *Staphylococcus* growth.

Staphylococcal
- Usually part of mixed blepharitis.
- Colonization of Zeis glands of lid margin and meibomian glands posterior to lashes with *S. aureus.*
- Impetigo contagiosa—*Staphylococcus.*
- Infectious eczematoid dermatitis—*Staphylococcus* is the hapten.
- *Staphylococcus* scalded skin syndrome—entire body involved (in young children).
- Angular blepharitis—*Staphylococcus* is bacterium most frequently involved.

Laboratory Studies

Cultures in atypical blepharitis only.

Cataract

Clouding of the cornea or lens. May be unilateral or bilateral. May be idiopathic scarring after injury or genetic-metabolic.

Etiologic Classification of Infantile and Developmental Cataracts

Inherited without Systemic Abnormalities

Autosomal dominant
Autosomal recessive
X-linked

Inherited as Part of Multisystem Disorders

Metabolic Disorders

See Table 1
Galactosemia (AR-230400)*
Galactokinase deficiency (AR-230200)
Fabry disease (XLR-301500)
Mannosidosis (AR-248500)
Refsum disease (AR-266500)
Wilson disease (AR-277900)
Diabetes mellitus
Pseudohypoparathyroidism
Hypocalcemia
Hypoglycemia
Multiple sulfatase deficiency (AR-272200)
Smith-Lemli-Opitz syndrome (AR-207400)

Renal Diseases

Lowe syndrome (XLR-309000)
Alport syndrome (AD-301050)

Musculoskeletal Disorders

Chondrodysplasia punctata (AD-118650, AR-215100, XLD-302960)
Myotonic dystrophy (AD-160900)
Marfan syndrome (AD-154700)
Osteopetrosis (AR-259700)
Weill-Marchesani syndrome (AR-277600)
Stickler syndrome (AD-108300)
Kniest syndrome (AD-156550)
Osteogenesis imperfecta (heterogeneous, AR-259410)
Albright hereditary osteodystrophy (AD-103580, XLD-300800)

Central Nervous System Syndromes

Zellweger syndrome (AR-214100)
Meckel-Gruber syndrome (AR-249000)
Sjögren-Larsson syndrome (AR-270200)
Marinesco-Sjögren syndrome (AR-248800)
Norrie disease (XLR-310600)

Dermatologic Diseases

Cockayne syndrome (AR-216400)
Goltz syndrome (XL-305600)
Rothmund-Thomson syndrome (AR-268400)
Atopic dermatitis
Incontinentia pigmenti (XL-308300)
Progeria (?AD-176670)
Werner syndrome (AR-277700)
Ichthyosis (heterogeneous)
Marshall ectodermal dysplasia

Craniofacial Syndromes

Hallerman-Streiff syndrome (AR-234100)
Crouzon disease (AD-123500)
Apert syndrome (AD-101200)
Engelmann syndrome (AD-131300)
Lanzieri syndrome

*Six-digit numbers are Mendelian Inheritance in Man catalog assignments. AD indicates autosomal dominant; AR, autosomal recessive; XL, X-linked; XLR, X-linked recessive.

Table 1. Ocular Findings in Metabolic Disorders

Disease	Cornea	Lens	Retina	Optic Nerve	Inheritance
Lysosomal storage disorders					
Sphingolipid storage					
Niemann-Pick A	+	+	CRS	+	AR
Niemann-Pick B	–	–	–	–	AR
Niemann-Pick C (D, E)	–	–	–	–	AR
Gaucher	–	–	+	–	AR
Fabry	+	+	V	–	XR
G_{M1} gangliosidosis 1	+	–	CRS	–	AR
Juvenile gangliosidosis (G_{M1} 2)	–	–	CRS	–	AR
Tay-Sachs (G_{M2} 1)	–	–	CRS	+	AR
Sandhoff (G_{M2} 2)	–	–	CRS	+	AR
Juvenile G_{M2} gangliosidosis (G_{M2} 3)	–	–	CRS	+	AR
Pelizaeus-Merzbacher (diffuse cerebral sclerosis)	–	–	–	+	XR
Krabbe	–	–	–	+	AR
Metachromatic leukodystrophy					
Infantile	–	–	CRS (?)	+	AR
Juvenile	–	–	–	+	AR
Adult	–	–	–	+	AR
Multiple sulfatase deficiency	–	–	D, CRS	+	AR
Oligosaccharide storage					
Fucosidosis	–	–	V	–	AR
Sialidosis (mucolipidosis I)	+	+	V	–	AR
Mannosidosis	+	+	–	–	AR
Mucopolysaccharidoses					
Hurler (IH)	+	–	D	+	AR
Scheie (IS)	+	–	D	+	AR
Hunter (III) (two types)	– (?)	–	D	+	XR
Sanfilippo (III) (four types)	–	–	D	+	AR
Morquio (IV)	+	–	–	+	AR
Maroteaux-Lamy (VI) (two types)	+	–	–	+	AR
VII	+	–	–	–	AR
Wolman	–	–	+	+	AR
Secondary lysosomal storage disorders					
Mucolipidoses					
Mucolipidosis II (I cell)	+	+	–	–	AR
Mucolipidosis III (pseudo–Hurler polydystrophy)	+	–	–	–	AR
Mucolipidosis IV	+	–	D	–	AR
Neuronal ceroid lipofuscinosis					
Hagberg-Santavuori	–	–	D	+	AR
Jansky-Bielschowsky	–	–	–	+	AR
Spielmeyer-Vogt	–	–	D	+	AR
Kufs	–	–	D	+	AR
Amino acid metabolism					
Cystinosis	+	–	D	–	AR
Gyrate atrophy (hyperornithinemia)	–	–	+	+	AR
Homocystinuria	–	+	–	–	AR

(continued)

Table 1. (continued)

Disease	Cornea	Lens	Retina	Optic Nerve	Inheritance
Hyperlysinemia	–	+	–	–	AR
Methylmalonic aciduria	+	–	–	–	AR
Molybdenum cofactor deficiency	–	+	–	–	AR
Sulfite oxidase deficiency	–	+	–	–	AR
Tyrosinemia	+	–	–	–	AR
Peroxisomal disorders					
Zellweger	+	+	D	+	AR
Neonatal adrenoleukodystrophy	–	–	D	+	AR
Infantile Refsum	–	–	D	+	AR
X-linked adrenoleukodystrophy	–	–	–	+	XR
Refsum	–	–	D	+	AR
Porphyria					
Congenital erythropoietic	+	–	–	–	AR
Acute intermittent	–	+	+	+	AD
Lipoprotein/lipid metabolism					
Abetalipoproteinemia	–	–	D	+	AR
Lecithin-cholesterol acyltransferase deficiency	+	–	–	–	AR
Tangier disease	+	–	–	–	AR
Carbohydrate metabolism—galactosemia					
Galactose-1-phosphate uridyltransferase deficiency	–	+	–	–	AR
Galactokinase deficiency	–	+	–	–	AR
Metal metabolism					
Acrodermatitis enteropathica	+	+	+	+	AR
Wilson	+	+	–	–	AR
Ceramidase deficiency					
Farber lipogranulomatosis	+	–	+	?	AR

–, unaffected; +, affected; CRS, cherry-red spot; D, retinal degeneration; V, vascular abnormality; AD, autosomal dominant; AR, autosomal recessive; XR, X-linked recessive.
Reproduced with permission from Bateman JB, Punnett HH, Harley RD. Genetics of eye disease. In: Nelson LB, Calhous JH, Harley RD, eds. *Pediatric ophthalmology,* 3rd ed. Philadelphia: WB Saunders, 1991:12.

Rubinstein-Taybi syndrome (268600)
Cerebro-oculofacioskeletal syndrome (AR-214150)
Nance-Horan syndrome (XLR-302350)

Associated with Chromosomal Abnormalities

Trisomy 21
Trisomy 13
Trisomy 18
Deletion 5p
Deletion 11p
Ring 4
10q+
Turner syndrome

Associated with Ocular Disease

Leber congenital amaurosis
Aniridia
Retinitis pigmentosa
Persistent hyperplastic primary vitreous
Peters anomaly

Posterior lenticonus
Microphthalmos
Anterior chamber cleavage syndrome
Coloboma
Persistent pupillary membrane

Associated with Intrauterine Infection

Rubella
Varicella
Toxoplasmosis
Rubeola
Poliomyelitis
Herpes simplex infection
Cytomegalovirus infection

Associated with Uveitis or Acquired Infection

Juvenile rheumatoid arthritis
Pars planitis
Toxocara canis infection

Drug-Induced

Corticosteroids
Others

Associated with Other Causes

Trauma
Radiation exposure
Prematurity

Diagnostic Testing for Infantile Cataract[1]

Tests for genetic-metabolic diseases (see Chapter 17, Metabolic and Hereditary Diseases).
Serum chemistry
- Glucose: diabetes, hypoglycemia
- High urea nitrogen level: renal disease
- Low calcium or high phosphorus level: hypoparathyroidism
- Low galactose enzyme level in red blood cells: galactosemia
- TORCH titer: rubella, toxoplasmosis, cytomegalovirus infection, herpes simplex virus infection, and varicella
- Electrolyte level: acidosis suggests Lowe syndrome
- High galactosyl-ceramide level: Fabry disease
- High phytanic acid level: Refsum disease
- High long-chain fatty acid level: Refsum disease, Zellweger syndrome
- High prostanoic and pipecolic acid level: Zellweger syndrome
- High cholestanol level: cerebrotendinous xanthomatosis

Urine studies
- Increased amino acid level: Lowe syndrome
- Hematuria: Alport syndrome

Cultured fibroblasts with a low α-mannosidase level: mannosidosis
Conjunctival biopsy with birefringent cellular inclusions: Fabry disease
Karyotyping: gross chromosomal abnormalities
Radiologic slides
- Skull radiographic films: abnormalities
- Calcifications: hypoparathyroidism, Albers-Schönberg disease, cytomegalovirus infection, toxoplasmosis
- Facial bone abnormalities: Hallermann-Streiff or Pierre Robin syndrome
- Craniostenosis: Crouzon disease, Apert syndrome
- Microcephaly: Smith-Lemli-Opitz syndrome, cerebrooculofacial-skeletal syndrome, Meckel syndrome

Skeletal survey
- Stippled epiphyses: chondrodysplasia punctata (Conradi syndrome)
- Dwarfism: Hallermann-Streiff or Rothmund-Thomson syndrome, progeria, Conradi syndrome, mannosidosis, Bardet-Biedl syndrome

[1]Eisenberg SJ. *The eye in infancy*, 2nd ed. St. Louis: Mosby, 1994.

Digital anomalies: Rubinstein-Taybi syndrome, oculodental-digital dysplasia, Bardet-Biedl syndrome

Audiologic evaluation

Deafness: rubella; Alport syndrome, Bardet-Biedl syndrome, and Cockayne syndrome; Refsum disease

Vestibular abnormalities: Alport syndrome

Mental retardation: Lowe syndrome, Cockayne syndrome, Down syndrome, rubella, Hallermann-Streiff syndrome, Bardet-Biedl syndrome, Rubinstein-Taybi syndrome, cerebral xanthomatosis

Chorioretinitis

Diagnosed by appearances of the retina. May be due to intrauterine infection, other infections (e.g., helminths), metabolic-genetic disorders, drugs, hypertension.

Laboratory Studies

In newborn, test for TORCHES (toxoplasma, rubella, cytomegalovirus, herpes virus, hepatitis, syphilis) antibodies. In others, test for toxins, drugs, hypertension, metabolic disease.

Conjunctivitis

Conjunctiva is red and edematous, with itching and pain. May be caused by infection (bacteria, *Mycoplasma*, helminths), allergy, increased intraocular pressure, drugs, chemical exposure. In newborns, exposure to chemicals used in chemoprophylaxis is the most common cause.

Laboratory Studies

Frequently no tests are necessary. Cultures, pressure measurement, tests for allergic sensitivity.

Frequency of Bacterial and Chlamydial Isolation in Infectious Ophthalmia Neonatorum[2]

Pathogen*	**Reported Incidence (%)**
Chlamydia trachomatis	10–43
Staphylococcus aureus	5–46
Neisseria gonorrhoeae	4–14
Streptococcus species, *viridans* group	1–29
Haemophilus species	5–14
Streptococcus pneumoniae	5–6
Escherichia coli	2–5
Branhamella catarrhalis	1–5
Mycoplasma hominis	3
Streptococcus species, group D	3
Corynebacterium species	2
Pseudomonas aeruginosa	1

*Includes pathogens isolated from cases of ophthalmia neonatorum in the absence of other organisms and pathogens that have been reported in more than one series, or identified in more than one patient in a single large series.

Ectopia Lentis (Dislocated Lens)

See Table 2.

Diagnosed by appearance, usually a fine line without magnification. Most commonly due to injury, may be due to metabolic-genetic disorder.

[2]Eisenberg SJ. *The eye in infancy*, 2nd ed. St. Louis: Mosby, 1994.

Table 2. Disorders Associated with Ectopia Lentis

Disorder/Inheritance	Systemic Findings	Ocular Findings	Lens changes
Ocular disorders			
Simple ectopia lentis			
Autosomal dominant	None	Lenticular myopia, glaucoma, retinal detachment	Microspherophakia, cataract, upward subluxation
Ectopia pupillae et lentis			
Autosomal recessive	None	Oval or slit-shaped pupil	Ectopia lentis
Microspherophakia			
Autosomal recessive or autosomal dominant	None	Lenticular myopia, glaucoma, microphthalmos	Spherophakia or microspherophakia, ectopia lentis
Ocular trauma			
None	None	Hyphema, glaucoma, choroidal rupture, retinal detachment, optic nerve injury	Subluxation, cataract luxation, torn zonules
Aniridia			
Autosomal dominant or sporadic	Wilms tumor in sporadic cases	Rudimentary iris, foveal hypoplasia, nystagmus, glaucoma, corneal opacity	Ectopia lentis, anterior polar cataract
Megalocornea			
X-linked recessive, autosomal dominant, autosomal recessive, or sporadic	None	Megalocornea, iris and angle abnormalities, ectopic pupil	Ectopia lentis, cataract
Buphthalmos			
None	None	Glaucoma	Ectopia lentis resulting from enlarged globe, stretched zonules
Systemic disorders			
Marfan syndrome			
Autosomal dominant	Tall stature, arachnodactyly, joint laxity, congenital heart disease, dissecting aortic aneurysm	High refractive errors, strabismus, amblyopia, retinal detachment, glaucoma	Upward subluxation, rarely cataract

(continued)

Table 2. (continued)

Disorder/Inheritance	Systemic Findings	Ocular Findings	Lens changes
Homocystinuria			
Autosomal recessive	Cystathionine β-synthetase deficiency, mental retardation, tall stature, thromboembolism, arachnodactyly, osteoporosis	Secondary glaucoma, retinal detachment, thickened zonules	Inferior subluxation, luxation into vitreous or anterior chamber
Weill-Marchesani syndrome			
Autosomal recessive	Short stature, stubby hands and feet, brachycephaly	Myopia, secondary glaucoma	Microspherophakia, ectopia lentis
Sulfite oxidase deficiency			
Autosomal recessive	Progressive muscular rigidity, decerebrate behavior, death in early childhood	—	Ectopia lentis
Hyperlysinemia			
Autosomal recessive	Hypotonia, mental retardation, seizure disorder, joint hyperextensibility	Strabismus	Ectopia lentis, spherophakia
Syphilis	Features of congenital or acquired forms	Interstitial keratitis, cloudy cornea	Ectopia lentis associated with ocular trauma
Crouzon syndrome			
Autosomal dominant	Multiple synostosis, midface hypoplasia, prognathism	Shallow orbits, exophthalmos, optic atrophy, microcornea, iris and choroidal colobomas, retinal detachment	Occasional ectopia lentis and cataract
Apert syndrome			
Autosomal recessive	Oxycephaly, midface hypoplasia, external ear defects, deafness	Antimongoloid slant of palpebral fissures, coloboma of lateral lower eyelid, microphthalmos	Rarely, ectopia lentis or cataract

Laboratory Studies

Tests for vision, refraction, metabolic disorders

Glaucoma

Due to increased intraocular pressure. May be unilateral or bilateral, associated with headache, irritability, conjunctivitis, triophthalmos (ox eye), due to anatomic abnormalities or genetic-metabolic disorders.

Shaffer-Weiss Classification of Congenital Glaucoma

Primary congenital glaucoma
Glaucoma associated with congenital anomalies
- Late-developing infantile glaucoma (late-developing primary congenital glaucoma)
- Aniridia
- Sturge-Weber syndrome
- Neurofibromatosis
- Marfan syndrome
- Pierre Robin syndrome
- Homocystinuria
- Goniodysgenesis (iridocorneal mesodermal dysgenesis: Rieger anomaly and syndrome, Axenfeld anomaly, and Peters anomaly)
- Lowe syndrome
- Microcornea
- Microspherophakia
- Rubella
- Chromosome abnormalities
- Broad-thumb syndrome
- Persistent hyperplastic primary vitreous

Secondary glaucoma in infants
- Retrolental fibroplasia
- Tumors
- Retinoblastoma
- Juvenile xanthogranuloma
- Inflammation
- Trauma

Laboratory Studies

Measurement of intraocular pressure. Tests for metabolic diseases (see Chapter 17, Metabolic and Hereditary Diseases).

Leukocoria

Retina appears white, commonly due to retinoblastoma. May be unilateral or bilateral and patient may be blind, associated with nystagmus. Other causes include metastatic tumors, infections, and retinal detachment.

Laboratory Studies

DNA or chromosome analysis (13q14). Computed tomographic scan or ultrasonography.

Orbital Disease in Infants, Classification

See Table 3.

Table 3. Classification of Orbital Disease in Infants

- Inflammation
  - Acute
    - Infections
      - Preseptal cellulitis
      - Orbital cellulitis
      - Orbital abscess
    - Idiopathic
      - Specific: Graves, Wegener, sarcoid
      - Nonspecific (pseudotumor)
    - Masquerade
      - Rhabdomyosarcoma, other neoplasms
      - Hemorrhage: lymphangioma, hematic cyst, bone cyst
  - Chronic
    - Idiopathic
    - Masquerade: neoplasm
- Mass
  - Soft tissue
    - Solid
      - Localized
        - Rhabdomyosarcoma
        - Metastatic neuroblastoma
        - Capillary hemangioma
        - Lymphangioma
        - Optic nerve glioma
        - Juvenile fibrosarcoma
        - Granulocytic sarcoma
        - Metastatic leukemia
        - Lymphoma
        - Peripheral nerve tumor
    - Diffuse
        - Metastatic leukemia
        - Idiopathic sclerosing orbititis (pseudotumor)
    - Cystic
      - Dermoid cyst
      - Teratoma
      - Mucocele
        - Lacrimal sac mucocele (dacryocele)
        - Paranasal sinus mucocele
      - Ocular cysts
        - Congenital cystic eye
        - Microphthalmos with cyst
      - Echinococcal cyst (hydatid cyst)
      - Hematocele
      - Lymphangioma
    - Bone
      - Osteosarcoma
      - Fibrous dysplasia and other idiopathic ossifying syndromes
      - Histiocytosis X
        - Eosinophilic granuloma
      - Osteoma
      - Ossifying fibroma
      - Xanthomatous bone lesions

(continued)

Table 3. (continued)

Structural
Encephalocele
Meningocele
Sphenoid wing hypoplasia (neurofibromatosis 1)
Congenital fibrosis
Orbital trauma in infants
Vascular
Dynamic lesions (pulsating or responding to changing venous pressure)
Orbital arteriovenous malformation
Cavernous sinus fistula
Varix
Cutaneous vascular change
Capillary hemangioma
Lymphangioma
Functional
Optic nerve glioma
Optic nerve leukemic metastasis
Fibrous dysplasia

From Eisenberg SJ. *The eye in infancy,* 2nd ed. St. Louis: Mosby, 2000.

Bibliography

Calhoun JH, Harley RD, eds. *Pediatric opthalmology,* 3rd ed. Philadelphia: WB Saunders, 1991: 208, 264.

Csonka GW, Coufalik ED. Chlamydial, gonococcal, and herpes virus infections in neonates. *Postgrad Med J* 1977;53:592–594.

Dobbins JG, Stewart JA, Demmler GJ. Surveillance of congenital cytomegalovirus disease, 1990–1991. Collaborating Registry Group. *MMWR Morb Mortal Wkly Rep* 1992;41:35–39.

Gilbert-Barness E, ed. *Potter's pathology of the fetus and infant.* St. Louis: Mosby–Year Book, 1997.

Gilbert-Barness E, ed. *Potter's atlas of fetus and infant pathology.* St. Louis: Mosby–Year Book, 1998.

Spencer WH. *Ophthalmic pathology.* Philadelphia: WB Saunders, 1996.

Stagno S, Whitley RJ. Herpesvirus infections of pregnancy. Part I: Cytomegalovirus and Epstein-Barr virus infections. *N Engl J Med* 1985;313:1270–1274.

23 Pleural, Pericardial, and Peritoneal Effusions

Body Fluid Examination

Prompt transport to the laboratory is essential.

Body Fluid Composition

Estimated electrolyte composition of body fluids

Fluid	Na (mEq/L)	K (mEq/L)	Cl (mEq/L)
Gastric	20–80	5–20	100–150
Pancreatic	120–140	5–15	40–80
Bile	120–140	5–15	80–120
Small bowel	100–140	5–15	90–130
Ileostomy	40–135	3–15	20–115
Diarrhea	10–90	10–80	10–110
Burn transudate	140	5	110

Effusion, Pleural

A pleural effusion occurs when excessive fluid is released into the pleural space or when lymphatic obstruction precludes normal drainage. Under normal conditions there is a small volume of pleural fluid in the pleural space, which functions as a lubricant. Under pathologic conditions, effusions develop and are classified as either transudates or exudates. Transudates are due to an imbalance between hydrostatic and oncotic pressures (as in hepatic cirrhosis, congestive heart failure, nephrotic syndrome, and obstruction of the superior vena cava). Exudates are secondary to a disturbance of the systems regulating pleural fluid formation and absorption and drainage (as in bacterial, viral, or fungal infection, rheumatologic disease, or malignancy). Distinguishing between these types of effusions can be helpful when cause is uncertain or when response to therapy is inadequate.

Signs and Symptoms

None in small volume effusion
Pleuritic chest pain and referred abdominal or shoulder pain
Cough, may be productive or nonproductive, depending on cause
Chest wall splinting
Dyspnea
Tachypnea, particularly with lung compression or more severe infections
Diminished chest wall excursion
Decreased tactile fremitus
Dullness to percussion over effusion
Diminished or absent breath sounds
Friction rub
Chills
Mediastinal shift (on chest radiograph)
Weight loss
Night sweats

Hemoptysis
Anorexia
General malaise

Normal Values for Pleural Fluid

Specific gravity	1.010–0.026
Total protein	
Albumin	0.3–4.1 g/dL
Globulin	50–70%
Fibrinogen	30–45%
pH	6.8–7.6

The underlying cause of an effusion is usually determined by first classifying the fluid as an exudate or a transudate (Table 1). A transudate does not usually require additional testing but exudates always do.

Exudate Occurs In

Pneumonia, malignancy, pulmonary embolism, and gastrointestinal conditions (especially pancreatitis and abdominal surgery, which cause 90% of all exudates)

Infection (causes 25% of cases)

- Bacterial pneumonia
- Parapneumonic effusion (empyema)
- Tuberculosis (TB)

Table 1. Differences between Transudates and Exudates

Test	Transudates	Exudates
Specific gravity[a]	<1.016	>1.016
Protein (g/dL)[b]	<3.0	>3.0
Pleural fluid/serum ratio[c]	<0.5	>0.5
LDH[d]		
IU	<200	>200
Pleural fluid/serum ratio[c]	<0.6	>0.6
Ratio pleural fluid/upper limit normal serum[c]	<2:3	>2:3
WBC count	<1,000/mm³	>1,000/mm³
	Mainly lymphocytes	May be grossly purulent
RBCs	Few	Variable; few or may be grossly bloody
Glucose	Equivalent to serum	May be decreased because of bacteria or many WBCs
Cholesterol (mg/dL)	<55	Usually >55
Pleural fluid/serum ratio	<0.32	>0.32
pH	Usually 7.4–7.5	Usually 7.35–7.45
Appearance	Clear	Usually cloudy
Color	Pale yellow	Variable

LDH, lactate dehydrogenase; RBCs, red blood cells; WBC, white blood cell.
[a]Long-standing transudates, however, can produce a high specific gravity.
[b]Protein level of 3.0 g/dL misclassifies 15% of effusions if it is the only criterion used.
[c]Each of these three criteria has been used to define pleural fluid exudate and transudate. Use of all three provides the best differentiation of exudate and transudate. Transudate meets none of these criteria, and exudate meets at least one criterion. Unequivocal presence of criteria for transudate precludes the need for pleural biopsy in most cases, unless two mechanisms are suspected (e.g., nephrotic syndrome with miliary tuberculosis, congestive heart failure with malignancy). It would be uncommon for use of diuretics in congestive heart failure to change characteristics of transudate to those of exudate.
[d]If nonhemolyzed, nonbloody effusion.
From Wallach J. *Interpretation of diagnostic tests,* 7th ed. Philadelphia: Lippincott Williams & Wilkins, 2000.

- Abscess (subphrenic, liver, spleen)
- Viral, mycoplasmal, rickettsial infection
- Parasitic infection (ameba, hydatid cyst, filaria)
- Fungal infection (*Coccidioides, Cryptococcus, Histoplasma, Blastomyces, Aspergillus*; in immunocompromised host, *Aspergillus, Candida, Mucor*)

Pulmonary embolism or infarction
Neoplasms (metastatic carcinoma, especially breast, ovary, lung; lymphoma; leukemia; mesothelioma; pleural endometriosis)
Trauma (penetrating or blunt)
- Hemothorax, chylothorax, empyema, associated with rupture of diaphragm

Immunologic mechanisms
- Rheumatoid pleurisy (5% of cases)
- Systemic lupus erythematosus (SLE)
- Other collagen vascular diseases occasionally cause effusions (e.g., Wegener granulomatosis, Sjögren syndrome, familial Mediterranean fever, Churg-Strauss syndrome, mixed connective tissue disease)
- After myocardial infarction or cardiac surgery
- Vasculitis
- Hepatitis
- Sarcoidosis (rare cause; may also be transudate)
- Familial recurrent polyserositis
- Drug reaction (e.g., nitrofurantoin hypersensitivity, methysergide maleate)

Chemical mechanisms
- Uremia

Diagnostic Studies

Tests for leukocytosis with bandemia
Tests for anemia
Tests for hypoalbuminemia
Antinuclear antibody titer
Rheumatoid factor assay
Pancreatic enzyme levels
Assay for cancer antigen 125
Assay for carbohydrate antigen 19-9
Creatinine/blood urea nitrogen ratio
Aerobic and anaerobic blood cultures
Microbial cultures of pleural effusions fluid

Special Tests

Evaluation of pleural fluid withdrawn by thoracentesis. Transudates and exudates must be distinguished. A transudate has none of the following characteristics; however, an exudate must show one:
Pleural fluid protein/serum protein ratio of >0.5
Pleural fluid lactate dehydrogenase/serum dehydrogenase ratio of >0.6
Pleural fluid dehydrogenase level higher than two-thirds the upper limit of that in serum

All exudates must be evaluated with
- Differential cell count
- Amylase level measurement
- Glucose level measurement
- Comprehensive microbiologic culturing and Gram staining
- Cytologic examination for tumor cells

Additional studies: pH, red blood cell (RBC) count (hemorrhagic effusion if >100,000/mL, consider trauma as cause for effusion).

Imaging Studies

Chest radiography: anteroposterior and lateral decubitus views
Thoracic ultrasonography
Computed tomographic scan

Other Diagnostic Procedures

Pleural biopsy if suspicion of TB or neoplasm
Thoracentesis
Thoracoscopy (provides direct view of both parietal and visceral aspects of pleura)

Clinical and Laboratory Findings

See Table 2.

Gross Appearance

Clear, straw-colored fluid is typical of transudate.

Cloudy, opaque appearance indicates more cellular components.

Bloody fluid suggests malignancy, pulmonary infarct, trauma, postcardiotomy syndrome; also uremia, asbestosis, pleural endometriosis. Bloody fluid from traumatic thoracentesis should clot within several minutes, but blood present more than several hours becomes defibrinated and does not form a good clot. Nonuniform color during aspiration and absence of hemosiderin-laden macrophages and some crenated RBCs suggest traumatic aspiration.

Chylous (milky) fluid is usually due to trauma (e.g., auto accident, surgery) but may be due to obstruction of thoracic duct (e.g., especially lymphoma, metastatic carcinoma, granulomas). Pleural fluid triglyceride level of >110 mg/dL or triglyceride pleural fluid/serum ratio of >2 occurs only in chylous effusions (seen especially within a few hours after eating). After centrifugation, supernatant is white due to chylomicrons, which also stain with Sudan III. With equivocal triglyceride levels (60–110 mg/dL), lipoprotein electrophoresis of fluid may be required to demonstrate chylomicrons.

Triglyceride level of <50 mg/dL excludes chylothorax.

Pseudochylous fluid is found in chronic inflammatory conditions (e.g., rheumatoid pleurisy, TB, chronic pneumothorax therapy for TB) due to either cholesterol crystals (rhomboid) in sediment or lipid-containing inclusions in leukocytes. Distinguish from chylous effusions by microscopy. Fluid may have lustrous sheen.

White fluid suggests chylothorax, cholesterol effusion, or empyema.

Black fluid suggests *Aspergillus niger* infection.

Greenish fluid suggests biliopleural fistula.

Purulent fluid indicates infection.

Anchovy (dark red-brown) color is seen in amebiasis, old blood.

Anchovy paste is seen in ruptured amebic liver abscess; amebas are found in <10% of cases.

Turbid and greenish yellow fluid is classical for rheumatoid effusion.

Turbidity may be due to lipids or increased white blood cells (WBCs); after centrifugation, a clear supernatant indicates WBCs as cause.

Very viscous (clear or bloody) fluid is characteristic of mesothelioma.

Debris in fluid suggests rheumatoid pleurisy; food particles indicate esophageal rupture.

Fluid the color of enteral tube food or central venous line infusion is due to tube or catheter entry into pleural space.

Odor

Putrid odor due to anaerobic empyema
Ammonia odor due to urinothorax

Glucose

Same concentration as serum in transudate.

Usually normal but 30–55 mg/dL or pleural fluid/serum ratio of <0.5 and pH <7.30 may be found in TB, malignancy, SLE; also esophageal rupture; lowest levels may occur in empyema and rheumatoid arthritis (RA). Therefore, only helpful if very low level (e.g., <30). A value of 0–10 mg/dL highly suspicious for RA.

pH

Low pH (<7.30) always means exudate, especially empyema, malignancy, rheumatoid pleurisy, SLE, TB, esophageal rupture. Esophageal rupture is only cause of pH close to 6.0; collagen vascular disease is only other cause of pH <7.0. A pH of <7.10 in parapneumonic effusion indicates need for tube drainage. In malignant effusion, pH <7.30 is associated with short survival time, poorer prognosis, and increased positive yield with cytology and pleural biopsy; tends to correlate with pleural fluid glucose level of <60 mg/dL.

Table 2. Pleural Fluid Findings in Various Clinical Conditions

Disease	Appearance	Total WBC (1,000/ mm^3)	Predominant Type WBC	Total RBC (1,000/mm^3)	pH	Glucose		Protein	LDH		Amylase	Comments
						(mg/dL)	PF/S	PF/S	PF/S	IU/L	PF/S	
Pulmonary embolus: infarction	Turbid to hemorrhagic Small volume	5–15	P May show many mesothelial cells	Bloody in one-third to two-thirds of patients	>7.3	>60	1	>0.5	>0.6		≤1	Occurs in 15% of patients; often no characteristic findings
Pneumonia	Turbid	5–40	P	<5	≥7.3	>60	1	>0.5	>0.6		≤1	Occurs in 15% of bacterial pneumonias and cases of legionnaires disease, 5–20% of viral and mycoplasmal pneumonias
Empyema[a]	Turbid to purulent	25–100	P	<5	5.50–7.29	<60	<0.5	>0.5	>0.6	May be >1,000/L	≤1	Most commonly due to anaerobic bacteria, *Staphylococcus aureus*, Gram-negative aerobic bacteria
Tuberculosis	Straw colored; serosanguineous in 15%	5–10	M	<10	<7.3 in 20%	30–60 in 20%	1	>0.5	>0.6		≤1	AFB stain positive in 15–20% and culture of fluid positive in 30% of cases. Histologic examination of biopsy specimen and culture of pleura are diagnostic in 85% of cases. Often presents as effusion; pulmonary disease may be present.
Malignancy[b]	Straw colored to turbid to bloody	<10	M	1 to >100	<7.3 in 30%	<60 in 30%	1	>0.5	>0.6		≤1	—

(continued)

Table 2. (continued)

Disease	Appearance	Total WBC (1,000/mm³)	Predominant Type WBC	Total RBC (1,000/mm³)	pH	Glucose (mg/dL)	Glucose PF/S	Protein PF/S	LDH PF/S	LDH IU/L	Amylase PF/S	Comments
RA effusion[c]	Turbid or green or yellow	1–20	P in acute M in chronic	<1	<7.3; usually 7.0	<30 in	>0.5	>0.6	—	Often >1,000/L	≤1	Biopsy is useful, especially in men with rheumatoid nodules and high RF titer
SLE	Straw colored to turbid		P in acute M in chronic	<7.3 in 30%	<60 in 30%	>0.5	>0.6	>2	—	—	—	PF may show LE cells, ANAs, and low complement. Usually found only when lupus is active

AFB, acid-fast bacillus; ANAs, antinuclear antibodies; LDH, lactate dehydrogenase; LE, lupus erythematosus; M, mononuclear cells; P, polynuclear leukocytes; PF, pleural fluid; PF/S, ratio of pleural fluid level to serum level; RA, rheumatoid arthritis; RBC, red blood cell; RF, rheumatoid factor; SLE, systemic lupus erythematosus; WBC, white blood cell.

Note: Blood specimens should always be drawn at the same time as serous fluid for determination of glucose, protein, LD, amylase, pH, etc. Pleural fluid for pH should be collected in the same way as arterial blood samples (i.e., heparinized syringe, maintained anaerobically on ice, analyzed promptly). Pleural fluid pH should normally be at least 0.15 greater than arterial blood pH. Normal pH is alkaline and may approach 7.6.

[a]pH <7.0 and glucose <40 mg/dL indicate need for closed chest tube drainage even without grossly purulent fluid.
pH of 7.0–7.2 is a questionable indication and should be repeated in 24 hr, but tube drainage is favored if pleural fluid LDH >1,000 IU/L. Tube drainage is also indicated if there is grossly purulent fluid or positive results on Gram stain or culture.

[b]Lung and breast cancer lymphomas cause 75% of malignant effusions; in 6%, no primary tumor is found. Pleural or ascitic effusion occurs in 20–30% of patients with malignant lymphoma.

[c]Decreased glucose level is the most useful finding clinically; may be 0.

From Wallach J. *Interpretation of diagnostic tests,* 7th ed. Philadelphia: Lippincott Williams & Wilkins, 2000.

Amylase

Increased in pancreatitis (pleural fluid/serum ratio >1.0 and may be >5, or pleural fluid higher than upper limit of normal for serum).

- In acute pancreatitis may be normal early with increase over time.
- Pancreatic pseudocyst is always increased, may be >100,000 U/L.
- Also increased in perforated ulcer, necrosis of small intestine (e.g., mesenteric vascular occlusion); 10% of cases of metastatic cancer and esophageal rupture.

Isoenzyme studies

- Pancreatic-type amylase is found in acute pancreatitis and pancreatic pseudocyst.
- Salivary-type amylase is found in esophageal rupture and occasionally in carcinoma of ovary or lung or salivary gland tumor.
- Type should be determined in undiagnosed left pleural effusions.

Cell Count

Total WBC count is almost never diagnostic.

Count of >10,000/mm^3 indicates inflammation, most commonly with pneumonia, pulmonary infarct, pancreatitis, postcardiotomy syndrome.

Count of >50,000/mm^3 is typical only in parapneumonic effusions, usually empyema.

Chronic exudates (e.g., malignancy and TB) contain <5,000/mm^3.

Transudates usually contain <1,000/mm^3.

Level of 5,000–6,000 RBCs/mm^3 is needed to give red appearance to pleural fluid.

This level may be caused by needle trauma producing 2 mL of blood in 100 mL of pleural fluid.

Count of >100,000 RBCs/mm^3 is grossly hemorrhagic and suggests malignancy, pulmonary infarct, or trauma, but occasionally it is seen in congestive heart failure alone.

Hemothorax (pleural fluid/venous hematocrit ratio >2) suggests trauma, bleeding from a vessel, bleeding disorder, or malignancy, but it may be seen in the same conditions as earlier.

Smears

Wright stain differentiates polymorphonuclear cells (PMNs) from mononuclear cells; cannot differentiate lymphocytes from monocytes.

Mononuclear cells predominate in transudates and chronic exudates (lymphoma, carcinoma, TB, rheumatoid conditions, uremia). A level >50% is seen in two-thirds of cases due to cancer. A level of >85–90% suggests TB, lymphoma, sarcoidosis, RA.

PMNs predominate in early inflammatory effusions (e.g., pneumonia, pulmonary infarct, pancreatitis, subphrenic abscess).

After several days, mesothelial cells, macrophages, lymphocytes may predominate.

Large mesothelial cells >5% are said to rule out TB (must differentiate from macrophages).

Lymphocytes

- Level of >85% suggests TB, lymphoma, sarcoidosis, chronic rheumatoid pleurisy, yellow nail syndrome, chylothorax.
- Level of 50–75% in >50% of cases of carcinoma.

Eosinophils in pleural fluid (>10% of total WBCs) is not diagnostically significant.

- May mean blood or air in pleural space [e.g., pneumothorax (most common) repeated thoracentesis, traumatic hemothorax].
- Is associated with asbestosis, pulmonary infarction, polyarteritis nodosa.
- Found in parasitic disease (e.g., paragonimiasis, hydatid disease, amebiasis, ascariasis).
- Found in fungal disease (e.g., histoplasmosis, coccidioidomycosis).
- May be drug related (e.g., nitrofurantoin, bromocriptine mesylate, dantrolene sodium).
- Found in idiopathic effusion (in approximately one-third of cases; may be due to occult pulmonary embolism).
- Uncommon with malignant effusions.
- Rare with TB.
- Not usually accompanied by striking blood eosinophilia. Many diseases associated with blood eosinophilia infrequently cause pleural effusion eosinophilia.

Basophils >10% only in leukemic involvement of pleura.

Occasionally presence of *lupus erythematosus cells* makes the diagnosis of SLE.

Gram stain for early diagnosis of bacterial infection.

Acid-fast smear findings are positive in 20% of cases of TB pleurisy.

Culture results are often positive in empyema but not in parapneumonic effusions.

Bacterial antigens may detect *Haemophilus influenzae* type b, *Streptococcus pneumoniae*, several types of *Neisseria meningitidis*. Useful when viable organisms cannot be recovered (e.g., due to prior antibiotic therapy).

Cytology

Positive findings in 60% of malignancies on first tap, 80% by third tap. Therefore, should repeat taps with cytologic examination if cancer is suspected. Is more sensitive than needle biopsy. High yield with adenocarcinoma, low yield with Hodgkin disease.

Rheumatoid effusions: cytologic triad of slender, elongated, and round giant multinucleated macrophages and necrotic background material with characteristically low glucose is pathognomonic. Mesothelial cells are nearly always absent.

Flow cytometry assay for DNA aneuploidy and staining with monoclonal antibodies (e.g., carcinoembryonic antigen, cytokeratin) to distinguish malignant mesothelioma, metastatic tumor, and reactive mesothelial cells can be performed.

Pleural Fluid Findings in Various Diseases

Congestive Heart Failure

Is predominantly right-sided or bilateral. If unilateral or left-sided in patients with congestive heart failure, rule out pulmonary infarct.

Empyema

Usually WBCs >50,000/mm^3, low glucose level, and low pH. Suspect clinically when effusion develops during adequate antibiotic therapy.

In *Proteus mirabilis* empyema, high ammonia level may cause a pH of 8.0.

Malignancy

Malignancies can cause effusion by metastasis to pleura, which leads to exudate-type fluid, or by metastasis to lymph nodes, which obstructs lymph drainage and giving transudate-type fluid. Low pH and glucose level indicate a poor prognosis with short survival time.

Characteristic effusion is moderate to massive, frequently hemorrhagic, with moderate WBC count and predominance of mononuclear cells; however, only half of malignant effusions have RBC counts >10,000/mm^3.

Cytologic examination establishes the diagnosis in 50% of patients.

Combined cytologic examination and pleural biopsy give positive results in 90%.

In some instances of suspected lymphoma with negative conventional test results, flow cytometric analysis of pleural fluid showing a monoclonal lymphocyte population can establish the diagnosis.

Mucopolysaccharide level may be increased in mesothelioma (normal is <17 mg/dL).

Pneumonias

Parapneumonic effusions (exudate type of effusion associated with lung abscess, bronchiectasis; 5% of bacterial pneumonias).

Infection with aerobic Gram-negative organisms (*Klebsiella, Escherichia coli, Pseudomonas*) is associated with a high incidence of exudates (with 5,000–40,000/mm^3, high protein, normal glucose, normal pH) and resolves with antibiotic therapy. Nonpurulent fluid with positive Gram stain or positive blood culture results or low pH suggests that effusion will become and behave like empyema.

Streptococcus pneumoniae causes parapneumonic effusions in 50% of cases, especially with positive blood culture results.

Staphylococcus aureus causes effusion in 90% of infants, 50% of adults; usually extensive bronchopneumonia.

Streptococcus pyogenes causes effusion in 90% of cases; massive effusion, greenish color.

H. influenzae causes effusion in 50–75% of cases.

Viral or *Mycoplasma* pneumonia—pleural effusions develop in 20% of cases.

Legionnaires disease—pleural effusion occurs in up to 50% of patients; may be bilateral.

Pneumocystis carinii pneumonia cases often have pleural effusion/serum lactate dehydrogenase ratio of >1.0 and pleural effusion/serum protein ratio of <0.5.

A pH <7.0 and glucose level <40 mg/dL indicate need for closed chest tube drainage, even without grossly purulent fluid.

A pH of 7.0–7.2 is a questionable indication and measurement should be repeated in 24 hours; however, tube drainage is favored if pleural fluid lactate dehydrogenase level is >1,000 U/L. Tube drainage is also indicated if fluid is grossly purulent or Gram stain or culture results are positive.

Normal pH is alkaline and may approach 7.6.

Pulmonary Infarct

Effusion occurs in 50% of patients with pulmonary infarct; it is bloody in one-third to two-thirds of patients; often no characteristic diagnostic findings occur.

Small volume, serous or bloody, predominance of PMNs, may show many mesothelial cells; this "typical pattern" is seen in only 25% of cases.

Rheumatoid Arthritis

Rheumatoid effusions found in 70% of RA patients at autopsy.

Exudate is frequently turbid and may be milky. Classic picture is cloudy greenish fluid with 0 glucose level. Level is <50 mg/dL in 80% and <25 mg/dL in 66% of patients; it is the most useful finding clinically. Failure of level to increase during intravenous glucose infusion distinguishes RA from other causes. Nonpurulent, nonmalignant effusions not due to TB or RA almost always have glucose level of >60 mg/dL.

Rheumatoid factor may be present but may also be found in other effusions (e.g., TB, cancer, bacterial pneumonia). Rheumatoid factor titer ≥1:320 or equal to or greater than serum level suggests rheumatoid pleurisy.

RA cells may be found.

Cytologic examination for malignant cells and smears and cultures for bacteria, tubercle bacilli, and fungi are negative.

Needle biopsy specimen usually shows nonspecific chronic inflammation but may show characteristic rheumatoid nodule microscopically. One-third of cases have parenchymal lung disease (e.g., interstitial fibrosis).

Other laboratory findings of RA are seen.

Protein level is >3 g/dL.

Table 3 compares pleural fluid findings in SLE and RA.

Systemic Lupus Erythematosus

Presence of lupus erythematosus cells is specific for SLE but test has poor sensitivity.

Antinuclear antibody titer ≥160 or pleural fluid/serum ratio >1.0 is suggestive but not diagnostic.

Table 3 compares pleural fluid findings in SLE and RA.

Tuberculosis

High protein content—almost always >4.0 g/dL.

Increased lymphocytes.

Acid-fast smears yield positive results in 20%, and culture results are positive in 67% of cases; culture combined with histologic examination establish the diagnosis in 95% of cases.

Table 3. Comparison of Pleural Fluid in Rheumatoid Arthritis and Systemic Lupus Erythematosus

Test	Rheumatoid Arthritis	Systemic Lupus Erythematosus
pH >7.2	≤7.2	>7.2
Glucose	<30 mg/dL	Normal
Lactate dehydrogenase	>700 IU/L	<700 IU/L
Rheumatoid factor	Strongly positive	Negative or weakly positive
Ratio pleural fluid to serum	>1.0	<1.0
Rheumatoid arthritis cells (ragocytes)	May be present	Absent
Epithelial cells	Present	Absent
C4	Markedly decreased (<10 × 10^5 g/g of protein)	Moderately decreased (<30 × 10^6 g/g of protein)
Clq-binding assay	Moderately positive	Weakly positive
Ratio pleural fluid to serum	>1.0	<1.0

Needle biopsy can be performed.

Large mesothelial cells >5% are said to rule out TB (must differentiate from macrophages).

TB often presents as effusion, especially in the young; pulmonary disease may be absent.

Effusion, Serous (Pleural, Peritoneal, and Pericardial)

Serous fluid specimens should be divided at the time of collection into several tubes, the number depending on the type of laboratory tests to be performed. Fluid from the last tube obtained should be used for cell counts and morphologic examination. Specimens should be examined promptly. If processing is delayed, storage at 4°C is advised to minimize deterioration of cells. Serous fluid specimens maintain satisfactory morphologic qualities up to 24 hours after fluid collection. Some pleural and peritoneal effusions clot unless fluid is drawn into syringes containing 1 mL of 1% heparin in saline solution. Serous fluids may be used for immunocytochemical, flow cytometric, molecular pathologic, and cytogenetic studies.

Cell concentration methods include cytocentrifugation and filter techniques. Papanicolaou stain and Wright-Giemsa stain have been used successfully.

If malignant lymphoma is suspected, cell blocks should be prepared in addition to cytocentrifuged or filtered specimens.

The majority of serous effusions in children are benign. Most malignant effusions are caused by lymphomas. Malignant serous effusions are usually clear or slightly blood stained; rarely, the effusions are chylous due to damage to thoracic duct or cisterna chyli.

Pericarditis

Acute pericarditis: an inflammatory process of the pericardium due to a wide spectrum of causes with or without associated effusion. The most common cause is idiopathic or nonspecific pericarditis.

Pericardial effusion may result in pericardial tamponade, which causes hemodynamic compromise and disruption of compensatory mechanisms.

Constrictive pericarditis results in thickening and adherence of the pericardium to the heart after chronic inflammation.

Signs and Symptoms

Acute pericarditis
- Chest pain, typically sharp, retrosternal with radiation to the trapezial ridge
- Pain frequently sudden in onset, with inspiration or movement
- Pain reduced by leaning forward and sitting up
- Splinted breathing
- Odynophagia
- Fever
- Myalgia
- Anorexia
- Anxiety
- Pericardial friction rub
- Cardiac arrhythmias often intermittent supraventricular tachycardia
- Tachypnea
- Localized rales

Pericardial tamponade
- Dyspnea
- Tachycardia
- Distended jugular neck veins
- Cyanosis
- Relative or absolute hypotension
- Quiet precordium with little palpable cardiac activity
- Pericardial friction rub
- Lungs clear

Ewart's sign—dullness and bronchial breathing between the tip of the left scapula and vertebral column
Rapid, thready pulse
Varying degrees of consciousness
Pulsus paradoxus: >10 mm Hg (1.33 kPa) decreased in systolic pressure with inspiration
Beck's triad—distended neck veins, hypotension, and muffled heart sounds

Constrictive pericarditis
Asymptomatic, early.
Dyspnea, pulmonary congestion.
Fatigue very common.
Peripheral edema.
Hepatomegaly.
Ascites.
Jugular venous distention—elevated, deep Y trough (not seen in tamponade).
Kussmaul's sign—inspiratory increase in jugular venous pressure.
Pericardial "knock"—follows S2 by 0.06–0.12 seconds, increases with squatting.
Hypovolemia may mask the signs of constriction.

Causes

Idiopathic
Viral infection: coxsackievirus, echo adenovirus, Epstein-Barr virus, mumps virus
Bacterial infection: *Haemophilus* (especially children), *Staphylococcus, Pneumococcus, Salmonella, Meningococcus, Borrelia burgdorferi* (Lyme disease), *Legionella, Mycoplasma*
Fungal infection: *Candida, Histoplasma, Aspergillus, Nocardia*
Mycobacterial infection: *Mycobacterium* TB
Parasitic, protozoal infestation
Neoplasia: breast, lung, lymphoma, mesothelioma
Drug effects: procainamide hydrochloride, hydralazine hydrochloride, bleomycin sulfate, phenytoin, minoxidil, mesalamine, azathioprine, and perhaps other
Connective tissue disease: SLE, RA, scleroderma, acute rheumatic fever
Dressler myocardial infarction
Radiation exposure
Postpericardiotomy
Uremia
Myxedema
Cholesterol pericarditis
Aortic dissection
Sarcoidosis
Pancreatitis
Inflammatory bowel disease
Acquired immunodeficiency syndrome
Chylopericardium
Familial, autosomal-recessive disorders (mulibrey nanism)

Risk Factors

Chest trauma

Laboratory Findings

Leukocytosis and increased erythrocyte sedimentation rate
May see elevated creatine kinase, lactate dehydrogenase, serum glutamic-oxaloacetic transaminase (aspartate aminotransferase)

Special Tests

Electrocardiogram—electrical alternans in tamponade
Echocardiogram—determines fluid, right atrial, or right ventricular collapse
Right heart catheterization—equalization of mean and diastolic pressure in all waveforms

Imaging Studies

Chest radiograph: small pleural effusion, transient infiltrates, "water bottle" silhouette in large associated pericardial effusion.
Chest computed tomography or magnetic resonance imaging in suspected constrictive pericarditis may reveal calcified or thickened pericardium; delineate effusions.

Other Diagnostic Procedures

Pericardiocentesis
Pericardial biopsy

Peritonitis, Acute

Acute inflammation of the visceral and parietal peritoneum.
Systems affected are gastrointestinal, endocrine and metabolic, and cardiovascular.

Signs and Symptoms

Acute abdominal pain
Fever
Nausea
Vomiting
Constipation
Abdominal pain exacerbated by motion
Abdominal distention
Dyspnea
Diffuse abdominal rebound
Generalized abdominal rigidity
Decreased bowel sounds
Abdominal hyperresonance on percussion
Hypotension
Tachycardia
Hippocratic facies
Tachypnea
Dehydration
Ascites

Causes

Primary
- Spontaneous bacterial peritonitis
- Ascites associated with cirrhosis, nephrotic syndrome

Secondary
- Abdominal trauma
- Penetrating wounds
- Continuous ambulatory peritoneal dialysis
- Perforation of bowel
- Appendicitis
- Infectious, inflammatory colitis
- Peptic ulcer perforation
- Gangrene of the bowel
- Diverticulitis
- Pancreatitis

Causes of Peritoneal Effusion

Acute cholecystitis
Neoplastic processes: mesothelioma from asbestos exposure, bronchogenic carcinoma, breast carcinoma, lymphoma, leukemia, metastatic disease
Rheumatic disease (SLE, RA)
Pancreatitis (left-sided exudate with high amylase concentration)

Esophageal rupture
Drug reaction, possibly accompanied by eosinophilia
Uremia
Meigs syndrome
Subdiaphragmatic abscess
Cirrhosis with ascites
Chylous or pseudochylous effusion (thoracic duct injury)
Trauma leading to intrapleural hemorrhage
Idiopathic

Risk Factors

Recent surgery
Advanced liver disease
Corticosteroid medication
Nephrotic syndrome
Continuous ambulatory peritoneal dialysis

Laboratory Findings

Positive results on culture of peritoneal aspirate
Leukocytosis
Increased blood urea nitrogen
Hemoconcentration
Positive results on blood culture
Metabolic acidosis
Respiratory acidosis
Elevated amylase level
Abnormal findings on ascitic fluid analysis

Pathologic Findings

Peritoneum—generalized fibrinopurulent exudate, PMN infiltration

Imaging Studies

Abdominal film: free air in peritoneal cavity, large-bowel dilatation, small-bowel dilatation, intestinal wall edema
Chest radiograph: elevated diaphragm
Computed tomographic scan: intraabdominal mass, ascites
Sonography: intraabdominal mass, ascites

Bibliography

Geisinger KR, Silverman RF, Wakely PE. *Pediatric cytopathology.* Chicago: American Society of Clinical Pathologists Press, 1994:161–202, 231–254.
Hallman JR, Geisinger KR. Cytology of fluids from pleural, peritoneal and pericardial cavities in children: a comprehensive survey. *Acta Cytol* 1994;38:209–217.
Kjeldsberg C, Knight J. *Body fluids.* Chicago: American Society of Clinical Pathologists Press, 1993:303–348.
Venrick MG, Sidawy MK. Cytologic evaluation of serous effusions: processing techniques and optimal number of smears for routine preparation. *Am J Clin Pathol* 1993;99:182–186.
Wallach J. *Interpretation of diagnostic tests*, 7th ed. Philadelphia: Lippincott Williams & Wilkins, 2000.

24 Connective Tissue Disorders and Vasculitis

Laboratory Tests for Connective Tissue Disorders and Vasculitis

Antinuclear Antibodies

Screening for Rheumatic Diseases

Connective tissue diseases represent a subgroup of rheumatic inflammatory diseases characterized by connective tissue damage. Systemic lupus erythematosus (SLE), mixed connective tissue disease (MCTD, or Sharp syndrome), scleroderma, myositis, and Sjögren syndrome are autoimmune diseases in this group. Many connective tissue diseases affect multiple organs, which makes the clinical diagnosis difficult. They all have in common the presence of specific antinuclear antibodies (ANAs) directed against various, primarily nuclear, proteins, nucleic acids, or nucleoprotein complexes.

An enzyme immunoassay method uses a cocktail of defined recombinant antigens that are targeted to the currently accepted clinically relevant ANAs.

Any samples giving positive results should then be assayed by indirect immunofluorescent assay (IFA).

Antinuclear Antibody Test

ANA testing by IFA should be ordered when warm-type autoimmune hemolytic anemia is diagnosed, particularly in young women, to determine whether SLE or another collagen vascular disease is the underlying cause. The hemolysis frequently precedes diagnosis of SLE by months or even years.

If ANAs are present, they bind to the cell nuclei and can be depicted with fluorescence.

The patient's serum is incubated with a source of nuclear antigen (e.g., tissue culture cells, rat kidney, human granulocytes). The antigen-antibody combination is demonstrated by an antiglobulin reagent tagged with a fluorescent dye. The patient's serum can then be titered.

Titers >1:20 are suspicious in most laboratories, and titers of 1:80 or greater are considered diagnostic of collagen vascular disease. Suspicious positive test results may be seen in up to 3% of older individuals.

Connective Tissue Diseases with Antinuclear Antibodies

SLE
Drug-induced lupus-like disorder
- Procainamide hydrochloride
- Hydralazine hydrochloride

MCTD
Sjögren syndrome
Scleroderma
Polymyositis-dermatomyositis
Rheumatoid arthritis

Disease Correlations with Fluorescent Antinuclear Antibody Patterns

Pattern	Correlation
Homogenous	SLE
Peripheral	SLE
Speckled	SLE
	MCTD
	Sjögren syndrome
	Polymyositis-dermatomyositis
	Scleroderma
Nucleolar	Scleroderma
	Sjögren syndrome

The peripheral pattern is relatively specific for SLE; the nucleolar pattern is found in scleroderma and Sjögren syndrome.

The speckled pattern is associated with a variety of nuclear antigens, including antibodies to a specific nuclear antigen—the centromere of chromosome spreads and ribonuclear protein (RNP) and nonhistone proteins.

Drugs that are associated with false-positive ANA test results are *p*-aminosalicylic acid, carbamazepine (Tegretol), chlorpromazine (Thorazine), ethosuximide (Zarontin), griseofulvin, hydralazine (Apresoline), isoniazid, mephenytoin (Mesantoin), methyldopa (Aldomet), penicillin, phenylbutazone (Butazolidin), phenytoin (Dilantin), hydantoin group, primidone (Mysoline), procainamide hydrochloride, propylthiouracil, and trimethadione (Tridione). Also some drugs in the following categories: heavy metals, iodides, oral contraceptives, tetracyclines, thiazide diuretics, and thiourea derivatives, including sulfonamides.

Pediatric Diseases Associated with a Positive Finding of Antinuclear Antibody

Rheumatic Diseases	Nonrheumatic Diseases
SLE	Drug-induced positivity
Juvenile rheumatoid arthritis (JRA)	Anticonvulsants (e.g., phenytoin)
Dermatomyositis	Antihypertensives (e.g., hydralazine)
Scleroderma	Antiarrhythmics (e.g., procainamide)
MCTD	Infections
	Syphilis
	Hepatitis
	Mononucleosis
	Malignancy (e.g., leukemia, lymphoma)
	Inflammatory bowel disease

Specific Antibodies Associated with Rheumatic Diseases

See Table 1.

Anti–Double-Stranded DNA

The anti–double-stranded DNA antibody is usually present in cases of positive ANA results that show a peripheral (rim) pattern and occasionally a homogenous pattern. This antibody is very specific for SLE and has prognostic significance in that high titers of anti–double-stranded DNA are associated with an increased risk of SLE nephritis.

Antihistone

The antihistone antibody is nearly always associated with a homogeneous ANA pattern and is most commonly seen in cases of drug-induced lupus.

Anti–Jo-1

The anti–Jo-1 antibody, associated with cytoplasmic staining of ANA substrate cells, is a marker for polymyositis. Testing for this antibody should be done in cases in which ANA results are negative but cytoplasmic staining is positive.

Table 1. Frequency of Specific Antibodies in Autoimmune Rheumatic Disease

Disorder	Antibody	%
SLE	Native DNA Abs	40–90
Patterns observed on IFA include homogenous, peripheral, and speckled	Histone Abs	70
	SM Abs	30
	RNP Abs	32
	SS-A (Ro) Abs	35
	SS-B (La) Abs	10–40
Drug-induced LE	Histone Abs	95
Patterns observed on IFA include homogenous and speckled		
Subacute Cutaneous LE	SS-A (Ro) Abs	65
Patterns observed on IFA include speckled		
MCTD	RNP Abs	95
Patterns observed on IFA include speckled		
Sjögren syndrome	SS-A (Ro) Abs	60
Patterns observed on IFA include speckled	SS-B (La) Abs	40–80
Scleroderma	Scl-70 Abs	70
Patterns observed on IFA include speckled, nucleolar		
Polymyositis	PM-Scl Abs	3
Patterns observed on IFA include centromere, speckled		
CREST syndrome	Centromere Abs	70–80
Patterns observed on IFA include centromere, speckled		
Polydermatomyositis	Jo-1 Abs	25–30
Patterns observed on IFA include speckled		

Abs, antibodies; CREST, *c*alcinosis, *R*aynaud phenomenon, *e*sophageal motility disorders, *s*clerodactyly, and *t*elangiectasia; IFA, immunofluorescent assay; LE, lupus erythematosus; MCTD, mixed connective tissue disease; PM-Scl, polymyositis-scleroderma; RNP, ribonuclear protein; Scl-70, scleroderma 70; SLE, systemic lupus erythematosus; Sm, smith; SS-A, Sjögren syndrome A; SS-B, Sjögren syndrome B.
The enzyme immunoassay method can determine immunoglobulin G antibodies directed against the human antigens of U1–small nuclear ribonucleoprotein, RNP-Sm, Sm, SS-A, SS-B, Scl-70, centromere antigens, Jo-1, double-stranded DNA, histone proteins, and PM-Scl-100. Interference by rheumatoid factors has not been observed.
From Quest Diagnostics Inc., Tampa, FL.

Antineutrophil Cytoplasmic Antibody Tests

Testing for antineutrophil cytoplasmic antibodies (ANCAs) has been found to be useful in establishing the diagnosis of suspected vascular diseases (Wegener granulomatosis, crescentic glomerulonephritis, microscopic polyarteritis and Churg-Strauss syndrome), bowel diseases (including Crohn disease, ulcerative colitis, primary sclerosing cholangitis, and autoimmune hepatitis), as well as other autoimmune diseases (including drug-induced lupus, SLE, Felty syndrome).

ANCA has classically been divided into c-ANCA (cytoplasmic) and p-ANCA (perinuclear) depending on the immunofluorescent pattern observed. More recently the specific antigens responsible for these patterns have been described and isolated. The antigen that gives the c-ANCA pattern is proteinase-3. Multiple antigens are responsible for p-ANCA pattern, the principle antigen being myeloperoxidase (MPO).

Patients with vascular diseases generally have either a c-ANCA pattern or p-ANCA pattern and results are positive in specific tests for proteinase-3 or MPO.

Patients with bowel disease have been shown to have antibodies that give a p-ANCA pattern. These antibodies, however, may not be directed toward MPO.

Patients with autoimmune SLE and drug-induced lupus often present with a p-ANCA pattern that is associated with antibodies against MPO.

Use in Diagnosis of Inflammatory Bowel Disease

For the diagnosis of bowel disease, the test is performed by an IFA procedure to detect all forms of p-ANCA.

Use in Diagnosis of Vasculitides

For the diagnosis of vascular and autoimmune disease, the test is performed by a semiquantitative enzyme immunoassay for detection of antibodies to proteinase-3 and MPO.

A 1-mL serum sample in a plastic screw-cap vial, serum separator tube, or red top tube is required.

Anti–Ribonuclear Protein

Antibodies to RNP may be identified by immunodiffusion; titers are determined by hemagglutination. The Smith (Sm) antigen is not destroyed by ribonuclease, whereas RNP is destroyed by ribonuclease; this fact is used to distinguish between antibodies to Sm and RNP in the hemagglutination test.

Sm and RNP antigens are obtained from rabbit thymus; these antigens are used to coat tanned sheep red blood cells. An aliquot of the coated cells is treated with ribonuclease. Then a hemagglutination test is done using the patient's serum. The antibody is associated with a speckled pattern of ANA immunofluorescence.

Very high titers of antibody to nuclear RNP are found in MCTD, occurring in 85–100% of cases at titers ≥1:10,000.

Antibodies to nuclear RNP may also be present in SLE and progressive systemic sclerosis (scleroderma).

This antibody, when present alone and with high titers, is quite specific for MCTD. Anti-RNP coexisting with other autoantibodies is not consistent with MCTD.

Anti–Scl-70

The anti–Scl-70 antibody, significantly associated with scleroderma, is related to the speckled and occasionally to the nucleolar pattern of ANA immunofluorescence. Anti–Scl-70 is present in a significant proportion of cases of diffuse scleroderma but is seen only rarely in the CREST (*c*alcinosis, *R*aynaud phenomenon, *e*sophageal motility disorders, *s*clerodactyly, and *t*elangiectasia) syndrome.

Anti-Smith Antibodies

Anti-Smith antibodies may be identified by immunodiffusion; titers are determined by hemagglutination. The Sm antigen is not destroyed by ribonuclease, whereas RNP is destroyed by ribonuclease; this fact is used to distinguish between antibodies to Sm and RNP in the hemagglutination test.

Sm and RNP antigens are obtained from rabbit thymus; these antigens are used to coat tanned sheep red blood cells. An aliquot of the coated cells is treated with ribonuclease. Then, a hemagglutination test is done using the patient's serum. The antibody is associated with a speckled pattern of ANA immunofluorescence.

Antibodies to Sm antigens are highly specific for SLE and are found in 20–30% of patients with SLE. They are found only rarely in other connective tissue disorders. Clinical data indicate that the presence of anti-Sm antibody is associated with a higher incidence of vasculitis, which results in peculiar visceral manifestations and poor response to therapy.

Anti–Smooth Muscle Antibody

Testing for Anti–Smooth Muscle Antibody

The IFA technique is used to detect anti–smooth muscle antibody. The patient's serum is diluted, usually 1:10, and added to fresh (frozen) tissue from mouse stomach or rat uterus or other appropriate tissue containing smooth muscle. The serum and tissue are incubated, and fluorescein-conjugated antiglobulin is added. The sections are examined by fluorescence microscopy.

This test is useful in differentiating chronic active hepatitis (lupoid hepatitis) from extrahepatic biliary obstruction, drug-induced liver disease, viral hepatitis, and other conditions involving the liver.

Conditions with Increased Anti–Smooth Muscle Antibody

Condition	% Positive Results at 1:10 Dilution	Titer Suggestive of Diagnosis
Chronic active hepatitis (lupoid hepatitis type)	50–80	Generally, titers >1:80
Viral hepatitis (acute)	1–2	Titers <1:80 and transient
Biliary cirrhosis	0–50	Titers between 1:10 and 1:40
Intrinsic asthma	20	Low titers

In chronic active hepatitis, lupoid hepatitis type, the titers of anti–smooth muscle antibody are generally high and persistent.

Most of the antibodies are fairly specific for the diseases with which they are associated. However, many of these antibodies, in low titers, can be seen in association with other autoimmune or connective tissue diseases. Because of this degree of nonspecificity and the relatively rare overlap of any two or more of these diseases, these assays are most useful in confirming clinical diagnoses.

When ANAs are absent or present in low titers (1:80 or less), follow-up testing for specific autoantibodies is not useful. Because ANAs are often absent or of low titer, it is not appropriate to construct panels that include tests that should be performed only if the ANA result is positive. The panels could be constructed so as to perform downstream tests reflectively, but the initial evaluation of connective tissue disorders should begin with ANA measurement alone.

If the ANA test is positive at a titer of ≥1:160, follow-up testing for more specific autoantibodies is indicated and is based on the pattern of immunofluorescence seen in the initial ANA test.

Anti–SS-A/Ro and Anti–SS-B/La

Both anti–SS-A/Ro and anti–SS-B/La antibodies show a significant association with Sjögren syndrome and are related to speckled pattern ANA immunofluorescence.

Other Nonnuclear Autoantibodies

In addition to the common antinuclear (and anticytoplasmic) antibodies, there are a number of other nonnuclear autoantibodies that are important in the diagnosis of certain other autoimmune disorders. These include

- Antimitochondrial antibodies, seen in primary biliary cirrhosis
- Smooth muscle antibodies, seen in autoimmune hepatitis
- Skeletal muscle antibodies, associated with certain cases of myasthenia gravis
- Myocardial antibodies, seen in cases of inflammatory cardiomyopathies
- Thyroid peroxidase antibodies, associated with immune thyroid disease
- Parietal cell antibodies, seen in cases of pernicious anemia
- Reticulin antibodies, associated with many cases of gluten-sensitive enteropathy

Rheumatoid Factor

Pediatric diseases associated with rheumatoid factor include the following:

Rheumatic Diseases	Nonrheumatic Diseases
JRA	Viral infection (e.g., Epstein-Barr virus)
SLE	Chronic active hepatitis
Scleroderma	Chronic infections (e.g., tuberculosis, malaria)
Vasculitis	Subacute bacterial endocarditis
	Malignancy (e.g., leukemia, lymphoma)
	Sarcoidosis
	Chronic pulmonary disease
	Postvaccination

Tests Used in the Diagnosis of Acute-Phase Reactants

Erythrocyte Sedimentation Rate

The rate of fall in milliliters per hour of red blood cells by the Westergren method (erythrocyte sedimentation rate, or ESR) is used to document inflammation and to follow the course of chronic rheumatic disorders such as JRA, SLE, juvenile-onset diabetes mellitus, and vasculitis. In inflammatory disorders, red blood cells tend to form stacks (rouleaux) that partly result from increased concentration of fibrinogen and thus sediment more rapidly. Falsely low sedimentation rates are found in sickle cell disease, anisocytosis, spherocytosis, polycythemia, and heart failure. Prolonged storage of blood or tilting of the calibrated tube will increase the ESR.

C-Reactive Protein Level

C-reactive protein (CRP) is an acute-phase reactant serum protein that is present in low concentration in normal serum and gives a precipitin reaction with pneumococcal C-polysaccharide. CRP concentrations rise rapidly under an inflammatory stimulus. In SLE and scleroderma, CRP concentrations are inappropriately low unless infection is present. CRP testing may be performed on freeze-stored serum, its major advantage compared to ESR testing.

Diseases of Connective Tissue and Vasculitis

See Tables 2–4.

Arthritis, Juvenile Psoriatic

Juvenile psoriatic arthritis is a chronic, recurrent, polyarthritis in children <16 years of age, preceded, accompanied, or followed within 15 years by psoriasis. Psoriasis affects 1–2% of the white population and has its onset in childhood in one-third of patients. Five percent to 7% of patients with psoriasis have arthritis. The onset of arthritis may be acute or insidious and is often preceded by skin disease.

Table 2. Serologic Test Findings in Rheumatoid Diseases

Disease	ANA Titer[a]	Cases with RF Present[b] (%)	Serum Complement Level
Systemic lupus erythematosus	>1:100	30–40	↓
Rheumatoid arthritis			
Adult	1:20–1:100	80–90	N or ↑
Juvenile	<1:5	15	N
Mixed connective tissue disease	1:100–1:200	50	N or ↑
Dermatomyositis	1:25	10–15	N
Scleroderma	1:25–40	33	N
Polyarteritis nodosa	<1:5 (L)	5–10	N or ↓

↑, increased; ↓, decreased; ANA, antinuclear antibodies; N, normal; RF, rheumatoid factor.
Anti-DNA antibodies correlate best with a diagnosis of systemic lupus erythematosus (SLE); they are found in <5% of patients with other immunologic diseases.
[a]Diagnosis of SLE is barely credible without a positive ANA test result.
[b]Positive RF test result shows a significantly higher titer in rheumatoid arthritis than in other collagen diseases, but diagnosis is primarily clinical rather than serologic. Serial titers are not helpful in following response to treatment because antiglobulins remain at constant levels despite clinical status. RF is frequently present at low to moderate titers in polyclonal hypergammaglobulinemia (e.g., SLE, sarcoidosis, cirrhosis, active viral hepatitis, some acute viral infections).

Table 3. Characteristics of Synovial Fluid in the Rheumatic Diseases

	Synovial Fluid			Mucin				
Group	Condition	Complement	Color/Clarity	Viscosity	Clot	WBC count	PMN %	Miscellaneous Findings
Noninflammatory	Normal	N	Yellow/clear	N	N	<200	<25	—
	Traumatic arthritis	N	Xanthochromic/ turbid	N	N	<2,000	<25	Debris
	Osteoarthritis	N	Yellow/clear	N	N	1,000	<25	—
Inflammatory	SLE	↓	Yellow/clear	N	N	5,000	10	LE cells
	Rheumatic fever	N or ↑	Yellow/cloudy	A	Fair	5,000	10–50	—
	Juvenile rheumatoid arthritis	N or ↓	Yellow/cloudy	A	Poor	15,000–20,000	75	—
	Reiter syndrome	↑	Opaque	A	Poor	20,000	80	Reiter cell
Pyogenic	Tubercular arthritis	N or ↑	Yellow/cloudy	A	Poor	25,000	50–60	Acid-fast organisms
	Septic arthritis	↑	Serosanguine-ous, turbid	A	Poor	80,000–200,000	75	Low glucose, bacteria

↑, increased; ↓, decreased; A, abnormal; LE, lupus erythematosus; N, normal; PMN, polymorphonuclear cell; SLE, systemic lupus erythematosus; WBC, white blood cell.

Table 4. Abnormal Laboratory Findings in Rheumatic Diseases of Childhood

	Juvenile Rheumatoid Arthritis							
Abnormality	Polyarthritis	Oligoarthritis	Systemic Onset	Systemic Lupus Erythematosus	Dermatomyositis	Scleroderma	Vasculitis	Rheumatic Fever
Anemia	+	–	+	+	+	+	+	+
Leukopenia	–	–	–	+++	–	–	–	–
Thrombocytopenia	–	–	–	+	–	–	–	–
Leukocytosis	+	–	+++	–	+	–	+++	+
Thrombocytosis	+	–	+	–	+	–	+	+
Antinuclear antibodies	+	+	–	+++	+	+	–	–
Anti-DNA antibodies	–	–	–	+++	–	–	–	–
Rheumatoid factors	+	–	–	+	–	+	+	–
Antistreptococcal antibodies	+	–	+	–	–	–	–	+++
Hypocomplementemia	–	–	–	+++	–	–	+	–
Elevated hepatic enzyme levels	+	–	+	+	+	+	+	–
Elevated muscle enzyme levels	–	–	–	+	+++	+	+	–
Abnormal urinalysis	+	–	+	+++	+	+	+	–

–, absent; +, minimal; ++, moderate; +++, severe.

Laboratory evaluation usually demonstrates an increased ESR, absence of rheumatoid factor, and ANA positivity in 17–50% of patients. Hyperuricemia is occasionally seen in patients with severe skin disease. Synovial fluid examination reveals a white blood cell count of 5,000–40,000/mL, predominately polymorphonuclear cells.

Arthritis, Juvenile Rheumatoid

JRA is the most common form of chronic arthritis in children and a major cause of musculoskeletal disability. Current evidence indicates an autoimmune pathogenesis. JRA is primarily a synovial disease (i.e., affecting the joint lining), with secondary pathologic changes occurring in the synovial fluid, cartilage, periarticular tissues, and bone. The synovium becomes inflamed, which causes pain and swelling in one or several peripheral joints. Fibroblasts, blood vessels, and chronic inflammatory cells proliferate, and the resulting granulation tissue pannus extends over the surface of the articular cartilage, eroding and destroying it. The destructive changes may extend to articular and periarticular bone and to periarticular soft tissue, leading to joint deformities.

The pathogenic process may extend beyond the border of synovia tissue and involve other tissues. Clinically, the patient may have overwhelming fatigue, morning stiffness lasting many hours, high fever, rash, swelling of joints, pericarditis, uveitis, and other signs of acute or chronic disease. There are three subtypes of the disease, determined by the clinical characteristics occurring within the first 6 months of illness.

Systemic JRA: occurs in 10–20% of affected children; usually characterized by a febrile onset and evanescent rash with multiple physical and laboratory abnormalities.

Polyarticular JRA: occurs in 30–40% of affected children; characterized by multiple (more than four) joint involvement and minimal systemic features.

Pauciarticular JRA: occurs in 40–50% of affected children; characterized by involvement of four or fewer joints, usually larger joints; a risk for chronic uveitis in young girls and axial skeletal involvement in older boys.

Genetics

HLA-B27 histocompatibility antigen is associated with risk of evolving spondyloarthropathy in older boys with pauci-type JRA. Weaker HLA associations exist for the other subtypes (HLA-DR5; HLA-DR8; HLA-DR4).

Signs and Symptoms

Systemic disease is characterized by arthralgia and arthritis, chest pain, pericardial friction rub, dyspnea, fatigue, fever, hepatosplenomegaly, lymphadenopathy, myalgias, rash, and weight loss.

Polyarticular disease is characterized by arthralgia and arthritis, cold intolerance, difficulty writing, fatigue, growth retardation, hand weakness, limitation of motion, malaise, morning stiffness, rheumatoid nodules, synovial cysts, synovial thickening, and weight loss.

Pauciarticular disease is characterized by abnormal gait, eye pain, redness, joint swelling, leg length abnormality, morning stiffness, photophobia.

Predominant age:	1–4 years and 9–14 years
Predominant sex:	Girls affected more than boys

Causes

Multifactorial, including abnormal immune response, genetic predisposition, and environmental triggers, possibly infectious.

Risk Factors

HLA-B27 in pauci-type JRA increases risk for development of spondyloarthropathy.
Rheumatoid factor positivity increases risk for severe arthritis in poly-type JRA.
ANA positivity increases risk for uveitis in pauci and poly JRA.

Laboratory Findings

White blood cell count normal or markedly elevated (systemic).
Hemoglobin level normal or low (especially in systemic JRA).
Platelet count normal or elevated.
ANA positivity in 40% of cases (poly or pauci JRA).
Rheumatoid factor positivity in 10–15% of cases (usually poly JRA).
HLA-B27 positivity in 70% of cases of pauci JRA in boys.
ESR elevated in most patients with active disease; >100 mL/hour (Westergren) in active systemic disease.

Drugs That May Alter Laboratory Results

Antiinflammatory therapy may alter complete blood count and ESR.

Disorders That May Alter Laboratory Results

Hemoglobinopathies may alter ESR.

Pathologic Findings

Synovium shows hyperplasia of synovial cells, hyperemia, and infiltration of small lymphocytes and mononuclear cells.

Special Tests

Echocardiography (pericarditis)
Radionuclide scans (infection, malignancy)

Imaging Studies

Early radiographic changes—soft tissue swelling, periosteal reaction, juxtaarticular demineralization; later changes—joint space loss, articular surface erosions, subchondral cyst formation, sclerosis, and joint fusion.
Computed tomography and magnetic resonance imaging are very helpful in delineating early erosions.

Diagnostic Procedures for Joints

Joint fluid aspiration and analysis are helpful in excluding infection.
Synovial biopsy is occasionally indicated in persistent, atypical monoarthritis.

Dermatomyositis, Juvenile

Pathogenic mechanisms of juvenile dermatomyositis (JDM) include abnormalities of cellular immunity resulting in T lymphocyte–mediated destruction of striated muscle and deposition of immune complexes in muscle tissue. JDM has also been described in association with immunodeficiency and infection. Immunoglobulin (Ig) G, IgM, and the third component of complement (C3) can be found deposited in the vessel walls of skeletal muscle.
Dermatomyositis usually presents in childhood with a combination of easy fatigue, malaise, muscle weakness, rash, and fever. Clinical expression and progression of the disease are variable.

Laboratory Findings

Routine laboratory studies are of little diagnostic help in evaluating the child with JDM. Nonspecific tests of inflammation such as the ESR and C-reactive protein level tend to correlate with the degree of clinical inflammation or to be of no clinical usefulness.
Leukocytosis and anemia are uncommon at the onset, except in the child with associated gastrointestinal (GI) bleeding. Results of urinalysis usually are normal, although a few children have microscopic hematuria. There are no specific abnormalities of serum immunoglobulin concentrations. Children with JDM usually lack circulating rheumatoid factor. ANAs have been reported in the serum at a frequency varying from 10% to 50% of cases.

The three most helpful abnormal laboratory findings are

- Increased serum concentrations of the muscle enzymes.
- Abnormal electromyographic changes.
- Specific histopathologic abnormalities on muscle biopsy. Creatinine kinase, aspartate aminotransferase, and aldolase levels should be measured. The height of increase is variable but ranges from 20 to 40 times normal for creatinine kinase and aspartate aminotransferase.

Inflammatory Bowel Disease

(See also Chapter 9, Gastrointestinal Diseases.)

Inflammatory joint disease constitutes one of the most common extraintestinal complications of both ulcerative colitis and Crohn disease, occurring in 10–20% of children with such disorders.

Two type of arthritis accompany inflammatory bowel disease: one is characteristically a nondeforming, nonerosive polyarthritis, and the other is inflammation of the sacroiliac joints. The former is correlated with activity of the gut inflammation and occurs slightly more frequently in girls than in boys. The latter is independent of enteric disease activity, is associated with HLA-B27, and occurs most frequently in teenage boys. In a child with arthritis in whom weight loss, unexplained fever, abdominal pain, hematochezia, marked abnormalities of inflammatory indices, or hypoalbuminemia occurs, the diagnosis of inflammatory bowel disease should be considered, because joint disease may precede other manifestations of bowel disease by many months.

Laboratory Tests

White blood cell count, ESR, C-reactive protein level. Anemia may be due to iron and vitamin B_{12} deficiency. Serum albumin is decreased, and γ-globulins are increased. Definitive diagnosis is by intestinal biopsy.

Lyme Disease

A spectrum of disease manifestations, including a characteristic skin lesion (erythema chronicum migrans), arthritis, and neurologic and cardiac abnormalities, is associated with infection with the tick-borne organism *Borrelia burgdorferi*. The serologic test for the antibody response to *B. burgdorferi* is a laboratory method for diagnosis of the disease.

Antibodies to *B. burgdorferi* can be identified by either IFA or enzyme-linked immunosorbent assay (ELISA). Sensitivity is 4–70% in early disease and 95% in late disease. Specific IgM titers to *B. burgdorferi* peak between the third and sixth weeks of the illness. IgG antibody is detected somewhat later, but may persist for years.

Cross reactivity of antibodies with antibodies to other species is a continuing problem. *Treponema pallidum* infection can be readily diagnosed by more specific tests. *Treponema denticola*, *Leptospiras*, and *Borrelia hermsii* may induce antibodies that cross-react with those to *B. burgdorferi*. Low-titer antibodies to *B. burgdorferi* occur in a variety of other rheumatic diseases (e.g., rheumatoid arthritis, SLE) and other illnesses (e.g., infective endocarditis, infectious mononucleosis, mumps, meningitis, Rocky Mountain spotted fever, and other rickettsial diseases).

Western blot analysis is reserved as a confirmatory test for children with low-titer positive ELISA results or with atypical clinical manifestations. Test results are rarely positive when ELISA testing yields normal or negative results. Criteria for interpretation of Western blot test results have not been established.

The results of serologic testing should not be relied on as the sole criteria in making the diagnosis of Lyme disease.

Lupus Erythematosus, Systemic

SLE is an episodic multisystem disease characterized by widespread inflammation of the blood vessels and connective tissue and the presence of circulating autoantibodies. SLE is believed to result from altered immunologic responsiveness on a background of a genetic predisposition to the disease.

The basic pathologic lesions of SLE are immune complex and autoantibody deposition in vessels and other tissues, which results in fibrinoid necrosis, inflammatory cellular infiltrates, and sclerosis of collagen. The fibrinoid material is eosinophilic with hematoxylin-eosin stain and is deposited within the interfibrillar ground substance of the connective tissues. Vascular endothelial thickening is another characteristic of SLE. Capillaries, venules, and arterioles are all involved. Secondary changes include vascular obstruction and development of thrombosis.

Presentations in children with SLE range from acute-onset disease that is rapidly fatal to disease of insidious onset with a long history of exacerbations. Any organ in the body may be involved. A single system may be affected at onset; however, it is more usual to find multisystem disease. A lupus-like syndrome may be induced by many drugs, especially antiarrhythmics (procainamide, quinidine), anticonvulsants, antihypertensive agents (hydralazine, methyldopa), and D-penicillamine.

Lupus Comprehensive Panel

Test	Reference Range	Methodology
ANA (Hep2)	<1:40	IFA
Double-stranded DNA (native) antibody	<35 IU/mL	EIA
RNP/Sm antibody	<0.91 index	Immuno
Smooth muscle antibody	<1.20	IFA
SS-A antibody	<0.91 index	Immuno
SS-B antibody	<0.91 index	Immuno
Scleroderma antibody	<0.91 index	Immuno
Thyroid peroxidase antibody	<0.3 U/mL	Immuno
C3	75–161 mg/dL	NEPH
C4	16–47 mg/dL	NEPH
Rheumatoid factor	<40 IU/mL	NEPH
Mitochondrial antibody	<1:20	IFA
Myocardial antibody	<1:20	IFA
Parietal cell antibody	<1:20	IFA
Reticulin antibody	None detected	IFA
Smooth muscle antibody	<1:20	IFA
Skeletal muscle antibody	<1:40	IFA
Ribosomal P antibody	<0.090	ELISA

EIA, enzyme immunoassay; IFA, immunofluorescent assay; Immuno, immunodiffusion; SS, Sjögren syndrome.
From SmithKline Beecham technical update.

The most appropriate workup is initial testing for ANA and subsequent follow-up testing. Rheumatoid factor is primarily used in diagnosing and determining prognosis for rheumatoid arthritis; rheumatoid factor is elevated in a number of other connective tissue diseases but nonspecifically. In connective tissue diseases, complement levels are used for monitoring disease activity, not for diagnosis.

Lupus Syndrome, Neonatal

Children of mothers who have SLE may develop manifestations of lupus in the neonatal period that are mediated by the transplacental passage of maternal IgG autoantibodies. Neonatal lupus syndrome is more common in girls than in boys.

The affected infant demonstrates a transiently positive ANA finding and diminished serum complement concentration. In the majority of these babies, there is no associated clinical disease, and the serologic abnormalities regress within several weeks to months after birth, in accordance with the normal half-life of maternal IgG (24–28 days). The clinical manifestations include rash, complete congenital heart block, hepatomegaly, thrombocytopenia, and neutropenia.

At least two specificities of Ro antigen have been identified. The highest risk for neonatal lupus syndrome appears to be associated with the presence of antibodies to the 48-kilodalton La/SS-B polypeptide and the 52-kilodalton Ro/SS-A polypeptide, but not to the 60-kilodalton Ro antigen. Because ELISA currently does not differentiate between the two Ro antigens, care must be exercised in interpreting test results. The Ro antigen is widely distributed in the fetal conduction system and myocardium. Antibodies to Ro are bound to the conduction system and myocardium of infants and are present in the conduction system of infants dying of complete congenital heart block.

Anti-Ro antibodies are most characteristic of the syndrome, although anti-La antibodies may be found in some individuals. The latter infants usually do not have complete congenital heart block.

Some cases can be mediated by antibodies other than anti-Ro (SS-A), anti-La (SS-B), or anti-U_1RNP, or perhaps by some factor or cofactor yet to be determined. In cases in which only anti-U_1RNP antibodies are found, only cutaneous disease has been reported.

Polyarteritis Nodosa

Polyarteritis nodosa represents one entity in a spectrum of inflammatory diseases involving arteries and veins. It is a multisystem disease characterized by acute inflammation and fibrinoid necrosis of small and medium-sized vessels. The etiology of the vascular inflammation is unknown, although infections and hypersensitivity mechanisms have been suggested. Similar arterial lesions are seen in serum sickness–like illnesses after allergic reactions to drugs, after bacterial infections, and in patients who have circulating hepatitis B surface antigen.

Polyarteritis nodosa presents pathologically as an ongoing segmental inflammatory response within the media of small and medium-sized muscular arteries.

Organ involvement includes kidney, GI tract, skin, muscles, joints, genitourinary tract, peripheral and central nervous system, heart, testes, epididymis, and ovaries. Severity varies from mild, self-limited skin lesions to severe, systemic isolated and combined multiorgan dysfunction and death. The disease is classified as a systemic necrotizing vasculitis. Hepatitis B antigens are found in 30% of cases.

Clinical and Laboratory Findings

	% of Cases
Fever	>50
Renal changes	
Microscopic hematuria	
Glomerulonephritis	
Hypertension	
Skin rashes (nonspecific)	30–50
Arthritis and arthralgia	
Neuropathy and mononeuritis, such as isolated cranial nerve palsy	
Myalgia and myositis	
Pulmonary changes[a]	
Hemoptysis	
Asthma	
Central nervous system changes (nonspecific)	<30
Cardiac changes	
Pericarditis	
Myocardial ischemia	
Intestinal changes (ischemia)	
Abdominal pain	
Diarrhea	
Perforation	
Hepatomegaly (painful)	
Hematologic abnormalities	>50
Anemia	
Leukocytosis and eosinophilia	
Thrombocytosis and thrombocytopenia	
Elevated erythrocyte and sedimentation rate	
Serum abnormalities	20–50
Hepatitis B surface antigen	

Rheumatoid factor
Cryoglobulins
Decreased complement factor

[a]Pulmonary changes do not occur in classic polyarteritis; they are seen in a variant form of the disease known as *allergic granulomatosis* and *angiitis of Churg and Strauss*.

Pathologic Findings

Necrotizing inflammation, in various stages, of small and medium-size muscular arteries. Segmental in distribution, often seen at bifurcations and branchings. Involvement of venules not seen in classic polyarteritis nodosa.
Acute lesions show infiltration of polymorphonuclear cells through vessel wall and perivascular area.
Subsequent proliferation, degeneration, appearance of monocytes, necrosis with thrombosis, and infarction of the involved tissue. Aneurysmal dilatations characteristic.
Aortic dissection reported attributed to necrotizing vasculitis of the vasa vasorum.

Special Tests

Angiographic demonstration of aneurysmal changes of small and medium-sized arteries involving renal hepatic and mesenteric arteries represents strong evidence supporting the diagnosis.

Imaging Studies

Angiography: mesenteric artery aneurysm, renal aneurysm, hepatic aneurysm, intestinal aneurysm.

Purpura, Henoch-Schönlein

A vasculitis of small vessels characterized by nonthrombocytopenic, usually dependent, palpable purpura, arthritis, abdominal pain, and nephritis.
Most cases occur between 2 and 8 years of age but can occur at any age.
Males more affected than females (2:1).

Signs and Symptoms

Onset can be acute or gradual.
Fifty percent of patients have malaise and low-grade fever.
One hundred percent of patients have skin lesions:
- Lesions appears on lower extremities and buttocks but may involve face, trunk, and upper extremities.
- Begin as small wheals or erythematous maculopapular lesions that blanch on pressure but later become petechial or purpuric.
- Lesions appear in crops.
- Angioedema of scalp, lips, eyelids, ears, dorsa of hands and feet, back, scrotum, and perineum may be seen.

Seventy percent of patients experience arthritis:
- Large joints (knees and ankles) are most commonly involved.

Thirty-five percent of patients experience GI symptoms:
- Colicky abdominal pain associated with vomiting is most common.
- Occult or gross blood in stool.
- Hematemesis.
- Intussusception, obstruction, or infarction occurs.
- Pancreatitis.

Twenty percent of patients have renal involvement:
- Hematuria, with or without casts or proteinuria

Other manifestations:
- Seizures, neuropathies
- Hepatosplenomegaly
- Lymphadenopathy

Cardiac involvement
Pulmonary hemorrhage
Rheumatoid-like nodules
Orchitis

Infantile Henoch-Schönlein purpura:
Children <2 years old
Rare
Edema and diffuse purpura of face and ears
Fewer GI and renal symptoms

Causes

Multiple infectious agents, drugs, and toxins have been investigated, with no firm link found. *Helicobacter pylori* infection has been implicated.

Laboratory Findings

Not diagnostic.
Sedimentation rate and white blood cell count may be elevated.
Coagulation studies, platelet count, and complement levels are normal.
Serum IgA elevated in 50% of cases.
Urinalysis shows protein, red blood cells, and white blood cells if renal involvement.

Pathologic Findings

Renal
Focal and segmental increases in mesangial cells and matrix.
IgA deposition in glomerular basement membrane.
A minority show generalized mesangial changes.
Rarely, diffuse necrotizing glomerulonephritis with crescent formation.

Skin
Small vessels are surrounded by an acute leukocytoclastic inflammatory reaction of neutrophils and round cells with IgA deposition.
GI vasculitis.

Imaging Studies

Abdominal radiographs may show ileus and segmental narrowing due to submucosal edema and hemorrhage.
Barium studies performed in acute condition may show large filling defects in the bowel wall, mimicking Crohn disease or neoplasm.

Diagnostic Procedures

Clinical diagnosis.
Renal biopsy rarely indicated except in cases of decreased renal function or development of nephrotic syndrome.

Reiter Syndrome

Reiter syndrome is a clinical triad consisting of arthritis, urethritis, and conjunctivitis. Fever, malaise, and weight loss occur commonly with acute arthritis. The urethritis is nonspecific and often asymptomatic. The conjunctivitis is mild, but 20–50% of patients develop iritis. Balanitis circinata, painless oral ulcerations, and keratoderma blennorrhagicum (thick keratotic lesions of the palms and soles) are mucocutaneous manifestations. Complications include spondylitis and carditis.

Most patients have a mild leukocytosis. The urethral discharge is purulent, and smear and culture results are usually negative. Synovial fluid is sterile, with a white cell count of 2,000–50,000/mL, mostly PMNs.

The cause of Reiter syndrome is not known. Some cases have been associated with sexual contact. Several infectious agents have been linked with Reiter syndrome. Eighty percent of patients with Reiter syndrome have HLA-B27.

Rheumatic Disorders in Children

Acute monoarthritis or oligoarthritis (affecting one or a few joints)
Acute polyarthritis
Chronic monoarthritis or pauciarthritis
Chronic polyarthritis
Arthritis with skin disease
Arthritis with GI disease
Arthritis with pleuropulmonary disease
Arthritis with infection
Arthritis with hematologic and neoplastic disorders
Systemic disease with vasculitis
Arthritis with endocrine, biochemical, or metabolic disorders
Hereditary diseases of connective tissue

Rheumatic Fever, Acute

(See also Chapter 7, Cardiovascular Diseases.)

Appears to be slightly more common in girls than in boys. A β-hemolytic streptococcal pharyngitis is followed 2–3 weeks later by migratory joint pain, fever, and palpitations or fatigue. Chorea may occur, but the onset is usually several months after the pharyngitis. The revised Jones criteria provide diagnostic guidance. Treatment usually involves penicillin prophylaxis, nonsteroidal antiinflammatory drugs, and, for severe cases, steroids. Phenothiazides may be used in children with chorea.

Diagnostic Studies

1. Increased antistreptolysin-O and antistreptococcal deoxyribonuclease B titers that later return to normal provide supporting evidence of a recent streptococcal infection.
2. Increased sedimentation rate or C-reactive protein level. A prolonged P-R interval on electrocardiogram is supportive evidence of rheumatic heart disease.

No test, however, is conclusively diagnostic of acute rheumatic fever.

Sclerosis, Progressive Systemic

Progressive systemic sclerosis is a disease of unknown cause characterized by abnormally increased collagen deposition in the skin and internal organs. The course is usually slowly progressive, but it can be rapidly progressive and fatal because of involvement of internal organs such as the lungs, heart, kidneys, and GI tract. There may be vascular abnormalities in the lungs and kidneys.

Biopsy of involved skin reveals thinning of the epidermis with loss of rete pegs, atrophy of the dermal appendages, hyalinization and fibrosis of arterioles, and a striking increase of compact collagen fibers in the reticular dermis. Synovial tissue findings range from an acute inflammatory lymphocytic infiltration to diffuse fibrosis with relatively little inflammation. The histologic changes seen in muscle include interstitial and perivascular inflammatory infiltration followed by fibrosis and myofibrillar necrosis, atrophy, and degeneration.

In patients with renal involvement, the histologic appearance of the kidney is similar to that of malignant hypertensive nephropathy, with intimal proliferation of the interlobular arteries and fibrinoid changes in the intima and media of more distal interlobular arteries and of afferent arterioles.

Polyclonal hypergammaglobulinemia is frequently present in patients with progressive systemic sclerosis. The fluorescent ANA test results are positive in 70% of cases and show a speckled or nucleolar pattern. A specific ANA found only in progressive systemic sclerosis is anti–Scl-70.

Spondylitis, Juvenile Ankylosing

Juvenile ankylosing spondylitis is a chronic, progressive, inflammatory disorder of unknown etiology involving the sacroiliac joints, spine, and large peripheral joints.

Ninety percent of cases occur in males, with onset usually occurring during the second or third decade of life. There is a strong genetic predisposition; 90% of patients with ankylosing spondylitis have HLA-B27. There is no specific immunologic diagnostic test.

The disease begins with insidious onset of low back pain and stiffness, usually worse in the morning. Symptoms of the acute disease include pain and tenderness in the sacroiliac joints and spasm of the paravertebral muscles; in advanced disease, ankylosis of the sacroiliac joints and spine, loss of lumbar lordosis, cervical kyphosis, and decreased chest expansion are present. Twenty-five percent of patients have iritis. Carditis, with or without aortitis, is seen in 10% of patients.

During phases of active disease, elevated sedimentation rate and a mild anemia may be observed but hypergammaglobulinemia, rheumatoid factor, and ANAs are not present.

Stevens-Johnson Syndrome

Erythema multiforme spectrum is not a single entity. The milder form, also known as erythema multiforme Hebra, either has no mucous membrane involvement or may involve one mucous membrane. The more severe form is erythema multiforme major, in which more than one mucous membrane is involved. In both these variants, it is a self limited hypersensitivity reaction, usually due to a preceding viral infection, and has an excellent prognosis.

Systems Affected

Skin, exocrine system, nervous system, cardiovascular system, renal/urologic system, hemic/lymphatic/immunologic system.

Signs and Symptoms

There was a preceding illness for which medication was given.

Sudden onset with rapidly progressive pleomorphic rash that includes petechiae, vesicles, bullae.

The condition is classified as Stevens-Johnson syndrom (SJS) if epidermal detachment affects <10% of the skin and as toxic epidermal necrolysis if epidermal detachment exceeds 30% or if it exceeds 10% in the absence of discrete skin lesions. Cases with discrete skin lesions and cases in which there is between 10% and 30% epidermal detachment are in the overlap between SJS and toxic epidermal necrolysis.

Vesicles and ulcers on the mucous membranes, especially of the mouth and throat.

Burning sensation of the skin and sometimes of the mucous membranes.

Usually no pruritus.

Fever 39–40°C (102–104°F).

Headache.

Arthralgias.

Epistaxis.

Crusted nares.

Conjunctivitis.

Corneal ulcerations.

Erosive vulvovaginitis.

Cough productive of thick purulent sputum.

Tachypnea and respiratory distress.

Albuminuria and hematuria.

Arrhythmias.

Pericarditis.

Congestive heart failure.

Mental status changes.

Electrolyte disturbance.

Seizures.

Coma.

Sepsis.

Causes

Often unknown
Medications–especially sulfonamides, penicillins, anticonvulsants, salicylates, nonsteroidal antiinflammatory drugs, methazolamide, carvedilol
Vaccines—diphtheria/typhoid, bacille Calmette-Guérin, oral polio vaccine
Mycoplasma pneumoniae, virus infection

Risk Factors

Patients with human immunodeficiency virus infection appear to be predisposed to developing SJS in response to their medications.
Previous history of SJS
Male sex

Laboratory Tests

Culture or serologic tests for suspected sources of infection.

Pathologic Findings

Compared with the mainly inflammatory changes in erythema multiforme, necrotic changes predominate in SJS and toxic epidermal necrolysis. There is a cell-poor infiltrate in which macrophages and dendrocytes predominate with a strong immunoreactivity for tumor necrosis factor-α.

Bibliography

Ansell BM, Falcini F, Woo P. Scleroderma in childhood. *Clin Dermatol* 1994;12:299–307.
Bisno AL. The resurgence of acute rheumatic fever in the United States. *Annu Rev Med* 1990;41:319–329.
Burgo-Bargas R. Spondyloarthropathies and psoriatic arthritis in children. *Curr Opin Rheumatol* 1993;5:634–643.
Buyon JP. Neonatal lupus. *Curr Opin Rheumatol* 1996;8:485–490.
Cassidy JT, Petty RE. *Textbook of pediatric rheumatology*, 3rd ed. Philadelphia: WB Saunders, 1995.
Gilbert-Barness E, ed. *Potter's pathology of the fetus and infant*. St. Louis: Mosby–Year Book, 1997.
Golightly MG. Lyme borreliosis: laboratory considerations. *Semin Neurol* 1997;17: 11–17.
Lipnick RN, Rsokos GC. Immune abnormalities in the pathogenesis of juvenile rheumatoid arthritis. *Clin Exp Rheumatol* 1990;8:177–186.
Luger SW, Krauss E. Serologic tests for Lyme disease. *Arch Intern Med* 1990;150:761–763.
Ozean S, Besbas N, Saatci U, et al. Diagnostic criteria for polyarthritis nodosa in childhood. *J Pediatr* 1992;120:206–209.
Pachman LM. Inflammatory myopathy in children. *Rheum Dis Clin North Am* 1994:919–942.
Provost TT, Watson R, Simmons-O'Brien E. Significance of anti-Ro (SS-A) antibody in evaluation of patients with cutaneous manifestations of a connective tissue disease. *J Am Acad Dermatol* 1996;35(2 Pt 1):147–169.
Reed A, Haugen M, Pachman LM, et al. 25-Hydroxyvitamin D therapy in children with active juvenile rheumatoid arthritis: short-term effects on serum osteocalcin levels and bone mineral density. *J Pediatr* 1991;119(4):657–660.
Southwood TR, Petty RE, Malleson PN, et al. Psoriatic arthritis in children. *Arthritis Rheum* 1989;32:1007–1013.
Wallach J. *Interpretation of diagnostic tests*, 7th ed. Philadelphia: Lippincott Williams & Wilkins, 2000.

25 Disorders Due to Poisons, Toxins, Other Physical and Chemical Agents, and Animal Bites

Physical and Chemical Agents

Acetaminophen Poisoning

Blood levels

- 200 μg/mL at 4 hours or <30–35 μg/mL at 12 hours predicts severe liver damage, and treatment with acetylcysteine should begin.
- <150 μg/mL at 4 hours or <30–50 μg/mL at 12 hours indicates that no liver damage will occur.
- Toxicity is dose dependent but is exaggerated by starvation and use of certain drugs, especially alcohol.
- Liver toxicity cannot be predicted from blood levels determined earlier than 4 hours after ingestion.
- Exact time of ingestion is often difficult to ascertain.
- Patients taking other drugs may develop liver toxicity at different blood levels.
- Toxicity is less common in children <5 years old, and changes in liver function test results may be mild when serum drug levels are in toxic range.

With hepatotoxicity

- During the first 12–24 hours, increased aspartate aminotransferase (AST) and alanine aminotransferase (ALT) levels are found in only 50% of patients, and serum drug levels are the chief guide to therapy; this is the only stage at which treatment can prevent liver damage.
- During the next 24–48 hours, AST, ALT, and serum bilirubin levels and prothrombin time are increased. AST and ALT levels are very high (typically >4,000 U/L, often >10,000 U/L). AST/ALT ratio is <2 in 90% of cases.
- On the third to fourth day, liver function abnormalities peak; hypoglycemia and secondary renal failure may occur.

Addiction (Narcotics) and Chronic Usage; Drugs of Abuse (Usually Heroin)

See Table 1.

Persistent absolute and relative lymphocytosis occurs, with lymphocytes, often bizarre and atypical, that may resemble Downey cells.

Eosinophilia is seen in 25% of patients.

Liver function tests commonly show increased serum AST and ALT (increased in 75% of patients). Higher frequency of positive test results is evident on routine periodic repeat of these tests, which probably represents a mild, chronic viral hepatitis. Serum protein electrophoresis results are usually normal.

Hepatitis B surface antigen is found in 10% of patients.

Liver biopsy specimen shows abnormal morphology in 25% of patients, and foreign particles are particularly suggestive.

Laboratory findings due to preexisting glucose-6-phosphate dehydrogenase (G-6-PD) deficiency may be precipitated by quinine, which is often used to adulterate heroin.

Table 1. Drugs of Abuse

Drug	Street Name	Route	Usual Dose	Toxic Dose	Half-life (hr)	Duration of Effect (hr)	% Not Changed in Urine
Stimulants							
Cocaine[a]	Coke, crack, snow	Nasal, smoked, IV, oral	1.5 mg/kg	>1.2 g	2–5	1–2	<10
Amphetamine[b] (Benzedrine, Dexedrine)	Bennies, dexies, uppers	Oral, IV	10 mg	30–500 mg	4–24	2–4	~30
Methamphetamine (Desoxyn, Methedrine)	Speed, meth, crystal	Oral, IV	5–10 mg	>1 g	9–24	2–4	10–20
Methylphenidate (Ritalin)		Oral, IV	5–20 mg	>2 g	2–3	2–4	<1
Phenmetrazine (Preludin)		Oral, IV	75 mg		8	12	15–20
Cannabis							
Marijuana,[c] hashish	Grass, Mary Jane, pot, THC, hash	Smoked, oral, IV		50–200 μg/kg	14–38	2–4	<1
Narcotics							
Heroin[d]	Horse, smack, white lady, scag	IV, smoked, nasal	5–10 mg	100–250 mg	1.0–1.5	3–6	<1
Codeine[e] (e.g., with aspirin)		Oral, IV, IM	15–60 mg	500–1,000 mg	2–4	3–6	5–20
Morphine[f] (morphine sulfate, Duramorph)	M, junk, morpho, white stuff	IV, IM, oral, smoked	5–10 mg	50–100 μg/kg	2–4	3–6	<10
Methadone[g] (Dolophine, Amidone)	Methadose	Oral, IV, IM	40–100 mg	100–200 mg	15–60	12–24	5–50
Meperidine (Demerol, Mepergan, Pethidine)		IV, IM, oral	25–100 mg	500–2,000 mg	2–5	3–6	5
Propoxyphene[h] (Darvon Darvocet, Dolene)	Yellow footballs	Oral	65–400 mg	500 mg	8–24	1–6	<1
Barbiturates[i]							
Pentobarbital (Nembutal)	Yellow jackets, yellows	Oral, IV, IM	50–200 mg	2–10 g	15–48	3–6	1
Amobarbital (Amytal, Tuinal)	Blues, bluebirds, rainbows	Oral, IV, IM	30–200 mg	1.5–10.0 g	12–60	3–24	<1

Secobarbital (Seconal, Tuinal)	Reds, red devils, M&Ms	Oral, IV, IM	100–200 mg	2–5 g	15–40	3–6	5
Butabarbital (Butisol)		Oral	15–100 mg	>2 g	30–40	3–6	5–10
Butalbital (Fiorinal)		Oral	50–100 mg	>1 g	30–40	3–6	5
Phenobarbital (Luminal)	Downers	Oral, IV, IM	50–200 mg	6–20 g	48–120	10–20	20–35
Benzodiazepines[j]							
Alprazolam (Xanax)		Oral	0.25–1.0 mg		7–13	4–8	20
Chlordiazepoxide (Librium)		Oral, IM	5–100 mg	>500 mg	6–27	4–8	<1
Diazepam (Valium)		Oral, IV, IM	5–30 mg	>250 mg	20–50	4–8	<1
Flurazepam (Dalmane)		Oral	15–30 mg	>500 mg	2–3	4–12	<1
Lorazepam (Ativan)		Oral, IV, IM	0.5–2 mg	25–100 mg	9–16	4–8	<1
Antidepressants							
Tricyclics, e.g., imipramine (Tofranil, Janimine)		Oral, IM	100–500 mg	>1 g	12–30		<1
Phenothiazines, e.g., chlorpromazine (Thorazine)		Oral, IV, IM, rectal	500–800 mg	>1 g	7–120		<1
Sedatives, depressants							
Ethanol		Oral		100 g	2–14	2–6	2–10
Methaqualone[k] (Quaalude)	'Ludes, soapers	Oral	150–500 mg	2 g	20–60	4–8	<1
Meprobamate (Equanil, Miltown, Pathibamate)		Oral	400–1,000 mg	2–5 g	6–16	4–8	5
Glutethimide (Doriden)		Oral	150–500 mg	5 g	5–22	4–8	<2
Chloral hydrate (Noctec)	Mickey Finn, joy juice	Oral, rectal	300–1,000 mg	3 g	<1	5–8	<1
Hallucinogens							
Phencyclidine[l]	PCP, angel dust, killer weed	Oral, nasal, smoked, IV	0.25 mg/kg	10–20 mg	7–16	2–4 (psychosis may last wk)	30–50

(continued)

Table 1. (continued)

Drug	Street Name	Route	Usual Dose	Toxic Dose	Half-life (hr)	Duration of Effect (hr)	% Not Changed in Urine
Lysergic acid diethylamide (LSD)	Acid, white lightning, microdots	Oral	1–2 μg/kg	100–200 μg	3–4	8–12	1
Amphetamine analogs	STP, DOM	Oral, IV	2 mg		4–8		20
Ketamine (Ketalar)		IV, IM	1.0–4.5 mg/kg	>500 mg	3–4	0.5–2.0	2–5
Mescaline	Peyote, mesc, buttons	Oral		200–700 mg	6	8–12	50–60

Detection Times in Urine with Enzyme-Multiplied Immunoassay Technique

[a]Cocaine	Up to 48 hr after a single dose.
[b]Amphetamines	Detectable within 24–48 hr after ingestion. Cold medicines that contain ephedrine, pseudoephedrine, or phenylpropanolamine may cause positive reaction.
[c]Marijuana	≤5 d after occasional use; 21–32 d after last dose in habitual users.
[d]Heroin	One 10-mg dose detectable for up to 24 h, 4–5 d in habitual users.
[e]Codeine	Excreted as morphine; 120-mg dose detectable for up to 48 hr.
[f]Morphine	Single 10-mg dose detectable for 24–48 hr.
[g]Methadone	Approximately 3 d. Interference from high levels of chlorpromazine, promethazine, and dextromethorphan may occur.
[h]Propoxyphene	Up to 48 hr.
[i]Barbiturates	Up to 9 d after one 250-mg dose of phenobarbital; other common barbiturates can be detected for 1–2 d.
[j]Benzodiazepine	Results not usually positive after one dose with normal renal function. Up to 5–7 d in habitual users.
[k]Methaqualone	≥5 d after a typical dose.
[l]Phencyclidine	1 wk after a single dose. Up to 2 wk after last dose in habitual users.

From Wilson J, comp. *Clin Chem News laboratory guide to abused drugs*. Roche Diagnostic Systems.

Laboratory findings due to malaria transmitted by common syringes. (Malaria is not frequent; may be suppressed by quinine used for adulteration of heroin.)
Laboratory findings due to active duodenal ulcer.
Laboratory findings due to tuberculosis, which develops with increased frequency in narcotics addicts.

Lower Limits of Detectability in Urine Screening for Drugs of Abuse[1]

Drug Abuse Screen (Urine)	Lower Limit of Detectability
Alcohol	300 μg/mL
Amphetamines	500 μg/mL
Barbiturates	1,000 ng/mL
Benzodiazepine	300 ng/mL
Benzoylecgonine	150 ng/mL
Cocaine	150 ng/mL
Opiates	300 ng/mL
Phencyclidine	25 ng/mL
Tetrahydrocannabinol carboxylic acid	15 ng/mL

Blood level measurements only detect recent ingestion and do not predict toxicity. Have no clinical value but can be used to calculate when drug was used. Higher ratio of cocaine to benzoylecgonine (cocaine metabolite) indicates more recent use.
Chewing of coca leaves (practiced by Peruvian Indians)—usually 300–400 ng/mL.
Snorting cocaine—600–800 ng/mL; snorting one line (25 mg) produces level of 50 ng/mL.
Intravenous cocaine—may reach 1,200–1,400 ng/mL.
Considerable overlap between lethal and recreational levels; death is not usually dose related.
Urine screen detection time (approximate)
  Alcohol: 6–12 hours
  Cocaine: 6–9 days in neonate; 2–4 days in adult
  Amphetamines: 2–4 days
  Cocaine and amphetamines are difficult to detect >48 hours after use.
  Opiates: 2–5 days
  Marijuana: ≤30 days
  Phencyclidine: ≤8 days

- Assay of hair permits estimate of cocaine use for previous several months and can indicate isolated or steady pattern [average hair growth = 1.3 cm (0.5 in) in 30 days]. Thus 8-cm length of hair can detect cocaine use over a period of 6 months.
- Radioimmunoassay of hair for cocaine or heroin has 100% specificity for both, 97% sensitivity for cocaine, and 83% sensitivity for heroin.

Interferences

Detection of adulteration of urine specimen:

- Appearance: Dark color may be caused by goldenseal tea. Cloudy appearance may be due to liquid soap.
- pH: Range of 4.6–8.0 for preliminary screening. Acidification of urine may speed elimination of phencyclidine or amphetamine before test. Alkalinization of urine may slow excretion during testing period.
- Creatinine level of <30 mg/dL or specific gravity of <1.003 may be due to external dilution of specimen, ingestion of large amounts of fluids, or use of diuretics. Creatinine level of <10 mg/dL may indicate replacement by water. Specific gravity of >1.035 may be due to sodium chloride contamination.
- Nitrite is present in some commercial adulterants composed of KNO.
- Pyridinium chlorochromate ("urine luck") is an effective adulterant for urine drug testing for opiates and delta-9-tetrahydrocannabinol (THC). Suspect if abnormally low pH or orange tint to urine. Can be identified with a spot test for this oxidant but test is not specific. Also produces a darker purple color with

[1]Leavelle DE, ed. *Mayo Medical Laboratories' test catalog*. Rochester, MN: Mayo Medical Laboratories, 1995.

nitrate dipstick. Confirm by direct gas chromatography or mass spectrometry for pyridine and colorimetric assay for chromate.

Positive subject identification and chain of custody should be assured.

The clinician should be aware of which drugs are included in the screen, causes of false reactions, and detection levels for the particular methodology.

False-negative immunoassay results may occur due to

- Adulteration by addition to urine of various substances, such as Drano, bleach, acids, bases, Visine (benzalkonium), glutaraldehyde, soap, or table salt.
- Brief time after drug use.
- Ibuprofen may interfere with gas chromatography and mass spectrometry confirmation for marijuana.
- In urine testing for cannabinoids (marijuana metabolites), use of a lower level of 100 ng/mL for enzyme-multiplied immunoassay technique (EMIT) failed to detect 25–40% of cases identified by thin-layer chromatography (lower levels of 25 ng/mL)
- Traces of marijuana may be found by EMIT up to 1 week after use or, in a heavy user, up to 4 weeks after use; 15% false-positive rate by EMIT and 2% by high-pressure liquid chromatography.
- Screening tests not generally available for designer drugs, lysergic acid diethylamide, mescaline, and psilocybin.

False-positive immunoassay results may occur due to

- Barbiturates and benzodiazepines: ibuprofen ingestion
- Opiates: ingestion of dextromethorphan, poppy seeds. Eating poppy seeds may cause a false-positive EMIT result for heroin confirmed by gas chromatography and mass spectrometry. Poppy seed ingestion as the only source of urinary morphine, and codeine can be ruled out if urine codeine level is >300 ng/mL, urine morphine level is >5,000 ng/mL, morphine level is >1,000 ng/mL when no codeine is present, and morphine/codeine ratio is <2.

Laboratory Findings Due to Complications of Cocaine Abuse

Catecholamine blood levels may reach several thousand nanograms per milliliter.

Sudden death due to acute myocardial infarction—may occur in relatively young persons (i.e., <40 years) and without evidence of coronary artery obstruction; for example, coronary artery spasm with arrhythmias.

Acute myocarditis, acute cardiomyopathy.

Bacterial endocarditis.

Aortic rupture.

Pneumopericardium.

Acute rhabdomyolysis that may cause acute renal failure and disseminated intravascular coagulation (DIC), and so on.

Cerebral vasculitis with cerebral and subarachnoid hemorrhage.

Hyperthyroidism.

Pulmonary hemorrhage and hemoptysis, pulmonary edema, “crack lung.”

Laboratory Findings Due to Complications of Phencyclidine Abuse

Massive ingestion may cause

- Rhabdomyolysis
- Acute tubular necrosis
- Hypoglycemia

Alcohol Intoxication

See Table 2.

Ethanol Breath Test

The ethanol breath test is a screening test. Expired air is blown directly into an instrument and is measured by spectrophotometry. The result is usually provided as a blood level, less commonly as the actual concentration in expired air.

Table 2. Stages of Acute Alcoholic Intoxication

Ethanol Concentration (% Weight/Volume) Blood Level	Urine Level	Stage of Alcohol Influence	Effects
0.01–0.05	0.01–0.07	Sobriety	Little effect on most persons
0.04–0.12	0.03–0.16	Euphoria	Decreased inhibitions, decreased judgment, loss of fine control, increased reaction time (≤20%)
0.09–0.20	0.07–0.30	Excitement	Incoordination, loss of critical judgment, memory loss, increased reaction time (≤100%)
0.15–0.30	0.12–0.40	Confusion	Disorientation, impaired emotional balance, slurred speech, disturbed sensation
0.25–0.40	0.20–0.50	Stupor	Paralysis, incontinence
0.30–0.50	0.25–0.60	Coma	Depressed reflexes, decreased respiration, possible death

If a positive result is of clinical significance, it is necessary to collect a blood specimen, as the blood level estimated from a breath specimen may be inaccurate.

Ethanol Level in Plasma or Blood

The venipuncture site must not be swabbed with alcohol. A 5-mL blood sample is drawn into a tube with lithium heparin (for plasma) or oxalate (whole blood). Medicolegal specimens require proof of identity, and ethanol is measured in a whole-blood specimen. Measurement is by gas liquid chromatography or spectrophotometry.

Interpretation

Level of 22–33 mmol/L (0.10–0.15 g/100 mL)—intoxicated
Level of 44–55 mmol/L (0.20–0.30 g/100 mL)—poisoned
Level of >88 mmol/L (>0.40 g/100 mL)—often fatal
Legal limits vary; for specific information contact local authorities. Commonly, the legal driving limit is "0.05%," that is, 11 mmol/L or 0.05 g/100 mL; in some locales it is "0.08%," that is, 18 mmol/L or 0.08 g/100 mL.

Interference

False-positive values of ≤690 mg/dL due to elevated lactate and LDH concentrations can occur using EMIT but not using protein-free ultrafiltrates or gas chromatography.
Laboratory findings due to alcohol ingestion.
Blood alcohol level of >300 mg/dL at any time or >100 mg/dL in routine examination. (Blood alcohol level of >150 mg/dL without gross evidence of intoxication suggests alcoholic patient's increased tolerance.) In high-dose coma, blood alcohol should be >300 mg/dL; otherwise, rule out other causes, especially diabetic acidosis and hypoglycemia.
Rules of thumb to estimate alcohol level:
- Peak is reached 0.5–3.0 hours after last drink.
- Each ounce of whiskey, glass of wine, or 12 oz of beer raises blood alcohol 15–25 mg/dL.
- Women absorb alcohol much more rapidly than do men and show a 35–45% higher blood alcohol level. During premenstrual period, peaks occurs more rapidly and reaches a higher level. Use of birth control pills causes a higher, more sustained level.
- Elderly become intoxicated more quickly than young persons.

Urine concentration is not well correlated with blood levels; cannot be used to determine level of intoxication or impairment.

Laboratory Findings

Hypoglycemia.
Hypochloremic alkalosis.
Low magnesium level.
Increased lactic acid level.
Metabolic acidosis with increased anion gap (AG).
Alcoholic ketoacidosis is preponderantly due to β-hydroxybutyrate, and therefore increased ketone levels in blood and urine often yield negative or only weakly positive results because nitroprusside test detects acetoacetic but not β-hydroxybutyric acid. As the patient improves, the ketone test may yield more strongly positive results (although total ketone level declines) because the improved liver function slows the conversion of acetoacetate to β-hydroxybutyrate.
Thrombocytopenia.
Anemia most often due to folic acid deficiency; less frequently due to iron deficiency, hemorrhage, and so on.
Alcohol is a common cause of ring sideroblasts.
Three types of hemolytic syndrome may occur (spur cell anemia, acquired stomatocytosis, Zieve syndrome).
Increase in the following blood values with no other known cause should arouse suspicion of alcoholism:

- Mean corpuscular volume (e.g., >97) (26% of cases) with round macrocytosis
- Serum γ-glutamyltransferase
- Uric acid (10% of cases)
- ALT, AST (48% of cases)
- Alkaline phosphatase (16% of cases)
- Bilirubin (13% of cases)
- Triglycerides

Alcohol (Isopropanol) Poisoning

Increased blood levels of isopropanol. In absence of acetone, usually indicates an artifact.
Serum levels

- Level of >400 mg/L—severe toxicity
- Level of >1,000 mg/L—coma

Presence of acetone in blood and urine, especially in high levels, suggests isopropanol poisoning.
Severe metabolic acidosis with increased AG is not a feature (as in ethanol poisoning but in contrast to methanol and ethylene glycol poisoning) unless lactic acid acidosis is present.
Osmolal gap increases 0.17 mOsm/L for every 1 mg of isopropanol; increase of 1 mOsm/L represents an isopropanol increase of 6 mg/dL.

Alcohol (Methyl) Poisoning

See Table 3.
Onset is 12–24 hours after ingestion.
Severe metabolic acidosis with increased AG and increased osmolar gap similar to that in ethanol intoxication and ethylene glycol poisoning.
Frequent concomitant acute pancreatitis.
Treat with ethyl alcohol to achieve blood alcohol level of 100–150 mg/dL and maintain until methyl alcohol level is <10 mg/dL, formate level is <1.2 mg/dL, AG is normal, and acidosis resolves.
Institute hemodialysis if blood methyl alcohol level is >50 mg/dL and severe resistant acidosis or renal failure is present. Lethal concentration = 80 mg/dL.

Allergic Disease

Increased serum total immunoglobulin (Ig) E is not a sensitive test result and is of limited clinical value, but extreme values may be helpful:

Table 3. Comparison of Poisoning by Various Alcohols

Alcohol[a]	Metabolic Acidosis with I AG	Urine Osmolal Gap	Serum Acetone	Urine Ketones	Oxalate Crystals
Ethanol	Var	I	Var	Var	–
Methanol	+	+	–	–	–
Isopropanol	–	I	+	+	–
Ethylene glycol	I	I	–	–	One-third of cases

+, present; –, absent; AG, anion gap; I, increased; Var, varies—findings depend on presence of lactic acidosis or alcoholic ketoacidosis.
[a]Measured by gas chromatography.

- Very low levels (<50 μg/L) help exclude atopic disease but not IgE sensitivity to special allergens such as penicillin or *Hymenoptera* venoms.
- If level is >900 μg/L, atopic disease is likely but tests for specific allergens are needed.
- Very high levels (2,000 to >60,000 μg/L) are found in asthma associated with severe atopic dermatitis, allergic bronchopulmonary aspergillosis, Buckley's syndrome (staphylococcal infections with hyper-IgE), systemic parasitic infestations, IgE myeloma, immune deficiency.
- Principal value in infants is to alert the clinician to the possibility of allergic disease when this is not the presumptive diagnosis.

Radioallergosorbent test (serum IgE antibodies specific for various allergens) measures IgE specific for individual allergies. Useful when skin testing cannot be done (e.g., in children, those at risk for anaphylaxis) or when skin testing is unreliable (e.g., in cases of generalized dermatitis, severe dermographism). Less sensitive than skin and bronchial provocation tests.

Blood eosinophil counts of >450/mm^3 in adults and >750/mm^3 in children suggest allergic disorders. Significant number of false-positive and false-negative results occur.

Nasal cytologic smears stained with Wright-Giemsa showing >5% eosinophils, >1% basophils, or >50% goblet/epithelial cells suggest allergic disease of respiratory tract. Findings do not correlate with blood eosinophilia. Presence of large numbers of neutrophils suggests infection. Presence of both eosinophils and neutrophils suggests chronic allergy with superimposed infection. Significant number of false-positive and false-negative results occur.

Measurement of serum complement level is not useful.

Aluminum Toxicity

May occur in chronic renal failure in patients on long-term dialysis treatment.

Serum aluminum level should always be <200 μg/L (7.4 μmol/L); frequent monitoring and close observation for toxicity are indicated if serum level is >100 μg/L. Can be prevented by treatment of dialysate water (e.g., by reverse osmosis) so that final aluminum concentration in dialysate is <15 μg/L.

Microcytic hypochromic anemia (non–iron-deficiency type) is seen.

Osteomalacic osteodystrophy is progressive, associated with a myopathy, resists treatment with vitamin D or its metabolites; may be associated with hypercalcemia. Metastatic calcification is common. Bone biopsy (special techniques) is most reliable test.

Dialysis encephalopathy may be present.

Chelation treatment with deferoxamine increases serum level with decrease in protein-bound fraction.

Arsenic Poisoning, Chronic

See Table 4.

Table 4. Normal and Toxic Levels of Some Common Toxic Substances and Trace Metals

Chemical	Specimen[a]	Normal Range	Toxic Concentration
Arsenic	Hair or nails	<1.0 μg/g	
	Serum	<0.07 μg/mL	
	Urine	<25 μg/specimen	>150 μg/specimen
Cadmium	Blood	<5.0 ng/mL	
	Urine	<3 μg/24 hr	
Carbon monoxide	Blood	<7% <15% in heavy smokers	>20%
Chromium	Serum	0.3–0.9 μg/L	
	Urine	<8.0 μg/specimen	
Copper	Serum	0.70–1.40 μg/mL (men) 0.80–1.55 μg/mL (women) 1.20–3.00 μg/mL (pregnant women) 0.80–1.90 μg/mL (children 6–12 yr) 0.20–0.70 μg/mL (infants)	
	Urine	15–60 μg/specimen	
	Liver tissue	10–35 μg/g dry weight	
Ethanol	Blood		>2,000 μg/mL
Ethylene glycol	Serum		Toxic >2 mmol/L, lethal >20 mmol/L
Lead	Blood	<0.2 μg/mL	
	Serum	0.8–2.5 ng/mL	
	Urine	<80 μg/specimen; abnormal, >400 μg/specimen; inconclusive, 80–400 μg/specimen	
	Hair and nails	<25 μg/g	
Manganese	Serum or plasma	0.4–1.1 ng/mL	
	Whole blood	7.7–12.1 ng/mL	
	Urine	<0.3 μg/specimen	
Mercury	Blood	<0.005 μg/mL	
	Urine	<0.3 μg/specimen	
	Hair or nails	<1.0 μg/g	
Selenium	Serum	46–143 ng/mL	
	Whole blood	58–234 ng/mL	
	Urine	7–160 μg/L	
	Hair	0.2–1.4 μg/g	
Silver	Serum	<0.2 μg/mL	
	Urine	<1.0 μg/specimen	
Thallium	Serum	<10 ng/mL	
	Urine	<10 μg/specimen	
Zinc	Plasma	0.70–120 μg/mL	
	Serum	5–15% higher than plasma	
	Urine	0.15–1.0 mg/d	

[a]Urine concentration is reported as per 7-mL aliquot of 24-hr urine collection.
From Jacob RA, Milne DB. Biochemical assessment of vitamins and trace metals. *Clin Lab Med* 1993;13:371.

Increased arsenic appears in urine (usually >0.1 mg/L; in acute cases may be >1.0 mg/L). Can be present for up to 10 days after a single exposure. With high industrial exposure, urine level may reach 1,600 μg/L. After large seafood meal, level may reach 400 μg/L in 4 hours.
Increased arsenic appears in hair (normal = 0.05 mg/100 g of hair; chronic toxicity = 0.1–0.5 mg/100 g of hair; acute toxicity = 1–3 mg/100 g of hair); may take several weeks to appear.
Increased arsenic appears in nails 6–9 months after exposure.
Moderate anemia is present; commonly normocytic, normochromic, basophilic stippling.
Moderate leukopenia occurs (2,000–5,000/mm^3), with mild eosinophilia.
Pancytopenia, aplastic anemia, and leukemia are associated with arsenic poisoning.
Liver function test results show mild abnormalities.
Abnormal renal function is frequent (oliguria, proteinuria, hematuria, casts).
Increased cerebrospinal fluid (CSF) protein (>100 mg/dL) is frequent; easily confused with Guillain-Barré syndrome.

Barbiturate Overdose

Correlation between serum concentrations of barbiturates and state of intoxication in patients who have taken only a short-acting barbiturate, who are not habitual drug users, and who have no medical complications:

<6 μg/mL	Alert
6–10 μg/mL	Drowsy
11–17 μg/mL	Stuporous
16–20 μg/mL	Coma 1
20–24 μg/mL	Coma 2
24–28 μg/mL	Coma 3
28–40 μg/mL	Coma 4

If the serum drug level is less than expected for the state of intoxication, look for medical complications (e.g., aspiration pneumonia, head trauma) or presence of other drugs.

Burns

Decreased plasma volume and blood volume. This decrease follows (and therefore is not due to) marked drop in cardiac output. Greatest fall in plasma volume occurs in the first 12 hours and continues at a much slower rate for only 6–12 hours more. In a 40% burn, plasma volume falls to 25% below preburn levels.
Infection—burn septic: Gram-positive organisms predominate until the third day, when Gram-negative organisms become dominant; reflects hospital's flora. By fifth day, untreated infection is active. Fatal burn wound sepsis shows no noteworthy spread of bacteria beyond the wound in half of cases. Before antibiotic therapy, burn sepsis caused 75% of deaths due to burns; it now causes 10–15% of deaths.
Diagnosis by quantitative biopsy of eschar showing >10^5 bacteria/g of tissue and histologic evidence of bacterial invasion in underlying unburned tissue. Cultures of surface specimens do not accurately predict incipient burn wound sepsis. Local and systemic infection due to *Candida* and *Phycomycetes*.
Laboratory findings due to pneumonia, which now causes most deaths that result from infection.

- Two-thirds of pneumonia cases are airborne infections. One-third are hematogenous infections and are often due to septic phlebitis at the sites of old cutdowns.

Laboratory findings due to smoke inhalation injury

- Carbonaceous sputum is pathognomonic; casts composed of mucin, fibrin, white blood cells (WBCs), cell debris may be present.
- Hypoxemia.
- Increased carboxyhemoglobin (>15%).

Cyanide toxicity should be suspected if metabolic acidosis is present with apparently sufficient oxygen delivery.

Laboratory findings due to renal failure. Reported frequency varies from 1.3% of total admissions to 1% of patients with burns involving >15% of body surface.

Laboratory findings due to gastrointestinal complications.

- Curling's ulcer. Occurs in 11% of burn patients. Gastric ulcer is more frequent in general, but duodenal ulcer occurs twice as often in children as in adults. Gastric lesions are seen throughout the first month with equal frequency in all age groups, but duodenal ulcers are most frequent in adults during the first week and in children during the third and fourth weeks after the burns.
- Other findings include acute pancreatitis, superior mesenteric artery syndrome, adynamic ileus.

Laboratory findings due to complications of topical antibacterial therapy.

- Mafenide acetate (Sulfamylon)—metabolic acidosis (carbonic anhydrase inhibition).
- Silver nitrate—methemoglobinemia due to conversion of nitrate to nitrite by some strains of *Enterobacter cloacae*. Agyria does not occur.
- Silver sulfadiazine (Silvadene)—hemolysis in patients with G-6-PD deficiency.

Blood viscosity rises acutely; remains elevated for 4–5 days although hematocrit (Hct) has returned to normal.

Fibrin split product levels are increased for 3–5 days.

Other findings that may occur in all types of trauma.

- Platelet count rises slowly, with increase lasting for 3 weeks.
- Platelet adhesiveness is increased.
- Fibrinogen falls during first 36 hours, then rises steeply for up to 3 months.
- Factors V and VIII may be at four to eight times normal level for up to 3 months.

Carbon Monoxide Poisoning, Acute

Displaces oxyhemoglobin dissociation curve to left.

Increased carboxyhemoglobin level is diagnostic. Pulse oximetry cannot distinguish carboxyhemoglobin from oxyhemoglobin.

Symptoms are correlated with the percentage of carbon monoxide in hemoglobin (%COHb):

% COHb	Symptoms
0–2	Asymptomatic
2–5	Found in moderate cigarette smokers; usually asymptomatic but may be slight impairment of intellect.
5–10	Found in heavy cigarette smokers; slight dyspnea with severe exertion
10–20	Dyspnea with moderate exertion; mild headache
20–30	Marked headache, irritability, disturbed judgment and memory, easy fatigability
30–40	Severe headache, dimness of vision, confusion, weakness, nausea
40–50	Headache, confusion, fainting, ataxia, collapse, hyperventilation
50–60	Coma, intermittent convulsions
>60	Respiratory failure and death if exposure is long continued
80	Rapidly fatal

Blood pH is markedly decreased (metabolic acidosis due to tissue hypoxia).

Arterial Po_2 is normal, although O_2 is significantly decreased.

Arterial Pco_2 may be normal or slightly decreased.

Increased carbon monoxide in patient's exhaled air or in ambient air at site of exposure can help confirm diagnosis if level of carbon monoxide in Hb has already fallen substantially.

Cigarette Smoking

Cotinine increased in plasma or urine. Used to assess compliance in smoking cessation programs and to identify passively exposed nonsmokers. Has a longer half-life than nicotine, is more sensitive and specific than other markers to distinguish smokers from nonsmokers.

The active and addictive agent is nicotine, although cigarette smoke contains numerous other toxic and carcinogenic agents.

	Cotinine Plasma	Urine
Nonsmoker or passive exposure	0–8 μg/L	0.0–0.2 mg/L
Smoker	>8 μg/L	>0.2 mg/L

Increased blood carbon monoxide

Diseases of increased incidence and severity in smokers (values in parentheses indicate increased risk compared to the nonsmoking population).

- Cancer of the lung (×10)
- Chronic obstructive pulmonary disease (×10) (chronic bronchitis and emphysema)
- Atherosclerotic arterial disease (×2)
- Ischemic heart disease (angina and infarction)
- Cerebral thrombosis and infarction
- Thromboangiitis obliterans (Buerger disease) (×100)
- Chronic peptic ulcer (×2–3)
- Cancer of the oral cavity and tongue (×5)
- Cancer of the urinary bladder (×5)
- Cancer of the larynx and pharynx (×5)
- Cancer of the esophagus (×5)

Cyanide Poisoning

Potassium cyanide is in rodenticides, insecticides, laboratory reagents, film developer, amygdalin, silver polish, and acetonitrile used to remove artificial fingernails.

Hydrogen cyanide is in insecticides and fumigants and is released by the burning of plastic and synthetics.

The Po_2 and oxygen saturation are normal except in severe cases when respiratory failure occurs.

- Patient may first have respiratory alkalosis due to hyperventilation caused by tissue hypoxia.
- Then severe lactic (metabolic) acidosis develops.
- With respiratory depression, respiratory acidosis may occur.

Increased venous oxygen with decreased arteriovenous oxygen difference due to decreased tissue extraction of oxygen.

Blood cyanide level is increased. Toxic concentration is >50 μg/dL.

Treat with nitrites to achieve methemoglobin level of >30%.

Drowning and Near-Drowning

Hypoxemia (decreased Po_2)

Metabolic acidosis (decreased blood pH)

In near-drowning in freshwater, often

- Normal serum sodium and chloride levels
- Variable serum potassium level
- Increased free plasma Hb; hemoglobinuria may occur.
- Fall in red blood cells (RBCs), Hb, and Hct in 24 hours.

In severe freshwater aspiration

- Decreased serum sodium and chloride
- Increased serum potassium
- Increased plasma Hb

In severe seawater aspiration

- Increased serum sodium and chloride
- Normal plasma Hb
- Hypovolemia

In near-drowning in seawater, often

- Moderate increase in serum sodium and chloride
- Normal or decreased serum potassium
- Normal Hb, Hct, and plasma Hb

Blood Hb may appear normal even when considerable hemolysis is present because usual methodology does not distinguish between Hb within RBCs and free Hb in serum.

Decrease in Hb and Hct may be delayed 1–2 days.

Electric Current and Lightning Injury

Increased WBC count with large immature granulocytes.
Albuminuria; hemoglobinuria in presence of severe burns.
CSF sometimes bloody.
Myoglobinuria and increased serum AST, creatine kinase (CK), and so on, indicate severe tissue damage.

Ethylene and Diethylene Glycol (Antifreeze) Poisoning

Severe metabolic acidosis with increased AG and osmolal gap.
Detection of ethylene glycol and its metabolite glycolic acid in serum.
Oxalate and hippurate crystals in urine.
Characteristic oxalate crystals in renal biopsy.
Urine may fluoresce under Wood lamp due to fluorescein added to antifreeze.
Institute dialysis if glycol level is >50 mg/dL or renal failure or persistent severe acidosis is present.
Treat by intravenous administration of ethyl alcohol to achieve level >100 mg/dL.

Exercise, Severe

May occur with variable severity and in variable number of persons.
Increased serum enzyme concentrations due to skeletal muscle injury, for example, CK total, CK-MB, lactate dehydrogenase (LDH), AST, aldolase, malate dehydrogenase.
Changes due to mechanical destruction of RBCs, for example, increased serum and urine myoglobin, increased serum indirect bilirubin.
Increased serum uric acid, decreased serum phosphate.

Heat Exhaustion and Heat Stroke

A continuum of increasingly severe heat illnesses caused by dehydration, electrolyte losses, and failure of the body's thermoregulatory mechanisms.
Heat exhaustion is an acute heat injury with hyperthermia due to dehydration.
Heat stroke is extreme hyperthermia with thermoregulatory failure and profound central nervous system dysfunction.
More likely in children or elderly.

Heat Exhaustion

Signs and Symptoms

Fatigue and lethargy
Weakness
Dizziness
Nausea, vomiting
Myalgias
Headache
Profuse sweating
Tachycardia
Hypotension, shock
Lack of coordination
Agitation
Intense thirst
Hyperventilation
Paresthesias
Core temperature elevated but <103°F (<39.4°C) or <96°F (<37°C)

Laboratory Studies

Serum electrolyte levels: urinalysis shows hyponatremia

Heatstroke

Multiorgan dysfunction.
Abnormal liver function and increased muscle enzyme values.
Exhaustion.
Confusion, disorientation.
Coma.
Hot, flushed, dry skin.
Core temperature >105°F (>40.5°C).

Uniformly increased serum AST (mean is 20 times normal), ALT (mean is 10 times normal), and LDH (mean is five times normal); reach peak on third day and return to normal by 2 weeks. Increased CK-MM. Lethal outcome is associated with significantly higher serum values that continued to increase in next 12–24 hours. Consecutive normal values rule out diagnosis of heatstroke.

Hemoconcentration.
Evidence of kidney damage may vary from mild proteinuria and slight abnormalities of urine sediment, to azotemia, to acute oliguric renal insufficiency.
Serum sodium level is often decreased but may be high, especially in exertional heatstroke.
Respiratory distress syndrome.
Respiratory alkalosis occurs early and lactic acidosis and hyperkalemia later.
Hypoglycemia may occur.
Increased WBC count is usual.
DIC is common in severe cases.
Rhabdomyolysis, DIC, and acute renal failure are relatively uncommon in elderly because exertional heatstroke is less common in elderly.
CSF, AST, ALT, and LDH are normal.

Causes

Failure of heat-dissipating mechanisms or an overwhelming heat stress leading to a rise in core temperature, dehydration, and salt depletion.

Risk Factors

Poor acclimatization to heat or poor physical conditioning
Salt or water depletion
Obesity
Acute febrile or gastrointestinal illnesses
Chronic illnesses—uncontrolled diabetes or hypertension, cardiac disease
Alcohol and other substance abuse
High heat and humidity, poor air circulation in environment
Heavy, restrictive clothing

Laboratory Studies

Used primarily to detect end-organ damage.
Electrolyte levels, urinalysis.
Creatinine, blood urea nitrogen levels.
Liver enzyme levels.
Complete blood count.
Urine specific gravity.
Results of the studies listed yield hypernatremia, hyperchloremia, hemoconcentration, and increased urine specific gravity.

Household Cleaning Products, Ingestion of Corrosive Agents In

Accidental ingestion usually occurs in children 1–3 years of age.
Most household cleaning agents are alkalis (70%).
Acids account for 20% and others, including bleaches, detergents, microwave-overheated baby bottles, and button mercuric acid batteries, account for 10%.
These agents cause an erosive esophagitis.
Alkalis produce a severe deep liquefactive necrosis.
Acid agents include toilet bowel cleaners, some drain declogging agents, and rust and stain removers. They contain hydrochloric, sulfuric, or oxalic acid sulfates.

The peak age for ingestion is before 5 years.
Alkaline agents cause severe burns of the mouth and oral mucosa. Ulceration and even esophageal perforation may occur, and esophageal strictures may develop over the following few weeks. Leukocytosis and fever occur.

Hypervitaminosis A

Acute intoxication after ingestion of 150–600 mg (500,000–2,000,000 U).
Chronic hypervitaminosis after ingestion of 7.5–90.0 mg/day (25,000–300,000 U) for minimum of 1 month up to 2 years.
Plasma vitamin A = 300–1,000 µg/dL.
Increased tissue levels of vitamin A and retinoic acid derivatives.
May also show
- Increased erythrocyte sedimentation rate
- Increased serum ALP, γ-glutamyltransferase, bilirubin
- Decreased serum albumin
- Decreased Hb
- Slight proteinuria
- Slightly increased serum carotene
- Increased prothrombin time

Abnormal liver biopsy findings.

Hypothermia, Accidental

Acid-base disturbances are very common.
Initial hyperventilation causes respiratory alkalosis followed by respiratory acidosis due to carbon dioxide retention.
Metabolic acidosis due to lactate accumulation. During rewarming, metabolic acidosis may become worse as lactic acid is mobilized from poorly perfused tissues.
Hemoconcentration is common.
WBC count frequently falls, but differential is usually normal.
DIC may occur during rewarming.
"Cold diuresis," glycosuria, and natriuresis may occur; oliguria suggests complicating hypovolemia, acute tubular necrosis, rhabdomyolysis, or drug overdose.
Pancreatitis is a frequent complication.
Marked abnormalities in liver function test results are unusual.
Extreme hyperkalemia (>6.8 mEq/L) is a good indicator of death during acute hypothermia.

Intoxications, Specific, Characteristics of (Toxidromes)[2]

Anticholinergics (Atropine, Tricyclic Antidepressants)

Fixed dilated pupils
Fever
Dry skin and mucous membranes
Rubor
Hallucinations, mania
Increased heart rate

Anticholinesterases (Organophosphates, Carbamates)

Constricted or pinpoint pupils
Profuse sweating and salivation
Bronchial secretions and bronchospasms
Muscle fasciculations

[2]Temple AR. *Poisoning I.* Leawood, KS: American Academy of Family Physicians, 1983. Monograph 52.

Coma
Bradycardia

Carbon Monoxide

Coma
Labored breathing
Cherry-red skin coloration (only rarely)
Possible involvement of multiple individuals

Cyanide

Coma
Rapid breathing
Hypotension
Odor of bitter almonds on breath

Narcotics and Other Central Nervous System Depressants

Pinpoint pupils
Decreased respiration
Coma
Hypotension
Decreased or absent reflexes

Salicylates

Vomiting
Deep, labored breathing
Lethargy or disorientation or both
Dehydration
Fever
Ringing in ears
Coma or convulsions

Iron Poisoning, Acute

(Occurs in children who have ingested medicinal iron preparations)

Increased serum iron. Peak usually occurs 2–4 hours after ingestion. Levels begin to fall after 6 hours. If the first sample was taken 1–2 hours after ingestion, a second sample should be obtained several hours later. Serum should be obtained after absorption is complete and before peak serum level falls due to protein binding and tissue distribution.

- Level of <350 μg/dL is rarely significant clinically; patient may have mild symptoms.
- Level of 350–500 μg/dL: patient frequently has symptoms but risk of serious abnormality is mild; prolonged chelation therapy usually not required. Ten percent of patients develop coma or shock.
- Level of >500 μg/dL within 6 hours of ingestion with severe intoxication: patient needs urgent chelation treatment in hospital. Twenty-five percent develop coma or shock.
- Level of >1,000 μg/dL may be lethal; patient may require hemodialysis or exchange transfusion. Seventy percent develop coma or shock.

Increased total iron-binding capacity itself is unreliable and not useful. Poor prognostic sign when serum iron level greatly exceeds total iron-binding capacity. Spuriously increased by deferoxamine chelation therapy.

Serum glucose level of >150 mg/dL or WBC count of >15,000/mm^3 and presence of radiopaque material on flat radiographic plate of abdomen correlate with increased serum iron level.

In deferoxamine challenge (50 mg/kg up to 1 g/kg administrated intramuscularly) deferoxamine chelates free iron in circulation (100 mg binds 9 mg of iron, chiefly ferric); later appears in urine bound to iron, causing light orange to dark red-brown ("vin rose") color. Parenteral chelation should continue until serum iron level is <100 μg/dL or urine loses vin rose color.

Renal changes may occur (e.g., acute renal failure, nephrotic syndrome, specific tubular defects).

Lead Poisoning (Plumbism)

Source of Lead

In children, lead poisoning usually due to pica or paint from old cribs, batteries.

In adolescents, may be due to gasoline sniffing.

In all groups, epidemics may be due to contamination of water supply, use of contaminated pottery, and so on.

Determination of Lead Level

Measurements of zinc protoporphyrin (hematofluorometer) and free erythrocyte protoporphyrin (FEP) in blood using rapid micromethods are more sensitive indicators of lead poisoning than measurement of δ-aminolevulinic acid in urine. Especially useful for screening children. Zinc protoporphyrin appears only in new RBCs and remains for life of RBC; therefore zinc protoporphyrin does not increase until several weeks after onset of lead exposure and remains high long after lead exposure has ended; therefore it is good indicator of total body burden of lead. FEP is sensitive measure of chronic exposure; increased whole-blood level is sensitive measure of acute exposure. After therapy or removal of exposure, blood lead level becomes normal weeks to months before RBC values. The Centers for Disease Control and Prevention (CDC) now recommends determination of whole-blood lead in children, because zinc protoporphyrin measurement is not reliable below approximately 25 μg/dL.

Classification of Lead Levels in Young Children

CDC classification of whole-blood lead in children 6–72 months of age for prevention and control[3]

Level (μg/dL)	Classification
≤9	Not considered lead poisoning
10[a]	Rescreening; intervention; search for source
>10–14	Need for more frequent tests
15–19	Rescreening; educational and nutritional intervention
20–44	Evidence of increased lead exposure; remediation of environment; chelation should be considered
45–69	Chelation therapy; environmental intervention
>70	Emergency treatment should begin immediately

[a]CDC has lowered the intervention level from 25 to 10 μg/dL.

Screening for Lead Poisoning in High-Risk Children

See Table 5.

Clinical and Laboratory Findings

Effects of lowest lead concentration on laboratory changes[4]

	Blood Lead Concentration (μg/dL)
Death	150
Encephalopathy	90
Nephropathy	75

[3]Centers for Disease Control and Prevention. *Preventing lead poisoning in young children*. Washington: U.S. Department of Health and Human Services, Public Health Service, 1994.

[4]Williams RH, Erickson T. Evaluating lead and iron intoxication in an emergency setting. *Lab Med* 1998;29:224.

Anemia	75
Colic	60
Decreased Hb synthesis	40
FEP increased	10–20
Developmental toxicity	
Decreased intelligence quotient, growth, hearing	10
Transplacental transfer	<10

The CDC regards all results ≥10 μg/dL as abnormal for children 1–5 years of age and all other individuals not known to be at risk.

The Occupational Safety and Health Administration workplace normal reference range is ≤40 μg/dL for industrial monitoring.

Submitted blood sample is 3 mL of whole blood collected in a certified lead-free (EDTA) tube.

Other causes of increased FEP are iron deficiency, anemia of chronic disease, sickle cell disease, erythropoietic protoporphyria. FEP of ≥190 μg/dL is almost always due to lead intoxication. Iron deficiency and thalassemia should be ruled out even if lead level is increased because iron deficiency and lead poisoning can occur together. Use blood lead and zinc protoporphyrin levels together to evaluate for possible lead poisoning, blood zinc protoporphyrin with serum iron and ferritin levels to evaluate for iron deficiency.

The level of δ-aminolevulinic acid in urine is increased. Because it is increased in 75% of asymptomatic individuals exposed to lead who have normal coproporphyrin in the urine, it can be used to detect early excess lead absorption. It is not increased until the blood lead is >40 μg/dL.

Confirm diagnosis with assay of blood lead level—a single determination cannot distinguish chronic from acute exposure. It reflects equilibrium between body com-

Table 5. Screening for Lead Poisoning in High-Risk Children

Lead (μg/dL)	FEP (μg/dL)[a] ≤34	35–109	110–249	≥250
≤24	Retest in 1 yr	Rule out other causes of increased FEP[b]; retest in 3 mo	Rule out iron deficiency; retest in 3 mo	Rule out erythropoietic protoporphyria; retest in 3 mo
25–49	Retest next visit	Retest in 1–3 mo, then every 3–6 mo[c]	Rule out iron deficiency; retest in 2–4 wk[c]	—
50–69	Usual pattern; retest to confirm	Retest in 2 wk, then every 1–3 mo[d]	Retest at once; rule out iron deficiency[d]	Retest at once; perform mobilization test or treat
≥70	Unusual pattern; retest to rule out contaminated specimen	Retest at once and treat	Retest at once and treat	Hospitalize at once

FEP, free erythrocyte protoprophyrin.
[a]Other causes of increased FEP are iron deficiency, anemia of chronic disease, sickle cell disease, and erythropoietic protoporphyria.
[b]Iron deficiency and thalassemia should be ruled out even if lead level is increased because iron deficiency and lead poisoning can occur together. Measure blood lead and zinc protoporphyrin (ZPP) levels together for possible lead poisoning; measure blood ZPP with serum iron and ferritin for iron deficiency.
[c]Consider mobilization test if lead is ≥35 μg/dL.
[d]Consider mobilization test if lead = 35–55 μg/dL. Treat if lead = 56–69 μg/dL.
From Westchester County (New York) Department of Health.

partments and therefore a relatively recent exposure. All blood and urine specimens for lead measurement must be collected in special (lead free) containers.

Urine lead level:

Level of <80 µg/L is normal for children.

Level of >500 µg/24 hours in children indicates excess mobile total body lead burden and suggests need for chelation therapy.

Lead mobilization test—administer 500 mg/m^2 (up to 1,000 mg) of edetate calcium disodium, then measure 8-hour urine excretion of lead. Ratio of total urine lead (in micrograms) to edetate infused (in milligrams) of >0.6 is considered positive finding. Difficulty in collecting urine frequently makes test invalid. Begin chelation therapy if blood lead level is >45 µg/dL.

Increased coproporphyrin in urine is a reliable sign of intoxication and is often demonstrable before basophilic stippling (but one should rule out a false-positive reaction due to drugs such as barbiturates and salicylates). This is a useful rapid screening test.

Mild anemia is common (rarely <9 g/dL) and is usually normochromic and normocytic but may be hypochromic and microcytic, especially in children. Mean corpuscular hemoglobin concentration is reduced only moderately. In acute lead poisoning, hemolytic crisis may occur. Anemia may be seen at blood lead levels of 50–80 µg/dL in adults and 40–70 µg/dL in children.

Anisocytosis and poikilocytosis may be found, and a few nucleated RBCs may be seen. Some polychromasia is usual.

Stippled RBCs occur later in approximately 2% of cases (due to inhibition of 5'-pyrimidine nucleotidase).

Basophilic stippling is not pathognomonic of lead poisoning. Amount of stippling is not correlated with severity of lead toxicity.

Bone marrow shows erythroid hyperplasia, and 65% of erythroid cells show stippling with some ringed sideroblasts (thus this may be considered a secondary sideroblastic anemia).

Osmotic fragility is decreased, but mechanical fragility is increased.

Hematologic changes of lead poisoning are more marked in patients with iron deficiency.

Urine urobilinogen and uroporphyrin levels are increased.

Porphobilinogen level is normal or only slightly increased in the urine (unlike in acute intermittent porphyria).

Renal tubular damage occurs, with Fanconi syndrome (hypophosphatemia, amino aciduria, and glycosuria), usually in very severe or chronic cases. Albuminuria, increased WBCs, and transient rising blood urea nitrogen may occur. With chronic exposure interstitial nephritis develops with increased serum uric acid (saturnine gout).

CSF protein level is increased, and frequently ≥100 mononuclear cells/mm^3 are present in encephalopathy, which is rare with blood lead levels <100 µg/dL.

In children, acute encephalopathy may be seen with blood lead level of ≥80 µg/dL; abdominal and gastrointestinal symptoms may occur with levels of 50 µg/dL but their presence usually indicates levels of ≥70 µg/dL.

Laboratory studies during dimercaprol (British anti-Lewisite) therapy:

- Check daily for hematuria, proteinuria, cast formation.
- Check every other day for hypokalemia and hypercalcemia.
- Rule out G-6-PD deficiency and liver disease before starting therapy.

Mercury Poisoning

Levels of mercury in serum, urine, and CSF are increased.

Ninety-five percent of asymptomatic healthy people (not exposed to mercury) have a urine value of <20 µg/L and a blood level of <3 µg/L. Urine and blood levels are nondiagnostic, because they vary among patients with symptoms, and daily urine levels vary in the same patient. The earlier values apply to mercury vapor and inorganic mercury salts.

Organic mercury (e.g., ethyl and methyl mercury) is more toxic; accumulates in RBCs and central nervous system. Most is slowly excreted in feces with half-life of 70 days. Only 10% is excreted in urine; urine levels may be normal even with significant exposure. Phenyl and methoxyethyl mercuries are less toxic and show higher urine levels.

Clinical correlation with organic mercury

	Whole-Blood Total Mercury (µg/L or ng/mL or ppm)
Safe level	<100
Probably no symptoms	100–200
Symptoms occasionally present	>650
Symptoms usually present	>1,000

Signs and Symptoms

Acrodynia (painful extremities)
Proteinuria, nephrotic syndrome, edema, renal failure

Metals, Heavy, Urine Examination

See Table 4.

A randomly obtained or 24-hour urine specimen is collected into a trace-element-free container. Special testing may be done after intravenous calcium EDTA infusion, particularly if the history of exposure was in the past.

Estimation of heavy metal content can be performed by atomic absorption spectrophotometry, inductively coupled plasma spectrometry, or spectrophotometry. Lead, mercury, arsenic, and cadmium are generally measured, whereas others such as thallium and uranium are usually assayed only on specific request.

These studies are done to monitor patients at risk from environmental exposure, in cases of suspected poisoning, or to evaluate patients with suspicious clinical features such as neuropathy, encephalopathy, renal failure, or Fanconi's syndrome.

Urine screening: Heavy metal poisoning causes proteinuria, glycosuria.

Mothball (Camphor, Paradichlorobenzene, Naphthalene) Poisoning

Paradichlorobenzene inhalation may cause liver damage.

Naphthalene ingestion may cause hemolytic anemia in patients with G-6-PD deficiency, liver damage.

Pesticide Exposure

Pesticides Commonly Found in the United States

Approximately 600 pesticide active ingredients, found in insecticides, herbicides, rodenticides, and fungicides, are registered with the United States Environmental Protection Agency (EPA). These compounds are mixed with one another and blended with inert ingredients to produce >20,000 commercial pesticide products. The EPA estimates that each year domestic users in the United States spend $8.5 billion for 1.1 billion pounds of pesticide active ingredients.

The principal classes of insecticides in use in the United States are the organophosphates, carbamates, and pyrethroids. Unlike earlier generations of pesticides, such as dichlorodiphenyltrichloroethane (DDT), these compounds are short lived in the environment and do not accumulate in human and animal tissues. The organophosphates and carbamates are toxic to the nervous system, and some of the pyrethroids may be toxic to the reproductive system and disruptive to endocrine function.

Sources of Children's Exposure to Pesticides

Children may be exposed to pesticides in schools, day care centers, parks, and gardens. Farm children can be exposed in the fields as well as at home, when pesticides are transported into the house. Pesticides from agricultural runoff can contaminate drinking water supplies. Diet is an important source of exposure.

The largest source of children's exposure is the use of pesticides in the home and on lawns and gardens. Approximately 90% of American households use pesticides.

Homeowners accounted for the purchase of an estimated 74 million pounds of the pesticides used in the United States in 1995. Multiple exposures may be additive in their effect on children's health.

Organochlorine pesticides, such as chlordane, DDT, dieldrin, and lindane, have been widely detected in residential air and on indoor surfaces in houses in U.S. cities. Many of these pesticides have been banned for decades, and they are found more often in older homes. Chlordane was used in an estimated 24 million U.S. homes, usually as a termiticide, and it has been detected in the home environment as long as 35 years after use.

Illegal pesticides (street pesticides) are of great concern in cities. For example, a very highly concentrated and illegal preparation of the carbamate insecticide aldicarb is available in inner-city communities under the name Tres Pasitos ("three little steps," the distance a rodent is said to be able to walk after ingesting this agent). A case report described a 2-year-old girl in New York City who had an acute toxic episode after eating Tres Pasitos. Another roach killer bought on urban street corners is Tiza China ("Chinese chalk"), which reportedly contains boric acid. A 1996 poisoning episode involved methyl parathion. Eleven hundred homes in Chicago and Cleveland and on the Gulf Coast were illegally sprayed with this highly toxic pesticide.

Effects of Pesticides

The effects of pesticide poisoning on children can be acute and obvious, or chronic, cumulative, and subtle. The Consumer Product Safety Commission collects data on acute pesticide poisonings in the United States, based on a statistical sample of emergency rooms in 6,000 selected hospitals. From 1990 to 1992, an estimated 20,000 emergency room visits were the result of pesticide exposure. The incidence was disproportionately high among children, who accounted for 61%, or >12,000, of these cases. Organophosphates were the class of compounds most frequently involved.

Acute high-dose exposure to organophosphate pesticides inhibits the enzyme acetylcholinesterase in the nervous system, which leads to a spectrum of cholinergic symptoms, including lacrimation, abdominal cramps, vomiting, diarrhea, miosis, and profuse sweating. The more severe cases progress to respiratory arrest and death. Studies in animals indicate that young animals are more susceptible than adults to this acute neurotoxic syndrome, probably because the young are less able to detoxify and excrete organophosphates.

Concern about the chronic effects of pesticides focuses on two particular areas: subclinical neurotoxicity and disruption of endocrine function.

Subclinical Injury

The mechanism of chlorpyrifos-induced neurotoxicity appears to involve injury to the adenylyl cyclase cascade, a system in brain cells that mediates cholinergic as well as adrenergic signals. Even at low levels of exposure, insufficient to compromise survival or growth, chlorpyrifos was found to produce cellular deficits in the developing brain that could contribute to behavioral abnormalities.

The EPA issued a ruling that bans the use of chlorpyrifos in schools, parks, and day care settings, and prohibits and phases out nearly all residential use. Prevention of developmental disability in children was the major reason for this ruling.

Endocrine Effects

Heavy exposure to DDT may disrupt estrogen cycles.

Concern about the endocrine toxicity of pesticides in humans has focused especially on the pyrethroids, a class of insecticides widely used as substitutes for chlorpyrifos and other organophosphate and carbamate pesticides. Pyrethroids have been used in pediatric practice to control body lice and scabies instead of more toxic agents such as lindane, and their acute toxicity is low. Hormonal activity has been reported for certain pyrethroids in laboratory systems, however, which suggests that their capacity to affect hormonal and reproductive development in children should be investigated further. The pyrethroid sumithrin (Anvil) has been used in spraying for mosquitoes to prevent the spread of West Nile virus.

In fetal life, even low-dose exposure to endocrine-disrupting pesticides can have devastating effects, because hormones play critical roles in shaping the early development of the immune, nervous, and reproductive systems. The developmental effects of exposure to endocrine function vary with age at exposure and sex.

The Food Quality Protection Act of 1996 requires that pesticides be tested for potential endocrine toxicity. The EPA has designed a screening protocol for testing pesticides for endocrine-disrupting potential and will be making recommendations for safety standards based on these tests.

Phenacetin, Long-Term Excessive Exposure

Laboratory findings due to increased incidence of peptic ulceration, often with bleeding, may be present.
Laboratory findings associated with increased incidence of papillary necrosis and interstitial nephritis may be present.
Proteinuria is slight or absent.
Hematuria is often present in cases of active papillary necrosis.
WBC count is increased in urine with absence of infection.
Papillae are passed in urine.
Creatinine clearance is decreased.
Renal failure may occur.
Anemia is common and frequently precedes azotemia.

Phenytoin Sodium (Dilantin) Therapy, Complications

Megaloblastic anemia may occur. It is completely responsive to folic acid therapy (even when phenytoin sodium therapy is continued) but not always to administration of vitamin B_{12}. Is the most common hematologic complication.
Rarely pancytopenia, thrombocytopenia alone, or leukopenia, including agranulocytosis, may occur.
Laboratory findings of hepatitis may be present.
Laboratory findings resembling those of malignant lymphomas may be present.
Laboratory findings resembling those of infectious mononucleosis may occur, but heterophil agglutination is not increased.
Increased triiodothyronine uptake, but radioactive iodine uptake, serum cholesterol level, and so on, are normal (because of competition for binding sites of thyroid-binding globulin).
Phenytoin sodium therapy may induce a lupus-like syndrome.

Phosphate (Organic) Poisoning (from Insecticides, e.g., Parathion, Malathion)

RBC and serum cholinesterase decreased by ≥50% due to inhibition of cholinesterase by organic phosphate pesticides (e.g., diazinon, malathion) and carbamates (e.g., carbaryl).
Decrease in serum of 40% when first symptoms of acute ingestion appear.
Decrease in serum of 80% when neuromuscular effects occur.
Patients with chronic low-level exposure may be symptomatic even with decreased levels.
RBC assay is a better reflection of cholinesterase activity in nerve tissue than is serum assay.
Worker experiencing industrial exposure should not return to work until these values rise to 75% of normal. RBC cholinesterase regenerates at rate of 1%/day and returns to baseline in 5–7 weeks. Serum cholinesterase regenerates at rate of 25% in 7–10 days and returns to baseline in 4–6 weeks.
Because of wide normal range patients may lose 50% of their cholinesterase activity and still be within normal range. Therefore baseline levels should be determined for all workers at risk due to organophosphates or carbamates. A decrease of 30–50% from baseline indicates toxicity even if value is still within normal range.
When baseline levels are not available, retrospective diagnosis is by serial measurements that increase after exposure.
Normal variation of ±20% in serum activity and ±10% in RBC activity prevents assessment of mild toxicity and recovery by only one or two assays.
Nonketotic hyperglycemia and glucosuria are common.

Serum amylase increase may reflect pancreatitis.
Serum cholinesterase may also be decreased in
- Liver diseases
  - Especially hepatitis (30–50% decrease). Lowest level corresponds to peak of disease, and level becomes normal with recovery.
  - Cirrhosis with ascites or jaundice (50–70% decrease). Persistent decrease may indicate a poor prognosis.
  - Some patients with metastatic carcinoma (50–70% decrease), obstructive jaundice, congestive heart failure.
- Congenital inherited recessive disorder. Such patients are particularly sensitive to administration of succinylcholine during anesthesia.
- Some conditions that may have decreased serum albumin levels (e.g., malnutrition, anemias, infections, dermatomyositis, acute myocardial infarction, pregnancy, recent surgery, liver diseases).
- Exposure to other drugs or chemicals [e.g., neostigmine methylsulfate (Prostigmin), quinine, fluoride, tetramethylammonium chloride, carbamate insecticides].

Phosphorus (Yellow) Poisoning (Rat Poison Ingestion)

Acute yellow atrophy of liver occurs.
Vomitus may glow in the dark.

Plant Poisoning or Milk Sickness (Trembles)

(Poisoning from goldenrod, snakeroot, richweed, and so on, or from eating poisoned animals)
Acidosis
Hypoglycemia
Increased nonprotein nitrogen (particularly guanidine)
Acetonuria

Polychlorinated Biphenyl Exposure

Polychlorinated biphenyls (PCBs) are a family of synthetic organic compounds with a common two-ring structure and one to ten substituted chlorine atoms. Commercial PCB products, which were used as insulating fluids and dielectrics in the manufacture of electrical capacitors and transformers, consisted of mixtures of isomers of varying degrees of chlorination. They were dispersed widely in the environment, and production of PCBs was halted in the United States in the 1970s because of concern about their extreme persistence. Low-level exposure to these chemicals via the food chain remains widespread even 25 years later.

Once ingested, PCBs concentrate in lipid-rich tissues, including brain and breast milk, and they readily cross the placenta from mother to fetus. The principal source of human exposure is consumption of fish and shellfish.

PCBs can have neurodevelopmental effects in young children at levels of exposure that are widely prevalent in the general population. Children exposed prenatally exhibit a variety of conditions, including low birth weight, abnormal skin pigmentation, delay in reaching developmental milestones, and lower intelligence quotients than unexposed siblings. The difference is 9 to 19 points during 6 years of annual testing. Exposed boys, but not girls, showed deficits in spatial reasoning compared with control subjects.

An association between transplacental PCB exposure and lower scores at 18 and 24 months on the Bayley Scales of Infant Development has been noted. Prenatal exposure to PCBs may be related to early onset of puberty.

Potassium Chloride (Enteric-Coated Pill) Poisoning

Laboratory findings due to small intestine ulceration, obstruction, or perforation.

Procainamide Therapy, Complications

Procainamide therapy may induce the findings of systemic lupus erythematosus.
Positive results on serologic tests for systemic lupus erythematosus are very frequent, especially at dosage of ≥1.25 g/day, and may precede clinical manifestations.
  Lupus erythematosus cell test results become positive in 50% of patients.
  Antideoxyribonucleoprotein test results becomes positive in 65% of patients.
  Anti-DNA test results become positive in 35% of patients.
  Results of one of these tests become positive in 75% of patients.
Serologic tests for systemic lupus erythematosus should be performed on all patients receiving procainamide.

Salicylate Intoxication

(Due to aspirin, sodium salicylate, oil of wintergreen, methylsalicylate)
Increased serum salicylate level (correlation does not apply to cases of long-term ingestion or ingestion of enteric-coated aspirin)
  Level of >10 mg/dL when symptoms are present.
  Level of 19–45 mg/dL when tinnitus is first noted.
  Level of >40 mg/dL when hyperventilation is present.
  At approximately 50 mg/dL, severe toxicity with acid-base imbalance and ketosis occurs.
  At 45–70 mg/dL, death occurs.
  For level of >100 mg/dL, hemodialysis is indicated.
Peak serum level is reached 2 hours after therapeutic and at least 6 hours after toxic dose.
Measurements of serum levels on blood drawn <6 hours after ingestion cannot be used to predict severity of toxic reaction using Done's nomogram, although they confirm salicylate overdose. Done's nomogram cannot be used with ingestion of enteric-coated aspirin.
Level of 15–30 mg/dL for optimal antiinflammatory effect; 5–27 mg/dL in patients with rheumatoid arthritis on dose of 65 mg/kg/day.
While laboratory measurements are being awaited, peak salicylate levels can be estimated as follows:

$$\text{mg/dL of salicylate} = \frac{(\text{mg of salicylate ingested})}{70\% \text{ of body weight (g)*}} \times 100$$

* = Total body water
In older children and adults, serum salicylate level corresponds well with severity; in younger children, correlation is more variable.
Gastric lavage may increase salicylate level by <10 mg/dL.
In early phase, serum electrolyte and carbon dioxide levels are normal.
Early respiratory alkalosis followed by metabolic acidosis; 20% of patients have either one alone.
Later, progressive decrease in serum sodium and $P\text{CO}_2$ occurs. Eighty percent of patients have combined primary respiratory alkalosis and primary metabolic acidosis; change in blood pH reflects the net result. (Infants may show immediate metabolic acidosis with the usual initial respiratory alkalosis. In older children and adults, the typical picture is respiratory alkalosis.)
Hypokalemia accompanies the respiratory alkalosis. Dehydration occurs.
Urine shows paradoxic acid pH despite the increased serum bicarbonate.
  Ferric chloride test gives positive results on boiled as well as unboiled urine (thus differentiating salicylate from ketone bodies); it may have a false-positive result because of phenacetin.
  Tests for glucose (e.g., Clinistix), reducing substances (e.g., Clinitest), or ketone bodies (e.g., Ketostix) give positive results. All positive urine screening test results should be confirmed by serum sample.
  RBCs may be present.
  Number of renal tubular cells is increased because of renal irritation.
Hypoglycemia occurs, especially in infants on restricted diet and in patients with diabetes.
Serum AST and ALT levels may be increased.

Hypoprothrombinemia after some days of intensive salicylate therapy is temporary and occasional; rarely causes hemorrhage.
Hydroxyproline is decreased in serum and urine.
Patient should be monitored by following blood glucose level, potassium level, pH.

Serum Sickness

Serum sickness is a hypersensitivity reaction that follows the administration of antitoxin. It may be caused by the reaction of the serum proteins of the animal in which the antitoxin was prepared. More commonly, however, serum sickness syndrome is due to drug allergy, particularly penicillin allergy. Symptoms occur 7–12 days after the injection of foreign protein and include urticaria due to IgE's reacting with horse serum proteins and joint symptoms due to deposition of antigen-antibody complexes of IgG and IgM. Histamine release from basophils and most cells mediated by IgE antibodies results in deposition of immune complexes. If there has been a previous reaction, the onset of symptoms is accelerated and anaphylaxis may occur. Carditis, glomerulonephritis rarely occur; Guillain-Barré syndrome of peripheral neuritis is the most serious complication.

Laboratory Findings

Increase in WBC count, especially eosinophils, and thrombocytopenia may occur.
Urine: mild proteinuria, hemoglobinuria, and microscopic hematuria.
Erythrocyte sedimentation rate is often increased.
Sheep cell agglutinin titer of the Forssman type is usually elevated.
Serum C3 and C4 levels are depressed; $C3_a$ anaphylatoxin usually increased, antibodies to IgG, IgM, IgA, and IgE against horse serum proteins increased.
Direct immunofluorescent assay of skin lesion specimen demonstrates IgM, IgA, IgE, or C3.

Steroids, Side Effects That Cause Laboratory Changes

Endocrine effects (e.g., adrenal insufficiency after prolonged use, suppression of pituitary or thyroid function, development of diabetes mellitus)
Increased susceptibility to infections
Gastrointestinal effects (e.g., peptic ulcer, perforation of bowel, infarction of bowel, pancreatitis)
Musculoskeletal effects (e.g., osteoporosis, pathologic fractures, arthropathy, myopathy)
Decreased serum potassium, increased WBCs, glycosuria, ecchymoses, and so on

Toxic Substances, Ingestion by Children

Ingestion of toxic substances by children is estimated to cause >4 million poisonings annually. Substances that are most accessible to children, such as cosmetics and personal care products, cleaning products, analgesics, and cough and cold preparations, account for 58% of the products listed in poisoning cases. The substances associated with the greatest risk of death to children include cocaine, anticonvulsant drugs, antidepressant drugs, and iron supplements.

Agents Most Commonly Ingested By Children Younger Than Six Years of Age[5]

Agent Ingested	No. of Children
Cosmetics and personal care products	568,856
Cleaning products	500,791
Analgesics	354,722
Plants	322,991

[5]From Litovitz T, Manoguerra A. Comparison of pediatric poisoning hazards: an analysis 3.8 million exposure incidents: a report from the American Association of Poison Control Centers. *Pediatrics* 1992;89:999–1006.

Cough and cold preparations	278,460
Foreign bodies	256,653
Topical agents	234,997
Pesticides	164,277
Vitamins	151,871
Hydrocarbons	106,269

Primary Agents Involved in Fatal Poisonings Among Children Younger Than Six Years of Age[6]

Category	Specific Agents
Analgesic drugs	Acetaminophen, ibuprofen, methadone hydrochloride, oxycodone hydrochloride, salicylates, morphine sulfate
Cleaning products	Corrosives, fluoride-based solutions
Electrolytes and minerals	Elemental iron
Hydrocarbons	Gasoline, paint thinner, lamp oil
Antidepressant drugs	Barbiturates, benzodiazepine, phenothiazine
Insecticides and pesticides	Propoxyphene organophosphates
Cosmetics and personal care products	Ethanol, baby oil
Anticonvulsant drugs	Carbamazepine, valproate sodium
Stimulants and illicit drugs	Crack cocaine, heroin
Plants	Cayenne pepper, pennyroyal tea
Foreign bodies	Activated charcoal
Sedatives and hypnotic drugs	Promethazine hydrochloride, chloral hydrate
Cardiovascular agents	Nifedipine
Tobacco	Cigarette butts
Cough and cold preparations	Phenylpropanolamine
Hormone and hormone antagonists	Glipizide
Chemicals	Diethylene glycol
Alcohols	Ethanol
Gastrointestinal preparations	Bismuth subsalicylate

Vitamin Toxicity

Ingestion of a large number of vitamin tablets usually occurs in infants, who may ingest children's chewable vitamins. Ingestion of vitamins A and D may result in toxic effects.

Vitamin A Toxicity

Acute hypervitaminosis A may occur in infants after ingesting 1,000 μg (20 tablets) or more. (Childrens vitamins contain 50 μg/tablet.) Symptoms are vomiting, drowsiness, and bulging of the fontanel. Diplopia, papilledema, cranial nerve palsies, and symptoms suggestive of brain tumor with cerebral edema may be present.

Vitamin D Toxicity

Ingestion of excessive amounts of vitamin D results in signs and symptoms similar to those of idiopathic hypercalcemia, which may be due to hypersensitivity to vitamin D. Symptoms develop 1–3 months after large intakes of vitamin D and include hypotonia, anorexia, irritability, constipation, polydipsia, polyuria, and pallor. Hypercalcemia and hypercalciuria are noted, and evidence of dehydration is seen. Aortic valvular stenosis, vomiting, hypertension, retinopathy, and clouding of the cornea and conjunctiva may occur. Proteinuria is usually present and renal damage with metastatic calcification may occur. Radiography of long bones shows metastatic calcification and generalized osteoporosis.

[6]From Litovitz T, Manoguerra A. Comparison of pediatric poisoning hazards: an analysis 3.8 million exposure incidents: a report from the American Association of Poison Control Centers. *Pediatrics* 1992;89:999–1006.

Bites and Stings

Insect Bites and Stings

There are literally thousands of species of insects capable of stinging.

Fire Ants

Extreme pain follows multiple bites. Blisters appear within 24 hours and become infected easily.
Symptoms may be mild to severe.

Vinegaroons

Sprays a vinegar-like substance that can be irritating to the eyes.
If eyes are sprayed, flush eyes with water for 15 minutes to relieve pain.

Florida Scorpions

Extreme pain followed by swelling and redness are associated with this bite.

Centipedes

Sting causes pain and sensitivity similar to that caused by bee stings. Treat affected area by applying an ice pack.

Giant Water Bugs

Grasps victim with strong front legs and, like the assassin bug, injects a tissue-dissolving venom that causes extreme pain and inflammation below the bite.

Blister Beetles

When disturbed, the blister beetle excretes juices that cause the skin to blister like a burn.

Caterpillars

(Saddleback caterpillar, Io caterpillar, Puss caterpillar)
The most common symptoms are redness, swelling, localized pain, itching, and rash.

Bees, Wasps, and Hornets

People who are extremely sensitive (allergic) to bee stings should wear a Medic Alert bracelet, and ask a physician for a bee sting allergy kit. If the skin becomes flushed, the face swells, or shortness of breath occurs, immediate medical attention should be obtained.

Honey Bees and Bumblebees

The muscle around the venom sac of the stinger continues to work for up to 20 minutes after the stinger has become detached from the insect's body. It is important to remove the stinger as soon as possible.

Wasps

Capable of stinging multiple times when disturbed.

Hornets and Yellow Jackets

May sting multiple times.

Marine Organism and Fish Stings

Portuguese Man-of-War

Stings usually occur when people brush against the man-of-war in the water or step on it on the beach.

Soak wound in seawater then in vinegar for 30 minutes. Baking soda (mixed with water to form a paste) may be applied to affected area. Do not rub area. Allergic symptoms can develop quickly.

Sea Nettle

Sting is moderately severe and painful. Stung area resembles an itchy, red, raised rash.

Stingray

Stings result in immediate sharp pain, redness, swelling, and bleeding. Symptoms last up to 48 hours. Symptoms progress quickly and can include welts, nausea and vomiting, diarrhea, and increased heart rate.

Irrigate wound immediately with cold water to dilute the venom. Then soak the injured area in hot (not scalding) water to relieve pain.

Catfish

Symptoms may include intense throbbing or scalding pain spreading upward from wounds and lasting 30–60 minutes. Area quickly swells and is easily infected. Muscle spasms usually follow, and victims may experience episodes of fainting, decreased heart rate, and slowed breathing.

Immerse wound immediately in hot (not scalding) water for 30 minutes to an hour.

Snakebites

(Mortality is <1% in United States; 95% of cases are due to rattlesnakes.)

Laboratory Findings

Increased WBC (20,000–30,000/mm^3).

Platelets decreased to 10,000/mm^3 within 1 hour; return to normal in 4 hours.

Burrs on almost all RBCs.

Clotting caused by some venoms; normal coagulation prevented by others, which destroy fibrinogen so that fibrin split products are detected, fibrinogen levels are very low or absent, and prothrombin time and a partial thromboplastin time are very high. As a screening test, failure of blood drawn into a modified Lee-White clotting tube to clot within a few minutes with constant agitation is a reliable indication of envenomization.

Albuminuria.

Pit Vipers

(Rattlesnakes, copperheads, water moccasins; in United States all native snakes with elliptical pupils are poisonous.)

These snakes also have large foldable fangs, and a facial pit for sensing heat. Their venom thins out the blood and can cause swelling, bruising, vomiting, weakness, bleeding, and shock after a bite. Physicians treat these bites by observing signs to see if antivenin is needed.

Elapidae

(Coral snakes, kraits, cobras)

The small teeth produce bites, leaving tiny marks that result in little or no swelling. The neurotoxic venom takes hold many hours after the bite and leads to difficulty speaking, swallowing, or breathing. Eventually, it can cause permanent paralysis or death. Physicians treat these bites by immediately administering antivenin to prevent symptoms from occurring.

Spider Bites

Approximately 20,000 species of spiders live in the United States. Almost all are capable of biting, but very few can penetrate human skin. Bites can be painful and may cause redness, swelling, and infection. In Florida, only the black widow and the brown recluse are considered potentially dangerous.

Black Widow Spider (Latrodectus mactans)

Bite may or may not be painful initially. Pain begins in 1–3 hours and may last up to 48 hours.
Symptoms include abdominal pain, dizziness, headache, sweating, leg cramps, weakness, and difficulty breathing.

Laboratory Findings

Moderately increased WBCs
Findings of acute nephritis

Brown Spider (Loxosceles reclusa)

Bite feels like a sting followed by intense pain. Wound looks like a blister and may take on a bull's-eye appearance. Eventually the wound may develop into a large ulcerated area. Symptoms develop within 36 hours.

Laboratory Findings

Hemolytic anemia with hemoglobinuria and hemoglobinemia
Increased WBCs
Thrombocytopenia
Proteinuria

Biologic Warfare Agents

See also Chapter 5, Infectious Diseases, sections on anthrax and plague.

Anthrax

See Fig. 1.
Persons who may have been exposed to anthrax are not contagious; therefore, quarantine is not indicated.

Signs and Symptoms

Skin—itchy bump turns into an ulcer.
Inhaled—acts like a cold at first but leads to respiratory failure.
Intestinal—nausea, fever, abdominal pain, diarrhea.

Inhalation Anthrax

A brief prodrome resembling a viral respiratory illness followed by development of hypoxia and dyspnea, with radiographic evidence of mediastinal widening. This, the most lethal form of anthrax, results from inspiration of 8,000–50,000 spores of *Bacillus anthracis*. The incubation period of inhalation anthrax among humans typically ranges from 1 to 7 days but may possibly be up to 60 days. Host factors, doses of exposure, and chemoprophylaxis may play a role. Initial symptoms include mild fever, muscle aches, and malaise. These symptoms may progress to respiratory failure and shock; meningitis frequently develops. Case-fatality rates for inhalation anthrax are extremely high even with all possible supportive care, including treatment with appropriate antibiotics.

Cutaneous Anthrax

The presentation of cutaneous anthrax is classic, beginning with a skin lesion evolving from a papule, through a vesicular stage, to a depressed black eschar. This is the most common naturally occurring type of infection (>95%) and usually occurs after skin contact with contaminated meat, hides, or leather from infected animals. Incubation period ranges from 1 to 12 days. Skin infection begins as a small papule, progresses to a vesicle in 1–2 days, followed by a necrotic ulcer. The lesion is usually painless, but patients may have fever, malaise, headache, and regional lymphade-

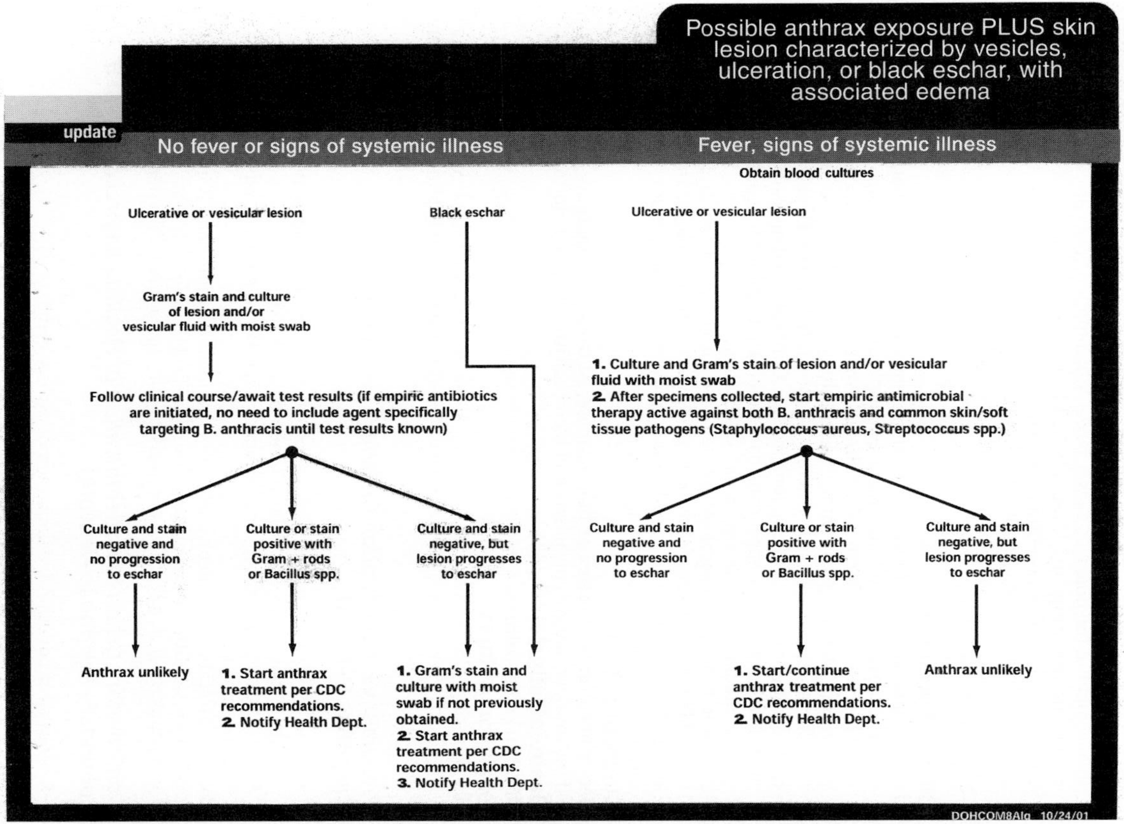

Fig. 1. Algorithm for diagnosis of anthrax. CDC, Centers for Disease Control and Prevention; spp., species. (Reproduced with permission from *Guidelines for healthcare providers.* Tallahassee: Florida Department of Health, 2001.)

nopathy. The case-fatality rate for cutaneous anthrax is 20% without antibiotic treatment and less than 1% with antibiotic treatment.

Gastrointestinal Anthrax

Severe abdominal pain followed by fever and signs of septicemia. This form of anthrax usually follows the consumption of raw or undercooked contaminated meat and is considered to have an incubation period of 1–7 days. An oropharyngeal and an abdominal form of the disease have been described. Lesions at the base of the tongue, sore throat, dysphagia, fever, and regional lymphadenopathy usually characterize involvement of the pharynx. Lower bowel inflammation typically causes nausea, loss of appetite, vomiting, and fever, followed by abdominal pain, vomiting of blood, and bloody diarrhea. The case-fatality rate is estimated to be 25–60%. The effect of early antibiotic treatment on the case-fatality rate is not established.

Laboratory Studies

Clinical Specimens

Only patients showing clinical signs consistent with anthrax or patients with a confirmed exposure should be tested. Suspect cases should be reported to the local county health department. Most clinical laboratories, including hospital laboratories with microbiology laboratories, can culture the anthrax bacteria. Cultures positive for anthrax-like bacilli should be forwarded to the Department of Health, State Laboratory for confirmatory testing. Confirm the diagnosis by obtaining the appropriate laboratory specimens based on the clinical form of anthrax that is suspected (inhalation, gastrointestinal, or cutaneous).

Nasal swab testing and serology are not used for clinical diagnostic purposes. Nasal swab and serologic testing for anthrax is used for epidemiologic and criminal investigations only. There is no reliable clinical screening test for the detection of anthrax infection in an asymptomatic person.

Cutaneous Anthrax

Bacterial cultures of vesicular fluid or material from ulcer margins. A Gram stain of fluid or ulcer margin specimens and blood cultures may be helpful.

Gastrointestinal Anthrax

Blood and stool cultures

Inhalation Anthrax

Blood testing; CSF testing (if meningeal signs are present); chest radiograph, which might show evidence of thoracic edema and a widened mediastinum; and sputum culture.

Presumptive Identification Criteria (Level A Laboratory Response Network)

- From clinical samples, such as blood, CSF, or skin lesion (vesicular fluid or eschar) material: encapsulated Gram-positive rods.
- From growth on sheep's blood agar: large Gram-positive rods, nonmotile and nonhemolytic.

Contact the state public health laboratory immediately and send it a culture for identification. Additional Laboratory Response Network level B laboratory criteria for confirmation of *B. anthracis* are available through state public health laboratories.

Confirmatory Criteria for Identification of Bacillus anthracis (Level B Laboratory Response Network)

- Capsule production (visualization of capsule), and
- Lysis by γ phage, or
- Positive result on direct fluorescent antibody assay

Rapid screening assays, such as nucleic acid signatures and antigen detection, which can be performed directly on clinical specimens and environmental samples, are being made available for restricted use in Laboratory Response Network B- and C-level laboratories.

State public health laboratories cannot accept whole-blood or serologic specimens for anthrax testing.

Environmental Testing

In Florida, samples are accepted at the state laboratory only after law enforcement and hazardous materials personnel have performed their assessment to rule out radiologic, explosive, and chemical agents.

Suspected samples such as swab, powder, liquid, or contaminated paper or letter should be submitted for testing.

Samples should be double-bagged and put in a container no larger than 1-gallon size with sample submission form.

No extraneous materials in need of decontamination should be included (towels, gloves, clothing). These materials should be placed in a biohazard bag and disposed of locally according to state and federal guidelines.

Specimen Handling

Packing of Specimens

Packing of specimens: Packaging and labeling of specimens are the same as for any infectious substance.

Nonclinical specimens: If the specimen is a dry powder or paper material, place it in a plastic ziplock bag and use a biohazard label.

Clinical specimens: If the specimen is a clinical specimen, place the biohazard label on the specimen receptacle; wrap the receptacle with an absorbent material.

The following steps should be followed for both clinical and nonclinical specimens:

1. Place the bag or specimen receptacle into a leakproof container with a tight cover, labeled "biohazard."
2. Place this container into a second leakproof container with a tight cover labeled "biohazard." The size of the second container should be no larger than a one-gallon paint can.
3. Place the second container into a third leakproof container with a tight cover labeled "biohazard." Nonclinical specimens do not require an ice pack. Clinical specimens do, however, to keep the specimen cold.
4. The third container should be no larger than a 5-gallon paint can.
5. Both outer containers should meet state and federal regulations for transport of hazardous materials and should be properly labeled.

Transporting of Specimens

Transporting of specimens must be coordinated with the state department of health and public health laboratories. State personnel of the Federal Bureau of Investigation may be used to transport specimens if bioterrorism is suspected or if the specimens are related to a criminal investigation. In cases in which the specimen is shipped by commercial carrier, ship according to state and federal shipping regulations.

Decontamination

Cleaning of Surfaces and Nonsterilizable Equipment

Work surfaces should be wiped before and after use with a sporicidal decontamination solution. All nonsterilizable equipment should be routinely cleaned with a decontamination solution.

Cleaning of Accidental Spills of Material Known or Suspected to Be Contaminated

For contamination involving a fresh clinical sample, flood with a decontamination solution and soak for 5 minutes before cleaning up.

For contamination involving laboratory samples (culture plates or blood cultures) or spills occurring in areas that are below room temperature, gently cover spill then liberally apply decontamination solution. Soak for 1 hour before cleaning up. Any materials soiled during the cleanup must be autoclaved or incinerated.

Botulism

Incubation period 1–5 days.

Signs and Symptoms

Early symptoms include double vision, slurred speech, and muscle weakness. The infection leads to paralysis of limbs and of the respiratory system.

Diagnostic Studies

Testing of serum for toxin if <3 days since exposure; culture and toxin testing of stool or gastric secretions; nerve conduction testing

Plague

Incubation period is 2–3 days.

Signs and Symptoms

Warning signs include swollen and sore lymph nodes, fever, headache, and extreme exhaustion.

Diagnostic Studies

Culture of GA, staining of blood, sputum, lymph node aspirate

Smallpox

Incubation period is 7–17 days.

Signs and Symptoms

High fever, headache, backache, rash on face, arms, and legs. Easy to misdiagnose as chickenpox in its early stage.

Diagnostic Studies

Culture of pharyngeal swab or lesion specimen

Bibliography

Baselt RC, Cravey RH. *Disposition of toxic drugs and chemicals in man*, 3rd ed. Chicago: Year Book Medical Publishers, 1989.

Committee on Environmental Health, American Academy of Pediatrics. *Handbook of pediatric environmental health.* Elk Grove, IL: American Academy of Pediatrics, 1999.

Krenzelok EP, McGuigan M, Lheur P. Position statement: ipecac syrup. American Academy of Clinical Toxicology; European Association of Poisons Centres and Clinical Toxicologists. *J Toxicol Clin Toxicol* 1997;35:699–709.

Levy BS. The teaching of occupational health in United States medical schools: 5-year follow-up of an initial survey. *Am J Public Health* 1985;75:79–80.

Litovitz T, Manoguerra A. Comparison of pediatric poisoning hazards: an analysis 3.8 million exposure incidents: a report from the American Association of Poison Control Centers. *Pediatrics* 1992;89:999–1006.

Litovitz TL, Klein-Schwarcz W, Dyer KS, et al. 1997 Annual report of the American Association of Poison Control Centers Toxic Exposure Surveillance System. *Am J Emerg Med* 1998;16:443–497.

Litovitz TL, Klein-Schwarcz W, Caravari EM, et al. 1998 Annual report of the American Association of Poison Control Centers Toxic Exposure Surveillance System. *Am J Emerg Med* 1999;17:435–487.

Litovitz TL, Smilkstein M, Felberg L, et al. 1996 Annual report of the American Association of Poison Control Centers Toxic Exposure Surveillance System. *Am J Emerg Med* 1997;15:447–500.

National Research Council. *Pesticides in the diets of infants and children*. Washington: National Academy Press, 1993.

Needleman HL, Landrigan PJ. Raising children toxic free: how to keep your child safe from lead, asbestos, pesticides and other environmental hazards. New York: Farrar, Strauss and Giroux, 1994.
Porter WH, Moyer TP. In: Burtis CA, Ashwood ER, eds. *Tietz textbook of clinical chemistry*, 2nd ed. Philadelphia: WB Saunders, 1994.
Shannon M. Ingestion of toxic substances by children. *N Engl J Me*d 2000;342:186–191.
Wallach J. *Interpretation of diagnostic tests*, 7th ed. Philadelphia: Lippincott Williams & Wilkins, 2000.

Web Site Bibliography

For additional information on anthrax, updates on developments in Florida, or information on other diseases likely to be associated with biologic agents, please consult the following Web sites:

http://www.myflorida.com: Updates on developments in Florida, guidelines for hospitals, prophylaxis and treatment.
http://www.bt.cdc.gov: CDC bioterrorism Web site. Detailed facts on specific diseases, laboratory protocols, prophylaxis and treatment; updates on developments around the country; mail guidelines from the U.S. Postal Service.
http://www.idsociety.org: Infectious Disease Society of America Web site. This site reviews the heightened surveillance recommended by the CDC when the World Trade Center event occurred.
http://www.acponline.org/bioterr/: American College of Physicians Web site. General information on bioterrorism agents and resources.
http://www.apic.org/bioterror: Association for Professionals in Infection Control and Epidemiology Web site. Reviews infection control guidelines and information on bioterrorism planning for hospitals.

Poison control centers can be contacted in all major cities and hospitals in the United States.

Index

Note: Page numbers followed by *t* indicate tables; those followed by *f* indicate figures.